Kammerer and Gross' Medical Consultation

The Internist on Surgical, Obstetric, and Psychiatric Services

Third Edition

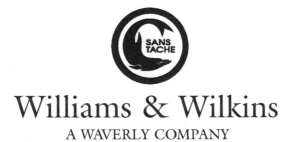

Williams & Wilkins

A WAVERLY COMPANY

BALTIMORE • PHILADELPHIA • LONDON • PARIS • BANGKOK
HONG KONG • MUNICH • SYDNEY • TOKYO • WROCLAW

Kammerer and Gross' Medical Consultation

The Internist on Surgical, Obstetric, and Psychiatric Services

Third Edition

Editors

Richard J. Gross, MD, FACP, ScM
Assistant Professor of Medicine
Division of General Internal Medicine
The Johns Hopkins University School of Medicine
The Johns Hopkins Hospital
The Johns Hopkins Bayview Medical Center
Sinai Hospital
Baltimore, Maryland

Gregory M. Caputo, MD, FACP
Associate Professor of Medicine
Chief, Division of General Internal Medicine
Pennsylvania State University College of Medicine
The Milton S. Hershey Medical Center
Hershey, Pennsylvania

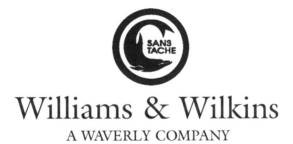

Williams & Wilkins

A WAVERLY COMPANY

BALTIMORE • PHILADELPHIA • LONDON • PARIS • BANGKOK
HONG KONG • MUNICH • SYDNEY • TOKYO • WROCLAW

Editor: Jonathan W. Pine, Jr.
Managing Editor: Leah Ann Kiehne Hayes
Marketing Manager: Daniell T. Griffin
Production Coordinator: Peter J. Carley
Project Editor: Kathy Gilbert
Designer: Artech Graphics II
Illustration Planner: Lorraine Wrzosek
Cover Designer: Artech Graphics II
Typesetter and Digitized Illustrations: Graphic World, Inc.
Printer/Binder: Walsworth Publishing Co.

Accurate indications, adverse reactions, and dosage schedules for drugs are provided in this book, but it is possible that they may change. The reader is urged to review the package information data of the manufacturers of the medications mentioned.

Printed in the United States of America

First Edition 1983
Second Edition 1990

Library of Congress Cataloging-in-Publication Data

Kammerer and Gross' medical consultation : the internist on surgical, obstetric, and psychiatric services / editors, Richard J. Gross, Gregory M. Caputo. —3rd ed.
    p.   cm.
    Rev. ed. of : Medical consultation. 2nd ed. c1990.
    Includes bibliographical references and index.
    ISBN 0-683-03639-4
    1. Internal medicine. 2. Medical consultation. 3. Internists. I. Gross, Richard J. (Richard Joseph), 1948– . II. Caputo, Gregory M. III. Kammerer, William S.
    [DNLM: 1. Referral and Consultation. 2. Internal Medicine. W 64 K15 1998]
RC48.M43 1998
616—dc21
DNLM/DLC
for Library of Congress   97-23571
                                              CIP

The publishers have made every effort to trace the copyright holders for borrowed material. If they have inadvertently overlooked any, they will be pleased to make the necessary arrangements at the first opportunity.

To purchase additional copies of this book, call our customer service department at **(800) 638-0672** or fax orders to **(800) 447-8438.** For other book services, including chapter reprints and large quantity sales, ask for the Special Sales department.

Canadian customers should call **(800) 665-1148** or fax **(800) 665-0103.** For all other calls originating outside the United States, please call **(410) 528-4223** or fax us at **(410) 528-8550.**

Visit Williams & Wilkins on the Internet: **http://www.wwilkins.com**, or contact our customer service department at **custserv@wwilkins.com**. Williams & Wilkins customer service representatives are available from 8:30 AM to 6:00 PM, EST, Monday through Friday, for telephone access.

          98 99 00
2 3 4 5 6 7 8 9 10

To Graham H. Jeffries, MB, ChB, DPhil,
Founding Chairman of the Department of Medicine
and, for 20 years, Professor of Medicine at the
University Hospital of The Pennsylvania State University.
Mentor and friend. Pre-eminent consultant.
He leads by example.

Foreword to the First Edition

When thou arte callde at anye time,
A patient to see;
And doste perceave the cure too grate,
And ponderous for thee;

See that thou laye disdeyne aside,
And pride of thyne owne skyll;
And thinke no shame counsell to take,
But rather wyth good will.

Gette one or two of experte men,
To help thee in that nede;
And make them partakers wyth thee,
in That worke to procede.

—John Halle, MD (1529 1566)
From *Goodlye Doctrine and Instruction*

The practicing internist is often called on to provide advice to colleagues. The time devoted to this endeavor during medical residency training varies from program to program to program but in general is not consonant with the need. A busy general internist may spend up to 40% of practice time providing consultations. The error made in most training programs is the assumption that, if a physician is competent to care for the diabetic on a medicine service, then he or she is competent to manage the diabetic through delivery or a surgical procedure. In fact, to give valuable service the consultant needs to understand the exigencies of anesthesia, the surgical procedure, the dynamics of pregnancy, labor, and delivery, and the disposition of colleagues.

The general internist is often in the best position to understand and work with these multiple variables. By virtue of their usual practice mix, general internists are faced daily with "interface medicine." Multiple medical problems in the same patient are the rule in general internal medicine, and the proper care of such patients requires knowledge of the effects of one disease on another, the hazards of polypharmacy, and the importance of the larger picture of health and disease.

Because these considerations and techniques are not the province of traditionally oriented textbooks, the editors felt the need to present this information in a composite form. Although chaptered and indexed in usual organ or disease entity ways, the information stresses the effects of surgery or pregnancy on a disease process or, conversely, the effects of a disease or pregnancy on the outcome of a surgery. Further, the editors and contributors provide specific practical management advice designed to minimize these effects.

Before launching into the specific portions of this text, we would offer some general recommendations regarding the conduct of consultations which experience has taught us are worth bearing in mind as you make your appointed rounds.

KNOW FOR WHOM YOU ARE PROVID-ING THE SERVICE. Different services may be looking for different kinds of advice. So, too, some individual physicians may routinely call for specific types of assistance.

KNOW WHY YOU ARE BEING CONSULTED. In general terms the request may be: "Help! What do I do now?"; "Come argue with another consultant"; or "Come see what a nice job I've done." More specifically, try to elicit the exact question being asked.

BE BRIEF–ALLOW FOR SELECTIVE READING OF YOUR NOTE. Long notes are not read. You should title sections of your note so that areas of interest for different readers will be readily identified. If you wish to record information for your own future review or to help a covering consultant, separate it from the rest of your text.

BE SPECIFIC WITH RECOMMENDA-TIONS. Therapeutic measures should be spelled out with respect to drug dose, route of administration, desired effect, and toxicity.

SUPPORT YOUR RECOMMENDA-TIONS AND IMPRESSIONS. Your text should include the data to warrant a diagnosis and the indications for diagnostic and therapeutic recommendations.

TEACH THE READER. You have been asked to provide a special service. This is an admission that the requestor seeks information. Your experience with similar cases and pertinent points from the literature are appropriate.

FOLLOW-UP. It is a rare consultation which should involve one visit. If that is the case, you should indicate that you will not return unless requested. Your note should include what progress you expect and should provide the opportunity to change your problem list as the database expands. Flow sheets which you can initiate might be a worthwhile venture. The follow-up visit is your best learning device.

BE CHARITABLE. You do not help the patient when you shame or anger his doctor.

ATTEMPT PERSONAL COMMUNICA-TION. This is a courtesy which allows you to amplify your note and reinforce your recommendations.

BE HONEST. You have been called in as an expert. Do not suggest diagnoses which are not supported by the data. Get help when you need it or recommend other consultants who can deal adequately with the situation.

The editors and contributors to this volume are from two training programs that endeavor to stress consultation skills as important educational components. All have wide experience in both providing and teaching consultations. Their contributions contain the science of the discipline and the wisdom of having done it many times.

J.W. Burnside

Preface to the Third Edition

"Each of us, however old, is still an under-graduate in the school of experience. When a man thinks he has graduated, he becomes a public menace."

John Chalmers DaCosta

"You must always be students, learning and unlearning till your life's end, and if, gentle-men, you are not prepared to follow your profession in this spirit, I implore you to leave its ranks . . ."

Joseph Lister

"A life so short, an art so long to learn."
Hippocrates

This edition embodies both continuity and change. The fundamental principles of consultative medicine have been constant over the past generation. A careful bedside examination with meticulous attention to details, measured interpretation of clinical data, assessment of perioperative risk, and close communication with the consulting physician and appropriate follow-up remain the cornerstones of excellence in medical consultation. These time-honored elements received continued emphasis in this third edition.

This edition brings a new co-editor to the process, but one who trained under former co-editor Dr. William Kammerer, owing him a great debt for stimulating an early interest in consultative medicine. We have maintained the tradition of blending the knowledge and experience of experts in Baltimore, a medical community steeped in tradition, and Hershey, a relative newcomer but nevertheless a major academic center committed to advancing the field of medical consultation.

Any new textbook edition needs to reflect the dynamic changes that are occurring both in medical science and in medical practice. This book is fortunate to have as contributors individuals who are at the cutting edge of academic medicine and who also are busy clinicians, and this perspective is invaluable. The book blends an evidence-based approach, based on an insistence on the best available scientific evidence before making firm recommendations, with the recognition that clinical judgement and experience are invaluable components of excellent medical practice. In addition, in several chapters (e.g., those on obstetrics, psychiatry, and pulmonary medicine), the viewpoint of a subspecialist is merged with that of a general internist to provide a unique perspective on the topic.

Powerful economic forces no doubt have challenged technologic ones as the prime movers of change in medicine. Cost-effective approaches are sought in this book, however, primarily because stream-lined diagnostic and therapeutic strategies most often are the best for the patient. The third edition also continues the trend of emphasizing developments in outpatient preoperative evaluation and ambulatory surgery.

Despite the gender bias reflective of their times, the quotations presented earlier emphasize the physician's dedication to lifelong learning. Every physician is a member of a profession committed to continuous scientific advancement as the foundation of an often humbling art. We have found it a privilege (and a great challenge) to contribute to the efforts of fellow physicians in keeping up with the ever-changing practice of consultative medicine.

Our goal continues to be providing the consulting internist with practical information from a scientific basis for the care of our most seriously ill and complex patients.

Richard J. Gross
Gregory M. Caputo

Preface to the First Edition

"Operating on someone who has no place else to go."

—Dr. John Kirklen, quoted by
Dr. C.B. Mullins, with permission.

What would motivate one to put together a multiauthored text on a subject traditionally learned through years of trial and error at the bedside and hours of labor in the library? We felt that, by bringing together the views of experienced internist consultants and a widely scattered literature, we could provide a nidus for an effective teaching program for residents, as well as a reference for continuing self-education for the practicing internist. Because medical consultations to nonmedical services make up a large part of an average working day for practicing internists and medical residents, most training programs now include a rotation on a general medical consultation service. However, teaching on such services is hampered by the lack of reference material, and the experience is often haphazard, isolated, and unsupervised. Many medical residents thus come to dread this activity and feel it is irrelevant and unscientific.

By categorizing the lessons learned from personal experience and the thinking of experienced internists, we hope that the prolonged floundering of trial and error learning will thereby be shortened and given direction. Consultation medicine is one of the few remaining areas in a subspecialty world where the venerable concept of the general internist as a master diagnostician of all ills "from the skin in" can come alive and allow the full utilization of all of his/her skills.

Recognizing that even the most complete general internist tends to become more proficient in one area than another, we felt a multiauthored approach, representing several institutions and styles of practice, would best serve the goals of this book. With few exceptions (e.g., anesthesiology, mechanical respiratory support, and dermatology) dictated by special skills and knowledge, all of the contributors are practicing general internists.

Undoubtedly, some subspecialists will find omissions or generalizations in the text which are unacceptable to them. However, rather than attempting an encyclopedic subspecialty reference text, our goal is to provide an approach as practiced by experienced general internists to specific perioperative problems and to medical problems in pregnancy and psychiatry. This approach emphasizes clinical decision making and practical management techniques rather than extended discussions of medical, surgical, and anesthetic pathophysiology. Due to the complex interrelationships at the interface of medical, surgical, and anesthetic problems and to the rapid changes in their relative importance through the pre-, intra-, and postoperative periods, pathophysiologic generalizations are often impossible to apply to the individual patient. Thus, we place the majority of our emphasis on clinical decision making based on well-designed empirical studies and extensive personal experience. However, in areas where a general understanding of current surgical or anesthetic pathophysiology cannot reasonably be expected of the general internist, it is incorporated in the appropriate clinical discussions. Obviously, this approach assumes a general familiarity with a wide range of medical and surgical problems.

While attempting to keep the general structure and organization of all sections reasonably uniform, the remaining diversity in styles tends to reemphasize the need for versatility and practicality in the approach to medical consultations to surgical and non-medical services.

Discerning readers will note that the bibliography occasionally appears dated, or even absent, for common consultation problems. Perhaps this observation will provide a stimulus to our readers to fill these gaps.

We hope the book will serve the needs of both medical residents and the consulting general internist and prove practical, educational, and stimulating.

W.S. Kammerer, MD
R.J. Gross, MD

Acknowledgments

The editors wish to acknowledge Drs. Kelly Warshel and Melissa Falk for their review of selected manuscripts. Ms. Donna Harris and Ms. Donna Ream provided invaluable secretarial and organizational support. Librarians Dianne Deck and Deborah Peters provided superb assistance. We also are deeply indebted to the editorial staff at Williams & Wilkins, particularly Leah Hayes, Jonathan Pine, David Retford, Katey Millet, Pete Carley, and Kathy Gilbert, for the commitment to moving this project steadfastly towards completion. We thank our wives, Kathleen and Leesa, and our children, David, Jonathan, Jennifer and Michael, for their understanding, patience, and laughter during the preparation of this book as well.

In addition, the editors wish to acknowledge the contributions to the first two editions of William S. Kammerer, Kermit Tantum, Barbara G. Ford, Joseph J. Trautlein, Thomas J. McGlynn Jr., David E. Kern, Harold Tucker, John W. Burnside, and Janet Woodcock. Their contributions will continue to serve as a basis for this text as it is updated.

Contributors

Mohamad Ghias Arar, MD
Chief Resident in Neurology
University of Louisville School of
   Medicine
Louisville, Kentucky

Stewart F. Babbott, MD
Assistant Professor of Medicine
Tufts University School of Medicine
Boston, Massachusetts
Director of Faculty Development
Department of Medicine
Baystate Medical Center
Springfield, Massachusetts

James O. Ballard, MD
Professor of Medicine
Division of Hematology and Oncology
Pennsylvania State University College
   of Medicine
The Milton S. Hershey Medical Center
Hershey, Pennsylvania

Noel Ballentine, MD
Assistant Professor of Medicine
Division of General Internal Medicine
Pennsylvania State University College
   of Medicine
The Milton S. Hershey Medical Center
Hershey, Pennsylvania

John Botti, MD
Professor and Vice Chairman
Department of Obstetrics and
   Gynecology
Director, Division of Maternal and Fetal
   Medicine
Pennsylvania State University College
   of Medicine
The Milton S. Hershey Medical Center
Hershey, Pennsylvania

Gary R. Briefel, MD
Associate Professor of Medicine
Division of Renal Medicine
The Johns Hopkins University School of
   Medicine
The Johns Hopkins Bayview Medical
   Center
Baltimore, Maryland

Gregory M. Caputo, MD
Associate Professor of Medicine
Division of General Internal Medicine
Pennsylvania State University College
   of Medicine
The Milton S. Hershey Medical Center
Hershey, Pennsylvania

Lourdes C. Corman, MD, FACP, FACR
Professor and Vice Chair
Department of Internal Medicine
University of Louisville School of
   Medicine
Louisville, Kentucky

Yousef Dairi, MD
Clinical Faculty
Department of Medicine
University of Louisville School of
   Medicine
Louisville, Kentucky

Sudhir K. Dutta, MD
Professor of Medicine
University of Maryland School of
   Medicine
Director, Division of Gastroenterology
Sinai Hospital of Baltimore
Baltimore, Maryland

Rita A. Falcone, MD
Assistant Professor of Medicine
Division of Cardiology
The Johns Hopkins University School of
    Medicine
The Johns Hopkins Bayview Medical
    Center
Baltimore, Maryland

John M. Field, MD
Associate Professor of Medicine
Division of Cardiology
Pennsylvania State University College
    of Medicine
The Milton S. Hershey Medical Center
Hershey, Pennsylvania

Kevin Gleeson, MD
Associate Professor of Medicine
Division of Pulmonary and Critical Care
    Medicine
Pennsylvania State University College
    of Medicine
The Milton S. Hershey Medical Center
Hershey, Pennsylvania

Robert A. Gordon, MD
Associate Professor of Medicine
Division of Hematology and Oncology
The Pennsylvania State University
    College of Medicine
The Milton S. Hershey Medical Center
Hershey, Pennsylvania

Richard J. Gross, MD, FACP, ScM
Assistant Professor of Medicine
Division of General Internal Medicine
The Johns Hopkins University School of
    Medicine
The Johns Hopkins Hospital
The Johns Hopkins Bayview Medical
    Center
Sinai Hospital
Baltimore, Maryland

Larry B. Grossman, MD
Anesthesiologist
Department of Anesthesiology
Northwest Hospital Center
Randallstown, Maryland

Gerald A. Hofkin, MD
Assistant Professor of Medicine
The Johns Hopkins University School of
    Medicine
Department of Medicine
Division of Gastroenterology
Sinai Hospital of Baltimore
Baltimore, Maryland

Howard T. Jacobs, MD
Chief, Division of Pulmonary Medicine
Northwest Hospital Center
Randallstown, Maryland

William S. Kammerer, MD
Executive in International Internal
    Medicine
Department of Medicine
Mayo Clinic Jacksonville
Jacksonville, Florida

Paul Kettl, MD
Associate Professor of Psychiatry
Pennsylvania State University College
    of Medicine
The Milton S. Hershey Medical Center
Hershey, Pennsylvania

Donald P. Lookingbill, MD
Professor of Medicine
Chief, Division of Dermatology
Pennsylvania State University College
    of Medicine
The Milton S. Hershey Medical Center
Hershey, Pennsylvania

Philip A. Masters, MD
Assistant Professor of Medicine
Pennsylvania State University College
    of Medicine
Hershey, Pennsylvania

Thomas J. McGlynn, Jr., MD
Professor of Medicine
Wayne State University School of
    Medicine
Dayton, Ohio

Brent G. Petty, MD
Associate Professor of Medicine
Divisions of Clinical Pharmacology and
  Internal Medicine
The Johns Hopkins University School of
  Medicine
Baltimore, Maryland

Richard J. Simons, MD
Associate Professor of Medicine
Associate Chairman for Education
Pennsylvania State University College
  of Medicine
Hershey, Pennsylvania

John Stuckey, MD
Section of Internal Medicine
Washington Hospital Center
Washington, DC

Luanne Thorndyke, MD
Assistant Professor of Medicine
Division of General Internal Medicine
Pennsylvania State University College
  of Medicine
The Milton S. Hershey Medical Center
Hershey, Pennsylvania

Paul E. Turer, MD
Chief of Nephrology
St. Agnes Hospital
Baltimore, Maryland

Roy C. Ziegelstein, MD
Assistant Professor of Medicine
Division of Cardiology
Deputy Director of Medicine
The Johns Hopkins University School of
  Medicine
The Johns Hopkins Bayview Medical
  Center
Baltimore, Maryland

Contents

Foreword to the First Edition vii
Preface to the Third Edition ix
Preface to the First Edition xi
Acknowledgments xiii
Contributors xv

1/ GENERAL MEDICAL CONSULTATION SERVICE: THE ROLE OF THE INTERNIST

– Richard J. Gross and Gregory M. Caputo

Initial Contact 2
Completion of the Consultation
   Report 3
Follow-up 5
Effectiveness of Consultations 5

2/ FUNCTION OF A GENERAL INTERNAL MEDICINE CONSULTATION SERVICE

– Gregory M. Caputo and Richard J. Gross

Attributes of a General Medicine
   Consultation Service 10
Description of a General Medicine
   Consultation Service 12
Risk Assessment 14
The Effect of Capitated Insurance
   Systems on General Internal
   Medicine Consultation 17

3/ EVALUATION OF MEDICAL RISKS IN THE SURGICAL PATIENT

– Richard J. Gross

Risk–benefit: General Principles ... 19
Approach to the Preoperative
   Evaluation.................................. 22

4/ EVALUATION OF HEALTHY PATIENTS AND AMBULATORY SURGICAL PATIENTS

– Richard J. Gross and Stewart F. Babbott

Evaluation of Healthy Patients 29
Evaluation of Ambulatory Surgical
   Patients 33

Selecting Preoperative Tests:
   An Overview 40
Specific Preoperative Tests:
   Evaluation.................................. 42

5/ ANESTHESIA: RISKS, TECHNIQUES AND AGENTS, ORGAN EFFECTS, AND SPECIFIC CONCERNS

– Larry B. Grossman

Risks and Mortality....................... 55
Spinal or Epidural Anesthesia
   versus General Anesthesia 57
Same-day Admissions 58
Outpatient Anesthesia.................... 58
Anesthesia Management................ 58
Anesthetic Agents 59
Effects on Organ Systems.............. 60
Drug Interactions 64
Specific Concerns 66

6/ THE RECOGNITION, CORRECTION, AND PREVENTION OF MALNUTRITION

– Sudhir K. Dutta

Rationale 71
Recognition.................................... 72
Correction of Malnutrition............. 77
Nutritional Intervention 79
Enteral Nutrition............................ 79
Parenteral Nutrition 85
Complications of Parenteral
   Nutrition 87
Nutritional Support and Clinical
   Conditions 89
Inflammatory Bowel Disease 90
Pancreatitis 90
Chronic Liver Disease 90

Renal Disease................................. 90
Chronic Lung Disease 91
Cardiac Disease 91
Cancer.. 91
Human Immunodeficiency Virus ... 91

7/ PREOPERATIVE PULMONARY EVALUATION

– Philip A. Masters and Kevin Gleeson

Postoperative Pulmonary
    Complications 94
Effects of Anesthesia and Surgery
    on Respiratory Function 94
Risk Factors for Pulmonary
    Complications 97
Preoperative Pulmonary Testing.. 101
Approach to the Surgical
    Patient...................................... 104
Postoperative Management 107

8/ BASIC MECHANICAL RESPIRATORY SUPPORT

– Larry B. Grossman and Howard T. Jacobs

Epidemiology 115
Indications for Intubation and
    Mechanical Support.................. 117
Sources of Information for
    Ventilatory Plans 118
Technical Aspects 119
Ventilatory Equipment and Its
    Management 120
Problems from Mechanical
    Ventilation................................ 125
Criteria for Extubation 126
Additional Modes of Mechanical
    Ventilation................................ 129

9/ INVASIVE PHYSIOLOGIC MONITORING IN THE INTENSIVE CARE UNIT: CONTROVERSIES AND CONSENSUS

– John M. Field

The Controversy 133
Historical Background.................. 134
The Issues 134
Consensus Indications.................. 135
Complications................................ 136
Clinical Competence..................... 136

10/ THROMBOEMBOLIC DISORDERS

– Brent G. Petty

Prevention of Deep Venous
    Thrombophlebitis...................... 141
Deep Venous Thrombophlebitis ... 144
Pulmonary Embolism 146

11/ CARDIOVASCULAR DISEASE AND HYPERTENSION

– Rita A. Falcone and Roy C. Ziegelstein

General Considerations................ 149
Assessment of the Patient 149
Effective Consultation 152
Risk and Prevalence of Myocardial
    Ischemia 153
Coronary Revascularization
    Procedures................................ 171
Treatment of Perioperative
    Arrhythmias.............................. 174
Perioperative Systolic and
    Diastolic Myocardial
    Dysfunction 177
Hypertension................................ 179
Valvular Heart Disease 188
Prosthetic Heart Valves 195
Hypertrophic Cardiomyopathy 197

12/ RENAL, FLUID, ELECTROLYTE, AND ACID-BASE DISORDERS

– Paul E. Turer and Gary R. Briefel

Preoperative Evaluation and
    Treatment of Patients with
    Normal Renal Function 207
Evaluation and Treatment of the
    Surgical Patient with Acute
    Renal Failure............................ 216
Evaluation and Treatment of
    Patients with Chronic
    Renal Failure............................ 229
Treatment of Renal Transplantation
    Donors and Recipients 236
Surgery in Renal Transplant
    Recipients................................. 239
Acid-Base Disorders 276

13/ GASTROENTEROLOGY

– Gerald A. Hofkin

Nutrition.. 297
Liver Disease 297
Pancreatitis.................................... 307
Postoperative Pancreatitis 308
Peptic Ulcer Disease..................... 309
Complications from Surgery 312
Postoperative Diarrhea 323
Treatment of "Ostomates"............ 323

14/ ENDOCRINE DISORDERS

– Thomas J. McGlynn, Jr. and Richard J. Simons

Diabetes Mellitus........................... 329
Hyperthyroidism............................ 334
Hypothyroidism 337
Adrenal Insufficiency..................... 340
Selective Aldosterone
    Deficiency 343
Primary Hyperaldosteronism 345
Pheochromocytoma 347
Syndrome of Inappropriate
    Antidiuretic Hormone 348
Diabetes Insipidus......................... 351
Pituitary Insufficiency.................. 354
Hyperparathyroidism and
    Hypercalcemia 355

15/ HEMATOLOGY

– James O. Ballard and Robert A. Gordon

The Preoperative Patient
    with Anemia.............................. 361
Postoperative Anemias.................. 364
The Transfused Patient................. 367
Special Operative Considerations
    in Patients with Erythrocyte
    Abnormalities 370
White Blood Cell Disorders.......... 377
Evaluation and Treatment of
    Hemostasis in Surgical
    Patients 380
Hypercoagulable States................ 393
Treatment of Platelet Disorders in
    Surgical Patients 396
Special Hematologic Treatment
    Issues in Surgical Patients...... 401

16/ ONCOLOGY

– Robert A. Gordon

Incidental Surgery in Patients
    with Cancer............................... 407
Therapeutic Surgery in Patients
    with Cancer............................... 411
Appendix: Staging Systems of
    Common Cancers....................... 443

17/ INFECTIOUS DISEASE

– John Stuckey and Richard J. Gross

Prophylactic Antibiotics 450
Postoperative Problems................ 476

18/ DERMATOLOGY

– Donald P. Lookingbill and Gregory M. Caputo

Rash and Fever............................. 519
Acquired Immunodeficiency
    Syndrome 527
Skin Signs of Malignancy 528
Skin Reactions Associated with
    Pregnancy 531
Pruritus 532
The Diabetic Foot 533
Cutaneous Complications of
    Hospitalizations....................... 534
Dermatologic Therapy 537
When to Consult a
    Dermatologist 538

19/ ORTHOPAEDICS AND RHEUMATOLOGY

– Richard J. Gross and Brent G. Petty

Hip Fractures............................... 541
Joint Replacements 544
Fat Embolization 547
Rheumatologic Considerations in
    Surgical Patients 547

20/ PERIOPERATIVE MANAGEMENT OF NEUROLOGIC CONDITIONS AND COMPLICATIONS

– Mohamad Ghias Arar, Yousef Dairi, and Lourdes C. Corman

Patients with Preexisting Neurologic
    Conditions 553

Seizure Disorders........................... 556
Dementia 558
Myasthenia Gravis 559
The Extrapyramidal Disorders.... 560
Myotonic Dystrophy..................... 563
Postoperative Neurologic
    Complications 563

21/ MEDICAL ILLNESS IN THE PSYCHIATRIC PATIENT

– Noel Ballentine and Paul Kettl

Management of Concomitant
    Medical Illness.......................... 569
Consultation to Surgical Services:
    Psychiatric Issues.................... 572
Preoperative Evaluation and
    Preparation for Surgery.......... 573
Postoperative Delirium 577
Medical Evaluation for
    Electroconvulsive Therapy....... 582
Medical Illness Presenting with
    Psychiatric Symptoms.............. 584
Alcohol Abuse 591
Eating Disorders and Their
    Medical Complications............. 592
Psychiatric Problems in Elderly
    Patients 595
Antipsychotic Drugs 597
Treatment of Anxiety Disorders .. 604
Appendix: Some Drugs that
    Cause Psychiatric
    Symptoms................................ 605

22/ SPECIAL TOPICS

– Richard J. Gross

Surgical Problems in Elderly
    Patients 615
Specific Organ System
    Disease 621

23/ MEDICAL ILLNESS DURING PREGNANCY

– John Botti and Luanne Thorndyke

Diabetes Mellitus.......................... 661
Pulmonary Disease....................... 663
Cardiovascular Disease 665
Hypertension................................ 673
Renal Disease............................... 675
Hematologic Disease.................... 676
Gastrointestinal, Hepatic,
    Biliary, and Pancreatic
    Disease 679
Thyroid Disease 687
Collagen Vascular Diseases 691
Infectious Diseases 694
Immunizations 697

24/ USEFUL EQUATIONS FOR THE CONSULTANT

– Richard J. Gross and William S. Kammerer

INDEX 711

1

General Medical Consultation Service: The Role of the Internist

Richard J. Gross and Gregory M. Caputo[1]

Little formal attention has been directed to the role of the internist as a consultant. Most authors have concentrated on a brief list of responsibilities or ethical constraints to prevent stealing patients or splitting fees. A few major figures in American medicine during the early 20th century commented briefly on the consultant's role, but none elucidated their philosophy in detail. The chapter outlines the consulting internist's role in relationship to the patient, the problem, and the consulting physician.

The opinions and reports of the Judicial Council of the American Medical Association contain the most comprehensive list of consultant responsibilities (1). The AMA document lists nine ethical principles of consultation. These include:

1. One physician should be in charge of the patient's care.
2. The attending physician has overall responsibility for the patient's treatment.
3. The consultant should not assume primary care of the patient without consent of the referring physician.
4. The consultation should be done punctually.
5. Discussions during the consultation should be with the referring physician and only with the patient by prior consent of the referring physician.
6. Conflicts of opinion should be resolved by a second consultation or withdrawal of the consultant; however, the consultant has the right to give his or her opinion to the patient in the presence of the referring physician.

The other three principles involve responsibilities of the referring physician for obtaining consultations:

1. Consultations are indicated "on request," in doubtful or difficult cases, or when they enhance the quality of medical care.
2. Consultations are primarily for the patient's benefit.
3. A case summary should be sent to the consulting physician unless a verbal description of the case has already been given.

A consultation should be differentiated from a referral, although these terms are often used interchangeably. A **consultation** is strictly defined as requesting another physician to give his or her opinion on diagnosis or management. A **referral** means to request another physician to assume direct responsibility for a portion

---

[1]William S. Kammerer contributed to this chapter in the first and second editions of this book.

(e.g., a specific problem) or for all of the patient's care.

Based on clinical experience, discussion with other internists, and review of available literature, we conceptualize the role of the consultant as outlined here. Performing a consultation involves the phases of initial contact, completion of the consultation report, and follow-up (Table 1.1).

INITIAL CONTACT

The Consultation Request (Statement of the Problem)

Commonly, consultations are submitted without a clear statement of the questions to be answered by the consultant. A consultation request stating the problem as "angina" might be submitted in the following greatly different situations: (a) a patient with atypical chest pain whose the referring physician wants confirmation of a noncardiac etiology, (b) a patient with refractory angina referred for cardiac catheterization before noncardiac surgery, (c) a patient with stable angina whose surgeon desires to know if further evaluation or therapy is necessary, (d) a patient with new chest pain and gallbladder disease whose physician needs to know the etiology of

Table 1.1.   Role of the Consultant

Initial Contact
1. Consultation request
2. Referring physician
3. The patient

Completion of the Consultation Report
4. Existing database (chart)
5. The consultation report
6. Timeliness
7. Relationship to other consultants

Follow-up
8. Follow-up
   a. Inpatient
   b. After discharge (primary medical physician)

---

the pain, or (e) a patient with symptomatic gallstones whose referring physician desires to know if the patient can withstand surgery. **A precise understanding of the reasons for a consultation** is imperative if the consultant is to provide optimal service to the referring physician and patient. Poorly defined reasons for consultation often lead to duplication of effort, increased cost to the patient, and most important, suboptimal care (as well an unsatisfied referring physician).

In addition, it is important for the consultant to know what procedure is planned, what alternatives the referring physician will or will not consider, what benefits the procedure or alternatives offer the patient, and the extent of the consultant's involvement in patient care and follow-up desired by the referring physician. Speaking with the referring physician for a few minutes before seeing the patient to clarify the reasons for a consultation will save time and result in more specific suggestions. The consultant should remember that he or she was called to help, not to be another burden by asking peripheral questions and making suggestions that are not pertinent to the problem at hand.

The Referring Physician

Conflicts over patient management between referring physicians and consultants are among the most difficult areas of interprofessional relationships. Factors contributing to these disagreements are differences in expertise between physicians as training becomes more specialized; differences in the approach to common problems between internists, anesthesiologists, and surgeons; and differences in philosophy between internists and surgeons about how closely the patient needs to be followed or the urgency for surgery. In academic institutions, the departmental structure also can foster conflicts between different services.

It serves no purpose to criticize the

referring physician because of differences in knowledge or philosophy of patient care. This only increases resistance to the consultant's recommendations or decreases appropriate consultation in the future, both of which depend on some goodwill. In our experience, the best way to prevent conflicts is communication before the consultation, as described earlier, and verbal as well as written transmission of recommendations, especially when some controversy is anticipated. Restricting recommendations to only those affecting diagnosis and therapy is appreciated by many surgeons and patients.

Methods of resolving conflicts vary in academic and community practice situations. In academic settings, a case conference including residents, consultants, and attending physicians is useful, especially if it is guided by a senior attending physician. Communication between senior attending physicians can often resolve problems that begin on the resident or fellow level. In community practice, personal verbal communications between the private internist and referring physician usually resolve the problem. In training or private practice settings, using persuasion by other consultants or obtaining a second formal consultation can be helpful.

The Patient

The following information should be explained to the patient at the beginning of the consultant's visit: *(a)* your name, *(b)* that you are a consultant requested by his or her physician, *(c)* the service that you represent, and *(d)* the reason for the consultation. If more than one person from the consulting service will see the patient (e.g., medical student, fellow), this should be explained, as should each person's role.

It is regarded by many physicians as discourteous, if not "unethical," for a consultant to discuss diagnostic and therapeutic recommendations with the patient before obtaining specific approval from the referring physician. The attending physician should be informed of the consultant's recommendations *first*, before the patient. The consultant should work out any differences of opinion with the referring physician before relating these to the patient. If important, irreconcilable differences of opinion exist, they should be cited specifically in the chart with a request for another opinion to help resolve the dilemma. If all else fails, the consultant should indicate to the patient his or her intention to withdraw from the case because of disagreement with the referring physician on a diagnosis or a management plan, and the consultant should explain that it is the patient's right to request that his or her physician seek another opinion.

COMPLETION OF THE CONSULTATION REPORT

The Existing Database (Chart)

A careful review of the patient's chart is necessary for a complete consultation. This review should include obtaining outside office or hospital records, unreturned laboratory data (especially those tests sent to bacteriology, serology, or out-of-hospital laboratories), and a personal review of electrocardiograms, radiographs, and other special studies such as echocardiograms and Gram-stained smears.

The Consultation Report

A consultation to a nonmedical service should include a very brief summary of the patient's history and hospital course. The aspects of the physical examination important to the problems for which the consultation was obtained should be detailed, particularly any differences from those recorded by the primary physician. Only pertinent laboratory data should be listed, preferably in a flow sheet. Emphasis should be placed on the consultant's impressions and recommendations, including a brief discussion of how the conclusions were reached and the reasons for the consultant's recommendations.

We have found the following format to be useful for recording consultations: Impressions, Recommendations, Discussion, References (see Figs. 2.1 and 2.2). Impression, Discussion, and Recommendations should specifically address the central question asked by the referring physician as well as more general problems.

Consultations to medical services will, in most instances, be somewhat longer and more detailed. References supporting recommendations are often appreciated, especially by academic services. These are generally interpreted as indicators of the enthusiasm of the consultant and often help to forestall disagreements based on opinions rather than fact.

A complete recording of a comprehensive history and physical examination for a hospitalized patient should not be necessary. This is the responsibility of the primary service. The consultant's report should be confined to the major and pertinent problems identified and to any differences in observations from those recorded by the primary physician.

Recommendations should be as specific as possible, because the referring physician may not be familiar with the performance of certain tests or the use of certain drugs. For example, one should not write to "digitalize the patient" but to give "digoxin 0.25 mg intravenously now, again in 6 hours, and then once a day." Large numbers of recommendations are less likely to be carried out by surgical services. There should be some balance between the desire to comprehensively cover all problems, no matter how unrelated or minor, and what can be practically achieved. Some nonacute recommendations may need to be deferred to later follow-up notes in complex cases to increase the likelihood that suggestions will be carried out. Critical or stat recommendations should be listed first and clearly labeled as urgent (2–9). It is useful to discuss specific impressions and recommendations with the referring service, and this is mandatory if recommendations are urgent or many.

The consultant should provide the surgeon with:

1. A clear, concise evaluation of medical risks.
2. Measures to improve or stabilize the patient preoperatively.
3. Postoperative medical considerations.
4. The role that the consultant will assume in the overall care of the patient (1, 10) (see Chapter 3).

Timeliness

Consultations are often asked for in a rushed manner, whether because of the patient's critical state or for the convenience of the referring physician. There is some truth to the saying that "consultations requested today were urgently needed yesterday, and should have been requested a week ago." Such "urgent" consultations should be seen promptly, regardless of whether they are mandated by the patient's condition or the physician's request. Elective consultations for surgery should be done so as not to postpone surgery, even if the request was received late. Patients will appreciate this courtesy, because it may often prevent costly hospitalization from being prolonged. In cases of repeated unnecessary requests for urgent consultation, a gentle reminder of the inconvenience is usually sufficient. An interesting protocol for identifying patients with "risk factors" for last-minute consultation regarding cardiac problems (11) might serve as an alternative strategy for reducing repeated urgent consultations. All consultations, however, should be seen for at least a brief triage assessment on the day they are received. The situation of unrecognized severity is just as important and common as the situation in which severity is known to the referring physician. If the consultation cannot be completed on the day it is received, the anticipated delay must be immediately and directly communicated to the referring physician.

Relationship to Other Consultants

The general internist is commonly one of several medical consultants for an individual patient; this situation occurs 60% of the time according to a study from the University of Chicago (9). A common mistake is to simply make suggestions for the specific problems relating to one's specialty. Conflicts with the suggestions of other consultants most often arise in this manner. These conflicts may include different advice for the same problem and recommendations for therapy that may adversely affect another problem or interfere with another consultant's recommendations. The consulting internist must keep abreast of any suggestions from other consultants and, in many cases, negotiate with them as needed. One function of the general internist should be to integrate the advice from subspecialists and help to resolve conflicting suggestions.

FOLLOW-UP

There are no specific data on how often follow-up visits need to be made by the consultant. The consultant's advice is more likely to be taken, however, if follow-up is more frequent and documented with a progress note (7, 12). The need for follow-up ranges from two to three visits per day for a critically ill patient (e.g., a myocardial infarction after surgery), two to three visits per week for a relatively stable patient (e.g., a resolving postoperative pneumonia), or one visit per week for a stable patient (e.g., awaiting return of a laboratory value for an elective workup). **The type and frequency of follow-up should be specifically listed** as part of the recommendations/plan in the initial consultation note.

Brief progress notes should usually be made for each visit and emphasize new data, changes in impressions, and suggested changes in tests or therapy. Problem-oriented flow sheets attached to the patient's original consultation report and updated on each visit are an efficient way of recording data. The frequency of or need for continued follow-up should be questioned if the consultant does not feel that follow-up notes need to be made on more than an occasional visit. Recommendations should be documented in follow-up notes as well as communicated to the referring physician verbally, because the written record provides the only means for reviewing the longitudinal course of the patient. Verbal interchange is quite useful for the same reasons as the initial consultation report. **A written note should document when the consultant will no longer follow the patient and that the consultation is complete.** One common and inexcusable practice by many consultants is to just stop seeing the patient with only a vague word to the referring service that follow-up is being discontinued. This can mislead the referring physician into thinking that everything is going well when in reality the patient is doing poorly and is not being followed.

A final job of the consultant is to assure continuity of the patient's care for medical problems after discharge. This is easily accomplished if the consultant is also the patient's primary physician. Minor problems are often adequately handled by mentioning to the surgeon what information should be communicated to the primary physician, either verbally or in the discharge summary. Contact between the consultant and the patient's primary physician is important for serious medical problems or complex patients; in this case, a letter to the primary physician is often indicated after the consultant coordinates his or her recommendations with the physician who requested the consultation. When the patient has no primary physician, the consultant should assist in making arrangements for medical follow-up care.

EFFECTIVENESS OF CONSULTATIONS

Considerable literature is available regarding the effectiveness of medical consultants on nonmedical services (2–10, 12–14). Using the principles listed earlier, certain aspects of the consultant's role can be identified that have the most influence on his or her recommendations being carried out by the referring physician (the "best" measure of consultation "quality").

The available literature is limited, however, because only one measure of consultation quality has been examined (i.e., the referring physician's compliance with the consultant's advice) and the data have been gathered mostly from academic institutions, in which the consulting and referring physicians may be attendings, residents, or medical students. The relevance of these data for private or group community practice has not been established (15).

Compliance with the consultant's advice ranged from 54 to 77% of his or her recommendations made in academic centers (Table 1.2). A study from a military teaching hospital (4) found that 90% of recommendations were followed, suggesting that compliance may be higher in nonacademic settings.

In studies of medical consultation on nonmedical services, the referring and consulting physicians disagreed in some manner about the major reason for the consultation in approximately 14 to 36% of cases (Table 1.3). Reasons for these disagreements varied among studies and included the referring physician never stating a reason for the consult, the consulting physician's note never answering the major question asked by the

Table 1.2.   Compliance with Advice from the Medical Consultant

Study	Compliance (%)[a]
Klein (2)	54
Sears (5)	77
Pupa (4)	90
Ballard (6)	72
Ferguson (13)	95

[a]Compliance = number of recommendations carried out/total number of recommendations by consultant.

Table 1.3.   Referring/Consulting Physician Disagreements on the Central Reason for Consultation

Study	Disagreement (%)[a]
Lee (8)	14
Horowitz (7)	18
Rudd (9)	36

[a]Disagreement was defined variously as different reasons, no stated reason for consult, or consult report not answering the question listed by the referring physician.

referring physician, or both physicians stating different reasons for the consult. Obviously, if the consultant does not answer the *"central question"* (3) for the consultation *specifically* in his or her report, the consultation has not served its intended purpose, no matter how much more important or interesting the other problems may be.

Several factors have been noted to improve compliance with the consultant's advice (Table 1.4) (4), and most are within the consultant's ability to change, except the severity of illness and type of recommendation (i.e., diagnostic versus therapeutic). The way the consultation is performed affects it outcome. **Improved compliance was found when the consult was performed promptly (i.e., within 24 hours), follow-up was frequent and noted in the chart, and the consultant discussed his or her findings with the referring physician. Aspects that improved the consultation included limiting the number of recommendations to five or fewer, keeping all recommendations tied to the central reason for the consultation, making the recommendations definite (i.e., written as "do today" versus "suggested"), and listing specific details, especially for drug recommendations (e.g., dose and route of administration).**

Performing a consultation following the advice in Table 1.4 improves compliance with the recommendations, but this advice cannot always be followed. Many patients have multiple serious problems other than the disease for which the consultation was requested that require recommendations. Severely ill patients tend to have more recommendations made by the consultant (i.e., 4–6); often, these cannot be reduced to five or fewer recommendations. There also is a need to document recommendations for unrelated problems affecting the patient's health for medicolegal reasons. An approach to take in handling consultations in which the points of Table 1.4 must be violated (e.g., a large number of recommendations) includes personal, verbal discussion with the referring physician (2, 3, 8, 16), often on a repeated basis during the follow-up period. More elective recommendations for peripheral problems can be deferred to follow-up notes once the critical recommendations have been carried out. There is a tendency to list every recommendation in the initial consultation report even if they involve long-term, nonacute prob-

lems, which may overwhelm the referring physician who is caring for an acutely ill patient and be forgotten later in the course.

Preliminary studies (17-19) have suggested that the yield (in terms of new problems identified) of perioperative medical consultation are found mostly in high-risk patients (e.g., those over 50 years of age or ASA Class III-IV). Another preliminary study (20) showed a decreased length of stay, less use of tests, and possibly lower mortality with routine perioperative medical consultation on all patients. This study was limited, however, because it was confined to male patients undergoing cardiac or thoracic surgery in a veterans hospital and did not have a randomized control group. Inadequate data exist to determine if perioperative medical consultation improves patient outcome (21), which is the ultimate measure of effectiveness of a consultation.

SUMMARY

Based on their experience as consultants and on the literature cited in this chapter, Burnside (22), Goldman and Rudd (23), and Merli and Weitz (24) have summarized a philosophy of consultation into the "Ten Commandments of Consultation" (Table 1.5). These serve as a brief (pocket) reminder of the important points of consultation listed here.

The skills and process of consultation are learned through experience and observing accomplished senior consultants. This analysis is not intended to supplant such experiences but to complement them by providing an outline for critical observation of patient care. A number of residency programs have established general medical consultation services with the aim of teaching these consultation skills.

In summary, the ideal consultant as described by Bates (25, 26) is one who "informs without patronizing, educates without lecturing, directs without ordering, and . . . solves the problem without making the referring physician look stu-

Table 1.4. Factors Improving Compliance with Recommendations of the Medical Consultant

	Reference
1. Consultation performed within 24 hours of request	7
2. Follow-up (frequent, follow-up notes more than two follow-up visits.	7, 12
3. Verbal contact with referring physician; positive attitude toward referring service.	4, 8, 9
4. Limited number of recommendations (≤5).	2–5
5. Recommendation related to "central reason" for consultation.	3, 5, 8
6. Definitiveness of recommendation.	2, 3, 7–9
7. "Crucial" (versus routine) recommendation.	4–6
8. Specific details for drug recommendations (dose, duration).	7, 9, 12
9. Medication/treatment (versus diagnostic) recommendation.	2–6
10. Severely ill patient.	5, 6

Table 1.5.   Ten Commandments for Consultations

1. Determine the question.
2. Establish urgency.
3. Obtain your own primary data.
4. Be brief in your report.
5. Be specific in your recommendations; support your impressions and recommendations. (Be honest.)
6. Provide contingency plans.
7. Respect the referring physician's prerogatives.
8. Teach.
9. Talk with the referring physician.
10. Provide follow-up.

Adapted from Burnside JW. Command for consultants. Hosp Physician 1973;7:53–54; Goldman L, Rudd P. Ten commandments for effective consultations. Arch Intern Med 1983;143:1753–1755; and Merli GJ, Weitz HH. The medical consultant. Med Clin North Am 1987;71:353–354.

pid." The consultant, then, should try always to support the referring physician, comfort the patient, and be specific.

REFERENCES

1. Opinions and reports of the judicial council. Chicago: American Medical Association, 1960.
2. Klein LE, Levine DM, Moore RD, et al. The preoperative consultation: response to internists' recommendations. Arch Intern Med 1983; 143:743–744.
3. Klein LE, Moore RD, Levine DM, et al. Effectiveness of medical consultations. J Med Educ 1983;58:149–151.
4. Pupa LE, Coventry JA, Hanley JF, et al. Factors affecting compliance for general medicine consultations to non-internists. Am J Med 1986;81: 508–514.
5. Sears CL, Charlson ME. The effectiveness of a consultation. Am J Med 1983;74:870–876.
6. Ballard W, Gold JP, Charlson ME. Compliance with the recommendations of medical consultants. J Gen Intern Med 1986;1:220–224.
7. Horwitz RL, Henes CG, Horwitz SM. Developing strategies for improving the diagnostic and management efficacy of medical consultations. J Chronic Dis 1983;36:213–218.
8. Lee T, Pappius EM, Goldman L. Impact of inter-physician communication on the effectiveness of medical consultations. Am J Med 1983; 74:106–112.
9. Rudd P, Siegler M, Byyny RL. Perioperative diabetic consultation: a plea for improved training. J Med Educ 1978;53:590–596.
10. Burke GR, Corman LC. The general medicine consult service in a university teaching hospital. Med Clin North Am 1979;63:1353–1358.
11. Dudley JC, Brandenburg JA, Hartley H, et al. Last-minute preoperative cardiology consultations: epidemiology and impact. Am Heart J 1996;131:245–249.
12. Mackenzie TB, Popkin MK, Callies AL, et al. The effectiveness of cardiology consultation. Chest 1981;79:16–22.
13. Moore RA, Kammerer WS, McGlynn TJ, et al. Consultations in internal medicine: a training program resource. J Med Educ 1977;52:323–327.
14. Robie PW. The service and educational contributions of a general internal medicine consultation service. J Gen Intern Med 1986;1:225–227.
15. Ferguson RP, Rubinstien E. Preoperative medical consultations in a community hospital. J Gen Intern Med 1987;2:89–92.
16. Charlson ME, Cohen RP, Sears CL. General medical consultation: lessons from a clinical service. Am J Med 1983;75:121–128.
17. Gluck R, Munoz E, Wise L. Preoperative and postoperative medical evaluation of surgical patients. Am J Surg 1988;155:730–734.
18. Levinson W. Preoperative evaluations by an internist—are they worthwhile? West J Med 1984;141:395–398.
19. Clelland C, Worland RL, Jessup DE, East D. Preoperative medical evaluation in patients having joint replacement surgery: added benefits. South Med J 1996;89:958–960.
20. MacPherson DS, Parenti C, Nee J, et al. An internist joins the surgery service: does comanagement make a difference? J Gen Intern Med 1994;9:440–444.
21. Massie BM, Mangano DT. Assessment of perioperative risk: have we put the cart before the horse? J Am Coll Cardiol 1993;21:1353–1356.
22. Burnside JW. Commandments for consultants. Hosp Physician 1973;7:53–54.
23. Goldman L, Rudd P. Ten commandments for effective consultations. Arch Intern Med 1983; 143:1753–1755.
24. Merli GJ, Weitz HH. The medical consultant. Med Clin North Am 1987;71:353–354.
25. Bynny RL, Siegler M, Taylor AR. Development of an academic section of general internal medicine. Am J Med 1977;63:493–498.
26. Bates RC. The two sides of every successful consultation. Med Econ 1979;7(56):173–180.

RECOMMENDED READINGS

Golden WE, Lavender RC. Preoperative cardiac consultations in a teaching hospital. South Med J 1989; 82:292–295.
Lee TH, Goldman L. Role of the consultant. In: Breslow MJ, Miller CF, Rogers M, eds. Perioperative management. St. Louis: CV Mosby, 1990:46–51.

2

Function of a General Internal Medicine Consultation Service

Gregory M. Caputo[1] and Richard J. Gross

The renewed prominence of the general internist on academic medicine faculties has prompted much discussion by students, residents, medical subspecialists, and general internists themselves as to their actual role. Therefore, much attention has been directed to their wide-ranging activities in patient care and resident teaching, primarily in the outpatient setting. The general internal medicine consultation service is a major additional activity that is often overlooked or misunderstood (1–6). The major role of consultation in general internal medicine has been emphasized by several studies of what the practicing internist does (6–10). From 20 to 50% of an internist's new patients are referred by other physicians for either problem-oriented consultation or ongoing total care. Thus, the relevance of the general medicine consultation service should be made clear to residents interested in practicing general internal medicine.

A wide spectrum of unfamiliar medical problems faces the resident during the general medical consultation experience. In addition, the resident must deal with the intricacies and nuances of the relationship between referring phy-

sician and consultant. Most of the medical problems dealt with by a general medicine consultation service differ categorically or in severity from those seen by the primary medicine inpatient service. These differences are becoming more pronounced with the increasing emphasis, driven by capitated systems, on efficiency and shortened lengths of stay. The practice of admitting "interesting" cases for teaching purposes has virtually disappeared. Admissions to university teaching hospital medical wards now involve predominately tertiary care problems demanding the multiple resources and technical apparatus associated with these institutions. For example, a patient with uncomplicated hyperthyroidism, rheumatoid arthritis, anemia, hypertension, diabetes mellitus, or systemic lupus erythematosus would not, in today's environment, be admitted to the medicine service. However, these problems are often seen on the various surgical services, even if they are typically unrelated to the surgical diagnosis. In addition, appropriate diagnostic techniques and care must be integrated with those of the underlying surgical illness. Understanding and managing the stress of surgery or childbirth on these illnesses demands important skills, information, and insight from the medical resident that are different from those learned on medical wards or in clinic (2, 3, 6).

[1]William S. Kammerer contributed to this chapter in the first and second editions of this book.

The goals of the educationally oriented general medical consult service should be:

1. Educate residents in the process of risk identification, assessment, and correction.
2. Expose residents to the concept and complexities of "interface medicine" (i.e., the relationship between consultant, consulting physician, and patient).
3. Develop the professional and social skills necessary for effective interdisciplinary communication and patient care.
4. Develop an attitude that fosters lifelong, independent, self-directed learning and professional development.
5. Emphasize and encourage attention to detail.
6. Develop an approach that stresses efficiency, specificity, and patient advocacy.
7. Provide the understanding an internist must have regarding the indications for surgery, likelihood of risks and benefit, and appropriate perioperative care.

ATTRIBUTES OF A GENERAL MEDICINE CONSULTATION SERVICE

When organizing an academic general internal medicine consultation service, one should carefully consider not just what services are provided but how it functions to accomplish its goals. It is far too easy to discuss only the patient's medical problems with a resident and not specifically discuss risk assessment or the interprofessional relationships involved in communicating about the case, thus losing much of the educational value of the situation. Paradoxically, **the goals of teaching interprofessional relationships, risk assessment, and style of consultation are the unique aspects of the general medical consultation service** and are those that require the most attention during organization. As-

pects that must be considered when creating a general medical consultation service are the patient base, role of the resident, role of the faculty, and means of teaching.

Patient Base

Most general medical consultation services function alongside subspecialty services. In a few hospitals, however, the general medical consultation service sees all consults initially and refers appropriate cases to subspecialty services. Either arrangement is satisfactory if adequate numbers of consultations are available for teaching purposes (e.g., 30–50 new consultations per month per resident on the service). The general consult service cannot gain credibility with residents if all cases that involve preoperative assessment go to subspecialty services and only routine care of nonoperative cases are referred to the service. An important role of the faculty is to attract and maintain an adequate number and variety of cases from surgical colleagues. In general, most requests come from the orthopedic, otorhinolaryngology, neurosurgery, urology, plastic surgery, psychiatry, and obstetrics/gynecology services. Lesser numbers come from the general and thoracic surgery services (2–4).

Role of the Resident

The resident's primary responsibility during his or her rotation must be to the consult service for it to function effectively. Institutions in which residents have primary responsibilities elsewhere and are only secondarily responsible for consultations typically cannot maintain the service's teaching function. A number of services have had great success when the resident has other secondary responsibilities within the Division of General Internal Medicine during this rotation, such as clinic responsibilities for seeing new patients, evaluating preoperative outpatients, performing emergency room consultations, and seeing referred patients together with faculty preceptors on a one-to-one basis. Increasing numbers of consult services make the resident responsible for a set number of sessions in the outpatient preoperative evaluation clinic. This outpatient experience must be carefully coordinated to avoid conflict with inpatient consults and to provide adequate supervision and teaching by the faculty. A multidisciplinary program including general internists, subspecialists, anesthesiologists, and surgeons can be very effective. The service must maintain 24-hour availability both for clinical service and resident teaching. It is impossible for a single resident to do this (and most services will only have one resident), so adequate cross-coverage for night call and weekends must be arranged. The service should be busy enough that it will not be viewed as an "easy" rotation spent mainly in the library, but it should allow adequate time for reading and assimilation of overall responsibilities. These factors must be considered when determining the number of residents on the service and their responsibilities.

Role of the Faculty

The role of the faculty preceptor is crucial to the proper functioning of the service. This faculty member must see all patients to provide bedside teaching, adequate role modeling, and supervise even senior residents who have little experience with or knowledge of preoperative evaluation. The faculty should emphasize: (a) approach to the patient in preoperative evaluation (see Chapters 1 and 3); and (b) review of the literature and its application to the individual patient. Aspects to be emphasized are preoperative risk assessment and the differential diagnosis and management of postoperative problems, because most residents will have an adequate background in the routine medical aspects by the time they reach the consult service. It is absolutely crucial, however, for the faculty to discuss the interprofessional relationships involved in most cases. This involves discussing how the resident will communicate with the consulting service and advising on management of difficulties in professional relationships, such as when the referring service ignores the consultant's advice. Having the faculty review and sign all consultation reports will also ensure feedback to the resident on the adequacy of his or her written communication.

Teaching Methods

Teaching should involve three methods. First, adequate literature resources and references should be available. Guidance on systematic, computerized literature reviews on this specialized topic should be given. We have given residents a packet of reprints with seminal articles addressing the most common consultation problems seen by our service (11), accompanied by a list of specific references and texts (12, 13) to be useful. Outlining goals and objectives at the beginning of the rotation is critical.

Second, conference-based teaching should be provided to efficiently teach residents the approach to common consultation problems. This can be done through either medicine grand rounds or conferences of the Division of General Internal Medicine. The essential topics that should be covered during the year include the approach to preoperative evaluation and the commonly seen organ system problems (i.e., cardiac, pulmonary, diabetes, thromboembolic disease).

Finally, most hospitals also provide several other opportunities for resident teaching. Examples are consultation to the psychiatry service in evaluating possible medical illnesses in psychiatric patients, joint medical–obstetric clinics for pregnant patients with high-risk medical disease, consultation to surgical specialty units (e.g., burn units), and evaluation of potential kidney donors. Such functions can be easily integrated into the more traditional inpatient consultation roles of the consultation service.

DESCRIPTION OF A GENERAL MEDICINE CONSULTATION SERVICE

At Penn State's Milton S. Hershey Medical Center, senior medical residents rotate for 1 month on the general internal medicine consultation service. Faculty members likewise have 1-month rotations on the service. Rounds with the attending internist are made daily, and every consultation is seen within 24 hours of the request, usually on the same day. Forty to fifty new consultations are completed each month. Two-thirds of the requests originate from the orthopedic, otorhinolaryngology, and psychiatric services; the remainder originate from the obstetrics/gynecology, neurosurgical, urology, and general surgery services. Urgent requests from the outpatient nonmedical practice sites are also seen, and the consult resident helps to coordinate care in the emergency room for patients with medical problems needing admission or medical follow-up.

Continued and direct faculty participation in the consultation process provides support and direction to the medical resident, improves the efficiency of patient care, and demonstrates the important interdisciplinary communication and professional skills that are necessary for a successful outcome. For example, in a review of 36 general medicine consultation services at university teaching hospitals in the 1970s, 50% were found to offer no ongoing faculty supervision. These were deemed by residents to have primarily service-oriented functions and little or no educational value. The other 50%, which had regular and formal faculty input, were reported to be educationally rewarding and satisfying rotations (2).

The use of a structured format (Figs. 2.1 and 2.2) for reporting the consultation both improves communication and provides the resident with an efficient means for clearly stating his impressions and recommendations. This format requires the consultant to focus clearly and specifically on the major issues, and it prevents obfuscation in a lengthy narrative that recounts the obvious and avoids answering the questions asked. We have found that using this format improves relations between medical and surgical residents, because both are forced to deal with facts and observations rather than with loosely formed opinions. In addition, the faculty will add comments or suggestions to indicate that they also have personally examined the patient and discussed specific impressions and recommendations with the resident. The faculty portion of the note must be sufficient to meet Medicare and other insurance billing documentation standards, and a brief faculty dictation is sometimes done to ensure adequate documentation.

Even the most senior residents at the beginning of the general medicine consultation service often find themselves having little basic factual information with which to support their opinions. This is a source of much frustration, especially when their recommendations are ignored or overridden in a contest of opinions. Therefore, we try to build into our teaching program as much specific published material as available and urge residents to research problems and complications that are new to them. While using didactic and conference-style teaching to a certain extent, we prefer to stress careful bedside observations, evidence-based support of recommendations, and the importance of close patient follow-up as effective learning techniques. Careful follow-up directly confronts the consultants with the consequences of their recommendations, thus reinforcing positive results as well as spotlighting mistakes or errors in judgment. With this approach, we hope to reinforce DaCosta's dictum that "diagnosis by intuition is a rapid method of reaching a wrong conclusion."[2] Systematic follow-up also provides an opportunity

---

[2]From DaCosta JC. Selections from the papers and speeches of John Chalmers DaCosta, MD, LLD. Philadelphia: WB Saunders, 1931:50.

Consultation   **From: General Surgery**   **To: General Internal Medicine**

REASON FOR CONSULTATION

75 year old white male with symptomatic cholelithiasis; plans underway for closed cholecystectomy in 2 weeks.

PROVISIONAL DX

Cholelithiasis

Assessment:

1. Symptomatic cholecystitis.
2. Systolic murmur. The bedside characteristics suggest moderate aortic stenosis.
3. Essential hypertension, with reasonable control.
4. Left ventricular hypertrophy by physical exam and electrocardiography.
5. Upper respiratory infection; most likely early, mild bacterial sinusitis.

Recommendations:

1. Transthoracic echocardiogram to further define valvular and left ventricular function.
2. Chest radiograph. No clear indication for pulmonary function tests or arterial blood gases.
3. Oral trimethroprim sulfamethoxazole DS po BID for 7 days plus oxymetozaline nasal spray BID for 3 days.
4. Antibiotic prophylaxis for subacute bacterial endocarditis (if A.S. confirmed by echo):
   - ampicillin 2 G IV
   - gentamicin 80 mg
   - cefazolin 1 G (for wound infection prophylaxis)

   Give each antibiotic one hour prior to surgery and 8 hours later.
5. Close attention postoperatively to fluid and volume status to avoid CHF—this patient may be at particular risk due to valvular heart disease and left ventricular hypertrophy.
6. Prophylaxis against deep venous thrombophlebitis—Heparin 5,000 units subcutaneously Q 12 hours until ambulatory.

   NB: I have ordered #1-3 as per our discussion.

Discussion:

This patient is at increased risk for general anesthesia due to his age and his aortic stenosis (if confirmed by echo). However, the risk should not be considered prohibitive, in our opinion. Close attention to volume status will be essential. He is at some increased risk for pulmonary complications due to the upper abdominal incision but there is no clear evidence that preoperative pulmonary function tests would be of value, given his lack of known pulmonary disease or symptoms.

His respiratory infection is mild but should be treated prior to surgery.

Figure 2.1.   The Milton S. Hershey Medical Center Hospital Consultation Report.

Figure 2.1. *(continued)*

History

HPI	This is an 86 year old man with a history of 4 episodes of colicky postprandial right upper quadrant pain and gall stones on ultrasound.
PMH	Systolic hypertension since 1979.
PSH	Negative
Medications	Enalapril 10 mg po QAM. NKDA
SH	Non-smoker. One beer per week. Walks 1 mile a day for exercise.
ROS	"Sinus congestion" for 3 days. Low grade fever (100 deg. po).

Physical Exam

Vitals	99.2 148/84 16 80
HEENT	Boggy nasal mucosa, moderate right maxillary tenderness, mucopurulent post-nasal drainage
Neck	No bruits; carotid upstrokes slightly delayed
Lungs	Clear
Heart	Prominent PMI, not displaced. Normal S1S2; 3/6 somewhat harsh SEM peaks in midsystole heard best in the aortic area radiating to the carotids. No gallop.

ABDOMEN, EXT, SKIN, NEURO, GENIT WNL

Gregory M. Caputo, M.D., F.A.C.P.

to identify common problems on which to concentrate our teaching, literature searches, and research topics.

RISK ASSESSMENT (SEE ALSO CHAPTER 3)

The most difficult aspect of the consultation process for many internists arises when attempting to specifically assess the risk to the patient of a proposed procedure. In large part, this develops from unfamiliarity with the physiologic stresses of anesthesia or of specific surgical procedures and from the unpredictability of intraoperative complications. Another key factor is the difficulty in predicting overall risk from anesthesia, surgical, and medical considerations, especially with the complex interactions of the physiologic stresses from these three areas and the different physiology of the pre-, intra-, and postoperative periods. In the past, this led internists to conclude their recommendations with the gratuitous and superficial reminder to "maintain blood pressure and oxygenation and avoid volume overload." Obviously, this kind of advice is rarely helpful to the physician requesting a consultation. Rather, most consultation requests are really asking the consultant to identify and define the severity of significant medical problems, to help optimally manage them preoperatively, and to be available for close follow-up postoperatively.

The ability to make reasoned judgments in the absence of complete data, to anticipate likely problems, and to provide accurate and efficient monitoring of the patient's postoperative course characterizes the mature consultant. Anesthesiologists and

MEDICAL CONSULTATION

Anna E. Smith
February 10, 1987

REF: Dr. John Jones

SUBJECTIVE: CC: Preoperative medical evaluation for cerebral arteriogram and craniotomy, because of multiple medical problems.

58-year-old white female with left falx meningioma discovered 6 weeks ago. Patient developed severe occipital headache, profound vomiting, and hypertension. An emergency CT scan showed the meningioma. Only physical finding was partial rt. homo. hemianopsia.

3 weeks ago: Early papilledema noted on opthal. evaluation and Decadron increased to 4 mg. q6h with improvement.

Medical problems include: 1. AODM on insulin; 2. Unstable angina 1/87 with finding of 30–50% LAD before 1st septal perforator, small rt. coronary & nl. LV fxn. on catheterization; 3. COPD No angina since prior hospitalization; some atypical pain (prob. noncardiac), but activity limited. No DOE, orthopnea, edema, sputum production. Insulin requirements have risen on steroids. 4. H/O pulmonary emboli.

No personal or family HX. of anesthesia problems, transfusion reaction, bleeding disorders, or family hx. thromboombolic disease.

PAST MEDICAL HISTORY		SOC. HX. 58-year-old married secretary
ALLERGIES: None		Smokes: 1PPD ×26 yrs. ETOH: Rare
ILLNESSES:	1. Angina (1987)	Drugs: None
	2. AODM	FAMILY HISTORY: +COPD, heart disease,
	3. COPD	cancer, diabetes
	4. Pulmonary Emboli	ROS: (Positives): Otherwise non-contributory.
	5. Lt. falx meningioma	
SURGERY:	1. T&A	
	2. Cholecystectomy, 1976	
	3. L5/S1 disectomy, 1986	
INJURIES:	1. Back	
MEDICATIONS:	1. Humulin-N insulin 45U AM 12U PM (Humulin-R coverage per schedule)	
	2. Nitrodur 0.4 mg/hr. Patch QAM	
	3. Cardiazem 60 mg. Q6H	
	4. Theodur 400 mg. Q12H	
	5. TNG 0.4 mg, sl PRN	

OBJECTIVE:

VITAL SIGNS: BP RT. Arm(lie) 140/80 Pulse 76 (reg.) RR 14 Temp: 98.6 WT: 180 lbs. HT: 5'6"

GEN: Obese
NODES: Non-felt
NECK: Nl thyroid without nodules.
HEENT: Ears: Nl EAC and drums   Eyes: Flat discs w/o H,E. PERRLA = 3mm.
      Oropharynx: Clear w/o lesions or inflammation/discharge
CHEST: Clear to P&A; Minimal wheezes.
COR: PMI = MCl. S1&S2 normal; no murmurs, gallops, clicks, NVD or edema. Pulses all 2+/2+ without bruits, including carotid and pedal pulses.
ABDOMEN: Nl bowel sounds, no organomegaly, masses or tenderness.
EXTREMITIES: No cords, calf tenderness, edema. Calf (9") = 32 cm./32 cm. R/L
NEURO: M.S. Normal   GAIT: Normal
      CN: 2/12 normal, except rt field hemi-   CEREBELLAR: Normal
      anopsia   DTR's: 1–2/1–2

Figure 2.2.   Alternative format for consultation report (Baltimore).

Figure 2.2.   *(continued)*
        MOTOR: 5 + /5 + all forur ext.
        SENSORY: Normal

LABORATORY: EKG: Normal. CXR: Normal. Hct: = 46; Na$^+$ = 140.K$^+$ = 4.4 CO2 = 25. U/A Normal

ASSESSMENT:
1. Angina
2. COPD; smoker
3. AODM
4. H/O Pulmonary emboli
5. Lt. falx meningioma

No medical contraindications to planned procedures, although increased, but acceptable risk.

DISCUSSION: Multiple problems seem stable; coronary disease not critical by catheterization. Would emphasize monitoring diabetes, prevention P.E., and monitor for CV symptoms.

RECOMMENDATIONS:
1. Humulin-N 24U & ½ usual coverage day of arteriogram; D5/¼NSS @ 50 cc/hr while NPO
2. Same dose day of surgery
3. Stat Astra, acetone AM of surgery & in recovery room—call physician
3. Leg compression cuffs during surgery
4. While NPO postop, Aminophyllin 25 mg/hr continuous IV drip
5. No smoking
6. Chemstix bG ac + HS (I will write coverage); monitor chemstix q2hrs intraoperatively

Richard J. Gross, M.D., F.A.C.P.

surgeons have developed their own techniques, skills, and judgment for assessing and classifying preoperative risk factors, and they basically desire from their medial consultant a physician capable of identifying and correcting both obvious and subtle medical problems that are relevant to the patient's optimum care. Nonetheless, the results of continuing research into the most frequent types of medical risks and complications in surgical patients now enable the internist to often make important recommendations regarding risk assessment and corrective measures based on clinical and physiologic observations. Listed below are some of the most frequently encountered problems and current approaches to evaluation and management. Much of the remainder of this book is devoted to a thorough analysis of these observations and principles:

Pulmonary disease

- Pulmonary preoperative evaluation: clinical evaluation versus pulmonary function testing; objective predictors of risk.
- Intensive preoperative regimens to improve pulmonary function.
- Improved techniques for management of secretions and atelectasis.
- Pulmonary embolism

Cardiovascular disease

- Assessment of cardiac risk via multifactorial clinical assessment, non-invasive testing, and invasive testing (e.g., cardiac catheterization).
- Timing of surgery relative to previous myocardial infarction.

- Controveries in right-heart Swan-Ganz catheterization.

Perioperative infections

- Prophylactic antibiotic regimens.
- Nutritional assessment and support.
- Closed-sterile drainage systems.
- Intravenous line care.

Diabetes mellitus

- Low-dose, constant insulin infusion regimens versus traditional regimens of subcutaneous insulin.
- Postoperative complications.

Hypertension

- Appropriate drug maintenance until surgery.
- Management of hypertensive crisis and postoperative hypertension.
- Postoperative management when patient is unable to take oral medications.

THE EFFECT OF CAPITATED INSURANCE SYSTEMS ON GENERAL INTERNAL MEDICINE CONSULTATION

The advent of capitated insurance coverage has affected the practice and teaching of medical consultation in several ways. First, it creates an environment in which unnecessary consultation is strongly discouraged and the consultation process is scrutinized, so it becomes increasingly important that medical residents are well-versed in medical consultation. Fewer subspecialty consultations and more general internal medicine consultations are likely to occur as managed care increases. Second, close scrutiny of diagnostic tests is likely to increase. Thus, a strong foundation in evidence-based medicine is more important than ever in providing excellent patient care, and the physician will be on solid ground in justifying needed tests (however expensive) while avoiding those with no clear support from the results of carefully designed studies. Finally, the coordination of services and communication between internist, surgeon, and anesthesiologist carries even greater importance during an era that demands both excellence and efficiency.

SUMMARY

The well-structured and supervised general medicine consultation service can provide residents with a variety of skills and experiences important to the practice of general internal medicine. Exposure to assorted surgical disorders, surgical judgment and decision making, and various common medical problems not often seen today in medicine ward services are features that make the consult service educationally rewarding for the resident.

A preoperative assessment clinic for high-risk patients, coordinating the skills of the surgeon, anesthesiologist, and internist, would appear to be a natural extension of this service. When feasible, the resulting improvements in patient and physician convenience; more efficient and orderly evaluations; more harmonious relations between internists, surgeons, and anesthesiologists; and optimally prepared patients would be only a few of the benefits from such an approach.

REFERENCES

1. Byyny RL, Siegler M, Tarlov AR. Development of an academic section of general internal medicine. Am J Med 1977;63:493–498.
2. Moore RA, Kammerer WS, McGlynn TJ, et al. Consultations in internal medicine: a training program resource. J Med Educ 1977;52:323–327.
3. Robie PW. The service and educational contributions of a general medicine consultation service. J Gen Intern Med 1986;1:225–227.
4. Deyo RA. The internist as consultant. Arch Intern Med 1980;140:137–138.
5. Bomalaski JS, Martin GH, Webster JR. General internal medicine consultation. Arch Intern Med 1983;143:875–876.

6. Devor M, Renvall M, Ramsdell J. Practice patterns and the adequacy of residency training in consultation medicine. J Gen Intern Med 1993;8:554–560.
7. Burnside JW. What the general internist does. Arch Intern Med 1977;137:1286–1288.
8. Burnum JF. What one internist does in his practice: implications for the internist's disputed role and education. Ann Intern Med 1973;78: 437–444.
9. Barondess JA. The training of the internist: with some messages from practice. Ann Intern Med 1979;90:412–417.
10. Johnson AC, Kroeger HH, Altman I, et al. The office practice of internists: III. Characteristics of patients. JAMA 1965;193:144–150.
11. Gross RJ. Preoperative planning for the ambulatory patient. In: Barker RL, Burton JR, Zieve PD, eds. Principles of ambulatory medicine. 4th ed. Baltimore: Williams & Wilkins, 1995:1275–1297.
12. Gross R, Kammerer WS. Medical consultation on surgical services: an annotated bibliography. Ann Intern Med 1981;95:523–529.
13. Caputo GM, Gross RG. Medical consultation on surgical services: an annotated bibliography. Ann Intern Med 1993;118:290–297.

3

Evaluation of Medical Risks in the Surgical Patient

Richard J. Gross

RISK–BENEFIT: GENERAL PRINCIPLES

Evaluation of preoperative risks involves an area of the literature and a decision-making process that is not covered in traditional ward rotations during internal medicine training and is different from that in the routine practice of ambulatory medicine. This chapter covers the decision-making process in the preoperative evaluation of surgical patients, which involves balancing the estimated risks against the anticipated benefits of the procedure.

An estimation of preoperative risk is based on a thorough patient history, physical examination, review of any relevant database, and selectively ordered laboratory and noninvasive tests. Using the information gathered from these sources, the literature on preoperative evaluation (1–3), and clinical judgment, the risk posed by the medical problems associated with surgery can be estimated. The benefits of surgery are available in standard medical and surgical texts and (very importantly) from referring surgical colleagues.

The decision to proceed, balancing the risks and the benefits, made on basis of five points (Table 3.1). These are:

1. Why was the consult really requested?
2. What is the benefit to the patient of the proposed procedure or therapy?

3. What are the real, well-documented risks?
4. What is the risk–benefit balance (including mortality and disability)?
5. What are the patient's values and desires?

This five-point scheme includes the total process of surgical decision making. In most cases, the consulting internist is mainly involved in steps 1 through 3, with the final decision and discussion with the patient reserved for the referring surgeon.

Why Was the Consult Really Requested?

The reason for a consultation often is written as a three- or four-word statement on the consultation request form, such as "angina" or "anemia, CHF, hip fracture." In each instance, the consultation could have been requested for numerous different purposes. The requesting physician might want approval of the patient for anesthesia or surgery, confirmation that a poor-risk patient can undergo lifesaving surgery, advice on medical management, approval of a treatment the patient already is receiving, a document for medicolegal reasons or to satisfy the anesthesiologist, or a plan for routine medical care and follow-up with no relation to the surgical procedure itself. In each case, the surgeon may be asking for confirmation that what he or she already is doing is correct, for advice on one or more specific

1. Why was the consult really requested?
2. What is the benefit to the patient of the proposed procedure versus no operation or an alternative procedure in terms of morbidity, disability, mortality?
3. What are the real, well-documented risks (estimated in order of magnitude)?
4. What is the risk–benefit balance including both mortality and disability?
5. What are the patient's desires?

points, or for the internist to assume total care of the patient's medical problems. It is not possible to ascertain these sometimes subtle differences from the routine three- or four-word request. Therefore, in most cases, the reason for a consultation should be discussed with the referring physician to clarify the "real" motive. The time involved in obtaining this information will be richly rewarded in time saved and the quality of the consultation that is provided.

What Is the Benefit to the Patient of the Proposed Procedure or Therapy?

An estimation of risk cannot be used in a vacuum. A given operation with a 25% mortality rate is viewed very differently if it is a necessary, lifesaving procedure than if it is an elective surgery that offers the patient only some minimal cosmetic benefit. The recommendation for surgery also may be different if an alternative procedure offering lower risk is available. The precise question usually is not "can" but "should" a patient undergo surgery.

The benefit of a planned operative procedure must be clearly understood by the consulting internist to accurately state whether the patient should undergo surgery and to interpret the preoperative risk (4–6). The consultant should know the benefits of the planned procedure, any possible alternative procedures, and the course the patient's problem will take if no

operation is performed. Also vital is an understanding of how the various medical risk factors relate to alternative procedures compared with the proposed procedure. Benefits of surgery often are stated in terms of mortality, for which the most data are available; however, the benefit to the patient in terms of morbidity and disability frequently is more important. Therefore the consultant should know and consider the benefits in terms of quality of life as well as mortality. The final decision to undergo surgery, made on the basis of benefit to the patient, usually is reserved for the patient's personal physician and the surgeon. The consultant should be tactful in communicating how the benefit of the procedure will affect his or her evaluation of the surgical risk. The subject of relative benefit to the patient, however, cannot be ignored in any accurate evaluation of preoperative risk or in the statement of the consultant's recommendations.

What Are the Real, Well-documented Risks?

The risks posed by medical problems need to be clearly stated and evaluated. Risks can be overstated, however, as commonly occurs with older patients who are thought to be poor risks simply because of their age. In addition, risks can be listed incorrectly, such as a patient who is thought to be a bad risk because of his age when a treatable problem (e.g., obstructive lung disease) is the major risk factor. Risks also can be understated, as occurs with patients having complicated conditions in whom one or two important problems are overlooked. It is important to evaluate the problems specifically in terms of preoperative risk, because many problems have a different level of severity in terms to preoperative risk than they do in terms of clinical severity (e.g., angina, hypertension). The specific problems that affect preoperative risk should be listed, and the consulting internist should mentally review both whether and how these will affect the patients' operative status.

Risk should be estimated in terms of an order of magnitude. The specific percentage risk is not accurate in a single patient, because statistical risks based on large groups of patients have wide variations when applied to single individuals. The risk for a given patient is a combination of the risk for a specific risk factor as found in large studies and the baseline risk (i.e., pretest probability) for the patient group or population from which the patient comes (i.e., Bayesian analysis). As an example, for a patient considered to be Cardiac Risk Index class II, Goldman (7) calculated that the risk of cardiac complications varied by from 1% for minor surgery (i.e., low-risk group) to 10% for high-risk or aortic aneurysm surgery (i.e., high-risk group). Multiple interacting factors, biologic variations among individuals, and differences in the technical skills of physicians lead to major differences in risk for "similar" patients. Thus we find it neither accurate nor useful to state that a 25% risk is better than a 20% risk. In 1997, the general order of magnitude of risk can be classified as:

Usual or "low" risk: 0–0.01% (?0.05%) mortality
Low but increased risk: 0.01–0.9% mortality
Significant risk: 1–5% mortality
Moderate risk: 5–10% mortality
High risk: >10% mortality
Very high risk: >20% mortality

These figures are vastly different than they were 10 or 20 years ago, when "low risk" represented 1 to 5% and high risk was on the order of 25% mortality. This reduction in risk has been attributed to general advances in anesthesia and surgical techniques.

What Is the Risk–benefit Balance (Including Mortality and Disability)?

When deciding whether to undertake surgery, the consulting internist should first establish the benefits of the procedure to the patient and then the effect of any increased risks due to unrelated conditions. This approach is comparable to that in medical patients, in whom benefits are considered before side effects when deciding on therapy. In preoperative consultations, the line of reasoning often is reversed, with risk being considered the primary concern and benefit a secondary issue.

In deference to the consulting surgeon, the internist often confines his or her comments to medical risk factors. Few medical disorders carry an absolutely prohibitive risk if the need for surgery is sufficiently great. The long-term benefits of the surgical procedure should be the basis against which any short-term risks are measured, not the reverse.

What Are the Patient's Values and Desires?

There are implicit value judgments in balancing risks and benefits. The value placed on life and a patient's ability to perform certain social functions varies. A coronary artery bypass graft that would render the patient asymptomatic and able to return to work might be viewed much differently than a palliative cancer operation that would leave the patient with continued pain and inability to work—even if both would provide an additional year of life. This balance of risk and benefit must take into account the patient's wishes. In most instances, this information should be obtained from the patient by his or her referring or personal physician rather than by the consulting internist. However, it is important for the consultant to be cognizant of the patient's wishes.

Patients' opinions should be excluded only in the rare cases when he or she patient is unable to communicate in any manner or suffers from a severe psychiatric disturbance. In these situations, the family should be interviewed for their opinion and perception of the patient's wishes.

APPROACH TO THE PREOPERATIVE EVALUATION

If the decision is made to proceed with surgery, as occurs in most cases, the risk–benefit decision must be carried over to the decision whether to delay surgery for medical stabilization or to proceed immediately. Decisions also need to be made regarding which diagnostic and therapeutic recommendations are appropriate given the allotted time before the surgery. Certain procedures and therapies ordinarily performed on medical patients may interfere with or increase the risk of the surgery; for example, an upper gastrointestinal series could not be done the afternoon before a colon resection because of residual barium in the colon and the preoperative bowel preparations.

A *useful approach to preoperative decision making balances the urgency of surgery against the risk for significant organ system impairment* (Table 3.2). The *urgency of the surgery* is *the key controlling factor* in allowing what can be done for medical problems preoperatively. Some surgical emergencies cannot be delayed for medical problems; examples include a rupturing abdominal aortic aneurysm or a perforated bowel. **Conversely,** remember that **elective surgery is always elective.** If the consulting internist feels that further evaluation is needed, a new problem is uncovered, or the patient is medically unstable, elective surgery should be delayed until adequate investigation is completed or stabilization has occurred, even in the face of pressures from the surgeon or patient's family to proceed with surgery for convenience or personal reasons.

Another important consideration is *whether preoperative "preparation" will reduce risk*. Often forgotten, but important, are *recommendations for intraoperative* and *perioperative care that may reduce risk*. This approach (Table 3.2) is useful when deciding whether to delay surgery and what diagnostic or therapeutic recommendations to make once a risk–benefit decision has been made in favor of surgery.

A *special case* exists when two surgical procedures are potentially required. A common example is a patient in whom a carotid endarterectomy (the first operation) may be required before a major abdominal surgery, such as for aortic aneurysm or colon cancer (the second surgery), when the abdominal surgery is the original problem. This dilemma can be approached by first establishing whether the patient would still require the first procedure (i.e., carotid endarterectomy) if the original abdominal surgery was not needed; in other words, is the carotid operation *purely prophylaxis* for the second surgery? If the patient would still require carotid surgery for *medical* reasons alone, then the issue is simplified to a patient who requires two operations for medical reasons and the decision becomes the priority of the two required operations. The priority of operations is decided on the basis of: *(a)* the more pressing indication, or which disease is more likely to worsen with a delay in surgery; *(b)* whether one operation, if done first, will lower or raise the risk of the second surgery; and *(c)* which surgery will postpone the second

Table 3.2. Approach to Preoperative Evaluation

---

1. What is the status of the patient's health?[a]
2. If there is evidence of major organ system impairment:[a]
   (a) How severe is the impairment?
   (b) Does the impairment affect or increase operative risk (is it relevant)?
3. *How urgent is the surgery?* (Can it wait?)[b]
4. Will the degree of impairment be less if the surgery is delayed and the patient treated?
5. If there is no reason to delay the surgery, what specific changes in intra- and perioperative care are appropriate for the individual patient?

Reprinted with permission from Dr. Lourdes C. Corman, University of Florida, Gainesville, unpublished (slightly adapted).
[a]From Table 3.1.
[b]This is considered to be *the* most important question.

operation for the least amount of time. Typically, the decision is fairly straight-forward.

A more difficult situation occurs when the patient would *not* require the first surgery (i.e., prophylactic carotid endar-terectomy) if it were not for the second surgery. Establishing the priority of op-erations would be much more difficult, because the first surgery usually raises operative risks significantly and there are little data on lowering operative risk by prophylactic surgery, such as in the com-mon example of carotid surgery cited here. The decision should be made on the basis of a careful review of the literature regard-ing the established benefit of the specific prophylactic procedure for the subsequent surgery, the local experience in terms of operative risks, and how urgent an indi-cation exists for the original surgery. In the example here, the evidence favors *not* performing prophylactic carotid endarter-

ectomy solely for abdominal surgery in most situations (see Chapter 20).

REFERENCES

1. Papper EM. Some reflections on mortality due to anesthesia. Anesthesiology 1964;25:454–460.
2. Rhoades JE, Allen JG, Harkins HN, et al. The assessment of operative risk. In: Surgery: prin-ciples and practice. 4th ed. Philadelphia: JP Lippincott, 1970:232–243.
3. Feigal DW, Blaisdell FW. The estimation of surgical risk. Med Clin North Am 1979;63:1135 1143.
4. Eisman B, ed. Prognosis of surgical disease. Philadelphia: WB Saunders, 1980.
5. Bunker JP, Barnes BA, Mosteller F. Costs, risks and benefits of surgery. New York: Oxford Uni-versity Press, 1977.
6. Norton LW, Steele G, Eisman B, eds. Surgical decision making. Philadelphia: WB Saunders, 1993
7. Goldman L. Multifactorial index of cardiac risk in noncardiac surgery: ten-year status report. J Cardiothorac Anesth 1987;1:237–244.

4

Evaluation of Healthy Patients and Ambulatory Surgical Patients

Richard J. Gross and Stewart F. Babbott

A consensus has not been reached on the appropriate, routine medical preoperative evaluation of the healthy patient and the ambulatory surgical patient. This results from both a lack of data and of clinical agreement (1–3). Additionally, it has been difficult to make general recommendations for an evaluation in which many important variables determine an individual's assessment. With as many as 70% of surgical patients having outpatient or same-day surgery (4), accurate, efficient, and cost-effective evaluations will enhance the perioperative course. General opinion holds that traditional, routine laboratory work has a low yield of valuable information, and that an accurate patient history and physical examination with selected testing will enhance both patient care and cost-cutting efforts (5–10). Others, however, disagree (11).

The purpose of any preoperative evaluation includes the assessment of known disease and screening for disease that may affect perioperative morbidity and mortality. The preoperative evaluation is not a time to perform routine health maintenance. Optimal treatment of a patient's disease can help to minimize the risks of anesthesia, surgery, and the underlying condition. The preoperative evaluation also can help the patient by decreasing his or her anxiety, augmenting the patient's understanding of the proposed anesthesia and surgery, and developing a baseline against which any postoperative changes may be assessed.

A preoperative evaluation should be considered for two types of patients: (a) those who are healthy (i.e., no known underlying disease), and (b) those with a specific disease (i.e., known disease). Many of the chapters in this book address disease specific issues regarding perioperative management, and the reader is referred to them for additional information. This chapter focuses on healthy patients and ambulatory surgical patients. The medical evaluation of preoperative patients as described in this chapter is based on the *limited* available data, expert consensus, and our own experience. We feel that a practical approach to this type of evaluation is needed by internists, even in the absence of definitive study results or expert consensus.

Traditionally, medical evaluation of surgical patients by the internists has included the basic components of a comprehensive patient history, physical examination, admission laboratory work, chest radiography, and electrocardiography (ECG). Recently, more limited approaches have been described, though little information is available (12). The patient history usually is obtained by personal interview and occasionally with computer assistance (13). While not in general use at present, automated, patient-completed histories are as accurate as physician questioning in a personal interview (14, 15). Most hospitals or clinics have developed a form for the history and physical (Fig. 4.1), and it is important for the internist to be familiar with it. Some centers also perform the initial history over the phone (13), which can increase patient satisfaction by potentially decreasing the number of preopera-

---

GREATER BALTIMORE MEDICAL CENTER
6701 North Charles Street, Towson, Maryland 21204
HISTORY AND PHYSICAL, PAT WITH NURSE PRACTITIONER

Sex M F	Exam. date	Medical Dr.	Age

CC/PI:

Family history: CA	CVA	Anesthesia rxn	MGP/PGP	Mother	Father	Siblings	Offspring
DM	Kidney dis.	Thromboembolic dis.					
HBP	Liver dis.	Bleeding					
Cardiac	Anemia	Txn. rxn.					

Meds:	Allergies:	Anesthesia complications:
	Tobacco:	Transfusion Rx:
	ETOH:	Coag hx: Bleeding; clotting Phlebitis, P.E.
	DRUGS:	

MEDICAL HISTORY	**SURGICAL HISTORY**
	MAJOR INJURIES:
LAST PAP	

Figure 4.1. Sample form for patient history and physical examination. Adapted and reproduced with permission of the Greater Baltimore Medical Center, Baltimore, Md., and Pat Dunning, CANP.

REVIEW OF SYSTEMS

EYES:	Glaucoma	
ENT:	Sinusitis, tinnitus, hearing loss, epistaxis, frequent sore throats, hoarseness	
CNS:	Seizures, dizziness, syncope, weakness, numbness, headaches	
ENDOCRINE:	Thyroid disease, recent weight change, thirst, DM	
BREASTS:	Lumps, pain, discharge	
CARDIOVASCULAR:	Chest pain, palpitations, edema, claudication, phlebitis	
PULMONARY:	SOB, hemoptysis, productive cough, wheezing, asthma, pneumonia	
GI:	Recent change in bowel habits, ulcer, HH, GB disease, colitis, hemorrhoids, dysphagia, abdominal pain, jaundice, blood in stools, melena	
GU:	Frequent UTIs, renal stones, dysuria, hematuria, frequency, nocturia	
GYN:	LMP, chance of pregnancy	

PHYSICAL EXAM

Pulse	Blood pressure Lying Sitting	Respiration	Temperature	Height	Weight
Integument: Skin, hair, nails					
Head/neck: Skull, thyroid, carotids					
Eyes: Pupils, conj. sclera					
ENT: Canals, TMs, mucosa					
Lymph nodes: Cervical, supraclavicular, axillary					
Breasts: Symmetry, palpation, nipples					
Lungs: Respirations, percussion, breath sounds					
Heart: PMI, rhythm, ectopics, murmur					
Peripheral vascular: Femoral, dorsalis pedis, distal					
Abdomen: Tenderness, masses, scars, inspection					
Extremities: Edema, varicosities, color					
Neuro: Motor, sensory, orientation					

Other pertinent findings:

Impression:

Recommendations:

Signed: _____

Figure 4.1 *(continued)*

tive visits and can benefit the center by identifying which patients need in-depth evaluation before the day of surgery.

Questions may arise regarding medicolegal issues, including the extent of the examination that is needed and whether more selective testing places the practitioner at risk. Merli and Weitz (16) stress "the importance of an orderly and in depth approach to patient evaluation, accurate documentation, and precise recommendations as well as ongoing communication with the surgical [and anesthesia] team." As discussed later, batteries of tests may yield false-positive results, thus requiring more investigation and increasing patient anxiety. Such broad testing and laboratory follow-up of false-positive results may place the practitioner at risk as well (10). As always, the reader should seek local legal advice for any specific questions.

Some references and algorithms refer to major versus minor surgery. Often, no firm distinction can be made, but some variables may help in this determination. Blery et al. (17) distinguish between no blood loss and blood loss greater than 500 mL. In assessing the overall degree of risk from surgery plus anesthesia, Smith et al. (18) note that higher-risk procedures are associated with unstable medical conditions, long operative times, large intra- and extravascular fluid shifts, or high-risk anatomic locations. Thoracic cavity, abdominal cavity, neurologic, and vascular surgery often are considered to involve higher-risk sites. Goldman et al. (19) provide good descriptions of procedures and implications, and the Johns Hopkins Medical Institutions Surgical Classification System, shown in Table 4.1, offers more detail for determining surgical risk

Table 4.1.   Johns Hopkins Medical Institutions Surgical Classification System[a]

Category	Risk to Patient Independent of Anesthesia	Invasiveness of Procedure[b]	Blood Loss Potential	Examples
			Criteria	
1	Minimal	Minimal	Little or no	Cystoscopy Breast biopsy Bronchoscopy
2	Mild	Minimal to moderate	<500 mL	Arthroscopy Laparoscopic choleycystectomy Inguinal hernia repair
3	Moderate	Moderate to significant	500–1500 mL	Hysterectomy Hip/knee replacement Major laparoscopic/ gastrointestinal procedures

4	Major	High	>1500 mL	Major orthopedic/spinal
				    reconstruction
				Major gastrointestinal/
				    genitourinary surgery
				Major vascular repair

5	Critical	High	>1500 mL	Cardiothoracic procedure Intracranial procedure Aortic and vascular

Courtesy of B. Rosenfeld.
[a]For any questions about a procedure, its alternatives, and its risks, ask the surgeon or anesthesiologist.
[b]*Invasiveness* refers to tissue trauma, neuroendocrine, and cytokine response to the procedure.

Table 4.2.   Comparison of History–Physical to Laboratory Tests in Preoperative Evaluation

Study	Laboratory Test	% Abn. H&P + Abn. Lab (Sensitivity)	% Nl. H&P + Abn. Lab (FN)	Significant False-Negative (FN)
Jakobsson and White (22)	ECG		8%	
Rucker et al. (23)	CXR		0.3%	0%
Tornebrandt and Fletcher (24)	CXR		37%	37%
Boghosian and Mooradian (25)	CXR	62%	34%	34%
Haubek (in Sox [26])	CXR		3%	0%
Thomsen (in Sox [26])	CXR		7%	0.2%
Eisenberg et al. (27)	PTT	18%	3%	0.2%
Kaplan et al. (28)	Admission lab tests[a]		0.4%	0.2%
Turnbull and Buck (12)	Admission lab tests[a]		22%	10%
Median		40%	7%	0.2%

Abn., abnormal; CXR, chest radiography; FN, false-negatives (see Table 24-17); H&P, history and physical examination; Lab, laboratory; Nl., normal; TP, true-positives.
[a]Admission lab tests included some combination of complete blood count, urinalysis, chemistry tests.

(20). Should you have concerns, it is best to call the surgeon regarding the planned procedure and any alternatives.

This chapter first discusses the basic evaluation of healthy patients, then discusses special aspects in the evaluation of patient admitted for ambulatory or same-day surgery. The chapter also summarizes current literature on the yield of preoperative diagnostic testing, thus allowing the reader to review the basis for our recommendations.

EVALUATION OF HEALTHY PATIENTS

The basic preoperative medical evaluation includes a core evaluation that is common both to patients who presumably are healthy aside from the primary surgical disease and to patients with multiple other illnesses. In healthy patients, the goal of this evaluation is to ensure an accurate patient history and physical examination and to screen for any disease that may contribute to perioperative morbidity. In patients with multiple nonsurgical illnesses, additional clinical examination and laboratory testing may be needed to further evaluate the extent of specific diseases' severity, but the core evaluation serves as a basic minimum for all other systems. This chapter discusses the core evaluation; evaluation of other nonsurgical diseases is discussed in the appropriate chapter. Decision making is discussed in Chapter 3, and organizational issues regarding evaluation are discussed later in this chapter.

Patient History and Physical Examination

The patient history and physical examination, as a general trend, are playing an increasingly important role in defining which patients need to undergo specific tests (21). Few objective studies are available (12), however, and there is no agreement among experts to guide recommendations on the extent of these examinations preoperatively. Table 4.2 addresses some relationships between the patient history, physical examination, and laboratory tests, but not the extent of the history or physical. Many institutions have a locally developed format for the preoperative history, physical, and laboratory evaluation (Figure 4.1). Numerous factors make general rules difficult to apply to determining the extent of examination for an individual patient. **Important factors that affect the extent of examination that is needed include the patient's age and functional status, the time interval since the last comprehensive physical examination, and the nature of the surgery (i.e., minor versus major).** Other considerations, such as establishing a baseline for anticipated postoperative changes or complications and the inability to obtain an adequate patient history or physical examination, are reviewed in Table 4.3.

Regarding chronologic age, several authors emphasize that functional status is a critical determinant and stress the importance of its assessment. Gerson et al. (29) showed in patients older than 65 years that if patients were unable to perform 2 minutes of supine bicycle exercise and achieve a heart rate of 99 bpm or

Table 4.3.   Considerations in Selecting Preoperative Laboratory Screening Tests (Other than Yield of Abnormal Results and Estimation of Anesthetic-Surgical Risk)

1. Interval since and quality of last physical examination; extent of preoperative exam
2. Inability to evaluate by history–physical in an individual patient (e.g., poor historian; distant heart sounds due to chronic obstructive pulmonary disease)
3. Efficient evaluation of patients with known medical disease
4. Evaluation of primary surgical problem
5. Nature of surgery (major/minor; inpatient/ outpatient)
6. Type of anesthesia (local, regional, spinal, general)
7. Other need for information:
   a. Estimate operative risk
   b. Rare, catastrophic abnormality (e.g., thrombocytopenia in a craniotomy patient)
   c. Baseline for postoperative change/ complication
   d. Determining drug levels; monitoring drug effects
   e. Medicolegal documentation
   f. Avoiding harm to others (e.g., tuberculosis)

greater, they had a much higher rate of cardiac complications. Additionally, the recent American College of Cardiology/ American Heart Association (ACC/AHA) guidelines for preoperative cardiovascular evaluation in patients undergoing noncardiac surgery emphasize functional status, as measured in metabolic equivalents, as one criterion for decisions about noninvasive testing (30). Geriatric related issues are addressed in Chapter 22, and several reviews (31, 32) may provide additional information for the assessment of elderly patients.

Decisions about the type of anesthesia to be used are primarily the anesthesiologist's. One recent review (33) or an anesthesia or surgical text may offer answers to specific questions. Some practitioners feel that patient evaluation before general anesthesia should be of greater depth than that in patients who will undergo other types of anesthesia (Tables 4.3 and 4.4). We recommend that if the internist is concerned about a patient's ability to tolerate a proposed anesthetic that he or she discuss this directly with the anesthesiologist.

The traditional evaluation has included a comprehensive patient history and physical examination, ECG, chest radiography, urinalysis, and blood work (i.e., complete blood count; tests of hemostasis, blood urea nitrogen [BUN], creatinine, glucose, electrolytes; liver function tests; and possibly automated panels of tests and serologic test for syphilis). As noted, this approach has been criticized for low yield and high cost, and it has been suggested that only very limited examination or testing is worthwhile (5, 10, 26, 34). It is important to understand that while the more limited approaches have been well described, they also have not been proved.

A practical approach is to **select one of two general types of preoperative evaluation, either a limited or a comprehensive history and physical** (Table 4.4) (35). Guidelines for choosing between these alternative work-ups

Table 4.4. General Preoperative History and Physical: Limited vs. Comprehensive Examination

Component of Workup	Limited Workup	Comprehensive Workup
History	HPI, past med. hx, past surg hx, allergies, medications; heart, lungs, hemostasis, endocrine, family hx of surgical/anesthesia problems, and new symptoms (especially upper respiratory infection)	HPI, past med hx, past surg hx, social hx, family hx, allergies, medications, brief review of all systems
Physical examination	Vital signs, oral cavity, chest, heart, and abdomen	Complete physical examination

HPI, history of present illness; hx, history.
Adapted from Gross RJ. Preoperative planning for the ambulatory patient. In: RL Barker, et al., eds. Principles of ambulatory medicine. Baltimore: Williams & Wilkins, 1995;1276.

Table 4.5. Guidelines for Selecting the Type of General Preoperative Evaluation

Limited Workup	Comprehensive Workup
Age <40 y	Age >40 y (especially >60 y)
Established patient, previously examined by physician	New patient, unknown to physician
Recent comprehensive physical examination	No, old, or inadequate data base
Well patient	Patient with moderate-severe major organ disease
Local, regional, or spinal anesthesia	General anesthesia
Minor procedure	Major procedure (especially thoracic, abdominal, neurosurgical, vascular)

Reprinted with permission
Adapted from Gross RJ. Preoperative planning for the ambulatory patient. In: RL Barker, et al., eds. Principles of ambulatory medicine. Baltimore: Williams & Wilkins, 1995;1277.

(Table 4.5) are outlined, but the multiple factors in individual patients listed earlier preclude rigid rules for choosing the type of work-up. Generally, limited work-ups are appropriate for patients who are between 18 and 40 years of age, with a recent (i.e., <1 year) complete physical examination, generally healthy without major organ-system disease, and having local or regional anesthesia for a minor procedure. The comprehensive examination is more appropriate for inpatient consultations or patients previously unknown to the internist. In borderline situations, we recommend the more extensive work-up, at least until more data are available on the adequacy of limited work-ups. Limited work-ups usually are not appropriate for patients with major organ-system disease (e.g., cardiac, pulmonary, renal, liver, central nervous system [CNS]), who are chronically ill, who are elderly and without recent physical examinations, who are undergoing major procedures, and who have major undiagnosed symptoms (e.g., chest pain).

Table 4.4 provides general areas to be included in the patient history. Questions about cardiac disease (including hypertension, coronary artery disease, congestive heart failure, and valvular disease), peripheral vascular disease, pulmonary disease (e.g., chronic obstructive pulmonary disease, bronchospastic disease, smoking), and underlying conditions (e.g., diabetes) are important. Additional questions that are not routinely asked or emphasized in the evaluation of routine

Table 4.6.   Supplemental Screening History in the Medical Preoperative Evaluation

1. Have you ever had abnormal bleeding, or been told you are a bleeder?
2. Have you ever had a blood transfusion? If yes, any reaction *including* fever?
3. Have you ever had any problem with anesthesia, including fever?
4. Is anyone in your family a bleeder; or had problems (including fever) with anesthesia, a blood transfusion, or thromboembolic disease?
5. What medications do you take? Do you take any nonprescribed (over-the-counter) drugs, including pills patients often don't consider medication (such as birth control pills/hormones, diet pills, vitamin pills, or aspirin)?
6. Any history of alcohol or illicit drug use?

medical patients need to be asked as part of the history in preoperative patients (Table 4.6). A few well-worded screening questions can cover these items quickly; an extensive list of questions is not needed unless something abnormal is present. Specific questions should include the patient's bleeding history, especially if clotting studies are not routinely obtained (see Chapter 15). A history of prior anesthesia should be obtained, with inquiry about any anesthetic problems, particularly high and unexplained fever (i.e., malignant hyperthermia) or jaundice postoperatively (i.e., halogenated hydrocarbon anesthesia hepatitis). A history of prior transfusion and any related reactions, especially fever (i.e., leukocyte sensitization), should be obtained as well. The family history should specifically ask about bleeding problems, thromboembolic disease, anesthesia problems as described earlier, and transfusion reactions. These questions ask about relatively rare problems, but the problems are potentially catastrophic and cannot be screened for by other means.

Bleeding histories can vary from a single question to a prolonged, time-consuming review. Relatively brief lists of screening questions have been developed (36, 37), but these have not been well validated. A reasonable, brief screening for a history of bleeding is reproduced in Table 4.7; similar questions have been incorporated into patient-completed questionnaires. An extensive bleeding history is described in Table 4.8. We feel that at least the abbreviated bleeding history should used for patients with all but very minor surgery, either by the physician or by patient questionnaire. History of medication use should emphasize recent aspirin and aspirin-containing compounds, over-the-counter and nonprescribed compounds, diuretics/hormones, and drugs that patients often do not consider to be "medications" (e.g., aspirin, diet, and birth control pills).

Alcohol and illicit drug use pose special problems for the anesthesiologist as well as for the consulting internist and surgeon postoperatively. Specific questions about their use should be included as well.

Laboratory Tests

More studies are available on the yield and benefit of preoperative laboratory tests than on those of the clinical exami-

Table 4.7.   Brief Screening Bleeding History

1. Do you develop large bruises without a good reason? Have you bled a long time after minor cuts or trauma to your tongue, cheek, or lip? If so, how old were you when this began?
2. Have you had teeth extracted? If so, which ones? How long did you bleed after extraction? Did bleeding start up again a day or so later?
3. What operations have you had? Was bleeding after surgery or childbirth hard to stop? Were transfusions necessary? Did your wounds heal well?
4. Have you had general medical problems? What are these and how are they being treated? Have you had kidney, liver, or arthritic diseases?
5. What medicines do you take? Do you use over-the-counter drugs for colds, allergy, headaches, arthritis, menstrual cramps, backaches, or other pains? Have you taken any medicines, including antibiotics within the last 7–10 days?
6. Do you have any blood relatives who have experienced prolonged or excessive bleeding?

Modified from Rappaport SI. Preoperative hemostatic evaluation: which tests, if any? Blood 1983;61: 229–231.

Table 4.8.   Extensive Bleeding History and Physical Examination

A. History
  1. Bleeding during childhood (circumcision, tonsillectomy and adenoidectomy, epistaxis, joints, soft tissues, lacerations)
  2. Extent of bruising from minor trauma; any spontaneous bruising (including minor lacerations, and biting mouth). Ask specifically about bruises on trunk or abdomen, quantitate size)
  3. Any delayed or delayed recurrent (more than 12–24 hours) postoperative bleeding; prolonged bleeding after surgery or procedures (more than 24 hours)
  4. Menses
  5. Dental extractions or work
  6. Procedures (cardiac catheterization, etc.)
  7. Prior surgery (abnormal or late bleeding)
  8. Predisposing diseases (uremia, liver disease, malabsorption, malnutrition, autoimmune disease)
  9. Medications (ASA, ASA-compounds, some NSAIDs, coumadin, heparin, medications high risk for thrombocytopenia, radiation therapy, chemotherapy)
  10. Transfusions
  11. Alcohol use
  12. Family history of bleeding disorder
B. Physical examination
  1. Signs of bleeding on skin and mucous membranes
  2. Telangectasia, skin signs of liver or renal disease
  3. Hepatosplenomegaly
  4. Lymphadenopathy

ASA, acetylsalicylic acid; NSAIDs, nonsteroidal anti-inflammatory drugs.

nation. Most studies, however, have only looked at one factor (i.e., positive tests that change therapy), not the many factors that influence a clinician's decision. The available literature provides general guidelines, but absolute rules cannot be given. Blery et al. (17) proposed and prospectively tested, and Roizen (38) modified, a grid for testing, incorporating the type of test on one axis and the indications for testing on the other. The general trend in laboratory testing is to do selected tests based on patient age, the underlying disease, and the current therapy or type of surgery; for healthy patients, this may mean no testing. Computerized algorithms also have been used

for deciding which tests to obtain (14, 39). For patients needing tests, Macpherson et al. (40) showed that if tests have been done within the past 4 months and the patient has not had any changes in health status, the tests do not need to be repeated. This may help to reduce the amount of testing performed in patients while ensuring that appropriate preoperative laboratory investigation is still completed.

Suggested laboratory testing is shown in Figure 4.2. Patients for whom there is low risk because of young age, type of surgery, and lack of comorbid disease generally would require no testing (5, 10). Narr et al. (5) suggested that no testing be done in American Society of Anesthesiologists (ASA) class 1 patients (see Chapter 5 for ASA classification). This is a change from the recommendations in the previous edition of this chapter and from those of Gross et al. (35), and it reflects the change in practice to more selective testing.

Non-invasive cardiac tests are covered in Chapter 10.

EVALUATION OF AMBULATORY SURGICAL PATIENTS

The number of surgical patients having their medical preoperative evaluation performed on an outpatient basis has increased dramatically over the last 25 years; in many hospitals, 50% or more of surgical cases currently are outpatients (41). This does not include the many patients who are admitted the same morning as inpatient major surgery and, hence, have an outpatient medical consultation. Surgeons may request outpatient medical consultation to avoid late cancellations and the resultant loss of operating room time (Table 4.9).

Only approximately 1% of outpatient surgical patients require unplanned inpatient admission following surgery (42, 43). Most of these admissions result from anesthesia-related problems (e.g., vomiting) or surgically related problems (e.g., pain or complications), not from medical problems. Consistent with this are data showing that preoperative medical prob-

Figure 4.2. Suggested laboratory testing.

Indication	Hgb	WBC	PT/PTT	PLT/BT	Electrolyte	Cr/BUN	Serum glu
Surgical procedure							
minor/no EBL							
EBL >500; <1500	X						
EBL >1500/JHH cat 5	X		X		X	X	X
GU procedure or recent GU infection							
orthopedic implant surgery							
Age							
<40	F#						
40–49	F#						
50–64	F#					C	
65–74	X					X	X
>75	X					X	X
Associated condition							
cardiovascular disease						X	
pulmonary disease							
malignancy	X	*	*				
chemotherapy	X				X	X	
radiation therapy		X					
hepatobiliary disease			X				
exposure to hepatitis							
renal disease	X				X	X	
bleeding disorder	X		X	X			
diabetes mellitus					X	X	X
smoking >20 pyr	C						
possible pregnancy							
CNS disease		X			X	X	X
Medications							
diuretics					X	X	
digoxin					X	X	
steroids					X		X
anticoagulants	X		X				

Note that not all diseases and tests are included here; therefore the physician should use his or her own judgment regarding patients with diseases or test indications not listed. *Symbols:* X, obtain; M, men only; F, women only; C, consider obtaining; #, lack of consensus for women in these age groups; *, obtain from leukemias only. *Abbreviations:* BT, bleeding time; Cr/BUN, creatinine/BUN; EBL, estimated blood loss; Elect, electrolytes (sodium, potassium, chloride, bicarbonate); GU, genitourinary; Hgb, hemoglobin; JHH, Johns Hopkins Hospital; PLT, platelet count; Preg Test, pregnancy test; serum glu, serum glucose.

Figure 4.2. Suggested laboratory testing *(continued)*.

SGOT/Alk	CXR	ECG	Preg test	T/S	Urinalysis
				X	
	X	X		X	X
					X
					X

SGOT/Alk	CXR	ECG	Preg test	T/S	Urinalysis
		M			
		X			
	C	X			
	C	X			

SGOT/Alk	CXR	ECG	Preg test	T/S	Urinalysis
	C	X			
	X	C			
	X				
	X	X			
X					
X					
		X			C
	C				
			X		
		X			

SGOT/Alk	CXR	ECG	Preg test	T/S	Urinalysis

SGOT/Alk; serum glutamic-oxaloacetic transaminase and alkaline phosphatase; T/S, type and screen; WBC, white blood cell count. (Adapted with permission from Roizen MF. Preoperative evaluation. In: Miller RD, ed. Anesthesia. 4th ed. New York: Churchill Livingstone, 1994;1:827–882. Additional data from Blery C, Szatan M, Fourgeaux B, et al. Evaluation of a protocol for selective ordering of preoperative tests. Lancet 1986;i:139–141; and Kaplan EB, Sheiner LB, Boeckmann AJ, et al. The usefulness of preoperative laboratory screening. JAMA 1985;253:3576–3581.)

Table 4.9.   Outpatient Preoperative Assessment—Why?

1. Better patient satisfaction
2. Better care
3. Eliminates inefficiency of last-minute surgical cancellation for patient, surgeon, hospital/operating room/anesthesiologist, insurance company (cost)
4. Same-day surgical centers (efficiency)
5. Inpatient surgery—no preoperative days covered by insurance

lems do not predict who will subsequently require admission (42, 43). The mortality related to medical complications has been low in initial studies (1:22,500). Of selected postoperative medical complications, approximately 60% occur within 48 hours of surgery, with the remaining 40% occurring over the next 28 days (44).

A number of important organizational points regarding the medical preoperative evaluation of surgical patients outpatients are discussed in the following subsections. The importance of factors such as timely communication, clear recommendations, and accurate coordination of care (with well-described responsibilities for the anesthesiologist, surgeon, and internist) is stressed. The two types of clinical evaluation and the guidelines for laboratory evaluation from the preceding section also apply in the outpatient setting (Table 4.4), and the differences in factors influencing the extent of the evaluation in the outpatient setting are discussed. Management issues unique to the outpatient setting are described as well.

This section includes as "ambulatory" surgical patients both those undergoing totally outpatient surgery and those admitted the morning of major inpatient surgery. This is not the usual definition of the term, which usually is applied to totally ambulatory surgery; however, both types of patients raise many similar issues for the internist (i.e., both have their preoperative medical evaluation performed on an outpatient basis).

This section assumes that the prior material on the evaluation of healthy patients has been read.

Organizational Issues

The organization of or rules for the preoperative medical evaluation of ambulatory surgical patients vary widely between hospitals. Because of the potential fragmentation of outpatient work-ups regarding timing and communication, several procedural issues should be firmly established in hospital policy and in the consulting internist's practice. A quality-improvement project showed that some of these barriers can be successfully overcome (45). Only an outline of recommendations can be given, however, because of the absence of a solid research base.

In some centers, the preoperative assessment service is run by the anesthesia department, with all evaluations being performed, done, or reviewed by this service (4, 46). Preoperative evaluations by internists are sent here, and at times, consultation by an internist is sought. Internal medicine services may run a preoperative clinic or see patients in an office setting (47). Increasingly, the multidisciplinary nature of such an evaluation is both evident and enhanced by the team approach (48). The surgeon generally is the member of the team with primary preoperative responsibility, but the internist and anesthesiologist both contribute to successful perioperative care.

The choice of which patients are candidates for ambulatory surgery without admission is based on medical considerations (Table 4.10) as well as on issues such as the patient's anesthetic risk, attitude toward having an operation out-of-hospital, and the social and family situation (49). These *medical* guidelines, however, must be adjusted in light of the type of surgery to be performed and the individual situation. Even some excluded types of patients may undergo outpatient surgery under certain conditions, such as if the surgery is very minor (e.g., minor abscess drainage), and the criteria for allowing outpatient surgery have continued to be liberalized over the past several years. Elderly patients initially were excluded from outpatient surgery, but there currently is no accepted maximum age limit (31, 32). Most centers will not allow ambulatory surgery on many ASA class III and any ASA class IV patients; some *stable* ASA class III patients can have outpatient minor surgery based on the individual circumstances. Patients with unstable, major organ medical disease generally need postoperative overnight observation. Recent acute myocardial infarction or unstable cardiovascular disease generally are considered to be contraindications to outpatient surgery. Patients with insulin-dependent, brittle diabetes usually require hospital admission for intravenous fluids and observation of glucose measurements.

The routine preoperative medical evaluation is performed by different practitioners in different settings, including the primary physician (e.g., internist or family practitioner), surgeon, anesthesiologist, and nurse practitioner or physician assistant. (This is separate from the preoperative medical consultation for a specific problem.) No specific data and insufficient experience exist to show whether one type of practitioner is preferable. The midlevel providers need physician super-vision; we feel they also should be trained specifically in preoperative assessment. Regardless of who does the *routine* preoperative evaluation, however, the internist should be involved on either a primary or a consultative basis for patients who are chronically ill, patients who have major organ-system disease or abnormal laboratory studies, and other high-risk patients.

Policies need to be established and disseminated regarding the *responsibility* for coordinating outpatient evaluation, treatment, and follow-up of medical problems (Table 4.11). Clear lines of responsibility should be delineated, because the internist may perform the preoperative physical, the surgeon may obtain the laboratory results, and the anesthesiologist may interview the patient about changes in his or her condition between the preoperative evaluation and the surgery. Clearly, there is a large possibility of loss of information (e.g., lab results) (45) or of poor coordination. Changes in patient condition and abnormal laboratory data need to be communicated between the surgeon, anesthesiologist, and internist. The patient must be given a clear understanding of which physician to contact should his or her condition change and of which physician will provide instruction regarding use of long-term medication during the perioperative period.

One person should be responsible for coordinating this multifaceted effort. We believe the surgeon is best positioned for this, because he or she is the only physician having contact with all parties from the preoperative evaluation through the postoperative visit. Other arrangements may exist, however, and are satisfactory if all parties agree.

A policy also must be established regarding the appropriate time before surgery for performance of the preoperative examination. Hospital policies often vary between 2 to 14 days. The longer interval makes administration of preoperative testing easier (i.e., results are obtained well before surgery), but it increases the chance of interval illnesses as well.

Table 4.10.   Suggested Guidelines on Patient Eligibility for Ambulatory Surgery Based on Medical Condition (*Not* Considering Type of Surgery)

1. ASA class I–II (some class III for minor procedures)
2. Stable, compensated chronic medical problems; absence of acute medical problems
3. No recent myocardial infarction, unstable cardiac disease, or decompensated lung disease
4. If diabetic, not on insulin; if on insulin, stable, not brittle; patient capable of and able postoperatively to do self-monitoring (insulin-dependent diabetics should be done *early* in the morning)

Table 4.11.   Recommended Hospital Policy Issues Regarding Administrative Aspects of Preoperative Evaluation

1. When should evaluation be done before surgery (<1–4 weeks)?
2. Who does the evaluation (internist, surgeon, anesthesiologist, nurse practitioner, or physician assistant)?
3. What laboratory, ECG, and radiography are routinely required by simple categories (age, presence/absence chronic disease). Where will lab work be done (? required at hospital)?
4. Who receives the laboratory, ECG, and radiography results. Need to establish mechanism for internist, surgeon and assistant to be routinely notified of abnormal results.
5. Who is responsible for compiling data on history/physical, lab, ECG, and radiography—making sure it was all completed, and making decisions regarding surgery based on results (surgeon, internist, anesthesiologist)?
6. What is the mechanism or who is responsible person to notify internist **routinely** if all abnormal results (#4) or changes in surgical plans (#5), if these are done by surgeon.
7. Who sends a copy of laboratory, ECG, and radiography results to consulting internist even if normal? (may go through normal channels or mail, as long as mechanism of notification of abnormal results)
8. Who is responsible for interviewing patient on day of surgery, to see if an interval illness or worsened chronic disease has developed since medical evaluation days before; how is this to be documented? (This **cannot** be the internist.)
9. Who is responsible for instructing patient on preoperative orders (e.g., NPO after midnight)? Does this person know he or she should instruct about medical considerations— AM medications, ASA use, patient to call if interval illness, etc. (see Table 4.12)?
10. Who is responsible for postoperative patient instructions? Does this person know to give medical instructions (e.g., resumption of preoperative medications, call internist if worsened chest pain, etc.) (see Table 4.12)?

ASA, acetylsalicylic acid; NPO, nothing per os.

Other issues include where the laboratory tests, ECG, and radiography are obtained (e.g., community laboratory or office versus hospital) and how the work-up is sent from the internist's office to the hospital. Currently, this information may transmitted by a dictated letter or a completed, preprinted form; use of computer networks to access central dictation services and labs can make information transfer more efficient (50, 51).

Diagnostic Activities and Approaches

The extent of evaluation (Tables 4.4 and 4.5) in the outpatient setting is influenced by the fact that the internist often knows the patient well. Most surgical procedures done on an outpatient basis are minor, and only local or regional anesthesia is required. Thus, for many similar ambulatory surgical patients, a limited work-up will suffice.

A compelling reason for a comprehensive work-up exists at the other end of the spectrum, when an outpatient is seen for the first time by the internist for a preoperative consultation. Thus, an elderly patient who is chronically ill with multiple diseases seen for the first time in a consultation for outpatient surgery or evaluation for same-day surgery needs more attention than the same patient who is having an inpatient procedure.

We have identified several aspects of the patient history, physical examination, and treatment that frequently are forgotten in the outpatient setting (Tables 4.12

Table 4.12.   Commonly Forgotten or Underestimated Items of History–Physical–Lab in Medical Evaluation of the Ambulatory Surgical Patient[a]

1. One disease (review the problem list)
2. The generally sick patient
3. Medications (include ASA, birth control pills, over-the-counter drugs)
4. Inquiry about recent steroid use (? need for stress dosing)
5. Evaluation of murmurs (? need for SBE prophylaxis)
6. Blood tests indicated by specific medical diseases or medications (e.g., drug levels, potassium for diuretics)
7. Pregnancy test (serum qualitative HCG)
8. Spirometry (in a pulmonary patient)
9. Echocardiogram (evaluation of murmur regarding SBE prophylaxis)

ASA, acetylsalicylic acid; HCG, human chorionic gonadotropin; SBE, subacute bacterial endocarditis.
[a]See also Table 4.6.

Table 4.13.   Commonly Forgotten Management Items in the Ambulatory Surgical Patient[a]

1. Tell patient to report to internist, surgeon, and anesthesiologist even **minor intercurrent illnesses** (including minor "colds"), between physical and day of surgery. Also, postoperative problems of potential medical interest after surgery.
2. Negotiate with patient to stop **smoking, alcohol,** illicit **drugs, over-the-counter medications** (no new over-the-counter medications).
3. **Medication (preop) review**—what to do the AM of surgery regarding taking medicines when NPO. Discontinuing medications such as ASA, coumadin if indicated (and when to restart postoperatively).
4. **Corticosteroids**—administer or increase dose to cover stress (including patients who have recently been on but have discontinued steroids).
5. **SBE prophylaxis.**
6. **Teach patients** "what" to expect pre- and postoperatively.
7. Tell surgeon to **notify internist** if medical problems outside certain limits postoperatively (e.g., blood pressure over 180/100), in certain situations or diseases.
8. **Medications (postop)**—when to restart postoperatively and what to do if unexpected problems arise (i.e., call internist).

ASA, acetylsalicylic acid; NPO, nothing per os; SBE, subacute bacterial endocarditis.
[a] See also Table 4.6.

and 4.13). The patient's problem list should be reviewed specifically for diseases with the potential to increase his or her operative risk (e.g., cardiovascular or pulmonary disease). The patient who appears to be generally ill from multiple diseases or malnutrition should not be underestimated because no one disease is severe. Medication history is important, including over-the-counter medications, recent corticosteroid use (i.e., within 1 year), aspirin, and anticoagulants. Frequently forgotten tests to consider are pregnancy tests, blood tests indicated by medications (e.g., potassium in a patient on diuretics, drug levels such as digoxin), spirometry in pulmonary patients (see Chapter 7), and echocardiogram for evalu-

ation of the need for subacute bacterial endocarditis prophylaxis (see Chapter 11).

Treatment

Additional potentially overlooked issues include instructions to patients on the discontinuation of habits affecting surgical risk (e.g., smoking) and the administration of medications immediately pre- and postoperatively (Tables 4.13 and 4.14). Prophylaxis for subacute bacterial endocarditis must be considered in advance, because special arrangements usually are required for intravenous antibiotics, especially if a second, postoperative dose is needed. The patient should be instructed to notify the *internist as well as the surgeon* about even minor changes in condition or intercurrent illnesses between the preoperative examination and surgery. Reasonable postoperative expectations in terms of the symptoms of medical diseases should be explained to the patient as well as when to call the internist because of a change in condition or the need for medical adjustment.

Smoking should be discontinued before surgery. Some data, mostly from coronary

Table 4.14.   Medical Consultation Report for Ambulatory Surgery: Additional Recommendations

Specific Recommendations:
1. Patient instructed to take all medications AM of surgery with sip of H_2O, except diuretic. Aspirin discontinued 7 days preop.
2. Please notify me if any intercurrent illnesses before surgery (patient also instructed).
3. Please notify me of any perioperative medical complications; if blood pressure under 120/60 or over 180/100; check postop Chemstix and notify me if under 100 or over 300 mg%.
4. Please instruct patient if he can resume aspirin day after surgery.
5. Please notify me of any abnormal laboratory data preoperatively.

General Points about Recommendations:
1. Limit to five or less.
2. Focus on therapy over diagnosis if possible.
3. Include dose, route, timing for medications.
4. Provide contingency plan.
5. Identify critical recommendations.

bypass artery graft operations (53, 54), suggest that discontinuation of cigarettes may need to be done 2 months before surgery to achieve the maximal benefit, but smoking should be stopped even if a shorter period of time before surgery is available. Nicotine patches can be of benefit to patients who will not quit but who will consider the change to avoid pulmonary complications.

Some patients will require temporary medication adjustment preoperatively, such as an adjustment of insulin dosage or of blood pressure medication. Both the surgeon and the patient should be given guidelines on when to notify the internist for dose adjustment, such as an unexpectedly prolonged time NPO for a diabetic or a lower-than-usual blood pressure at the time of discharge from the recovery room.

The consultation report should contain guidelines for the surgeon on notifying the internist if certain limits are exceeded for select diseases (e.g., blood pressure). Effective methods of communication have been described (52, 55, 56), and the report should be transmitted in a timely fashion. Recommendations for the assessment of risk, suggested tests and rationale, and specific treatment should be specific. Pupa et al. (52) noted increased compliance with recommendations if the consultant: *(a)* identifies critical recommendations; *(b)* makes early, direct contact with the referring physician; *(c)* limits the number of recommendations (i.e., five or less); and *(d)* renders definite recommendations. Medication recommendations should contain dose, route, and frequency. A straightforward explanation to the patient usually will suffice, and supplementation by a simple, written sheet of instructions, similar to that shown in Table 4.14, will encourage patient understanding and compliance. Especially because of short turnaround times, prompt transmission of the report using a central dictation service or a completed, preprinted form (or fax transmission of a dictated note) will be beneficial.

Remember, elective surgery is elective. If the internist feels that further evaluation is needed, a new problem is uncovered, or the patient is unstable, then elective surgery should be delayed until the diagnostic investigation or period of observation is complete.

SELECTING PREOPERATIVE TESTS: AN OVERVIEW

Interest continues in defining which preoperative laboratory tests should be routinely performed on all surgical patients. Most of the information accumulated has been on then yield of selected tests. **The reader should understand that available data are limited. Clinical circumstances vary widely, as do local community practices. Thus, general recommendations should be adapted to the physician's individual setting and patient.**

The methodology for deciding on a "good" screening laboratory test is crucial in understanding the recommendations that follow. Recommendations for individual tests are based on studies from the literature (where available), expert consensus, and our own clinical experience.

Most of the literature analyzes only one factor: the cost–benefit (or yield) of preoperative laboratory testing; however, many other important factors affect the clinical decision to perform preoperative tests. These include nature of the surgery (i.e., major versus minor) (17, 38), estimation of operative risk in the decision for surgery (internists generally do not do this), baseline for postoperative changes and complications, and any rare but catastrophic abnormality in the surgical setting (e.g., thrombocytopenia in craniotomy patients). The high cost of such rare catastrophes has not been considered in most cost–benefit studies. Individualized testing should be based on a broader set of guidelines, such as that in Figure 4.2.

Most studies evaluating laboratory testing have assumed a highly complete patient history, physical examination, or clinical data retrospectively sought with the patient outcome already known. The necessity for an accurate history and physical cannot be overemphasized as the trend toward more selective testing continues. Clinical information may not be complete, and laboratory testing may serve a larger, back-up function in actual practice. Complicating factors are the multiple indications for selected testing (e.g., 30 indications for chest radiography alone in one study [23]) and the needs of multiple physicians (i.e., anesthesiologist, surgeon, and internist). The immense practical difficulty in considering all of these factors in an individual patient on a daily basis is obvious, particularly if no local consensus has been developed, and is magnified by the number tests that can potentially be ordered. One practical solution was proposed by Bleary et al. (17), who developed by consensus and prospectively tested an algorithm that allowed for individual patient needs; they showed that according to predetermined criteria, 0.4% of nonordered tests would have been potentially helpful.

Whereas the preceding discussion has been limited to laboratory tests, this same type of analysis could be applied to parts of the patient history and physical examination. Keep in mind, however, that again, even cost–benefit data are limited by the small number and quality of studies available. Allison and Bromley (9) used a cost analysis of preoperative laboratory evaluation of ambulatory surgical patients before and after a revised surgical service preoperative investigation policy was instituted, and they showed significant savings with no added morbidity.

Standard criteria have been developed to select a good screening test (Table 4.15). Additional factors in preoperative patient include: (a) the disease should not be easily detectable by routine patient history and physical examination, (b) the test result should affect the risk of surgery or anesthesia; and (c) early knowledge of the disease should affect the perioperative treatment.

Table 4.15.   Criteria for Screening Tests

1. Treatable disease whose natural history is known
2. Important problem (high incidence/prevalence; clinically significant)
3. Screening test available (sensitivity, specificity, predictive value)
4. Arrangements for treatment and follow-up

Modified from WHO criteria. World Health Organization: Mass health examination. PUBLIC Health Paper No. 45, Geneva, World Health Organization, 1971.

Screening tests can be further selected by knowing their sensitivity, specificity, and predictive value (Table 4.16). *Sensitivity* is the number of patients with a positive test and the disease divided by the total number of patients with the disease (i.e., patients correctly identified as having the disease). *Specificity* is the number of patients with a negative test and no disease divided by the total number of patients without the disease (i.e., patients correctly identified as having no disease).

It is important to recognize that in populations having a low prevalence of the condition being screened for, the predictive value of these tests will be low. Therefore, accurate definition of specific subpopulations requiring screening is critical to the preoperative evaluation. Increasingly, the patient history and physical examination play the key role in defining these populations. *Predictive value positive* is the probability of a patient with a positive test actually having the disease, and *predictive value negative* is the probability of a patient with a negative test actually being free of the disease. Bayes' theorem states that the probability of a patient with a positive test actually having the disease depends in part on the prevalence of the disease in the population or group to which the patient belongs. The predictive value of a positive test is higher in patient populations

Table 4.16. Evaluation of Screening Tests for Preoperative Evaluation

		DISEASE[a]	
		+	−
TEST[b]	+	True-positive (TP)	False-positive (FP)
	−	False-negative (FN)	True-negative (TN)

$$\text{Sensitivity} = \frac{TP}{TP + FN} \quad \text{(correctly identify patients with disease)}^c$$

$$\text{Specificity} = \frac{TN}{TN + FP} \quad \text{(correctly identify patients with \textbf{no} disease)}^c$$

Predictive value of **Positive** (+) test[c,d] $= \dfrac{TP}{TP + FP}$ (probability an individual patient with a positive test has the disease)

[a]+ = disease patient; − = disease absent in patients.
[b]+ = test positive; − = test negative in patients.
[c]Sensitivity and specificity given overall accuracy for a large study population of patients; to obtain the value for an individual patient, the prevalence of the condition in the population must be calculated in (= predictive value). A simplified method of calculating predictive value is given.
[d]Predictive value of **Negative** test not shown in table $\left(= \dfrac{TN}{TN + FN} \right)$ (= probability individual patient with a negative test is disease-free).

among whom the prevalence of the disease is higher (26).

Other factors influencing the selection of screening tests include the selection of cut points for determining abnormal tests results, the method used for the test, and the precision of the individual hospital laboratory.

SPECIFIC PREOPERATIVE TESTS: EVALUATION

Patient History and Physical Examination

Little information is available on the yield of the patient history and physical examination in preoperative evaluation. If the laboratory is used as the standard of accuracy (despite limitations in such a use), there are few and conflicting data on the accuracy of the history–physical in identifying abnormalities (Table 4.2). There seems to be reasonable sensitivity when the clinical evaluation is abnormal, however. Johnson et al. (34) found that most abnormalities in a prospective study of preoperative evaluations could be explained by the patient history and physical examination. A wide variation in results is obtained when the negative history–physical is examined for false-negative results, whether the laboratory criterion is any abnormal test or only abnormal tests that are clinically significant. The reasons for this variation in results is not clear but may include different quality of clinical examinations, study criteria, and type of test being considered. Studies have not looked at the yield of individual portions of the history–physical.

Recommendations: Guidelines for selection of the comprehensive versus the limited history–physical are given in Tables 4.4 and 4.5 (based on limited studies and clinical experience). It is important to know your institution's preoperative procedures as well as its patient history and physical examination form (Figure 4.2). An accurate history–physical is critical to selection of appropriate laboratory tests.

Laboratory Tests

The overall yield of the traditional battery of admission laboratory tests (i.e., complete blood count, clotting studies, chemistries) has been low in most studies (Fig. 4.3) (12, 17, 28, 57). This has lead most authors to advise against such batteries, especially in healthy patients (10, 17, 38). Individual tests are considered here. Additionally, see Figure 4.2.

Electrocardiography

The number of preoperative ECGs found to be abnormal is significant, but the number that are unpredicted by history–physical is less (10%) (Table 4.17) (10). Only a small number of unexpected ECGs result in changes to therapy or surgical plans.

The percentage of unexpected abnormal ECGs in surgical patients rises with age; few are found before the age of 35 years (22, 26, 58). The AHA Task Force report on electrocardiography (65) found that in healthy patients, there was general agreement on routine preoperative ECGs being recommended over age 40, disagreement on their being recommended between the ages of 30 and 40, and general agreement on their not being indicated below the age of 30. Blery et al. (17) recommended ECGs for all such patients older than 40 years. Roizen (38), Allison and Bromley (9), as well as local guidelines suggest ECG for male patients

beginning at age 40 and for all patients over age 50.

Expert consensus (26, 65–68) indicates that routine ECGs in all patients are not indicated. Routine ECGs are indicated preoperatively in patients over the ages of 35 to 40. There is no agreement on the age cutoff, and it may be higher for women. (The AHA recommendations were noted earlier.)

Recommendations: Routine preoperative ECGs should be obtained in male patients over age 40 and in all patients over age 50. ECGs in patients between ages 30 and 40 remain an area of controversy. Condition-specific indications include cardiovascular disease (e.g., hypertension, coronary artery disease, vascular disease), diabetes, renal disease, high-risk surgery, and history of radiation therapy or CNS disease.

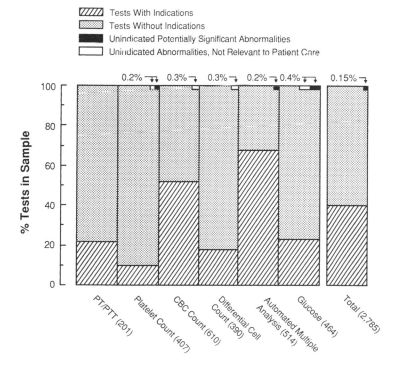

Figure 4.3. Proportions of indicated and unindicated preoperative tests, drawn to scale. Numbers in parentheses represent sample sizes used. Automated multiple analysis is six factor. CBC, complete blood cell. (Reprinted with permission from Kaplan EB, Sheiner LB, Boeckmann AJ, et al. The usefulness of preoperative laboratory screening. JAMA 1985;253:3576–3581.)

Table 4.17.   Routine Preoperative ECGs: Yield

Study	Patients (n)	All Patients: Abnormals	Normal Patients by H&P	
			Abnormals	Abnormal *and* Change Management or Surgical Plans
Jakobsson and White (22)	731		8%	
Ferrer (58)	1068	19%		
Paterson et al. (59)	267	31%	16%	2%
			(3% major abnormality)	
Rabkin and Horne (60)	812	21%		0%
Seymour et al. (61)[a]	222	79%		
Turnbull and Buck (12)	632	16%	(0.4% major abnormality)	
Charpak et al. (62)	1610	38%		
Catchlove et al. (63)	60	20%	—	—
Gold et al. (67)	751	43%	—	—
Median		31%	10%	0.7%
			(2% major abnormality)	

H&P, history and physical.
[a]Study restricted to patients over age 65.

Chest Radiography

Ordering chest radiography and changes in treatment based on its results have been inconsistent (69). The number of chest radiographs found to be abnormal in preoperative patients is high, but the number found to be abnormal in patients without clinical indicators of chest disease is much smaller (10). A meta-analysis of studies involving preoperative chest radiography showed that on average, abnormalities were found in 10% of routine preoperative films (Table 4.18) (70). In only 1.3% were the abnormalities unexpected (i.e., not known or would not otherwise have been detected), and only 0.1% of patient had their treatment changed on the basis of their radiographs. The authors concluded that when a reliable patient history and physical examination were done, no routine chest radiography was needed. The number of chest radiographic findings that change medical or surgical treatment in patients with a normal history–physical is almost zero, except for one study involving a small number of elderly patients. The overall yield of chest radiography is small among healthy patients in the available studies, but the total number of well-studied patients also is small. These numbers of patients may not be adequate to define risk and to identify high-risk subgroups. Some of the studies referenced in Archer et al. (70) are included this reference list (12, 23, 24–26, 62, 63, 71, 72); for the remainder, please consult Archer et al.'s reference list.

The percentage of abnormal radiographic findings increases with age in a general hospital population (i.e., from age 30 [2%] to over age 70 [45%]). Whether a baseline chest radiograph is helpful for comparison in the diagnosis of postoperative pulmonary complications cannot be decided on the basis of the one small study presently available (26).

Expert consensus (26, 75) has advised against routine chest radiography solely because the patient is having surgery. Chest radiography is indicated on the basis of findings in the history–physical, because of the high incidence of concomitant disease, for cardiothoracic surgery, and for surgery with a high risk of chest complications. Specific examples are chronic obstructive pulmonary disease or asthma that is disabling, has had changes in symptoms over the past 6 months, or has had an acute episode in the last 6 months (20). Chest radiography has been proposed for elderly patients, but no firm age recommendations are available. Boghosian and Mooradian (25) have reported abnormal radiographs in patients older than 60 years but significantly fewer postoperative complications in the 60- to 70-year-old group versus patients older than 70. They suggested age 70 and developed high- and low-risk groups based on the patient history (e.g., cardiovascular, pulmonary, tobacco, diabetes, cancer) and physical examination. Even with these clinical predictors and significantly more abnormal findings in the high-risk group, however, there was no significant difference in postoperative complication rates between groups. Others (23, 74, 76) have used risk factors as well and found that the clinical history was associated with abnormal chest radiographs. As discussed earlier, functional status and "biologic" rather than chronologic age are important determinants in test selection.

Table 4.18.   The Frequency of Abnormalities on Routine Preoperative Chest Radiographs

| | | Study Group | | All Abnormalities | | Unsuspected Abnormalities | | | |
| | | | | | | Total | | Influencing Management | |
Author	Study Design	Age (y)	n	n	%	n	%	n	%
Sane	P	0–19	1500	111	7.4	41	2.7	0	0
Wood	R	0–19	749	35	4.7	9	1.21	3	0.4
Farnsworth	R	1–14	350	31	8.9	1	0.3	0	0
Maigaard	P	>30	1256	57	4.5	2	0.2	0	0
Lamers	P	>40	810	5	0.6	1	0.1	0	0
Wyatt	R	>49	388	4	1.0	1	0.4	1	0.4
Gagner	R	All	1000	74	7.4	6	0.6	0	0
Jeavons	P	Adults	500	33	6.6	11	2.2	4	0.8
Rucker	P	All	872	115	13.2	1	0.3	0	0
Thomsen	R	>40	1823	241	13.0	42	2.3	4	0.2
Haubek	P	1–94	400	24	6.0	6	1.9	0	0
Tape	R	24–90	341	20	5.9	—	—	0	0
Catchlove	R	40–>70	79	5	6.3	—	—	0	0
Petterson	P	All	1530	134	8.8	—	—	2	0.1
Loder	R	9–30	437	5	1.1	1	0.2	—	—
Turnbull	R	Adults	691	38	5.5	10	1.4	—	—
Törnebrandt	P	70–94	91	43	47.3	10	11	—	—
Seymore	P	>65	233	93	40.0	—	—	—	—
Mendelson	P	All	369	62	17.0	—	—	—	—
Wiencek	P	Adults	237	101	42.6	—	—	—	—
Weibman	R	0–90	734	213	29.0	—	—	—	—
All studies			14,390	1,444		140		14	
Weighted mean[a]					10.0		1.3		0.1
95% CI					8.6–11.3		0.0–2.8		0.0–0.6
Weighted mean (exluding Törnebrandt)							1.0		
95% CI							0.0–2.5		

Reprinted with permission from Archer C, Levy AR, McGregor M. Value of routine preoperative chest x-rays: a meta-analysis. Can J Anaesth 1993;40:1022–1028.

P, prospective; CI, confidence interval; R, retrospective.

[a]Weighted according to the number of study subjects.

Table 4.19.   Routine Preoperative Hematocrit/Hemoglobin: Yield

Study	Patients (n)	All Patients: Abnormals	Normal Patients by H&P	
			Abnormals	Abnormal *and* Change Management or Surgical Plans
Kaplan et al. (28)	610	3.6%	0.3%	0%
Turnbull and Buck (12)	1005	0.7%	0.7%	0.2%
Charpak et al. (62)	2138	32%		
Johnson et al. (34)	212	9.0%		0%
Narr et al. (5)	3282	0.8%		
McKee and Scott (81)	397	3.3%		
Median		3.4%	0.5%	0.6%

H&P, history and physical.

Recommendations: Routine chest radiography need not be ordered solely because the patient is having surgery. Until more definitive studies are available, use of routine preoperative chest radiography depends on clinical judgment, with additional important factors being the patient's age, results of the history–physical, and type of surgery. Factors indicating the need for chest radiography include, but are not limited to, pulmonary disease that has changed in the last 6 months or is debilitating and surgery with a high risk of postoperative thoracic complications (see Chapter 7). While age alone is not a criterion for chest radiography, some preoperative testing centers may set a specific age beyond which chest radiography is suggested; in this case, the reader is referred to his or her local policy.

Hematology

Few studies (10, 26, 77–79) are available on the yield of the complete blood count and differential in routine perioperative assessment. Preliminary, small studies have found a low incidence of abnormal hematocrit or hemoglobin measurements in otherwise healthy surgical patients (Table 4.19). Small degrees of anemia may not increase surgical risk (77), as once was thought. Kaplan et al. (28) used an "action limit" of hemoglobin of 10 mg/dL. Carson et al. (80) showed that for surgical patients who declined blood transfusions for religious reasons, no patient who had a hemoglobin level of 8 mg/dL or higher and an operative blood loss of less than 500 mL died. Expert consensus (77, 81) once held that a hematocrit or hemoglobin test was indicated routinely because of the risk of anemia during anesthesia and of further lowering of the hematocrit by intraoperative bleeding, but dissenting views have been raised (26). Blery et al. (17) did not include routine hemoglobin testing unless blood loss of greater that 500 mL anticipated, and no age criterion was used. In addition to estimated blood loss, however, it is important to consider the underlying disease, including anemia and anticoagulation therapy. Some testing recommendations include hemoglobin determination for all menstruating women.

The yield of routine white blood cell counts in healthy preoperative patients has been 0.2%, and no white blood cell count has been reported to have changed medical or surgical treatment (12, 28). Expert consensus has not been reached for the routine white blood cell counts in surgical patients, again because of inadequate data (26), but it has been suggested that the utility of this routine test is low unless leukopenia or leukocytosis is suspected (10).

The yield of the routine differential white blood cell count in preoperative patients is low. In two studies of preoperative healthy patients and one study of a general hospital population (12, 78, 83), no screening differential led to a significant new diagnosis or therapy. Expert consensus is that routine differential white blood cell counts are not needed in preoperative screening (26).

Recommendations: Routine hematocrit or hemoglobin counts should be obtained on preoperative patients with an estimated blood loss of greater than 500 mL; an underlying disease that may be associated with anemia, anticoagulation therapy (warfarin or aspirin); receiving long-term chronic medications, including aspirin-containing compounds and non-steroidal anti-inflammatory drugs; or patients with a predisposition or risk for anemia. Condition-specific indications include bleeding disorder, renal disease, malignancy, or chemotherapy. For healthy patients with only minimal expected blood loss, a reasonable age to consider measuring the hemoglobin level is 65 years. Routine hemoglobin determination in healthy women younger than 65 years remains an area of debate. Routine white blood cell counts and differentials are not needed in preoperative patients, other than in those with leukemia, or when other causes of leukopenia or leukocytosis are suspected.

Clotting Studies

Studies of common preoperative coagulation tests, such as partial thromboplastin time (PTT), prothrombin time (PT), platelet count, and bleeding time, in otherwise low-risk patients have found low yields of abnormal results and little effect on patient outcome (Table 4.20) (10, 26, 84–86). The PTT has been best studied; inadequate numbers of patients have been involved in studies of the PT and platelet count. Two studies (17, 86) found low yield to routine bleeding times in surgical patients (1.5% abnormal, 0 to 0.1% significantly abnormal), and a recent study confirmed this (87). The bleeding history may

not be as accurate as most clinicians assume (23, 36). The low incidence of clotting disorders not identified by the patient history makes the best-case, theoretic predictive value of routine preoperative clotting studies very low, as already demonstrated for the PTT (85). Houry et al. (88) showed that for all four tests, routine testing was of no value in patients with a normal history and physical examination. Expert consensus is uniform in stating that these tests are not routinely indicated in preoperative testing (26, 37, 84, 85).

Recommendations: Routine hemostasis studies are not recommended for perioperative testing, except in the setting of high-risk surgery (e.g., neurosurgery), in patients receiving anticoagulation or in whom anticoagulation will be used intraoperatively, or in patients who provide a history or have physical findings suggestive of a hemostatic abnormality.

Serum Glucose

Little data are available on the yield of routine serum glucose screening for undiagnosed diabetes in surgical patients; what is known must be derived from the yields of multitest chemistry screening. The incidence of unexpected abnormal glucose levels in routine preoperative testing generally has been from 1 to 5% (10, 12, 28) but may be as low as 0.3% (82). Changes in management have occurred in 0.5% of patients screened (12, 17, 28). The risk for occult, adult-onset diabetes probably is lower than that for juvenile diabetes in surgical patients. Expert consensus is not available for glucose screening. An alternative screening test is urinalysis with testing for glycosuria. This is less sensitive and specific than serum glucose screening, but comparative figures are not available for surgical patients.

Recommendations: The serum glucose level should be checked in patients older than 65 years. Urinalysis with a chemical test for glucose could be a substitute. A fasting serum glucose level should be obtained in patients undergoing major surgical procedures or prolonged anesthe-

Table 4.20.   Routine Preoperative ECGs: Yield

Study	Patients (n)	All Patients: Abnormals	Normal Patients by H&P	
			Abnormals	Abnormal *and* Change Management or Surgical Plans
Partial thromboblastic time (PTT)				
Robbins and Mushlin (82)	1,000	14%		
Eisenberg et al. (27)	480	2.7%	2.7%	0%
Suchman and Mushlin (84)	2134	16.3%		*a*
Kaplan et al. (28)	199	.5%	0%	0%
Turnbull and Buck (12)	210	1.4%		0%
Charpak et al. (62)	952	8%	—	0%
Rohrer et al. (91)	282	5%	2.4%	
Median		5%	2.4%	0%
Prothrombin time (PT)				
Kaplan et al. (28)	201	1%	0%	0%
Turnbull and Buck (12)	213	0%	0%	0%
Charpak et al. (62)	935	13%		
Rohrer et al. (91)	282	.7%	.8%	—
Median		.8%	0%	0%
Platelet count				
Turnbull and Buck (12)	1005	0%	0%	0%
Rohrer et al. (91)	282	12%	.8%	
Johnson et al. (34)	212	0%		
Kaplan et al. (28)	407	.7%		
Median		.4%	.4%	0%

H&P, history and physical.
[a]No difference in bleeding complications between patients with and without elevated PTT.

sia when the underlying disease or medications would lead to hyperglycemia or hypoglycemia.

BUN, Creatinine, Urinalysis

Little information is available on the routine preoperative testing of renal function. The yield of unexpected abnormalities in BUN and creatinine among otherwise healthy preoperative patients has been 0.2% in limited studies (10, 12, 17, 26, 28). The yield of preoperative urinalysis varies depending on what is called "abnormal"; minor abnormalities (e.g., a few white cells) are common but have little effect on treatment (89, 90). Expert consensus is not available for renal function tests. Urinalysis is important for patients who will undergo genitourinary procedures, who have had a recent genitourinary infection, or who will have orthopaedic implantation surgery (19).

Recommendations: A urinalysis is not routinely recommended other than for high-risk procedures, genitourinary procedures, a recent genitourinary infection, or an orthopaedic implant surgery. A creatinine level should be obtained before major surgical procedures and in all patients older than 65 years, and it should be considered in patients between 50 and 64 years of age. A BUN is redundant, less accurate, and not needed (unless for diagnostic purposes).

Electrolytes

Routine preoperative electrolytes in normal patients have yielded unexpected abnormalities of potassium in 0.0 to 1.5%

of patients and of sodium in 0.0 to 0.5% of patients (2, 15, 20, 21). Data are not available for abnormalities of chloride or carbon dioxide, but the yields would presumably be low. Expert consensus is not available.

Recommendations: Routine electrolyte measurements should not be obtained in patients undergoing minor surgery. Until data are available on the safety of omitting a full set of electrolytes, this test should be obtained in those undergoing major procedures. Patients with renal disease, diabetes, CNS disease, or who have had chemotherapy also should have electrolyte levels obtained. Patients undergoing high-risk procedures or on diuretics, digoxin, or steroids should have electrolytes obtained as well.

Liver Enzymes

The yield of liver enzyme tests in routine preoperative screening is not available. One study found that approximately 1 in 700 healthy patients were found to have "significant" elevations of liver enzymes, and that approximately 1 in 2500 later became clinically jaundiced (92). Another study showed that 12 of 3782 patients had abnormal aspartate transaminase levels, and that no patient had a change in therapy because of this result (5). A review of several other studies found that 0.5% of liver enzyme tests were abnormal. Whether these figures can be generalized, however, is not known; theoretic calculations indicate the yield would be low. The risk of occult hepatitis to the operating room team must be considered (82), but liver enzyme tests will have an uncertain effect on reducing this risk.

Recommendations: Routine testing of healthy preoperative patients for liver enzymes is not recommended. High-risk groups, including alcoholics, patients practicing unsafe sex, intravenous drug abuser, patients on prescribed drugs with a high risk of causing liver abnormalities, and patients whose history and physical examination suggests one of these risk groups, should be tested.

Multiphasic Chemistry Batteries

Routine multiphasic chemistry panels have been investigated in general hospital populations and in a small number of studies involving surgical patients (12, 26, 28, 93–98). Data on the yield in healthy surgical patients, however, are difficult to extract from the available publications. In general hospital populations, abnormal chemistry tests may be found in from 10 to 40% of patients, but they lead to a new diagnosis in only 0.2 to 10.0% of patients and result in treatment changes in only a small percentage. The number of false-positive tests is significant, because 20 tests are run (each with a false-positive rate of 2.5%) in most laboratories; hence the false-positive rate approaches the total gross yield of these tests (26). Most of other positive tests can be accounted for by known diseases in the patients. Many of the unexpected abnormal results were ignored by the clinicians; no follow-up or action was taken.

Expert consensus generally recommends not obtaining routine multiple biochemical chemistry panels on healthy preoperative patients. These chemistry panels frequently are ordered in clinical practice.

Recommendations: Multiphasic chemistry batteries are not routinely indicated for healthy preoperative patients. A reasonable use for such panels is the patient requiring multiple individual chemistry tests (as described earlier), in whom the battery would be less expensive.

Nutritional Testing

Nutritional testing is discussed in Chapter 5.

Pregnancy Testing

Quantitative data on the incidence of unsuspected pregnancy in surgical patients are not available, but clinical experience suggests that the incidence is low. Surgery during pregnancy carries some risk to the fetus. Expert consensus is not available on the indications for pregnancy testing in healthy preoperative patients, but Malviya et al. (99) showed that in adolescent patients with a detailed history, serum pregnancy testing appeared to be indicated only when suggested by the patient history.

Recommendations: A serum pregnancy test (qualitative human chorionic gonadotropin) should be obtained preoperatively on women of childbearing age who are uncertain of their pregnancy status, who have signs of pregnancy on physical examination, or for whom pregnancy might complicate the surgery.

Serologic Testing for Syphilis

Expert consensus is that routine testing for syphilis no longer is indicated. This recommendation is made on the basis of the low incidence of syphilis in most hospital populations.

Recommendations: Routine testing of all preoperative surgical patients for syphilis is not indicated.

Human Immunodeficiency Virus

Consideration of routine testing in surgical patients for the human immunodeficiency virus (HIV) has been raised because of concerns for the safety of the operating team and for operating room precautions (100). The prevalence of undiagnosed HIV infection in surgical patients is not known, and it probably varies by hospital depending on patient population.

Routine testing of surgical patients for HIV infection raises the ethical questions of consent and of the high ratio of false- to true-positive tests among low-prevalence populations. Large logistical problems also are raised, including the time required for testing, retesting of the false-positive results (with potential cancellation of surgery), and required counseling of patients with positive results. The adverse effect of false-positive results on the patient must be considered as well. Most surgeons in one study favored HIV testing, but the ethical and

logistical issues outweigh this indication at present.

The current expert recommendation is not to screen routinely for HIV in all healthy surgical patients (101–103). The internist should keep abreast of recent developments in this controversial area, however.

Recommendations: Routine HIV testing of all healthy preoperative patients is not currently recommended.

Pulmonary Function Tests and Arterial Blood Gases

Pulmonary function tests and arterial blood gases are discussed in Chapter 6.

Noninvasive Cardiac Evaluation

Noninvasive cardiac evaluation is discussed in Chapter 10.

REFERENCES

1. Bass EB, Steinberg EP, Luthra R, et al. Do ophthalmologists, anesthesiologists and internists agree about preoperative testing in healthy patients undergoing cataract surgery? Arch Ophthalmol 1995;113:1248–1256.
2. Bellan L. Preoperative testing for cataract surgery. Can J Ophthalmol. 1994;29:111–114.
3. Cataract Management Guideline Panel. Cataract in adults: management of functional impairment. Agency for Health Care Policy and Research publication AHCPR 93-0542. Clinical Practice Guideline No. 4. Rockville, MD: U.S. Dept of Health and Human Services, Public Health Service; February 1993.
4. Fischer S. Development and effectiveness of an anesthesia preoperative evaluation clinic in a teaching hospital. Anesthesiology 1996;85: 196–206.
5. Narr BJ, Hansen RT, Warner MA. Preoperative laboratory screening in healthy Mayo patients. Mayo Clin Proc 1991;66:155–159.
6. Narr BJ, Warner ME, Schroeder DR, Warner MA. Outcomes of patients with no laboratory assessment before anesthesia and a surgical procedure. Mayo Clin Proc 1997;72:505–509.
7. Perez A, Planell J, Bacardaz C, et al. Value of routine preoperative tests: a multicentre study in four general hospitals. Br J Anaesth 1995; 74:250–256.
8. Velanovich V. Preoperative laboratory evaluation. J Am Coll Surg 1996;183:79–85.
9. Allison JG, Bromley HR. Unnecessary preop-

erative investigations: evaluation and cost analysis. Am Surg 1996;62:686–689.

10. Macpherson DS. Peroperative laboratory testing: should any tests be 'routine' before surgery? Med Clin North Am 1993;77:289–308.

11. Clelland C, Worland RL Jessup DE, et al. Preoperative medical evaluations in patients having joint replacement surgery: added benefits. South Med J 1996;89:958–960.

12. Turnbull JM, Buck C. The value of preoperative screening investigations in otherwise healthy individuals. Arch Intern Med 1987;147:1101–1105.

13. Vitkun SA, Gage JS, Anderson DH, et al. Computerization of the preoperative anesthesia interview. Int J Clin Monitoring Computing 1995;12:71–76.

14. Roizen MF, Coalson D, Hayward RSA, et al. Can patients use an automated questionnaire to define their current health status? Med Care 1992;30:S74–S84.

15. Lutner RE, Roizen MF, Stocking CB, et al. The automated inteview vs. the personal interview: do patient responses to preoperative health questions differ? Anesthesiology 1991; 75:394–400.

16. Merli GJ, Weitz HH. Medical care of the surgical patient. Philadelphia: WB Saunders, 1992:3.

17. Blery C, Szatan M, Fourgeaux B, et al. Evaluation of a protocol for selective ordering of preoperative tests. Lancet 1986;i:139–141.

18. Smith R, Osterweil D, Ouslander JG. Perioperative care in the elderly urologic patient. Urol Clin North Am 1996;23:27–41.

19. Goldman DR, Brown FH, Guarnieri DM, eds. Perioperative medicine: the medical care of the surgical patient. 2nd ed. New York: McGraw-Hill, 1994.

20. Rosenfeld B. Johns Hopkins Medical Institutions Guidelines for preoperative evaluation of the ambulatory and same day admission patient. Personal communication, 1997.

21. Arvidson S. Preparation of adult patients for anesthesia and surgery. Acta Anaesthesiol Scandinavica 1996;40:962–970.

22. Jakobsson A, White T. Routine preoperative electrocardiograms. Lancet 1984;i:972.

23. Rucker L, Frye EB, Staten MA. Usefulness of screening chest roentgenograms in preoperative patients. JAMA 1983;250:3209–3211.

24. Tornebrandt K, Fletcher R. Pre-operative chest x-rays in elderly patients. Anaesthesia 1982; 37:901–902.

25. Boghosian SG, Mooradian AD. Usefulness of routine preoperative chest roentgenograms in elderly patients. J Am Geriatr Soc 1987;35:142–146.

26. Sox HC, ed. Common diagnostic tests: use and interpretation. 2nd ed. Philadelphia: American College of Physicians, 1990.

27. Eisenberg JM, Clarke JR, Sussman SA. Prothrombin and partial thromboplastin times as preoperative screening tests. Arch Surg 1982; 117:48–51.

28. Kaplan EB, Sheiner LB, Boeckmann AJ, et al. The usefulness of preoperative laboratory screening. JAMA 1985;253:3576–3581.

29. Gerson MC, Hurst JM, Hertzberg VS, et al. Predicition of cardiac and pulmonary complications related to elevtive abdominal and non cardiac thoracic surgery in geriatric patients. Am J Med 1990;88:101–107.

30. Eagle KA and colleagues for the ACC/AHA Task Force on Practice Guidelines. Guidelines for perioperative cardiovascular evaluation for noncardiac surgery. J Am Coll Cardiol 1996;27:910–948.

31. Thomas DR, Ritchie CS. Preoperative assessment of older adults. J Am Geriatr Soc 1995; 43:811–821.

32. Cheng EY, Wang-cheng RM. Impact of aging on preoperative evaluation. J Clin Anesth 1991;3:324–343.

33. Appleby J, Lawrence VA. Anesthesia: clinical review. J Gen Intern Med 1994;9:635 617.

34. Johnson H Jr, Knee-Ioli S, Butler TA, et al. Are routine preoperative laboratory screening tests necessary to evaluate ambulatory surgical patients? Surgery 1988;104:639–645.

35. Gross RJ, Barker LR, Spees EK. Preoperative planning for the ambulatory patient. In: Barker RL, Burton J, Zeve P, eds. Principles of ambulatory medicine. Baltimore: Williams & Wilkins, 1995:1275–1298.

36. Borzotta AP, Keeling MM: Value of the preoperative history as an indicator of hemostatic disorders. Ann Surg 1984;200:648–652.

37. Rapaport SI. Preoperative hemostatic evaluation: which tests, if any? Blood 1983;61:229–231.

38. Roizen MF. Preoperative evaluation. In: Miller RD, ed. Anesthesia. 4th ed. New York: Churchill Livingstone, 1994;1:827–882.

39. Davies JM, Pagenkopf D, Todd K, et al. Comparison of selection of preoperative laboratory tests: the computer vs. the anaesthetist. Can J Anaesth 1994;41:1156–1160.

40. Macpherson DS, Snow R, Lofgren RP. Preoperative screening: value of previous tests. Ann Intern Med 1990;113:969–973.

41. Laffaye HA. The impact of an ambulatory surgical service in a community hospital. Arch Surg 1989;124:601–603.

42. Gold BS, Kitz DS, Lecky JH, et al. Unanticipated admission to the hospital following ambulatory surgery. JAMA 1989;262:3008–3010.

43. Freeman LN, Schachat AP, Manolio TA, Enger C. Multivariate analysis of factors associated with unplanned admission in 'outpatient' ophthalmic surgery. Opthalmic Surg 1988;19:719–723.

44. Warner MA, Shields SE, Chute CG. Major morbidity and mortality within 1 month of ambulatory surgery and anesthesia. JAMA 1993;270:1437–1441.

45. Palladoro VA, Dent JN, Strong DT. Ensuring that preoperative test results are available at the time of surgery: a quality improvement project at Strong Memorial Hospital. Quality Letter for Health Care Leaders 1993;5:18–20.

46. Pollard JB, Zboray AL, Mazze RI. Economic benefit attributed to opening a preoperative evaluation clinic for outpatients. Anesth Analg 1996;83:407–410.

47. Macpherson DS, Lofgren RP. Outpatient internal medicine preoperative evaluation: a randomized clinical trial. Med Care 1994:32:498–507.

48. Swan BA. A collaborative ambulatory preoperative evaluation model: implementation, implications and evaluation. AORN J 1994;59:430–437.

49. Davis JE, Ugioka K. Selecting the patient for major ambulatory surgery: surgical and anesthesiology evaluations. Surg Clin North Am 1987;67:721–732.

50. Nicol ST, Dyle JA. Innovations in anesthesia prescreening through data systems and communications. Healthcare Information Management 1993;7:33–39.

51. Nicol ST, Dyle JA. Improving the surgical screening process. Plast Surg Nurs 1996;16:35–40.

52. Pupa LE, Coventry JA, Hanley JF, et al. Factors affecting compliance for general medicine consultations to non-internists. Am J Med 1986;81:508–514.

53. Gomez MN, Tinker JH. Smoking, anesthesa, and coronary bypass operation: a witches' cauldron? Mayo Clin Proc 1989;64:708–711.

54. Pearce AC, Jones RM. Smoking and anesthesia: preoperative abstinence and perioperative morbidity. Anesthesiology 1984;61:576–584.

55. Lee T, Pappius EM, Goldman L. Impact of inter-physician communication on the effectiveness of medical consultations. Am J Med 1983;74:106–112.

56. Goldman L, Lee T, Rudd P. Ten commandments for effective consultations. Arch Intern Med 1983;143:1753–1755.

57. Durbridge TC, Edwards F, Edwards RG, et al. Evaluation of benefits of screening tests done immediately on admission to hospital. Clin Chem 1976;22:968–971.

58. Ferrer MI. The value of obligatory preoperative electrocardiograms. J Am Med Wom Assoc 1978;33:459–469.

59. Paterson KR, Caskie JP, Galloway DJ, et al. The pre-operative electrocardiogram: an assessment. Scott Med J 1983;28:116–118.

60. Rabkin SW, Horne JM. Preoperative electrocardiography: effect of new abnormalities on clinical decisions. Can Med Assoc J 1983;128:146–147.

61. Seymour DG, Pringle R, Maclennan WJ. The role of the routine pre-operative electrocardiogram in the elderly surgical patient. Age and Ageing 1983;12:97–104.

62. Charpak Y, Blery C, Chastang C, et al. Usefulness of selectively ordered preoperative tests. Med Care 1988;26:95–104.

63. Catchlove BR, Wilson RM, Springs S, et al. Routine investigations in elective surgical patients. Med J Aust 1979;2:107–110.

64. Gold BS, Young ML, Kinman JL, et al. The utility of preoperative electorcardiograms in the ambulatory surgical patient. Arch Intern Med 1992;152:301–305.

65. Schlant RC, Adolph RJ, DiMarco JP, et al. Guidelines for electrocardiography. Circulation 1992;85:1221–1228.

66. Diagnostic and therapeutic technology assessment: mandatory ECG before elective surgery. JAMA 1983;250:540.

67. Goldberger AL, O'Konski M. Utility of the routine electrocardiogram before surgery and on general hospital admission. Ann Intern Med 1986;105:552–557.

68. Paraskos JA. Who needs a preoperative electrocardiogram? Arch Intern Med 1992;152:261–263.

69. National Study by the Royal College of Radiologists. Preoperative chest radiology. Lancet 1979;ii:83–86.

70. Archer C, Levy AR, McGregor M. Value of routine preoperative chest x-rays: a meta-analysis. Can J Anaesth 1993;40:1022–1027.

71. Tape TG, Mushlin AI. How useful are routine chest x-rays of preoperative patients at risk for postoperative chest diseases? J Gen Intern Med 1988;3:15–20.

72. Tape TG, Mushlin AI. The utility of routine chest radiographs. Ann Intern Med 1986;104:663–670.

73. Rees AM, Roberts CJ, Bligh AS, et al. Routine preoperative chest radiography in non-cardiopulmonary surgery. BMJ 1976;1:1333–1335.

74. Charpak Y, Blery C, Chastang C, et al. Prospective assessment of a protocol for selective ordering of preoperative x-rays. Can J Anaesth 1988;35:259–264.

75. National Center for Devices and Radiological Health. The selection of patients for x-ray examinations: chest x-ray screening examinations. HHS publ. no. (FDA) 83-8204. Rockville, MD: U.S. Food and Drug Administration, 1983.

76. ACAPEM, Bouillot J-L, Fingerhut A, Paquet J-C, et al. Are routine preoperative chest radiographs useful in general surgery? Eur J Surg 1996;162:597–604.

77. Consensus conference: perioperative red blood cell transfusion. JAMA 1988;260:2700–2703.

78. Connelly DP, McClain MP, Crowson TW, et al. The use of the differential leukocyte count for inpatient casefinding. Hum Pathol 1982;13: 294–300.

79. Shapiro MF, Greenfield S. The complete blood count and leukocyte differential count: an approach to their rational application. Ann Intern Med 1987;106:65–74.

80. Carson JL, Spence RK, Poses RM, et al. Severity of anaemia and operatiave morbidity and mortality. Lancet 1988;1:727–729.

81. McKee R, Scott EM. The value of routine preoperative investigations. Ann R Col Surg England 1987;69:160–162.

82. Robbins JA, Mushlin AI. Preoperative evaluation of the healthy patient. Med Clin North Am 1979;63:1145–1156.

83. Shapiro MF, Hatch RL, Greenfield S. Cost containment and labor-intensive tests: the case of the leukocyte differential count. JAMA 1984; 252:231–234.

84. Suchman A, Mushlin AI. How well does the activated partial thromboplastin time predict postoperative hemorrhage? JAMA 1986;256: 750–753.

85. Clarke JR, Eisenberg JM. A theoretical assessment of the value of the PTT as a preoperative screening test in adults. Med Decision Making 1981;1:40–43.

86. Barber A, Green D, Galluzzo T, et al. The bleeding time as a preoperative screening test. Am J Med 1985;78:761–764.

87. Gerwitz AS, Kottke-Marchant K, Miller ML. The preoperative bleeding time test: assessing its clinical usefulness. Cleve Clin J Med 1995; 62:379–382.

88. Houry S, Georgeac C, Hay J-M, et al. A prospective multicenter evaluation of preoperative hemostatic screening tests. Am J Surg 1995;170:19–23.

89. Kroenke K, Hanley JF, Copley JB, et al. The admission urinalysis. J Gen Intern Med 1986; 1:238–242.

90. Lawrence VA, Kroenke K. The unproven utility of preoperative urinalysis. Arch Intern Med 1988;148:1370–1373.

91. Rohrer MJ, Michelotti MC, Nahrwold DL. A prospective evaluation of the efficacy of preoperative coagulation testing. Ann Surg 1988; 208:554–557.

92. Schemel WH. Unexplained hepatic dysfunction. Anesth Analg 1976;55:810–814.

93. Durbridge TC, Edwards F, Edwards RG. An evaluation of multiphasic screening on admission to hospital. Med J Aust 1976;1:703–705.

94. Belliveau RT, Fitzgerald JE, Nickerson DA. Evaluation of a routine profile chemistry screening of all patients admitted to a community hospital. Am J Clin Pathol 1970;53: 447–451.

95. Whitehead TP, Woolton IDP. Biochemical profiles for hospital patients. Lancet 1974;ii:1439–1443.

96. Bradwell AR, Carmalt MHB, Whitehead TP. Explaining the unexpected abnormal results of biochemical profile investigations. Lancet 1974;ii:1071–1074.

97. Campbell IT, Gosling P. Preoperative biochemical screening. BMJ 1988;2:803–804.

98. Cebul RD, Beck JR. Biochemical profiles: applications in ambulatory screening and proadmission testing of adults. Ann Intern Med 1987;106:403–413.

99. Malviya S, D'Errico C, Reynolds P, et al. Should pregnancy testing be routine in adolescent patients prior to surgery? Anesth Analg 1996; 83:854–858.

100. Chapman K, Meadows J, Catalan J, et al. Testing patients for HIV before surgery: the views of doctors performing surgery. AIDS Care 1995;7:125–128.

101. Bayer R, Levine C, Wokf SM. HIV antibody screening: an ethical framework for evaluating proposed programs. JAMA 1986;256:1768–1771.

102. DeVita VT, Hellman S, Rosenberg SA. AIDS: etiology, diagnosis, treatment and prevention. Philadelphia: JB Lippincott, 1988.

103. Hagen MD, Meyer KB, Pauker SG. Routine preoperative screening for HIV: does the risk to the surgeon outweigh the risk to the patient? JAMA 1988;259:1357–1359.

5

Anesthesia: Risks, Techniques and Agents, Organ Effects, and Specific Concerns

Larry B. Grossman[1]

The scope of anesthesiology is continually broadening and becoming more complex. Some anesthesiology departments have added the term *perioperative medicine* to their name to better define the responsibilities of this specialty both inside and outside the operating room and during the preoperative, intraoperative, and postoperative periods (1).

Information provided by the consulting internist about the patient's medical problems and therapies helps the anesthesiologist to select the appropriate anesthetic agents and techniques. Not uncommonly, however, misunderstandings occur between physicians regarding their respective roles in the treatment of patients to be anesthetized for therapeutic interventions. Anesthesiologists have considered a medical consult that recommends "avoiding hypoxia and hypertension" to be a "medical insult," because good anesthetic management would, of course, provide such care. In general, the anesthesiologist expects the consultant to diagnose disease processes, to optimize organ function, and to estimate any increased risks for anesthesia and surgery posed by concomitant medical problems.

The anesthesiologist is responsible for selecting those drugs and techniques that

will have the least deleterious effects and result in the most favorable outcome. During surgery, the anesthesiologist must continuously address the needs of both the surgeon and the patient. Optimal patient care requires the close cooperation of internists, surgeons, and anesthesiologists during the perioperative period.

RISKS AND MORTALITY

When an internist is requested to give "medical clearance" for a patient about to undergo a therapeutic or a diagnostic intervention (e.g., surgery, arteriography, endoscopy), he or she actually is being asked to estimate the risk of anesthesia in that patient. In answering this request, **the hazards of anesthesia cannot be considered independently of many other factors.** The overall risk is determined by the delicate balance of anesthetic agents and techniques, the surgical procedure, patient monitoring, diseases, preoperative preparation, and postoperative care.

One extensively used system of risk assessment is the American Society of Anesthesiologists (ASA) classification of physical status before anesthesia. This classification (Table 5.1) is based on the presence of systemic disturbances that may be absent (class 1), mild (class 2), moderate (class 3), severe (class 4), or

---

[1]Kermit Tantum wrote this chapter in the first and second editions.

Table 5.1.   American Society of Anesthesiologists Physical Status Measure

Class 1	There is no physiologic, biochemical, or psychiatric disturbance. The pathologic process for which operation is to be performed is localized and not conducive to systemic disturbance. Examples: a fit patient with inguinal hernia; fibroid uterus in an otherwise healthy woman.
Class 2	Mild to moderate systemic disturbance caused either by the condition to be treated surgically or by other pathophysiologic processes. Examples: presence of mild diabetes, essential hypertension, or anemia.
Class 3	Rather severe systemic disturbance or pathology from whatever cause, even though it may not be possible to define the degree of disability with finality. Examples: severe diabetes with vascular complications; moderate to severe degrees of pulmonary insufficiency; angina pectoris or healed myocardial infarction.
Class 4	Indicative of the patient with a severe systemic disorder already life-threatening and not always correctable by the operative procedure. Examples: advanced degrees of cardiac, pulmonary, hepatic, renal, or endocrine insufficiency.
Class 5	This category embraces the moribund patient who has little chance of survival but is submitted to operation in desperation. Examples: the burst aneurysm with the patient in profound shock; major cerebral trauma with rapidly increasing intracranial pressure; massive pulmonary embolus.
Emergency operation (E)	Any patient in one of the classes listed above who is operated on as an emergency is considered to be in somewhat poorer physical condition. The letter E is placed beside the numerical classification.

mean almost certain death (class 5). The letter E designates an emergency procedure. The assumption is that an emergency patient has had less preparation, may have a full stomach, and may have more severe pathology. The ASA physical status measure is a rather crude classification of the patient's physical condition and not of his or her total surgical risks; all the factors associated with the operation are ignored.

The ASA classification allows a simple comparison of patients undergoing various anesthetics. Several studies have correlated outcome with the ASA physical status, and patients in the lower-numbered classes generally have better outcomes. Emergency operations have a higher overall morbidity than elective procedures (2, 3). One recent study (4), consisting of 97% class 1 and 2 patients who had no preoperative laboratory tests, had no deaths or perioperative morbidity.

A more specific evaluation of physical status relative to cardiac patients, in the form of a multifactorial index of cardiac risks in patients undergoing noncardiac operations, has been developed by Goldman et al. (5). They identified nine factors associated with severe or fatal cardiac complications (see Chapter 11). Intraoperative factors were not included in this index.

Risk assessment for noncardiac procedures often has been based on the time between a myocardial infarction (MI) and surgery. Risk of reinfarction was felt to increase if the surgery was performed within 6 months of the initial infarction; however, with newer treatment modalities (e.g., angioplasty, thrombolytics), this 6-month interval no longer may be valid (6). An American Heart Association/American College of Cardiology task force listed a recent MI (i.e., <30 days) in the highest-risk category; after that period, risk is based on the status of the disease and on exercise tolerance (7).

Considerable attention has been devoted to the preventable morbidity and mortality that is related to "critical incidents" in anesthesiology (8). A critical incident is a human error or equipment failure that could have led—or did lead—to an undesirable outcome, ranging from an increased length of hospital stay to death. To decrease such preventable situations, considerable attention has been focused on improved patient monitoring. The ASA has set standards for basic intraoperative monitoring (9), which include monitoring of oxygenation, ventilation, circulation, and body temperature. Therefore pulse oximeters and capnographs now are routinely used.

Anesthesia safety has improved from approximately 25,000 deaths per 10^8 hours of anesthesia exposure in the 1950s to 500 deaths per 10^8 hours of exposure today (10). Increased training, new drugs and monitors, improved surgical techniques, and better perioperative planning all help to improve patient outcomes.

SPINAL OR EPIDURAL ANESTHESIA VERSUS GENERAL ANESTHESIA

The belief that spinal or epidural anesthesia is inherently safer than general anesthesia is prevalent among physicians. This concept is difficult to study, however, because many high-risk procedures (e.g., cardiac or neurologic surgery) cannot be performed with use of regional anesthesia. In addition, many outcome studies are poorly designed, interpret morbidity differently, use different monitors, and have subtle differences in techniques.

The choice of regional versus general anesthesia depends on many factors: *(a)* site, type, position, and duration of surgery; *(b)* specific medical concerns; and *(c)* personal preference of the patient, surgeon, or anesthesiologist. Whereas spinal anesthesia could be useful in a patient with severe chronic pulmonary disease, in whom a low dermatome level is adequate (e.g., lower extremity or prostate surgery), the high levels required for intraabdominal surgery could have a more deleterious effect on respiration than a carefully performed general anesthesia. A patient with morbid obesity and severe gastric reflux who is undergoing a procedure in the lithotomy position, Trendelenburg position, or both may require intubation to protect the airway and to provide adequate ventilation. Each individual patient and procedure must be evaluated for their unique requirements.

Many studies have shown no difference in cardiac morbidity or mortality rates between patients receiving general and patients receiving regional anesthesia when both are properly managed (11–13). An editorial in *Anesthesiology* reviewed an article (14) that compared regional and general anesthesia in patients undergoing peripheral vascular surgery and showed no difference in cardiac outcomes; the editorial (15) concluded that additional studies comparing cardiac outcomes are not needed. One study that evaluated an elderly population undergoing elective total knee replacement found that the type of anesthesia did not affect cognitive dysfunction or major cardiovascular complications (16). The advantages of regional anesthesia may be specific for select patient populations, such as patients at increased risk for vaso-occlusive events, or procedures (17).

Hypotension and bradycardia are the most frequent physiologic changes associated with spinal or epidural blockade. The higher the level of the block by the sympathetic efferents, the more evident the hypotension. Treatment of the hypotension is directed at a decreased cardiac output, decreased peripheral vascular resistance, or both (18). There also have been reports of sudden, unexplained, severe bradycardia and asystole during spinal or epidural anesthesia (19, 20).

Neurologic sequelae can range from the often-discussed postdural puncture headache to the rare, serious neurologic injury, such as cauda equina syndrome. The incidence of headache decreases with increasing patient age and use of smaller-gauge spinal needles with noncutting tips. Treatment of the cerebral spinal fluid leak can be as conservative as bed rest and analgesia or as invasive as an epidural blood patch. Central neuraxial blockade generally is contraindicated in the presence of neurologic disease, hypovolemia, increased intracranial pressure, coagulation problems, sepsis, and localized infections at the puncture site.

The decision to use either a spinal or an epidural technique is based on the requirements of the procedure and the patient. Spinal anesthesia usually requires less time to perform, has a faster onset of action, and generally provides a better-quality block. An epidural with a catheter can extend the time of the block and provide postoperative analgesia. Epidurals require larger amounts of local anesthetic to achieve their effects, so the risk of an adverse reaction increases if the local agent is injected intravenously or into the subarachnoid space (18).

SAME-DAY ADMISSIONS

The percentage of surgical patients admitted to the hospital on the day of their surgery has increased dramatically. This has been encouraged—and sometimes even mandated—by third-party payers. Many earlier concerns about increased risk have been ameliorated by increased efforts to prepare the patient before arrival, including preadmission instructions, continuing medications, and obtaining appropriate tests and consultations. The development of "critical paths" (i.e., practice guidelines) have helped to facilitate the preoperative preparation of these patients.

OUTPATIENT ANESTHESIA

Over half of all surgical procedures now are performed in an outpatient setting (see Chapter 4). Initially, this setting was restricted to patients in ASA class 1 and 2, but most centers now accept patients in ASA class 3 if they are stable and the proposed procedure would create minimal postoperative impairment. Most complications and unplanned admissions result from anesthetic–surgical problems, such as urinary retention, postoperative bleed-

ing, nausea, and vomiting, or from more extensive surgery than was planned. Major developments in shorter-acting anesthetic agents have helped to expand the outpatient population (21, 22).

ANESTHESIA MANAGEMENT

Anesthesiologists refer to their management plan using three terms: *(a)* general anesthesia, *(b)* regional anesthesia, and *(c)* monitored anesthesia care (MAC). Often, however, there may be a blurring of the exact definition. For example, an ophthalmic block is a type of regional anesthesia, but the anesthesiologist might refer to MAC when the surgeon administers the local anesthetic and the anesthesiologist provides the sedation and monitoring.

General anesthesia provides a loss of sensation with the loss of consciousness. The airway usually is maintained with a mask and, possibly, an oropharyngeal airway, an endotracheal tube, or a laryngeal mask airway. Other devices used to establish an airway are required for specific situations. Ventilation can be spontaneous, assisted, or controlled. General anesthesia can be provided by inhaled agents, a combination of inhaled and intravenous drugs, or by a totally intravenous anesthetic technique. The selection of agents is determined by numerous factors, such as the patient's health, requirements for the procedure and the surgeon, anticipated hemodynamics, and drug interactions.

Regional anesthesia uses a local anesthesia to produce insensitivity over a certain, specific area. Epidurals, spinals, axillary blocks, intravenous regional blocks, ankle blocks, and caudals are a few of the techniques more frequently used. Generally, some degree of sedation is administered in addition to the regional anesthesia, but this is not absolutely necessary. The degree of sedation varies with the needs of the patient, the procedure, and the quality of the regional anesthetic. One must always be prepared, however, to convert an inadequate or problematic block into a general anesthetic.

MAC anesthesia occurs when an anesthesiologist provides specific services to a patient and is responsible for the patient's medical care during a procedure. Infiltration of a local anesthetic may or may not be used during a MAC procedure. The patient may receive intravenous sedation, antiemetics, narcotics, other analgesics, vasopressors, antihypertensives, or other pharmacologic therapy as required. The term *MAC* refers both to an awake, monitored patient and to a deeply sedated patient. Often, terms such as *intravenous sedation*, *standby*, and *local with sedation* are used in this category. Sometimes there is a fine line between the deeply sedated, unconscious MAC patient and a patient undergoing general anesthesia.

Rather than dictating a specific anesthetic technique, the consulting internist is most helpful when he or she clearly defines the patient's status and anticipated treatment plans. Then, the anesthesiologist's experience and training will be used to determine the anesthetic plan.

ANESTHETIC AGENTS

The obvious goal in developing new anesthetic agents is fast onset, fast dissipation, predictable effects, and few side effects. The anesthetic drugs include opioids, specific induction agents, sedatives, amnestics, inhaled gases, muscle relaxants, reversal agents, local anesthetics, and a number of varied medications. An entire review is beyond the scope of this chapter, but a few comments concerning some specific agents should be noted.

In the opioid category, alfentanil is a synthetic narcotic with a rapid onset and brief duration of action. Over the years, fentanyl and the more potent sufentanil

have shown their versatility. Remifentanil is a new, ultrashort-acting opioid that has no accumulation with repeated doses or infusion. Future experience with this agent will determine if the predictability and reversibility of its actions are as useful as expected.

Midazolam is a water-soluble, intravenous benzodiazepine with sedative and amnestic qualities of relatively short duration and little or no pain with intravenous injection (as compared to diazepam). This drug has been used as a premedicant, as a component of general anesthesia, and to provide conscious sedation.

The intermediate-duration muscle relaxants vecuronium and atracurium have come into widespread use, especially during outpatient surgery. Because atracurium uses the Hoffman degradation process, this drug is not dependent on renal or liver function for elimination. Mivacurium was introduced as a relaxant of short duration and rapid recovery. Rocuronium, which was introduced in 1994, has a faster onset than the intermediate agents presently in use.

Propofol has become a popular drug because it is useful as an induction agent, as a major component in a general anesthetic, and as an infusion for sedation. This agent provides prompt awakening, which is useful in outpatient anesthesia. The cardiac and respiratory depressant aspects of propofol, however, require careful monitoring.

The newest inhalation agents, sevoflurane and desflurane, have rapid onset, awakening, and adjustment of effect. This improved control allows better predictability of the agent's effects. Sevoflurane is well tolerated during mask inductions, especially with children. (The liver and renal concerns of these agents are reviewed in this chapter under the appropriate headings.)

Although not used specifically for anesthesia, flumazenil is useful as a selective benzodiazepine antagonist (i.e., to reverse the effects of benzodiazepines). Ondansetron now is being used in anesthesia to prevent or to treat nausea and emesis. The small doses of 4 mg intravenously are considered to be expensive, but the drug is very effective.

EFFECTS ON ORGAN SYSTEMS

This section discusses the effects of an anesthetic agent or technique on a specific organ system, but one must realize that the anesthetic rarely is used alone. The other drugs can cause additive effects or even counteract an action; therefore the comments here are broad generalizations.

The Respiratory System

Effects of Anesthesia

Most anesthetic agents have the potential to adversely affect respiration. These effects include alteration of respiratory control, lung volumes, distribution of ventilation and perfusion, and respiratory muscle function (23).

Increasing the concentration of inhaled agents alters the normal central nervous system response to carbon dioxide. The usual increase in minute ventilation is blunted as the arterial carbon dioxide tension rises. Narcotics also diminish this response, primarily by slowing the respiratory rate. In addition, there is a loss of the hypoxic drive, and the normal cough reflex is either depressed or abolished.

During general anesthesia, there is a reduction of the functional residual capacity, which persists until the recovery period. Abnormalities in the distribution of ventilation and perfusion occur regularly during anesthesia, with resulting abnormalities of oxygen and carbon dioxide exchange. The distribution of ventilation within the lung varies according to the mode of ventilation. With spontaneous ventilation, the dependent portions of the lung are preferentially ventilated; with controlled ventilation, the upper portions are affected.

Paralysis of the respiratory muscles routinely is produced by neuromuscular blocking agents. Adequate reversal of the muscle paralysis, either by drugs or spontaneously, must be carefully evaluated. Various tests have been devised to assess this recovery, such as use of an electrical nerve stimulator, the patient's ability to support his or her head off the bed for 5 seconds unaided, and measurement of vital capacity (i.e., >10 mL/kg).

The various alterations of respiratory function can extend into the postoperative period as well. This so-called *anesthetic tail* can be of special importance in those patients with preexisting cardiopulmonary disorders.

Anesthesia Management

There is no one anesthesia technique of choice for patients with pulmonary problems. Instead, it is useful to think of the choices as ranging between "minimal interference" and "maximum support." Minimal interference usually involves regional or local anesthetics or general anesthesia without an endotracheal tube. These methods generally are used for lower abdominal and lower extremity procedures with spontaneous or assisted ventilation. Even these techniques can interfere with respiration to varying degrees, however. Many patients with respiratory disease cannot lie flat or cease coughing for the time required for the procedure. Maximal support involves a general anesthetic with tracheal intubation, mechanical ventilation, suctioning, and positive pressure ventilation as required in the postoperative period.

Anesthesia management in patients with reactive airways presents special problems (24). These patients should continue their bronchodilators (i.e., β-adrenergic agonists, corticosteroids, theophylline) up to the time of the procedure, and the anesthesiologist must achieve an adequate level of anesthesia before instrumenting the airway to prevent precipitating a severe bronchospasm. During intubation, intravenous lidocaine often is used to prevent reflex bronchospasm. Drugs stimulating histamine release (e.g., curare) generally are avoided. Inhalation anesthetics such as halothane, isoflurane, and sevoflurane are used for their bronchodilator qualities (25).

Anesthesiologists always are concerned about the risk of aspirating gastric contents into the lung. Patients who are predisposed to aspiration include those who are morbidly obese, who have recently ingested food, who have a bowel obstruction, who are pregnant, and who have reflux or a hiatal hernia. These patients might benefit from preoperative antacids, histamine-receptor antagonists, and special intubating techniques.

The Cardiovascular System

Effects of Anesthesia

Currently used inhalation agents are myocardial depressants due to a combination of hemodynamic changes. Heart rate is increased by isoflurane, desflurane, and sevoflurane, but not by halothane. However, sevoflurane increases the heart rate only at very deep levels. Halothane is associated with ventricular dysrhythmias when endogenous or exogenous catecholamines are increased, and cardiac output is decreased in a dose-dependent fashion by this agent. The decreases in systemic vascular resistance by isoflurane, sevoflurane, and desflurane are dose-dependent as well. All the inhaled agents will decrease left ventricular stroke volume (26).

Opioids are used in anesthesia to provide analgesia and to blunt or eliminate dangerous hemodynamic responses to stimuli. Opioids produce minimal cardiac depression and modest to no decreases in preload and afterload. The decreases in heart rate caused by narcotics are useful in patients with ischemic heart disease. Hypotension and bradycardia are noted more frequently with morphine than with fentanyl (27).

Ketamine has unique cardiovascular actions. It stimulates the cardiovascular system; increases blood pressure, heart rate, cardiac output; and increases oxygen consumption. Therefore ketamine is used for situations in which its unique properties are useful (e.g., hypovolemia, cardiac tamponade) (28).

Caution must be exercised during major regional blocks requiring large doses of potent local anesthetics. An accidental intravascular injection of a medication such as bupivacaine could cause a rapid and profound cardiovascular depression.

Anesthesia Management

Increasing numbers of patients with MI need to undergo anesthesia. In these patients, the balance between oxygen supply and demand must be appreciated. By maintaining the appropriate heart rate, blood pressure (i.e., afterload), ventricular volume (i.e., preload), and contractility, one tries to avoid MI. Other factors to be considered are the hematocrit, coronary blood flow, and oxygen saturation. Manipulations such as laryngoscopy, intubation, and surgical stimulation elicit autonomic responses, and opioids are used to reduce the stress response and the increased heart rate. Nitroglycerin may be given intravenously to improve coronary circulation. Antihypertensive and antianginal agents should be maintained until the time of the procedure (29). (The section on regional versus general anesthesia reviews selecting a technique for cardiac patients undergoing noncardiac surgery.)

The treatment of postoperative pain is important in stabilizing the patient's postoperative hemodynamics. Epidural narcotics, intravenous patient-controlled analgesia, and the addition of nonsteroidal anti-inflammatory drugs should be considered in appropriate patients. In addition, the patient should be kept normothermic during the perioperative period. Frank et al. (30) concluded that in patients with cardiac risk factors, maintenance of normothermia was associated with a decreased incidence of cardiac events and ventricular tachycardia.

Optimal control of heart failure is mandatory before the induction of anesthesia. Certainly, active congestive heart failure is a contraindication to elective procedures. Careful titration or avoidance of intravenous agents causing cardiovascular depression is necessary, and depending on the patient's fluid status, invasive monitoring may be required. The postoperative period is important, because many factors can precipitate congestive heart failure in this period (e.g., fluid replacement or fluid shifts, acute MI, peripheral vasoconstriction) (29).

Antihypertensive medications should be given to patients on the day of surgery. Discontinuation of drug therapy is more dangerous and stressful than continuation. Generally, with extra care and awareness of hypovolemia as a possibility, the anesthesiologist can avoid serious hypotension.

The Liver

Effects of Anesthesia

Anesthetic techniques and agents may affect the liver to different degrees. Abnormalities in hepatic function could result from the direct action of an agent or the indirect effect on oxygen and blood flow to the liver. All inhaled anesthetics depress portal blood flow, but they vary in their effect on hepatic arterial flow and hepatic oxygen uptake. Isoflurane, sevoflurane, and desflurane appear to have the least effect on hepatic flood flow and hepatic oxygen delivery if an approximately normal blood pressure and cardiac output are maintained. Intravenous and regional anesthetics alter liver function by the degree to which they change the systemic hemodynamics. When mechanical ventilation increases intrathoracic pressure, the change in venous return and cardiac output can affect the hepatic blood flow (31, 32).

Surgical stress probably is the most important factor determining liver dysfunction. Several studies have found that postoperative liver abnormalities mainly result from the operative site and procedure rather than from a specific anesthetic (33–35).

Because two chemically related substances, chloroform and carbon tetrachloride, are toxic to the liver, other halogenated hydrocarbons that are used as general anesthetics have been closely monitored. Halothane has received the most publicity. Halothane-induced hepatic necrosis is a very rare (36) but often fatal immune response initiated by halothane metabolism and the formation of antibodies in susceptible patients. With reexposure to halothane, the antibodies mediate the hepatic necrosis (37). Because of decreased metabolism, enflurane and isoflurane hepatitis is far less common than with halothane hepatitis. Well-documented cases of hepatotoxicity with the newer inhaled agents are rare. Desflurane is the least metabolized, but only one case has been reported (38). An immune response–initiated hepatitis after sevoflurane has not yet been reported (37).

Anesthesia Management

In selecting an anesthetic for patients with liver disease, the effects of altered metabolism and protein binding must be considered. All medications should be carefully titrated to achieve the desired effect, because their duration and intensity of action could be prolonged. One also may decide to use agents that are not metabolized by the liver; with attention to detail, an inhaled agent such as isoflurane and a narcotic such as fentanyl can be used successfully in this situation. The muscle relaxant atracurium is a theoretically appropriate choice, because elimination is by Hoffman degradation and therefore is relatively independent of liver and renal function. Regional anesthesia can be used if there are no coagulation abnormalities and cardiovascular stability can be maintained (32).

The Kidney

Effects of Anesthesia

All general anesthetic agents tend to decrease the glomerular filtration rate (GFR) and the intraoperative urine flow. Inhaled agents affect the kidney by their action on the renal circulation, with mild to moderate reduction in both renal blood flow (RBF) and GFR. Opioids generally have a minimal effect on GFR and RBF, and regional anesthesia does not alter RBF and GFR as long as adequate renal perfusion pressure is maintained. Hypotension will result in decreased urine flow, but urine output will be reestablished with normotension unless the kidneys are abnormal or hypovolemia is prolonged. Vasoconstriction and salt-retaining stress responses to surgical stimulation (i.e., catecholamines, renin, ADH) also must be considered. The decrease in cardiac output by positive pressure ventilation ultimately will decrease the RBF, GFR, sodium excretion, and urine flow (39).

The concern with possible nephrotoxicity of inhaled, fluorinated anesthetics stems from the metabolic production of free fluoride ions. Historically, methoxyflurane produced a high-output renal failure when used at high concentrations for extended periods of time. Renal damage corresponded to fluoride levels. Enflurane generally is not nephrotoxic, but it probably should not be used in prolonged cases or if there is kidney dysfunction. Because of their metabolic patterns, isoflurane, halothane, and desflurane have not been shown to have adverse renal effects. Sevoflurane requires the same precautions as enflurane due to fluoride production (40). In addition, sevoflurane is degraded by the strong bases in carbon dioxide absorbents to a product referred to as *Compound A*, which is a dose-dependent nephrotoxin in rats. Sevoflurane currently is recommended for use at gas flow rates of 2 L/min or greater to reduce the formation of Compound A.

There is still a question as to whether flow recommendations are necessary, however (41–43).

Anesthesia Management

The importance of preoperative dialysis in improving the risk and safety of anesthesia in patients with uremia cannot be overemphasized. Agents and techniques are selected to avoid further damage in patients with diminished renal function. An important factor to be considered in patients with chronic renal failure is proper fluid balance, especially the avoidance of hypovolemia resulting in intraoperative hypotension and organ damage. In patients undergoing long-term dialysis with no significant renal function, the intraoperative concern is to avoid hypervolemia, which could contribute to hypertension and cardiac failure. Because these patients do not tolerate either over- or underhydration, the appropriate monitors should be selected (i.e., urine output, systemic blood pressure, and possibly, central venous or pulmonary wedge pressures).

Equally important is the electrolyte balance, with an emphasis on normal serum potassium levels. A low serum potassium level may cause arrhythmia, and a high level can be increased by succinylcholine, cold bank blood, hypoventilation, and tissue destruction. Electrocardiography is an additional monitor reflecting potassium abnormalities.

Some drugs are converted by the liver to water-soluble, ionized derivatives that have no pharmacologic activity and are excreted by the kidney. These agents can be used if there is renal failure (e.g., induction doses of propofol and ketamine). Drugs that rely on renal excretion for termination of their action include several older, long-acting muscle relaxants, atropine, and neostigmine. Reduced protein binding in chronic renal failure affects the action of thiopental and benzodiazepines.

Isoflurane often is selected as the inhalation agent. Fentanyl is useful in end-stage renal disease because of its lack of active metabolites. Sufentanil, however, does have an active metabolite that is excreted by the kidney, which can prolong narcosis. Because atracurium undergoes Hoffman degradation, it is not affected by renal failure (39).

DRUG INTERACTIONS

Patients frequently will be taking numerous over-the-counter and prescription medications. With the additional 5 to 10 agents used during a procedure, the possibility of a drug interaction must be anticipated. **It is essential that the anesthesiologist be informed of all medications currently or recently used by the patient.**

With the exception of monoamine oxidase inhibitors, it rarely is mandatory for drugs to be discontinued before anesthesia if they are a necessary part of medical treatment. This long-held concern for monoamine oxidase inhibitors had been

Table 5.2.   Anesthetic/Drug Interactions

Drug Class and Prototype	Anesthetic/Drug Interaction	Problem	Anesthetic Management
ACE inhibitors (Catopril)	Chronic use of ACE inhibitors	Hypotension in the postcardiopulmonary bypass period	Vassopressors
Antiarrhythmics Quinidine	Muscle relaxants	Prolonged	Reduced relaxant dose; monitor with nerve stimulator
Amiodarone	Volatile anesthetics	Bradydysrhythmias, low cardiac output and systemic vascular resistance	Careful monitoring
Antibiotics Tetracyclines	Methoxyflurane	Renal toxicity	Avoid concomitant use
Aminoglycoside antibiotics	Muscle relaxants	Prolonged action	Monitor with a nerve stimulator
Anticoagulants	Regional techniques	Bleeding	Avoid regional techniques; check PT/PTT
Anticonvulsants Phenobarbital	Volatile anesthetics	Increased biotransformation due to enzyme inductions	Avoid agents with toxic metabolites
Phenytoin	Nondepolarizing muscle relaxants	Resistance to the muscle relaxants	Monitor carefully
Antihypertensives Methyldopa	Volatile anesthetics	Hypotension	Fluids, pressors, titrate anesthetic concentration
Antiparkinson drugs Levodopa	Thorazine droperidol	Extrapyramidal symptoms	Avoid droperidol and phenothiazine
β-Blockers Propranolol	Volatile anesthetics	Cardiac depression, bradycardia, hypotension	Isoproterenol, atropine
Calcium channel blockers Verapamil Nifedipine	Volatile anesthetics	Enhances cardiac depression	Regulate the concentrations of volatile agents

Table 5.2 *(continued)*.   Anesthetic/Drug Interactions

Drug Class and Prototype	Anesthetic/Drug Interaction	Problem	Anesthetic Management
Cocaine	Volatile anesthetics, sympathomimetics	Dysrhythmias, exaggerated response to vassopressors	Avoid dysrythmogenic drugs (halothane) and sympathomimetics
Digitalis		Arrhythmia	Avoid alkalosis and hypokalemia
Diuretics	Volatile anesthetics	Hypokalemia, hypovolemia	Monitor carefully, check potassium level
Fenfluramine (Pondimin)	General anesthesia	Cardiac arrest, catecholamine-depleting effect	Discontinue 1–2 wks preoperatively; if not, cardiac monitoring
Lithium	Pressors, muscle relaxants	Exaggerated response, prolonged action	Monitor with a nerve stimulator
MAO inhibitors Nardil Phenzeline Isocarboxazid	Opiates (especially meperidine), sympathomimetics	Hypertension, hypotension, convulsion, coma, death	Discontinue 2 wks, avoid opiates and pressors; nitroprusside for hypertension; direct-acting pressors for hypotension
Myasthenia gravis drugs Pyridostigmine	Muscle relaxants	Prolonged action	Avoid or reduce dose, monitor with a nerve stimulator
Organophosphates Echothiophate	Succinylcholine, mivacurium, ester-type local anesthetics	Prolonged action	Avoid or use reduced doses with caution
Phenothiazines Chlorpromazine	Opiates and other CNS depressants	Augment CNS depression	Use less CNS depressants
Tricyclic antidepressants Imipramine Nortriptyline	Volatile anesthetics	Hypotension tachycardia	Titrate the anesthesia, monitor
Vasodilators Nitroglycerin Isosorbide		Hypotension	Titrate the anesthesia, monitor

ACE, angiotensin-converting enzyme; CNS, central nervous system; MAO, monoamine oxidase; PT/PTT, prothrombin time/partial thromboplastin time.

questioned (44–46), but the potential for complications should not be understated (47). Most antihypersensitivity and cardiac medications should be continued; in fact, clonidine should be maintained up to the time of surgery due to the risks of rebound hypertension (47).

The frequent use of fenfluramine in diet plans has brought that medication to the attention of anesthesiologists. One article and the manufacturer's information suggest that fenfluramine should be discontinued 1 to 2 weeks before use of an elective anesthetic (48, 49). Additional studies, however, are needed to decide this issue.

Table 5.2 lists commonly used drugs that could affect anesthetic management.

The interaction, anesthetic drug, resulting problem, and suggested management are briefly outlined.

SPECIFIC CONCERNS

A few medical problems are unique to anesthesia, either because of the agents used or their occurrence during a procedure.

Malignant Hyperthermia

Malignant hyperthermia (MH) is a potentially lethal (10%) disorder that is triggered by exposure to anesthetic agents. It is a hypermetabolic response to potent, inhaled agents and succinylcholine and is characterized by increased carbon dioxide production, oxygen consumption, and muscle membrane breakdown. These changes result in tachycardia, muscle rigidity, hyperkalemia, rhabdomyolysis, myoglobinuria, and arrhythmias. The elevated body temperature is a dramatic but often late sign (50).

This inherited disorder of skeletal muscle affects humans, certain strains of swine, and other animals. In humans, the inheritance is autosomal dominant, with variable expression. The incidence varies by region due to the differences in the gene pools. One study reported the incidence to be 1 in 50,000 adults undergoing anesthesia and 1 in 15,000 children undergoing anesthesia. There also has been a reported association with myopathic disorders, such as Duchenne's muscular dystrophy (51).

An MH treatment protocol must be available wherever general anesthesia is provided. Dantrolene is the essential medication in the treatment of MH and must be available. A patient who is susceptible to MH can be anesthetized with nontriggering agents, monitored appropriately (e.g., temperature, end-tidal carbon dioxide), and isolated from contamination by potent, inhaled agents.

The history, both the patient's and the family's, is the first step in determining whether the patient is MH susceptible. Suggestive histories include a history of MH, an unexplained intraoperative death, unexpected adverse events with anesthesia, myopathies, and muscle abnormalities such as strabismus and scoliosis. A history of succinylcholine-induced masseter muscle rigidity has been associated with MH in 50% of patients tested (52). The only accepted test for MH is the exposure of biopsied vastus lateralis muscle to halothane and caffeine and observation for an abnormal contracture response. Presently, there are 11 testing centers in North America; the MH-Hotline number is: 1-800-MH-HYPER (50).

Abnormal Plasma Cholinesterase

Plasma cholinesterase, pseudocholinesterase, or nonspecific cholinesterase degrades acetylcholine released at the neuromuscular junction. Inherited variants are important to the anesthesiologist, because the enzyme **affects the duration of two neuromuscular-blocking agents: succinylcholine and mivacurium.** Patients with low or absent activity of pseudocholinesterase or enzyme variants will have no symptoms except for prolonged apnea after administration of succinylcholine (53).

The qualitative and quantitative differences of the enzyme can be evaluated by use of various tests. Patients who are homozygous for the condition have prolonged paralysis (i.e., 3–6 hours) after the usual doses of succinylcholine. The duration of action is only slightly prolonged in heterozygous patients. The failure to identify abnormal phenotypes with basic testing will be improved as more mutations (>20 so far) are identified (54). Although many exogenous and endogenous factors (e.g., pregnancy, liver disease, uremia, malnutrition, echothiophate iodine, and plasmapheresis) can reduce the activity of the enzyme, the level must decrease by approximately 75% for prolongation with succinylcholine to be observed.

Mivacurium is a nondepolarizing relaxant that is metabolized to a significant extent by plasma cholinesterase. In the atypical homozygote, there is little or no metabolism of mivacurium, and the block can persist for hours. The genetic frequency is 1 in every 2500 to 4000 patients (i.e., the same for succinylcholine) (55, 56).

Controlled, mechanical ventilation is the treatment for prolonged muscle relaxation and apnea after succinylcholine. Reversal agents are unpredictable in the reversal and should be avoided.

Latex Allergy

A type I hypersensitivity latex allergy implies that a patient's immune system responds to proteins found in natural rubber products with an immunoglobulin E–mediated response. The possibility of an anaphylactic reaction to an unknown latex allergy during anesthesia is of particular concern. Anaphylaxis in the operating room requires rapid differential diagnosis and skillful resuscitation.

Identifying susceptible patients by a screening history is the first step. Individuals who appear to be at high risk include children with multiple surgeries; patients with spina bifida, fruit allergies, or congenital urologic anomalies, or who are atopic; and health care workers (57). Testing, evaluation, and interpretation should be done by an experienced allergist (58).

Patients with latex allergy require a latex-free environment. **Everyone involved in the care of such patients must be alerted to the situation so that all precautions can be taken**. By scheduling latex-allergic patients for the first procedure of the day, the allergen level should be at its lowest point. All items that come in contact with these patients or the health workers involved should be without latex (59).

A facility needs to formulate a comprehensive plan for the entire institution, not just the operating room. A premedication protocol of diphenhydramine, prednisone, and ranitidine often is used in susceptible patients (58).

REFERENCES

1. Alpert CC, Conroy JM, Roy CR. Anesthesia and perioperative medicine: a department of anesthesiology changes its name. Anesthesiology 1996;84:712–715.
2. Beecher HK, Todd DP. A study of the deaths associated with anesthesia and surgery based on a study of 599,548 anesthestics in ten institutions, 1948–1952 inclusive. Ann Surg 1954; 140:2–34.
3. Dripps DR, Lamont A, Eckenhoff JE. The role of anesthesia in surgical mortality. JAMA 1961; 178:261–266.
4. Narr BJ, Warner ME, Schroeder DR, et al. Outcomes of patients with no laboratory assessment before anesthesia and a surgical procedure. Mayo Clinic Proc 1997;72:505–509.
5. Goldman L, Caldera DL, Nussbaum SR, et al. Multifactorial index of cardiac risk in noncardiac surgical procedures. N Engl J Med 1977;297: 845–850.
6. Fleisher LA. Perioperative management of the cardiac patient undergoing noncardiac surgery. In: Annual refresher course lectures by the American Society of Anesthesiologists. Philadelphia: JB Lippincott, 1996.
7. Eagle KA, Brundage BH, Chaitman BR, et al. Guidelines for perioperative cardiovascular evaluation for noncardiac surgery: an abridged version of the report of the American College of Cardiology /American Heart Association Task Force on Practice Guidelines. Mayo Clinic Proc 1997;72:524–531.
8. Cooper JB, Newbower RS, Kitz RJ. An analysis of major errors and equipment failures in anesthesia management: consideration for prevention and detection. Anesthesiology 1984;60: 34–42.
9. The American Society of Anesthesiologists House of Delegates. Standards for basic anesthesia monitoring. Approved Oct. 21, 1986; amended Oct. 25, 1995.
10. Ward DS. The anatomy of anesthesia monitors: what they can do and cannot do, and what if they do nothing. In: Annual refresher course lectures by the American Society of Anesthesiologists. Philadelphia: JB Lippincott, 1996.
11. Cook PT, Davies MJ, Cronin KD, et al. A prospective randomised trial comparing spinal anesthesia using hyperbaric cinchocaine with general anesthesia for lower limb vascular surgery. Anaesth Intensive Care 1986;14:373–380.
12. Damask MD, Weissman C, Todd G. General versus epidural anesthesia for femoral popliteal bypass surgery. J Clin Anesth 1990;2:71–75.
13. Rivers SP, Scher LA, Sheehan E, et al. Epidural versus general anesthesia for infrainguinal arterial reconstruction. J Vasc Surg 1991;14: 764–768.
14. Bode RH, Lewis KP, Zaroich SW, et al. Cardiac

outcome after peripheral vascular surgery: Comparison of general and regional anesthesia. Anesthesiology 1996;84:3–13.

15. Go AS, Browner WS. Cardiac outcomes after regional or general anesthesia. Do we have the answer? Anesthesiology 1996;84:1–2.

16. Williams-Russo P, Sharrock NE, Mattis S, et al. Cognitive effects after epidural vs. general anesthesia with older adults: a randomized trial. JAMA 1995;274:44–50.

17. Liu S, Carpenter RL, Neal JM. Epidural anesthesia and analgesia: their role in postoperative outcome. Anesthesiology 1995;82:1475–1506.

18. Bernards CM. Epidural and spinal anesthersia. In: Barash PG, ed. Clinical anesthesia. 3rd ed. Philadelphia: Lippincott-Raven, 1996:645–668.

19. Mackay DC, Carpenter RL, Thompson GE, et al. Bradycardia and asystole during spinal anesthesia: a report of three cases without morbidity. Anesthesiology 1989;70:866–868.

20. Caplan RA, Ward RJ, Posner K, et al. Unexpected cardiac arrest during spinal anesthesia: a closed claims analysis of predisposing factors. Anesthesiology 1988;68:5.

21. Ostman PL, White PF. Outpatient anesthesia. In: Miller RD, ed. Anesthesia. New York: Churchill Livingstone, 1994:2213–2246.

22. Twersky R, Fishman D, Homel P. What happens after discharge? Return hospital visits after ambulatory surgery. Anesth Analg 1997;84:319–324.

23. Rehderk, Sessler AD, Marsh M. State of the art: general anesthesia and the lung. Am Rev Respir Dis 1975;112:541–563.

24. Warner DO, Warner MA, Barnes RD. Perioperative respiratory complications in patients with asthma. Anesthesiology 1996;85:460–467.

25. Bishop MJ. New perspectives in the patient with reactive airways. In: The 1997 international Anesthesia Research Society review course lectures. Anesth Analg 84(supplement), March 1997:14–18.

26. Calahan MK. Hemodynamic effects of inhaled anesthetics. In: The International Research Society review course lectures. Anesth Analg supplement, March 1996:14–17.

27. Bailey PL, Stanley TH. Intravenous opioid anesthetics. In: Miller RD, ed. Anesthesia. New York: Churchill Livingstone, 1994:303–312.

28. Reves JG, Glass PSA, Lubarsky DA. Nonbarbituate intravenous anesthetics. In: Miller RD, ed. Anesthesia. New York: Churchill Livingstone, 1994:259–264.

29. Leslie JB. Prevention and treatment of intraoperative myocordial ischemia. In: The 1997 International Anesthesia Research Society course lectures. Anesth Analg, supplement, March 1997:79–89.

30. Frank SM, Fleisher LA, Breslou MJ, et al. Perioperative maintenance of normothermia reduces the incidence of morbid cardiac events: a randomized clinical trial. JAMA 277:1127–1134.

31. Gelman S. Anesthesia and the liver. In: Barash PG, ed. Clinical anesthesia. 3rd ed. Philadelphia: Lippincott-Raven, 1996:1003–1019.

32. Coursin DB. Anesthetic concerns for the patient with liver disease. In: Annual refresher course lectures by the American Society of Anesthesiologists. Philadelphia: JB Lippincott, 1996.

33. Viegas O, Stoelting RK. LDH5 changes after cholecystectomy or hysterectomy in patients receiving halothane, enflurane, or fentanyl. Anesthesiology 1979;51:556.

34. Zinn SE, Fairley HB, Glen JD. Liver function in patients with mild alcoholic hepatitis, after enflurane, nitous oxide-narcotic, and spinal anesthesia. Anesth Analg 1985;64:487.

35. Loft S, Boel J, Kyst AA, et al. Increased hepatic microsomal enzyme activity after surgery under halothane or spinal anesthesia. Anesthesiology 1985;62:11.

36. Subcommittee on the National Halothane Study of the Committee on the Anesthesia, National Academy of Science: Report: National Halothane Study (1966) possible association between halothane anesthesia and postoperative hepatic necrosis. JAMA 1966;197:775–788.

37. Kharasch ED. Inhalation anesthetic toxicity: current controversies. In: Annual refresher course lectures by the American Society of Anesthesiologists. Philadelphia: JB Lippincott, 1996.

38. Martin JL, Plevak DJ, Flannery KD, et al. Hepatotoxicity after desflurane anesthesia. Anesthesiology 1995;83:1125–1125.

39. Sladen RN. Renal physiology. In: Miller RD, ed. Anesthesia, NewYork: Churchill Livingstone, 1994:663–668.

40. Kharasch ED. Inhalation anesthetic toxicity: current controversies. In: Annual refresher course lectures by the American Society of Anesthesiologists. Philadelphia: JB Lippincott, 1996.

41. Bito H, Ikeachi Y, Ikeda K. Effects of low-flow sevoflurane anesthesia on renal function. Anesthesiology 1997;86:1231–1237.

42. Kharasch ED, Frink EJ, Zager R, et al. Assessment of low-flow sevoflurane and isoflurane effects on renal function using sensitive markers of tubular toxicity. Anesthesiology 1997;86:1238–1253.

43. Mazze RI, Jamison RL. Low-flow sevoflurane: is it safe? Anesthesiology 1997;86:1225–1227.

44. Michaels I, Serrins M, Shier NQ, et al. Anesthesia for cardiac surgery in patients receiving monamine oxidase inhibitors. Anesth Analg 1984;63:1041–1044.

45. Hirshman CA, Lindeman K. MAO inhibitors: must they be discontinued before anesthesia? JAMA 1988;260:3507.

46. El-Gahzoure AR, Ivankovich AD, Braverman B, et al. MAO inhibitors: should they be discontinued preoperatively? Anesth Analg 1985;64:592.

47. Cullen BF. Drug interactions for the anesthesi-

ologist. In: Annual refresher course lectures by the American Society of Anesthesiologists. Philadelphia: JB Lippincott, 1996.

48. Lockhart AC. Fen/Phen and anesthesia—fact, fiction and other concerns. Am Soc Anesthesiologists Newsletter 1997;61(4):19–20.

49. Bennett JA, Eltringham RJ. Possible dangers of anesthesia in patients receiving fenfluramine. Results of animal studies following a case of human cardiac arrest. Anaesthesia 1997;37:8–13.

50. Rosenberg H. Malignant hyperthermia and other anesthesia induced myodystrophies. In: Annual refresher course lectures by the American Society of Anesthesiologists. Philadelphia: JB Lippincott, 1996.

51. Wedel DJ. Current understanding and treatment of malignant hyperthermia. In: The 1997 International Anesthesia Research Society review course lecture. Anesth Analg supplement, March 1997:140-144.

52. Rosenberg II, Fletcher JE, Stevenson D. Pharmacogenetics. In: Barash PG, ed. Clinical anesthesia. 3rd ed. Philadelphia: Lippincott-Raven, 1996:489–505.

53. Rosenberg H, Fletcher JE, Steitman D. Pharma-

cogenetics. In: Barash PG, ed. Clinical anesthesia. 3rd ed. Philadelphia: Lippincott-Raven, 1996:505–508.

54. Bevin DR, Donoti F. Muscle relaxants. In: Barash PG, ed. Clinical anesthesia. 3rd ed. Philadelphia: Lippincott-Raven, 1996:380.

55. Savarese JT. Reversal and monitoring of neuromuscular blockade: changing attitudes. In: The 1997 International Anesthesia Research Society review course lectures. Anesth Analg supplement, March 1994:102.

56. Peterson RS, Bailey PL, Kalameghan R, et al. Prolonged neuromuscular block after mivacurium. Anesth Analg 1993;76:194.

57. Porri F, Pradal M, Lemiere C, et al. Association between latex sensitization and repeated latex exposure in children. Anesthesiology 1997;86:599–602.

58. Mostello L. The clinical significance and management of latex allergy. In: Annual refresher course lectures by the American Society of Anesthesiologists. Philadelphia: JB Lippincott, 1996.

59. Randel G. Latex allergy: who is next? Am Soc Anesthesiologists Newsletter 1997;61(5):14–17.

6

The Recognition, Correction, and Prevention of Malnutrition

Sudhir K. Dutta

Several lines of evidence suggest that recognition and correction of the malnutrition that accompanies a variety of diseases may play a significant role in providing optimal patient care. Furthermore, as we move toward the 21st century, it becomes increasingly clear that optimal nutrition to prevent and correct nutritional deficiencies is critical in controlling the ever-increasing cost of health care. In this environment, every primary care physician should be able to recognize nutritional deficiencies and apply appropriate corrective measures by delivering various nutrients to the sick patient by new methods. Furthermore, the ability of primary care physicians to prevent various nutritional deficiencies in chronically ill, elderly, and surgical patients will be a key factor in providing optimal health care to all patients. This chapter discusses the rationale for nutritional intervention, methods of nutritional assessment before and after the intervention, and various modalities of delivering nutrients to the patient.

RATIONALE

The rationale for providing proper nutritional assessment and support to our patients is based on well-recognized observations suggesting that presence of protein-energy malnutrition is associated with increased morbidity and mortality in most disease processes as well as in surgical operations. Furthermore, active intervention to correct malnutrition as well as its prevention can lead to shorter lengths of hospitalization and a reduction in the morbidity and mortality associated with a given disease process or surgical procedure. Improved modalities of delivering nutrients to sick patients by parenteral and enteral routes have significantly enhanced our ability to provide adequate nutritional support to critically ill patients. It has been estimated that in the United States, approximately $8.5 billion were spent on 18 million patients in hospitals, nursing homes, and homes for parenteral and enteral nutrition (1). It is generally believed that similar to cardiac monitoring, respiratory support, and dialysis treatment, customized nutritional support provided according to a patient's needs is important for a favorable outcome in various illnesses. The cost-effectiveness of nutritional support in the intensive care or perioperative setting has not been proven by well-designed, prospective, controlled clinical trials. Such carefully planned trials are needed to prove the significance of nutritional support in the successful outcome of complicated and major surgical intervention as well as of severe illnesses.

It is important that primary care physicians recognize that most well-nourished patients can tolerate 7 to 10 days of marginal postoperative nutrition provided by intravenous fluids; however, this may not be applicable to malnourished patients. This is particularly relevant because protein-energy malnutrition has been reported in approximately 20 to 40% of hospitalized patients. As primary care physicians, it is important to recognize these patients early and initiate appropriate steps to assess and correct their nutritional deficiencies.

RECOGNITION

Malnutrition should be suspected in any patient who has lost 10 to 20 pounds of weight in the last few months and demonstrates signs of cachexia and laboratory evidence of hypoalbuminemia. However, the diagnosis should be based on several detailed pieces of information, which include: (a) clinical and dietary history, (b) underlying clinical disorder, (c) anthropometric measurements, and (d) laboratory tests. These pieces of information can help to promptly assess the degree of malnutrition in a given patient.

Clinical and Dietary History

During a nutritional assessment, the following key observations may help:

1. Magnitude and rate of weight loss.
2. Reduction in appetite.
3. Impaired ability to chew and swallow foods.
4. Presence of associated gastrointestinal (GI) disorders, such as nausea, vomiting, or diarrhea.
5. History of excessive alcohol consumption.
6. Information about social conditions, such as whether the patient lives alone or prepares his or her own meals.
7. Insight into economic conditions that may restrict the patient's ability to buy, refrigerate, and cook appropriate foods.
8. Assessment of the patient's mental status (e.g., presence of depression may reduce caloric intake).
9. Ethnic, cultural, or religious beliefs that may influence food intake.

Besides these questions, a dietary history is an important part of the nutritional assessment. In addition, a physician may be able to perform a rough dietary evaluation by inquiring about the intake of major food items, such as dairy products, meat, poultry, fish, and eggs. Information about the intake of fresh fruits, vegetables, and cereal and butter is also important. Although 24-hour recall of food intake is not considered to be accurate, this measure should provide a rough guide to the physician in his or her office about the amount and composition of food intake by the patient. Furthermore, a physician may seek a consultation from a dietician who can be involved in assessing the protein-caloric intake and its composition in a given patient.

The physician should also be able to perform a clinical evaluation regarding the development of malnutrition. Clinical evaluation will include detecting the presence of catabolic states (e.g., fever, burns, trauma) or presence of conditions such as diarrhea, malabsorption, hyperthyroidism, diabetes mellitus, and so on. Both the dietary and the clinical history should be corroborated, preferably by a member of the patient's family.

Anthropometric Measurements

Although a large number of anthropometric measurements have been recommended for nutritional assessment, the most important are height (in centimeters), weight (in kilograms), triceps skinfold thickness (in millimeters), and mid-arm muscle circumference (in centimeters). Accurate measurement of these parameters requires a lever-balance scale, vertical measurement rod, skinfold caliper, and measuring tape.

Interpretation of the height/weight

data requires height/weight reference tables based on actuarial data obtained from the metropolitan tables between the ages of 20 to 55 years. For people older than 55, specific weight for height-median values obtained from National Health and Nutritional Examination Surveys (NHANES) are recommended (2) (Tables 6.1 and 6.2) (3). Thus, in a given patient, current body weight as well as ideal body weight from the metropolitan tables should be recorded. An important caveat, however, is that these reference weights cannot be applied to patients with peripheral edema or ascites, although a 20% variation from the ideal clearly suggests significant malnutrition or obesity in a patient without edema.

Another measure for assessing relative body weight is the body mass index (i.e., weight/height^2). Body mass index partially compensates for the shrinkage in height that occurs in elderly people, and Table 6.1 provides a nomogram for determining and interpreting body mass index. Other anthropometric measures include triceps skinfold and mid-arm muscle circumference (MAMC), which is equal to the mid-arm muscle circumference less the triceps skinfold thickness multiplied by 0.314. Mid-arm muscle circumference is a good marker of somatic proteins. The mid-arm circumference ranges between 25 to 27 cm in healthy adult males and between 21 to 23 centimeters in females. Interpretation of these data requires age- and gender-specific tables that have been developed based on combined data sets from the NHANES I and NHANES II studies. It is important to recognize that

Table 6.1. Reference Weights for Height Derived from Actuarial (Mortality Experience) Data for Ages 20 to 55^a

Height		Weight			
		Male		Female	
in	cm	lb	kg	lb	kg
58	147.3	—	—	114.0	51.7
59	149.9	—	—	116.5	52.8
60	152.4	—	—	119.0	53.9
61	154.9	—	—	122.0	55.3
62	157.5	133.0	60.3	125.0	56.7
63	160.0	135.0	61.2	128.0	58.0
64	162.6	137.5	62.4	131.0	59.4
65	165.1	140.0	63.5	134.0	60.8
66	167.6	143.0	64.9	137.0	62.1
67	170.2	146.0	66.2	140.0	63.5
68	172.7	149.0	67.6	143.0	64.9
69	175.3	152.0	68.9	146.0	66.2
70	177.8	155.0	70.3	149.0	67.6
71	180.3	158.5	71.9	152.0	69.0
72	182.9	162.0	73.9	—	—
73	185.4	166.0	75.3	—	—
74	188.0	169.5	76.9	—	—
75	190.5	174.0	78.9	—	—

Adapted from Russell RM. Nutritional assessment. In: Wyngaarden JB, Smith LH, and Bennett JC, eds. Cecil's textbook of medicine. 19th ed. Philadelphia: WB Saunders, 1992:1151–1154.
^{a}Weights represent the midpoint of the middle frame for each height. These values correct the 1983 Metropolitan Tables to nude weights and heights.

Table 6.2.   Median Weights for Height for Ages 55 to 74 from Combined NHANES I and II Data Sets

Height		Weight			
		Male		Female	
in	cm	lb	kg	lb	kg
58	147	—	—	125.4	57
59	150	—	—	136.4	62
60	152	—	—	143.0	65
61	155	—	—	140.8	64
62	157	149.6	68	140.8	64
63	160	154.0	70	143.0	65
64	163	156.2	71	145.2	66
65	165	158.4	72	158.4	67
66	168	162.8	74	154.0	66
67	170	171.6	78	158.4	72
68	173	171.6	78	154.0	70
69	175	169.4	77	160.6	72
70	178	176.0	80	—	73
71	180	184.8	84	—	—
72	183	178.2	81	—	—
73	185	193.6	88	—	—
74	188	209.0	95	—	—

Adapted from Russell RM. Nutritional assessment. In: Wyngaarden JB, Smith LH, and Bennett JC, eds. Cecil's textbook of medicine. 19th ed. Philadelphia: WB Saunders, 1992:1151–1154.

the amount of weight loss as well as the rate at which it has been lost are both important in assessing nutritional status. Unintentional weight loss of 10% or greater over a period of longer than 4 to 6 months is generally considered to indicate malnutrition. The measurement of triceps skinfold thickness provides an estimate of a body's fat reserve. This is primarily used for calculating mid-arm muscle circumference, which is an indicator of somatic proteins.

Clinical Signs of Malnutrition

Protein-energy malnutrition manifests in a variety of clinical disorders. Generalized wasting and skinny appearance are indicative of protein-energy malnutrition. Clinical signs and symptoms of nutrient deficiencies and their specific manifestations are listed in Tables 6.3 and 6.4. Eczematous scaling in the nasolabial fold and/or perianal area indicates zinc deficiency. Skin pallor may suggest anemia from iron, folic acid, or vitamin B_{12} defi-

ciency. Upper keratosis may suggest vitamin A depletion or deficiency. Flaking dermatitis may indicate riboflavin, niacin, and zinc deficiency. Frequent bruising of the skin may suggest vitamin C and vitamin K deficiencies. Skin thickening and dryness may indicate essential fatty acid deficiency. Hair loss and skin depigmentation may indicate overall protein deficiency, and night blindness may indicate vitamin A deficiency. Xerosis, Bitot's spots, and keratomalacia also suggest severe vitamin A deficiency.

Examination of the oral cavity is also very informative about specific nutrient deficiencies. Diffuse glossitis may indicate riboflavin or folic acid deficiency. Bleeding gums generally suggest vitamin C deficiency. Angular stomatitis may suggest riboflavin depletion, and fissuring or atrophy of the tongue may indicate riboflavin or niacin deficiency. A large thyroid gland in the form of a goiter generally indicates iodine deficiency. Thoracic cage rosary on chest examination suggests vitamin D deficiency, and spooning of the nail as well as transfer lines suggest protein and iron deficiencies. Bone softening or tenderness may suggest vitamin D deficiency. Paraesthesias may suggest thiamine (B_1) or cyanocobalamin (B_{12}) deficiency, whereas tetany may indicate calcium and magnesium depletion.

Anemia and hemolysis would suggest deficiencies of iron, folic acid, vitamin B_{12}, phosphorus, or some combination of these.

Biochemical Measurements

Salient biochemical or laboratory markers of malnutrition include serum albumin, prealbumin, serum transferrin, and retinol-binding protein (Table 6.5). Total lymphocyte count and delayed hypersensitivity index are generally not very helpful because of the associated disorders in a given patient with malnutrition. Serum albumin can be low for reasons other than malnutrition, such as cirrhosis and nephrotic syndrome, but it is considered to be an important marker of visceral proteins. Since serum albumin is considered to have a half-life of 10 to 14 days, rapid turnover proteins such as transferrin and retinol-binding proteins are more sensitive indicators of patient response to nutritional intervention by parenteral or enteral routes.

Table 6.3.   Clinical Signs and Symptoms of Protein–energy Malnutrition in Adults

	Clinical Sign or Symptom	Nutrient
General	Wasted, skinny	Calorie
	Loss of appetite	Protein–energy
Skin	Psoriasiform rash, eczematous scaling	Zinc
	Pallor	Folate, iron, vitamin B_{12}, copper
	Follicular hyperkeratosis	Vitamin A
	Perifollicular petechiae	Vitamin C
	Flaking dermatitis	Protein energy, niacin, riboflavin, zinc
	Bruising	Vitamin C, vitamin K
	Pigmentation changes	Niacin, protein–energy
	Scrotal dermatosis	Riboflavin
	Thickening and dryness of skin	Linoleic acid
Head	Temporal muscle wasting	Protein–energy
Hair	Sparse and thin, dyspigmentation	Protein
	Easy to pull out	
Eyes	History of night blindess	Vitamin A, zinc
	Photophobia, blurring, conjunctival inflammation	Riboflavin, vitamin A
	Corneal vascularization	Riboflavin
	Xerosis, Bitot's spots, keratomalacia	Vitamin A
Mouth	Glossitis	Riboflavin, niacin, folic acid, vitamin B_{12}, pyridoxine
	Bleeding gums	Vitamin C, riboflavin
	Cheilosis	Riboflavin
	Angular stomatitis	Riboflavin, iron
	Hypogeusia	Zinc
	Tongue fissuring	Niacin
	Tongue atrophy	Riboflavin, niacin, iron
	Scarlet and raw tongue	Niacin
	Nasolabial seborrhea	Pyridoxine

Adapted from Russell RM. Nutritional assessment. In: Wyngaarden JB, Smith LH, and Bennett JC, eds. Cecil's textbook of medicine. 19th ed. Philadelphia: WB Saunders, 1992:1151–1154.

The level of somatic proteins in a patient can also be estimated roughly by measurement of urinary creatinine excretion. It is generally accepted that the amount of creatinine in the urine over 24 hours is proportional to the muscle mass of an individual. Creatinine height index usually complements anthropometric measures of mid-arm muscle area. Creatinine height index is calculated by dividing measured urinary creatinine (μg/dl) by ideal urine creatinine and then multiplying it by 100. A crude standard for creatinine can be derived by multiplying the individual's reference weight for height by 23 for males or by 18 for females. A measurement 20% below these derived values may represent muscle protein depletion. It is noteworthy, however, that kidney disease, strenuous exercise, and fever can significantly alter urinary creatinine excretion.

The nitrogen balance can be calculated by dividing the total protein intake (in grams) in 24 hours with 6.25 and then subtracting urinary urea nitrogen (gms), plus a factor of 4. Nitrogen balance is important in assessing response to nutritional intervention.

Although the number of circulating lymphocytes as well as delayed hypersensitivity to common skin antigens such as mumps, candida, and tuberculin have been used to determine protein-energy malnutrition, these tests are generally difficult to interpret because of associated anergy as well as metabolic factors that may cause alterations in these measures.

Table 6.4. Clinical Signs and Symptoms of Nutritional Inadequacy in Adults

	Clinical Sign or Symptom	Nutrient
Neck	Goiter	Iodine
	Parotid enlargement	Protein
Thorax	Thoracic rosary	Vitamin D
Abdomen	Diarrhea	Niacin, folate, vitamin B_{12}
	Distention	Protein–energy
	Hepatomegaly	Protein–energy
Extremities	Edema	Protein, thiamine
	Softening of bone	Vitamin D, calcium, phosphorus
	Bone tenderness	Vitamin D
	Bone ache, joint pain	Vitamin C
	Muscle wasting and weakness	Protein, calorie, vitamin D selenium, sodium chloride
	Muscle tenderness, muscle pain	Thiamine
	Hyporeflexia	Thiamine
	Ataxia	Vitamin B_{12}
Nails	Spooning	Iron
	Transverse lines	Protein
Neurologic	Tetany	Calcium, magnesium
	Paresthesias	Thiamine, vitamin B_{12}
	Loss of reflexes, wrist drop, foot drop	Thiamine
	Loss of vibratory and position sense	Vitamin B_{12}
	Dementia, disorientation	Niacin
Blood	Anemia	Vitamin E, vitamin B_{12}, folate, iron, pyridoxine
	Hemolysis	Phosphorus
	Thickening and dryness of skin	Linoleic acid

Adapted from Russell RM. Nutritional assessment. In: Wyngaarden JB, Smith LH, and Bennett JC, eds. Cecil's textbook of medicine. 19th ed. Philadelphia: WB Saunders, 1992:1151–1154.

Table 6.5.   Assessment of Nutritional Status

Method of Assessment	Degree of Malnutrition		
	Normal	Moderate	Severe
Routine Methods			
Ideal weight (%)[a]	100	60–80	<60
Creatinine height index	100	60–80	<60
Triceps skinfold thickness (mm)	M 12.5	7.5–11.3	<7.5
	F 16.5	9.9–14.9	<9.9
Mid-arm muscle circumference (cm)	M 29.3	17.6–26.4	<17.6
	F 28.5	17.1–25.7	<17.1
Serum albumin (g/dL)	3.5–5.0	2.1–3.0	<2.1
Serum prealbumin (mg/dL)	>20	10–15	<10
Serum transferrin (mg/dL)	200–400	100–150	<100
Retinol-binding protein (mg/dL)	3–6	2–3	<2
Total lymphocyte count (10^6/L)	1.8–3.0	0.8–1.2	<0.8
Delayed hypersensitivity index[b]	2	1	0
Functional Tests			
Prognostic nutritional index (%)	<40	40–50	>50
Subjective global assessment	A	B	C
Grip strength/skeletal muscle function	82	65	50

Adapted from Malone M, Howard L. Parenteral and enteral nutrition. In: Bayless T, ed. Current therapy in gastroenterology and liver disease. 4th ed. St. Louis: Mosby–Year Book, 1994; 261–272.
[a]Male = 50 kg + 2.3 kg for each inch over 60; female = 45.5 kg + 2.3 kg for each inch over 60.
[b]Quantitates the amount of induration elicited by skin testing with common antigens such as *candida*, PPD, or mumps. Induration grade: 0 = <0.5 cm, 1 = 0.5 cm, 2 = 1.0 cm.

The value of nutritional assessment parameters in predicting patient outcomes from a disease process remains unproven, but a prognostic nutritional index (PNI) has been developed using various indices. These indices include serum albumin, transferrin, triceps skinfold, and delayed hypersensitivity responses, as listed in Table 6.6. A PNI greater than 50% is associated with high risk for postoperative complications in a given setting. In one study, higher PNI was correlated with greater postoperative problems.

All in all, careful measurement of clinical, anthropometric, and biochemical parameters provides a reliable assessment of a patient's nutritional status.

tion is necessary. This information includes: *(a)* fluid requirements, *(b)* caloric requirements, and *(c)* protein requirements.

Table 6.6.   Prognostic Nutritional Index (PNI)

$PNI = 158\% - 16.6\,(Alb) - .78\,(TSF) - .2\,(Transferrin) - 5.8\,(DH)$

  Alb = Albumin (gm/dL)
  TSF = Triceps skinfold thickness (mm)
  Transferrin (gm/dL)
  DH = 0, nonreactive
     1, <5 mm
     2, >5 mm

>50% High risk
40–49% Intermediate risk
<40% Low risk

Adapted from Malone M, Howard L. Parental and enteral nutrition. In: Bayless T, ed. Current therapy in gastroenterology and liver disease. 4th ed. St. Louis: Mosby–Year Book, 1994; 261–272.

CORRECTION OF MALNUTRITION

To develop a strategy to correct protein-energy malnutrition, some basic information

Fluid Requirements

Fluid requirements can be estimated for most patients as 35 to 40 mL/kg per day or, alternatively, 1500 mL for the first 20 kg of body weight and then 20 mL/kg per day for the remainder. A rough estimate of additional abnormal fluid losses in feces, sweat, and breath should also be added to this estimate. On average, most adults drink approximately about 2000 to 2500 mL per day. This includes water present in solid and soft foods as well.

Caloric Requirements

Caloric requirements can be calculated based on a patient's energy expenditure. For practical purposes, caloric requirements can be calculated using the estimates provided in Table 6.7. For instance, the normal maintenance caloric requirement after elective surgery is approximately 25 kcal/kg per day. On the other hand, for patients with severe inflammatory bowel disease, pancreatitis, or trauma, the requirement may increase to 30 kcal/kg per day. Patients with burns, sepsis, or severe trauma may require as much as 35 to 40 kcal/kg per day. The other reliable method for calculating resting energy expenditure is based on the Harris-Benedict Equation (Table 6.8). Most of these estimates are available in a number of handbooks on clinical nutrition. These estimates are also fairly crude, although clinically very useful, because

Table 6.7.   General Calorie Requirements

Normal maintenance/elective surgery	25
Trauma, acute pancreatitis, inflammatory bowel disease	30
Sepsis, minor burns	35
Major burns, severe trauma	40

Adapted from Malone M, Howard L. Parenteral and enteral nutrition. In: Bayless T, ed. Current therapy in gastroenterology and liver disease. 4th ed. St. Louis: Mosby–Year Book, 1994; 261–272.

Table 6.8.   Formula for Determining Basal Metabolic Rate by Harris-Benedict Equation[a]

$$\text{Men} = 66 + (13.7 \times W) + (5 \times H) - (6.8 \times A)$$
$$\text{Women} = 655 + (9.6 \times W) + (1.8 \times H) - (4.7 \times A)$$

[a]Basal metabolic requirement in kilocalories, where W is ideal body weight in kilograms; H is height in centimeters, and A is age in years.

they provide quantitative guidelines for providing the magnitude of supplementation in a given patient. It is noteworthy that this equation underestimates BMR (basal metabolic rate) in malnourished patients by approximately 10% and overestimates BMR in patients who are obese.

Protein Requirements

Besides caloric requirements, protein needs must be estimated for a given patient. Protein needs are influenced by metabolic rate, caloric intake, nutritional status, age, and body protein reserves. A positive nitrogen balance can generally be achieved when 7 to 8% of the required calories are provided as proteins. In the hypermetabolic patient, as much as 15 to 20% of calories may be provided as proteins. In the case of inadequate protein and caloric intake, a reduction in body weight generally occurs and is associated with a loss of lean body mass. For hospitalized patients receiving proteins of high biologic value, such as in milk, eggs, and meats, only 0.6 g/kg per day is adequate for mild illness. For ambulatory patients, this becomes 0.8 to 0.9 g/kg per day; however, in severely ill patients with markedly depleted body stores, protein requirements may exceed 1.2 to 1.5 g/kg per day. It should be emphasized, however, that the patients who are ill cannot assimilate large amounts of proteins, because a large number of nonprotein calories are also needed. It now is generally agreed that calorie and protein requirements for such patients were previously overestimated.

Carbohydrate and Fat Requirements

Carbohydrates generally constitute approximately 50 to 60% of total caloric intake. They are administered as glucose or in oral feeding preparations in form of oligosaccharides or lactose. Carbohydrates generally contribute significantly to increased osmolality of the preparation. Fat is generally provided in form of an emulsion that does not add to osmolality and provides a greater number of calories (i.e., each gram of fat is capable of providing nine calories). In the oral preparations, fat can be obtained from butter (i.e., long-chain fat) or coconut (i.e., medium-chain fat). Approximately 30 to 40% of total caloric intake comes from fat. In addition, minerals and vitamins are generally added to oral preparations according to the recommended daily allowance.

NUTRITIONAL INTERVENTION

After obtaining the clinical history and assessing the degree of malnutritional, the primary care physician must determine the modality and duration of nutritional support to be provided by dietary intervention, enteral nutrition, or parenteral nutrition. In general, if the degree of malnutrition is mild and the GI tract is intact, oral or enteral supplementation may suffice. However, if the degree of malnutrition is moderately severe and the anticipated duration of support is quite long, then intensive therapy may be needed, requiring parenteral nutrition. Intactness of the GI tract is generally evaluated through the patient history, which should indicate the presence of diarrhea or malabsorption. In certain situations such as pancreatitis, Crohn's disease, and GI surgery, in which the bowel needs rest, total parenteral nutritional (TPN) may be the only viable option.

In patients with an intact GI tract, the physician may consider one or more of the following options: *(a)* dietary supplementation by selecting specific diet and adding oral supplementation, *(b)* enteral feeding via nasogastric feeding tube in a patient with swallowing disorders or dysphagia; *(c)* enteral feeding via gastrostomy tube placed endoscopically in a patient who does not tolerate a nasogastric tube; *(d)* enteral feeding via nasoenteral tube in a patient with gastric stasis and gastroesophageal reflux; or *(e)* enteral feeding via jejunostomy feeding tube placed through a gastrostomy tube or by direct jejunostomy tube placement. Indications for enteral nutrition include all patients with a partially or totally functional GI tract. A very large group of patients can tolerate enteral feeding. Furthermore, a small amount of enteral feeding is encouraged even in patients receiving TPN therapy to avoid multiorgan system failure. Patients with anorexia nervosa, eating disorders, esophageal problems, and GI cancers generally do well with enteral feeding. In addition, patients with marginal nutritional status who are being prepared for open GI surgery also benefit from enteral feeding.

The principle indication for parenteral nutrition is a nonfunctional GI tract because of disease or surgery.

ENTERAL NUTRITION

Diet and Table Foods

If the patient's GI tract is functional and his or her appetite is reasonable, table foods can be recommended for protein and caloric supplementation. Without doubt, table foods remain an excellent choice for oral supplementation simply because they are tasty, socially appealing, and easily available at a reasonable cost. A prescription for table foods requires some basic information regarding the availability of proteins and carbohydrates. Generally, each ounce of meat, fish, poultry, or cheese contains approximately 7 g of protein, an egg contains approximately 6 to 7 g, and a cup of milk provides approximately 6 to 8 g. One-half cup of nuts, beans, and peas provides approximately 5 to 7 g. According to some experts, certain proteins in various vegetables and nuts have a lower biologic value and may not be therapeutically useful in nutritionally depleted patients. Milk proteins are exceedingly useful if the patient does not have milk intolerance. Each tablespoon of peanut butter contains approximately 4 g of protein and is considered to be a good, concentrated source of calories.

As a matter of patient education about food and caloric intake, the physician may provide a copy of the U.S. Food Guide Pyramid (Figure 6.1). This pyramid clearly shows that carbohydrates present in bread, cereal, rice and pasta, and so on constitute the staple of an individual's daily diet. Fruits and vegetables provide vitamins, minerals, and fibers, and they should be taken on a regular basis in smaller quantities than rice and bread. Certainly, proteins from both vegetable and animal sources are important, but they should be taken in still smaller amounts and are placed just before the tip of the pyramid, which is occupied by fats and oils. In my opinion, the concept of

providing this kind of information to patients and their relatives who are involved in cooking for the patient is an important one. It should be emphasized to the patients that long-term dietary guidelines include: *(a)* ingestion of a variety of foods rather than one special kind, *(b)* maintaining a healthy body weight, *(c)* ingestion of a diet reasonably low in saturated fat and cholesterol, and *(d)* incorporating plenty of vegetables, fruits, and grain products. Salt and sugar are recommended only in small quantities and in great moderation.

Patients generally have many questions related to the efficacy of ingesting fiber, various vitamins, and minerals that are available through heath food stores. The scientific information in this area is frequently incomplete, and most physicians have very limited knowledge as well. Depending on the interest and knowledge of a given patient and their relatives, information should be provided to them as needed.

Physicians should also be familiar with the various diets used to manage specific disorders. In general, these diets restrict one or more dietary elements to control

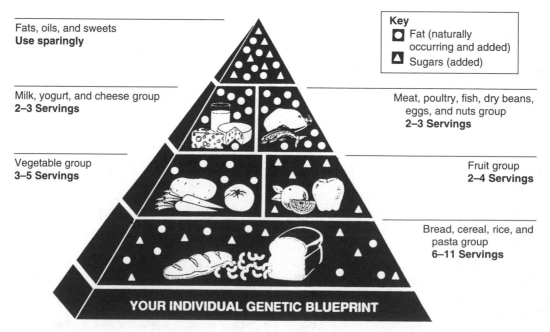

Figure 6.1. The U.S. Food Guide Pyramid, modified to account for genetic variability.

Table 6.9.   Therapeutic Diets Characterized by Restriction of Dietary Components

Diet	Typical Indication
Low fat (60–75 g/day)	Steatorrhea, mild
Low fat (40–60 g/day)	Steatorrhea, severe
Low oxalate	Enteric hyperoxaluria
Low lactose	Lactose intolerance
Gluten free	Celiac sprue
Low fiber	Acute diarrhea, bowel preparation
Low proteins	Hepatic encephalopathy
	Chronic renal failure
Elimination	Food allergies
Controlled carbohydrate	Diabetes mellitus
Calorie restricted	Obesity
Low sodium	Edematous states
Low fat, cholesterol, or carbohydrate according to type	Hyperlipidemia
Low copper	Wilson's disease
Low phosphate	Chronic renal failure

Adapted from Alpers DH, Clouse RE, Stenson MD. In: Manual of nutritional therapeutics. 2nd ed. Boston: Little, Brown, 1991:193–332.

symptoms (Table 6.9) (4). For example, a lactose-free diet is used to control symptoms of abdominal cramping, bloating, and diarrhea in patients with lactase deficiency. Low-fat diets are useful in patients with small intestinal disease and pancreatic biliary disorders. Gluten-free diets are helpful in celiac sprue. Similarly, carbohydrates may be restricted in patients with diabetes mellitus, and a low-sodium diet may be recommended to most patients with peripheral edema and hyponatremia. A low-protein diet is generally recommended for patients with hepatic encephalopathy; in these patients, the estimated daily protein allowance is reduced to 0.4 to 0.6 g/kg per day. Similarly, low-protein diets are also important in the management of chronic renal failure. It has been suggested that when the renal glomerular filtration rate (GFR) falls below 25 mL/min, the protein allowance should be 1 g/kg of ideal body weight per day, and if the GFR falls below 10 mL/min, the protein intake may be reduced to 0.6 g/kg of ideal body weigh per day. It is noteworthy that over 50% of the dietary protein should include proteins of high biologic value (i.e., proteins containing high amounts of essential amino acids). Because amino acids are lost in dialysis, patients with chronic failure undergoing hemodialysis or peritoneal dialysis may require 1 g of protein per each kg of body weight.

Some of the diets used for therapy actually modify the content of macronutrients rather than restricting them. For instance, successful management of an obese patient with diabetes mellitus combines weight reduction with caloric restriction and also reduction in carbohydrate content. A prudent diet recommended by American Diabetes Association suggests 40 to 50% of calories be carbohydrates, with less than 10% being simple sugars and 35 to 40% being starch. Several studies have shown that high-starch diets that control total caloric intake are reasonably well tolerated by patients with diabetes.

Supplemental Diets

Therapeutic diets characterized by the supplementation of certain dietary components are becoming increasingly important. These diets primarily include high fiber, high protein, and high caloric content in specific clinical situations. Table 6.10 outlines the various diets and their typical indications.

A high-fiber diet is frequently recommended in patients with irritable bowel syndrome, constipation, and prevention of recurrent diverticulitis. Although efficacy in these clinical settings has not been proven by controlled, randomized trials, most clinicians find high-fiber diets to be helpful in ameliorating symptoms and reducing complications from these diseases. Different components of dietary fiber include cellulose, hemicellulose, pectin, mucilage, and gums. It has been estimated that daily average dietary fiber intake in the United States is approximately 10 to 12 g or less. Most often, fiber supplementation is recommended in the form of fruits, vegetables, or commercial preparations such as psyllium, seed powders, or bran. Psyllium is rich is hemicellulose, whereas bran contains mostly cellulose. Two tablespoons of psyllium or bran generally provide approximately 10 g of fiber. An additional benefit from a high-fiber diet is reduced sugar absorption, which is particularly helpful in patients with diabetes mellitus. Furthermore, fiber supplementation reduces caloric intake and lowers dietary cholesterol absorption, and it is also used in chronic diarrheal illnesses to provide more solid consistency to stool. Low-fiber or fiber-free diets are used in bowel prepa-

ration before barium enema, colonoscopy, and intestinal surgery. High-calcium diets containing milk products are recommended for postmenopausal women to prevent osteoporosis. A modest positive effect of dietary calcium on cortical bone mass has been demonstrated in some published reports. Most studies in this area have only had a 2-year duration, however, so the long-term effects of calcium supplementation on osteoporosis are not known.

Potassium supplementation is frequently recommended for patients who are receiving diuretic therapy and at risk of potassium deficiency or depletion because of diuretic therapy. Potassium is usually present at high concentrations in fruits, vegetable, and juices. For instance, 8 oz of orange or tomato juice may contain as much as 10 to 12 mEq of potassium. A banana may contain as much as 6 to 8 mEq. Milk is also considered to be a reasonably good source of potassium; however, its high sodium content may be a limiting factor in patients receiving diuretic therapy for hypertension. Protein supplements may be needed for patients who are losing high amounts of proteins to fistulas or malabsorption (e.g., patients with gastrocolic fistulas, jejunocutaneous fistula, burns, or undergoing dialysis). For these patients, each gram of protein should be provided with approximately 25 calories from nonprotein sources for

Table 6.10.   Therapeutic Diets Characterized by Supplementation of Dietary Components

Diet	Typical Indication
High fiber	Irritable bowel, prevention of recurrent diverticulitis
High calcium (milk products, $CaCO_3$, or combination)	Postmenopausal osteoporosis
High protein (high biologic value)	Chronic hemodialysis or peritoneal dialysis
High protein	Malabsorption
Supplemental potassium	Diuretic use
High calorie	Weight loss because of illness

Adapted from Alpers DH, Clouse RE, Stenson MD. In: Manual of nutritional therapeutics. 2nd ed. Boston: Little, Brown, 1991:193–332.

proper assimilation of amino acids in the protein.

Other types of diets used in hospitalized patients include liquid diets, which provide appropriate hydration because of the presence of water in such diets. Clear-liquid diets include bouillons and gelatins and require minimal digestion and intestinal motility. However, such diets are useful only for short-term management of patients undergoing bowel surgery, colonoscopy, or barium enema preparations. These diets may also be useful in patients recovering from GI surgery or pancreatitis, but they do not provide adequate amounts of calories or nutrients. For long-term management, a full-liquid diet may be provided that includes not only appropriate water but also milk and other dairy products, cereals, and eggs. These diets can be enriched with commercial supplements, nutritionally complete, and be used on a long-term basis in patients with significant esophageal swallowing problems. Bland diets are generally recommended in patients with peptic ulcer disease or gastritis to prevent irritation of the GI tract. Objective scientific data to support the widespread use of bland diets are not available, however, and restriction of seasoning and spices can make foods less palatable and diminish a patient's ability to take them on a long-term basis.

Commercial supplements should be used in patients with diminished appetite and who need additional calories as well as specific nutrients. Patients with malnutrition who are being prepared for surgical intervention, cancer chemotherapy, or radiation therapy are candidates for these commercial supplements. The total amount of supplements to be taken on a daily basis should be adjusted according to the patient's caloric and overall nutritional needs. These commercial supplements are available as sources of single macronutrients, such as predominantly protein, carbohydrates, or lipids, or in the form of nutritionally complete supplements containing all necessary micronutrients and macronutrients. Most of these products have a high caloric density and well-defined nutrient composition, and most are available in flavors to make them more palatable and appealing.

The limitations of these preparations include taste "fatigue" because of constant use two or three times a day by the patient. Furthermore, diarrhea and nausea can frequently occur in some patients. Cost is an additional factor restricting use of these supplements in chronically ill patients on a long-term basis. It is worth emphasizing that each gram of protein should be provided with nonprotein calories, because assimilation of each gram of protein requires approximately 30 to 40 kcal of nonprotein origin to maintain a positive nitrogen balance. Without adequate nonprotein calories, the amino acids in proteins are converted to carbohydrates to provide the energy needed for amino acid assimilation.

In recommending commercial supplements to patients, the physician should be aware of the following major characteristics of the supplements available:

1. Presence or absence of lactose in the preparation. Lactose-free preparations are generally better tolerated by most patients.
2. Osmolality of the solution. Most solutions may be hypertonic and hyperosmolar, and they may require dilution before drinking to avoid diarrhea.
3. The source and nature of the protein present in the preparation, whether it is whole protein or hydrolyzed protein. Patients with chronic small bowel disease may tolerate hydrolyzed protein better than whole protein.
4. The presence of large amounts of fat as a caloric source. In general, lactose-free isotonic preparations are better tolerated by patients who are chronically ill.

Enteral Feeding by Intubation

A variety of feeding tubes to provide antral nutrition are available for patients who are unable to eat because of difficulty in swallowing, gastric emptying, or mechanical obstructions from cancer or surgery of the upper GI tract. Thin, pliable nasogastric feeding tubes are used to deliver calories in the stomach provided that gastric emptying is normal. Most intensive care units use nasoenteric feeding tubes to administer calories as well as macronutrients and micronutrients directly into the small intestine without exposing the patient to the risk of regurgitation and aspiration of gastric contents. Most of these tubes are soft, pliable, thin, easily removed, and replaceable. Placement of a feeding tube in the small bowel, however, can be difficult in patients with gastric emptying problems from diabetes or recent surgery. Endoscopic placement of nasoduodenal tubes is performed in some patients if necessary. Patients requiring enteral feeding on a long-term basis are candidates for gastrostomy feeding tubes placed endoscopically. These tubes are placed in the upper abdominal area by percutaneous endoscopy and prevent constant irritation to the nasopharyngeal, oropharyngeal, and esophageal area by intubation. In patients with gastric stasis or gastroesophageal regurgitation, an endoscopically placed or surgically placed jejunostomy feeding tube may be necessary.

The primary care physician must decide which modality is most suitable for the administration of enteral feedings in a given patient. In general, patients requiring enteral supplemental for 4 weeks or less are probably best served with nasoduodenal, nasogastric, or nasoenteral feeding; however, patients requiring enteral feeding for longer periods of time may require an endoscopically placed gastric feeding tube. Gastrostomy tubes can also be placed under computed tomographic guidance in those patients with a history of upper GI surgery and in whom endoscopic placement is not feasible.

Selection of Enteral Formulas

A variety of enteral formulas are available to meet the nutritional needs of patients. In these formulas, carbohydrates are present in the form of glucose, maltodextrins, or lactose. Protein may be present in the form of an intact protein from milk, protein hydrolysate, or free amino acids. Approximately 10 to 20% of calories are provided by proteins in most enteric formulas. Enteral formulas with intact protein taste much better than preparations with hydrolyzed protein or amino acids; however, this is relevant only for patients who are ingesting supplemental nutritional formulas orally. Butter fat (i.e., long-chain fatty acids) and coconut oil (i.e., medium-chain fatty acids) provide the usual sources of fat calories, and vitamins and minerals are added to meet the recommended dietary allowance. Factors to consider in choosing an enteral formula include:

1. The patient's general condition.
2. The underlying medical disorder.
3. The patient's nutritional status.
4. Status of the patient's GI system and its efficiency in absorbing various nutrients.
5. The patient's renal function.
6. Route of administration based on underlying medical problems and anticipated duration of nutritional supplement.

Palatability is also important for formulas to be consumed orally. A physician selecting a given formula for enteral feeding should be aware that these commercially available preparations are frequently milk based, with high lactose content and an osmolality ranging from 500 to 700 mOsm/L. Certainly, patients with lactase deficiency do not do well with these preparations, and lactose-free formulas are frequently selected in these cases. Their osmolality is lower, ranging from 300 to 400 mOsm/L, and their viscosity is also low.

Elemental diets are designed for patients with impaired absorption capacity resulting from short-gut syndrome, malabsorption, or diseases of the small bowel. Protein is supplied in the form of oligopeptide or amino acids. Fat is supplied in the form of triglyceride and carbohydrate in form of glucose or oligosaccharide. In these preparations, viscosity is high, and osmolality ranges from 600 to 800 mOsm/kg. These formulas should preferably be started on a half-strength basis and given slowly while monitoring the patient's tolerance.

Complications of Enteral Feeding

The most common side effect of enteral feeding is diarrhea, which is primarily induced because of increased osmolarity or the presence of lactose. Diluting the preparation or reducing the rate of delivery is helpful in this situation. It should be remembered that with a gastrostomy and a jejunostomy feeding tube, patients can receive up to 100 to 150 mL of enteral feedings per hour. Gastric stasis and regurgitation resulting in tracheobronchial aspiration and esophagitis are problems that must be carefully monitored. After each feeding, gastric residual should be checked to prevent the accumulation of large amounts of enteral feeds in the stomach and their regurgitation. Aspiration is best prevented by monitoring the gastric residual periodically, using pump infusion, avoiding bolus feedings, and positioning the feeding tube appropriately in the distal stomach or, preferably, the duodenum.

PARENTERAL NUTRITION

Patients who are unable to digest or absorb orally or enterally administered dietary supplements because of a host of clinical conditions require nutritional support by the parenteral route. Two methods of parenteral nutrition are available: peripheral and total.

For patients who are expected to resume oral nutrition within 7 to 10 days, administration of 3% crystalline amino acids combined with glucose for protein sparing significantly improves nitrogen balance compared with the administration of routine intravenous fluids containing dextrose only. Peripheral parenteral nutrition can supply calories and amino acids with protein-sparing properties for a select group of patients (i.e., well-nourished patients undergoing elective GI surgery). As many as 2000 kcal can be provided with the help of peripheral parenteral nutrition when fat emulsions are also administered. Thus, peripheral parenteral nutrition is a short-term method to provide a positive nitrogen balance and meet the caloric needs of the patient. Because peripheral solutions are hyperosmolar and given intravenously in a peripheral vein, the risk of developing phlebitis is significant. These peripheral parenteral nutrition formulas contain 3% crystalline amino acid solution along with 10% dextrose. One liter of 10% dextrose, 1 L of 7% amino acid, and 1 L of 10% fat can provide up to 2000 kcal and 70 g of protein with an osmolality of 500 to 900 mOsm/kg.

The principle source for calories in parenteral nutrition is carbohydrates or lipids. Dextrose in form of dextrose monohydrate can be used as the sole nonprotein calorie source; however, dextrose in most intravenous solutions provides only 3.4 kcal/g in contrast to lipid emulsions, which provide 9 kcal/g. Lipid emulsions also provide a source for essential fatty acids such as linoleic acid and as much as 50 to 70% of the daily caloric requirement. Lipid emulsions also reduce the likelihood of hyperglycemia as well as the volume of fluid needed to provide a certain number of calories. Furthermore, lipids provide a lower respiratory quotient (0.7) as compared to carbohydrates which have respiratory quotient of 1.0. Respiratory quotient is calculated by dividing V_{CO_2} by V_{O_2}, where V_{O_2} is oxygen consumption and V_{CO_2} is carbon dioxide production (Table 6.11). In the normal state, the respiratory quotient is 0.9 to 1.0. However,

Table 6.11.   Interpretation of Respiratory Quotient (RQ) Values

RQ	Interpretation	Recommended Action
0.7	Fat catabolism	Increase calories
0.8	Protein catabolism	Increase calories
0.9	Normal state	Maintain
1.0	Carbohydrate catabolism	Maintain
>1.0	Fat synthesis	Decrease calories

Adapted from Malone M, Howard L. Parenteral and enteral nutrition. In: Bayless T, ed. Current therapy in gastroenterology and liver disease. 4th ed. St. Louis: Mosby–Year Book, 1994; 261–272.

during protein or fat catabolism, the respiratory quotient is 0.7 to 0.8, suggesting an increase in calories as most desirable action. A respiratory quotient of greater than 1.0 is suggestive of endogenous fat synthesis; therefore, caloric administration should be reduced (Table 6.11). The principle source of lipid emulsions is droplets of soybean or safflower oil. Lipid emulsions are generally available in 10 or 20% solutions. Ten-percent lipid solution generally provides 1.0 kcal/mL, and 20% solution generally provides 2.0 kcal/mL. A contraindication to lipid emulsions, however, is preexisting hyperlipidemia in the form of triglyceridemia or development of triglyceridemia, and it should be remembered that proper energy balance and nitrogen balance can be achieved with dextrose alone if adequate amino acids are supplied with it. This is particularly important in patients who are intolerant to lipid emulsions or suffer from lipid metabolic disorders.

In parenteral nutrition, protein requirements are generally met by the infusion of amino acids in crystalline form. The amino acid profiles of standard commercial products are based on normal plasma amino acid concentration with slight modifications. For patients with renal failure, liver failure, and undergoing metabolic stress, amino acid ratios are altered in specialized commercial products. Since patients with chronic renal failure but without dialysis have a lower concentration of essential amino acids in their plasma profiles, a large percentage of their protein requirements are in the form of essential amino acids. A preparation with a higher proportion of essential amino acids may provide the necessary amino acids and prevent worsening of uremia in these patients. In patients on dialysis, however, a more balanced, standard amino acid concentration can be used. As stated previously, dextrose in appropriate quantities inhibits gluconeogenesis from amino acids and thereby reduces urea formation.

In patients with liver disease, plasma branched-chain amino acids (BCAAs) are reduced, and blood levels of aromatic amino acids are elevated. Parenteral formulations with increased ratios of BCAAs to aromatic amino acids, in which the percentage of BCAAs is increased to 40% (from the 20% in standard solutions), are administered. It is noteworthy that BCAAs do not require hepatic processing as metabolic substrates, and they can be oxidized extrahepatically in skeletal muscles, heart, and kidney. They can also serve as potential fuel for muscle in a sick patient. BCAAs reportedly prevent protein degradation and stimulate protein synthesis; therefore, these amino acids have been recommended in clinical conditions associated with extreme metabolic stress (i.e., sepsis, severe burns, major trauma).

In general, the final parenteral solution that provides appropriate energy and proteins needs to be administered through a central vein because of its high osmolality. The problem of hyperosmolality primarily occurs with dextrose and amino acid solutions. Furthermore, major minerals such as sodium and potassium salts also add to the final osmolality. Addition of isotonic lipid emulsion reduces osmolality, volume, and helps to provide the necessary total calories. For all practical purposes, central venous access is uniformly employed for the administration of TPN. A central venous catheter generally lasts for approximately 10 days to 2 weeks, and they must be changed regularly to prevent infection. Patients requiring long-term (i.e., longer than 1 month) TPN generally receive specialized catheters surgically placed through the chest wall.

Indications for Total Parenteral Nutrition

Indications for TPN primarily include conditions in which the intestines cannot be used for digestion or absorption of nutrition delivered through an enteral feeding tube. Such conditions include: (a) short-gut syndrome resulting from mesenteric vascular thrombosis; (b) Crohn's disease with extensive small bowel involvement; (c) trauma of the small bowel; (d) patients with acute, severe pancreatitis; (e) malnourished patients before and after GI surgery; (f) patients with intra-abdominal abbesses; and (g) patients with severe ulcerative colitis involving the entire colon. Several large, well-designed clinical studies have also demonstrated the value of 10 days of preoperative TPN in malnourished patients undergoing surgery for GI malignancies, bone marrow transplantation, severe trauma, and extensive burns.

Home TPN therapy should be considered for patients with irreversible GI disease or short-gut syndrome, and it is particularly relevant for patients who are stable and need TPN therapy for longer than a month. Patients who may benefit from home TPN therapy include those with severe inflammatory bowel disease and multiple complications, severe GI motility disturbances related to sclero-

derma, or short-bowel syndrome from trauma or ischemic insult to the bowel. A cyclic method of delivering calories with the help of long central catheters burrowed through the subcutaneous tunnel of the anterior chest walls is usually employed for this purpose.

A typical example of daily nutrient requirements during TPN for stable adult patients is provided in Table 6.12. It should be emphasized that mineral requirements may vary from patient to patient, and in the same patient over time to time. Trace elements such as zinc, copper, chromium, selenium, and iodine should also be added. Deficiencies of trace elements do occur in patients who have been on TPN for some time, and they can be easily avoided by supplementing TPN with these trace elements. Similarly, vitamins should also be supplemented in the parenteral solutions; quantities of vitamins generally provided in TPN solutions are also provided in Table 6.12 (5).

Essential fatty acids such as linoleic, linolenic, and arachidonic acids cannot be synthesized in human subjects, and their deficiencies can occur in patients on TPN. Fatty acid deficiency generally manifests clinically with dry skin, dry hair, hair loss, and impaired wound healing. Deficiency of essential fatty acids can be prevented by supplying adequate quantities of these acids in lipid emulsions. Presence of essential fatty acids in the adipose tissue of human subjects has been well demonstrated; however, the high level of insulin usually present with TPN administration prevents its mobilization. Therefore, 500-mL lipid emulsions (i.e., 10% solution) should be administered three times a week in every patient to prevent the development of essential fatty acid deficiency.

COMPLICATIONS OF PARENTERAL NUTRITION

Tables 6.13 and 6.14 list the complications of parenteral nutrition, which can be divided into two categories: complications related to problems of the central venous

Table 6.12.   Daily Nutrient Requirements During Total Parenteral Nutrition for Stable Adult Patients

Calories	Dextrose	60–80% of requirement
	Lipid emulsion	20–40% of requirement
Protein	Crystalline amino acids	100% of requirement
Minerals	Sodium	90–120 mEq
	Potassium	90–150 mEq
	Chloride	90–150 mEq
	Calcium	12–16 mEq
	Phosphorus	20–40 mmol
	Magnesium	12–16 mEq
	Iron[a]	
	Zinc[b]	2.5–4.0 mg
	Copper	300–500 μg
	Chromium	10–20 μg
	Manganese	0.15–4.0 mg
	Selenium[c]	40–80 μg
	Iodine[c]	70–140 μg
	Molybdenum[c]	100–200 μg
Vitamins	A	3000 IU
	D	200 IU
	E	10 IU
	B_1 (thiamine)	3.0 mg
	B_2 (riboflavin)	3.6 mg
	Pantothenic acid	15.0 mg
	Niacin	40.0 mg
	B_6 (pyridoxine)	4.0 mg
	Biotin	60.0 μg
	Folic acid	400.0 μg
	B_{12} (cobalamin)[d]	5.0 μg
	C (ascorbic acid)	100.0 mg[e]
	K	5 mg/wk[f]
Essential fatty acids[g]	Linoleic acid	4% of total calories

Adapted from Clouse RE. Parenteral nutrition. In: Wyngaarden JB, Smith LH, and Bennett JC, eds. Cecil's textbook of medicine. 19th ed. Philadelphia: WB Saunders, 1992:1189–1193.

[a]The daily requirement (not taking phlebotomy losses into consideration) is approximately 1.5 mg and can be met by giving 1 mL (50 mg Fe) of iron–dextran solution intramuscularly per month. Replacement is usually dictated by indices of iron stores.

[b]Requirements are increased if intestinal fluid losses are great.

[c]Additive usually reserved for patients on long courses of TPN.

[d]May be given by monthly intramuscular injection.

[e]Daily provision often increased to 500 mg or more during periods of catabolic stress.

[f]Not provided by multivitamin preparation; given by separate injection.

[g]Provided by lipid emulsions on a biweekly or triweekly basis. Linolenic acid is also present in some emulsions and may be required during long-term TPN.

catheter, and metabolic complications. Catheter-related problems include pneumothorax resulting from placement of a central or peripheral venous catheter, thrombosis at the tip of the catheter after insertion, thrombophlebitis from the hyperosmolar solutions, and catheter-related sepsis. Catheter-related sepsis occurs in as many as 5% of all patients receiving TPN. Contamination of the catheter hub is generally responsible for this infection; culturing the material and periodic removal of the catheter helps to eradicate this problem.

Metabolic complications of TPN include:

1. Hyperglycemia resulting from concentrated doses of dextrose through a central vein. Regular insulin adminis-

tration is needed to correct this problem and keep the serum glucose level below 200 mg/dL. Hypoglycemia can occur when TPN is abruptly terminated or insulin is administered by a subcutaneous route. It is recommended that TPN be terminated slowly, over a period of 2 or 3 days.

2. Hepatic dysfunction generally manifests through elevated levels of transaminases (ALT, AST), transpeptidases (GGT), and alkaline phosphatase. Significant (i.e., more than twice the upper limit of normal) as well as persistent elevations frequently indicate fat accumulation from excessive caloric carbohydrate. Reduction in caloric intake may be necessary to correct this problem. Another suspected mechanism is overgrowth of microorganisms in the GI tract during TPN, as is passage of toxic byproducts of these microorganisms in the portal stream, which can be reduced by giving small amounts of enteral solutions.

3. Long-bone pain and back pain have been described in patients receiving long-term TPN. The underlying cause is unclear but is thought to relate to

Table 6.13. Catheter-related Complications of Parenteral Nutrition

---

Central-vein Catheter Related
Infection
Pneumothorax
Hemothorax
Air embolus
Venous thrombosis
Arterial injury
Brachial plexus injury
Catheter fragmentation and embolization
Peripheral-vein Catheter
Thrombophlebitis
Infection

Adapted from Clouse RE. Parenteral nutrition. In: Wyngaarden JB, Smith LH, and Bennett JC, eds. Cecil's textbook of medicine. 19th ed. Philadelphia: WB Saunders, 1992:1189–1193.

Table 6.14. Catheter-related Metabolic Complications of Parenteral Nutrition

---

Frequent
Hyperglycemia and hyperosmolarity
Hypoglycemia
Electrolyte disturbances
Liver dysfunction
Fatty liver
BUN elevation
Hypercapnia
Hyperlipidemia from lipid emulsion
Cholelithiasis (long-term treatment)
Rare
Vitamin and trace mineral deficiency
Essential fatty acid deficiency
Metabolic bone disease
Hyperammonemia

Adapted from Clouse RE. Parenteral nutrition. In: Wyngaarden JB, Smith LH, and Bennett JC, eds. Cecil's textbook of medicine. 19th ed. Philadelphia: WB Saunders, 1992:1189–1193.

altered vitamin D metabolism as characterized by the presence of hypercalciuria. Hypercalciuria is frequently observed in patients on TPN, presumably related to increased glucose or organic sulfate load. Discontinuation of TPN or removal of vitamin D from the TPN fluid is frequently helpful in ameliorating bone pain.

4. Hyperlipidemia resulting from lipid infusion and triglyceridemia is observed in 1 to 2% of patients receiving TPN. Discontinuation of lipid infusion as a principle source of calories is generally efficacious in correcting the problem.

NUTRITIONAL SUPPORT AND CLINICAL CONDITIONS

Perioperative Nutrition

A large Veterans Administration cooperative study as well as a meta-analysis of 18 smaller studies have shown that preoperative nutrition is only beneficial in patients who are severely malnourished.

In patients with mild-to-moderate malnutrition, nutritional support has not been shown to have any benefit; however, 7 to 10 days of preoperative parenteral nutrition before major surgery of the GI tract may reduce postoperative complications, duration of hospitalization, and mortality in severely malnourished patients. Furthermore, recent studies have also shown that multiorgan system failure in postoperative and trauma patients as observed in the intensive care unit may relate to bacterial translocation from an unused bowel, and that small amounts of enteral feeding via a jejunostomy tube can reduce postinflammatory cytokines and bacterial translocation.

INFLAMMATORY BOWEL DISEASE

Crohn's disease as well as severe ulcerative colitis constitute major indications for TPN in a variety of patients. However, the decision to provide TPN rather than enteral nutrition should be based on the extent of disease in the bowel and the patient's history of previous surgery. Nutritional support helps to restore growth in children with Crohn's disease. Furthermore, no difference has been found between responses to elemental and polymeric diets in patients with inflammatory bowel disease. The possible roles of soluble fiber in providing short-chain fatty acids in the colon, which may be the preferred fuel for colonocytes, and of glutamine as the preferred fuel for enterocytes are under investigation at present.

PANCREATITIS

Patients with severe pancreatitis are helped by parenteral nutrition. Special attention should be given to the triglyceride levels, and patients with hypertriglyceridemia should not be given lipid infusions in presence of pancreatitis. Enteral feedings can be tolerated in most patients after 4 weeks of an acute attack of severe pancreatitis.

CHRONIC LIVER DISEASE

Patients with chronic liver disease have low plasma levels of BCAAs, and supplementation with BCAA-enriched formulas has been recommended. However, BCAA-enriched formulas are expensive and should be reserved only for select patients who cannot tolerate adequate protein intake and easily develop hepatic encephalopathy. Most patients with chronic liver disease can do without these formulations. Recent data also suggest that aggressive pre– and post–liver transplantation nutritional support is beneficial in patients with chronic liver disease.

RENAL DISEASE

Acute renal failure in patients with major trauma is generally associated with a high mortality rate because of multiorgan system failure. These patients have complex nutritional support needs. Randomized clinical trials have not shown any benefit from special amino acid formulas, which have been recommended to replenish plasma essential amino acids. In general, patients with acute renal failure who are not on dialysis require reduced fluid and protein intake, and their nutritional needs should be carefully monitored on a daily basis.

In malnourished patients with chronic renal failure requiring dialysis, parenteral nutrition has been recommended with the idea of improving nutritional parameters; however, postinfusion hypoglycemia may be observed with the abrupt discontinuation of parenteral nutrition at the end of dialysis. It is recommended that glucose administration in these patients not exceed 1.2 g/kg per dialysis treatment. Similarly, lipid infusion should not exceed more than 1 g/kg per hour in these patients (i.e., those with chronic renal failure requiring dialysis).

CHRONIC LUNG DISEASE

Patients with severe lung disease have increased energy expenditure resulting from the increased work of breathing. This increased expenditure should be accounted for when assessing the caloric needs of a patient with chronic lung disease. Excessive weight loss impairs respiratory muscle strength, ciliary clearance function, and immunocompetence, and it places the patient at increased risk for acute exacerbation. Furthermore, carbohydrate calories produce more carbon dioxide by increasing the metabolic rate and stimulating lipogenesis. Therefore, lipids should be considered as the principle source of calories in these patients, but they should not provide more than 40% of the total nonprotein calories because of concerns for the development of impaired lung diffusion. Short-term studies have shown improved respiratory muscle function with improved nutritional support. Patients with cystic fibrosis and chronic lung disease as well as malabsorption also benefit from nutritional support. Enteral nutrition delivered through a gastrostomy or jejunostomy tube is exceedingly helpful in some malnourished patients with cystic fibrosis.

CARDIAC DISEASE

Nutritional wasting in patients with severe, advanced cardiac disease is well recognized. Enteral nutritional support in these patients is complicated, however, because of associated edematous states. Excessive fluid intake or feeding may aggravate or compound the cardiac and metabolic problems, and diuretic therapy generally increases the loss of potassium, calcium, and magnesium. Extra supplementation of these minerals may be necessary to prevent their deficiencies. Selenium deficiency has been reported to result in congestive cardiomyopathy in patients receiving long-term TPN. Supplementation of the TPN solution with selenium (80–100 mg/day) is essential to prevent this complication. Hyperlipidemia, which is often present in this population, generally requires modification in the use of lipids infusion as well.

CANCER

Although enteral and parenteral nutrition are frequently provided to patients with cancer who are being prepared for surgery or receiving either chemotherapy or radiation therapy, no data indicate a significant nutritional or survival benefit in these patients. Therefore, routine use of parenteral nutrition in patients with cancer is not recommended. However, nutritional support may be justified for a well-defined period of time in select patients during aggressive chemotherapy and radiation therapy.

HUMAN IMMUNODEFICIENCY VIRUS

The role of nutritional support in patients infected with human immunodeficiency virus has not been clearly defined. Nutritional status is a major influence on immune function, and patients with acquired immunodeficiency syndrome have impaired an nutritional system resulting from intestinal malabsorption, lactose deficiencies, zinc depletion, protein losses, and vitamin B_{12} deficiency. Nutritional supplementation administered parenterally or through an enteral tube may help select patients. Data showing a benefit from nutritional intervention in this group are currently lacking, and large, multicenter studies are needed to define the best use of nutritional support in these patients.

REFERENCES

1. Malone M, Howard L. Parenteral and enteral nutrtition. In: Bayless T, ed. Current therapy in gastroenterology and liver disease. 4th ed. St. Louis: Mosby–Year Book, 1994:261–272.
2. Frisancho AR. New standard of weight and body

composition by frame size and height for assessment of adults and the elderly. Am J Clin Nutr 1984;40:808–819.

3. Russell RM. Nutritional assessment. In: Wyngaarden JB, Smith LH, and Bennett JC, eds. Cecil's textbook of medicine. 19th ed. Philadelphia: WB Saunders, 1992:1151–1154.

4. Alpers DH, Clouse RE, Stenson MD. In: Manual of nutritional therapeutics. 2nd ed. Boston: Little, Brown, 1991:193–332.

5. Clouse RE. Parenteral nutrition. In: Wyngaarden JB, Smith LH, and Bennett JC, eds. Cecil's textbook of medicine. 19th ed. Philadelphia: WB Saunders, 1992:1189–1193.

7

Preoperative Pulmonary Evaluation

Philip A. Masters and Kevin Gleeson

Interest in preoperative pulmonary assessment of surgical patients developed following the observation that postoperative respiratory complications were a major cause of morbidity and mortality. Subsequent advances in our understanding of the effects of anesthesia and surgery on respiratory function, recognition of specific pulmonary risk factors, and the evolution of interventions to prevent complications further highlighted the value of preoperative pulmonary assessment for improving surgical outcome.

Internists may be involved in preoperative pulmonary evaluation and postoperative management in several ways. First, consultants are frequently asked to assist in the estimation of surgical risk related to either suspected or known pulmonary dysfunction. This may include diagnosis of previously unknown lung disease or evaluation of preexisting pulmonary abnormalities along with an assessment of their potential effect on surgical outcome. Preoperative identification of patients at increased risk thereby allows more accurate assessment of overall surgical risk, which in turn aids in surgical decision making and further defining the group of patients who may benefit from alternative treatments or intensive pulmonary management in the perioperative period. Second, internists sometimes participate in the perioperative management of high-risk patients to decrease the occurrence of pulmonary complications and provide assistance when they do. Finally, with patients being considered for lung resection, the consultant may be involved in the estimation of postoperative pulmonary function and its potential effect on postsurgical survival and quality of life, thus contributing to often difficult decisions regarding the feasibility of surgery. Therefore, a thorough preoperative pulmonary evaluation, performed in concert with the surgeon and anesthesiologist and coupled with careful perioperative management of those patients considered to be at risk for complications, would be expected to provide the best opportunity to avoid serious respiratory problems during necessary surgical intervention.

Unfortunately, there are few definitive data concerning the optimal preoperative pulmonary assessment and perioperative management of surgical patients. Many studies of this process have been flawed by small sample sizes, differing definitions of outcome, and other significant methodologic limitations. As a result, many commonly held assumptions in this area lack a foundation in the literature, thus making evidence-based clinical evaluation difficult. **This chapter focuses on the information available to guide perioperative pulmonary assessment and management and attempts to develop a rational approach for use by the consulting internist.**

POSTOPERATIVE PULMONARY COMPLICATIONS

Studies in general surgical populations have shown an overall occurrence of pulmonary complications ranging from 6 to 35% of cases (1–11). This remarkably broad range of incidence results largely from differing definitions of what constitutes a pulmonary complication in the postoperative period and whether it is considered to be clinically significant (e.g., "major" or "minor"). Researchers commonly disagree about what degree of routine postoperative occurrences such as atelectasis, cough, subjective dyspnea, subclinical hypoxia, leukocytosis, low-grade fever, and small pleural effusions constitutes a "complication," thus leading to highly variable complication rates and ambiguity in the interpretation study results. Clearly, bacterial pneumonia, ventilatory failure, need for prolonged respiratory support, and death are the most important pulmonary complications that are associated with anesthesia and surgery. Although relatively uncommon in most populations that have been studied, their profound influence on clinical outcome makes identification of those patients at risk extremely important to making informed surgical decisions and planning perioperative management. Unfortunately, and despite considerable investigation, the goal of reliably identifying those in whom major pulmonary complications are likely to occur has been elusive, and this remains a central challenge to the consulting internist.

EFFECTS OF ANESTHESIA AND SURGERY ON RESPIRATORY FUNCTION

Anesthesia and surgery lead to well-described and relatively predictable changes in respiratory function. Specific alterations depend on the type of anesthesia employed as well as the nature and location of the surgery. Knowledge of these effects is important to understanding the pathophysiology underlying the development of respiratory complications, assists in recognizing clinical settings that may place patients at higher risk, and forms the foundation on which preventive measures are based.

Anesthesia

General Anesthesia

General anesthesia may be induced by use of inhaled anesthetic gases, intravenous narcotics, intravenous barbiturates, or some combination. Regardless of the particular drugs or means of delivery, induction of general anesthesia is associated with a reduction in the patient's functional residual capacity on the order of 15% (12). The mechanism for this decrease is disputed, but it appears to result mostly from alterations in the relative positions of the hemidiaphragms and the chest wall, an effect that is independent of changes in posture. Whatever its cause, however, it is associated with radiographically visible atelectasis (primarily depicted by CT) in dependent lung zones in 95% of patients (13, 14) (Fig. 7.1).

Individual anesthetic agents may influence ventilatory mechanics. Ketamine, for example, is a well-known bronchodilator. Nearly all drugs that produce effective general anesthesia alter ventilatory control by decreasing the ventilatory response to hypoxia, hypercapnia, or changing the pattern of breathing. Most relevant, however, may be the effect of general anesthetics on mucociliary clearance. Reduction in the velocity of the normal cephalad mucociliary flow persisting for as long as 6 days has been observed with several general anesthetics (15), and if a cuffed endotracheal tube is employed as well, it has similar and compounding effects. Some general anesthetic drugs also may reduce mucociliary clearance by altering the composition of the respiratory mucus, thereby increasing its viscosity (16).

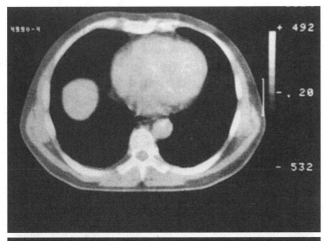

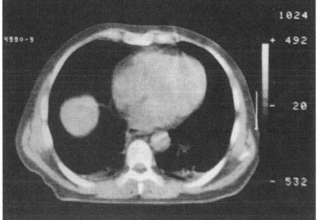

Figure 7.1. Computed tomographic images in an identical plane taken before (top) and during (bottom) general anesthesia without surgical intervention. Opacities in the dependent lung zones reflect atelectasis resulting from the anesthesia process alone. (Reprinted with permission from Brismar B, Hendenstierna G, Lunquist H, et al. Pulmonary densities during anesthesia with muscular relaxation—a proposal of atelectasis. Anesthesiology 1985;62:422–428.)

Regional Anesthesia

Neural blockade that is adequate for major surgical procedures is produced by the application of a local anesthetic to the spinal cord, a nerve plexus, or to one or several individual nerves. Barring local complications of the anesthetic injection (e.g., pneumothorax during brachial plexus blockade), only spinal or epidural anesthesia would appear likely to have an effect on the breathing apparatus. Because nerve roots innervating the diaphragm originate in the neck, even high spinal anesthesia has no large effect on either diaphragm function or lung volume. As a result, respiratory rate, timing, and arterial blood gases are usually not altered by spinal or epidural anesthesia. The paralysis or weakness of the anterior abdominal muscles that accompanies these forms of anesthesia may reduce a patient's ability to expire forcefully, however, and thus compromise the effectiveness of cough for the duration of the anesthesia.

Type of Surgery

Thoracic Procedures Without Lung Resection

Thoracotomy without lung resection produces postoperative reductions in lung volume on the order of 60%. This results from multiple factors, including alterations in chest wall function related to intercostal muscle transection, pain from the incision and chest tubes, and measures aimed to relieve pain. Consequently, pulmonary atelectasis, primarily in the lower lobes, is routinely seen following thoracotomy, as are small pleural effusions and restrictive pulmonary physiology. Previous problems with phrenic nerve injury resulting from cold cardioplegia or internal mammary artery mobilization during coronary artery bypass grafting (CABG) surgery have been mostly eliminated through the use of appropriate preventive measures during surgery (17).

Thoracotomy with Pulmonary Resection

Pulmonary resection produces changes in pulmonary function similar to those from any other thoracotomy as well as the unique effects of lung removal. Postoperative lung function is reduced, as would be expected. Other potential adverse effects are the removal of functioning lung tissue and producing a space in the chest that is largely occupied by overdistension of the remaining lung tissue, contraction of the hemithorax, or both. Fortunately, this appears to have only a minor effect on either acute or chronic pulmonary function.

Abdominal Surgery

Abdominal surgery is associated with a decrease in lung function that varies inversely with the distance of the operative site from the diaphragm. Thus, open biliary tract and gastric procedures routinely produce a decrease in vital capacity to below 50% of baseline. Decreased diaphragm function appears to be primarily responsible for the respiratory changes that follow upper abdominal surgery (Fig. 7.2), and this impairment results in reduced inspiratory transdiaphragmatic pressures, recruitment of the nondiaphragm muscles of breathing (e.g., intercostal and neck muscles), substantial and prolonged decrease in forced vital capacity and forced expiratory volume in 1 second (FEV_1), and a corresponding degree of hypoxemia as well as rapid, shallow breathing.

The mechanisms underlying this alteration in diaphragm function have not been fully elucidated, but experimental and clinical evidence suggests that upper abdominal surgery produces a reflex inhi-

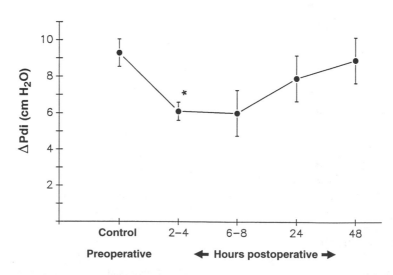

Figure 7.2. The strength of diaphragmatic contraction during normal tidal breathing, represented here by the difference between inspiratory and expiratory transdiaphragmatic pressure or △Pdi, is reduced following upper abdominal surgery in man. *Difference from baseline, $P < .05$ (two-way ANOVA). (Modified from Ford GT, Whitelaw WA, Rosenal TW, Cruse PJ, Guenter CA. Diaphragm function after upper abdominal surgery in humans. Am Rev Resp Dis 1983;17:431–436.)

bition of diaphragm function that is mediated by intra-abdominal neuronal activation, and this is postulated to be an integrated reflex that immobilizes the abdomen in response to injury (18). Phrenic nerve activation in patients with intraoperative diaphragm dysfunction produces normal diaphragm contraction; thus, the malfunctioning diaphragm appears to be structurally and physiologically intact. It malfunctions, however, because the neural traffic that normally activates it is now diminished (19) (Fig. 7.3). Similar changes in lung function and gas exchange can be found following abdominal surgery regardless of whether spinal or general anesthesia is employed, which suggests that some factor independent of the anesthesia is responsible (20). Also, meticulous efforts to control pain do

not alter the time course of the recovery of diaphragm function postoperatively, apparently indicating that these changes are not related to postoperative pain alone (21).

Nonabdominal, Nonthoracic Procedures

Operations that do not violate the pleura or peritoneum alter pulmonary function only minimally beyond the effects of anesthesia alone and their influence on normal respiratory protective mechanisms (e.g., inhibition of cough resulting from pain).

RISK FACTORS FOR PULMONARY COMPLICATIONS

Multiple prospective and retrospective studies have sought to identify specific clinical factors predisposing patients to the development of postoperative respiratory complications. Several risk factors have been relatively well-established, but others remain less clearly defined (Table 7.1).

Surgical and Anesthetic Considerations

As expected, the site and type of operation significantly influence the risk of developing pulmonary complications (Fig. 7.4). Thoracic, lung resection, and upper abdominal surgeries pose the greatest risk, followed by lower abdomi-

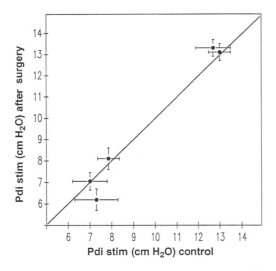

Figure 7.3. The strength of diaphragmatic contraction produced by experimental bilateral phrenic nerve stimulation is similar before and after upper abdominal surgery. Values for transdiaphragmatic pressures (Pdi stim) measured before and 4 hours after surgery for five different subjects fall very near the identity line. These data suggest that postoperative diaphragm dysfunction results from decreased phrenic nerve activation rather than from impaired functional integrity of the diaphragm itself. (Reprinted with permission from Dureuil B, Viires N, Cantineau JP, Aubier M, Desmonts JM. Diaphragmatic contractility after upper abdominal surgery. J Appl Physiol 1986; 61:775–780.)

Table 7.1.   Risk Factors for the Development of Postoperative Pulmonary Complications

---

Established Risk Factors
Type of operation
Surgical site
Cigarette smoking
Underlying pulmonary disease
   Chronic obstructive pulmonary disease
   Asthma
Potential Risk Factors
Age
Obesity
Duration of surgery

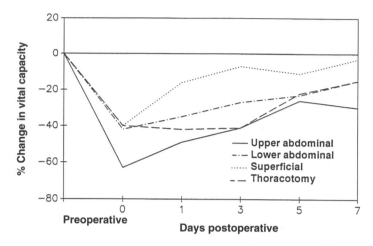

Figure 7.4. Percentage change in postoperative vital capacity plotted as a function of the site of surgery. Reduction in vital capacity is greatest and most prolonged following upper abdominal surgery. (Data from Ali J, Weisel RD, Layug AB, et al. Consequences of postoperative alterations in respiratory mechanics. Am J Surg 174;128:76–382.)

nal surgeries (2–6, 8, 9). Nonthoracic, nonabdominal operations carry the lowest risk, and this finding has been documented for gynecologic, urologic, orthopaedic, head and neck, and ophthalmologic surgeries (2, 8).

The type of surgical incision may influence the complication rate as well. More rapid recovery of normal pulmonary function has been associated with use of a median sternotomy than with use of a lateral intercostal approach in thoracic procedures and is thought to be secondary to decreased pain with this approach (22). Vertical laparotomies have been associated with more atelectasis, hypoxemia, and pneumonia than horizontal incisions, which are also thought to result from increased pain caused by these incisions (23, 24). In open cholecystectomy, patients with subcostal incisions show less pulmonary dysfunction by spirometry, improved oxygenation, and fewer overall complications when compared to those with midline incisions (25, 26). Early studies of abdominal laparoscopic procedures suggest that this approach produces less compromise of pulmonary function, reduced postoperative pain, and decreased atelectasis and hypoxia compared with an open cholecys-

tectomy, potentially leading to fewer pulmonary complications (27–30). The ability of this technique to effectively lower the rates of major complications, however, remains to be determined. Thoracoscopic resective techniques have been recently introduced, but their potential to avoid the known complications of thoracotomy also remains to be established.

The commonly held assumption that spinal or epidural anesthesia carries a lower risk than general anesthesia for the development of pulmonary complications is not well supported in the literature. Clinical studies do not suggest a clear advantage in terms of clinical outcome with these types of anesthesia (31–35). In contrast, the pulmonary risks of peripheral regional anesthesia have been noted to be considerably less than with general, spinal, or epidural anesthesia (33).

Smoking

Smoking causes multiple alterations in respiratory function, including changes in the respiratory epithelium, decreased tracheobronchial clearance, increased sputum production, small airway dysfunction, and decreased closing volumes, thus increasing the possibility of pulmonary complications (36–39). Smoking also elevates the level of carboxyhemoglobin, which may theoretically increase risk by impairing tissue oxygen delivery (40).

Cigarette smoking is the major cause of chronic obstructive pulmonary disease and emphysema, thus raising the likelihood of baseline preoperative pulmonary dysfunction (an additional risk factor). Multiple studies have shown that cigarette smoking also elevates the risk for atelectasis in the postoperative period, and there is evidence that the risk of postoperative pneumonia is significantly increased in smokers as well (3, 5–7, 9, 33, 41).

Several studies have attempted to relate the degree of smoking to the rate of complications. In one, smoking at the rate of at least one pack per day was associated with increased purulent sputum production postoperatively (42). In another, smokers with a greater than 20 pack-year (defined as the number of packs smoked per day multiplied by the total number of years smoked) history of tobacco use had at least a 10% higher rate of complications than those who smoked less (41).

There is evidence suggesting that reversal of smoking-related pulmonary effects, with a resulting decrease in the complication rate, requires at least 8 weeks of not smoking. Physiologically, reversal of tobacco-induced pulmonary changes occurs slowly, over a period of weeks, after smoking cessation (37–39). Clinically, an 8-week cessation period has been associated with decreased purulent sputum production postoperatively (42). A retrospective review of patients who underwent CABG surgery showed that those who had stopped smoking for fewer than 8 weeks had a threefold increase in the complication rate compared to those who had stopped for longer periods (41). A prospective trial in a similar population of patients also undergoing CABG found consistent results,

with those abstaining for fewer than 2 months before surgery having an almost fourfold increase in the complication rate relative to those who had stopped for a longer time period (57.1 versus 14.5%, respectively). Also, patients who stopped smoking at least 6 months before CABG surgery had complication rates similar to those who had never smoked (43).

Underlying Pulmonary Disease

Chronic obstructive pulmonary disease has been well established as a risk factor for the development of postoperative pulmonary complications (3, 8, 44–47). In contrast, patients with restrictive lung dysfunction appear to manifest fewer complications, likely because of the relative preservation of pulmonary flow rates and other protective mechanisms (48).

Attempts have been made to gauge the relative increase in risk based on the degree of obstruction as assessed through spirometry. Various parameters suggesting increased risk have been proposed (Table 7.2); however, no single test or combination of studies has proven

Table 7.2. Pulmonary Function Criteria Associated with Increased Risk in Nonresective Procedures

	Value	Reference
FEV_1	<60–70% predicted	42, 43
FVC	<70–80% predicted	6, 8, 100
FEV_1/FVC	<65%	6
	<60% predicted	100
$FEF_{25\%-75\%}$	<50% predicted	8
MEFR	<200 L/min	1
MVV	<50% predicted	8
$Paco_2$	>45 mm Hg	1, 46

Modified from Gass GD, Olsen GN. Preoperative pulmonary function testing to predict postoperative morbidity and mortality. Chest 1986;89:127–135. $FEF_{25\%-75\%}$, forced expiratory flow in the midexpiratory phase, *FVC*, forced vital capacity, *MEFR*, maximum expiratory flow rate, *MVV*, maximum voluntary ventilation, $Paco_2$, arterial partial pressure of carbon dioxide.

to be effective in delineating a group of patients who are more likely to experience problems. **Thus, the presence of obstructive disease clearly imparts an elevated likelihood of respiratory complications, and it seems certain that increasingly severe disease would be directly associated with a proportional elevation in risk. Thus far, however, studies have been unable to reliably quantitate this risk or allow for the accurate prediction of respiratory problems in a given patient.**

Asthma places patients at higher surgical risk, primarily because of possible bronchospasm in the perioperative period (49, 50). **There is good reason to believe that control of bronchospasm preoperatively and careful pulmonary follow-up will allow surgery to be performed safely in most patients with asthma** (51).

Age

Age-related changes in pulmonary function include decreased static lung volumes, oxygenation, elastic recoil and maximal expiratory flow, and decreased sensitivity of upper airway reflexes (33). Coupled with the increase in overall mortality associated with surgery in elderly patients, these changes have led to the consideration of an age greater than 60 to 70 years as a risk factor for perioperative pulmonary complications (52). Several studies have supported this concept, but others have failed to identify age as an independent risk factor for pulmonary complications (9, 11, 34, 42, 52–56). **In general, the underlying medical condition and pulmonary status of older patients appear to be the primary determinants of operative risk in this group, just as they are in young patients, thus suggesting that the preoperative evaluation focus on these variables.**

Obesity

Establishing obesity as a pulmonary risk factor has been difficult because of a lack of uniformity among study definitions of obesity and postoperative complications. Multiple physiologic and clinical considerations suggest a higher potential risk in patients who are obese, including reduced total respiratory compliance, functional residual capacity, and expiratory reserve volume. Abnormalities in standard pulmonary function tests are not evident, however, unless body weight is at least twice the predicted ideal, and spirometric evaluation alone does not appear to be helpful in assessing risk for these patients (57–60). Preoperative oxygenation and the respiratory response to hypoxia and hypercapnia may be diminished, with exaggerated postoperative hypoxia in patients who are obese relative to controls (7, 24, 58, 61). Additionally, studies of these patients have noted both increased volume and acidity of gastric contents preoperatively, thus raising the issue of increased risk of perioperative aspiration (62). Technical aspects of the intubation of obese patients and difficulty in mobilization postoperatively are additional factors thought to increase operative risk from a pulmonary perspective (63). **Documentation of significant operative risk attributable to obesity alone, however, has been difficult.** Overall surgical mortality has been noted to increase only among patients who are very obese (64, 65). The well-known mechanical alterations associated with increased weight would be expected to negatively influence lung volumes, thus leading to atelectasis, which is more prevalent in obese patients postoperatively and is reduced in those patients who lose weight preoperatively (6, 7, 66, 67). The rates of pneumonia and other clinically significant pulmonary complications, however, do not appear to be markedly increased in overweight patients (3, 57, 66–69).

An additional consideration in obese patients is the increased prevalence of obstructive sleep apnea and the obesity-hypoventilation syndrome. Potential postoperative problems associated with upper airway instability, arterial hypoxia and hypercapnia, and the influence of anesthetics and analgesics on these factors highlight the need to identify such patients preoperatively.

Duration of Surgery

There is conflicting evidence regarding the duration of surgery (i.e., operative time) as an independent risk factor. However, several studies do suggest that operations lasting longer than 3 or 4 hours have a higher risk of pulmonary complications (6, 9, 32, 34, 42, 49).

PREOPERATIVE PULMONARY TESTING

In addition to a careful patient history and physical examination, multiple studies are available to provide information on pulmonary function. The appropriate application of preoperative pulmonary function testing remains controversial, however. Rational use of such tests requires an understanding of their ability to provide clinically relevant information.

Chest Radiography

There is little evidence supporting the routine use of chest radiography as a preoperative screening tool in low-risk patients (70, 71). A thorough history and physical examination are likely to be more valuable for identifying those patients in whom active pulmonary disease may be present and chest radiography beneficial. In patients with known cardiopulmonary disease or identifiable risk factors, abnormalities on chest radiography are common; however, their effects on management appears to be minimal. In these patients, decisions regarding the usefulness of preoperative chest radiography need to be individualized based on specific clinical consider-

ations such as the type of proposed surgery and anesthesia and the nature and extent of pulmonary dysfunction. Use of chest radiographs to establish a preoperative baseline in otherwise low-risk patients is also not well supported, with the exception of those undergoing thoracic surgery (in whom delineation of anatomic structures before operation may be helpful).

Spirometry and Lung Volume Measurement

The information generated by spirometry allows the assessment of a variety of pulmonary parameters obtained under dynamic conditions. These data are often coupled with static measurements of lung volumes and compared to population-based reference information to assess ventilatory function. This type of testing is simple, noninvasive, relatively inexpensive, and readily available. Thus, it is an attractive means of evaluating pulmonary function. Recent refinements, such as the use of radionuclide scanning to define the contribution of each lung lobe or segment (discussed later) to the overall pulmonary function, have increased its potential use in certain clinical settings.

Since the development of spirometry and lung volume measurement, attempts have been made to define its best use in preoperative evaluation. Because of its attractiveness as a *screening* test, it has been applied routinely to general surgical patients to identify those at potential risk for pulmonary complications who might benefit from further evaluation. **However, the results of multiple trials in a variety of surgical settings have failed to establish the efficacy of preoperative pulmonary function screening.** Spirometry has also been used as a screening test in those with known lung disease or those undergoing potentially high-risk surgeries from a pulmonary perspective (e.g., nonresective thoracic and upper abdominal) to select patients who are likely to encounter respiratory problems postoperatively. Again, no single measurement or combination of tests has been shown to provide the adequate sensitivity, specificity, or predictive power to justify routine use in this manner (72, 73). The overlap in preoperative values obtained from those with and those without complications most likely reflects the multifactorial nature of respiratory complications in surgical settings, which simple spirometry and lung volume determination cannot delineate.

Thus, there is little support for this type of preoperative testing on a *routine* basis in most patient populations. Spirometry and lung volume measurement do appear to have a significant role in assessing patients undergoing resective pulmonary surgery, however, as discussed later. The greatest value of spirometry and lung volume measurement continues to be in the diagnosis of previously unknown lung disease and further characterization of the type and degree of pulmonary impairment in those with known but poorly defined respiratory dysfunction, information which may ultimately affect management decisions.

Arterial Blood Gas Analysis

The usefulness of preoperative arterial blood gas analysis has not been thoroughly studied, and existing data are somewhat conflicting. For example, arterial hypoxemia appears to be inconsistent in predicting postoperative complications, because many patients with resting hypoxemia do well during the operation as well as postoperatively (8, 45, 46). Additionally, nonreversible preoperative elevations of carbon dioxide, particularly above a level of 45 mm Hg, remain controversial as a predictor of postoperative complications or mortality in resective surgery (44, 46, 73, 74). Therefore, routine testing is not likely to be helpful, although in selected patients, hypoxia and hypercarbia may aid in the diagnosis (e.g., as in the obesity-hypoventilation syndrome) or indicate the degree of pulmonary dysfunction at baseline.

Diffusing Capacity

Diffusing capacity measures the adequacy of gas exchange and is affected by diseases of the lung and pulmonary vasculature. It has been studied primarily in pulmonary resective surgery, and it makes a useful contribution to the assessment of postoperative function (Tables 7.3 and 7.4). Its use in other clinical settings, however, has not been well established.

Regional Lung Function Assessment

Several tests are available to evaluate the specific contribution of each lung, lobe, or lung segment to overall pulmonary function. At present, their role is generally limited to second-level assessment of candidates for pulmonary parenchymal resection to ascertain whether adequate lung function will remain after operation.

Split-perfusion lung scanning is a readily available and highly accurate means of evaluating focal lung function. It is performed in a manner similar to routine nuclear medicine perfusion scanning. The percentage perfusion to each lung is determined, as are the contributions of each lobe and lung segment (75). Although this information is easily gathered in individual patients, testing in larger populations has led to the development of "standard" contributions from each lung area, thus allowing the potential functional lung loss for a given, planned resection to be estimated based on these data. This information may then be applied to other measures, such as spirometry, lung volumes, diffusing capacity, or exercise capacity to estimate the remaining function after resection. For example, estimates of postoperative forced vital capacity, diffusing capacity, and exercise capacity obtained in this manner correlate reasonably well with actual, measured values (76, 77). Although this approach is quite promising as a means for estimating residual pulmonary function in resective surgery, its effectiveness in predicting outcome and complications, as well as its use in

Table 7.3. Preoperative Pulmonary Function Criteria Suggesting Increased Risk in Pulmonary Resective Surgery

		Specified Extent of Resection			
	Resection	Pneumonectomy	Lobectomy	Segmentectomy	Reference
FEV_1	<2 L	<2 L	<1 L	<0.6 L	56, 101
	<1.2 L				102
		<1.65 L			103
		<65% predicted			
	<60% predicted				104
FVC	<2 L				105
	<1.7 L				102
	<70% predicted				106
		<2.13 L			103
		<64% predicted			
FEV_1/FVC	<35%				102
	<50%				56
	<55%				107
$FEF_{25\%-75\%}$		<1.6 L	<0.6 L	<0.6 L	101
MVV	<59% predicted				54
	<50% predicted				105, 106, 108
		<55% predicted	<40% predicted	<35–45% predicted	101
	<45 L/min				106
	<28 L/min				102
DLCO	<50% predicted				109
Exercise $\dot{V}O_2$ max	<1 L/min associated with increased mortality				110
	<15 mL/kg per min associated with high risk of complications; >20 mL/kg per min demonstrated lower risk				78
	<10 mL/kg per min associated with high morbidity and mortality; <20 mL/kg per min but >10 mL/kg per min associated with increased morbidity				79
	Decreasing values associated with increased complications after lobectomy				111
	<1.25 L associated with increased complications				104
	≥15 mL/kg per min in high risk patients associated with acceptable operative mortality				73
PVR	>190 dynes/sec per cm^{-5} with exercise				77

Modified from Gass GD, Olsen GN. Preoperative pulmonary function testing to predict postoperative morbidity and mortality. Chest 1986;89:127–135.
DLCO, diffusing capacity of carbon dioxide, $FEF_{25\%-75\%}$, forced expiratory flow in the midexpiratory phase, *FVC,* forced vital capacity, *MEFR,* maximum expiratory flow rate, *MVV,* maximum voluntary ventilation, *PVR,* pulmonary vascular resistance, $\dot{V}O_2max$, maximum oxygen consumption.

other types of surgery, remains to be established.

Pulmonary vascular resistance during exercise has shown some promise for predicting outcome in thoracic surgery (78). However, only small numbers of patients have been studied, and practical difficulties associated with performing this test generally confine its use to specialized centers.

Exercise Capacity

Exercise testing similar to that used in cardiac diagnosis has been developed using various indicators of pulmonary function, such as the level of dyspnea or ability to achieve a specific level of physical exertion. The clinical usefulness of testing exercise capacity has varied, particularly in assessing those undergoing resective

Table 7.4.   Predicted Postoperative Pulmonary Function Criteria Suggesting Increased Risk in Pulmonary Resection

	Value	Reference
FEV_1	<40% predicted best predictor of postoperative mortality in pneumonectomy	75, 111
	<1.65 L or <58% of preoperative value associated with higher operative mortality	112
	<1 L best predictor of postoperative complications	87
	<0.89 L or <34% predicted associated with increased operative mortality	103
FVC	<2.5 L or <60% of preoperative value associated with higher operative mortality	112
	<1.31 L or <41% predicted associated with higher operative mortality	103
DLCO	Inverse relationship with pulmonary morbidity and overall mortality	113, 114
	<40% predicted best predictor of respiratory failure and is associated with high mortality	75, 111
	<40% predicted associated with high morbidity and mortality	75
Exercise Vo_2max	Lower values associated with increased morbidity and mortality; <10 mL/kg per min associated with 100% mortality; <40% predicted associated with 50% mortality	75

DLCO, diffusing capacity of carbon dioxide, *FVC,* forced vital capacity, Vo_2max, maximum oxygen consumption.

surgery. Results of two small studies using maximum oxygen consumption (Vo_2max) during exercise suggest that a reduction in this value may be useful for predicting outcome in resective surgery (79, 80), but further study is required before routine use of this methodology is appropriate.

APPROACH TO THE SURGICAL PATIENT

General Surgical Patients

A thorough patient history and physical examination, with evaluation of the patient's overall medical condition and level of function, should be the starting point for all preoperative pulmonary assessments. The presence or absence of pulmonary risk factors and examination findings suggestive of significant underlying pulmonary disease should be particularly emphasized. Concurrent medical conditions and the patient's nutritional status should be reviewed in terms of their potential effect on pulmonary function both during and after surgery. **In those patients with no identifiable risk factors and a normal physical examina-tion, there is no indication for further pulmonary evaluation.**

In patients with risk factors or evidence of previously undiscovered respiratory disease on history or physical examination, further diagnostic evaluation is warranted. In general, chest radiography, and spirometry and lung volume determination should be adequate in defining the presence and nature of most significant pulmonary abnormalities. Furthermore, determination of arterial blood gases in patients with abnormal studies may further clarify the degree of baseline respiratory dysfunction. If these studies fail to suggest the presence of significant pulmonary disease, no further evaluation is necessary before surgery.

In those patients who are found to have risk factors or newly discovered pulmonary dysfunction, their potential influence on the overall surgical risk and on perioperative management must be assessed. This information should be carefully reviewed with the surgeon and the anesthesiologist. In selected patients, postponing surgery (if possible) pending optimization of the patient's respiratory status may be beneficial. Alternative procedures may also be available in certain cases to minimize potential pulmonary effects. For example, in high-risk patients, peripheral regional anesthesia may be preferable to general anesthesia, and other surgical considerations such as the type and location of incision and the duration of the operation can be addressed as well. Anesthesiologists should be aware of the nature and degree of the underlying pulmonary disease, which may significantly alter their approach to management. Furthermore, preoperative consultation with both the surgeon and the anesthesiologist allows for early planning of postoperative management strategies with those directing care to anticipate potential respiratory problems.

If possible, an attempt should be made to reverse pulmonary risk factors (Table 7.5). Smoking should be discontinued at least 8 weeks (or as long as possible) before the operation. Obese patients should be counseled on weight loss, and those with a clinical history suggestive of obstructive sleep apnea or obesity-hypoventilation syndrome should be considered for further evaluation using arterial blood gas determination and polysomnography.

All patients undergoing surgery at high-risk sites (e.g., thoracic and upper abdominal) should be instructed in lung-expansion maneuvers (discussed later)

before surgery, and they should be encouraged to continue these maneuvers postoperatively. Alternative lung-expansion methods should be planned preoperatively for those who are unable to perform these maneuvers voluntarily.

Patients with Existing Pulmonary Disease

In patients with chronic obstructive pulmonary disease, maximization of pulmonary function prior to operation is a central goal of preoperative care; careful management of patients with even severe obstructive disease allows a majority of operations to be performed safely (81).

It is helpful to establish the patient's baseline pulmonary function through clinical evaluation and review of previously obtained spirometric and arterial blood gas data. If such information is not available, testing in selected patients may assist in evaluating the preoperative respiratory status and guide attempts to maximize pulmonary function postoperatively.

Aggressive bronchodilator therapy with inhaled β-agonists and anticholinergic agents is indicated to decrease bronchospasm and increase pulmonary flow rates, and this therapy should be implemented early during the preoperative period in all

Table 7.5. Preoperative Management of Pulmonary Risk Factors

Risk Factor	Management Recommendations
Smoking	Discontinue at least 8 weeks, or as soon as possible, before the operation.
Obesity	Weight loss if possible before the procedure; assessment for evidence of obstructive sleep apnea or obesity-hypoventilation syndrome; careful instruction in postoperative lung expansion maneuvers.
Asthma	Avoidance of known exacerbating factors; maximal use of inhaled bronchodilators and steroids, consideration of systemic steroids based on preoperative clinical status; adjustment of theophylline level and determination of need for perioperative aminophylline if clinically indicated.
Chronic obstructive pulmonary disease	Aggressive bronchodilator therapy to maximize respiratory status before the operation; judicious use of antibiotics for overlying bronchitis; consideration of steroid use in responsive patients; adjustment of theophylline level and determination of need for perioperative aminophylline if clinically indicated.

patients with significant obstructive disease. Supplemental corticosteroids are helpful in those patients who are considered to have an inflammatory component to their bronchospasm, although the benefits of their use must be weighed against the potential detrimental effects on immune function, wound healing, blood pressure, glucose metabolism, fever, and fluid balance. Preoperative use of antibiotics is indicated in those with purulent sputum production or other evidence of chronic bronchitis or bronchiectasis. Additionally, chest physical therapy and postural drainage may be useful in those with high levels of sputum production. Although theophylline is less commonly used now for obstructive disease and bronchospasm than in the past, it does exert a positive inotropic effect on diaphragmatic function, which may theoretically be helpful in patients undergoing high-risk surgery (82). Therefore, in patients currently on theophylline, serum levels should be checked preoperatively to assure appropriate oral dosing, and post-operative intravenous aminophylline should be considered when circumstances warrant. In those with known marginal oxygenation, supplemental oxygen should be provided, with perioperative oxygenation being monitored closely in anticipation of potential hypoxemic changes associated with anesthesia and surgery. Aggressive treatment of any underlying obstructive disease should be continued postoperatively until the patient's preoperative baseline is achieved.

Patients with poorly controlled asthma should be aggressively treated before the operation to minimize bronchospasm and maximize respiratory function. Inhaled bronchodilator therapy as well as inhaled and possibly systemic corticosteroids should be administered preoperatively, with their intensity based on the results of clinical and spirometric assessment (83). Similar consideration regarding the use of theophylline should be given in this situation as in obstructive disease. **The need for aggressive treatment with bronchodilators, anti-inflammatory agents, and prophylactic measures throughout the postoperative period must be emphasized.**

Candidates for Pulmonary Resection

Resective surgery involves the removal of functional lung tissue, and this loss of respiratory capacity must be considered in terms of the adequacy of pulmonary function following surgery. Thus, a central goal of preoperative evaluation in this setting involves estimating the expected postoperative functional lung capacity and assessing its potential effect on both the survivability of surgery and the quality of life after the surgery.

Unfortunately, this is a complex task, and it is complicated by multiple factors. For example, in patients undergoing resection for malignant lesions, the possibility of unplanned resection for occult metastasis discovered at surgery will obviously have a marked effect on postoperative pulmonary capacity. Although lobectomy is most commonly performed, these patients may ultimately need pneumonectomy during surgery, which requires consideration of this possibility during the preoperative evaluation. Additionally, it has been estimated that up to 90% of patients with lung cancer who are being considered for resective surgery have signs and symptoms of obstructive lung disease, and up to 20% may have severe pulmonary dysfunction, thus adding further risk to surgery and potential limitations on postoperative function (84). However, because most pulmonary malignancies carry an extremely high mortality rate if left untreated, the risks of surgery must be kept in perspective. **The predictive capabilities of preoperative pulmonary evaluation are imperfect, which makes determination of "prohibitive" lung function difficult in light of an otherwise extraordinarily poor prognosis.**

Preoperative evaluation generally includes spirometry and determination of diffusing capacity. Those patients in whom these studies are well within the normal range are generally considered to be reasonable surgical candidates from a pulmonary perspective.

In those patients with abnormalities discovered through these tests, a decision must be made regarding further evaluation. As with use of this type of testing in other surgical settings, there is controversy regarding the "cutoff" points to establish either a need for further testing or that a patient has a level of lung function that would preclude surgery. As Table 7.3 shows, multiple parameters have been proposed to suggest increased risk in this patient population. Whereas the quality of these data varies and multiple studies have used absolute parameters (e.g., spirometric values determined in adult men that may not apply to all patients), general criteria may be reasonably inferred. For example, multiple clinicians use an FEV_1 of less than 2 L or less than 60% of that predicted, or a diffusing capacity of less than 60% predicted, as indicators for further testing (48, 84, 85).

In these patients, regional lung function studies are usually performed to estimate postoperative spirometric and diffusing capacity. Criteria suggesting increased risk based on predicted measures are listed in Table 7.4. Unfortunately, however, these values are generally based on small studies. Also, a significant number of these patients had complications with test results indicating only moderate pulmonary dysfunction, and others with severe disease by these criteria did well. Even the commonly held assumption that a predicted postoperative FEV_1 of less than 800 mL constitutes "inoperability" has been disputed. This value was established by the observation that most patients with obstructive lung disease suffer significant dysfunction at this level (86). Whereas the concept that those with significantly impaired lung function are more likely to experience increased morbidity and mortality has been generally supported in some subsequent studies,

others have demonstrated acceptable survivability in carefully selected and managed patients with this degree of predicted lung dysfunction (87, 88). Therefore, patients who are considered to be at high risk under these criteria and in whom operation would still otherwise be considered may benefit from further testing with an assessment of exercise capacity or determination of pulmonary vascular resistance. Pulmonary consultation is often helpful in these circumstances to assist in further evaluative efforts and clinical decision making.

POSTOPERATIVE MANAGEMENT

Several prophylactic interventions have been developed for use in the postoperative period to decrease the incidence of postsurgical respiratory complications. Their use should be viewed as a direct continuation of preoperative efforts at avoiding pulmonary problems. Preventive measures should be planned according to the patient's risk-factor profile before the operation and applied aggressively throughout the postoperative period. Even in relatively low-risk patients, routine preventive interventions such as early mobilization and prophylaxis for deep-vein thrombosis should not be overlooked.

Lung-expansion Maneuvers

The goal of lung-expansion maneuvers is to increase the functional residual capacity and stimulate the reflexively inhibited diaphragm, thereby decreasing atelectasis and encouraging return to more normal pulmonary dynamics. These maneuvers improve postoperative pulmonary mechanics, and there is evidence that their use in high-risk patients may decrease the rate of pulmonary complications (32, 89, 90). Several lung-expansion modalities of varying complexity and cost are available.

Deep-breathing exercises are programmed maneuvers that are performed periodically by the patient. Although several protocols are available, most involve inhalation to total lung capacity on a prescribed schedule. Effective use requires a cooperative and motivated patient, carefully instructed and observed in properly performing the exercises, coupled with encouragement and assessment of compliance postoperatively.

Incentive spirometry encourages patients to perform lung-expansion activities similar to deep-breathing exercises using an inexpensive, handheld, disposable spirometer. This offers the advantage of direct feedback to the patient concerning the adequacy of his or her performance and a visual reminder that may encourage use.

Intermittent positive-pressure breathing (IPPB) assists with lung expansion through delivering positive pressure by face mask to the airways during inspiratory efforts and is administered periodically during the postoperative period. This method requires specialized equipment and trained personnel, may cause abdominal distension, and is clearly more expensive than either deep-breathing exercises or incentive spirometry. Thus, its routine use has declined recently. It does have a potential role, however, when a patient may not be physically able to perform lung-expansion maneuvers voluntarily, such as in those with severe skeletal abnormalities or alterations in mental status.

Continuous positive airway pressure (CPAP) has also recently been applied as a postoperative lung expansion method. A predetermined constant pressure is applied to inhaled air through a face mask. It increases lung volumes relatively rapidly after surgery compared with voluntary maneuvers, and it may also aid in oxygenation and carbon dioxide removal (91, 92). However, its effectiveness in preventing postoperative complications remains to be established (93, 94). Similar to IPPB, CPAP also requires specialized equipment and personnel trained in its use; therefore, it is more complicated

and expensive relative to other measures.

Multiple studies have compared the efficacy of available lung-expansion maneuvers. Their results suggest that no single method is superior in terms of improving clinical outcome (32, 95–99). Lung expansion may likely be achieved most effectively through various means. Therefore, choice of methodology should rest on the individual needs of the patient and the available resources (Figure 7.5).

Lung-expansion maneuvers appear to be more effective when they are taught and practiced preoperatively, when the patient is awake, alert, and not in pain (100). Although data on the ideal frequency and duration of postoperative treatment are lacking, it is reasonable to continue lung-expansion maneuvers for at least 3 to 4 days after high-risk surgery or until full mobilization and a return to the patient's clinical baseline is achieved.

Cough

Coughing is an expiratory maneuver that does not directly expand lung volume; however, it does aid in clearance of secretions and stimulation of the diaphragm. Additionally, the deep breathing before a cough likely does provide significant lung expansion. Cough maneuvers are often coupled with deep-breathing exercises to enhance the removal of secretions along with lung expansion. More effective coughing may be encouraged by adequate pain control and splinting of the surgical site.

Early Mobilization

The supine position is associated with lower lung volumes, which have been shown to improve with an upright position such as sitting or standing. Thus, upright positioning and early mobilization of the patient appear to aid lung expansion, although their direct effect on preventing pulmonary complications has not been well studied. It is reasonable to attempt upright positioning and mobilization as early as possible after the operation, particularly in patients who are at an increased risk for pulmonary complications.

Pain Reduction

Great strides have been made in controlling postoperative pain. Many options are available, including periodic bolus doses of analgesic agents, patient-controlled analgesia with or without a baseline continuous infusion of pain medication, and epidurally administered analgesics delivered either in bolus fashion or via continuous infusion.

Epidural analgesia provides better control of postoperative pain compared with systemic analgesics, and it has been thought to potentially decrease postoperative complications through various mechanisms, such as superior pain relief, improved pulmonary dynamics, and reduced severity of postoperative hypoxia. Interestingly, however, current data are equivocal concerning the ability of postoperative epidural analgesia to reduce pulmonary complication rates relative to other forms of analgesia, although some benefit has been suggested in high-risk patients (31).

From a pulmonary perspective, ideal pain control allows the patient to aggressively engage in lung-expansion activities, cough, and early mobilization without suppressing respiratory drive and protective reflex mechanisms such as cough and gag. Careful, individualized attention to pain management may therefore increase the effectiveness of other efforts to avoid postoperative complications.

Prophylaxis for Deep-vein Thrombosis

Meticulous attention should be directed to prophylaxis for deep-vein thrombosis in all surgical patients, particularly as patients at the highest risk for this complication (e.g., in pelvic or orthopaedic procedures) may otherwise be considered to be at low risk for pulmonary complications.

CONCLUSION

Identifying those patients who are at increased pulmonary risk before an operation plays a key role in reducing surgical morbidity and mortality. Despite the lack

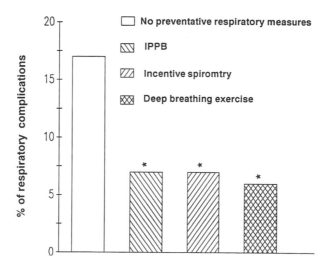

Figure 7.5. Incidence of clinical respiratory complications following abdominal surgery comparing no preventive measures (control), intermittent positive-pressure breathing therapy, incentive spirometry, and deep-breathing exercises. All methods for generating deep breaths postoperatively are effective, but none is superior to the others. (Data from Celli BR, Rodriguez KS, Snider GL. A controlled trial of intermittent positive pressure breathing, incentive spirometry and deep breathing exercises in preventing pulmonary complications after abdominal surgery. Am Rev Respir Dis 1984;130:12–15.)

of definitive data to guide this process, a careful clinical assessment of pulmonary risk factors and function, judicious use of testing, and comprehensive planning for perioperative respiratory care will maximize the effectiveness of the consulting internist.

REFERENCES

1. Stein M, Koota GM, Simon M, Frank HA. Pulmonary evaluation of surgical patients. JAMA 1962;181:765–770.
2. Anderson WH, Dossett BE, Hamilton GL. Prevention of postoperative pulmonary complications: use of isoproterenol and intermittent positive pressure breathing on inspiration. JAMA 1963;186:763–766.
3. Wightman JAK. A prospective survey of the incidence of postoperative pulmonary complications. Br J Surg 1968;55:85–91.
4. Collins CD, Darke CS, Knowelden J. Chest complications after upper abdominal surgery: their anticipation and prevention. BMJ 1968;1:401–406.
5. Forthman HJ, Shepard A. Postoperative pulmonary complications. South Med J 1969;62:1198–1200.
6. Latimer RG, Dickman M, Day WC, et al. Ventilatory patterns and pulmonary complications after upper abdominal surgery determined by preoperative and postoperative computerized spirometry and blood gas analysis. Am J Surg 1971;122:622–632.
7. Hansen G, Drablos PA, Steinert R. Pulmonary complications, ventilation and blood gases after upper abdominal surgery. Acta Anesthesiol Scand 1977;21:211–215.
8. Gracey DR, Divertie MB, Didier EP. Preoperative pulmonary preparation of patients with chronic obstructive pulmonary disease. Chest 1979;76:123–129.
9. Garibaldi RA, Britt MR, Coleman ML, Reading JC, Pace NL. Risk factors for postoperative pneumonia. Am J Med 1981;70:677–680.
10. Williams-Russo P, Charlson ME, MacKenzie CR, Gold JP, Shires GT. Predicting postoperative pulmonary complications. Arch Intern Med 1992;152:1209–1213.
11. Spivack SD, Shinozaki T, Albertini JJ, Deane R. Preoperative prediction of postoperative respiratory outcome: coronary artery bypass grafting. Chest 1996;109:1222–1230.
12. Strandberg A, Tokics L, Brismar B, Lundquist H, Hedenstierna G. Atelectasis during anesthesia and in the postoperative period. Acta Anesth Scand 1986;30:154–158.
13. Hedenstierna G, Tokics L, Strandberg A, Lundquist H, Brismar B. Correlation of gas exchange impairment to development of atelectasis during anesthesia and muscle paralysis. Acta Anesthesiol Scand 1986;30:183–191.
14. Brismar B, Hedenstierna G, Lundquist H, et al. Pulmonary densities during anesthesia with muscular relaxation—a proposal of atelectasis. Anesthesiology 1985;62:422–428.
15. Gamsu G, Singer MM, Vincent HH, Berry S, Nadil JA. Postoperative impairment of mucous transport in the lung. Am Rev Respir Dis 1976;114:673–679.
16. Pizov R, Takahashi M, Hirshman CA, Croxton T. Halothane inhibition of ion transport of the tracheal epithelium. Anesthesiology 1992;76:985–989.
17. Markand DN, Moorthy SS, Mahomed Y, King RD, Brown JW. Postoperative phrenic nerve palsy in patients with open-heart surgery. Ann Thorac Surg 1985;39:68–73.
18. Ford GT, Rosenal TW, Clerque F, Whitelaw WA. Respiratory physiology in upper abdominal surgery. Clin Chest Med 1993;14:237–252.
19. Dureuil B, Viires N, Cantineau JP, Aubier M, Desmonts JM. Diaphragmatic contractility after upper abdominal surgery. J Appl Physiol 1986;61:1775–1780.
20. Boutros AR, Weisel M. Comparison of effects of three anesthetic techniques on patients with severe chronic obstructive disease. Can Anesthesiol Soc J 1971;18:286–292.
21. Simoneau G, Vivien A, Sartene R, et al. Diaphragm dysfunction induced by upper abdominal surgery: role of postoperative pain. Am Rev Respir Dis 1983;128:899–903.
22. Cooper JD, Nelems JM, Pearson FG. Extended indications for median sternotomy in patients requiring pulmonary resection. Ann Thorac Surg 1978;26:413–418.
23. Becquemin JP, Piquet J, Becquemin MH, Melliere D, Harf A. Pulmonary function after transverse or midline incision in patients with obstructive pulmonary disease. Intensive Care Med 1985;11:247–251.
24. Vaughan RW, Wise L. Choice of abdominal operative incision in the obese patient. Ann Surg 1975;181:829–835.
25. Ali J, Khan TA. The comparative effects of muscle transection and median upper abdominal incisions on postoperative pulmonary function. Surg Gynecol Obstet 1979;148:863–866.
26. Halasz NA. Vertical versus horizontal laparotomies. Arch Surg 1964;88:911–914.
27. Couture J, Chartrand D, Gagner M, Bellemare F. Diaphragmatic and abdominal muscle activity after endoscopic cholecystectomy. Anesth Analg 1994;78:733–739.
28. McMahon AJ, Russell IT, Ramsay G, et al. Laparoscopic and minilaparotomy cholecystectomy: a randomized trial comparing postoperative pain and pulmonary function. Surgery 1994;115:533–539.

29. Schauer PR, Luna J, Ghiatas AA, Glen ME, Warren JM, Sirinek KR. Pulmonary function after laparoscopic cholecystectomy. Surgery 1993;114:389–397.
30. Rademaker BM, Ringers J, Odoom JA, deWit LT, Kalkman CJ, Oosting J. Pulmonary function and stress response after laparoscopic cholecystectomy: comparison with subcostal incision and influence of thoracic epidural anesthesia. Anesth Analg 1992;75:381–385.
31. Liu S, Carpenter RL, Neal JM. Epidural anesthesia and analgesia: their role in postoperative outcome. Anesthesiology 1995;82:1474–1506.
32. Celli BR, Rodriguez K, Snider GL. A controlled trial of intermittent positive pressure breathing, incentive spirometry and deep breathing exercises in preventing pulmonary complications after abdominal surgery. Am Rev Respir Dis 1984;130:12–15.
33. Tisi GM. Preoperative evaluation of pulmonary function. Am Rev Respir Dis 1979;119:293–310.
34. Tarhan S, Moffit EA, Sessler AD, et al. Risk of anesthesia and surgery in patients with chronic bronchitis and chronic obstructive pulmonary disease. Surgery 1973;74:720–726.
35. Ravin MB. Comparison of spinal and general anesthesia for lower abdominal surgery in patients with chronic obstructive pulmonary disease. Anesthesiology 1971;35:319–322.
36. Chalon J, Tayyab MA, Ramanathan S. Cytology of respiratory epithelium as a predictor of respiratory complications after operation. Chest 1975;67:32–35.
37. Camner P, Phillipson K. Some studies of tracheobronchial clearance in man. Chest 1973;63(Suppl):23S.
38. Buiste AS, Sexton GJ, Nagy JM, et al. The effect of smoking cessation and modification on lung function. Am Rev Respir Dis 1976;114:115–122.
39. Bode FR, Dosman J, Martin RR, et al. Reversibility of pulmonary function abnormalities in smokers. Am J Med 1975;59:43–52.
40. Kaubam JR, Chen LH, Hyman SA. Effect of short term smoking halt on carboxyhemoglobin levels and P-50 values. Anesth Analg 1986;65:1186–1188.
41. Warner MA, Divertie MB, Tinker JH. Preoperative cessation of smoking and pulmonary complications in coronary artery bypass patients. Anesthesiology 1984;60:380–383.
42. Mitchell C, Gamaby P, Peake P. Post-operative respiratory morbidity: identification and risk factors. Aust N Z J Surg 1982;52:203–209.
43. Warner MA, Offord KP, Warner ME, Lennon RL, Conover MA, Jansson-Schumacher U. Role of preoperative cessation of smoking and other factors in postoperative pulmonary complications: a blinded prospective study of coronary artery bypass patients. Mayo Clin Proc 1989;64:609–616.
44. Stein M, Cassara EL. Preoperative pulmonary evaluation and therapy for surgical patients. JAMA 1970;211:787–790.
45. Cain HD, Stevens PM, Adaniya R. Preoperative pulmonary function and complications after cardiovascular surgery. Chest 1979;76:130–135.
46. Milledge JS, Nunn JF. Criteria of fitness for anaesthesia in patients with chronic obstructive lung disease. BMJ 1975;3:670–673.
47. Williams CD, Brenowitz JB. "Prohibitive" lung function and major surgical procedures. Am J Surg 1976;132:763–766.
48. Jackson CV. Preoperative pulmonary evaluation. Arch Intern Med 1988;148:2120–2127.
49. Gold MI, Helrich M. A study of the complications related to anesthesia in asthmatic patients. Anesth Analg 1963;42:283–293.
50. Fowkes FGR, Lunn JN, Farrow SC, et al. Epidemiology in anaesthesia: mortality risk in patients with co-existing physical disease. Br J Anaesth 1982;54:819–825.
51. Oh SH, Patterson R. Surgery in corticosteroid-dependent asthmatics. J Allergy Clin Immunol 1974;53:345–351.
52. Mohr DN. Estimation of surgical risk in the elderly: a correlative review. J Am Geriatr Soc 1983;31:99–102.
53. Lewin I, Lerner AG, Green SH, Del Guercio LRM, Siegel JH. Physical class and physiologic status in the prediction of operative mortality in the aged sick. Ann Surg 1971;174:217–231.
54. Didolkar MS, Moore RH, Takita H. Evaluation of the risk in pulmonary resection for bronchogenic carcinoma. Am J Surg 1974;127:700–703.
55. Jezek V, Ourednik A, Lichtenberg J, Mostecky H. Cardiopulmonary function in lung resection performed for bronchogenic cancer in patients above 65 years of age. Respiration 1970;27:42–50.
56. Boushy SF, Billig DM, North LB, et al. Clinical course related to preoperative and postoperative pulmonary function in patients with bronchogenic carcinoma. Chest 1971;59:383–391.
57. Strauss RJ, Wise L. Operative risks of obesity. Surg Gynecol Obstet 1978;146:286–291.
58. Luce JM. Respiratory complications of obesity. Chest 1980;78:626–631.
59. Ray CS, Sue DY, Bray G, Hansen JE, Wasserman K. Effects of obesity on respiratory function. Am Rev Respir Dis 1983;128:501–506.
60. Crapo RO, Kelly TM, Elliott CG, Jones SB. Spirometry as a preoperative screening test in morbidly obese patients. Surgery 1986;99:763–767.
61. Vaughan RW, Englehart RC, Wise L. Postoperative hypoxemia in obese patients. Ann Surg 1974;180:877–882.

62. Vaughn RW, Bauer S, Wise L. Volume and pH of gastric juice in obese patients. Anesthesiology 1975;43:686–689.

63. Catenacci AJ, Anderson JD, Boersma D. Anesthetic hazards of obesity. JAMA 1961;175:657–665.

64. Prem KA, Mensheha NM, McKelvey JL. Operative treatment of adenocarcinoma of the endometrium in obese women. Am J Obstet Gynecol 1965;92:16–21.

65. Putnam L, Jenicek JA, Allen CR, Wilson RD. Anesthesia in the morbidly obese patient. South Med J 1974;67:1411–1417.

66. Postlethwait RW, Johnson WD. Complications following surgery for duodenal ulcer in obese patients. Arch Surg 1972;105:438–440.

67. Meyers JR, Lembeck L, O'Kane H, et al. Changes in functional residual capacity of the lung after operation. Arch Surg 1975;110:576–583.

68. Pemberton LB, Manax WG. Relationship of obesity to postoperative complications after cholecystectomy. Am J Surg 1971;121:87–89.

69. Bermudez-Gomez M, Rose L, Celli B. Is weight an independent risk factor in the development of post-operative pulmonary complications after abdominal surgery [abstract]? Am Rev Respir Dis 1987;135:A211.

70. Rucker L, Frye EB, Staten MA. Usefulness of screening chest roentgengrams in preoperative patients. JAMA 1983;250:3209–3211.

71. Tape TG, Mushlin AI. The utility of routine chest radiographs. Ann Intern Med 1986;104:663–670.

72. Gass GD, Olsen GN. Preoperative pulmonary function testing to predict postoperative morbidity and mortality. Chest 1986;89:127–135.

73. Zibrak JD, O'Donnell CR, Marton K. Indications for pulmonary function testing. Ann Intern Med 1990;112:763–771.

74. Morice RC, Peters EJ, Ryan MB, et al. Exercise testing in the evaluation of patients at high risk for complications from lung resection. Chest 1992;101:356–361.

75. Wernly JA, DeMeester TR, Kirchner PT, Myerowitz PD, Oxford DE, Golomb HM. Clinical value of quantitative ventilation-perfusion scans in the surgical management of bronchogenic carcinoma. J Thorac Cardiovasc Surg 1980;80:535–543.

76. Bolliger CT, Wyser C, Roser H, Soler M, Perruchoud AP. Lung scanning and exercise testing for the prediction of postoperative performance in lung resection candidates at increased risk for complications. Chest 1995;108:341–348.

77. Corris PA, Ellis DA, Hawkins T, et al. Use of radionuclide scanning in the preoperative estimation of pulmonary function after pneumonectomy. Thorax 1987;42:285–291.

78. Fee JH, Holmes EC, Gewirtz HS, et al. Role of pulmonary vascular resistance measurements in preoperative evaluation of candidates for pulmonary resection. J Thorac Cardiovasc Surg 1975;75:519–524.

79. Smith TP, Kinasewitz GT, Tucker WY, et al. Exercise capacity as a predictor of postthoracotomy morbidity. Am Rev Respir Dis 1984;129:730–734.

80. Bechard D, Wetstein L. Assessment of exercise oxygen consumption as preoperative criterion for lung resection. Ann Thorac Surg 1987;44:344–349.

81. Kroenke K, Lawrence VA, Theroux JF, Tuley MR. Operative risk in patients with severe obstructive pulmonary disease. Arch Intern Med 1992;152:967–971.

82. Dureuil B, Desmonts JM, Mankikian B, et al. Effects of aminophylline on diaphragmatic dysfunction after upper abdominal surgery. Anesthesiology 1985;62:242–246.

83. Kingston HGG, Hirshman CA. Perioperative management of the patient with asthma. Anesth Analg 1984;63:844–855.

84. Marshall MC, Olsen GN. The physiologic evaluation of the lung resection candidate. Clin Chest Med 1993;14:305–320.

85. Mohr DN, Jett JR. Preoperative evaluation of pulmonary risk factors. J Gen Intern Med 1988;3:277–287.

86. Olsen GN, Block AJ, Swenson EW, Castle JR, Wynne JW. Pulmonary function evaluation of the lung resection candidate: a prospective study. Am Rev Respir Dis 1975;111:379–387.

87. Miller JI, Hatcher CR. Limited resection of bronchogenic carcinoma in the patient with marked impairment of pulmonary function. Ann Thorac Surg 1987;44:340–343.

88. Kearney DJ, Lee TH, Reilly JJ, DeCamp MM, Sugarbaker DJ. Assessment of operative risk in patients undergoing lung resection. Chest 1994;105:753–759.

89. Roukema J, Carol E, Prins J. The prevention of pulmonary complications after upper abdominal surgery in patients with noncompromised pulmonary status. Arch Surg 1988;123:30–34.

90. Morran C, Findlay I, Mathieson M, et al. Randomized controlled trial of physiotherapy for postoperative pulmonary complications. Br J Anesth 1983;55:1113–1116.

91. Lindner KH, Lotz P, Ahnefeld FW. Continuous positive airway pressure effect on functional residual capacity, vital capacity and its subdivisions. Chest 1987;92:66–70.

92. Katz JA, Marks JD. Inspiratory work with and without continuous positive airway pressure in patients with acute respiratory failure. Anesthesiology 1985;63:598–607.

93. Ricksten S, Bengtsson A, Soderberg C, et al. Effects of periodic positive airway pressure by mask on postoperative pulmonary function. Chest 1986;89:774–781.

94. Stock MC, Downs JB, Gauer PK, et al. Prevention of postoperative pulmonary complications with CPAP, incentive spirometry, and conservative therapy. Chest 1985;87:151–157.

95. Christensen EF, Schultz P, Jensen OV, et al. Postoperative pulmonary complications and lung function in high-risk patients: a comparison of three physiotherapy regimens after upper abdominal surgery in general anesthesia. Acta Anesthesiol Scand 1991;35: 97–104.

96. Hall JC, Tarala R, Harris G, et al. Incentive spirometry versus routine chest physiotherapy for prevention of pulmonary complications after abdominal surgery. Lancet 1991;337: 953–956.

97. Oikkonen M, Karjalainen K, Kahara V, Kuosa R, Schavikin L. Comparison of incentive spirometry and intermittent positive pressure breathing after coronary artery bypass graft. Chest 1991;99:60–65.

98. Jenkins SC, Soutar SA, Loukota JM, Johnson LC, Moxham J. Physiotherapy after coronary artery surgery: are breathing exercises necessary? Thorax 1989;44:634–639.

99. Jung R, Wight J, Nusser R, Rosoff L. Comparison of three methods of respiratory care following upper abdominal surgery. Chest 1980;78: 31–35.

100. Thorens L. Postoperative pulmonary complications: observations on their prevention by means of physiotherapy. Acta Chir Scand 1954; 107:194–205.

101. Calligaro KD, Azurin DJ, Dougherty MJ, et al. Pulmonary risk factors for elective abdominal surgery. J Vasc Surg 1993;18:914–921.

102. Miller JI, Grossman GD, Hatcher CR. Pulmonary function test criteria for operability and pulmonary resection. Surg Gynecol Obstet 1981;153:893–895.

103. Lockwood P. Lung function test results and the risk of post-thoracotomy complications. Respiration 1973;30:529–542.

104. Putnam JB, Lammermeier DE, Colon R, McMurtrey MJ, Ali MK, Roth JA. Predicted pulmonary function and survival after pneumonectomy for primary lung carcinoma. Ann Thorac Surg 1990;49:909–915.

105. Dales RE, Dionne G, Leech JA, Lunau M, Schweitzer I. Preoperative prediction of pulmonary complications following thoracic surgery. Chest 1993;104:155–159.

106. Gaensler EA, Cusell DW, Lindgren I, Verstraeten JM, Smith SS, Streider JW. The role of pulmonary insufficiency in mortality and invalidism following surgery for pulmonary tuberculosis. J Thorac Cardiovasc Surg 1955;29: 163–187.

107. Mittman C. Assessment of operative risk in thoracic surgery. Am Rev Respir Dis 1961;84: 197–207.

108. Patel RL, Townsend ER, Fountain SW. Elective pneumonectomy: factors associated with morbidity and operative mortality. Ann Thorac Surg 1992;54:84–88.

109. Boysen PG, Block AJ, Moulder PV. Relationship between preoperative pulmonary function tests and complications after thoracotomy. Surg Gynecol Obstet 1981;52:813–815.

110. Candler L. Physiologic assessment and management of the preoperative patient with pulmonary emphysema. Am J Cardiol 1963;12: 324–326.

111. Eugene J, Brown SE, Light RW, et al. Maximum oxygen consumption: a physiologic guide to pulmonary resection. Surg Forum 1982;33: 260–262.

112. Markos J, Mullan BP, Hillman DR, Musk AW, Centico VF, Lovegrove FT. Preoperative assessment as a predictor of mortality and morbidity after lung resection. Am Rev Respir Dis 1989; 129:730–734.

113. Wahi R, McMurtrey MJ, DeCaro LF, et al. Determinants of perioperative morbidity and mortality after pneumonectomy. Ann Thoraac Surg 1989;48:33–37.

114. Ferguson MK, Little L, Rizzo L, et al. Diffusing capacity predicts morbidity and mortality after pulmonary resection. J Thorac Cardiovasc Surg 1988;96:894–900.

8

Basic Mechanical Respiratory Support

Larry B. Grossman and Howard T. Jacobs

Mechanical respiratory support is generally considered during one or more of four basic situations compromising the patient. These situations occur when the patient is unable to: *(a)* secure the quantity of oxygen required, *(b)* adequately remove carbon dioxide, *(c)* protect the airway, or *(d)* clear secretions. This chapter deals with the technical aspects of mechanical ventilation in some detail and emphasizes the "how to" aspects. Complications also are discussed, with concern for their prevention and prompt recognition. Because of the breadth of this chapter's topic, specifics and mechanics rather than theory are emphasized. Common abbreviations are presented in Table 8.1.

EPIDEMIOLOGY

Respiratory failure requiring mechanical ventilation is more likely to occur in several specific situations. An appreciation of the most common risk factors leading to hypoxemia or hypercarbia will aid in both recognition and prompt corrective action.

An obstructive airway abnormality could result from increased large-airway resistance due to tumor or tracheal stenosis, or it could result from small-airway resistance, as seen with asthma or chronic obstructive pulmonary disease. The **flow-volume loop,** which presents data graphically, is useful in determining whether the obstruction is in the large or the small airway. Pulmonary function tests provide quantitative information that can determine the degree of impairment, response to bronchodilators, and progressive changes in the patient's chronic ailment. Clinically, the compromised patient exhibits an increased effort to ventilate, increased heart rate, decreasing Pao_2 with an increasing $Paco_2$, and decreasing pH. **The pH** is an indicator of the progressive severity of the clinical situation. To avoid intubation in the patient with small-airway obstruction, bronchodilators are usually the first line of therapy, but if the situation deteriorates, mechanical support is often required.

Inadequate gas exchange due to an acute parenchymal disease may require respiratory support. A high oxygen gradient and low compliance are characteristic of processes such as pneumonia, atelectasis, and pulmonary edema. Generally, oxygenation is more of a problem than ventilation, but both are seen. In any case, the patient must dramatically increase his or her work of breathing.

Ventilatory failure (i.e., hypercarbia) can result from several different (or combined) situations. Hypoventilation can result from a neurologic problem, as in the case of muscle weakness or central depression (1). Preoperative evaluations and the patient's clinical history can alert one to possible postoperative respiratory compromise in patients with neuromuscular weakness, and Guillain-Barré syndrome is but one example of a diagnosis that can be followed by serial measurements to

Table 8.1.   Abbreviations

A-aDO_2	Alveolar-arterial oxygen tension difference
ABG	Arterial blood gas
CPAP	Continuous positive airway pressure
CVP	Central venous pressure
f/V_T	Ratio of the spontaneous ventilatory rate or frequency to the tidal volume
FiO_2	Inspired oxygen fraction
IMV	Intermittent mandatory ventilation
NIF	Negative inspiratory force
$PaCO_2$	Arterial carbon dioxide tension
PaO_2	Arterial oxygen tension
PEEP	Positive end expiratory pressure
SIMV	Synchronized IMV
VC	Vital capacity
V_D/V_T	Ratio of dead space to tidal volume

indicate whether ventilatory support is necessary. A vital capacity of less than 1 L or a 50% decrease from the initial vital capacity predicts ventilatory failure.

An iatrogenic cause of muscle weakness is the use of muscle relaxants in the operative period. One must check the anesthesia report for documentation, as well as check the patient for clinical signs, that the muscle relaxants have been adequately reversed. A basic evaluation would be to examine the patient's grip and ability to lift his or her head for 5 seconds. In addition, a nerve stimulator is often used by the anesthesiologist to evaluate the effect of neuromuscular-blocking agents. For cases in which succinylcholine or mivacurium chloride has been used, postoperative muscle weakness possibly could result from a pseudocholinesterase deficiency. Whatever the cause, however, mechanical respiratory support should be used as long as the patient's respiratory status is compromised.

Cranial surgery or trauma may alter the respiratory pattern and level of consciousness. Artificial hyperventilation to a $PaCO_2$ of approximately 30 mm Hg can decrease cerebral blood flow and aid in decreasing cerebral edema. The neurologist or neurosurgeon may request that the patient be ventilated to a lowered $PaCO_2$ as

a treatment modality; this is often fine tuned by monitoring intracranial pressures. Because medication may be used to sedate neurologic patients, respiratory support also may be required. If the patient is obtunded, one must protect the airway from the risk of aspiration or obstructed breathing.

Classically, narcotics are the medications that cause a patient to hypoventilate or even obstruct the airway. Narcotics will alter the carbon dioxide response curve so that a higher carbon dioxide tension is required to promote a ventilatory response, and other sedatives may act with narcotics to further alter the response curve and cause hypoventilation. When reversing a narcotic with an antagonist, it is important to remember that the duration of the reversal agent and of the narcotic may differ. If the effect of the antagonist dissipates before that of the narcotic, the patient may become "renarcotized."

The specific type of surgery or trauma also is a major factor in the need for respiratory support, as previously noted with cranial surgery. The chest can be affected by pneumothorax, hemothorax, or hydrothorax. Similarly, chest wall instability can cause hypoxia, decreased vital capacity, hypoventilation, and increased work of breathing. Upper abdominal surgery may affect ventilation by impairing diaphragmatic excursions. In addition, incisional pain and the requirement for narcotics can be major factors resulting in shallow breathing and atelectasis.

The respiratory problems of obese patients will be magnified after surgery. Because the work of breathing is increased for these individuals, addition of drugs, position in bed, and incisional pain will compound the problem. Obese patients generally ventilate more easily in a sitting position because of their large abdomen and its contents not pressing against the diaphragm.

Poor nutrition is often the factor that upsets a marginal situation. With further postoperative deterioration in nutrition, a marginal patient may not be able to maintain the work of breathing.

In addition, there is the problem of **restrictive diseases** that limit the ventilatory capacity. Patients with significant scoliosis, ankylosing spondylitis, and so on must be protected from all factors that might compromise their already decreased vital capacity. A restrictive abnormality can be temporarily improved by removing ascites or effusion.

Surgery can add factors that cause a marginal patient to require mechanical respiratory support as well. Kofke (2) described why pulmonary dysfunction is seen after major abdominal and thoracic surgery. Significant reduction in the functional residual capacity is accompanied by the loss of expiratory reserve volume and inspiratory reserve. There is also a decrease in the forced vital capacity and the maximal expiratory flows. This situation of low lung volume results in small-airway closure and atelectasis.

One study specifically sought to identify risk factors associated with postoperative respiratory morbidity (3). The authors concluded that these factors were a productive cough, purulent sputum, low 1-second forced expiratory volume, upper abdominal surgery, previous history of postoperative respiratory problems, and presence of a nasogastric tube.

When a high probability of respiratory failure is evident, the patient should remain intubated and be given respiratory support postoperatively. The patient can be extubated when it will not be deleterious (e.g., the patient after heart surgery who should have a stable cardiovascular system before extubation).

INDICATIONS FOR INTUBATION AND MECHANICAL SUPPORT

Indications for intubation and mechanical support will be discussed together, because intubation requires mechanical support of varying degrees. One must evaluate for **oxygenation, ventilation, pulmonary toilet, airway protection, and airway obstruction.** The criteria for intubation (or for mechanical ventilatory support) are essentially the opposite of those for weaning a patient from ventilatory support and extubation.

Whereas patients with apnea obviously require intubation and mechanical support, those with lesser degrees of respiratory failure must be individually evaluated. To determine the **adequacy of oxygenation,** one uses arterial blood gas (ABG) values, alveolar-arterial oxygen tension differences (A-aDO_2), or comparison of inspired oxygen (FIO_2) to Pao_2. An increase in the A-aDO_2 is detrimental and can result from right-to-left shunting of blood past alveoli that are perfused but not ventilated (i.e., true shunt) or from incomplete oxygenation of blood passing by alveoli that are poorly ventilated (i.e., a ventilation-perfusion inequality). When a patient is being followed with pulse oximetry, a sudden and pronounced decrease in the oxyhemoglobin saturation may indicate an event requiring additional respiratory support. The section on "Technical Aspects" presents values and data concerned with oxygenation.

Ventilation can often be assessed using ABG values. A severe, uncompensated respiratory acidosis would require mechanical support. A patient with a relatively normal Pao_2 and pH, however, may require urgent intervention if he or she is experiencing ventilatory muscle fatigue. In this situation, the patient will no longer be able to accomplish the work of breathing, and fatigue and abrupt decompensation may ensue if this aspect is not evaluated or anticipated. Clinical signs include a rapid, shallow pattern of ventilation and the presence of paradoxical respirations (i.e., inward inspiratory movements of the abdomen without active abdominal muscle contractions and use of accessory muscles).

A depressed level of consciousness identifies a patient who is not able to **protect his or her airway** from obstruction or aspiration. Because aspiration can precipitate a rapid respiratory arrest, the obtunded patient must be carefully evaluated for laryngeal reflexes. One must be aware that if a nasogastric tube in an obtunded patient becomes obstructed or active emesis develops, the nasogastric tube can cause the cardioesophageal sphincter to be less competent, thus making aspiration a significant risk. In these situations, an endotracheal tube is an effective way to protect the airway.

The endotracheal tube also provides a means for satisfactory **pulmonary toilet** in the patient who cannot cough adequately. The patient with thick or copious secretions may not be able to clear them if he or she cannot generate a negative inspiratory force of at least 25 cm H_2O or has a vital capacity of less than 15 mL/kg of body weight. If the patient cannot take a deep breath, he or she will be at risk for not keeping the alveoli expanded and not clearing secretions. The chest radiograph should be examined for areas of atelectasis and pneumonia, and fiberoptic bronchoscopy is sometimes required in addition to routine suctioning.

In summary, an increasing Pa_{CO_2}, decreasing Pa_{O_2} and pH, respiratory fatigue, risk of aspiration or airway obstruction, and ineffective cough would each suggest the need to carefully evaluate for intubation and mechanical respiratory support (4, 5).

SOURCES OF INFORMATION FOR VENTILATORY PLANS

The individual undertaking the patient's postoperative ventilatory care can gather considerable information by consulting the anesthesiologist's preoperative evaluation note and the anesthesia record from the operation. These will provide data on whether the patient is a likely candidate for respiratory failure and any immediate indications for mechanical ventilation. The pertinent preoperative information will often mention any preexisting respiratory problems, responses to

therapies, chest radiography reports, results from pulmonary function tests and ABG measurements, and previous surgical experiences. The prior records may reveal past surgical and postoperative respiratory complications as well as any successful or unsuccessful treatment of problems. They may also alert the physician to anticipate (or prevent) adverse situations during the present admission. Based on the preoperative evaluation, recommendations might include prescribing bronchodilators or chest physiotherapy, alerting the patient to the possibility of postoperative intubation, and instructing the patient in postoperative respiratory plans.

The anesthesia record should note the surgical procedure and complications, fluid replacement, the ventilation technique with volumes and rate, type of anesthetic, intubation approach and difficulties, intraoperative laboratory tests ordered, the reversal of muscle relaxants or narcotics, and the stability of various organ systems. It is important to know which agents have been used for the anesthetic because of their different actions and durations. A patient with asthma may have had clear breath sounds during the surgery because of the bronchodilator effects of a halogenated gas, but postoperatively, the patient's intrinsic disease and irritation of the endotracheal tube may require that bronchodilators be used immediately. When reviewing an anesthetic using a narcotic approach, both length of action and the amount used are key concerns. The patient's temperature during and after the procedure may affect the oxygen consumption, metabolism, and reversibility of the relaxants as well. Table 8.2 lists some pertinent information that may be available by reviewing the preanesthesia evaluation sheet, past records, patient chart, and the anesthesia record. Verbal communication with the anesthesiologist is an excellent approach, but the records should always be reviewed. In addition, communication with the respiratory therapists and nurses is essential.

Table 8.2. Preoperative and Operative Information that Might be Useful Postoperatively

---

Anesthesia Preoperative Evaluation Database

History and Physical
Orders
Laboratory results
Chest x-ray reports
ABG results
Pulmonary function tests: with and without
  bronchodilators
Respiratory problems: treatment and response to
  treatment
Previous anesthetics: operative and postoperative
  problems

Anesthesia Record

Operative procedure
Complications
Ventilator settings: FiO$_2$, volumes, rates.
Intubation: difficulties, size of endotracheal tube.
Anesthetic technique and agents: halogenated
  agents, narcotics, muscle relaxants.
Fluids
Invasive monitors
Nasogastric tube
Temperature
Operative laboratory tests

TECHNICAL ASPECTS

The technical aspects of mechanical ventilation can be approached by considering the specific indications requiring mechanical support. Although various needs will overlap and must be integrated into the overall plan, this approach at least provides a starting point.

Oxygenation is a priority in the postoperative period. Traditionally, the color of the skin, mucous membranes, and nailbeds provide the basic clinical signs. Cyanosis is an unreliable indicator of hypoxemia, however, because a sufficient amount of reduced hemoglobin must be available, the finding is subjective, and peripheral cyanosis may result from the patient simply being cold postoperatively. Therefore, a high index of suspicion and clinical signs will alert the physician to gather more information. A Pao$_2$ or pulse oximetry will further delineate the situation. Because the patient is usually receiving supplemental oxygen, the FIo$_2$ and Pao$_2$ can be compared to determine if the FIo$_2$ is adequate. When the patient arrives from the operating room with an endotracheal tube in place, one usually starts with the FIo$_2$ used in the operating room, with changes being made according to the Pao$_2$ or pulse oximeter measurements. The pulse oximeter is often useful as a noninvasive means to monitor oxyhemoglobin saturation serially, but the accuracy of the pulse oximeter may be compromised by significant levels of dysfunctional hemoglobins (e.g., carboxyhemoglobin, methemoglobin). Continued intubation is usually required if the Pao$_2$ is less than 60 to 70 mm Hg or the oxyhemoglobin saturation is less than 90% with supplemental oxygen. Of course, the clinical impressions and signs must be correlated with the laboratory values, and the FIo$_2$ should be analyzed to be certain that the cardiovascular system is actually delivering the oxygen concentration desired.

One must check intubated patients for proper positioning of the endotracheal tube. Bilateral breath sounds and, possibly, a chest radiograph will determine that one is not ventilating only one lung (generally the right) and causing a massive shunt because of the perfusion of both lungs from the ventilation of only one. When listening for bilateral breath sounds, one must listen along the midaxillary lines to determine that the breath sounds are equal for both lungs. If the endotracheal tube impinges on the carina, the patient may continue to cough and be uncomfortable. Also, one will not be able to satisfactorily suction both lungs. The endotracheal tube should be 3 to 5 cm above the carina. If for any reason fiberoptic bronchoscopy is necessary, the tube position can be verified during the procedure as well.

Because one would like to achieve a PaO_2 that permits nearly full hemoglobin saturation, a minimum value of 60 mm Hg is required in patients who are acutely ill. In light of the concern over oxygen toxicity, one attempts to decrease the FIO_2 as long as the PaO_2 is not a problem. **Oxygen toxicity** resulting from prolonged high inspired oxygen tensions causes deterioration of pulmonary function (6). There is an increased right-to-left shunt, decreased pulmonary compliance, and decreased functional residual capacity. Structurally, there is a loss of capillary endothelial integrity, interstitial edema, hemorrhage, and fibrosis. Patient tolerance to an increased FIO_2 varies, and there are no definite limits for safety. Generally, however, clinically significant changes are believed to occur if a patient with normal lungs receives 48 hours of exposure to an FIO_2 of 0.6 or greater at one atmosphere. An FIO_2 greater than 0.5 in a critically ill patient, however, has the potential of causing significant damage. The safest elevated FIO_2 for continuous administration has not been clearly defined, so we usually seek an FIO_2 of less than 0.5 and preferably 0.4. Register and coworkers (7) studied the results of mechanically ventilating patients with an FIO_2 of 0.5 for 16 to 24 hours and found that there may be an impairment of pulmonary gas exchange after extubation. They recommended that supplemental oxygen be administered at the lowest possible level that will still provide an oxyhemoglobin saturation greater than 90%.

By using positive end-expiratory pressure (PEEP) or continuous positive airway pressure (CPAP), one can generally decrease the FIO_2 to safer levels. Most patients can be started on PEEP at 5 cm H_2O because PEEP is useful in intubated patients at risk for developing decreased lung volume. **The contraindications to PEEP** are (a) an unstable cardiovascular system in which impeding venous return could be deleterious, (b) emphysematous bullae, or (c) increased intracranial pressure. PEEP is titrated against the cardio-vascular effects and the desired oxygenation. In difficult cases, one may need to consider cardiac output, PaO_2, and mixed venous PO_2. Because the PEEP can have a negative effect on cardiac output, the "best" PEEP should be determined by titration. This means that a PEEP of 10 cm H_2O may not be better than 5 cm. The "more is better" concept does not work in this situation. One seeks the lowest PEEP that enables use of a "safe" FIO_2 to provide a satisfactory PaO_2. If the mixed venous oxygen tension decreases with PEEP, the problem of tissue hypoxia may not be improved until cardiac output is improved, and one must then work to improve the cardiovascular hemodynamics with appropriate therapies (i.e., vasopressors, fluids, and so on). The basic goal is to lower the FIO_2 to 0.4 or less while achieving an acceptable PaO_2 (8).

In patients with obstructive lung disease, intrinsic or Auto-PEEP may develop from progressive air trapping. This could result in a precipitous drop in venous return and cardiovascular collapse. In addition, it might increase the burden on the ventilatory muscles, thereby hampering attempts at weaning the patient from mechanical ventilation. Auto-PEEP can be decreased by carefully adjusting the ventilator to allow more exhalation time and cautiously adding extrinsic PEEP (9).

Often, preoperative pulmonary function tests with and without bronchodilators will suggest that one consider intravenous or nebulized agents in the postoperative period to optimize bronchodilation. With an endotracheal tube in place, the airway that preoperatively was normal and minimally reactive may now require a bronchodilator.

VENTILATORY EQUIPMENT AND ITS MANAGEMENT

There are two basic types of ventilators. The **pressure-cycled ventilator** delivers an inflation until the direct, preset pressure is achieved, and then a passive expiration ensues. Because the tidal volume is determined by the inspired gas flow, preset pressure, and the patient's compliance, tidal volume can vary with this type of ventilator.

The **volume-limited ventilator** delivers a preset volume regardless of the pressure, although a peak-pressure pop-off valve is included as a safety measure. The volume-limited ventilator is generally preferred because it maintains a constant tidal volume. One can set the ventilator

with a tidal volume of 12 mL per kilogram of body weight (range, 10–15 mL/kg) and observe the movement of the chest wall to be certain the initial volume appears to be adequate. The exact tidal volume and rate can be fine tuned with ABGs.

The four approaches to the respiratory rate are *(a)* **controlled,** *(b)* **assist/control,** *(c)* **intermittent mandatory ventilation (IMV), and** *(d)* **synchronized IMV (SIMV).** Table 8.3 compares the various modes. Controlled ventilation is a set

Table 8.3. Basic Comparison of Mechanical Ventilation Methods

I. Pressure Determined
1. Pressure-Cycled
- Inflation to preset pressure and passive expiration
- tidal volume can vary
2. Pressue Control Ventilation (PCV)
- pressure cycled, but the pressure is maintained for a set time
- may improve gas distribution
3. Pressure Support Ventilation (PSV)
- requires spontaneous ventilation
- airway pressure is selected according to effects on rate and tidal volume
- weaning can be accomplished by gradually reducing the level of pressure
II. Volume Determined
- preset volume, and a constant tidal volume
- peak-pressure pop-off valve
1. Controlled
- preset rate and no spontaneous ventilation
2. Assist/control
- preset rate and a full tidal volume with patient initiated inspiration
3. Intermittent Mandatory Ventilation (IMV)
- spontaneous ventilation of variable volume between mandatory ventilations
- advocates point out use in weaning
- can provide full and partial ventilatory support
- less disruption of cardiopulmonary physiology
4. Synchronized IMV
- synchronizes the positive-pressure inspiration with the spontaneous breaths
- can provide full and partial ventilatory support
III. High Frequency Ventilation (HFV)
- lower mean airway pressure
1. High Frequency Positive Pressure Ventilation (HFPPV)
- 60-120 breaths/minute
2. High Frequency Jet Pressure Ventilation (HFJV)
- 80-300 breaths/min
3. High Frequency Oscillation (HFO)
- 600-3000 breaths/minute
IV. Inverse Ratio Ventilation (IRV)
- usually combined with PCV in order to provide gas exchange at a lower FiO_2 and mean airway pressure
- requires paralysis and sedation

rate with no spontaneous ventilation permitted by the patient. Although the assist/control mode allows a full tidal volume whenever the patient initiates an inspiration, it guarantees a preset rate even if an inspiration is not initiated by the patient. IMV allows spontaneous ventilation of variable volume between the mandatory ventilations, and SIMV synchronizes the positive-pressure inspiration with the patient's spontaneous breaths. No physiologic advantages to the SIMV concept have been shown, but some advocates point to the greater ease of weaning the patient from ventilatory support with this approach. Those individuals advocating the assist control mode see this method as a safeguard, because full volumes are guaranteed or generated with less effort.

Cane and Shapiro (10) have published an excellent review that logically presents and compares the four modes of ventilation by their ability to minimize disruption of cardiopulmonary physiology. As they point out, full ventilatory support (i.e., the ventilator provides all of the energy for effective alveolar ventilation) can be provided by each mode, but partial ventilatory support (i.e., both the patient and the ventilator provide the effective alveolar ventilation) can only be managed by IMV or SIMV. They also show that partial ventilatory support produces less disruption of cardiac output and ventilation-perfusion relationships, that it is very effective in conjunction with PEEP, and that less sedation may be needed. There is some concern, however, that the demand valve used with SIMV may increase the work of breathing at ventilator rates of four or less per minute.

One technique is to start with an IMV rate of 10 per minute and wean as tolerated. This provides full support until the patient's status allows increased spontaneous ventilations. The inspiration:expiration ratio is usually set initially as 1:2, but the patient with chronic obstructive pulmonary disease or asthma may require a longer expiratory phase. By checking an ABG approximately 20 minutes after changing the setting, one can aggressively titrate as required and wean as permitted. One seeks a normal pH with a $Paco_2$ of 35 to 40 mm Hg. Obviously, the vital signs should be monitored during the changes, and a pulse oximeter is a useful continuous monitor of oxyhemoglobin saturation. If the patient is not in phase with or is struggling with the ventilator in any way, it is important to check immediately that the circuit is not the cause of hypoxia or hypoventilation, and decide whether sedation is necessary.

In the very special circumstances when muscle relaxants are deemed to be necessary, total vigilance must be maintained, with ventilator alarms, appropriate monitors, and notification of participating staff. One such situation would be the use of neuromuscular blocking agents in head trauma to reduce intrathoracic pressure and venous pressure and thereby decrease intracranial pressure. One must be constantly concerned about inadequate analgesia or sedation in patients receiving neuromuscular blocking agents. Paralysis puts the patient at risk for disconnection from the ventilator, pulmonary emboli from immobility, lack of a cough reflex, and peripheral nerve injury from careless positioning (11). Muscle relaxants can be administered by bolus or infusions and monitored by a nerve stimulator, and the Society of Critical Care Medicine has developed practice parameters for neuromuscular blockade in the adult patient who is critically ill (12). Although pancuronium was the preferred neuromuscular blocking agent for most critically ill patients, vecuronium has been recommended for patients with cardiac disease or hemodynamic instability in whom tachycardia would be deleterious.

Often, sedation can be used to enable a patient to tolerate mechanical respiratory support and the intensive care environment. Lorazepam (for long-term use) and midazolam (for short-term use) can be administered by bolus or infusion. Usually, the effects of benzodiazepines are allowed to dissipate, but if the patient must be evaluated before the sedation has worn off, flumazenil can be used carefully to antagonize the action of the agents.

Propofol is an intravenous sedative-hypnotic that can be used as a short-term infusion for intensive care sedation. The advantage of this drug is the relatively rapid awakening of the patient after it has been discontinued. Patients must be monitored closely for hypotension and cardiovascular depression, and because the agent is not an antimicrobially preserved product under USP standards, strict aseptic techniques should be maintained in its handling. The tubing and any unused portions must be discarded after 12 hours. The use of disodium edetate, which is a chelator of trace metals, in propofol requires practitioners to consider those patients who are predisposed to zinc deficiency, such as those with burns, diarrhea, and/or sepsis. At high doses of 2 to 3 g/day, one should monitor for renal impairment and urine sediment. Propofol is formulated in an oil-in-water emulsion; therefore, serum triglyceride levels should be followed if it is administered for an extended period. There is 0.1 g of fat in each milliliter of propofol, and this should be considered in patients receiving lipids.

When using infusion agents for intensive care sedation, the physician and staff must be aware of their precautions, warnings, side effects, interactions, and adverse effects. Developing protocols for these infusions aids the physician in their selection and dosing, the pharmacy in preparation, and the nursing staff in administration, monitoring, and weaning. The Society of Critical Care Medicine has published practice parameters for intravenous analgesia and sedation for adults in the intensive care setting (13). The paper discusses preferred analgesic agents in specific situations and the selection of sedative agents based on short-term or long-term use. The reasons for not selecting certain agents are also reviewed.

Although analgesia can be provided by bolus administration, some physicians have found that by using the infusion settings of a patient-controlled analgesia technique, less agent is used, fewer hemodynamic changes occur, and weaning the patient from mechanical respiratory support is often easier. Also, in the appropriate surgical patients, epidural narcotics and local anesthetics are often useful in early weaning.

Because the obtunded patient cannot communicate, he or she is dependent on alarms and monitors to indicate faulty ventilation. Conversely, one can help an alert patient to communicate concerns for comfort by providing writing implements or word charts and appropriate sedation or pain medication. The patient with a tracheostomy might benefit from a "talking tracheostomy tube," using an external airflow directed to the larynx for speech, or from an electric artificial larynx device or other artificial voicing systems.

Proper pulmonary toilet is essential in the intubated patient, because he or she will be unable to clear secretions. When appropriate, the patient must be turned to different positions as tolerated and percussed to mobilize the secretions. Hourly hyperinflation with an anesthesia bag and suctioning with sterile techniques is essential for satisfactory pulmonary toilet. Hyperinflation was also thought to be necessary because the endotracheal tube prevents patients from sighing effectively. In patients with otherwise normal lungs, hyperventilation will reverse the deterioration of lung function caused by prolonged mechanical ventilation; however, this routine clinical practice has no value in patients with respiratory failure on prolonged ventilation (14). Suctioning must be done carefully to avoid complications; **endotracheal suctioning** can cause bradycardia and hypotension in some individuals. A study by Winston and coworkers (15) compared the prophylactic use of either nebulized (0.05 mg/kg) or parenteral (1 mg) atropine to prevent cardiovascular problems. Both preparations prevented hypotensive response, but more tachycardia occurred with parenteral use. At no time should the catheter be down the endotracheal tube for a prolonged period. A safe method for accomplishing this task is to manually ventilate with oxygen, place the suction catheter into position, apply suction on withdrawal, and then resume ventilation. Also available is a double-lumen suction catheter that simultaneously insufflates oxygen at 10 L/min while suctioning (16). One may instill 1 to 2 mL of sterile saline between ventilations if the secretions are particularly thick. If a routine for pulmonary toilet is not maintained, the patient is at risk for atelectasis, pneumonia, and inspissated secretions. Chest radiography will assist the physician to order chest physiotherapy in the best position to drain affected areas of the lungs (17). Fiberoptic bronchoscopy is useful for diagnosis, suctioning, and lavaging in difficult or persistent situations as well.

Because the endotracheal or tracheostomy tube bypasses the patient's humidification system and dry gases affect ciliary action, gas must be humidified to prevent the secretions from drying and causing mucosal irritation. Devices for bubble diffusion, jet nebulization, or passover humidification can be used to provide heated humidification.

The choice of an oral endotracheal tube versus a nasal endotracheal tube depends on several factors. Generally, the nasal tube is better tolerated by the patient for longer periods. It has less movement on the trachea and less accidental extubations. One must take care to prevent nasal necrosis, however. The oral tube must be securely taped to the upper lip to decrease mobility. The nasal tube would be contraindicated when there is risk of nasal hemorrhage (e.g., in anticoagulated patients), risk of sinus infection, or leakage of cerebral spinal fluid from the nose. One usually seeks an endotracheal tube that is large enough to prevent airway resistance, is small enough not to apply excessive pressure to the laryngeal area, and has a cuff of the high-compliance/low-pressure type. Cuff pressures need to be checked daily (<25 cm H_2O). The cuffs on

the endotracheal tube must have just enough volume for a seal, which can be accomplished by letting volume out of the cuff until a small leak is heard with positive-pressure ventilation, then adding a small volume to just seal the system. If a tracheostomy tube is in place, it can be changed weekly once the stoma is developed. Elective change of any tube should not be scheduled to take place after a feeding, however, because one is then risking a possible emesis and aspiration.

When to **convert from an endotracheal to a tracheostomy tube** has often been primarily a question of time. The "appropriate" length of time for an endotracheal tube to be in place is changing, however, because of the low-pressure cuffs now being used. Bishop (18) noted that a tracheostomy is best used in the patient who will require prolonged intubation and will benefit from the increased comfort, because it is no longer routine to perform a tracheostomy after 1 week of intubation. Direct fiberoptic visualization of the cuff site is now also possible. Generally, one might wait approximately 10 to 12 days before considering a tracheostomy, but if the patient might be extubated in a few days, one would probably delay the tracheostomy and weigh the relative risks.

Before removing a tracheostomy tube, it is important to determine that there is no requirement for positive pressure to augment oxygenation and ventilation, that pulmonary toilet can be accomplished without the tracheostomy, and that the patient can protect his or her airway. Certainly, a patient lacking a gag reflex will have difficulty protecting the airway. A simple test for determining protection of the airway can be accomplished by deflating the cuff, having the patient sip some very dilute methylene blue (i.e., a drop in a glass of water), and then checking to see if any blue has been suctioned from the trachea. If blue is noted, the patient has failed the test. However, if no blue is noted, this is still no guarantee that aspiration could not occur. If the patient fails the test, he or she should be encouraged to exercise the laryngeal apparatus by talking while the cuff is deflated, and then the test can be administered again. When the patient qualifies for removal of the tracheostomy tube, one can then insert a fenestrated tracheostomy tube, which does not have a cuff but does have an opening to allow free exchange from the oropharynx to the lungs. In this way, one can determine if the patient can handle the added dead space by plugging the exterior part of the tube. This allows the stoma to remain patent while testing the added dead space. Once the patient shows that he or she can handle both the dead space and secretions, the fenestrated tube can be removed and a dressing applied.

PROBLEMS FROM MECHANICAL VENTILATION

The endotracheal tube can create problems if one is not attentive to details. Proper placement must be checked by auscultation and, if necessary, chest radiography to prevent intubation of the right mainstem bronchus or obstruction of the right upper lobe orifice. If the tube encroaches on the carina, the patient may cough and struggle because of discomfort. The tube must be patent to function properly, so one must order humidification and suctioning to prevent inspissated secretions. Also, the tube should be observed for compression or kinking. The cuff on the endotracheal tube must be checked for leaks or overinflation as well, as previously discussed.

Generally, an endotracheal tube with an internal diameter of 7.5 to 8.5 mm will be adequate for an adult. Laryngeal damage is usually related to large tube size, mobility of the tube, duration of intubation, local sepsis, and decreased vascularity in the area resulting from decreased cardiac output. Irritation and pressure cause edema, erosion, ulceration, and occasionally fibrosis when healing. Hoarseness or stridor can be caused by edema of the vocal cords, and obstruction can de-

velop from subglottic edema. A flow-volume loop pulmonary function test may aid in this diagnosis. The severity of the obstruction will determine whether conservative treatment, reintubation, or tracheostomy is required. Conservative treatment may entail humidification or administration of oxygen and possibly nebulized racemic epinephrine (0.5 mL in 1.5 mL of normal saline) every 2 hours. A 21% oxygen and 79% helium gas mixture (i.e., heliox) may improve laminar gas flow, reduce the work of breathing, and provide the opportunity for more definitive treatment of the airway narrowing (19, 20). Some authors have also recommended steroids for edematous obstruction. If the vocal cords or subglottic areas develop granulation or fibrosis, surgical treatment may be required.

Tracheal complications result from irritation and pressure causing edema, erosion, ulceration, and fibrosis. Irritation results from high cuff pressures and tube mobility. Erosion can cause a fistula or erode a major vessel with resulting catastrophic hemorrhage. Severe problems with ventilation develop when tracheomalacia causes collapse of the airway and obstruction. Tracheal stenosis is usually noted within 2 months of decannulation. **Generally, stridor indicates an airway that has been narrowed to 5 mm or smaller.** In summary, the complications of intubation can be decreased by using low-pressure cuffs and securing the tube.

The patient who does not receive satisfactory nutrition may not be able to maintain the work of breathing. When tolerated, nasogastric or gastrostomy feedings are preferable to total parenteral nutrition, which may increase production of carbon dioxide and therefore cause respiratory distress in patients with already compromised ventilation. Increased ventilatory demands because of total parenteral nutrition can be alleviated by using more fat emulsion and less glucose than are contained in the standard hyperalimentation formulas. By measuring carbon dioxide production in expired gases or by indirect calorimetry, appropriate changes in glucose could be made and followed.

The patient in an intensive care unit is at risk for stress gastritis and gastrointestinal hemorrhage, and use of steroids adds to these concerns. Although the exact mechanism by which stress ulceration occurs has not been defined, the basic approach to prevention has been to decrease the gastric acidity. High-potency antacids and H_2-receptor antagonists are used to achieve a gastric pH of greater than 4 to decrease the incidence of bleeding from stress gastritis. When Noseworthy and coworkers (21) evaluated medications for controlling the gastric pH, they concluded that intravenous ranitidine hydrochloride in a dosage of 200 mg/day was as effective as antacids (Maalox and Amphojel) in reducing acidity. Increasing the dose of ranitidine did not provide additional control. Certainly, any clinician using H_2-receptor antagonists should be aware of the side effects and contraindications, and some studies suggest that the colonization rates of the gastrointestinal and the respiratory tracts are increased as the gastric pH is increased. Additional studies have reported that sucralfate may decrease colonization and subsequent nosocomial pneumonia, but this has not been a consistent finding (22, 23).

Many authors have detailed the psychologic problems of being in an intensive or a critical care environment. Some patients undergoing lengthy periods of mechanical ventilation are described as becoming **"ventilatory dependent."** The patient may hyperventilate or become agitated without the familiar sense of a functioning ventilator providing assistance. This problem often requires consultation with a psychiatrist, emotional support by the staff, and subtle variations in using the ventilator. One advantage of the IMV technique is to allow a gradual decrease in the mechanical rate. To provide the patient with a psychologic sense

of security, however, one may be required to artificially cycle the machine while the patient is actually breathing spontaneously and unassisted.

Although oxygen toxicity was discussed previously, it is worthwhile repeating here that it is best to use the least amount of F_{IO_2} required. In addition, one must be prepared to evaluate and treat the patient for a pneumothorax resulting from barotrauma or misplacement of central intravenous lines.

Because infection of the respiratory tree can result from instrumentation of the airway, sterile techniques must be strictly adhered to during suctioning or bronchoscopy. Infection is also a consideration with invasive monitors, such as arterial lines, central intravenous lines, and Foley catheters.

One cannot orchestrate ventilatory support without a concern for fluid management. By following serial body weights, central venous pressures, pulmonary capillary wedge pressures, and fluid input and output, one can make an educated estimate about changing the variables. Although the kidneys and lungs often appear to have opposite requirements, the data will usually enable one to respond appropriately.

CRITERIA FOR EXTUBATION

Criteria for extubation involve various clinical and laboratory evaluations. Clinical judgment will ultimately be based on experience with the criteria. The physician must ascertain that the clinical situation is stable or improving before considering extubation. The patient's level of consciousness must also be considered, because the comatose or obtunded patient will not be able to protect the airway from obstruction or aspiration. The confused patient may not be able to cooperate with voluntary coughing and deep breathing to prevent atelectasis, and the patient who cannot clear thick and copious secretions could be at risk for postextubation decompensation. The timing of sedation or analgesia may need to be considered as well. Stability of the cardiovascular system should be evaluated by noting the need for medications, arrhythmias, abnormalities of blood pressure or pulse rate, elevated central venous pressures, and the related renal status. Certainly, a chest radiograph should be examined for areas of atelectasis so that the problem can be treated before extubation: it is embarrassing to extubate a patient and then, on reviewing a postextubation radiograph, realize a condition exists that could have been improved before removing the tube. If bronchospasm is a problem, one should consider the timing of the bronchodilator treatment to optimize the extubation process. **Nutrition** should be carefully considered in patients who are difficult to extubate, because decreased nutrition and increased caloric intake both can be problems. Use of enteral or parenteral alimentation can prevent the consequences of starvation. However, excessive calories on the day of weaning may lead to an increased respiratory effort to handle the carbon dioxide that is produced, and this may not be well tolerated by some patients. Therefore, before weaning, calories might need to be decreased and carbohydrates limited to decrease the production of carbon dioxide (24).

Table 8.4 presents the **"classical" guidelines that can be used for weaning and extubation** and is divided into three categories. **Category I** lists the basic criteria that should be met before a patient undertakes the weaning process leading to extubation. **Category II** lists the evaluations at the end of weaning that will be met by most patients who can be extubated. **Category III** lists the more sophisticated criteria that may be useful in difficult cases or those of academic interest.

The "classical" criteria determine whether the patient can clear secretions and maintain expanded alveoli. They also

Table 8.4. "Classical" Guidelines for Extubation

Category I: Criteria to Qualify for Weaning

Vital capacity (ml/kg body weight)	>15
Inspiratory force (cm H_2O)	>25
PaO$_2$ (mm Hg or torr) with FiO$_2$ ≤0.4	65–75
PaCO$_2$ (mm Hg or torr)	<55 with normal pH
pH	7.35–7.45
Resting minute ventilation	<10 L
Ability to double the minute ventilation	

Category II: Criteria to Qualify for Extubation After Weaning

PaO$_2$ (mm Hg or torr) with FiO$_2$ at 0.6	>80
PaCO$_2$ and pH as listed in category I	
Respiratory rate	<35; preferably <25

Category III: Additional Criteria

V_D/V_T (normal 0.3)	<0.6
A-aDO$_2^{1.0}$ (mm Hg or torr)	<350

evaluate the strength of the respiratory muscles, guarantee sufficient arterial hemoglobin saturation, and assess adequate ventilatory reserves.

Most patients, however, can be evaluated using the approach of Yang and Tobin (25). They found that if a ratio of the spontaneous ventilatory rate (f as breaths per minute) to the tidal volume (V_T in liters) was determined to be greater than 100 (i.e., $f/V_T > 100$), then there was a 95% probability that extubation would fail. Therefore, it is reasonable to check the f/V_T ratio before the weaning trial. Clinically, one can also observe for shallow, rapid breathing.

Weaning should be started early in the day, after the patient has had the night to rest. The patient should be sitting up rather than supine. Figure 8.1 further explains the process of weaning and extubation. If the initial evaluation of the patient's clinical status and ABGs is satisfactory, then the f/V_T ratio

is determined. If the ratio is less than 100, then a T-piece trial is begun with an F_{IO_2} of 0.40. After 30 minutes, the f/V_T ratio is again determined. If it is still below 100, then an ABG is evaluated. With a Pao_2 greater than 65 mm Hg and

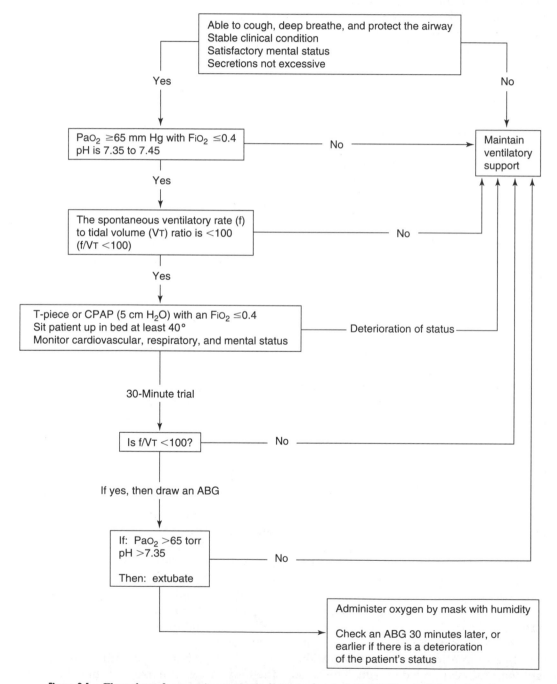

Figure 8.1.   Flow chart for weaning patients from mechanical ventilation and for extubation.

a pH greater than 7.35, the patient is a candidate for extubation. During the trial period, the patient is continuously observed for cardiovascular stability, level of consciousness, and ventilatory fatigue, and a pulse oximeter is used to follow oxyhemoglobin saturation during the weaning process.

If the patient does not meet the criteria or one's clinical judgment is negative, ventilator support is resumed until the situation improves. If the patient has been receiving 5 cm or less of PEEP during the weaning, the PEEP or CPAP does not have to be removed for the trial. In fact, maintaining 5 cm or less of CPAP during the trial has been considered to be advantageous. Before extubation, the patient is hyperinflated and suctioned. By giving a positive-pressure ventilation while removing the tube, one can often successfully cause any secretions lying above the cuff to be blown upward into the pharynx, where they can be removed by oral suctioning. **Someone skilled in intubation should be present at all extubations.**

When weaning a patient has been unsuccessful, mechanical ventilation should be resumed while the physician considers what might have caused the failure and possible therapies to improve the situation. One must evaluate the initial indications for the mechanical support and any problems that developed during intubation (e.g., infections, psychologic concerns, nutrition, cardiovascular hemodynamics, and so on).

The period after extubation requires several specific activities and orders. The patient should not be fed for a period of time (e.g., 8–24 hours) to prevent aspiration because of laryngeal incompetence that develops from having a tube in place for an extended period. In addition, if the patient requires reintubation, delaying oral intake will prevent the problem of intubating a patient with a full stomach, who is at increased risk of vomiting and aspiration. The patient can be started on an incentive spirome-

ter if his or her vital capacity is adequate ($\geq$15 mL/kg body weight). To prevent atelectasis, orders are written for deep breathing, percussion, coughing, and position changes, and supplemental oxygen with humidification is provided as necessary.

ADDITIONAL MODES OF MECHANICAL VENTILATION

High-frequency ventilation is a form of mechanical ventilatory support that is still being investigated. The original investigations were conducted while searching for an improved method of ventilation for laryngoscopy and bronchoscopy. The technique was then adapted for general mechanical ventilation. There are three basic types of ventilation included in the concept of high-frequency ventilation: (a) high-frequency positive-pressure ventilation, (b) high-frequency jet ventilation (HFJV), and (c) high-frequency oscillation.

The method that is most used clinically is HFJV, and only HFJV has been approved by the U.S. Food and Drug Administration (FDA), with the limit of a frequency less than 150 breaths per minute. The FDA has stated that the specific uses for HFJV are, at present, bronchopleural fistula, bronchoscopy, and tracheal or laryngeal surgery. HFJV has been tried in other clinical situations, but these other uses remain limited and investigative (26).

Inverse-ratio ventilation (IRV) requires positive-pressure ventilation to deliver a tidal volume with an inspiratory phase that is longer than the expiratory phase. This method improves oxygenation at a lower F_{IO_2} and lower airway pressures; however, it also requires paralysis and sedation.

Pressure-control ventilation (PCV) is a method that considers inspiration as a function of time rather than of flow. The preset pressure level is achieved during inspiration and maintained for a set time. In patients with acute respiratory distress syndrome, volume-cycled mechanical ventilation could result in airway pressures of such magnitude that barotrauma may occur. This situation is addressed when PCV is combined with IRV to provide an airway pressure that will not be exceeded and an inspiratory time that provides improved gas distribution. There is no evidence, however, that the use of PCV-IRV in patients with acute respiratory distress syndrome alters outcome.

Pressure-support ventilation (PSV) is a technique that augments a patient's respiratory efforts by supplying passive pressure during inspiration. The patient determines the respiratory rate, inspiratory and exhalatory times, and flow. Tidal volume becomes a function of respiratory compliance with each breath. By providing better synchronization between the patient and ventilator, the overall work of breathing may decrease. Weaning is accomplished by gradually decreasing the level of pressure, which is somewhat analogous to gradually decreasing the rate during SIMV weaning (27).

Positive-pressure ventilation provided by nasal mask or face mask may obviate endotracheal intubation in patients with acute respiratory failure. This method requires a patient who is alert, can protect his or her airway, and can tolerate a tight-fitting face mask. The weaknesses of this technique include noncompliance because of discomfort from the mask, pressure sores on the face (particularly on the bridge of the nose), and difficulty supplying nutrition orally or by nasogastric tube (28).

A technique of deliberately hypoventilating patients with severe airway obstruction who are on mechanical ventilation to minimize air trapping and dynamic hyperinflation is referred to as *permissive hypercarbia.* Dynamic hyperinflation may lead to hypotension or pneumothorax in these patients. Occasionally, an infusion of bicarbonate is needed to correct severe acidemia associated with the increase in Pao_2. This method should not be used in patients with suspected or documented increased intracranial pressure (29).

REFERENCES

1. O'Donohue WJ, Baker JP, Bell GM, et al. Respiratory failure in neuromuscular disease. JAMA 1976;235:733–735.
2. Kofke A. Postoperative respiratory care techniques. In: Kofke A, Levy JH, eds. Postoperative critical care procedures of the Massachusetts General Hospital. Boston: Little, Brown, 1986:32.
3. Mitchell C, Garrahy P, Peake P. Postoperative respiratory morbidity: identification and risk factors. Aust N Z J Surg 1982;52:203–209.
4. Lecky JH, Ominsky AJ. Postoperative respiratory management. Chest 1972;2:50S–57S.
5. Pontoppidon H, Geffin B, Lowenstein E. Acute respiratory failure in the adult (three parts). N Engl J Med 1972;287:690–698, 743–752, 799–806.
6. Otto CW. Respiratory intensive care. In: Lebowitz PW, ed. Clinical anesthesia: procedures of the Massachusetts General Hospital. Boston: Little, Brown, 1978:384–414.
7. Register SD, Downs JB, Stock MC, et al. Is 50% oxygen harmful? Crit Care Med 1987;6:598–601.
8. Annual refresher course lectures by the American Society of Anesthesiologists. Philadelphia: JB Lippincott. Some specific lectures are: (a) John B. Downs, Physiologic alterations of mechanical ventilation, #230, 1979; Physiological effects of mechanical ventilatory support, #133B, 1977; Weaning the ventilator-dependent patient, #142, 1984. (b) H. Barrie Fairley, Adult ARDS: Clinical aspects, #117, 1976; Respiratory "fine tuning": PEEP, CPAP, IMV, etc., #103A, 1978. (c) Robert Kirby, Respiratory "fine tuning": PEEP, CPAP, IMV, etc., #103B, 1978; Indications for and appropriate uses of PEEP/CPAP, #141, 1984. (d) Jerome Modell, Patterns of respiratory support aimed at pathophysiology, #223A, 1976; Update on means of mechanical ventilatory support, #401, 1984. (e) Barry A. Shapiro, PEEP therapy in acute lung injury, #173, 1985; Clinical management of the patient with ARDS, #412, 1987. (f) Ronald A. Harrison, Ventilation of the critically ill patient, #243, 1987.
9. Corbridge TC, Hall JB. Techniques for ventilating patients with obstructive pulmonary disease. J Crit Illness 1994;9:1027–1036.
10. Cane RD, Shapiro BA. Mechanical ventilatory support. JAMA 1985;254:87–92.
11. Willatta SM. Paralysis for ventilated patients? Yes or no? Int Crit Care Dig 1985;4:9–10.
12. Shapiro BA, Warren J, Egol AB, et al. Practice parameters for sustained neuromuscular blockade in the adult critically ill patient: an executive summary. Crit Care Med 1995;23:1601–1605.

13. Shapiro BA, Warren J, Egol AB, et al. Practice parameters for intravenous analgesia and sedation for adult patients in the intensive care unit: an executive summary. Crit Care Med 1995;23:1596–1600.

14. Novak RA, Shumaker L, Snyder JV, et al. Do periodic hyperinflations improve gas exchange in patients with hypoxemic respiratory failure? Crit Care Med 1987;12:1081–1085.

15. Winston ST, Gravelyn TR, Sitrin RG. Prevention of bradycardic responses to endotracheal suctioning by prior administration of nebulized atropine. Crit Care Med 1987;11: 1009–1011.

16. Kelly RE, Yao FSF, Artusio JF. Prevention of suction-induced hypoxemia by simultaneous oxygen insufflation. Crit Care Med 1987;9: 874–875.

17. Scanlan CL, ed. Fundamentals of respiratory care. St. Louis: Mosby–Year Book, 1995.

18. Bishop MJ. Endotracheal tubes and tracheotomies: risks and benefits in the OR and ICU, #262. In: Annual refresher course lectures by the American Society of Anesthesiologists. Philadelphia: JB Lippincott, 1987.

19. Orr JB. Helium-oxygen gas mixtures in the management of patients with airway obstruction. Ear Nose Throat J 1988;67:866–869.

20. Schmidt GA, Hall JB, et al. Management of the ventilated patient. In: Murray JF, Nadel JA, eds. Textbook of respiratory medicine. Philadelphia: WB Saunders, 1994:2640.

21. Noseworthy TW, Shustack A, Johnston RG, et al. A randomized clinical trial comparing ranitidine and antacids in critically ill patients. Crit Care Med 1987;9:817–819.

22. Driks MR, Craven DE, Celli BR, et al. Nosocomial pneumonia in intubated patients given sucralfate as compared with antacids or histamine type 2 blockers. N Engl J Med 1987;317: 1376–1382.

23. Hall JB, Schmidt GA, et al. Principles of critical care for the patient with respiratory failure. In Murray JF, Nadel JA, eds. Textbook of respiratory medicine. Philadelphia: WB Saunders, 1994:2578.

24. Beaton N, Bone CB. Criteria for weaning your patients from respirators. J Respir Dis 1985; April:80–83.

25. Yang KL, Tobin MJ. A prospective study of indexes predicting the outcome trials of weaning from mechanical ventilation. N Engl J Med 1991;324:1445–1450.

26. Gallagher TJ. Current status of high frequency ventilation, #171. In: Annual refresher course lectures by the American Society of Anesthesiologists. Philadelphia: JB Lippincott, 1986.

27. Tobin MJ, ed. Principles and practice of mechanical ventilation. New York: McGraw-Hill, 1994:Chapters 9, 11, 12, 16.

28. Meduri GU, Turner RE, Abou–Shala N, et al. Noninvasive positive pressure ventilation via face mask. First-line intervention in patients with acute hypercapnic and hypoxemic respiratory failure. Chest 1996;109:179–193.

29. Dariol R, Perret C. Mechanical controlled hypoventilation in status asthmaticus. Am Rev Respir Dis 1984;129:385–387.

9

Invasive Physiologic Monitoring in the Intensive Care Unit

Controversies and Consensus

John M. Field

Right-heart catheterization and monitoring of pulmonary artery pressure with balloon-tipped catheters has significantly advanced our knowledge and understanding of the pathophysiology of seriously ill patients. Therapeutic plans and patient response to treatment can now be objectively assessed, obviating the clinical "trial and error" technique that is not always optimal in patients who are hemodynamically or clinically unstable.

Controversy has developed, however, concerning the effective use of this technique and the patient data it generates. In addition to reviewing the principles of bedside heart catheterization, this chapter defines the current areas of concern and controversy for the practicing internist.

Initially, use of the Swan-Ganz catheter was directed at the complicated cardiac patient, but the current widespread use of this monitoring method, as well as its application to other medical and surgical conditions, make familiarity a necessity for the consulting internist. Any physician using hemodynamic monitoring should be able to answer two patient-related questions. First, what data will be obtained to discriminate between alternate treatment modalities, either of which may benefit or adversely affect the patient if undertaken? Second, what is the risk–benefit ratio and specific complications to which the patient will be exposed?

THE CONTROVERSY

After the introduction of bedside right-heart catheterization, the technique rapidly became perceived as a necessary adjunct to the treatment of critically ill patients in coronary care units. It also became identified as a tool for monitoring the physiologic status of high-risk or potentially unstable patients with a wide variety of critical illnesses. This assumed that early diagnosis or changes in physiologic parameters could prompt an intervention to eliminate or attenuate a patient's hemodynamic deterioration. Alternatively, a potentially catastrophic complication could have early and immediate recognition hemodynamically, with appropriate intervention reducing the morbidity and potential mortality of the untoward event.

Unfortunately, no study to date has proved that invasive physiologic monitoring improves patient outcome. In fact, some have suggested that patients who are subjected to this procedure have an adverse clinical course, including a higher mortality rate, lengthier stays in the ICU, and higher complication and comorbidity rates. Substantial issues remain to be studied and resolved.

HISTORICAL BACKGROUND

Frossman (1) was the first physician to catheterize the right side of the heart in a living person (himself). Perhaps foreshadowing today's controversy, however, he abandoned further study of the technique after criticism focusing on its danger, and he finally ended his career as a urologist (still a "tube man" of sorts). It was several decades until Richards (2) and Courand et al. (3) defined basic right-heart physiology through catheterization. Next, Dexter et al. (4, 5) recognized the significance of the pulmonary "wedge" pressure, and they demonstrated the usefulness of this measure in the diagnosis of congenital heart anomalies. Then, in 1970, Swan et al. (6) introduced a practical, balloon-tipped catheter (i.e., the Swan-Ganz catheter) that could guide the right-heart catheter to the pulmonary artery and wedge positions without use of fluoroscopy. This method was quickly and widely accepted by physicians caring for critically ill patients.

In 1986, it was estimated that 500,000 catheters were placed, including 100,000 in patients with acute myocardial infarction (7). The Worcester Heart Attack Study (8) analyzed the use of pulmonary artery catheters in patients with acute myocardial infarction from 1975 through 1984, and they found that use had tripled, from 7.2% in 1975 to nearly 20% in 1984. However, in this retrospective, observational study, use of the pulmonary artery catheter was associated with an increased length of hospital stay and no beneficial effects. Today, it is estimated that catheter sales in the U.S. market exceed 1 million units per year, and that a $2 billion industry exists (compliments of the pulmonary artery) (7).

THE ISSUES

During the introduction period of the Swan-Ganz catheter, it was recognized that mortality from acute myocardial infarction had reached a plateau following the development of the coronary care unit and the cardiac defibrillator. That this mortality resulted largely from hemodynamic impairment and congestive heart failure was confirmed, and Killip and Kimball (9) demonstrated that a clinical classification based on the degree of left ventricular failure was both useful and tied to mortality. Their classification did not define the exact hemodynamic status, however, and Forrester et al. (10) proposed medical therapy based on hemodynamic subsets. A logical, critical, and subsequently perceived diagnostic tool was the bedside right-heart catheter, which became indispensable for the treatment of complicated myocardial infarction. Early studies suggested that pharmacologic or mechanical support would improve the mortality rate (11, 12).

Unfortunately, the era of large, randomized, clinical trials would call these assumptions and early results into question. For example, death rates from cardiogenic shock remained high and were unaffected by hemodynamic interventions incorporating physiologic monitoring. In a community-based study, Goldberg et al. (13) reported that the incidence, prognosis, and mortality rate from cardiogenic shock had not changed from 1975 through 1988. Earlier, these same investigators had reported another community observational study on the use of pulmonary artery catheters in patients with acute myocardial infarction, which resulted in several critical reviews and editorials concerning use of the Swan-Ganz catheter (14). Robin (15, 16) even called for a moratorium on the use of these catheters pending controlled, clinical trials.

Subsequently, a randomized, controlled, clinical trial was attempted in Ontario (17), but the results were inconclusive. Only 22% of the initial 148 eligible patients were randomized, and 52 patients were excluded—because their attending physician believed it would be unethical to withhold a pulmonary artery catheter! Another recent observational study (18) not only questioned the efficacy of the pulmonary catheter but showed that right-heart catheterization was associated with an increased mortality rate and greater use of resources. A multivariate analysis failed to identify any specific related variable, but the authors noted that a missing covariable would have to increase the risk of death sixfold, and the risk of right-heart catheterization sixfold, for a truly beneficial effect to be misrepresented as harmful. These findings have again raised questions concerning the use of pulmonary catheters in the absence of controlled, clinical trials (19). The Canadian Critical Care Trials Group is currently enrolling patients in a randomized, prospective clinical trial that will evaluate use of the pulmonary artery catheter in those undergoing major surgical procedures.

CONSENSUS INDICATIONS

In the context of the data discussed here, there are no *routine* indications for pulmonary artery catheterization in the intensive care unit (ICU). This parallels the position of the American Heart Association and American College of Cardiology (AHA/ACC) Ad Hoc Task Force on Cardiac Catheterization. The AHA/ACC position statement notes that:

Although right heart catheterization is commonly considered a low risk procedure, it carries considerable risk when performed at the bedside by an inexperienced and perhaps over-confident operator . . . right heart catheterization must be conducted by physicians with expertise in the management of critically ill patients and experience in general catheterization. . . . (20)

Table 9.1. Indications for Physiologic Evaluation

I.   Establish or clarify a specific diagnosis affecting treatment or prognosis
II. Direct or initially monitor a treatment strategy known to affect outcome
III. Assist in the treatment of high-risk surgical patients in the operative/immediate postoperative period

In addition, the task force felt that routine study of the right heart in the catheterization laboratory clearly was not indicated.

The major consensus indications for bedside physiologic monitoring emphasize diagnostic uncertainty preventing the development of a specific management plan. That is, pending the results of right-heart catheterization, decisions regarding treatment will be made and acted on by the critical care team (Table 9.1). The AHA/ACC Task Force recently published guidelines for the treatment of patients with acute myocardial infarction (21) (Table 9.2).

Table 9.2. ACC/AHA Recommendations for Balloon Floatation Right-heart Catheter Monitoring in the Patient with Acute Myocardial Infarction

Class 1 (Indicated)
Severe or progressive congestive heart failure or pulmonary edema
Cardiogenic shock or progressive hypotension
Suspected mechanical complications of acute infarction
Class 2 (Possibly Indicated)
Hypotension that does not promptly respond to fluid administration in a patient without pulmonary edema
Class 3 (Not Indicated, Possibly Harmful)
Patients with acute infarction without evidence of cardiac or pulmonary complications

Adapted from Ryan TJ, Anderson JL, Antman EM, et al. ACC/AHA guidelines for the management of patients with acute myocardial infarction: a report from the American College of Cardiology/American Heart Association Task Force of Practice Guidelines (Committee on Management of Acute Myocardial Infarction). J Am Coll Cardiol 1996;28:1328–1428.

Table 9.3.   Major Complications

I.   Misinterpretation of data or waveform
II.   Access-related complications
III. Catheter-related complications

COMPLICATIONS

Complications are usually not life-threatening and, in experienced hands, occur in 3 to 5% of patients (22–24). These complications can be minimized if all members of the critical care team are experienced and familiar with the basic principles of physiologic monitoring, aware of the important preventive measures, and sensitive to the early indications of developing complications. A novice or self-fashioned interventionist as well as new members of the critical care team should be directly supervised at all times.

Fortunately, major complications (Table 9.3) are infrequent and can usually be minimized by experienced physicians. The literature is filled with case reports and reviews of minor complications that occur more often but can be amplified by an inexperienced physician. Although access and catheter complications are emphasized, perhaps the most significant "complication" is inability to interpret the physiologic data obtained and to appropriately apply these parameters to the clinical, pathophysiologic condition at hand. *An important and critical first step is cognitive validation of the clinical credibility of the data obtained.* The physician is ultimately responsible for the acquisition and integrity of this hemodynamic data, and he or she should realize that the most frequent cause of an unexpected change in hemodynamic status is shift recalibration of equipment by ICU personnel.

More frequent, major access complications include pneumothorax (especially in patients on ventilators) and hemorrhage from venous (i.e., impaired coagulation) or arterial sites (i.e., inadvertent arterial puncture). Access-sheath positioning in many novel sites has been reported, and no guide wire or dilator/sheath should be advanced against resistance or uncertainty of position. Pulmonary hemorrhage is perhaps the most catastrophic and lethal complication, and predisposing situations should be thoroughly familiar to the operator. In addition, a skilled pulmonologist or thoracic surgeon are usually essential to the patient's survival if this complication occurs.

CLINICAL COMPETENCE

It is again important to realize that mastery of cognitive skills must precede the technical attempt at positioning a pulmonary artery catheter. It then is important to recognize that successful placement initiates the intellectual-validation phase of data acquisition and its proper application to the patient. Failure to link these important steps will subject a patient to the risks of catheter placement and monitoring and the possibility of therapeutic misadventure, all for little clinical benefit.

In conjunction with the AHA and the ACC, the American College of Physicians has published guidelines for clinical competence and the "privileging" of physicians in hemodynamic monitoring (25). The necessary cognitive and technical skills are summarized in Tables 9.4 and 9.5.

CONCLUSIONS

Bedside catheterization of the pulmonary artery and thermodilution cardiac-output techniques have significantly advanced our understanding of the pathophysiology of critical illness. To date, however, the widespread use of this procedure in a heterogeneous patient population has not been shown to affect outcome in observational studies. In nonrandomized studies, the findings that patients with pulmonary artery catheters have an increased mortality rate,

Table 9.4.   Cognitive Skills Needed to Perform Hemodynamic Monitoring

I.   Knowledge of indications, with emphasis on the subtleties involved. Data obtained should be needed to make treatment decisions and to improve outcome. Obtaining high-quality hemodynamic data, even though abnormal and sometimes contrary to clinical judgment, does not of itself constitute an adequate indication.

II.   Knowledge of the anatomy of the neck, central venous system, peripheral arterial tree, heart, and lungs.

III.   Knowledge of and ability to recognize pulse waveforms for the wide array of hemodynamic conditions indicating the procedure.

IV.   Knowledge of and ability to perform the hemodynamic calculations that are possible and necessary (e.g., cardiac output, peripheral and pulmonary vascular resistance, derived measurements such as stroke volume, ventricular stroke work).

V.   Understanding the importance of and ability to recognize artifacts and clinical circumstances under which data may be misleading or difficult to obtain (e.g., situations when pulmonary capillary wedge pressure does not appropriately reflect left ventricular end-diastolic pressure, effect of pulmonary ventilation/ventilators on measurements).

VI.   Knowledge of fluid and electrolyte balance and their roles in altered hemodynamics.

VII.   Knowledge of the pharmacologic effects of drugs that alter preload, afterload, and the inotropic state.

VIII.   Knowledge of the complications of hemodynamic monitoring and appreciation of the approaches and techniques to minimize their occurrence, recognize their presence, and treat them promptly.

IX.   Knowledge of the interaction of multiple pathophysiologic states and diseases in many critically ill patients undergoing hemodynamic monitoring.

X.   Knowledge of the importance of and approach to assessing blood gases, pulmonary ventilation, and metabolic derangements.

XI.   Ability to communicate and document the examination results to the patient, the medical record, and other physicians.

Adapted from Freisinger GC, Williams S. Clinical competence in hemodynamic monitoring. A statement from the ACP/ACC/AHA Task Force on clinical privileges in cardiology. J Am Coll Cardiol 1990;15:1460–1464.

lengthier stays in the ICU, and no change in prognosis are troublesome. These do not appear to be attributable to patients who are more seriously ill receiving pulmonary artery catheters. On the other hand, the low overall complication rate cannot by itself be identified as significantly increasing morbidity and mortality.

Until additional data from clinical trials are available, it is prudent to follow the recommendations of the American College of Chest Physicians and the American

Table 9.5.   Technical Skills Needed to Perform Hemodynamic Monitoring

I.   Ability to perform surgical sterile technique.

II.   Ability to perform venous access from two (or multiple) sites with the percutaneous technique. Ability to do cut downs is also desirable.

III.   Ability to perform arterial access (primarily radial artery puncture) although ability to do arterial cutdown is desirable.

IV.   Ability to operate the instrumentation involved in hemodynamic monitoring, including catheters, introducers, and strain gauges. Ability to perform calibration, balancing, and zeroing techniques.

V.   Knowledge and ability to correct ("trouble shoot") common artifacts and technical problems with recording instrumentation and catheter/ tubings.

Adapted from Freisinger GC, Williams S. Clinical competence in hemodynamic monitoring. A statement from the ACP/ACC/AHA Task Force on clinical privileges in cardiology. J Am Coll Cardiol 1990;15:1460–1464.

Thoracic Society. In summary, these call for: *(a)* randomized trials of the catheter; *(b)* insertion of the catheter based on the specific clinical circumstances, weighing the risks and benefits; *(c)* informed patient consent, when possible; and *(d)* physicians who are proficient in the use and insertion of the catheter as well as in the anticipation, recognition, and appropriate intervention for resulting complications (26).

A focused, randomized trial such as that underway in Canada may allow us to define guidelines for the use of pulmonary artery catheterization in a specific subpopulation of critical care patients. It may also provide us with some insight into the risk–benefit issues of a larger, more heterogeneous group of patients. Until then, careful selection of patients is mandatory. The physician should have a specific diagnostic question that will impact clinical care, a therapeutic plan based on the data obtained, and a firm cognitive basis to apply this information. Once initial therapy has begun and serial measurements reflect either stabilization or improvement, pulmonary artery measurements should be discontinued. In most patients, discontinuation after 24 to 48 hours will help to minimize complications, shorten the length of stay in the ICU, and avoid bridging therapy with "routine" monitoring.

REFERENCES

1. Frossman W. Die Sondierung des rechten Herzens. Klin Wochenschr 1929;8:2085–2087.
2. Richards DW. Cardiac output by the catheterization technique in various clinical conditions. Fed Proc 1945;4:215.
3. Cournand AF, et al. Measurement of the cardiac output in man using the technique of catheterization of the right auricle or ventricle. J Clin Invest 1945;24:106–115.
4. Dexter L, Haynes FW, Burwell CS, et al. Studies of congenital heart disease. II: the pressure and oxygen content of the blood in the right auricle, right ventricle, and pulmonary artery in control patients, with observations on the oxygen saturation and source of pulmonary capillary blood. J Clin Invest 1947;26:554–560.
5. Dexter L, Haynes FW, Burwell CS, et al. Studies of congenital heart disease. I: technique of venous catheterization as a diagnostic tool. J Clin Invest 1947;26:547–553.
6. Swan HJC, et al. Catheterization of the heart in man with use of a flow directed balloon-tipped catheter. N Engl J Med 1970;283:447.
7. Gore JM, Zwenner PL. Hemodynamic monitoring of acute myocardial infarction. In: Alpert J, Francis G, eds. Coronary care. Boston: Little, Brown, 1995.
8. Gore JM, Goldberg RJ, Spodick DH, et al. A community-wide assessment of the use of pulmonary artery catheters in patients with acute myocardial infarction. Chest 1987;92:721–727.
9. Killip T III, Kimball JT. Treatment of myocardial infarction in a coronary care unit: a two year experience with 250 patients. Am J Cardiol 1967;20:457–464.
10. Forrester JF, Diamond G, Chatterjee K, Swan HJ. Medical therapy of acute myocardial infarction by the application of hemodynamic subsets (parts I & II). N Engl J Med 1976;295:1356–1362,1404–1413.
11. Held PH, Corbeij HMA, Dunselman P, et al. Hemodynamic effects of metoprolol in acute myocardial infarction. A randomized, placebo-controlled multicenter study. Am J Cardiol 1985;56:47G–54G.
12. Jugdutt BI, Warnica JW. Intravenous nitroglycerin therapy to limit myocardial infarct size, expansion, and complications. Circulation 1988;78:906–919.
13. Goldberg RJ, Gore JM, Alpert JS, et al. Cardiogenic shock after acute myocardial infarction. Incidence and mortality from a community wide perspective, 1975 to 1988. N Engl J Med 1991;325:1117–1122.
14. Eisenberg PR, Jaffe AS, Schuster DP. Clinical evaluation compared to pulmonary artery catheterization in the hemodynamic assessment of critically ill patients. Crit Care Med 1984;12:549–553.
15. Robin ED. The cult of the Swan-Ganz cather. Overuse and abuse of pulmonary flow catheters. Ann Intern Med 1985;103:445–449.
16. Robin ED. Death by pulmonary artery flow-directed catheter. Time for a moratorium [editorial]. Chest 1987;92:727–730.
17. Guyatt G, The Ontario Intensive Care Study Group. A randomized control trial of right-heart catheterization in critically ill patients. J Intensive Care Med 1991;6:91–95.
18. Connors AF, Speroff T, Dawson N, et al. for the SUPPORT Investigators. The effectiveness of right heart catheterization in the initial care of critically ill patients. JAMA 1996;276:889–897.

19. Dalen JE, Bone RC. Is it time to pull the pulmonary artery catheter? JAMA 1996;276: 916–918.

20. Pepine CJ, Allen H, Bashore T, et al. for the Ad Hoc Task Force on Cardiac Catheterization. ACC/AHA guidelines for cardiac catheterization and cardiac catheterization laboratories. Circulation 1991;84:2213–2247.

21. Ryan TJ, Anderson JL, Antman EM, et al. ACC/AHA guidelines for the management of patients with acute myocardial infarction: a report from the American College of Cardiology/American Heart Association Task Force of Practice Guidelines (Committee on Management of Acute Myocardial Infarction). J Am Coll Cardiol 1996;28:1328–1428.

22. Boyd KD, Thomas SJ, Gold J, Boyd AD. A prospective study of complications of pulmonary artery catheterization in 500 consecutive patients. Chest 1983;84:245–249.

23. Chatterjee K. Hemodynamic monitoring in critical care units. In: Hurst JW, ed. The heart. New York: McGraw-Hill, 1994:444–456.

24. Damen J, Bolton D. A prospective analysis of 1400 pulmonary artery catheterizations in patients undergoing cardiac surgery. Acta Anaesthesiol Scand 1986;30:386–392.

25. Freisinger GC, Williams S. Clinical competence in hemodynamic monitoring. A statement from the ACP/ACC/AHA Task Force on clinical privileges in cardiology. J Am Coll Cardiol 1990;15: 1460–1464.

26. Chernow B. Pulmonary artery flotation catheters. A statement by the American College of Chest Physicians and the American Thoracic Society. Chest 1997;111:261.

10

Thromboembolic Disorders

Brent G. Petty

Surgery predisposes patients to deep venous thrombophlebitis (DVT) of the lower extremities and, secondarily, to pulmonary embolism. The mechanisms for this predisposition include a direct effect of anesthesia and release of tissue thromboplastin, which induces a relatively hypercoagulable state, and reduced leg muscle contraction and venous pooling during perioperative immobility and lengthy surgery (1). Certain host factors also contribute to thrombophlebitis (1, 2), including oral contraceptives, pregnancy, obesity, age greater than 60 years, malignancy, trauma, congestive heart failure, congenital or acquired hypercoagulable states (3), or a past history of thrombophlebitis.

The risk of perioperative thrombophlebitis in patients undergoing surgery varies. It is highest in those undergoing hip surgery, knee surgery, urologic procedures, and in patients with several of the host factors listed earlier as contributing to thrombophlebitis. It is lowest in those undergoing brief procedures with small degrees of tissue disruption that are conducted in an outpatient setting (e.g., cataract surgery). In some cases, the type of anesthesia also affects risk. For example, patients undergoing hip surgery have a lower risk of DVT with regional anesthesia than with a general anesthetic (4, 5).

PREVENTION OF DEEP VENOUS THROMBOPHLEBITIS

A reasonable approach to the problem of perioperative thrombophlebitis is to assume that all patients undergoing surgery should receive prophylaxis against DVT unless the risk is very low. The physician should determine which prophylactic measures to use based on the patient's underlying medical illness, type of surgery, other risk factors, cost, and perceived safety of the prophylactic measures (6). Such an approach would improve the current underuse of accepted prophylactic strategies (7).

There are two main categories of DVT prophylaxis: pharmacologic and mechanical. The major types of pharmacologic prophylaxis include: (a) low-dose (e.g., "minidose") subcutaneous heparin, (b) adjusted-dose heparin, (c) adjusted-dose warfarin, and (d) low-molecular-weight heparins. Aspirin has been reported to be effective in preventing DVT in patients undergoing hip surgery (8). This experience has not been consistently positive, however, and aspirin has little or no efficacy in DVT prophylaxis in other surgical settings (1, 2). Dextran is not widely used because it must be given intravenously, costs more than other effective methods, and has the potential to cause or contribute to congestive heart failure. Pharmacologic prophylaxis appears to be most effective when started preoperatively, but even if started postoperatively, it is better than no treatment at all.

Mechanical prophylaxis includes graduated compression stockings and intermittent pneumatic compression devices. In all cases, however, ambulation as early as possible after surgery will decrease the risk of thromboembolic complications.

Pharmacologic Prophylaxis

Minidose subcutaneous heparin (5000 U given 2 hours before surgery and then postoperatively every 8–12 hours) has been used for many years in the prophylaxis of perioperative DVT and been the subject of many clinical trials. A particularly good meta-analysis of over 70 randomized trials involving nearly 16,000 patients showed that minidose heparin prevented approximately two-thirds of deep-vein thromboses and approximately one-half of all pulmonary emboli (9). The benefit was seen in patients undergoing general, orthopaedic, and urologic surgery (Fig. 10.1). Minidose heparin not only reduced the incidence of all pulmonary emboli but significantly reduced the incidence of fatal pulmonary emboli. Because there was no increase in mortality from other causes with minidose heparin, it produced a significant reduction in overall mortality (Fig. 10.2). Whereas minidose

heparin did increase the risk of bleeding, the absolute increase was quite small. Furthermore, the difference in bleeding between heparin and control groups was less in blinded studies than in open-label studies. This difference also was less when the analyses were limited to placebo-controlled trials. The risk of bleeding did not appear to differ when heparin was given every 8 hours compared with every 12 hours, and more-frequent dosing seems to be reasonable for heavier patients or those at higher risk and may be more effective based on meta-analysis (10). The concern about bleeding as a complication of minidose heparin prophylaxis for DVT is especially great in patients undergoing neurosurgery, in whom even a small amount of bleeding in the central nervous system can have drastic consequences. Studies have shown, however, that the rate of significant bleeding after DVT prophylaxis using postoperative minidose heparin is low and the reduction of postoperative thromboembolism substantial when minidose heparin is used in combination with pneumatic compression boots (11).

Adjusted-dose subcutaneous heparin appears to be superior to a fixed-dose regimen, but it requires more frequent monitoring and dose adjustment. In a randomized study of patients undergoing elective hip replacement (12), those randomized to 3500 U of heparin every 8 hours had a 39% incidence of DVT, whereas those whose dose was adjusted upward to achieve and maintain an activated partial thromboplastin time of 31.5 to 36.0 seconds had a 13% incidence of DVT (P <.01). The incidence of proximal vein thrombi also was reduced, from 13 of 41 patients to 2 of 38 patients (P = .003). No increased bleeding was noted in the adjusted-dose group. Despite the inconvenience for both patients and care givers, the adjusted-dose approach appears to be reasonable in patients at high risk for perioperative DVT.

Adjusted-dose warfarin therapy appears to be extremely effective in reducing

Type of surgery	Odds ratio (and 95% confidence interval)	Risk reduction (± standard deviation)
General		67% ± 4
Orthopedic		68% ± 7
Urologic		75% ± 15
Any type		68% ± 3

0.0   0.5   1.0
Heparin better │ Heparin worse
Odds ratio (heparin:control)

Figure 10.1. Apparent effects of perioperative subcutaneous heparin on reported rates of DVT in randomized trials involving patients undergoing general, orthopaedic, and urologic surgery. (Reprinted with permission from Collins R, Scrimgeour A, Yusuf S, Peto R. Reduction in fatal pulmonary embolism and venous thrombosis by perioperative administration of subcutaneous heparin: overview of results of randomized trials in general, orthopedic and urologic surgery. N Engl J Med 1988;318:1162–1173.)

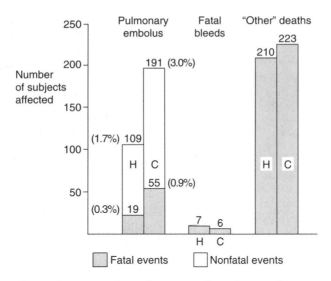

Figure 10.2. Apparent effects of perioperative subcutaneous heparin on pulmonary emboli and mortality rates in evenly randomized trials of patients undergoing general, orthopaedic, and urologic surgery. A total of 6366 patients were assigned to receive heparin (H), and 6426 were assigned as controls (C). (Reprinted with permission from Collins R, Scrimgeour A, Yusuf S, Peto R. Reduction in fatal pulmonary embolism and venous thrombosis by perioperative administration of subcutaneous heparin: overview of results of randomized trials in general, orthopedic and urologic surgery. N Engl J Med 1988,318:1162–1173.)

the incidence of perioperative thromboembolism, especially in high-risk patients such as those undergoing hip surgery (13, 14). When possible, warfarin should be started 10 to 14 days before surgery, with the prothrombin time regulated to from 1.5 to 3.0 seconds longer than control (INR, ≈1.5). Then, immediately after surgery, the dose is increased to prolong the prothrombin time to 1.5 times control (INR, ≈2.5), which is usually reached by 2 days after surgery. Using this regimen, bleeding complications affected only 4% of patients, and these patients had excessive prolongation of the prothrombin time (13).

As of August 1996, only two low-molecular-weight heparin products were marketed in the United States: enoxaparin and dalteparin. Even though these drugs are in the same class, they and other low-molecular-weight heparins that may be marketed in the future are sufficiently different in composition that it may be hazardous and inappropriate to extend the conclusions of clinical trials involving one of these agents to any of the others (15).

Enoxaparin and dalteparin have been shown to be effective in reducing the incidence of perioperative thromboembolism, including that among patients at high risk, such as those undergoing hip surgery (16–20). The approved dose of enoxaparin is 30 mg given subcutaneously every 12 hours, but clinical trials documenting its efficacy and safety also have used doses of 40 mg once daily and 20 mg every 12 hours (17, 18). The approved dose of dalteparin is 2500 U once daily. The first dose of either agent should be given 1 to 2 hours before surgery. The primary advantage of enoxaparin or dalteparin over adjusted-dose heparin or warfarin is absence of a need for monitoring the activated partial thromboplastin time or prothrombin time, respectively. Since the acquisition cost of enoxaparin or dalteparin is much greater than that of heparin or warfarin, the total cost of enoxaparin or dalteparin prophylaxis compared with adjusted-dose treatments depends primarily on assumptions or calculations of the labor costs involved in the monitoring tests during adjusted-dose therapy (21).

Mechanical Prophylaxis

Graduated compression stockings reduce venous stasis and the incidence of DVT by themselves or, more effectively, in combination with minidose heparin (22). The efficacy of intermittent pneumatic compression rivals that of minidose heparin in preventing DVT in patients undergoing general or orthopaedic surgery (2). Mechanical approaches to prophylaxis are especially popular in patients undergoing neurosurgery (23), in whom even a small increase in bleeding risk is felt to be unacceptable. Even though the mechanical methods of prophylaxis avoid the bleeding complications associated with the pharmacologic agents, they are not without risk. Peroneal nerve palsy (24), pressure necrosis (25), and dislodgment of preexisting subclinical thrombus leading to pulmonary embolism (26) have been reported following pneumatic compression.

Comparison of Prophylaxis Methods

Table 10.1 compares the pharmacologic and mechanical approaches to DVT prophylaxis in patients undergoing general surgery. The figures are based on pooled data from over 130 clinical trials involving approximately 18,000 patients. The baseline incidence of DVT in untreated control

patients, as demonstrated by fibrinogen uptake, was approximately 25%. The incidence falls by 60 to 80% with minidose heparin, low-molecular-weight heparin, warfarin, and mechanical methods. Aspirin is inadequately effective.

An even greater challenge is with hip surgery, which is possibly the most severe test of DVT prophylaxis. Table 10.2 shows pooled data from 50 clinical trials involving approximately 4000 patients in whom postoperative venography was required to confirm the diagnosis. In this group, all methods of prophylaxis except aspirin reduced the incidence of DVT, with adjusted low-dose heparin and low-molecular-weight heparin the most effective. Whereas some trials using other methods of diagnosing DVT have shown aspirin to be effective, it should be used only if the other, more effective measures are contraindicated. Table 10.3 summarizes some of the important issues involved when comparing the various approaches to DVT prophylaxis in hip surgery.

DEEP VENOUS THROMBOPHLEBITIS

In the absence of the prophylactic measures described earlier, and sometimes even when those measures are properly employed, DVT may occur in the postoperative period. DVT remains a challenging

Table 10.1.   Prevention of DVT After General Surgery[a]

	Incidence of DVT (%)	Reduction of Relative Risk (%)
Untreated controls	25	—
Minidose heparin	8	68
Low-molecular-weight heparin	5	80
Warfarin	10	60
Aspirin	20	20
Intermittent pneumatic compression	10	60
Elastic stockings	9	64

Adapted from Clagett GP, Anderson FA Jr, Heit J, Levine MN, Wheeler HB. Prevention of venous thromboembolism. Chest 1995;108(Suppl 4):3125–3345.
[a]Percentages are based on pooled data from clinical trials.

Table 10.2.   Prevention of DVT After Total Hip Replacement[a]

	Incidence of DVT (%)	Reduction of Relative Risk (%)
Untreated	51	—
Minidose heparin	34	32
Adjusted-dose heparin	11	78
Low-molecular-weight heparin	15	74
Two-step warfarin	28	45
Aspirin	56	0
Intermittent pneumatic compression	22	57
Graduated compression stockings	38	25

Adapted from Clagett GP, Anderson FA Jr, Heit J, Levine MN, Wheeler HB. Prevention of venous thromboembolism. Chest 1995; 108(Suppl 4):3125–3345.
[a]Percentages are based on pooled data from clinical trials.

diagnosis for the internist. While some patients develop classic symptoms and signs of DVT, such as unilateral leg pain, swelling, warmth, erythema, and a palpable venous cord, most develop few or even none. A high index of suspicion and early use of diagnostic testing can enhance the likelihood of identifying thrombosis of the leg veins, if present. Noninvasive tests such as Doppler ultrasonography or impedance plethysmography are fairly good at revealing the presence of proximal DVT (1). The best test to assess the leg veins for clot is venography, but this invasive test involves the systemic administration of iodinated dye, which can cause acute renal failure. In addition, venography may actually induce DVT in a small proportion of patients.

Treatment of DVT in the perioperative period is reasonably straightforward. Continuous administration of intravenous heparin to achieve an activated partial thromboplastin time of 40 to 70 seconds (1.5–2.5 times control) should be instituted. Because of recent surgery, the patient must be monitored carefully for bleeding. Those with thrombophlebitis involving only the lower leg (i.e., below the popliteal fossa) may not require anticoagulation, because the risk of pulmonary embolism in such patients is small. Regardless of the extent of the thrombosis, fibrinolytic therapy is contraindicated by

Table 10.3.   Comparison of Thrombophlebitis Prophylaxis in Patients Undergoing Hip Surgery

	Effective?	Advantages	Disadvantages
Minidose heparin	Inadequately	—	—
Adjusted-dose heparin	Yes	Inexpensive	Requires repeated aPTT tests and dose adjustment
Adjusted-dose warfarin	Yes	Inexpensive	Requires repeated PT tests and dose adjustment
Enoxaparin	Yes	No monitoring needed	Expensive
Aspirin	Inconsistent results	Inexpensive, no monitoring needed	Less effective than other methods, should be used only when other methods are contraindicated

aPTT, activated partial thromboplastin time; PT, prothrombin time.

recent surgery. Recent studies have determined that low-molecular-weight heparin appears to be as safe and effective as traditional intravenous heparin therapy for the treatment of DVT (27, 28), finding no significant difference between the two treatments in the incidence of pulmonary embolus, bleeding, or death. At least some of the patients studied were postoperative (27).

As soon as therapeutic levels of intravenous heparin have been achieved, oral therapy with warfarin should be initiated, which is usually possible the same day. Treatment with warfarin may begin with 5 to 10 mg/day for 2 to 3 days, with dose adjustments based on daily measurements of the prothrombin time. The therapeutic target for warfarin therapy is a prothrombin time of 1.5 to 2.0 times control (INR, 2.0–3.0). Because factor II levels/activity are the most resistant to warfarin therapy and factor II activity must be reduced for the patient to be truly anticoagulated with warfarin, the warfarin therapy should be administered concurrently with intravenous heparin for at least 4 to 5 days, and the prothrombin time should be in the therapeutic range before intravenous heparin therapy is discontinued. Warfarin therapy for DVT should be continued for 3 months after the patient is fully ambulatory, unless it is contraindicated by serious bleeding, a need for invasive diagnostic testing, or another surgical procedure.

PULMONARY EMBOLISM

Pulmonary embolism is the most serious and feared complication of DVT. When DVT is identified and adequately treated with anticoagulation, very few patients develop pulmonary embolism. Thus, it is critical to realize that pulmonary embolism is a preventable condition in most surgical patients.

Pulmonary embolism can be a difficult diagnosis to make if the physicians caring for the patient are not vigilant. Because of

anesthesia, sedation, or analgesia, postoperative patients may be unable to report the early, classic symptoms of pulmonary embolism, such as dyspnea or chest pain. Subtle indications, such as unexplained sinus tachycardia or low-grade fever, may be the first clues. Any patient who develops new dyspnea, tachypnea, respiratory distress, unexplained hypotension, atrial flutter or fibrillation, or persisting atelectasis should have pulmonary embolism high on their differential diagnosis. A reduced arterial oxygen saturation on pulse oximetry or reduced oxygen tension on arterial blood-gas measurement, especially in the absence of pulmonary infiltrate or pneumothorax on chest radiography, would support the diagnosis of pulmonary embolism, and preoperative measurements of either parameter could be a valuable baseline.

Ventilation-perfusion scanning is usually the first specific radiographic test for pulmonary embolism (1). A high-probability scan in a clinical setting moderately to highly suggestive of emboli is sufficient to make the diagnosis. When the test is of low or intermediate probability but the clinical suspicion remains high, pulmonary angiography may be required. This procedure generally carries a fairly low risk to the patient, and it may be important to confirm the diagnosis before subjecting the patient to the risks of anticoagulation therapy. Alternatively, positive testing for evidence of DVT (at the presumed site of clot leading to pulmonary embolism) may be sufficient corroboration of the clinical suspicion to initiate therapy.

Treatment for pulmonary embolism is similar to that for DVT, but because the patient has already sustained a serious complication of DVT and has less pulmonary reserve for subsequent embolism, the targets for anticoagulation are slightly higher. Heparin therapy should be dosed high enough to achieve an activated partial thromboplastin time of 50 to 80 seconds (2–3 times control), followed by warfarin therapy sufficient to achieve a prothrombin time of 1.75 to 2.25 times control (INR, 2.5–3.5). Warfarin therapy is generally continued for at least 6 months after the patient is ambulatory.

Sometimes, anticoagulation therapy in patients who have had postoperative pulmonary emboli is contraindicated because of active bleeding. In such patients, the physician may be forced to use mechanical measures to prevent thrombi from reaching the lungs again while trying to eliminate the cause of the bleeding and thereby allow reinstitution of anticoagulation (29). Mechanical measures include plication of the inferior vena cava or placement of an indwelling filter in the inferior vena cava. Often, however, these measures are only temporarily effective, because collaterals sufficient to allow embolism to recur may form around the site of iatrogenic obstruction. Thus, mechanical measures should be considered temporary solutions to bleeding in a patient for whom anticoagulation is desired but currently contraindicated.

REFERENCES

1. Hirsh J, Hoak J. Management of deep vein thrombosis and pulmonary embolism. Circulation 1996;93:2212–2245.
2. Clagett GP, Anderson FA Jr, Heit J, Levine MN, Wheeler HB. Prevention of venous thromboembolism. Chest 1995;108(Suppl 4):312S–334S.
3. Nachman RL, Silverstein R. Hypercoagulable states. Ann Intern Med 1993;119:819–827.
4. Sorenson RN, Pace NL. Anesthetic techniques during surgical repair of femoral neck fractures. Anesthesiology 1992;77:1095–1104.
5. Prins MH, Hirsch J. A comparison of general anesthesia and regional anesthesia as a risk factor for deep vein thrombosis following hip surgery. Thromb Haemost 1990;64:497–500.
6. Petty BG. Medical assessment and management of patients undergoing surgery. In: Stobo JD, Hellmann DB, Ladenson OW, Petty BG, Traill TA, eds. The principles and practice of medicine. 23rd ed. Norwalk: Appleton & Lange, 1996.
7. Anderson FA, Wheeler HB, Goldberg RJ, et al. Physician practices in the prevention of venous thromboembolism. Ann Intern Med 1991;115:591–595.
8. Powers PJ, Gent M, Jay RM, et al. A randomized trial of less intense postoperative warfarin vs.

9. Collins R, Scrimgeour A, Yusuf S, Peto R. Reduction in fatal pulmonary embolism and venous thrombosis by perioperative administration of subcutaneous heparin: overview of results of randomized trials in general, orthopedic and urologic surgery. N Engl J Med 1988;318:1162–1173.
10. Clagett GP, Reisch JS. Prevention of venous thromboembolism in general surgical patients: results of a meta-analysis. Ann Surg 1988;208:227–240.
11. Frim DM, Barker FG, Poletti CE, Hamilton AJ. Postoperative low-dose heparin decreases thromboembolic complications in neurosurgical patients. Neurosurgery 1992;30:830–833.
12. Leyvraz P, Richard J, Bachmann F, et al. Adjusted vs. fixed-dose subcutaneous heparin in the prevention of deep-vein thrombosis after total hip replacement. N Engl J Med 1983;309:954–958.
13. Francis CW, Marder VJ, Evarts CM, Yaukoolbodi S. Two-step warfarin therapy: prevention of postoperative venous thrombosis without excessive bleeding. JAMA 1983;249:374–378.
14. Francis CW, Pellegrini VD Jr, Marder VJ, et al. Comparison of warfarin and external pneumatic compression in prevention of venous thrombosis after total hip replacement. JAMA 1992;267:2911–2915.
15. MacFarlane LL, Weart CW. An introduction to low-molecular-weight heparins and their use in the treatment of deep venous thrombosis. Am J Therapeutics 1995;2:569–580.
16. Leclerc JR, Gurts WH, Desjardins L, et al. Prevention of venous thromboembolism after knee arthroplasty. A randomized double-blind trial comparing enoxaparin with warfarin. Ann Intern Med 1996;124:619–626.
17. Spiro TE, Johnson GJ, Christie MJ, et al. Efficacy and safety of enoxaparin to prevent deep venous thrombosis after hip replacement therapy. Ann Intern Med 1994;121:81–89.
18. Planes A, Vochelle N, Ferru J, et al. Enoxaparine low molecular weight heparin: its use in the prevention of deep venous thrombosis following total hip replacement. Haemostasis 1986;16:152–158.
19. Albada J, Nieuwenhuis HK, Sixma JJ. Treatment of acute venous thromboembolism with low-molecular-weight heparin (fragmin). Circulation 1989;80:935–940.
20. Bratt G, Aberg W, Johansson M, et al. Two daily subcutaneous injections of fragmin as compared with intravenous standard heparin in the treatment of deep venous thrombis (DVT). Thromb Haemost 1990;64:506–510.
21. Saltiel E, Sahe R. Evaluating costs of a

pharmacist-run thromboprophylaxis program. Formulary 1996;31:276–290.

22. Wille-Jorgensen P, Thorup J, Fischer A, et al. Heparin with and without graded compression stockings in the prevention of thromboembolic complications of major abdominal surgery: a randomized trial. Br J Surg 1985;72:579–581.

23. Turpie AGG, Hirsh J, Gent M, et al. J. Prevention of deep vein thrombosis in potential neurosurgical patients. A randomized trial comparing compression stockings alone or graduated compression stockings plus intermittent compression with control. Arch Intern Med 1989;149: 679–681.

24. Pittman GR. Peroneal nerve palsy following sequential pneumatic compression. JAMA 1989; 261:2201–2202.

25. Parra RO, Farber R, Feigl A. Pressure necrosis from intermittent-pneumatic-compression stockings. N Engl J Med 1989;321:1615.

26. Dwek JH, Buff DB. External pneumatic calf compression in patients with malignancy. Ann Intern Med 1988;108:344–345.

27. Levine M, Gent M, Hirsh J, et al. A comparison of low-molecular-weight heparin administered primarily at home with unfractionated heparin administered in the hospital for proximal deep-vein thrombosis. N Engl J Med 1996;334: 677–681.

28. Koopman MMW, Prandoni P, Piovella F, et al. Treatment of venous thrombosis with intravenous unfractionated heparin administered in the hospital as compared with subcutaneous low-molecular-weight heparin administered at home. N Engl J Med 1996;334:682–687.

29. Bell WR. Venous thrombosis and pulmonary embolism. In: Stobo JD, Hellmann DB, Ladenson PW, Petty BG, Traill TA, eds. The principles and practice of medicine. 23rd ed. Norwalk: Appleton & Lange, 1996.

11

Cardiovascular Disease and Hypertension

Rita A. Falcone and Roy C. Ziegelstein

GENERAL CONSIDERATIONS

The preoperative evaluation of a patient undergoing noncardiac surgery may be his or her initial entry into the medical system. The consulting internist evaluating the patient with possible cardiovascular disease therefore may be in a position not only to assess the patient's risk of perioperative cardiac morbidity and mortality but also to affect the his or her overall health care. For example, a patient with multiple cardiovascular risk factors may come to the physician's office because of leg claudication, but this patient may be of greater concern to the consultant due to symptoms or signs of myocardial ischemia.

Appropriate assessment of the patient should focus not only on the perioperative period but also on determining and reducing the risk of lifetime cardiovascular events. For this reason, the cardiovascular assessment should include a thorough patient history and physical examination, an assessment of cardiac risk factors, and baseline electrocardiography (ECG). These are important considerations for determining not only perioperative cardiac risk but also optimal long-term health care. In addition, the preoperative assessment should include factors specific to the surgical procedure, such as the type and anticipated duration of surgery, method of anesthesia, and urgency of the proposed operation; it should also determine the patient's medical comorbidities.

ASSESSMENT OF THE PATIENT

History and Physical Examination

A thorough patient history focusing on cardiovascular risk factors and symptoms or signs of myocardial ischemia, congestive heart failure (CHF), valvular heart disease, and significant cardiac arrhythmias should be obtained. Based on the results of numerous epidemiologic studies performed over the last few decades, several clinical factors have been identified as increasing the risk of cardiovascular disease (Table 11.1). These include the presence of hypertension, diabetes mellitus, cigarette smoking, a family history of premature cardiovascular disease or myocardial infarction, advanced age, and hyperlipidemia (1). In addition, results from several studies indicate that obesity and postmenopausal status increase the risk of cardiovascular events (2, 3). The patient history also should assess the patient's use of alcohol, illicit drugs, cancer chemotherapeutic agents, or other substances that may affect the heart. A past history of heart murmur, mitral valve prolapse, rheumatic heart disease, and previous cardiac surgery or cardiac diagnostic or interventional procedures should be elicited.

Symptoms of cardiovascular disease should be carefully sought. It is important to determine the characteristics of chest pain if this history is elicited. Chest pain due to myocardial ischemia (Table 11.2) typically is substernal in location and may be described as a pressure or a heaviness. It may radiate to the arm, jaw, or between the scapulae. It often is associated with shortness of breath, diaphoresis, light-headedness, nausea, and palpitations. Typically, angina pectoris is precipitated by exertional or emotional stress, and it is relieved by rest or use of nitroglycerin. Certain individuals (e.g., the elderly, women, and diabetics) may present with more atypical features. Bayer et al. (4) found that chest pain was a presenting feature of myocardial infarction only in approximately 40% of individuals over 85 years of age.

In addition to any aspects of the history that are suggestive of cardiovascular disease, the consultant should characterize the presence of other medical conditions likely to affect perioperative care and outcome. The patient's functional status should be assessed by detailed questioning of his or her activities of daily living, work habits, and involvement in and regularity of exercise. It may be useful to determine both the patient's usual activity level and the most strenuous activity within the months before surgery. The patient's activity level may be important not only as a predictor of perioperative mortality (5) but also because inactivity may mask clinically important symptoms of myocardial ischemia or other cardiovascular disease.

A complete physical examination is appropriate, but it is important to emphasize any aspects that may detect the presence of cardiopulmonary disease. Blood pressure and heart rate should be

Table 11.1.   Risk Factors for Cardiovascular Disease

Hypertension
Diabetes mellitus
Hyperlipidemia
Cigarette smoking
Family history
Age

Table 11.2.   Characteristics of Angina Pectoris

Substernal location
Quality of pressure or heaviness
Precipitation by physical activity
Relief with rest or nitroglycerin
Associated features of dyspnea, diaphoresis, and
   nausea

determined in both the supine and the standing positions to assess the intravascular volume and the possibility of autonomic dysfunction. Examination of the peripheral arterial pulses may suggest valvular disease or a secondary cause of hypertension (like coarctation of the aorta), or it may reveal vascular bruits, which may suggest the presence of atherosclerotic disease. The prevalence of coronary artery disease is as high as 70% in patients with evidence of early peripheral vascular disease (6). The jugular venous pressure, pulmonary examination, and evaluation of leg edema can help to determine clinical volume status and suggest the presence of decompensated heart failure. Careful auscultation of the heart should be performed as well to detect clinically important murmurs, gallops, and pericardial friction rub.

Factors Related to the Surgical Procedure

In addition to issues related to the physical condition of the patient, the consultant must understand any factors related to the surgical procedure so that preoperative risk can be determined and the patient's clinical status can be optimized for the proposed operation. It is important to know specific aspects of the intended operation, including the urgency of the procedure, possible alternatives to surgery, the type of surgical procedure, its anticipated duration, expected blood loss and volume shifts, and the method of anesthesia. There also may be issues specific to certain types of surgical procedures that call for preoperative measures to prepare the patient for surgery; for example, patients with prosthetic heart valves, previous episodes of infective endocarditis, cyanotic congenital heart disease, and specific valvular abnormalities (Table 11.3) require antibiotic prophylaxis against endocarditis before some surgical procedures likely to induce bacteremia (7) (Table 11.4). In addition, issues regarding

Table 11.3.   Cardiac Conditions Associated with Endocarditis

Endocarditis Prophylaxis Recommended

High-risk category
  Prosthetic cardiac valves, including bioprosthetic and homograft valves
  Previous bacterial endocarditis
  Complex cyanotic congenital heart disease (e.g., single ventricle states, transposition of the great arteries, tetralogy of Fallot)
  Surgically constructed systemic pulmonary shunts or conduits
Moderate-risk category
  Most other congenital cardiac malformations (other than listed above and below)
  Acquired valvar dysfunction (e.g., rheumatic heart disease)
  Hypertrophic cardiomyopathy
  Mitral valve prolapse with valvar regurgitation and/or thickened leaflets

Endocarditis Prophylaxis Not Recommended

Negligible-risk category (no greater risk than the general population)
  Isolated secundum atrial septal defect
  Surgical repair of atrial septal defect, ventricular septal defect, or patent ductus arteriosus (without residua beyond 6 mo)
  Previous coronary artery bypass graft surgery
  Mitral valve prolapse without valvar regurgitation
  Physiologic, functional, or innocent heart murmurs
  Previous Kawasaki disease without valvar dysfunction
  Previous rheumatic fever without valvar dysfunction
  Cardiac pacemakers (intravascular and epicardial) and implanted defibrillators

Reprinted with permission from Dajani AS, Taubert KA, Wilson W, et al. Prevention of bacterial endocarditis. Recommendations by the American Heart Association. JAMA 1997;277:1794–1801.

Table 11.4.   Other Procedures and Endocarditis Prophylaxis

Endocarditis Prophylaxis Recommended

Respiratory tract
  Tonsillectomy and/or adenoidectomy
  Surgical operations that involve respiratory mucosa
  Bronchoscopy with a rigid bronchoscope
Gastrointestinal tract[a]
  Sclerotherapy for esophageal varices
  Esophageal stricture dilation
  Endoscopic retrograde cholangiography with biliary obstruction
  Biliary tract surgery
  Surgical operations that involve intestinal mucosa
Genitourinary tract
  Prostatic surgery
  Cytoscopy
  Urethral dilation

Endocarditis Prophylaxis Not Recommended

Respiratory tract
  Endotracheal intubation
  Bronchoscopy with a flexible bronchoscope, with or without biopsy[b]
  Tympanostomy tube insertion
Gastrointestinal tract
  Transesophageal echocardiography[b]
  Endoscopy with or without gastrointestinal biopsy[b]
Genitourinary tract
  Vaginal hysterectomy[b]
  Vaginal delivery[b]
  Cesarean section
  In uninfected tissue:
    Urethral catheterization
    Uterine dilatation and curettage
    Therapeutic abortion
    Sterilization procedures
    Insertion or removal of intrauterine devices
Other
  Cardiac catheterization, including balloon angioplasty
  Implanted cardiac pacemakers, implanted defibrillators, and coronary stents
  Incision or biopsy of surgically scrubbed skin
  Circumcision

Reprinted with permission from Dajani AS, Taubert KA, Wilson W, et al. Prevention of bacterial endocarditis. Recommendations by the American Heart Association. JAMA 1997;277:1794–1801.
[a]Prophylaxis is recommended for high-risk patients but optional for medium-risk patients.
[b]Prophylaxis is optional for high-risk patients.

anticoagulation may be relevant to patients with chronic atrial fibrillation, cardiomyopathy, or prosthetic heart valves.

EFFECTIVE CONSULTATION

Formulating the Assessment

After the appropriate evaluation of both patient- and surgery-related factors, the consultant can formulate an assessment to include the estimated level of perioperative cardiac risk, specific measures to reduce this risk, and recommendations for perioperative treatment. The 1996 American College of Cardiology/American Heart Association (ACC/AHA) Guidelines for Perioperative Cardiovascular Evaluation for Noncardiac Surgery (8) established clinical predictors of increased perioperative cardiovascular risk (Table 11.5) and also classified noncardiac surgical procedures as either high, intermediate, and low cardiac risk (Table 11.6). The consultant should formulate his or her final assessment by combining these risk-stratifying tools with information specific to the patient and the intended surgical procedure.

Communicating the Assessment

Effective communication of the consultant's assessment should be timely, concise, specific, and supportive. The consultant should address the questions asked and discuss the relevant evidence used to make his or her specific recommendations. The consultant should avoid making broad generalizations unsupported by clinical evidence. For example, simply "clearing" a patient for surgery and not specifically communicating the cardiac risk and recommendations for perioperative treatment has little usefulness. It is more helpful to clearly stratify cardiac risk as either low, intermediate, or high based on the available clinical evidence. Recommendations to delay or postpone surgery so that additional diagnostic tests can be obtained or perioperative cardiac morbidity and mor-

Table 11.5. Clinical Predictors of Increased Perioperative Cardiovascular Risk

Major

Unstable coronary syndromes
  Recent myocardial infarction[a] with evidence of important ischemic risk by clinical symptoms or noninvasive study
  Unstable or severe[b] angina (Canadian class III or IV)[c]
Decompensated congestive heart failure
Significant arrhythmias
  High-grade atrioventricular block
  Symptomatic ventricular arrhythmias in the presence of underlying heart disease
  Supraventricular arrhythmias with uncontrolled ventricular rate
Severe valvular disease

Intermediate

Mild angina pectoris (Canadian class I or II)
Previous myocardial infarction by history or pathological Q waves
Compensated or previous congestive heart failure
Diabetes mellitus

Minor

Advanced age
Abnormal ECG (left ventricular hypertrophy, left bundle-branch block, ST-T abnormalities)
Rhythm other than sinus (e.g., atrial fibrillation)
Low functional capacity (e.g., inability to climb one flight of stairs with a bag of groceries)
History of stroke
Uncontrolled systemic hypertension

Reprinted with permission from Guidelines for perioperative cardiovascular evaluation for noncardiac surgery: Report of the American College of Cardiology/American Heart Association Task Force on Practice Guidelines (Committee on Perioperative Cardiovascular Evaluation for Noncardiac Surgery). J Am Coll Cardiol 1996;27:910–948.
[a]The ACC/National Database Library defines *recent MI* as greater than 7 days but less than or equal to 1 month (30 days).
[b]May include "stable" angina in patients who are unusually sedentary.
[c]Campeau L. Grading of angina pectoris. *Circulation* 1976;54:522–523.

tality can be minimized should be explicitly described. In addition, the assessment should be organized so that it clearly delineates the following:

1. Perioperative cardiac risk,
2. Suggestions to reduce the perioperative cardiac risk, and
3. Specific measures for perioperative management and follow-up.

RISK AND PREVALENCE OF MYOCARDIAL ISCHEMIA

General Considerations

Over 30 million patients undergo noncardiac surgery each year in the United States, 4 million of whom are at risk of coronary artery disease based on clinical risk factors (9). More than 1 million patients have cardiovascular complications postoperatively, thus increasing their risk for poor long-term cardiac outcome (10, 11, 12). More than 20,000 pa-

tients die of cardiac causes during the perioperative period, and 250,000 have nonfatal myocardial infarctions, CHF, or serious dysrhythmias. The health care costs associated with these adverse cardiac outcomes are significant and estimated to be in excess of $10 billion annually in the United States (13).

Cardiac complications remain an important cause of morbidity and mortality in high-risk patients after noncardiac surgery despite improvements in surgical techniques, anesthetic agents, and perioperative medical treatment. Possibly the most frequent assessment performed by the consulting primary care physician and cardiologist is quantifying a patient's risk of significant perioperative cardiac events before noncardiac surgery. This stratification of risk, especially in patients with known or suspected coronary artery disease, requires the consultant to understand both the overall condition of the patient and the risks of the proposed surgical procedure itself. This knowledge will assist the consultant in determining not only which patient is at highest risk but also which patient may benefit from alterations in treatment perioperatively.

The term *noncardiac surgery* covers a broad spectrum of operative settings, variable patient demographics and comorbid states, anesthetic techniques, institutional referral patterns, and surgical expertise, all of which need to be considered by the consultant. Assessment of surgical risk should include both the urgency and anticipated length of the proposed surgical procedure.

High-risk noncardiac surgical procedures include major emergency surgery, aortic and major vascular surgery, peripheral vascular surgery, and prolonged procedures associated with major fluid shifts (Table 11.6). Of these high-risk surgeries, vascular surgery accounts for over 500,000 procedures annually (12). The type of vascular surgical procedure planned is important in risk stratification as well. For example, the average mortality rate for vascular procedures is gener-

Table 11.6. Cardiac Risk Stratification for Noncardiac Surgical Procedures[a]

High (>5%)	Emergent major operations, particularly in elderly patients
	Aortic and other major vascular
	Peripheral vascular
	Anticipated prolonged surgical procedures associated with large fluid shifts and/or blood loss
Intermediate (<5%)	Carotid endarterectomy
	Head and neck
	Intraperitoneal and intrathoracic
	Orthopaedic
	Prostate
Low (<1%)	Endoscopic and superficial procedures
	Cataract
	Breast

Reprinted with permission from Guidelines for perioperative cardiovascular evaluation for noncardiac surgery: Report of the American College of Cardiology/American Heart Association Task Force on Practice Guidelines (Committee on Perioperative Cardiovascular Evaluation for Noncardiac Surgery). J Am Coll Cardiol 1996;27:910–948.
[a]Combined incidence of cardiac death and nonfatal myocardial infarction.

ally less than 2%, but it increases to 7% for procedures such as abdominal aortic aneurysm repair (14).

Intermediate-risk noncardiac surgical procedures are considered to include carotid endarterectomy, head and neck surgery, intraperitoneal and intrathoracic procedures, orthopaedic surgery, and prostate surgery. Low-risk noncardiac surgical procedures include endoscopy, breast surgery, as well as cataract and dermatologic procedures.

Coronary artery disease is the leading cause of both early and late mortality and morbidity following noncardiac surgery. The prevalence of atherosclerotic coronary artery disease in this population is estimated to be from 38 to 55% (14–17). The absolute risk of cardiac complications in patients with (or who are at risk for) coronary artery disease and are undergoing noncardiac surgery has been reported to be from 5 to 15% (18–22). Myocardial infarction may account for nearly 50% of postoperative mortality and morbidity in patients who undergo vascular surgery (23). Symptoms of coronary disease may be masked by a sedentary lifestyle in patients with severe peripheral vascular disease because of lower extremity claudication or previous limb amputation, thus limiting the predictive value of their clinical symptoms in determining increased cardiac risk (14). For these higher-risk procedures, risk stratification with use of noninvasive stress testing has been advocated in the hope that patients with evidence of myocardial ischemia and who are believed to be at the highest perioperative cardiac risk may benefit from further cardiac interventions, whether medical or invasive.

The lack of adequate randomized clinical trials to identify which patients benefit most from preoperative antianginal therapy or coronary revascularization limits an evidence-based approach to perioperative risk stratification with use of noninvasive cardiac stress testing. This is especially true for situations in which the surgical procedure itself is considered to be low risk, even in patients with multiple cardiac risk factors.

Preoperative Testing

General Comments

Preoperative evaluation to assess the cardiac risk of a patient before noncardiac surgery involves not only a careful history and physical examination but also an assessment of the risk of the specific surgical procedure. The consultant also must consider use of noninvasive cardiac stress testing. The sensitivity, specificity, and accuracy of the technique (along with the cost of the test) must be considered when choosing between available stress-testing modalities (Table 11.7). The prevalence of disease in the population is important as well. For example, female gender, absence of angina pectoris, and younger age can identify a population in which the prevalence of coronary artery disease may be low. A positive stress test may not have the same meaning in this population as in a population of elderly male patients with angina, in whom a high risk for coronary disease exists. In a low-prevalence population, a negative test result would more likely be correct than a positive result, and the converse would be true for a high-prevalence population. This type of risk stratification should be considered for all patients so that stress testing will be applied to those in it is most appropriate and useful (24) (Table 11.8).

The optimal approach for cardiac risk stratification in patients undergoing noncardiac surgery is still being debated. Several algorithms for systematically approaching preoperative cardiac risk assessment have been published (25–28), and in many studies (12, 19, 23), the presence of stress-induced myocardial ischemia is a significant predictor of perioperative risk. The negative predictive values of the specific stress-testing modalities studied in these patient populations are high; therefore, in a patient with

Table 11.7. Validity Measures of a Diagnostic Test

	Disease Present	Disease Absent
Test Positive	True Positive (TP)	False Positive (FP)
Test Negative	False Negative (FN)	True Negative (TN)

Sensitivity (TP/TP + FN)
  True-positive rate: percentage of patients with disease and with an abnormal test
Specificity (TN/TN + FP)
  True-negative rate: percentage of patients without disease and with a normal test
True-positive rate
  Percentage of abnormal tests in patients with the disease
False-positive rate
  Percentage of abnormal tests in patients without the disease
True-negative rate
  Percentage of normal tests in patients without the disease
False-negative rate
  Percentage of normal tests in patients with the disease
Positive predictive value
  Percentage of patients with a specific disease among a group in whom the test results are positive
Negative predictive value
  Percentage of patients without a specific disease among a group in whom the test results are negative

---

a negative stress test for myocardial ischemia, the risk of a perioperative cardiac event is relatively low. On the other hand, the positive predictive values of these same stress tests are consistently low. A patient with evidence of stress-induced myocardial ischemia may be at higher risk, but this does not always predict a poor perioperative outcome. There also is a lack of evidence that intensive, antianginal therapy or coronary revascularization lowers the postoperative risk in patients

Table 11.8. Prevalence of Coronary Artery Disease by Age and Symptoms[a]

Age (years)	Asymptomatic (% ± SD)	Typical Angina (% ± SD)
35–44		
Male	3.7 ± 2.4	80.9 ± 10.4
Female	0.7 ± 0.6	45.4 ± 18.6
45–54		
Male	0.7 ± 4.0	90.7 ± 4.9
Female	2.1 ± 1.8	67.7 ± 16.7
55–64		
Male	11.1 ± 4.9	93.9 ± 2.9
Female	5.4 ± 4.2	83.9 ± 10.8
65–74		
Male	11.3 ± 5.0	94.3 ± 2.6
Female	11.5 ± 7.8	94.7 ± 5.5

Adapted with permission from Rozanski A, Diamond GA. Cardiac stress testing: who should have it? J Cardiovasc Med 1984;293–300.
[a]Mean disease probability ± standard deviation.

with evidence of stress-induced myocardial ischemia.

Some studies raise questions about the usefulness of preoperative noninvasive stress testing before noncardiac surgery (29–32), but others suggest that it is helpful in certain patient populations (2, 18, 23, 25, 33–37). Myocardial infarction or unstable angina pectoris in the general population may be caused by an "unstable"—but not flow-limiting—coronary artery plaque. The precise mechanism of perioperative myocardial ischemia and infarction is unknown, but the presence of an unstable coronary artery plaque may play a role in this setting as well (13, 38, 39). Stress testing demonstrates myocardial ischemia by unmasking flow-limiting coronary artery stenoses (typically >70%). Myocardial infarctions may not always occur in areas of previously documented flow-limiting coronary artery stenoses (40); therefore the relatively poor positive predictive value of preoperative stress testing may be secondary to the fact that whereas existing coronary lesions are identified by stress testing, they may serve only as markers for less critical unstable coronary stenoses. Perioperative changes in adrenergic tone, plasma catecholamine levels, body temperature, fluid balance, and pain control fluctuate and may precipitate myocardial ischemia as well. Many cardiac events may be less clinically evident in the perioperative period due to an altered pain threshold, so monitoring for silent ischemia and more intensive control of postoperative hemodynamic changes may be more critical in the prevention of postoperative cardiac events.

Preoperative Clinical Predictors of Cardiac Disease

In early studies, clinical parameters suspected to be associated with coronary artery disease were proven predictors of perioperative morbidity. In the landmark prospective study of Goldman et al. (41) of patients older than 40 years undergoing noncardiac surgery, there were nine independent correlates of cardiac complications as confirmed by use of multivariate analysis:

1. Preoperative S3 or jugular venous distention;
2. Recent myocardial infarction (within 6 months);
3. More than five premature ventricular contractions per minute as documented on ECG at any time preoperatively;
4. Rhythm other than sinus or presence of premature atrial contractions preoperatively;
5. Age older than 70 years;
6. Intraperitoneal, intrathoracic, or aortic operation;
7. Emergency operation;
8. Significant aortic stenosis; and
9. Poor general medical condition.

Of note, only 80 patients (8%) underwent arterial reconstructive operations in this study. A point system, named the *Goldman Cardiac Risk Index*, was applied retrospectively to these predictors to help stratify those patients at highest risk for postoperative cardiac complications (Table 11.9).

Detsky et al. (42) validated the Goldman criteria a decade later in a series of 455 consecutive patients examined before noncardiac surgery. These authors used a modified version of the Goldman index that included other clinical parameters such as severity of angina pectoris and history of pulmonary edema. To date, this modified index has not been validated in a large series, and the disadvantage with the both indices is that many cardiac events occur even in patients with low-risk scores (43), thereby lowering the sensitivity of these methods.

Preoperative Noninvasive Stress-Testing Predictors of Cardiac Disease

Early studies only assessed clinical parameters associated with coronary artery disease, such as the Goldman and Detsky indices (41, 42), which were de-

Table 11.9.   Computation of Goldman Cardiac Risk Index

	Points
I. *History*	
Age >70 years	5
Recent myocardial infarction (<6 mo)	10
II. *Physical examination*	
S_3 gallop of jugular-vein distention	11
Important valvular aortic stenosis	3
III. *ECG*	
Rhythm other than sinus rhythm or PACs on the last preoperative ECG	7
>5 PVCs/min preoperatively	7
IV. *General status*	3
Po_2 <60 mm Hg or Pco_2 >50 mm Hg	
K <3 mEq/L or HCO_3 <20 mEq/L	
BUN >50 mg/dL or creatinine >3 mg/dL	
Abnormal SGOT	
Signs of chronic liver disease	
Bedridden state from noncardiac causes	
V. *Operation*	
Intraperitoneal, intrathoracic, or aortic	3
Emergency	4
Total possible score	53

Adapted with permission from Goldman L, Caldera DL, Nussbaum SR, et al. Multifactorial index of cardiac risk in noncardiac surgical procedures. N Engl J Med 1977;297:845–850.
PACs, premature atrial contractions; PVCs, premature ventricular contraction; SGOT, serum glutamic oxalacetic transaminase.

rived from populations with relatively low risk of coronary artery disease. Applying these clinical indices to patients undergoing vascular surgery, in whom the prevalence of coronary artery disease is high but exercise capacity is limited, may not be as reliable (43). This has led to the development of multiple preoperative, noninvasive cardiac stress-testing modalities. The ultimate goal of any preoperative stress test is to identify patients with myocardial ischemia in whom further cardiac interventions will significantly lower the perioperative cardiac risks associated with a given surgical procedure. In patients undergoing elective major vascular surgery, which carries the highest perioperative cardiac risk, noninvasive cardiac testing is helpful with cardiac risk stratification (18, 21, 23, 25, 33–37). Unfortunately, there are few prospective, randomized studies that establish the value of preoperative testing and how therapy based on

these test results affects perioperative outcomes. In most studies, biases have been present because test results were known preoperatively and may have had lead to further preoperative cardiac interventions that might have altered postoperative outcomes. Also, definitions of perioperative events and preoperative risk factors, clinical predictors, and determination of abnormal test results have varied among studies, thus limiting their applicability to more generalized patient populations.

Optimal Approach to Preoperative
Risk Stratification

Again, the main strength of most stress-testing modalities used in most studies is their high negative predictive value. Large, randomized trials are needed to assess the utility and indications for preoperative cardiac testing, however, to determine how the information is best utilized. Further studies also are needed to assess the impact of different preoperative interventions, such as coronary revascularization, in reducing both perioperative and long-term postoperative cardiac morbidity and mortality.

It is a challenging and complex task for the consultant to synthesize all the available clinical data to adequately stratify the risk for an individual patient of a specific surgical procedure. For a patient who has never had a cardiac or medical evaluation before this preoperative assessment, the benefits of such a detailed preoperative evaluation should include continued optimal, long-term medical treatment.

Summary

The 1996 ACC/AHA Task Force defined practice guidelines for perioperative cardiovascular evaluation before noncardiac surgery based on expert analysis of available data (8). These recommendations are based on a Medline search of the literature from 1975 through 1994 and a review of selected journals from 1995. These recommendations are noted in the following sections when applicable.

Noninvasive Preoperative Testing

Resting Electrocardiography

Every patient older than 40 years undergoing preoperative evaluation for noncardiac surgery should have a resting ECG performed. The baseline ECG has limited applicability in the assessment of myocardial ischemia, but it may be useful in the diagnosis of electrolyte abnormalities, significant conduction disturbances, and arrhythmias. In the AHA/ACC Task Force guidelines (8), arrhythmias such as high-grade atrioventricular block, symptomatic ventricular arrhythmias in the presence of underlying heart disease, and supraventricular arrhythmias with uncontrolled ventricular rate are major predictors of perioperative cardiac risk, and they mandate intensive treatment before surgery. Pathologic Q waves are in-

termediate predictors of risk. The presence of left ventricular hypertrophy, left bundle-branch block, ST-segment abnormalities, and rhythm other than sinus are minor predictors of risk.

Ambulatory Electrocardiography

General Comments The incidence of postoperative myocardial ischemia and infarction peaks at 48 to 72 hours after surgery, is often clinically silent, and can predict adverse perioperative outcomes (22). Ambulatory ECG can be an important tool for documenting silent or symptomatic perioperative myocardial ischemia. One limitation to this approach, however, is that many patients do not manifest these ECG changes, and many baseline ECG changes preclude interpretation of the ambulatory ECG. Preoperatively, the frequency of abnormal ST-segment changes on ambulatory ECG has been estimated to range from 9 to 39% (8). In subsequent studies, postoperative ischemic ST-segment changes on ambulatory ECG have been the strongest independent predictors of perioperative cardiac events. To date, there are no studies evaluating the perioperative and long-term effect of aggressive interventions when these ischemic changes are noted during the perioperative period (44–48).

Incidence of Perioperative Ischemia Using Continuous Ambulatory Electrocardiography The value of preoperative ischemia detected by continuous ECG monitoring in predicting postoperative events was evaluated by Raby et al. (19) in 176 consecutive patients. Of 32 patients with preoperative ischemia, 38% had postoperative cardiac events, but only one postoperative event occurred among those without preoperative ischemia. Preoperative ischemia was the most significant independent predictor of postoperative cardiac events, which suggests that continuous preoperative ECG monitoring is a significant contribution to clinical preoperative risk assessment. The absence of ischemia documented by this method carried a very high negative predictive value (99%). Other authors support these results (46).

Preoperative ischemia detected on ECG was again shown to be a major predictor of postoperative cardiac events by Raby et al. (49) in a study of 115 patients who underwent continuous ECG monitory before vascular surgery, preoperative, perioperatively, and postoperatively. There were 16 cardiac events (14%), 15 of which occurred within 48 hours of surgery, and at least 53 minutes of documented postoperative ischemia occurred before the adverse cardiac event in 88% of these patients. Those patients with cardiac events had a higher peak postoperative heart rate and had a history of diabetes, clinical manifestations of coronary artery disease, and age of 70 years or older more often than those patients without cardiac events. Of note, increases in heart rate did not correlate with episodes of ischemia, thus suggesting that ischemia often may occur at heart rates below those obtained with treadmill testing. Preoperative ischemia was the only independent correlate of postoperative cardiac events, and intraoperative ischemia was detected in only 18% of all patients. Intraoperative ischemia was a significant but relatively weak predictor of postoperative events, especially in patients with a low prevalence of coronary disease. Postoperative ischemia was more common (30% of patients) and occurred significantly more often in those with a history of diabetes and known coronary artery disease. All patients with preoperative ischemia who went on to have cardiac events had postoperative ischemia, which most often occurred in the first 24 hours postoperatively, thereby suggesting the need for more aggressive measures to lower immediate postoperative stressors.

In later studies, postoperative ischemia was determined to be the strongest independent predictor of perioperative cardiac events for both nonvascular and vascular surgical procedures, especially if the ischemic events were prolonged (44, 45, 50). In one study, periods of ST-segment depression lasting less than 30 minutes were not associated with perioperative cardiac events (45).

Postoperative ischemia has been found to be common and to have the greatest incidence and severity, but it is difficult to detect as it often is silent (22). Postoperative tachycardias have been noted to peak on postoperative days 1 and 2 and to occur before maximum ST-segment depression occurs during postoperative continuous ECG monitoring (44). Postoperative ischemia possibly is most associated with postoperative tachycardias, and extended monitoring and aggressive therapy for pain control and heart rate may be indicated during this period (22). The only variable that has been shown to predict postoperative cardiac events is ECG-documented ischemia during the early postoperative period (<48 hours). This was associated with a ninefold increase in the risk of ischemic cardiac event. Of interest, preoperative clinical variables such as hypertension, previous myocardial infarction, and a high cardiac risk index (41) failed to predict ischemic events.

Clinical Predictors of Perioperative Ischemia Using Continuous Ambulatory Electrocardiography To limit use of ambulatory ECG monitoring to those patients who would derive the most benefit, studies have been performed to identify which parameters predict those patients with the highest perioperative risk for cardiac ischemia. In a prospective study of 474 men undergoing major noncardiac surgery and who had continuous perioperative ECG monitoring to identify predictors of perioperative myocardial ischemia (51), multivariate analysis revealed five major, independent preoperative clinical predictors of postoperative myocardial ischemia:

1. Left ventricular hypertrophy by ECG,
2. Diabetes mellitus,
3. Definite coronary artery disease,
4. Use of digoxin, and
5. History of hypertension.

The risk of postoperative myocardial ischemia increased to 77% if four clinical predictors were present, and the first postoperative ischemic event occurred within the first 12 hours in 53% of patients. It must be noted, however, that the criteria used to define ischemic episodes on ambulatory ECG recordings can be less reliable in patients with ECG evidence of left ventricular hypertrophy and associated ST-segment abnormalities (52). Also, coronary revascularization procedures were performed in 24% of patients studied before noncardiac surgery, which may have improved their perioperative outcomes. The results of this study suggests that more aggressive perioperative continuous ECG monitoring may be warranted in a select group of patients with specific clinical predictors.

Long-term Postoperative Outcomes Using Continuous Ambulatory Electrocardiography There are limited data regarding the influence of perioperative ischemia on long-term postoperative outcome. One prospective study evaluated predictors of cardiac risk in male patients over a 2-year period following noncardiac surgery who had perioperative ambulatory ECG monitoring (12). Major cardiovascular complications occurred in 11% of patients. The overall mortality rate was 5%. Nearly one-third of the adverse cardiac outcomes occurred within 6 months, and two-thirds occurred within 1 year, of surgery. Five independent clinical predictors of long-term outcome were identified:

1. Known vascular disease,
2. History of CHF,
3. Known coronary artery disease,
4. Myocardial infarction and unstable angina postoperatively, and
5. Postoperative myocardial ischemia.

Patients who survived a postoperative myocardial infarction in-hospital had a 28-fold increase in the rate of subsequent cardiac complications within 6 months of surgery. Long-term adverse cardiac outcomes were preceded by in-hospital postoperative ischemia detected during ambulatory ECG monitoring in 70% of cases. The incidence of long-term adverse cardiac outcomes after noncardiac surgery is substantial; patients with acute perioperative ischemic events are at the highest risk.

Accuracy of Perioperative Continuous Ambulatory Electrocardiographic Monitoring Although the results of early studies were encouraging and suggested that preoperative monitoring for silent ischemia was accurate in predicting of cardiac risk after vascular surgery, recent data show that its sensitivity may be limited in some groups of patients. One major limitation to the more widespread use of ambulatory ECG monitoring in patients undergoing noncardiac surgery is that a significant percentage of these patients cannot be evaluated because of baseline ECG abnormalities. It is important to note that many patients were excluded from studies because of this. Also, protocols have varied, limiting the application of findings to larger groups of patients, and the lead systems used can be relatively insensitive in detecting myocardial ischemia (45). Further studies are needed to evaluate the effect of various treatment strategies on postoperative cardiac outcomes after noncardiac surgery in patients with perioperative ambulatory ECG documented ischemia.

Summary The 1996 ACC/AHA Task Force Guidelines (8) recommend that preoperative ambulatory ECG monitoring be restricted to high-risk patients in whom additional surveillance or medical intervention might be beneficial before noncardiac surgery. It should not be the only noninvasive study used before referring a patient for cardiac catheterization. During the intraoperative and postoperative period, ST-segment analysis should be reserved for high-risk patients who may benefit from further postoperative and long-term interventions.

Assessment of Left Ventricular Systolic Function

Echocardiography, radionuclide angiography, and contrast ventriculography are most often used to estimate baseline left ventricular systolic function. Left ventricular ejection fraction has been correlated with both short- and long-term prognosis in multiple studies of patients undergoing noncardiac surgery (8, 53, 54). The greatest risk of perioperative ischemic events is believed to be in patients with a resting left ventricular ejection fraction of less than 35%, but this has not been a consistent predictor (8). Some recent studies have shown that ejection fraction measurements do not predict cardiac complications after vascular surgery (8, 43, 48, 55)

A few small studies have examined the usefulness of nuclear-gated blood pool scanning for the prediction of perioperative cardiac risk in patients undergoing vascular surgery. A reduced left ventricular ejection fraction identified patients at high risk for myocardial infarction and with a reduced long-term survival after vascular surgery (8, 55, 56).

The 1996 ACC/AHA Task Force Guidelines (8) recommend that preoperative assessment of left ventricular systolic function before noncardiac surgery be limited to patients with poorly controlled, decompensated CHF (Table 11.10). In patients with a history of CHF and with dyspnea of unknown cause, however, the indications are less clear. Generally, it should not be used in patients who have not had previous CHF. Following this guideline would limit the unnecessary cost of these tests in patient populations for whom no benefit from this information is known.

Specialized Testing

General Comments Before proceeding to evaluation for myocardial ischemia with noninvasive stress-test modalities, the pretest probability (i.e., estimated prevalence) of coronary artery disease in each patient must be considered (10, 57). This

Table 11.10. Recommendations of the ACC/AHA for Preoperative Assessment of Left Ventricular Systolic Function Before Noncardiac Surgery

General agreement
  Current or poorly controlled CHF
Divergence of evidence
  History of CHF
  Dyspnea of unknown cause
Not indicated
  Routine test in patients without history of CHF

Adapted with permission from Guidelines for perioperative cardiovascular evaluation for noncardiac surgery: Report of the American College of Cardiology/American Heart Association Task Force on Practice Guidelines (Committee on Perioperative Cardiovascular Evaluation for Noncardiac Surgery). J Am Coll Cardiol 1996;27:910–948.

concept is referred to as *Bayes' theorem*, which addresses not only the sensitivity and specificity of the test being used to determine the presence of disease but also the prevalence of disease for the entire group of patients under consideration before the test is performed; this is to help determine the posttest risk of the disease. Bayes' theorem states that the predictive value of the test is predetermined by the incidence of disease in the population being evaluated. The prevalence of disease varies among clinical settings and cannot be estimated accurately from the noninvasive test result alone. For example, a false-positive result is most likely to occur in a patient group among which the particular disease is very uncommon. This Bayesian approach should be applied in the evaluation of each patient.

Predictive Value of Preoperative Stress Testing In the past 30 years, various stress-testing modalities for estimating perioperative cardiac risk in patients having noncardiac surgery have been evaluated. It also must be kept in mind that the likelihood of an adverse cardiac event occurring after noncardiac surgery, even in the subset of patients with evidence of coronary artery disease, is estimated to be less than 10% (38, 58). Stress testing is sensitive to the presence of coronary artery disease, and it often is used in the preoperative assessment. For all the stress-testing modalities studied, the positive predictive value is poor, ranging from 10 to 30%, so that a patient with a positive study result often will not have a postoperative cardiac event (even though the estimated cardiac risk is high). On the other hand, the negative predictive value for all stress-testing modalities studied has been high, ranging from 93% to 100%, so that patients without evidence of ischemia are at the lowest risk for an adverse perioperative outcome. Therefore, universal screening of all patients with stress testing before noncardiac surgery is not warranted, because potentially, the findings would not alter the postoperative prognosis in a large subset of patients.

A limited number of prospective studies have investigated the predictive value of noninvasive stress tests in determining the risk of postoperative cardiac events. Theoretically, there are significant therapeutic implications when myocardial ischemia is documented by any of these technologies, but there are no data comparing the impact of intensive medical therapy with that of coronary revascularization procedures based on the findings of these tests. Specialized cardiac testing should be limited to patients in whom the risk of significant coronary disease is high and to those undergoing the highest-risk surgical procedures; thus the test result would modify perioperative treatment both selectively and accurately. Imaging procedures such as echocardiography and nuclear scintigraphy often are incorporated, especially in patients who are unable to exercise. The cost of these procedures can be high, however, so their use must be strategically optimized.

The 1996 ACC/AHA Task Force Guidelines (8) state that the specialized testing of choice during the preoperative evaluation for noncardiac surgery in ambulatory patients is exercise ECG to determine functional capacity and to detect myocardial ischemia. In patients with ECG abnormalities or who are unable to ambulate, the choice of specialized testing using nuclear scintigraphic or echocardiographic imaging should depend on the expertise of the laboratory performing the study. If local expertise is good, then dobutamine stress echocardiography and dipyridamole-thallium have the same positive and negative predictive value, sensitivity, and specificity (59–62) (Table 11.11). Recommendations for the general use of dipyridamole-thallium can be found in the 1995 ACC/AHA Guidelines for clinical use of cardiac radionuclide imaging (63); guidelines for the use of echocardiography stress testing are currently being developed.

Exercise Stress Testing

The frequency of an abnormal exercise response depends on pertinent data from the preoperative clinical history. In patients with a normal baseline ECG and no

Table 11.11.   Sensitivity, Specificity, and Predictive Values for Noninvasive Stress-testing Modalities (60, 61, 62)

	Detection of Coronary Disease		Predictive Value (%) for Cardiac Events	
	Sensitivity	Specificity	Positive	Negative
Exercise stress testing	68–86	53–77	5–25	91–100
Dipyridamole-thallium scintigraphy	85–100	60–70	4–20	95–100
Dobutamine stress echocardiography	88–95	83–85	17–30	93–100

Table 11.12.   Cardiac Risk Stratification Using Level of Ischemic Response to Treadmill Exercise Testing

| Risk | ST Segment | | METs | PHR (%) | ECG Leads with Ischemia | Symptoms |
	Depression	Elevation				
Low	>0.1 mV	none	>7	>85	1–2	Angina
Intermediate	>0.1 mV	none	4–6	70–80	3–4	Angina
High	>0.1 mV	>0.1 mV	<4	<70	≥5	Angina

Adapted with permission from Guidelines for perioperative cardiovascular evaluation for noncardiac surgery: Report of the American College of Cardiology/American Heart Association Task Force on Practice Guidelines (Committee on Perioperative Cardiovascular Evaluation for Noncardiac Surgery). J Am Coll Cardiol 1996; 27:910–948.
PHR, Age-predicted maximal heart rate; METs, metabolic equivalents.

history of coronary disease, the exercise ECG response is abnormal in up to 25%, and it increases up to 50% in those with a history of myocardial infarction or an abnormal resting ECG (52). If an abnormal ischemic response occurs at a low cardiac workload, the positive predictive value of the test for determining a population at high cardiac risk is further increased (64–66). Most studies have shown that reduced treadmill exercise duration and exercise-induced ST-segment depression correlate with an increased likelihood of postoperative cardiac events (18, 64) (Table 11.12). Some investigators have found that the results of preoperative exercise tests are not independent predictors of cardiac risk, especially for nonvascular surgical procedures (8, 67).

In the general population being evaluated for the presence of coronary artery disease, an exercise ECG test has somewhat limited usefulness. The mean sensitivity and specificity are 68 and 77%, respectively, for detection of single-vessel disease, 81 and 66% for detection of multivessel disease, and 86 and 53% for detection of three-vessel or left main coronary disease, respectively (8). The older age of the patients undergoing noncardiac and, especially, vascular surgery reduces the sensitivity and prognostic utility of exercise stress testing in this group (52, 68). Often, these patients will have a submaximal treadmill exercise study, be-

cause they are not able to achieve their maximum predicted heart rate due to comorbid states, which can limit the study results. Patients with intermediate- to high-risk profiles who reach a cardiac workload of greater than 5 metabolic equivalents (METs) or a heart rate of greater than 75 to 85% of the maximum predicted for their age with a nonischemic ECG response are at low-risk for postoperative cardiac events (68). The results of these tests must be analyzed taking into account clinical parameters and knowledge regarding the risk of the proposed surgery for each individual patient to maximize the information obtained.

Estimation of Functional Capacity Functional capacity, or cardiac workload, can be estimated by the aerobic demands during activities of daily living and is expressed in METs (52) (Table 11.13). A 40-year-old, 70-kg man at rest has an oxygen consumption of 1 MET, or 3.5 mL of oxygen per kilogram per minute. Perioperative cardiac risk is increased in patients who are unable to achieve a 4-MET demand during normal daily activities (5, 8). Each exercise stress-testing protocol includes predetermined, estimated MET levels for each stage of exertion.

Prediction of Postoperative Events Several studies have evaluated the predictive usefulness of exercise ECG stress tests in pa-

Table 11.13. Estimated Energy Requirements of Selected Activities (MET)^{a}

Mild	Moderate	Vigorous
Horseback riding, 2.3	Mow lawn (power mower), 3.0	Cycling (moderate), 5.7
Golf (with cart), 2.5	Walking (3 mph), 3.3	Tennis (doubles), 6.0
Walking (2 mph), 2.5	Cycling, 3.5	Skiing (downhill), 6.8
	Gardening, 4.4	Climbing hills, 6.9
	Swimming (slow), 4.5	Swimming (fast), 7.0
	Walking (4 mph), 4.5	Jogging (10 min/mile), 10.2
	Golf (without cart), 4.9	Rope skipping, 12.0

Adapted with permission from Guidelines for perioperative cardiovascular evaluation for noncardiac surgery: Report of the American College of Cardiology/American Heart Association Task Force on Practice Guidelines (Committee on Perioperative Cardiovascular Evaluation for Noncardiac Surgery). J Am Coll Cardiol 1996; 27:910–948.
^{a}1 MET = 3.5 mL/kg per minute of oxygen uptake.
MET = metabolic equivalent.

tients undergoing major noncardiac surgery (8). Cutler et al. (66) studied 130 patients who underwent lower extremity peripheral vascular surgery. They found a 7% incidence of postoperative cardiac death or myocardial infarction in the entire population, which increased to 16% with evidence of stress-induced ischemia. A negative stress test for ischemia reduced the probability to 1%. Over 35% of patients were unable to reach 75% of their age-predicted maximal heart rate, and 13% of these patients had postoperative cardiac complications, one of which was fatal. Therefore, a positive ECG stress test added supplemental information even in those patients unable to achieve adequate heart-rate responses, and a negative ECG stress test had a high negative predictive value.

A patient's performance on a treadmill or bicycle ergometer also may be predictive of postoperative cardiac outcomes (69). Degree of ischemia alone on exercise ECG stress tests did not predict outcome in a study by McPhail et al. (65) of 100 consecutive patients undergoing major vascular surgery. Patients who could not reach 85% of their maximum age-predicted heart rate had a significantly higher postoperative cardiac complication rate compared with those who could reach that target heart rate (24%

versus 7%, respectively). In addition, if the exercise ECG was positive for ischemia, those who could not achieve their predicted heart rate had a 33% complication rate, whereas those who could had no cardiac complications, thereby making them a low-risk group. Only 30% of patients actually were able to achieve their maximum age-predicted heart rate, which limits the positive predictive value of exercise stress tests.

Exercise ECG stress testing alone seems to have only limited value as a preoperative screening test in patients undergoing vascular surgery and who are unable to maximally exercise, but the information obtained from the test often is useful. The level at which ischemia is evident can be used to estimate an "ischemic threshold" for a given patient to guide their perioperative medical treatment. The results of one study suggest this may support further intensification of perioperative medical therapy in high-risk patients, which may affect the incidence of perioperative cardiovascular events (70).

The ACC/AHA Guidelines for the use of preoperative exercise ECG stress testing apply to the use of ECG stress testing in the general population for determining the presence of cardiac ischemia. These indications have been summarized by the

ACC/AHA Task Force Subcommittee on Exercise Testing (52) (Table 11.14).

Nonexercise (Pharmacologic) Stress Testing

The exercise tolerance of many patients scheduled for noncardiac surgery may be limited by both comorbid diseases and symptomatic peripheral vascular disease. In this population, pharmacologic stress testing has been advocated for preoperative assessment of myocardial ischemia.

Pharmacologic stress testing techniques have been developed to either increase myocardial oxygen demand (dobutamine) or to produce coronary vasodilatation leading to a hyperemic response and coronary flow redistribution (dipyridamole or adenosine). These pharmacologic stress tests employ either echocardiographic or nuclear scintigraphic imaging. The pharmacologic stress-testing modalities that have been studied extensively in preoperative cardiac risk assessment for noncardiac, and especially vascular, surgery are dipyridamole-thallium scintigraphy and dobutamine stress echocardiography (8).

Nuclear Scintigraphy: Dipyridamole-thallium

General Comments Nuclear scanning techniques to predict adverse cardiac events after noncardiac surgery typically use dipyridamole-thallium scintigraphy (8). An abnormal preoperative dipyridamole-thallium scan is a sensitive marker of patients likely to have a postoperative cardiac event (8, 18, 21, 23, 34, 37, 54, 71–74). Pooled data show that the positive predictive value for adverse cardiac outcomes of this technique ranges from 36 to 45%. The negative predictive value, however, is high (approximately 97%); therefore, patients without redistribution defects have the lowest postoperative cardiac risk. In several studies, presence of a fixed defect had no predictive value for adverse postoperative cardiac outcomes (18, 21, 23, 34, 37, 71, 75, 76), but in two studies, there was a higher risk for a perioperative event compared with that in patients with no thallium defect (10, 58). Evidence also exists that long-term cardiac event rates are indistinguishable between fixed and reversible thallium defects (36, 77, 78).

Use of intravenous dipyridamole is contraindicated in patients with significant bronchospasm or who are dependent on theophylline preparations. Use of caffeine or other methylxanthines within 24 hours of the study, or of theophylline within 72 hours, is contraindicated as well. Both are adenosine-receptor antagonists, and they may abolish the coronary vasodilatation that is induced by dipyridamole and lead to a false-negative result.

Predicting Postoperative Cardiac Risk Boucher et al. (21) first described use of dipyridamole-thallium imaging as a predictor of adverse postoperative cardiac

---

Table 11.14.   Guidelines for Use of Preoperative Exercise ECG Stress-testing to Predict Perioperative Cardiac Outcomes

General agreement
Assist in diagnosis of coronary artery disease in male patients with atypical chest pain
Assess functional capacity and aid in assessing prognosis of patients with known coronary artery disease
Evaluate prognosis and functional capacity of patients with coronary artery disease soon after an uncomplicated myocardial infarction
Divergence of opinion
Evaluate asymptomatic male patients older than 40 years with special occupations
Evaluate asymptomatic males older than 40 years with two or more risk factors for coronary artery disease
Assist in diagnosis of coronary artery disease in women with a history of typical or atypical angina pectoris
Evaluate patients with baseline ECG changes that limit the value of the exercise testing
Evaluate response to therapy with cardiovascular drugs in patients with coronary artery disease or CHF

Adapted with permission from Clinical competence in exercise testing: a statement for physicians from the ACP/ACC/AHA Task Force on Clinical Privileges in Cardiology. J Am Coll Cardiol 1990;1061–1065.

outcomes in noncardiac surgery. Fifty-four patients were studied before elective abdominal aortic or lower extremity vascular surgery. High-risk patients with unstable coronary syndromes and low-risk patients with no clinical history of coronary disease were excluded. Abnormal thallium scans were present in 63% of patients. Among the 17% of patients with postoperative ischemic events, there was one cardiac death and two acute myocardial infarctions. Half of these patients had an abnormal dipyridamole-thallium scan. No adverse cardiac events occurred in those patients with a normal thallium scan or with a thallium scan without redistribution. Clinical factors did not predict adverse cardiac outcomes, but thallium redistribution identified high-risk patients with a sensitivity of 100% and a specificity of 73%. Preoperative dipyridamole-thallium scintigraphy therefore was superior to the clinical assessment alone in determination of cardiac risk. Patients with a negative scan were at the lowest risk for postoperative cardiac events. Of all patients with an abnormal thallium scan, six underwent coronary angiography before vascular surgery, and all had multivessel coronary disease. Coronary artery bypass graft (CABG) surgery was performed in four of these 6 patients, who then proceeded to undergo elective vascular surgery without complications.

The results of many studies support use of preoperative dipyridamole-thallium scintigraphy, in combination with clinical parameters, to identify patients at high risk for adverse cardiac outcomes after noncardiac surgery. In a study by Eagle et al. (23) of 61 patients before major vascular surgery, a preoperative abnormal dipyridamole-thallium scan was the most significant predictor of postoperative ischemic events, estimating the likelihood of an event at 45% (compared with 7% if the scan was negative). The only clinical predictors of postoperative events were pathologic Q waves on ECG and evidence of thallium redistribution. Patients with

no clinical predictors were stratified into the lowest perioperative cardiac risk group. Because their perioperative outcomes were not affected by the results of the scan, the authors believed these patients may not have needed preoperative dipyridamole-thallium scintigraphy. Dipyridamole-thallium scintigraphy more accurately stratified patients with multiple clinical predictors into higher-risk groups. Notably, a large subset of patients with a reversible thallium defect did well postoperatively, thus suggesting that occult coronary disease did not have a significant clinical impact perioperatively in this group.

In a second observational study, Eagle et al. (25) evaluated clinical variables and results of dipyridamole-thallium studies retrospectively in 254 consecutive patients undergoing vascular surgery. Fifteen percent of these patients had postoperative cardiac ischemic events. There was a 3% mortality rate and a 5% nonfatal myocardial infarction rate. Five clinical variables were found to be predictors of postoperative cardiac events:

1. Age older than 70 years,
2. Q waves on baseline ECG,
3. History of angina,
4. Ventricular ectopic activity requiring therapy, and
5. Diabetes mellitus.

Dipyridamole-thallium scintigraphy was found to be most useful in further stratifying patients who were considered at be at intermediate clinical risk. In this group, a redistribution defect was associated with a 30% event rate, compared with a 3% rate in patients without thallium redistribution. Both the Goldman and the modified Goldman indices (41, 79) were not independent predictors of adverse outcome. The combination of a thorough clinical evaluation and dipyridamole-thallium scintigraphy was important in determining cardiac risk. In more than half the patients, however, dipyridamole-thallium stress test did not add incremental information to the preoperative assessment after the clinical variables were evaluated. Other studies support these findings (18).

Lette et al. (68) have challenged the findings of Eagle et al. (25), finding that clinical criteria were not useful in estimating postoperative risk. Using 18 clinical parameters and several scoring systems, including the Eagle clinical criteria discussed earlier), 10% of patients undergoing vascular surgery had adverse cardiac outcomes postoperatively. Clinical parameters were not predictors of these events. The dipyridamole-thallium scans were the only predictors of postoperative cardiac events. Adverse cardiac outcomes occurred in 21% of patients with thallium redistribution and in no patients without thallium evidence of ischemia or with only a fixed thallium defect.

Number and Extent of Redistribution Defects Dipyridamole-thallium scans with an increased number and size of redistribution defects, presence of left ventricular dilatation after stress, or pulmonary radiotracer uptake are predictive of a higher postoperative risk (37, 68, 71, 75).

Dipyridamole-thallium scintigraphy in patients undergoing abdominal aortic surgery has been studied prospectively (34), and postoperative myocardial infarctions occurred in 26% of patients with abnormal thallium scans. The presence of ischemia in two or more myocardial territories was a significant predictor of adverse outcomes; those patients had a 12-fold increased likelihood of a postoperative ischemic event. In the 53% of patients with normal thallium scans, there were no events. Therefore, the dipyridamole-thallium scan provided a sensitivity of 100% and a specificity of 61%. Significant coronary artery disease was noted in all patients who had cardiac angiography, and 35% of patients underwent CABG before noncardiac surgery. Only those patients with an abnormal preoperative dipyridamole thallium scan were felt to warrant further cardiac evaluation before elective vascular surgery.

Accuracy of Evaluation The accuracy of dipyridamole-thallium in the preoperative evaluation of patients undergoing noncardiac surgery recently has been challenged (31, 32, 80, 81). In one study, intraoperative myocardial ischemia was assessed with use of continuous ECG monitoring and transesophageal echocardiography in patients during vascular surgery (31). All underwent dipyridamole-thallium scintigraphy preoperatively, and all treating physicians were blinded to the results. Thirty-seven percent of patients had redistribution defects, 30% had fixed defects, and 33% had normal scans. There was a 5% incidence of adverse postoperative cardiac outcomes and no association between redistribution defects and adverse cardiac outcomes or perioperative ischemia. The sensitivity of thallium scintigraphy for all adverse outcomes ranged from 40 to 54%, specificity from 65 to 71%, positive predictive value from 27 to 47%, and negative predictive value from 61 to 82%. These results show a lower sensitivity than previous studies, and the authors proposed that routine preoperative screening with dipyridamole-thallium scintigraphy may not be warranted in those patients scheduled for vascular surgery. A study by Baron et al. (32) using a different scanning technique confirmed these findings.

Single-photon Emission Computed Tomography More recently, single-photon emission computed tomography (SPECT) has been found to have increased sensitivity in the detection of detect coronary artery disease when compared with that of planar studies (73, 76). There is conflicting evidence, however, regarding whether redistribution defects as determined using this method are predictive of adverse cardiac outcomes in patients being evaluated before vascular surgery.

In a prospective study, there was an additive predictive value of reinjection thallium SPECT over clinical risk factors in patients undergoing aortic abdominal surgery (76). The presence of a fixed defect conferred a lower perioperative risk, and these findings have been supported by those of other studies (72, 73). In contrast, results of preoperative dipyridamole-thallium SPECT did not accurately predict adverse postoperative events in a similar population of patients undergoing aortic abdominal surgery (32), and use of dipyridamole-thallium SPECT for screening before aortic abdominal surgery was not believed to have prognostic value. Larger, prospective studies are necessary to determine if this technique provides equivalent prognostic information to that from dipyridamole-thallium scintigraphy and other stress-testing modalities.

Long-term Prognosis Following Noncardiac Surgery   Few studies have evaluated the long-term postoperative outcomes of patients with abnormal dipyridamole-thallium scans. In one such study, event rates were reported over a follow-up period of 18 months after peripheral vascular surgery (36). An abnormal dipyridamole-thallium scan was associated with a significantly increased risk of cardiac death in the perioperative period (7%) and late follow-up period (17%) compared with risk in patients with a normal scan. A reversible thallium defect was the only predictor of death or myocardial infarction during late follow-up, and it was associated with a risk of a cardiac event twofold greater than that with a fixed defect. The number of perfusion defects, history of angina, and the presence of chest pain during the dipyridamole study were independent predictors of perioperative cardiac events.

Newer Myocardial Perfusion Tracers   Initial data on use of technetium-99m sestamibi (a newer myocardial perfusion tracer) indicate it has the same diagnostic accuracy as thallium-201 for the detection of myocardial ischemia (82). Further stud-

ies are necessary, however, to determine if this technique provides prognostic information in the preoperative evaluation of patients before noncardiac surgery equivalent to that from other stress-testing modalities.

Summary   The ACC/AHA Guidelines concerning indications for stress testing with myocardial perfusion imaging apply to use of dipyridamole-thallium scintigraphy in the general population, and there are no additional, specific recommendations for patients undergoing noncardiac surgery (63). Use of pharmacologic or exercise perfusion imaging for risk stratification before noncardiac surgery is considered to be a class I recommendation (i.e., usually appropriate and considered to be useful).

Recently, the ACC/AHA Task Force algorithm for perioperative cardiovascular risk stratification before noncardiac surgery was applied to high-risk patients before major vascular surgery (83). An evaluation of functional status was incorporated to stratify patients after clinical variables had been assessed. Patients were then stratified into low-, intermediate-, and high-risk groups. Use of dipyridamole-thallium scintigraphy was randomized in the higher-risk patients and in intermediate-risk patients with a low functional capacity (<5 METs). The overall mortality for all groups combined was 3.5%, whereas the cardiac mortality rate was 1%. Two patients in the intermediate-risk group died of cardiac causes; no cardiac deaths occurred in the other groups. The cardiac morbidity rate was 12.4%, and there was no statistically significant difference between groups. There was no single independent predictor of morbidity. Cardiac risk stratification using a modified version of the proposed ACC/AHA Task Force Guidelines algorithm for high-risk patients has demonstrated an excellent clinical outcome and proved to be a safe and economical strategy in this protocol.

Dobutamine Stress Echocardiography

General Comments Dobutamine stress echocardiography involves the identification of new or worsening myocardial wall motion abnormalities using two-dimensional echocardiography during the intravenous infusion of dobutamine. It has the same accuracy as dipyridamole-thallium scintigraphy for the detection of coronary artery disease (29, 62, 84, 85), and it is sensitive for the assessment of preoperative cardiac risk in patients undergoing noncardiac surgery (8, 60, 86, 87). The estimated positive predictive value (17–43%) and negative predictive value (93–100%) are similar to those for dipyridamole-thallium scintigraphy (21, 23, 31, 34, 60, 62, 88). Dobutamine stress echocardiography has several advantages, however, over dipyridamole-thallium scintigraphy (Table 11.15): *(a)* left ventricular function and valvular abnormalities also are assessed, *(b)* the cost of the procedure is significantly lower (60, 62), *(c)* there is no exposure to radiation, *(d)* the duration of the study is significantly shorter, and *(e)* results are immediately available.

Use of dipyridamole echocardiography for the prediction of perioperative events after vascular surgery, which is reported to have high specificity for the detection of coronary artery disease, has been evaluated as well (89). Preliminary results suggest it has similar sensitivity and specificity but potentially higher positive predictive value than dobutamine, echocardiography, dipyridamole, thallium, scintigraphy, or ambulatory ECG. Further studies are needed to confirm the results of this study and to assess its safety profile in patients undergoing noncardiac surgery.

Several studies have examined the value of dobutamine stress echocardiography in preoperative risk assessment. In one of the first such studies, postoperative cardiac events were noted in 21% of 57 patients undergoing noncardiac surgery with evidence of preoperative dobutamine stress-induced myocardial ischemia, whereas no patient had a cardiac event if ischemia was not observed on the preoperative test (35). Similar findings have been reported by other authors: a high sensitivity (100%) (61, 62) and negative predictive value (100%) (61, 62, 90) for early postoperative cardiac events. The results of dobutamine stress echocardiography add significantly to the assessment of clinical risk in patients undergoing major vascular surgery (62), particularly in patients with intermediate clinical risk (90). As with other forms of preoperative risk assessment, however, dobutamine stress echocardiography has

Table 11.15.   Advantages and Disadvantages of Preoperative Evaluation Using Dipyridamole-Thallium Scintigraphy and Dobutamine Stress Echocardiography for Noncardiac Surgery

	Advantages	Disadvantages
Dipyridamole-thallium scintigraphy	Safe Validated	Higher cost Radiation exposure Long duration of test Side effects
Dobutamine stress echocardiography	Safe Validated Assessment of left ventricular function Assessment of valvular abnormalities Short duration of test Lower cost No radiation exposure	Side effects

a relatively low positive predictive value (61), and many patients with abnormal test results do not have postoperative cardiac events.

The predictive value of dobutamine stress echocardiography may extend beyond the immediate postoperative period, however. In one study, 20% of patients undergoing aortic surgery had a cardiac event within the first 30 postoperative days, including cardiac deaths in 5% and nonfatal myocardial infarctions in 10% (87). Over 90% of these events occurred in patients with dobutamine stress-induced ischemia. Only one cardiac event occurred among patients without stress-induced ischemia. The high negative predictive value (95%) and relatively low positive predictive value (29%) are similar to those reported for use of dipyridamole-thallium scintigraphy in patients undergoing major vascular surgery (Table 11.11).

Long-term Risk Assessment after Noncardiac Surgery Few studies have evaluated long-term outcomes after non-cardiac surgery in patients with abnormal preoperative dobutamine stress echocardiograms. In one study, 98 patients underwent dobutamine stress echocardiography before major vascular surgery and were followed for up to 2 years (60). Among those with a negative dobutamine stress echocardiogram, there were two cardiac events (3%). Among patients with a positive dobutamine stress echocardiogram, however, 68% underwent subsequent coronary revascularization before the non-cardiac surgery was performed, and there were no perioperative events in this group. Among patients with a positive dobutamine stress echocardiogram who did not have coronary revascularization, 40% had an adverse perioperative cardiac outcomes. Long-term complications were noted in 3% of those with a negative dobutamine stress echocardiogram and in 15% of those with a positive study. Dobutamine stress echocardiography was found to be safe and to predict both perioperative and long-term outcome in patients undergoing major vascular surgery; a negative dobutamine stress echocardiogram was found to be a strong predictor of low perioperative cardiac morbidity and mortality.

In a second study, patients undergoing major vascular surgery were evaluated with use of clinical parameters and results of dobutamine stress echocardiography and followed for an average of 19 months postoperatively (91). Cardiac events occurred in 10% of these patients. Extensive dobutamine-induced wall motion abnormalities and a history of myocardial infarction independently predicted late cardiac events, increasing the estimate of risk up to sixfold. Patients with these findings may need more intensive perioperative treatment to decrease the chance of long-term, adverse cardiac outcomes.

Summary Dobutamine stress echocardiography is both safe and accurate for preoperative cardiac risk stratification in patients undergoing noncardiac surgery. The negative predictive value is high; therefore patients without evidence of inducible ischemia are at low risk for adverse cardiac outcomes. The positive predictive value remains low, however, similar to that for dipyridamole-thallium scintigraphy. A meta-analysis of 15 studies to compare dipyridamole-thallium and dobutamine echocardiography for risk stratification before vascular surgery in intermediate-risk patients found the prognostic value of both noninvasive stress imaging techniques to be comparable but the accuracy to vary with the prevalence of coronary artery disease (88). Indications for use of dobutamine stress echocardiography before noncardiac surgery are similar to those for stress testing in the general population. Formal ACC/AHA Guidelines and indications for use of echocardiographic stress testing are pending.

CORONARY REVASCULARIZATION PROCEDURES

Coronary Angiography

Historically, some physicians have advocated routine use of coronary angiography in all patients as a screening procedure before elective peripheral vascular surgical procedures (92). This has been recommended on the basis of the high perioperative mortality rate and the prevalence of asymptomatic coronary artery disease among this group (approximately, 30–50%) (36). There is some evidence that preoperative revascularization may decrease postoperative cardiac risk by two- to fourfold in patients undergoing elective vascular surgery (93–95). Hertzer et al. (92), in a study of 1000 patients undergoing preoperative coronary angiography, found that 40% had no or insignificant coronary artery disease, 29% had disease not requiring coronary revascularization, 25% had severe disease warranting revascularization, and 6% had severe inoperable disease. CABG was performed in 96% of patients with correctable coronary disease before noncardiac surgery; the mortality rate among these patients was 5.2%. Only one postoperative death (0.07%), however, occurred in the patients who survived CABG and went on to have vascular surgery, whereas the overall operative mortality rate for cardiac and noncardiac procedures combined was 2.6%. This indicates that a significant proportion of patients had inoperable or severe coronary artery disease, and that the risk of adverse cardiac outcomes after noncardiac surgery in these patients may be reduced when a prior CABG procedure is successful (but with the added risk of morbidity and mortality from the CABG surgery) (92).

Many argue that performing cardiac catheterization on all patients scheduled for major vascular surgery is too costly and places patients at still-further risk due to the cumulative risks of these procedures. This has led to increased interest in preoperative noninvasive stress testing to assist in the risk stratification of these patients (96). It generally is assumed that coronary angiography should be performed preoperatively in patients with a redistribution defect on dipyridamole-thallium scintigraphy or inducible ischemia on dobutamine stress echocardiography (21, 23, 34, 36), but the results of no published, randomized trials support this approach. In addition, even when stress tests reveal evidence of myocardial ischemia, noncardiac surgery can be performed safely. On the other hand, coronary angiography may be considered when a stress test is negative in a patient with significant risk factors and a history that is suggestive of angina, because this may represent a false-negative stress test result.

The current indications for use of coronary angiography in the perioperative evaluation before noncardiac surgery are adapted from the ACC/AHA Guidelines and indications for coronary angiography in the general population (97) (Table 11.16). It generally is agreed that coronary angiography should be considered in patients with unstable symptoms of angina pectoris, high risk or equivocal preoperative noninvasive stress test results, or high-risk clinical parameters who are undergoing a high-risk, noncardiac surgical procedure. It also generally is agreed that coronary angiography is not indicated in patients with low-risk results of preoperative noninvasive testing, in those who are asymptomatic up to 5 years after previous coronary revascularization if they exhibit excellent exercise capacity (>7 METs), or for screening for coronary artery disease without a previous noninvasive test.

Coronary Artery Bypass Graft Surgery

Coronary artery disease significantly increases the risk for a cardiac event perioperatively in patients undergoing

Table 11.16.   Indications for Coronary Angiography in Perioperative Evaluation Before Noncardiac Surgery

General agreement
  High-risk results of stress test
  Refractory angina
  Unstable angina
  Equivocal noninvasive test results in high-risk patients undergoing high-risk surgery
Divergence of evidence
  Intermediate stress test results
  Equivocal noninvasive test in low-risk patients undergoing high-risk surgery
  Urgent surgery after acute myocardial infarction
  Perioperative myocardial infarction
Procedure not indicated
  Low-risk surgery with low-risk stress test results
  Screening without stress test
  Asymptomatic after coronary revascularization with excellent (>7 METs) functional capacity
  Mild, stable angina with good left ventricular function and low-risk noninvasive test results
  Previous cardiac catheterization within 5 years
  Left ventricular ejection fraction <20%, patient not a candidate for revascularization

Adapted with permission from Guidelines for perioperative cardiovascular evaluation for noncardiac surgery: Report of the American College of Cardiology/American Heart Association Task Force on Practice Guidelines (Committee on Perioperative Cardiovascular Evaluation for Noncardiac Surgery). J Am Coll Cardiol 1996; 27:910–948; and Guidelines for coronary angiography: a report of the American College of Cardiology/American Heart Association Task Force on Assessment of Diagnostic and Therapeutic Cardiovascular Procedures (Subcommittee on Coronary Angiography). J Am Coll Cardiol 1987;10:935–950.

noncardiac surgery (14–16, 98–100). The results of many studies support the notion that evidence of myocardial ischemia on preoperative stress testing determines a higher postoperative risk, but no prospective, randomized trials have assessed whether CABG surgery lowers the perioperative cardiac risk in patients undergoing noncardiac surgery (101). Many patients who are referred for noncardiac surgery, and for especially vascular surgery, are elderly and have comorbid conditions, and it is these patients in whom the risks of CABG surgery itself are significant (4.6–9.5%) (92, 102). Several nonrandomized and uncontrolled studies suggest that CABG surgery can reduce the postoperative risk following vascular surgery if the patient is believed to be at low risk for the CABG itself (15, 92, 103–107).

The influence of CABG on perioperative cardiac risks before noncardiac surgery was studied in a subset of patients in the Coronary Artery Surgery Study (CASS) Registry enrolled from 1978 to 1981 (107). The operative mortality rate for noncardiac surgery in patients without significant coronary artery disease was 0.5%. The operative mortality rate for patients who had CABG surgery before noncardiac surgery was 0.9%, but it was significantly higher (2.4%) in patients with significant coronary artery disease who did not have CABG prior to noncardiac surgery. There was a 1.4% mortality rate associated with the CABG procedure itself, however (101).

Another early study evaluated the proper timing and both the early and long-term outcomes of patients who had undergone both CABG and major vascular surgery between 1976 and 1984 (108). Among these patients, 23% had the procedures performed simultaneously, 26% had both operations performed during the same hospitalization, and 51% had the procedures performed during different hospitalizations. The overall postoperative mortality rate for each group was 4, 4, and 0.2%, respectively. There was a cardiac mortality rate of 3% in those with simultaneous surgery, 2.2% in the groups undergoing both surgeries in the same hospitalization, and no cardiac deaths in the group who had separate hospitalizations for the procedures. Late (5-year) survival rates did not differ among the groups. CABG surgery was found to be protective in all patient groups, especially when peripheral vascular operations were performed at a later date.

In summary, few data support the use of CABG surgery solely to improve perioperative outcomes in patients undergoing noncardiac surgery. The indications for CABG surgery are based on the 1991 ACC/AHA Task Force Guidelines and indications for CABG for the general population (109) (Table 11.17). Indications include patients with significant left main stenosis (>50%), three-vessel coronary artery disease with left ventricular dysfunction, two-vessel disease with severe proximal left anterior descending artery disease, and intractable ischemia after maximal medical therapy. Timing of CABG surgery before noncardiac surgery is an individualized decision, and there are no prospective, randomized data to suggest the optimal strategy.

Percutaneous Transluminal Coronary Angioplasty

The benefit of percutaneous transluminal angioplasty (PTCA) before noncardiac surgery to reduce the incidence of perioperative cardiac events has not been studied in a prospective, randomized fashion. Huber et al. (110) performed a small, retrospective study of patients considered to be at high risk for coronary artery disease. All patients underwent PTCA before noncardiac surgery, and 10% required urgent CABG surgery. The noncardiac surgery perioperative myocardial infarction rate was 5.6%, and the cardiac mortality rate was 1.9%. Successful preoperative PTCA in high-risk patients was associated with a low perioperative cardiac risk during noncardiac surgery.

In a large, 10-year study of patients who underwent PTCA, CABG surgery, or both before elective abdominal aortic aneurysm surgery from 1980 to 1990, there were no perioperative deaths in patients with previous coronary revascularization, compared with a 2.9% perioperative mortality rate within 1 year following the surgery for the group as a whole (111). The cause of death was cardiac in 60%. Of note, the trend to perform coronary revascularization preoperatively increased as the decade progressed. CABG did delay the

Table 11.17. Pertinent 1991 ACC/AHA Task Force Guidelines and Indications for CABG in Patients Undergoing Noncardiac Surgery

CABG indicated
  Asymptomatic patients with noninvasive test results indicative of myocardial ischemia
    with:
    Significant left main disease, or
    Significant three-vessel coronary artery disease with proximal stenosis of a large left anterior
      descending coronary artery
  Chronic stable angina (class III–IV)
  Unstable (rest or postinfarction) angina when intensive medical therapy fails
  Myocardial infarction with hemodynamic compromise
Divergence of opinion on indication
  Uncomplicated acute Q-wave myocardial infarction
CABG not indicated
  Asymptomatic patients with no myocardial ischemia on noninvasive testing

time to aortic abdominal aneurysm repair, but this was not statistically significant. The 3-year survival rate was the same with either revascularization procedure (92% with PTCA versus 83% with CABG surgery), but patients undergoing PTCA had significantly more late events at 3 years (56.5% versus 27.3%, respectively). This may result from the increased rate of coronary restenosis in this time period and to the small number of patients undergoing PTCA, and the results of this study may suggest that in a select group of patients undergoing abdominal aortic aneurysm surgery, preoperative coronary revascularization may improve perioperative outcomes.

The results of several observational studies suggest that the cardiac mortality rate is low in patients undergoing PTCA before noncardiac surgery, but there is evidence that the risk of significant complications during PTCA limits the generalized use of this procedure (110–112). The 1996 ACC/AHA Task Force Guidelines consider the indications for PTCA before noncardiac surgery to be similar to the 1993 ACC/AHA Guidelines for use of PTCA in the general population (113).

TREATMENT OF PERIOPERATIVE ARRHYTHMIAS

Perioperative Tachycardia

Increases in heart rate, especially among patients with known coronary artery disease, are associated with increases in myocardial oxygen demand that can worsen or precipitate myocardial ischemia. The results of many studies support a causal relationship between tachycardia and intraoperative myocardial ischemia in anesthetized patients (28). Both attenuation of the heart-rate response and control of exaggerated sympathetic responses during the perioperative period may limit the development of cardiac ischemia and subsequent myocardial infarction. The effect of intensive perioperative β-blockade on postoperative ischemia in high-risk patients undergoing noncardiac surgery has been evaluated (70), and the incidence of postoperative cardiovascular events was reduced by up to 2 years with use of β-adrenergic blockade throughout the in-hospital perioperative course (up to 1 week). There was a 15% increase in the event-free survival rate among patients on β-blockers compared with that among the placebo group (83% versus 68%, respectively), and the reduction in number of deaths from cardiac causes during the first 6 to 8 months was the principal effect. The results of this study support the safety and efficacy of β-blockers used perioperatively in patients undergoing noncardiac surgery.

Perioperative Atrial and Ventricular Arrhythmias

Atrial and ventricular arrhythmias are common and usually benign in patients without known heart disease. In the presence of coronary artery disease or left ventricular dysfunction, arrhythmias increase a patient's perioperative cardiac risk (8). This is especially true for elderly patients, in whom arrhythmias and conduction disturbances can be a marker of underlying cardiopulmonary disease. The incidence of arrhythmias during noncardiac surgery varies widely and is estimated from 0.9% to 70% (70), and controversy continues over whether these intraoperative arrhythmias are predictors of perioperative cardiac risk.

Goldman et al. (41) demonstrated that the presence of specific preoperative arrhythmias predicted an increased cardiac risk in patients undergoing noncardiac surgery. The prognostic importance of perioperative arrhythmias is not known, however, because the incidence of arrhythmias during the preoperative period has not often been studied (114). Also, very limited periods of preoperative ECG monitoring have been performed in most studies, so it could not be determined whether perioperative arrhythmias were new or related to preexisting arrhythmias. In addition, most patients studied have been at low risk for coronary artery disease.

The treatment of both intra- and postoperative ventricular arrhythmias in patients undergoing noncardiac surgery also has not been well studied.

Treatment of significant perioperative arrhythmias is similar to that in nonsurgical patients. Reversible factors, such as electrolyte disturbances, acid-base abnormalities, and decompensated CHF, should be corrected, and a search for underlying cardiac or pulmonary disease or potential drug toxicity is essential. Significant perioperative ventricular arrhythmias, including premature ventricular contractions or nonsustained ventricular tachycardia, do not often require therapy unless they are associated with ongoing cardiac ischemia, significant valvular disease, left ventricular dysfunction, or hemodynamic compromise (8). Postoperative arrhythmias often result from metabolic and sympathetic causes. Correction of any underlying reversible disorder is recommended before further therapy, such as cardioversion, is performed. To date, no studies provide evidence that suppression of preoperative arrhythmias with antiarrhythmic agents reduces surgical morbidity and mortality. The perioperative use of β-blockers has been evaluated, however, and may be beneficial regarding short- and long-term outcomes (70).

The most recent—and largest—prospective study of perioperative ventricular arrhythmias was performed with high-risk male patients undergoing noncardiac surgery (114). Patients underwent continuous ambulatory ECG monitoring for at least 12 hours preoperatively, intraoperatively, and 12 hours postoperatively. Major ventricular arrhythmias (>30 ventricular ectopic beats/hour or ventricular tachycardia) occurred in 44% of patients (21% preoperatively, 16% intraoperatively, and 36% postoperatively). Only 11% of these arrhythmias were clinically detected by routine ECG, and most occurred without clinical symptoms. Patients with CHF, ECG evidence of myocardial infarction, or a history of tobacco use had a higher incidence of preoperative arrhyth-

mias. Severity of the preoperative arrhythmia increased in only 1% of patients intraoperatively but in 10% postoperatively. Nonfatal myocardial infarction or cardiac death occurred in 4% of patients but did not occur more frequently in patients with previous perioperative arrhythmias. No adverse ischemic outcomes were associated with these arrhythmias. Based on these observations, such arrhythmias may not require aggressive treatment during the perioperative period.

Use of Digoxin

Certain subsets of patients are at increased risk for postoperative supraventricular tachyarrhythmias, and prophylactic digitalis may be useful preoperatively. Such patient subsets include elderly patients undergoing pulmonary surgery, patients with subcritical valvular stenosis, and patients with a history of supraventricular tachyarrhythmias, but the data from which these indications are derived were reported over three decades ago (115). It would be reasonable to use alternative medications, such as β-blockers, and calcium channel blockers, such as verapamil or diltiazem, to control the rate of supraventricular arrhythmias, especially in those patients with low-normal or normal left ventricular systolic function (116).

Perioperative Transvenous Pacemakers

More than 460,000 individuals in the United States are estimated to have permanent cardiac pacemakers, 85% of which are in persons older than 65 years (117). It is important for the consultant to know, if possible, the type of pacemaker implanted to guide treatment if further issues arise concerning the device. Major pacemaker manufacturers provide technical support for particular devices if specific problems occur, and if the cardiologist who implanted the device is available, he or she should be able to provide assistance. Indications for use of preoperative or intra-operative, temporary or permanent transvenous pacemakers and treatment of preexisting devices generally are based on expert opinion; no established, evidence-based guidelines are available.

In general, pacemakers are indicated for high-grade conduction abnormalities (e.g., complete atrioventricular block) and intraventricular conduction delays with associated symptoms. When dealing with patients with no symptoms and no intraventricular conduction delay, easy access to temporary transvenous pacing equipment in the operating room is advised. As with all invasive procedures, the risks of pacemaker placement, such as ventricular irritability, pneumothorax and hemothorax, infection, and myocardial perforation, must be considered. In general, noncardiac surgery should be delayed for 48 hours after the implantation of a permanent pacemaker, if possible, to minimize the risk of acute dislodgment of the leads. Recommendations for temporary or permanent pacemaker implantation are the same as those for elective pacemaker implantations in patients not undergoing surgical procedures (118).

Perioperative Treatment of Patients with Preexisting, Permanent Pacemakers

Potential difficulties exist in patients with permanent pacemakers when electrocauterization is used. Electrocauterization may interfere with pacemaker function by causing "oversensing" in patients with unipolar and, rarely, bipolar systems due to electrical activity that can simulate the intrinsic electrical cardiac activity. If electrocauterization is to be employed, it is recommended that the electrode be kept at least 4 to 6 inches from the pacemaker itself to minimize any electrical interference (119). In addition, the pacemaker could be programmed to a fixed-rate mode to avoid the potential for accidental reprogramming due to electrical interference. During emergent surgery or situations in which the pacemaker is not able to be

interrogated with a programmer, a magnet should be placed over the pacemaker preoperatively and an ECG recorded to evaluate the back-up mode and function of the pacemaker. The lack of pacing spikes on an ECG in response to application of a magnet indicates battery malfunction. A conservative recommendation is that a pacemaker be interrogated at least 2 months before an elective procedure. Interrogation after a procedure depends on whether there has been use of cautery, defibrillation, or cardioversion of arrhythmias, or a noted change in the function and pacing mode of the pacemaker.

Pacing thresholds may be decreased because of hypoxia and myocardial ischemia and increased because of hyperkalemia and acid-base disturbances. Monitoring for these conditions is essential so that pacemaker programming can be altered if needed (119). If possible, the necessary programming device should be available in the operating room when the potential for electrocautery interference is high or the use of defibrillation or cardioversion is expected. Prophylaxis for endocarditis in patients with permanent pacemakers before noncardiac surgery is not recommended in most cases (7).

Automatic Implantable Cardiac Defibrillators

Management of automatic implantable cardiac defibrillators (AICDs) in the perioperative setting also is based predominantly on expert opinion. No standards are available. It is advisable for the consultant to know the manufacturer of the device, and in general, the device should be inactivated and the appropriate resuscitation equipment available in the operating room. If the electrophysiologist who implanted the device is available, he or she should be able to provide expert assistance; in addition, technical support staff at the major AICD manufacturers may provide specific recommendations. The AICD can be left in the inactivated mode until the patient is transferred to an unmonitored hospital bed. Prophylaxis for endocarditis in patients with implanted defibrillators before noncardiac surgery is not recommended in most cases (7).

PERIOPERATIVE SYSTOLIC AND DIASTOLIC MYOCARDIAL DYSFUNCTION

A proven predictor of perioperative cardiac risk before noncardiac surgery is decompensated CHF. The two larger studies that evaluated CHF in this population were conducted in the late 1970s to early 1980s (41, 120), and the presumptions at the time were that certain factors played a role in precipitating CHF. These factors included regional or global myocardial ischemia and infarction as well as perioperative stressors such as catecholamine surges and changes in preload and afterload due to fluid shifts.

Clinical Predictors of Perioperative Congestive Heart Failure

It is recommended that the cause of cardiomyopathy be thoroughly investigated, and that if possible, any reversible causes be treated before elective surgery. Dyspnea of unknown origin warrants a careful preoperative assessment to determine if it has a cardiac or a pulmonary cause. Goldman et al. (41) identified clinical signs of CHF such as an S3 and jugular venous distention as prognostic indicators of increased postoperative risk. Other variables, such as significant valvular disease and arrhythmias, low functional capacity, and previous myocardial infarction, also were noted to be important, and

these may serve as markers for abnormal cardiac function. Evaluating these clinical variables before elective noncardiac surgery is critical. In the 1996 ACC/AHA Guidelines (8) of clinical predictors for perioperative risk, decompensated CHF is considered to be a major predictor, and compensated CHF and a history of CHF are considered to be intermediate predictors (Table 11.5).

Physical Examination Findings of Congestive Heart Failure

A thorough physical examination is critical, but in many patients, physical signs of CHF may be elusive and difficult to elicit. The physical examination alone has a low sensitivity for detecting systolic left ventricular dysfunction, even in patients with a significantly elevated pulmonary artery wedge pressure (121–123). Another indicator of myocardial dysfunction is a poor functional status. Functional status may be defined by the New York Heart Association functional classification (Table 11.18), but its use can be interpreter dependent. Eliciting symptoms of orthopnea or paroxysmal nocturnal dyspnea can be helpful but are much less specific for ventricular dysfunction.

Etiology

It is important to distinguish if CHF results from diastolic or systolic left ventricular dysfunction. Diastolic dysfunction caused by hypertrophic cardiomyopathy (discussed later) is important, because intravenous fluids, blood losses, and use of

Table 11.18.   New York Heart Association Functional Classification in Patients with Cardiac Disease

Class I	Ordinary physical activity does not cause fatigue, palpitation, dyspnea, or anginal pain.
Class II	Ordinary physical activity causes fatigue, palpitation, dyspnea, or anginal pain.
Class III	Less-than-ordinary physical activity causes fatigue, palpitation, dyspnea, or anginal pain. Patient is comfortable at rest.
Class IV	Inability to carry out any physical activity without discomfort.

Adapted with permission from Braunwald E. Valvular heart disease. In: Braunwald E, ed. Heart disease: a textbook of cardiovascular medicine. 5th ed. Philadelphia: WB Saunders, 1997:1007–1076.

catecholamines during the surgical procedure could lead to detrimental shifts in both preload and afterload. If systolic left ventricular dysfunction is diagnosed, then appropriate, optimal medical treatment is essential to stabilize the patient before the proposed noncardiac surgical procedure.

Treatment of Perioperative Congestive Heart Failure

It is critical to optimize the medical treatment of CHF before an elective noncardiac surgical procedure. For systolic left ventricular dysfunction, this often involves use of diuretics and angiotensin-converting enzyme inhibitors. These medications can alter hemodynamic and metabolic parameters, which may affect the perioperative cardiac risk, so their use must be carefully monitored. Patients at risk for CHF postoperatively are those with a history of dysrhythmia and diabetes (41, 107). In addition, prolonged surgical and vascular procedures have specifically been associated with a higher risk for postoperative CHF, possibly secondary to the increased use of intravenous fluids. It also has been noted that patients who develop CHF during the postoperative period have a better long-term prognosis than those patients in whom a significant postoperative myocardial ischemic event occurs (44). Patients with poorly controlled CHF should not proceed to surgery unless the condition requiring surgery is life-threatening.

Use of Intraoperative Pulmonary Artery Catheterization

One of the first groups in whom routine pulmonary artery catheter use was recommended were patients undergoing surgical procedures who had a history of a recent myocardial infarction or clinical evidence of CHF, because the postoperative mortality rate was high in this group (124). Use of intraoperative pulmonary artery catheterization to optimize hemodynamics in patients with CHF has been assessed in only a few prospective, randomized trials (125, 126) of patients undergoing vascular surgery, however, and it remains controversial.

In a study by Berlauk et al. (125) of 89 patients who were prospectively randomized and undergoing peripheral vascular surgery, two groups received a pulmonary artery catheter preoperatively at 3 and 12 hours, respectively. A third group had only a central line placed. Only 37% of patients with the pulmonary artery catheter met specific, predefined hemodynamic guidelines; in the remaining patients, further interventions (predominantly the administration of intravenous fluids) were used to meet these criteria. Patients receiving a preoperative pulmonary artery catheter were more stable intraoperatively, with less tachycardia, hypotension, and arrhythmias. This group also had a significantly lower incidence of postoperative cardiac morbidity and less early limb-graft thrombosis than the control group. Mortality was lower among the group in whom the pulmonary artery catheter was used, but this did not achieve statistical significance. There was no difference in outcome between the two groups who had pulmonary artery catheters placed at different times preoperatively.

In contrast, a recent study by Bender et al. (126) randomized 104 patients to pulmonary artery catheterization on the day of major vascular surgery or only if clinically indicated. There was no difference in intraoperative and postoperative complications or mortality between the two groups, and there was no difference in the overall length of stay in the hospital or intensive care unit. Routine pulmonary artery catheterization in patients undergoing elective vascular surgery showed no improvement in morbidity or mortality in this population.

In 1990, an American College of Physicians (ACP)/ACC/AHA Task Force statement on clinical competence in hemodynamic monitoring included an extensive list of common indications (127). Certain noncardiac surgical procedures were listed as being those in which hemodynamic monitoring is believed to be indicated to assist in the treatment of these

Table 11.19.   Common Indications for Hemodynamic Monitoring with Pulmonary Artery Catheters in Patients Undergoing Noncardiac Surgery

Vascular procedures
   Dissecting aneurysm
   Resection of thoracic aneurysm
   Abdominal aortic aneurysm
Nonvascular procedures
   High-risk obstetric patients with known cardiac
     disease
   Prolonged orthopaedic procedures in elderly
     patients
   Prostatic resection
   Extensive intra-abdominal resection (tumor)

Adapted with permission from Clinical competence in hemodynamic monitoring. A statement for physicians from the ACP/ACC/AHA task force on clinical privileges in cardiology. J Am Coll Cardiol 1990; 15:1460–1464.

patients (Table 11.19). Use of pulmonary artery catheterization preoperatively may be recommended (124) in patients with known cardiac disease in the following groups (Table 11.20):

1. Recent myocardial infarction (<6 months),
2. Unstable angina,
3. Refractory or easily treated CHF, and
4. Symptomatic valvular disease.

In the postoperative setting, use of pulmonary artery catheterization may be considered in patients with known cardiac disease and either acute, significant blood losses (>10 U) or early postoperative hypoxia. Care must be exercised in the use of pulmonary artery catheters because of their low (but potential) risk of complications such as pneumothorax, infection, and arrhythmias.

HYPERTENSION

Prevalence and Risk

Systemic arterial hypertension, which is defined as blood pressure ≥ 140/90 mm Hg, is common, and its prevalence increases with age (128). According to the Third National Health and Nutrition Examination Survey (NHANES III), 24% of all U.S. adults have hypertension (129). By age 70, the prevalence of hypertension increases to more than 60% (128), and a history of hypertension was found in 28% of the 1001 patients older than 40 years undergoing noncardiac surgical procedures in the large prospective study by Goldman et al. (41).

Postoperative hypertension occurs in approximately 5% of all patients after noncardiac surgery, but it is much more likely to occur in patients undergoing major vascular surgery, especially abdominal aortic aneurysm repair and carotid endarterectomy, in whom the incidence is approximately 50% (130). Several factors relate to the development of postoperative hypertension. Emergence from anesthesia is associated with a sympathetic nervous response resulting in a transient increase in both heart rate and systemic blood pressure (131). This pressor response is exaggerated in patients with hypertension (132, 133). The major risks of significant postoperative hypertension, which often is defined as systolic blood pressure ≥ 200 mm Hg, diastolic blood pressure ≥ 120 mm Hg, or both, include myocardial ischemia, stroke (especially in patients undergoing carotid endarterectomy), and bleeding (Table 11.21).

The relationship between chronic hypertension and vascular disease is well established (134), but the impact of hypertension on perioperative morbidity and mortality is controversial. Hypertension is

Table 11.20.   Guidelines for Use of Perioperative Pulmonary Artery Catheterization (124)

Intraoperative
   Recent myocardial infarction (<6 mo)
   Unstable angina
   Refractory CHF
   Symptomatic valvular disease
Postoperative
   Acute, significant blood losses (>10 units)
   Hypoxia

Table 11.21.   **Major Risks of Significant**
Postoperative Hypertension

Risk	Group
Myocardial ischemia	Patients with coronary artery disease
Stroke	Patients after cartoid endarterectomy
Bleeding	All patients

a known risk factor for coronary artery disease and stroke, increasing the risk for both these conditions by several-fold (1). As a result, patients with hypertension might be expected to be at greater risk of perioperative myocardial ischemia and infarction. The large, multivariate analysis by Goldman et al. (41, 135), however, did not establish mild-to-moderate hypertension as an independent predictor of postoperative cardiac complications. In that study, even patients with untreated hypertension and those who remained hypertensive despite treatment did not have an increased risk of perioperative infarction or cardiac death (135). This landmark study suggested that intraoperative hypotension is the biggest threat to patients with hypertension undergoing general anesthesia and noncardiac surgery. Those patients with a history of hypertension in the series of Goldman et al. and who had any intraoperative decrease in blood pressure of more than 50% or whose blood pressure fell by 33% for longer than 10 minutes had an increased risk of cardiac complications.

In agreement with the Goldman et al. study, the 1996 ACC/AHA Guidelines (8) also noted that mild-to-moderate hypertension is not an independent risk factor for perioperative cardiac morbidity. As a result of these studies (41, 135) and the ACC/AHA Guidelines (8), treatment of mild-to-moderate hypertension (diastolic blood pressure, 90–110 mm Hg) in those scheduled to undergo general anesthesia is controversial. More severe hypertension (diastolic blood pressure, >110 mm Hg)

should certainly be controlled before elective noncardiac surgery (8).

Mild-to-moderate elevations in blood pressure during the perioperative period may not increase the risk of cardiovascular events, but a hypertensive crisis during the postoperative period poses a definite risk of myocardial infarction and cerebrovascular accident. A hypertensive crisis is diagnosed when a patient has severe hypertension (diastolic blood pressure, >120 mm Hg) and clinical evidence for an immediate threat of irreversible damage to the cardiovascular system, brain, or kidneys if the blood pressure is not promptly lowered (136). Evidence for impending or actual end-organ damage includes papilledema or other evidence of increased intracranial pressure, myocardial ischemia, or acute renal failure. The most common cause of hypertensive crisis is an abrupt increase in blood pressure in a patient with preexisting hypertension, but it also can occur in a previously normotensive patient who develops an abrupt, severe increase in blood pressure.

Several potential causes of hypertensive crises have been identified (136), including some that may be particularly relevant to the perioperative setting (Table 11.22). These include obstetric patients with preeclampsia or eclampsia, patients whose clonidine has been abruptly withdrawn before surgery (137), patients with pheochromocytomas (138), and patients on chronic monoamine oxidase inhibitor therapy for the treatment of severe depression. Severe hypertension has been reported in patients receiving sympathomimetic drugs in combination with monoamine oxidase inhibitors, because

Table 11.22.   **Individuals at Risk of Perioperative**
Hypertensive Crisis

Preeclampsia
Pheochromocytoma
Clonidine withdrawal
Use of monoamine oxidase inhibitors

inhibition of intraneuronal monoamine oxidase impairs the degradation of sympathomimetic amines and increases adrenergic stimulation (139). It is appropriate to be aware of the possibility of hypertension in perioperative patients receiving long-term therapy with monoamine oxidase inhibitors, but anesthesia may be employed without adverse cardiovascular effects (139, 140).

In addition to diagnosing and treating hypertensive crisis once it develops, recognizing secondary causes of hypertension may be important in both the perioperative setting and the patient's long-term care. Causes of secondary hypertension should be investigated in patients with severe hypertension (systolic blood pressure, ≥ 200 mm Hg; diastolic blood pressure, ≥ 120 mm Hg; or both), particularly if it is of recent onset or was previously controlled with antihypertensive therapy but now has becomes poorly controlled.

Risk of Perioperative Myocardial Ischemia

The view that mild-to-moderate hypertension is not an independent predictor of perioperative cardiac morbidity arises from the conclusions of many studies (25, 79, 96, 141) and, in particular, from the frequently cited series of 1001 noncardiac surgical procedures reported by Goldman et al. (41, 135), in which preoperative hypertension was not an independent predictor of cardiac death, postoperative myocardial infarction, heart failure, or arrhythmias. In the series of Goldman et al. (135), those patients with a history of hypertension were more likely to develop intra- or postoperative hypertension, particularly if undergoing major vascular surgery. Postoperative hypertension, however, was not an independent predictor of cardiac complications.

Some authors have indicated that whereas increases in blood pressure do not affect the risk of perioperative myocardial ischemia, increases in heart rate have a greater effect. Slogoff and Keats (142) studied 1023 patients undergoing CABG

surgery to determine the predictors of postoperative myocardial infarction. This population may be particularly useful in examining the relationship between hemodynamic instability and perioperative myocardial ischemia/infarction, because by definition, all of these patients have significant, flow-limiting coronary artery disease. Not surprisingly, these authors found that the incidence of perioperative ischemia as detected by ischemic ST-segment depression on continuous ECG monitoring was relatively high in this group (36.9%). Both this study and a subsequent series of 495 patients reported by the same authors (143) emphasized the relationship between tachycardia, but not hypertension or hypotension, and perioperative myocardial ischemia.

Despite study results indicating that hypertension is not an independent risk for perioperative cardiac morbidity, coronary artery disease clearly is more prevalent among patients with chronic hypertension, especially in combination with other well-recognized cardiac risk factors such as diabetes mellitus, advanced age, hyperlipidemia, family history of premature coronary artery disease, and cigarette smoking. Because patients with hypertension are more likely to have coronary disease than patients without cardiac risk factors, chronic hypertension may indirectly predispose to perioperative myocardial ischemia due to fixed luminal narrowing of one or more coronary arteries combined with increased metabolic demand. Even without coronary artery disease, patients with chronic hypertension may have episodes of myocardial ischemia (144), perhaps due to impaired coronary vasodilator reserve. Chronic hypertension also may result in impaired coronary autoregulation (145) by producing structural changes in the arterial wall so that higher arterial pressures are required to maintain adequate perfusion of vital organs (i.e., brain, heart, kidney). Patients with chronic hypertension, particularly in combination with left ventricular hypertrophy and coronary artery disease, may be prone to subendocardial myocardial ischemia because of abrupt falls in blood pressure (145). Patients with hypertension and known atherosclerotic peripheral and coronary vascular disease should have their blood pressure maintained near preoperative levels both to avoid myocardial or cerebrovascular ischemia and to limit postoperative renal dysfunction.

The Study of Perioperative Ischemia Research Group (5, 51) examined 474 men who underwent elective non-cardiac surgery with general anesthesia, 407 of whom were continuously monitored by ECG in the pre-, intra-, and postoperative periods. In the first 48 hours postoperatively, 41% had at least one episode of myocardial ischemia. Patients with a history of hypertension had almost twice the risk of developing postoperative myocardial ischemia (51) and almost four times the risk of postoperative death (5) than patients without hypertension. Multivariate analysis showed that a history of hypertension was one of five independent predictors for postoperative ischemia (51) and one of three independent predictors for increased postoperative mortality (5); severely limited activity level and renal insufficiency also were independent predictors. The in-hospital mortality rate among those with two or more of these risk factors was 20%.

The link between systemic hypertension and perioperative cardiac complications may relate to an increased risk of silent myocardial ischemia, and it may be particularly important in patients whose blood pressure is not controlled by antihypertensive therapy. Allman et al. (146) studied 325 patients without angina who were scheduled to undergo elective non-cardiac surgery by use of ambulatory ECG monitoring to determine the incidence of preoperative silent myocardial ischemia. Twenty percent of these patients had at least one episode of ST-segment depression that was consistent with silent ischemia. Patients with hypertension despite antihypertensive therapy were at

particularly high risk, with more than a 50% incidence of silent myocardial ischemia. Only hypertension predicted the presence of preoperative silent ischemia, whereas male gender, previous myocardial infarction, history of angina pectoris, peripheral vascular disease, cigarette smoking, obesity, diabetes mellitus, and age 70 years or older did not (146).

Preoperative myocardial ischemia in patients undergoing peripheral vascular surgery also has been found to be more common in patients with hypertension (19). In that same study, it was one of two clinical variables (along with a history of coronary artery disease) that was associated with development of postoperative cardiac events (i.e., cardiac death, nonfatal myocardial infarction, unstable angina, ischemic pulmonary edema).

This apparent link between hypertension and silent myocardial ischemia is clinically important, because silent ischemia is a major predictor of postoperative cardiac morbidity (49, 142). In two studies of patients undergoing elective peripheral vascular surgery, Raby et al. (19, 49) examined silent myocardial ischemia with various clinical predictors of cardiac risk. These authors found that perioperative ischemia as detected by continuous ECG monitoring was the most important predictor of adverse cardiac events, with a high sensitivity (88–92%) and specificity (88–91%).

Shackelford et al. (147) examined the predictive value of both the Goldman Cardiac Risk Index (41) and the New York Heart Association functional classification of heart disease in identifying the risk of cardiac morbidity among 406 women undergoing vaginal surgical procedures, 168 of whom were postmenopausal. Eight of these women (all postmenopausal) had perioperative cardiac morbidity. Neither the Goldman Index nor the New York Heart Association functional classification was useful in predicting postoperative cardiac morbidity; in contrast, a history of hypertension or ischemic heart disease was a significant risk factor (147). Patients with hypertension had a risk of perioperative cardiac events almost six-fold greater than in those without hypertension.

This discrepancy between the classic work of Goldman et al. (41, 135) and the results of other studies discussed here (5, 19, 51, 146, 148) regarding the prognostic importance of hypertension may relate to the method used for monitoring and diagnosing cardiac events. In the series of Goldman et al., an ECG was obtained on approximately the fifth postoperative day and when clinically indicated. ECGs were considered to be clinically indicated if a patient had "any postoperative cardiac signs or symptoms or was considered by his physicians to have any potential cardiac problem" (41). Routine postoperative continuous ECG monitoring was not performed, and no attempt was made to rigorously determine the incidence of intraoperative myocardial ischemia. Thus, asymptomatic episodes of myocardial ischemia—and even ECG undetectable myocardial infarction—may have gone undiagnosed. The incidence of cardiac events therefore may have been underestimated in the series of Goldman et al. On the other hand, more recent studies linking hypertension to postoperative myocardial ischemia as diagnosed by continuous ECG monitoring (146, 148) may have overestimated the incidence of perioperative myocardial ischemia, particularly in patients with hypertension and left ventricular hypertrophy, in whom the criteria used to define episodes of myocardial ischemia by ECG monitoring may be less reliable (52).

Some authors (51) have attempted to control for this by analyzing data using more stringent criteria to define ischemic episodes. Even with this adjustment, however, hypertension remained a significant independent predictor of postoperative myocardial ischemia. Furthermore, the effects of left ventricular hypertrophy on the ECG, which may affect the ascertainment of "myocardial ischemia" by continuous ECG monitoring, could not explain the findings of Browner et al. (5), who reported an increased risk of postoperative death in those with a history of hypertension.

Thus, whether patients with mild-to-moderate hypertension should be considered to have a greater-than-average risk of perioperative myocardial ischemia remains uncertain, because the results of reports from the last 20 years often are in conflict. The operative risk for a patient with a history of hypertension should be determined on the basis of concomitant cardiac risk factors, symptoms and history of cardiac disease, and the patient's general medical condition. A suggested approach to the perioperative treatment of patients with a history of hypertension follows:

1. A thorough patient history and physical examination should be performed and focus on the presence of symptoms (e.g., angina, dyspnea, orthopnea, palpitations, claudication) and signs (e.g., peripheral pulses, vascular bruits, jugular venous distention, edema, pulmonary rales) of cardiovascular disease;
2. Preoperative testing should be performed on the basis of the history and physical examination findings, but it should include an ECG, measurement of serum electrolytes, assessment of renal function, and possibly, chest radiography (149);
3. Surgery should not be postponed or canceled in a patient with mild-to-moderate hypertension but no other complications (8);
4. If the patient is already on antihypertensive medication, it should be continued perioperatively (8);
5. Blood pressure should be maintained near preoperative levels to reduce the risk of myocardial ischemia, because patients with a history of chronic hypertension may require higher arterial pressures to maintain adequate perfusion of vital organs (145);

6. More severe hypertension (diastolic blood pressure, >110 mm Hg) should be optimally controlled before elective noncardiac surgery is performed (8);

7. Because patients with hypertension may have an exaggerated pressor response during tracheal intubation and emergence from anesthesia (132, 133), careful monitoring during these critical periods is appropriate; and

8. Particular care is warranted in patients with hypertension undergoing major vascular surgery, because postoperative hypertension is particularly common in this setting.

Diastolic Dysfunction

Chronic hypertension causes a variety of changes in the heart and vasculature that may affect a patient's response to the stress of general anesthesia and noncardiac surgery. The "hypertensive heart" is characterized by concentric left ventricular hypertrophy, normal or above-normal systolic function, and abnormalities of diastolic relaxation (i.e., diastolic dysfunction) (150) (Table 11.23). In some patients, particularly older individuals with severe concentric left ventricular hypertrophy and small end-systolic chamber sizes, diastolic dysfunction may be so severe that dyspnea from pulmonary congestion can develop (151). The typical patient with chronic systemic hypertension therefore may be particularly sensitive to factors that affect diastolic filling of the left ventricle, such as increased heart rate, atrial fibrillation, or volume depletion.

Table 11.23.   Characteristics of Patients with Diastolic Dysfunction

Chronic hypertension
Left ventricular hypertrophy on ECG/
 echocardiogram
Exertional dyspnea
Normal or above-normal left ventricular systolic
 function
Low peak filling velocity and decreased E : A ratio
 on transmitral Doppler echocardiography

These issues may be particularly relevant in the perioperative setting, and identifying patients with chronic hypertension and diastolic dysfunction would be expected to help guide optimal perioperative fluid and blood pressure treatment to reduce the development of perioperative CHF.

Two-dimensional, M-mode, and pulsed-wave Doppler echocardiography may be used to reliably diagnose left ventricular hypertrophy and to assess diastolic filling of the left ventricle (152–154). Routine echocardiography as part of the perioperative assessment of patients with hypertension cannot be routinely recommended, however, because of its relative cost. Rather, echocardiography should be considered for use in patients with chronic hypertension and a history of exertional or stress-induced dyspnea, particularly if there is evidence of left ventricular hypertrophy on the ECG. Patients with chronic hypertension, left ventricular hypertrophy, and diastolic dysfunction have abnormal responses to exercise (155), which may produce a suboptimal increase (or even a decrease) in the left ventricular ejection fraction of these individuals. This appears to result from impaired diastolic filling (155). The hemodynamic response to the stress of anesthesia and surgery might be expected to produce a similar response in these patients.

In addition to the effects of surgery and the stress of tracheal intubation, the consulting internist needs to understand issues relevant to patients with hypertension in the immediate postoperative period. Increased sympathetic nervous system activity, producing increases in both blood pressure and heart rate, may occur as the patient emerges from anesthesia (156). This response may compromise diastolic filling in patients with reduced left ventricular compliance resulting from chronic hypertension and left ventricular hypertrophy. It therefore is critical to assess volume status at this time, but this may be extremely difficult in certain patients without continuous, invasive hemodynamic monitoring. Large volume shifts can occur during the early postoperative period, especially in patients emerging from major vascular surgery, who characteristically receive large amounts of volume replacement therapy intraoperatively and often are hypertensive on arrival at the recovery room (157). The consultant who must determine intravascular volume during this critical period may face the task of assessing a "moving target." A pulmonary artery (Swan-Ganz) catheter cannot be routinely recommended, but its use may provide important information and pinpoint directional changes in volume assessment that may not otherwise be attained clinically.

Treatment of Postoperative Hypertension

Preventive Strategies

Transient elevations of blood pressure and heart rate are common during the immediate postoperative period, particularly as patients emerge from anesthesia. Episodes of postoperative hypertension are more common, however, in patients with a history of chronic hypertension (135). Increased sympathetic nervous system activity may result from pain and anxiety, and careful attention to these issues is of great importance (Table 11.24). Major vascular surgery is associated with large amounts of volume replacement therapy, and hypervolemia may contribute to elevations of blood pressure in this setting. Unintentional postoperative hypothermia is extremely common, occurring in more than 50% of patients (158, 159) and even more frequently during surgery (158). It is associated with markedly increased levels of circulating catecholamine (160, 161) as well as with peripheral vasoconstriction and shivering (156), which may increase blood pressure and oxygen consumption (162), respectively. Maintenance of normothermia by placing a forced-air warming cover over patients intraoperatively and during the first 2 hours postoperatively is associated with decreased postoperative shivering

Table 11-24.   Potentially Preventable Causes of Postoperative Hypertension and Their Treatment

Cause	Treatment
Pain	Effective analgesia
Anxiety	Sedation
Hypervolemia	Diuretics
Hypothermia/shivering	Forced-air warming cover; sedation
Hypoxia	Oxygen

and fewer hours with an abnormally elevated systolic blood pressure (163). These changes appear to influence perioperative cardiac morbidity, because perioperative hypothermia is an independent predictor of unstable angina/ischemia, cardiac arrest, or myocardial infarction during the first 24 hours postoperatively (163).

Continuation of Antihypertensive Therapy

The most recent ACC/AHA Guidelines for the perioperative cardiovascular evaluation of patients undergoing noncardiac surgery (8) emphasize the importance of continuing antihypertensive therapy throughout this period. Discontinuation of certain antihypertensive agents, particularly clonidine and β-blockers, may result in significant "rebound" hypertension and therefore should be avoided. In certain circumstances, discontinuation of diuretic agents may be appropriate to avoid volume contraction, which could exaggerate the hypotensive effects of blood loss, perioperative cessation of oral intake, third spacing of fluids, and the vasodilating effects of certain anesthetic agents (164).

Pharmacologic Treatment

Sodium Nitroprusside Sodium nitroprusside is a direct-acting, intravenous vasodilator with a rapid onset of action (1–2 min) (136) that is useful in perioperative treatment of hypertension. Because perioperative increases in arterial blood pressure often result from systemic vasoconstriction that in turn results from sympathetic nervous system stimulation, a direct arteriolar vasodilator such as nitroprusside often is quite useful. Nitroprusside is easily titrated to the desired mean arterial blood pressure. The potential for thiocyanate toxicity should be considered in all patients, however, and plasma levels should be monitored. This is particularly important in patients with renal insufficiency or who are receiving nitroprusside for more than 72 hours (136). Nitroprusside often is associated with reflex tachycardia as well, which may require combined therapy with β-blockers (165).

Hydralazine As a potent, direct-acting arterial vasodilator, hydralazine shares many of the advantages of sodium nitroprusside in the treatment of perioperative hypertension. The onset of the antihypertensive effect is not as rapid as that of sodium nitroprusside, however, but hydralazine does have a longer duration of action. When given orally, the onset of action is from 30 to 60 minutes, and its duration of action is from 6 to 12 hours. Intravenously, the antihypertensive effect occurs within 10 to 20 minutes (136). In contrast to nitroprusside, hydralazine is not associated with thiocyanate toxicity. It may be converted from a continuous, intravenous infusion to the oral form once the patient is able to take food and medication by mouth. Caution is advised when using hydralazine in patients with coronary artery disease, because hydralazine is associated with reflex tachycardia and increased cardiac output and therefore may have the potential for causing subendocardial myocardial ischemia or infarction (136).

Phentolamine and Phenoxybenzamine Phentolamine and phenoxybenzamine are direct α-adrenoreceptor blockers that are most useful in perioperative treatment of patients with pheochromocytoma (165), antihypertensive withdrawal syndrome, or interactions with monoamine oxidase inhibitors (136).

Nitroglycerin Although nitroglycerin is available in several forms, continuous, intravenous infusions of nitroglycerin are most useful in treatment of perioperative hypertension. Postoperative patients with CHF, ischemic heart disease, or both may benefit from the venodilating effects of nitroglycerin, which not only may lower blood pressure but also reduce preload and improve the myocardial oxygen supply. It also is easily titrated to the systemic arterial pressure. Prolonged use should be avoided, however, because it may be associated with tachyphylaxis.

Clonidine Clonidine may be useful in treatment of postoperative hypertension, because it is available for both oral and transdermal use. Clonidine stimulates central α_2-receptors and thereby decreases sympathetic nervous outflow to the vasculature, thus producing vasodilation and lowering the blood pressure (136). It is particularly appropriate for patients who take clonidine preoperatively to avoid the clonidine withdrawal syndrome (137). Clonidine should not be used in patients with conduction disturbances, especially sick sinus syndrome, significant bradycardia, or advanced or high-degree atrioventricular block (166).

β-Blockers During the early 1970s, β-blockers typically were withdrawn before surgery (167–170) because of a concern over excessive bradycardia or hypotension in the perioperative period. Several subsequent studies during the late 1970s, however, indicated that β-blockers could be safely continued preoperatively, often resulting in a reduced incidence of myocardial ischemia (171). These studies as well as the concern over β-blocker withdrawal–induced tachycardia, hypertension, and myocardial ischemia (172, 173) led to the recommendation that β-blockers be continued before surgery (174).

Use of β-blockers to treat patients with hypertension who are undergoing surgery has several theoretic advantages. By decreasing adrenergic stimulation of the heart, β-blockers have the potential to lower the incidence of perioperative tachycardia and reduce the incidence of both perioperative arrhythmias and myocardial ischemia. In a study of 128 unmedicated patients with mild-to-moderate hypertension (blood pressure, 160–200/90–100 mm Hg) undergoing general anesthesia, a single, low dose of an oral β-blocker produced reduced the incidence of ECG-detected intraoperative myocardial ischemia by thirteenfold (148). Ischemia was detected in 11 of 39 patients (28.2%) who did not receive β-blocker therapy, and all episodes occurred either during tracheal intubation or emergence from anesthesia. In those who received β-blocker therapy, only 2 of 89 (2.2%) had evidence of myocardial ischemia. Those who received β-blockers more frequently had bradycardia (and some therefore received atropine), had a greater fall in the mean arterial pressure during premedication, and had a lower pressor response during tracheal intubation and emergence from anesthesia.

The prophylactic use of β-blockers has been studied in patients considered to be at high risk for postoperative cardiac complications, and such use appears to be both safe and effective. Pasternack et al. (175) treated 32 patients undergoing abdominal aortic aneurysm repair with oral metoprolol before and with intravenous metoprolol after surgery. These patients were compared with 51 similar control patients who also underwent abdominal aortic aneurysm repair. Only one of the 32 patients who received β-blockers sustained a perioperative myocardial infarction (3%), compared with nine of the 51 patients (18%) who did not. A significant reduction in perioperative cardiac arrhythmias (both ventricular and supraventricular) in patients receiving β-blockers also was observed (12.5% vs. 56.9%). No β-blocker–related hypotension, significant bradycardia, bronchospasm, or CHF was observed.

The effect of atenolol recently was examined in a randomized, double-blind, placebo-controlled study of 200 patients either with or at risk for coronary artery disease who were undergoing noncardiac surgery (70). These patients received placebo or intravenous atenolol before and immediately after the surgical procedure and oral atenolol for the duration of their hospitalization. Most of these patients (66%) had a history of hypertension. Six patients died during the hospitalization (four in the atenolol group and two in the placebo group), but three of these deaths were from non-cardiac causes. Treatment with atenolol during the hospitalization was associated with a reduced mortality rate and reduced incidence of cardiovascular complications for the 2-year follow-up period. The effect was particularly prominent during the first 6 months of follow-up, when the overall mortality rate was 8% in the placebo group and 0% in the atenolol group (70).

Not all studies, however, have found an association between β-blockers and a reduced incidence of postoperative myocardial ischemia. In the Perioperative Ischemia Research Group study of 407 men (51), use of β-blockers before surgery (78 patients [19.2%]) did not relate to the development of postoperative myocardial ischemia. These authors also examined the relationship of β-blockers to postoperative myocardial ischemia in those patients with a definite history of coronary artery disease, because β-blockers may have been given to some patients for treatment of hypertension. In those patients, β-blockers also did not affect the development of postoperative myocardial ischemia.

In summary, β-blockers should not be discontinued before surgery. They are effective antihypertensive agents and may be used orally during the preoperative period and intravenously thereafter. The relationship between preoperative use of β-blockers and perioperative myocardial ischemia is not clear, but both intra- and postoperative use appear to be well tolerated and may lower the incidence of perioperative myocardial ischemia or infarction in certain high-risk patients.

Labetalol Labetalol hydrochloride is a combined α- and ß-adrenoreceptor blocker with a theoretic advantage in states of sympathetic nervous system stimulation, which are typical in the postoperative period. Labetalol is available in both intravenous and oral forms. Intravenous labetalol is appropriate for achieving prompt reductions in postoperative arterial pressure (176) and may be useful in patients with pheochromocytomas or to treat the antihypertensive withdrawal syndrome (136).

Calcium Channel Blockers The calcium channel blockers also may be useful in treatment of postoperative hypertension. These agents lower arterial blood pressure by reducing afterload, but they may produce reflex tachycardia. This is particularly true of the dihydropyridine compounds such as nifedipine (165). Recently, use of sublingual nifedipine capsules in the treatment of hypertensive emergencies has been questioned after numerous reports of drug-induced cerebrovascular ischemia and infarction, acute myocardial infarction, and death (177). Because numerous other antihypertensive agents are available for the treatment of postoperative hypertension, use of sublingual nifedipine in this setting should be avoided.

Diuretics Diuretics may be useful in the treatment of patients with hypertension and evidence of volume overload, which may be particularly common in the postoperative setting because of intraoperative volume replacement. They may be used both intravenously and orally. Diuretics should be used with particular care in patients with hypertension and left ventricular hypertrophy, who may be more susceptible to the effects of volume depletion or to electrolyte disturbances.

Epidural Morphine Epidural morphine has been used to decrease the incidence of postoperative hypertension in patients undergoing abdominal aortic surgical procedures (178). It may have particular usefulness in attenuating the sympathetic nervous system activation that is typical in the postoperative period.

VALVULAR HEART DISEASE
Prevalence and Risk

Valvular heart disease frequently is encountered in patients undergoing surgical procedures. In the large, prospective study by Goldman et al. (135), 5.5% had grade II/VI or louder murmurs of mitral regurgitation, 2.3% had significant aortic stenosis, and smaller percentages of patients had either aortic regurgitation or mitral stenosis. Because these diagnoses often were made on the basis of a physical examination alone, the reported prevalence of these conditions likely is greater today considering the more widespread use of echocardiography. The consulting internist must be familiar with all forms of stenotic and regurgitant valvular lesions, but particularly with those affecting the mitral and aortic valves. Left-sided (i.e., mitral and aortic) valvular disease is both more common than right-sided valvular disease and more likely to be associated with perioperative cardiac events. In addition, the consultant must be familiar with specific issues that may need to be addressed during the care of patients with mechanical prosthetic cardiac valves undergoing noncardiac surgery, particularly perioperative anticoagulation.

The 1996 ACC/AHA Task Force Guidelines (8) indicate that "severe valvular disease" is a major clinical predictor of increased perioperative cardiovascular risk. Severe aortic stenosis is considered to be the most serious valvular lesion predicting perioperative cardiac risk (8, 41). In the series of Goldman et al. (41), multivariate analysis identified "important valvular aortic stenosis" as a significant, independent predictor of postoperative life-threatening or fatal cardiac complications. The importance of aortic stenosis in predicting cardiac risk is based largely on the results of Goldman et al. (41, 135), but this finding is based on only 23 patients (2.3% of those studied) who were considered to have aortic stenosis, only some of whom had echocardiographic or cardiac catheterization data available to support the diagnosis. The results of a later study (179), in which all patients underwent Doppler echocardiography, found that selected patients with moderate-to-severe aortic stenosis can undergo noncardiac surgical procedures at relatively low risk.

Patients with other left-sided valvular lesions (e.g., mitral regurgitation, mitral stenosis, aortic regurgitation) may have an increased risk of developing new or worsening heart failure (135), but they do not appear to have an increased risk of perioperative cardiac mortality. In the series of Goldman et al. (135), mitral regurgitation was a significant univariate correlate of perioperative myocardial infarction and postoperative cardiac death, but the predictive value of mitral regurgitation did not persist after the presence of other criteria for heart disease were controlled for in a multivariate analysis. Mitral stenosis does not have the same prognostic importance as aortic stenosis, but it is important to recognize because of its hemodynamic effect. Patients with mitral stenosis have impaired diastolic filling, which may be clinically insignificant at normal heart rates but may result in the increased left atrial and pulmonary vascular pressures that occur during tachycardia. Patients with valvular heart disease may have an increased risk of developing infective endocarditis and therefore may require antibiotic prophylaxis for specific surgical procedures. These patients should undergo careful monitoring of volume status and may benefit from afterload reduction (8). Patients with mechanical prosthetic heart valves may need antibiotic prophylaxis for endocarditis and require careful treatment of perioperative anticoagulation.

Specific Types

A detailed description of all types of valvular heart disease is beyond the scope of this chapter. The major forms, however, are generally described, and treatment issues specific to the perioperative period are addressed. The consulting internist must have a general knowledge of all the common types of valvular disease, but mitral and aortic stenosis may present particular problems perioperatively and therefore are described in more detail.

Mitral stenosis most often results from rheumatic heart disease (180) and more often is found in women than in men. Typically, it results in increased left atrial and pulmonary vascular pressures. Over time, the left atrium increases in size, and atrial fibrillation may develop. Because diastolic filling of the left ventricle is impaired by the narrowed mitral valve orifice, the hemodynamic abnormalities of mitral stenosis are worsened by factors that further compromise diastolic filling, reduce cardiac output, and increase both left atrial and pulmonary vascular pressures.

The major issues of concern in patients with mitral stenosis undergoing noncardiac surgery are:

1. Maintaining adequate diastolic filling and cardiac output;
2. Decreasing the incidence of perioperative arrhythmias, particularly atrial fibrillation; and
3. Prevention of infective endocarditis (Table 11.25).

Increases in heart rate reduce the time available for the left ventricle to fill across the stenotic mitral valve and increase the transmitral pressure gradient (181). It therefore is not surprising that patients with mitral stenosis often become symptomatic with exercise, emotional stress, or

Table 11.25.   Important Issues in Patients with Mitral Stenosis Undergoing Noncardiac Surgery

Pain control
Avoiding volume depletion
Reducing anxiety
Prophylaxis for endocarditis
Prevention and prompt treatment of infection
Maintaining a normal body temperature
Avoiding drugs that increase heart rate

other daily activities associated with tachycardia. Similarly, patients with mitral stenosis may develop pulmonary edema during the perioperative period, when the heart rate may increase because of volume depletion, hypothermia, blood loss, pain, anxiety, fever, or the effects of particular pharmacologic agents or anesthesia methods. Patients with mitral stenosis who develop perioperative pulmonary edema may require therapy with β-blockers to reduce the heart rate to prolong diastolic filling times and to reduce both left atrial and pulmonary vascular pressures.

It is important to recommend measures to decrease the likelihood of hypovolemia, pain and anxiety, and fever, all of which may increase the heart rate and further compromise diastolic filling. β-Blockers may be used to reduce the ventricular rate in atrial fibrillation or to control the heart rate in sinus rhythm. Antiarrhythmic agents may be used to prevent development of atrial fibrillation among patients in whom this is particularly likely, such as those with frequent premature atrial contractions (116). Patients with mitral stenosis and chronic atrial enlargement not only have greater risk of developing atrial fibrillation than patients without these conditions, they also may be particularly sensitive to the hemodynamic effects of atrial fibrillation once this occurs. Because of the impaired diastolic filling that occurs in mitral stenosis, these patients depend more than healthy individuals on the atrial contribution to ventricular filling. Cardiac symptoms therefore typically

occur at the time that atrial fibrillation develops as a result of cessation of the atrial contribution to ventricular filling and because of the increase in heart rate that generally occurs when this arrhythmia ensues. The consultant also must include previously unrecognized mitral stenosis in the differential diagnosis of (apparently) previously healthy patients who abruptly develop pulmonary edema perioperatively. As discussed earlier, antibiotic prophylaxis may be indicated as well in patients with mitral stenosis who are undergoing specific surgical procedures.

Mitral regurgitation is common and has many causes, including rheumatic heart disease, papillary muscle dysfunction, and mitral valve prolapse. When the regurgitation is severe, left ventricular function often is reduced, left atrial and pulmonary vascular pressures are elevated, and atrial fibrillation may occur. While mitral regurgitation is more common than mitral stenosis, it is less likely to cause abrupt clinical deterioration in the perioperative period unless there are associated valvular lesions (e.g., aortic stenosis) or left ventricular dysfunction. Patients with significant mitral regurgitation or with mitral valve prolapse and regurgitation should receive antibiotic prophylaxis against infective endocarditis for certain surgical procedures as outlined earlier (Tables 11.3 and 11.4).

Valvular aortic stenosis, in contrast to mitral stenosis, is more common in men, is a condition of older individuals in particular, and usually results from degenerative calcific aortic disease (182). Another important cause of aortic stenosis, particularly in patients younger than 70 years, is calcification of a congenitally bicuspid valve (182). Typically, patients with moderate-to-severe valvular aortic stenosis develop concentric left ventricular hypertrophy and therefore may have clinical manifestations of diastolic dysfunction as described earlier. Although cardiac output may increase normally with exercise in asymptomatic patients with aortic stenosis, stroke volume may actually decrease slightly (183). Thus, even without symptoms, a normal hemodynamic response to exercise (and by extension to the stress of the perioperative period) may be critically dependent on an increase in heart rate. In patients with symptomatic and more severe aortic stenosis, cardiac output may be normal or slightly reduced at rest but not increase normally with increasing metabolic demand. In patients with the most severe cases of aortic stenosis, resting left ventricular systolic function is impaired.

Patients suspected of having aortic stenosis on the basis of physical examination findings merit further evaluation before surgery, because patients with severe aortic stenosis are considered to be at high risk for noncardiac surgery (8, 41, 135). In the large, prospective study by Goldman et al. (41), "important valvular aortic stenosis" was one of nine preoperative factors related to the development of postoperative life-threatening or fatal cardiac complications by as determined by multivariate analysis, and it was one of eight correlates of cardiac death (135). As noted, this important (but now 20-year-old) observation was based on only 23 patients. Aortic stenosis was defined by physical examination criteria (i.e., grade II/VI systolic ejection murmur with other consistent findings on carotid and cardiac examination) and by other supportive data (e.g., echocardiography, cardiac catheterization, aortic valve calcification on chest radiography or fluoroscopy) when available (41). Largely—or perhaps solely—because of the results of this study, severe aortic stenosis has subsequently been considered to be a major preoperative cardiac risk factor (8, 174). The 1996 ACC/AHA Guidelines (8) recommend that elective noncardiac surgery be postponed or canceled until aortic valve replacement can be performed in patients with severe, symptomatic aortic stenosis, and some authors (184) suggest that asymptomatic patients with significant aortic stenosis also be considered for

valve replacement before noncardiac surgery.

A more recent report (179) indicates that selected patients with aortic stenosis, and even with severe aortic stenosis, may be able to safely undergo noncardiac surgery. This may result from greater awareness of potential complications in this population and to closer perioperative monitoring and more meticulous perioperative care. In this report, 48 patients with moderate-to-severe aortic stenosis (all of whom were examined with Doppler echocardiography) underwent noncardiac surgical procedures without any intraoperative or early perioperative mortality. Most of these patients were elderly (mean age, 73 years), symptomatic (75% had either CHF, angina, or syncope), and had severe aortic stenosis (mean peak instantaneous gradient, 76 mm Hg; calculated aortic valve area [in 22 of the patients], 0.61 cm^2). Of the 22 patients who underwent general anesthesia, 17 had severe aortic stenosis. Hypotension was noted intraoperatively in four patients receiving general anesthesia and in the only patient who received spinal anesthesia. No patient who underwent local anesthesia developed perioperative hypotension. In one patient who received general anesthesia and developed hypotension, borderline elevation of the MB fraction of creatine kinase was noted, but a definite myocardial infarction was not diagnosed.

While the consulting internist may consider individuals with critical aortic stenosis for aortic valve replacement before noncardiac surgery, this is not feasible in some patients. For example, the noncardiac surgical procedure may be considered to be relatively urgent, and it may be thought that surgery cannot be safely delayed to allow the patient to undergo cardiac surgery and recuperate. Alternatively, the patient may decline surgery or be considered to have an unacceptably high risk to undergo valve replacement. The long-term outcome of patients who undergo aortic balloon valvuloplasty generally is poor, at least in part due to early restenosis (185, 186), but this procedure may be used for palliation of aortic stenosis before noncardiac surgery (187). Patients with asymptomatic mild aortic stenosis are believed to tolerate noncardiac surgery without any increased cardiac risk. General anesthesia may be preferable to spinal anesthesia in these patients, however, because the hemodynamic effects of spinal anesthesia (i.e., hypotension and tachycardia) may be undesirable in these patients (184).

Aortic regurgitation may result from disease of the valve itself (e.g., infective endocarditis, congenitally bicuspid valve, rheumatic heart disease) or from dilatation of the ascending aorta. Patients with chronic aortic regurgitation may have marked degrees of left ventricular hypertrophy and dilatation, and they eventually may develop left ventricular systolic dysfunction. As with patients experiencing mitral regurgitation, those with isolated, chronic aortic regurgitation typically do not deteriorate abruptly in the perioperative period as a result of their valvular heart disease. As discussed, patients with chronic aortic regurgitation require antibiotic prophylaxis against infective endocarditis for certain surgical procedures.

Evaluation

Patient History and Physical Examination

The consulting internist should inquire about a history of rheumatic fever or rheumatic heart disease, previously diagnosed valvular heart disease or known heart murmur, infective endocarditis, mitral valve prolapse, heritable disorder of connective tissue (especially Marfan syndrome), previous valve surgery, and intravenous drug use (Table 11.26). This information should help the consultant to determine whether a risk for a specific valvular lesion exists. In addition, a history of cardiac symptoms, especially chest pain, dyspnea, and syncope, should be determined.

Table 11.26. History Relevant to Valvular Heart Disease

Rheumatic fever/rheumatic heart disease
Previous infective endocarditis
Past history of valvular disease
Heritable disorder of connective tissue
Mitral valve prolapse
Previous valve surgery
Intravenous drug use
Known heart murmur

A diastolic murmur should alert the consultant to the possibility of aortic regurgitation or mitral stenosis. Systolic murmurs are more common and may be normal or of minimal concern; however, they also may signal a more important abnormality, such as aortic stenosis, hypertrophic cardiomyopathy, or mitral regurgitation. The consultant often must judge the significance of a systolic murmur on the basis of the physical examination and then decide whether further diagnostic testing to distinguish aortic stenosis from other causes is warranted. The proper clinical evaluation of systolic murmurs is important not only to avoid unnecessary and costly diagnostic studies but also to help in the decision of whether to postpone surgery so that additional cardiac testing can be performed. The most useful findings on physical examination for identifying aortic stenosis (Table 11.27) are a delayed carotid pulse, mid-to-late peak intensity of the systolic murmur, and decreased intensity of the aortic component of the second heart sound (188).

In addition to aortic stenosis, important causes of systolic murmurs include mitral

Table 11.27. Clinical Signs of Aortic Stenosis

Maximal intensity of systolic murmur in second right intercostal space
Radiation of systolic murmur to right carotid artery
Delayed carotid pulse
Mid-to-late peaking of systolic murmur
Decreased aortic component of S_2

regurgitation (with or without mitral valve prolapse), hypertrophic cardiomyopathy, tricuspid regurgitation, and ventricular septal defect. Patients without structural heart disease also may have "innocent" systolic murmurs, particularly during increased heart rate or cardiac output such as occurs with pregnancy, anemia, sepsis, or thyrotoxicosis (188).

Cardiac Diagnostic Studies

Noninvasive Assessment of Severity Echocardiography should be considered in patients with clinical evidence suggesting significant valvular aortic stenosis or mitral stenosis, and it may be appropriate in other situations as well. Several authors have reported that two-dimensional and Doppler echocardiography reliably assess both the pressure gradient and the severity of valvular aortic stenosis compared with cardiac catheterization (189, 190). Noninvasive assessment may be most useful for distinguishing those patients with severe aortic stenosis (aortic valve area, <0.75 cm^2) from those with noncritical aortic stenosis (191). Cardiac catheterization may be indicated in patients with intermediate transvalvular aortic gradients or to document the presence of concomitant coronary artery disease.

The echocardiogram may be used to accurately assess the severity of mitral stenosis, and results with this modality correlate well with measurements performed at cardiac catheterization in many patients (192). The correlation between mitral valve area calculated by the Doppler pressure half-time method as determined by echocardiography and the mitral valve area as determined by cardiac catheterization may not be as good in patients with atrial fibrillation or significant mitral (193) or aortic (192) regurgitation.

Noninvasive Assessment of Myocardial Ischemia General indications for preoperative exercise and pharmacologic stress testing were discussed earlier. Because aortic stenosis most commonly is a disease of older individuals, it is common to evaluate a patient with known or suspected aortic stenosis in whom exercise or pharmacologic stress testing may be indicated before noncardiac surgery. It also is common for patients with aortic stenosis to have symptoms compatible with the diagnosis of either valvular disease, coronary artery disease, or both. Without appropriate preoperative testing, it may be difficult to distinguish whether a patient's chest pain or dyspnea result from significant valvular aortic stenosis or from myocardial ischemia.

The safety of performing exercise stress testing in patients with aortic stenosis has been questioned, however, because exercise-induced cardiac events (particularly effort syncope) have been described (194). Indeed, the ACP/ACC/AHA Task Force statement on exercise testing (52) lists severe aortic stenosis as a general contraindication to exercise testing. Nevertheless, the result of some studies have indicated that patients with varying degrees of valvular aortic stenosis may safely undergo treadmill exercise stress testing (183, 195–197). The consultant may decide that alternative methods to assess myocardial ischemia are necessary if treadmill exercise is thought to be contraindicated because of particular patient characteristics (e.g., history of syncope, chest pain, or heart failure in a patient with known aortic stenosis or asymptomatic but severe aortic stenosis) or characteristics of the exercise stress-testing laboratory (e.g., insufficiently trained personnel, physician inexperience, office setting rather than referral center). In these situations, pharmacologic stress testing may be indicated. Even though only a small number of patients have been studied (198), adenosine myocardial perfusion imaging with nuclear scintigraphy can be safely performed in patients with moderate-to-severe aortic stenosis, and it may be an alternative to treadmill exercise testing. Dobutamine echocardiography has been safely performed in patients with severe aortic stenosis, even without invasive hemodynamic monitoring (199), and may be another alternative.

Cardiac Catheterization Cardiac catheterization may provide important information about the severity of valvular heart disease and both the presence and severity of coronary artery disease. It may be particularly useful in patients under consideration for valve surgery before noncardiac surgery to document coexistent coronary artery disease. The ACC/AHA Guidelines for coronary angiography (97) list this procedure as a class I recommendation when valve surgery is being considered:

1. In adult patients with chest discomfort, ECG changes, or both suggesting the presence of coronary artery disease;
2. In men 35 years and older; or
3. In postmenopausal women (97).

It also may be useful in patients with equivocal results of noninvasive studies but with symptoms or signs of significant coronary artery or valvular heart disease.

Treatment

General Measures

Patients with valvular heart disease may require antibiotic prophylaxis against infective endocarditis as described earlier (Tables 11.3 and 11.4). Data are limited, but spinal anesthesia may be less desirable than general anesthesia in patients with significant aortic stenosis because of the greater risk of hypotension (184). Patients with moderate-to-severe aortic stenosis also may benefit from close postoperative hemodynamic monitoring in an intensive care unit to limit periods of hypotension and to avoid volume depletion. Some patients may require constant monitoring of left ventricular filling pressures with use of a pulmonary artery catheter, but indications for this intervention have not been clearly defined. Treat-

ment of hypotension with use of volume replacement rather than sympathomimetic agents is preferable in patients with mitral stenosis.

Also as discussed, aortic valve replacement may be considered for some patients with severe aortic stenosis thought to have an excessively high risk for elective noncardiac surgery, particularly if it is believed these patients might benefit from aortic valve replacement even if the noncardiac surgery were not being considered. Careful attention should be given to patients with mitral stenosis to limit perioperative increases in heart rate (discussed earlier). Treatment of pain and anxiety is particularly important in this setting, and measures to reduce the risk of postoperative infections (e.g., limiting indwelling urinary catheters, use of incentive spirometry and early mobilization) as well as prompt treatment of any infectious complications (e.g., with use of antibiotics and antipyretics) may limit the risk of tachycardia. As with patients having chronic, systemic arterial hypertension (discussed earlier), most cardiac medications should be continued, if possible, during the perioperative period. This is particularly true for β-blockers and chronic antiarrhythmic therapy, both of which may reduce the incidence of perioperative tachycardia or hemodynamically significant tachyarrhythmias.

Balloon Valvuloplasty before Noncardiac Surgery

Balloon aortic valvuloplasty lessens the severity of aortic stenosis in most of patients (185, 186), but the procedure is not without risk. Fatal cardiac arrest has been reported as a complication in approximately 3% of patients (200), but the procedural mortality rate may be even higher. In a report by Holmes et al. (201) of 492 patients who underwent balloon aortic valvuloplasty, 4.9% died within 24 hours after the procedure, and 7.5% died during the hospitalization. Acute catastrophic complications, including ventricular perforation, acute severe aortic regurgitation, cerebrovascular accident, and limb amputation, have been reported in approximately 6% of patients (200). Thus balloon aortic valvuloplasty may decrease the severity of aortic stenosis in most patients, but the considerable procedure-related risk of morbidity and mortality risk must be carefully considered before recommending it to lower a patient's risk of noncardiac surgery.

The consulting internist also must be aware of the relatively poor long-term results of balloon aortic valvuloplasty in most patients, primarily because of restenosis (202). In a study of 55 elderly patients who underwent balloon aortic valvuloplasty for severe aortic stenosis (186), Doppler echocardiograms showed that the aortic valve mean gradient decreased significantly after the procedure, from 48 to 33 mm Hg, but that it increased again to 46 mm Hg approximately 6 months later.

Unlike balloon aortic valvuloplasty, balloon mitral valvuloplasty often is a reasonable alternative to mitral valve surgery. Results have been favorable, especially in younger patients with mitral stenosis but without severe mitral valve leaflet thickening or significant subvalvular fibrosis and calcification (203, 204).

PROSTHETIC HEART VALVES

In addition to patients with native valvular disease, the consulting internist may evaluate patients with either mechanical or bioprosthetic heart valves during the perioperative period, because more than 60,000 cardiac valve replacements are performed each year in the United States (205). Several issues are important in the perioperative evaluation and treatment of patients with prosthetic heart valves. The consultant must assess the function of the valve to address the possibility of prosthetic valve dysfunction, and other issues include managing long-term anticoagulation therapy, reducing the risk

of infective endocarditis, preventing valve thrombosis, and ruling out significant valve-related hemolysis (Table 11.28). Among these issues, management of anticoagulation in patients with mechanical prosthetic heart valves is the most difficult and is discussed later.

There are two major types of mechanical prosthetic heart valves: the caged-ball valve, and the tilting-disk valve. The St. Jude valve (St. Jude Medical), which is a type of tilting-disk valve, is the most commonly used prosthetic valve in the world (116). Mechanical prosthetic valves have greater durability than bioprosthetic valves, but they are more thrombogenic. The risk of valve thrombosis is greatest in patients with caged-ball prosthetic valves (Starr-Edwards) (205). Single-tilting-disk prosthetic valves (Bjork-Shiley; Medtronic-Hall and Omnicarbon) carry an intermediate risk of valve thrombosis, and bileaflet tilting-disk prostheses (St. Jude; Carbomedics, Edwards Duromedics) pose the lowest risk of the mechanical prosthetic valves (205). Obviously, the relative risk of prosthetic valve thrombosis is important in making decisions about management of anticoagulation. The possibility of prosthetic valve dysfunction may be suggested by new cardiac symptoms and abnormal auscultatory findings on physical examination, particularly with patients in whom the valve is nearing the time of its expected failure. The valve may be evaluated with use of cinefluoroscopy (for mechanical prosthetic valves) or echocardiography; cardiac catheterization may be warranted in some situations (205).

Table 11.28.   Important Issues in Perioperative Evaluation of Patients with Prosthetic Heart Valves

Valve dysfunction
Risk of infective endocarditis
Management of anticoagulation therapy
Preventing valve thrombosis
Hemolysis

Perioperative management of long-term anticoagulation therapy using warfarin is an issue in the care of patients with many forms of heart disease, including chronic atrial fibrillation and cardiomyopathy, but it is of major importance in patients with mechanical prosthetic heart valves. When making recommendations about anticoagulation therapy in patients with mechanical prosthetic heart valves who are being evaluated for elective noncardiac surgery, the consultant must weigh the risk of temporarily discontinuing anticoagulation, decide whether administration of heparin should be maintained while administration of warfarin is stopped, and specifically address whether it is necessary to promptly resume anticoagulation therapy following surgery. When evaluating the risk of interrupting long-term anticoagulation therapy, the relative benefit of warfarin in the patient's specific type of valvular heart disease must be considered. In general, however, the incidence of thromboembolism in patients with valvular heart disease (Table 11.29) depends on the valve involved, the presence and type of prosthetic heart valve (i.e., bioprosthetic versus mechanical prosthetic), the existence of concomitant heart disease (i.e., cardiomyopathy, known intracardiac mural thrombus), the presence of left atrial enlargement, and whether atrial fibrillation is present (206).

If the patient will undergo a minor surgical procedure without the potential for significant blood loss, the consultant may recommend continuing warfarin an-

ticoagulation without interruption. Some authors have recommended briefly reducing the level of warfarin anticoagulation to the low-therapeutic or subtherapeutic range for minimally invasive surgical procedures (207), then resuming the usual dose after the procedure. This recommendation can only be made, however, with knowledge of the specific plan for surgery, information about the usual risk of bleeding, and details about the potential for blood loss if the surgery does not go as planned. For most noncardiac surgical procedures in which blood loss is anticipated to be significant, it generally is recommended that patients maintained on warfarin anticoagulation discontinue this therapy several days (approximately 3–5) before surgery (205) if the planned operation can safely be delayed. Oral anticoagulation should be reversed prior to an emergency surgical procedure (208).

As Table 11.29 notes, the risk of thromboembolism varies by which heart valve is involved. Mechanical prosthetic mitral valves appear to pose a greater risk of thromboembolism than prosthetic aortic valves, and caged-ball valves are more thrombogenic than tilting-disk valves (205). It may be reasonable simply to stop anticoagulation therapy for several days before a surgical procedure without beginning intravenous administration of heparin, but those patients with the greatest risk of thromboembolism should be anticoagulated with intravenous heparin in therapeutic doses during the 3 to 5 preoperative days in which warfarin is discontinued (208). Thus, patients who are considered to be at high risk (Table 11.29) should have intravenous heparin started when warfarin is discontinued, and the heparin infusion should be continued until several hours before surgery (205, 206, 208). Subcutaneous heparin may be used both during and soon after the operation (206). Warfarin should be restarted as soon as possible following surgery, however, and intravenous heparin should be resumed and continued until oral anticoagulation is in the therapeutic range.

Table 11.29.   Determinants of the Risk of Thromboembolism in Patients with Valvular Heart Disease

Heart valve involved
Biomechanical versus mechanical prosthetic valve
Type of mechanical prosthesis
Left ventricular dysfunction
Left atrial size
Atrial fibrillation
Intracardiac mural thrombus
Previous systemic embolization

HYPERTROPHIC CARDIOMYOPATHY

Hypertrophic cardiomyopathy (also known as *idiopathic hypertrophic subaortic stenosis*) is not encountered in the general population or in the perioperative setting as frequently as the other forms of heart disease described in this chapter. In the series by Goldman et al. (41) of 1001 patients undergoing noncardiac surgery, hypertrophic cardiomyopathy was not present with enough frequency to be analyzed statistically.

A complete description of hypertrophic cardiomyopathy and its treatment is beyond the scope of this chapter. Hypertrophic cardiomyopathy is important to identify preoperatively, however, because patients with this condition may be at increased risk of hemodynamic compromise in the perioperative period. These individuals typically have marked degrees of left ventricular hypertrophy (often disproportionately involving the interventricular septum), reduced ventricular compliance, hyperdynamic left ventricular systolic function, and systolic anterior motion of the mitral valve with or without a dynamic pressure gradient in the subaortic area.

Patients with hypertrophic cardiomyopathy may have a family history of cardiomyopathy or of sudden, unexpected death at a young age. As with other forms of heart disease, a history of cardiac symptoms, especially chest pain, dyspnea, and syncope, should be determined. On physical examination, the systolic murmur of hypertrophic cardiomyopathy is quite characteristic and can readily be recognized. It generally is harsh and is best heard best in the left fifth intercostal space between the apex and the left sternal border, and it often radiates to the lower left sternal border. Dynamic auscultation during passive leg elevation or with the patient changing from the standing to the squatting position typically demonstrates a decrease in murmur intensity (188). Patients with hypertrophic cardiomyopathy also may have a precordial lift,

S_4 gallop, systolic thrill, prominent a wave in the jugular venous pulse, and bisferiens carotid pulse. Two-dimensional and Doppler echocardiography are useful in evaluating patients with known or suspected hypertrophic cardiomyopathy and can determine the degree of left ventricular hypertrophy and evidence of a dynamic subaortic pressure gradient (if one exists).

Little published information concerns the perioperative risk of patients with hypertrophic cardiomyopathy. In a review of 35 patients who underwent 56 noncardiac surgical procedures (209), the reported risk of general anesthesia and major surgery was low, with no deaths or significant ventricular tachyarrhythmias reported and only one patient with myocardial infarction and heart failure. Of note, one-third of these patients (who underwent almost half the reported surgical procedures) were asymptomatic before surgery, and it therefore is difficult to know whether these results are applicable to patients with more severe and symptomatic disease. It has been recommended (on limited evidence) that spinal anesthesia be avoided in patients with hypertrophic cardiomyopathy (209, 210), because such anesthesia can decrease systemic vascular resistance and increase venous capacitance.

Because of the pathophysiology of hypertrophic cardiomyopathy, these patients are particularly susceptible to factors that alter left ventricular filling, such as diminished intravascular volume, alterations in systemic vascular resistance, and increases in heart rate. Special care should be taken in these patients to maintain adequate intravascular volume, to minimize pain and anxiety, and to avoid treatment with catecholamines (8). Patients with hypertrophic cardiomyopathy also may benefit from close, postoperative hemodynamic monitoring in an intensive care unit to limit periods of hypotension and to avoid volume depletion. The role of pulmonary artery catheter monitoring has not been established, but some patients with hypertrophic cardiomyopathy may require close and constant monitoring of left ventricular filling pressures during the perioperative period.

REFERENCES

1. Castelli W, Anderson K. A population at risk. Prevalence of high cholesterol levels in hypertensive patients in the Framingham study. Am J Med 1986;80(2A):23–32.
2. Hubert HB, Feinleib M, McNamara PM, Castelli WP. Obesity as an independent risk factor for cardiovascular disease: a 26-year follow-up of participants in the Framingham Heart Study. Circulation 1983;67:968–977.
3. Lerner DJ, Kannel WB. Patterns of coronary heart disease morbidity and mortality in the sexes: a 26-year follow-up of the Framingham population. Am Heart J 1986;113:383–390.
4. Bayer AJ, Chadha JS, Farag RR, Pathy MSJ. Changing presentation of myocardial infarction with increasing old age. J Am Geriatr Soc 1986;34:263–266.
5. Browner WS, Li J, Mangano DT. In-hospital and long-term mortality in male veterans following noncardiac surgery. JAMA 1992;268: 228–232.
6. Valentine RJ, Grayburn PA, Eichhorn EJ, Myers SI, Clagett GP. Coronary artery disease is highly prevalent among patients with premature peripheral vascular disease. J Vasc Surg 1994;19:668–674.
7. Dajani AS, Taubert KA, Wilson W, et al. Prevention of bacterial endocarditis. Recommendations by the American Heart Association. JAMA 1997;277:1794–1801.
8. Guidelines for perioperative cardiovascular evaluation for noncardiac surgery: report of the American College of Cardiology/American Heart Association Task Force on Practice Guidelines (Committee on Perioperative Cardiovascular Evaluation for Noncardiac Surgery). J Am Coll Cardiol 1996;27:910–948.
9. Mangano DT. Perioperative cardiac morbidity. Anesthesiology 1990;72:153–184.
10. L'Italien GJ, Paul SD, Hendel RC, et al. Development and validation of a Bayesian model for perioperative cardiac risk assessment in a cohort of 1,081 vascular surgical candidates. J Am Coll Cardiol 1996;27: 779–786.
11. Paul SD, Eagle KA, Kuntz KM, Young JR, Hertzer NR. Concordance of preoperative clinical risk with angiographic severity of coronary artery disease in patients undergoing vascular surgery. Circulation 1996;94:1561–1566.
12. Mangano DT, Browner WS, Hollenberg M, Li J, Tateo IM. Long-term cardiac prognosis following noncardiac surgery. JAMA 1992;268: 233–239.

13. Massie BM, Mangan DT. Assessment of perioperative risk: have we put the cart before the horse? J Am Coll Cardiol 1993;21:1353–1356.
14. Jamieson WRE, Janusz MT, Miyagishma RT, Gerein AN. Influence of ischemic heart disease on early and late mortality after surgery for peripheral occlusive vascular disease. Circulation 1982;66(Suppl I):I-92–I-97.
15. Hertzer NR. Basic data concerning associated coronary disease in peripheral vascular patients. Ann Vasc Surg 1987;1:616–620.
16. Roger VL, Ballard DJ, Hallett JW, Osmundson PJ, Puetz PA, Gersh BJ. Influence of coronary artery disease on morbidity and mortality after abdominal aortic aneurysmectomy: a population-based study, 1971–1987. J Am Coll Cardiol 1989;14:1245–1252.
17. Gersh BJ, Rihal CS, Rooke TW, Ballard DJ. Evaluation and management of patients with both peripheral vascular and coronary artery disease. J Am Coll Cardiol 1991;18:203–214.
18. Leppo J, Plaja J, Gionet M, Tumolo J, Paraskos JA, Cutler BS. Noninvasive evaluation of cardiac risk before elective vascular surgery. J Am Coll Cardiol 1987;9:269–276.
19. Raby KE, Goldman L, Creager MA, et al. Correlation between preoperative ischemia and major cardiac events after peripheral vascular surgery. N Engl J Med 1989;321: 1296–1300.
20. Fleisher LA, Rosebaum SH, Nelson AH, Barash PG. The predictive value of preoperative silent ischemia for postoperative ischemic cardiac events in vascular and nonvascular surgery patients. Am Heart J 1991;122:980–986.
21. Boucher CA, Brewster DC, Darling C, Okada RD, Strauss HW, Pohost GM. Determination of cardiac risk by dipyridamole-thallium imaging before peripheral vascular surgery. N Engl J Med 1985;312:389–394.
22. Mangano DT, Hollenberg M, Fegert G, et al. Perioperative myocardial ischemia in patients undergoing noncardiac surgery—I: incidence and severity during the 4 day perioperative period. J Am Coll Cardiol 1991;17:843–850.
23. Eagle KA, Singer DE, Brewster DC, Darling RC, Mulley AG, Boucher CA. Dipyridamole-thallium scanning in patients undergoing vascular surgery. JAMA 1987;257:2185–2189.
24. Rozanski A, Diamond GA. Cardiac stress testing: who should have it? J Cardiovasc Med 1984;293–300.
25. Eagle KA, Coley CM, Newell JB, et al. Combining clinical and thallium data optimizes preoperative assessment of cardiac risk before major vascular surgery. Ann Intern Med 1989; 110:859–866.
26. Fleisher LA, Barash PG. Preoperative cardiac evaluation for noncardiac surgery: a functional approach. Anesth Analg 1992;74:586–598.
27. Gerson MC. Cardiac risk evaluation and man-

agement in noncardiac surgery. Clin Chest Med 1993;2:263–281.

28. Mangano DT, Goldman L. Preoperative assessment of patients with known or suspected coronary disease. N Engl J Med 1995;333: 1750–1756.

29. Marwick T, Willemart B, D'Hondt A-M, et al. Selection of the optimal nonexercise stress for the evaluation of ischemic regional myocardial dysfunction and malperfusion. Circulation 1993;87:345–354.

30. Fleisher LA, Hawes AD, Rosenbaum SH. The limited predictive value of dipyridamole thallium imaging in noncardiac surgery patients (abstract). Anesthesiology 1990;73:A75.

31. Mangano DT, London MJ, Tubau JF, et al. Dipyridamole thallium-201 scintigraphy as a preoperative screening test. Circulation 1991; 84:493–502.

32. Baron JF, Mundler O, Bertrand M, et al. Dipyridamole-thallium scintigraphy and gated radionuclide angiography to assess cardiac risk before abdominal aortic surgery. N Engl J Med 1994;330:663–669.

33. McPhail NV, Ruddy TD, Calvin JE, Davies RA, Barber GG. A comparison of dipyridamole-thallium imaging and exercise testing in the prediction of postoperative cardiac complications in patients requiring arterial reconstruction. J Vasc Surg 1989;10:51–56.

34. Cutler BS, Leppo JA. Dipyridamole thallium-201 scintigraphy to detect coronary artery disease before abdominal aortic surgery. J Vasc Surg 1987;5:91–100.

35. Lane RT, Sawada SG, Segar DS, et al. Dobutamine stress echocardiography for assessment of cardiac risk before noncardiac surgery. Am J Cardiol 1991;68:976–977.

36. Younis LT, Aguirre F, Byers S, et al. Perioperative and long-term prognostic value of intravenous dipyridamole thallium scintigraphy in patients with peripheral vascular disease. Am Heart J 1990;119:1287–1292.

37. Levinson JR, Boucher CA, Coley CM, Guiney TE, Strauss HW, Eagle KA. Usefulness of semiquantitative analysis of dipyridamole-thallium-201 redistribution for improving risk stratification before vascular surgery. Am J Cardiol 1990;66:406–410.

38. Bodenheimer MM. Noncardiac surgery in the cardiac patient: what is the question? Ann Intern Med 1996;124:763–766.

39. Goldman L. Cardiac risk for vascular surgery. J Am Coll Cardiol 1996;27:799–802.

40. Little WC, Constantinescu M, Applegate RJ, et al. Can coronary angiography predict the site of a subsequent myocardial infarction in patients with mild-to-moderate coronary artery disease? Circulation 1988;78:1157–1166.

41. Goldman L, Caldera DL, Nussbaum SR, et al. Multifactorial index of cardiac risk in noncar-

diac surgical procedures. N Engl J Med 1977; 297:845–850.

42. Detsky AS, Abrams HB, McLaughlin JR, et al. Predicting cardiac complications in patients undergoing noncardiac surgery. J Gen Intern Med 1986;1:211–219.

43. Wong T, Detsky AS. Preoperative cardiac risk assessment for patients having peripheral vascular surgery. J Intern Med 1992;116:743–753.

44. Mangano DT, Browner WS, Hollenberg M, London MJ, Tubau JF, Tateo IM. Association of perioperative myocardial ischemia with cardiac morbidity and mortality in men undergoing noncardiac surgery. N Engl J Med 1990; 323:1781–1788.

45. Fleisher LA, Nelson AH, Rosenbaum SH. Postoperative myocardial ischemia: etiology of cardiac morbidity or manifestation of underlying disease. J Clin Anesth 1995;7:1–6.

46. Pasternack PF, Grossi EA, Baumann FG, et al. The value of silent myocardial ischemia monitoring in the prediction of perioperative myocardial infarction in patients undergoing peripheral vascular surgery. J Vasc Surg 1989;10: 617–625.

47. Ouyang P, Gerstenblith G, Furman WR, Golueke PJ, Gottlieb SO. Frequency and significance of early postoperative silent myocardial ischemia in patients having peripheral vascular surgery. Am J Cardiol 1989;64:1113–1116.

48. McCann RL, Wolfe WG. Resection of abdominal aortic aneurysm in patients with low ejection fractions. J Vasc Surg 1989;10:240–244.

49. Raby KE, Barry J, Creager MA, Cook EF, Weisberg MC, Goldman L. Detection and significance of intraoperative and postoperative myocardial ischemia in peripheral vascular surgery. JAMA 1992;268:222–227.

50. Mangano DT, Wong MG, London MJ, Tubau JF, Rapp JA. Perioperative myocardial ischemia in patients undergoing noncardiac surgery—II: incidence and severity during the first week after surgery. J Am Coll Cardiol 1991;17: 851–857.

51. Hollenberg M, Mangano DT, Browner WS, London MJ, Tubau JF, Tateo IM. Predictors of postoperative myocardial ischemia in patients undergoing noncardiac surgery. JAMA 1992; 268:205–209.

52. Clinical competence in exercise testing: a statement for physicians from the ACP/ACC/AHA Task Force on Clinical Privileges in Cardiology. J Am Coll Cardiol 1990;16:1061–1065.

53. Pasternack PF, Imparto AM, Bear G. The value of radionuclide angiography as a predictor of perioperative myocardial infarction in patients undergoing abdominal aortic aneurysm resection. J Vasc Surg 1984;1(2):320–325.

54. Takase B, Younis LT, Byers SL, et al. Comparative prognostic value of clinical risk in-

dexes, resting two-dimensional echocardiography, and dipyridamole stress thallium-201 myocardial imaging for perioperative cardiac events in major nonvascular surgery patients. Am Heart J 1993;126:1099–1106.

55. Franco CD, Goldsmith J, Veith FJ, et al. Resting gated pool ejection fraction: a poor predictor of perioperative myocardial infarction in patients undergoing vascular surgery for infrainguinal bypass grafting. J Vasc Surg 1989;10:656–661.

56. Pasternack PF, Imparato AM, Riles TS, et al. The value of the radionuclide angiogram in the prediction of perioperative myocardial infarction in patients undergoing lower extremity revascularization procedures. Circulation 1985;72(Suppl II):13–17.

57. Patterson RE, Horowitz SF. Importance of epidemiology and biostatistics in deciding clinical strategies for using diagnostic tests: a simplified approach using examples from coronary artery disease. J Am Coll Cardiol 1989; 13:1653–1665.

58. Younis L, Stratmann H, Takase B, Byers S, Chaitman BR, Miller DD. Preoperative clinical assessment and dipyridamole thallium-201 scintigraphy for prediction and prevention of cardiac events in patients having major noncardiovascular surgery and known or suspected coronary artery disease. Am J Cardiol 1994;74:311–317.

59. Mantha S, Roizen MF, Barnard J, Thisted RA, Ellis JE, Foss J. Relative effectiveness of four preoperative tests for predicting adverse cardiac outcomes after vascular surgery: a meta-analysis. Anesth Analg 1994;79:422–433.

60. Dávila-Román VG, Waggoner AD, Sicard GA, Geltman EM, Schechtman KB, Perez JE. Dobutamine stress echocardiography predicts surgical outcome in patients with an aortic aneurysm and peripheral vascular disease. J Am Coll Cardiol 1993;21:957–963.

61. Eichelberger JP, Schwarz KQ, Black ER, Green RM, Ouriel K. Predictive value of dobutamine echocardiography just before noncardiac vascular surgery. Am J Cardiol 1993;72:602–607.

62. Poldermans D, Fioretti PM, Forster T, et al. Dobutamine stress echocardiography for assessment of perioperative cardiac risk in patients undergoing major vascular surgery. Circulation 1993;87:1506–1512.

63. Guidelines for clinical use of cardiac radionuclide imaging: a report of the American College of Cardiology/American Heart Association Task Force on Assessment of Diagnostic and Therapeutic Cardiovascular Procedures (Committee on Radionuclide Imaging), developed in collaboration with the American Society of Nuclear Cardiology. J Am Coll Cardiol 1995;25: 521–547.

64. Arous EJ, Baum PL, Cutler BS. The ischemic exercise test in patients with peripheral vascular disease: implications for management. Arch Surg 1984;119:780–783.

65. McPhail N, Calvin JE, Shariatmadar A, Barber GG, Scobie TK. The use of preoperative exercise testing to predict cardiac complications after arterial reconstruction. J Vasc Surg 1988;7: 60–68.

66. Cutler BS, Wheeler HB, Paraskas JA, Cardullo PA. Applicability and interpretation of electrocardiographic stress testing in patients with peripheral vascular disease. Am J Surg 1981; 141:501–506.

67. Carliner NH, Fisher ML, Plotnick GD, et al. Routine preoperative exercise testing in patients undergoing major noncardiac surgery. Am J Cardiol 1985;56:51–58.

68. Lette J, Waters D, Lassonde J, et al. Multivariate clinical models and quantitative dipyridamole-thallium imaging to predict cardiac morbidity and death after vascular reconstruction. J Vasc Surg 1991;14:160–169.

69. Weiner DA, Ryan TJ, McCabe CH, et al. Prognostic importance of a clinical profile and exercise test in medically treated patients with coronary artery disease. J Am Coll Cardiol 1984;3:772–779.

70. Mangano DT, Layug EL, Wallace A, Tateo I. Effect of atenolol on mortality and cardiovascular morbidity after noncardiac surgery. N Engl J Med 1996;335:1713–1720.

71. Lette J, Waters D, Lapointe J, et al. Usefulness of the severity and extent of reversible perfusion defects during thallium-dipyridamole imaging for cardiac risk assessment before noncardiac surgery. Am J Cardiol 1989;64: 276–280.

72. Shaw L, Miller DD, Kong BA, et al. Determination of perioperative cardiac risk by adenosine thallium-210 myocardial imaging. Am Heart J 1992;124:861–869.

73. McFalls EO, Doliszny KM, Grund F, Chute E, Chesler E. Angina and persistent exercise thallium defects: independent risk factors in elective vascular surgery. J Am Coll Cardiol 1993;21:1347–1352.

74. Coley CM, Field TS, Abraham SA, Boucher CA, Eagle KA. Usefulness of dipyridamole-thallium scanning for preoperative evaluation of cardiac risk for nonvascular surgery. Am J Cardiol 1992;69:1280–1285.

75. Brown KA, Rowen M. Extent of jeopardized viable myocardium determined by myocardial perfusion imaging best predicts perioperative cardiac events in patients undergoing noncardiac surgery. J Am Coll Cardiol 1993;21: 325–330.

76. Vanzetto G, Machecourt J, Blendea D, et al. Additive value of thallium single-photon emis-

sion computed tomography myocardial imaging for prediction of perioperative events in clinically selected high cardiac risk patients having abdominal aortic surgery. Am J Cardiol 1996;77:143–148.

77. McEnroe CS, O'Donnell TF, Yeager A, Konstam M, Mackey WC. Comparison of ejection fraction and Goldman risk factor analysis to dipyridamole-thallium 201 studies in the evaluation of cardiac morbidity after aortic aneurysm surgery. J Vasc Surg 1990;11:497–504.

78. Dilsizian V, Rocco TP, Freedman NMT, Leon MB, Bonow RO. Enhanced detection of ischemic but viable myocardium by the reinjection of thallium after stress-redistribution imaging. N Engl J Med 1990;323:53–60.

79. Detsky AS, Abrams HB, Forbath N, Scott JG, Hilliard JR. Cardiac assessment for patients undergoing noncardiac surgery: a multifactorial clinical risk index. Arch Intern Med 1986; 146:2131–2134.

80. Marwick TH, Underwood DA. Dipyridamole-thallium imaging may not be a reliable screening test for coronary artery disease in patients undergoing vascular surgery. Clin Cardiol 1990;13:14–18.

81. Eisenberg MJ, London MJ, Leung JM, et al. Monitoring for myocardial ischemia during noncardiac surgery. JAMA 1992;268:210–216.

82. Wackers FJT. Comparison of thallium-201 and technetium-99m methoxyisobutyl isonitrile. Am J Cardiol 1992;70:30E–34E.

83. Bartels C, Bechtel JFM, Hossmann V, Horsch S. Cardiac risk stratification for high-risk vascular surgery. Circulation 1997;95:2473–2475.

84. Sawada SG, Segar DS, Ryan T, et al. Echocardiographic detection of coronary artery disease during dobutamine infusion. Circulation 1991; 83:1605–1614.

85. Cohen JL, Greene TO, Ottenweller J, Binenbaum SZ, Wilchfort SD, Kim CS. Dobutamine digital echocardiography for detecting coronary artery disease. Am J Cardiol 1991;67:1311–1318.

86. Langan EM III, Youkey JR, Franklin DP, Elmore JR, Costello JM, Nassef LA. Dobutamine stress echocardiography for cardiac risk assessment before aortic surgery. J Vasc Surg 1993;18:905–913.

87. Lalka SG, Sawada SG, Dalsing MC, et al. Dobutamine stress echocardiography as a predictor of cardiac events associated with aortic surgery. J Vasc Surg 1992;15:831–842.

88. Shaw LJ, Eagle KA, Gersh BJ, Miller DD. Meta-analysis of intravenous dipyridamole–thallium-201 imaging (1985 to 1994) and dobutamine echocardiography (1991 to 1994) for risk stratification before vascular surgery. J Am Coll Cardiol 1996;27:787–798.

89. Tischler MD, Lee TH, Hirsch AT, et al. Prediction of major cardiac events after peripheral vascular surgery using dipyridamole echocardiography. Am J Cardiol 1991;68:593–597.

90. Poldermans D, Arnese M, Fioretti PM, et al. Improved cardiac risk stratification in major vascular surgery with dobutamine-atropine stress echocardiography. J Am Coll Cardiol 1995;26:648–653.

91. Poldermans D, Arnese M, Fioretti PM, et al. Sustained prognostic value of dobutamine stress echocardiography for late cardiac events after major noncardiac vascular surgery. Circulation 1997;95:53–58.

92. Hertzer NR, Beven EG, Young JR, et al. Coronary artery disease in peripheral vascular patients: a classification of 1000 coronary angiograms and results of surgical management. Ann Surg 1984;199:223–233.

93. Toal KW, Jacocks MA, Elkins RC. Preoperative coronary artery bypass grafting in patients undergoing abdominal aortic reconstruction. Am J Surg 1984;148:825–829.

94. Mahar LJ, Steen PA, Tinker JH, Vliestra RE, Smith HC, Pluth JR. Perioperative myocardial infarction in patients with coronary artery disease with and without aorta–coronary artery bypass grafts. J Thorac Cardiovasc Surg 1978;76:533–537.

95. Mason JJ, Owens DK, Harris RA, Cooke JP, Hlatky MA. The role of coronary angiography and coronary revascularization before noncardiac vascular surgery. JAMA 1995;273:1919–1925.

96. Ashton CM, Petersen NJ, Wray NP, et al. The incidence of perioperative myocardial infarction in men undergoing noncardiac surgery. Ann Intern Med 1993;118:504–510.

97. Guidelines for coronary angiography: a report of the American College of Cardiology/American Heart Association Task Force on Assessment of Diagnostic and Therapeutic Cardiovascular Procedures (Subcommittee on Coronary Angiography). J Am Coll Cardiol 1987;10: 935–950.

98. Hertzer NR. Fatal myocardial infarction following abdominal aortic aneurysm resection: three hundred forty-three patients followed 6–11 years postoperatively. Ann Surg 1980;192: 667–673.

99. Blombery PA, Ferguson IA, Rosengarten DS, et al. The role of coronary artery disease in complications of abdominal aortic aneurysm surgery. Surgery 1987;101:150–155.

100. Rihal CS, Gersh BJ, Whisnant JP, et al. Influence of coronary heart disease on morbidity and mortality after carotid endarterectomy: a population-based study in Olmsted County, Minnesota (1970–1988). J Am Coll Cardiol 1992;19:1254–1260.

101. Domanski M, Ellis S, Eagle K. Does preoperative coronary revascularization before noncardiac surgery reduce the risk of coronary events in patients with known coronary artery disease? Am J Cardiol 1995;75:829–831.

102. Rihal CS, Eagle KA, Mickel MC, Foster ED, Sopko G, Gersh BJ. Surgical therapy for coronary artery disease among patients with combined coronary artery and peripheral vascular disease. Circulation 1995;91:46–53.

103. Crawford ES, Morris GC Jr, Howell JF, Flynn WF, Moorhead DT. Operative risk in patients with previous coronary artery bypass. Ann Thorac Surg 1978;26:215–221.

104. Diehl JT, Cali RF, Hertzer NR, Beven EG. Complications of abdominal aortic reconstruction: an analysis of perioperative risk factors in 557 patients. Ann Surg 1982;197:49–56.

105. Reigel MM, Hollier LH, Kazmier FJ, et al. Late survival in abdominal aortic aneurysm patients: the role of selective myocardial revascularization on the basis of clinical symptoms. J Vasc Surg 1987;5:222–227.

106. Hertzer NR, Young JR, Beven EG, et al. Late results of coronary bypass in patients with peripheral vascular disease. I: five-year survival according to age and clinical cardiac status. Cleve Clin Q 1986;53:133–143.

107. Foster ED, Davis KB, Carpenter JA, Abele S, Fray D. Risk of noncardiac operation in patients with defined coronary disease. The Coronary Artery Surgery Study (CASS) Registry experience. Ann Thorac Surg 1986;41:42–50.

108. Reul GJ, Cooley DA, Duncan JM, et al. The effect of coronary bypass on the outcome of peripheral vascular operations in 1093 patients. J Vasc Surg 1986;3:788–798.

109. Guidelines and indications for coronary artery bypass graft surgery: a report of the American College of Cardiology/American Heart Association Task Force on Assessment of Diagnostic and Therapeutic Cardiovascular Procedures (Subcommittee on Coronary Artery Bypass Graft Surgery). J Am Coll Cardiol 1991;17:543–589.

110. Huber KC, Evans MA, Bresnahan JF, Gibbons RJ, Holmes DR Jr. Outcome of noncardiac operations in patients with severe coronary artery disease successfully treated preoperatively with coronary angioplasty. Mayo Clin Proc 1992;67:15–21.

111. Elmore JR, Hallett JW, Gibbons RJ, et al. Myocardial revascularization before abdominal aortic aneurysmorrhaphy: effect of coronary angioplasty. Mayo Clin Proc 1993;68:637–641.

112. Allen JR, Helling TS, Hartzler GO. Operative procedures not involving the heart after percutaneous transluminal coronary angioplasty. Surg Gynecol Obstet 1991;173:285–288.

113. Guidelines for percutaneous transluminal coronary angioplasty: a report of the American College of Cardiology/American Heart Association Task Force on Assessment of Diagnostic and Therapeutic Cardiovascular Procedures (Committee on Percutaneous Transluminal Coronary Angioplasty). J Am Coll Cardiol. 1993;22:2033–2054.

114. O'Kelly B, Browner WS, Massie B, Tubau J, Ngo L, Mangano DT. Ventricular arrhythmias in patients undergoing noncardiac surgery. JAMA 1992;268:217–221.

115. Burman SO. The prophylactic use of digitalis before thoracotomy. Ann Thor Surg 1972;14(4):359–368.

116. Braunwald E. Valvular heart disease. In: Baunwald E, ed. Heart disease: a textbook of cardiovascular medicine. 5th ed. Philadelphia: WB Saunders, 1997:1007–1076.

117. Silverman BG, Gross TP, Kaczmarek RG, Hamilton P, Hamburger S. The epidemiology of pacemaker implantation in the United States. Public Health Reports 1995;110(1):42–46.

118. Guidelines for implantation of cardiac pacemakers and antiarrhythmia devices: a report of the American College of Cardiology/American Heart Association Task Force on Assessment of Diagnostic and Therapeutic Cardiovascular Procedures (Committee on Pacemaker Implantation). J Am Coll Cardiol 1991;18:1–13.

119. Furman S, Hayes DL, Holmes DR. Electromagnetic interference, drug-device interactions, and other practical considerations. A practice of cardiac pacing. Mount Kisco, NY: Futura, 1993:665–684.

120. Rao TLK, Jacobs KH, el-Etr AA. Reinfarction following anesthesia in patients with myocardial infarction. Anesthesiology 1983;59:499–505.

121. Stevenson LW, Perlott JK. The limited reliability of physical signs for estimating hemodynamics in chronic heart failure. JAMA 1989;261:884–888.

122. Butman SM, Ewy GA, Standen JR, Kern KB, Hahn E. Bedside cardiovascular examination in patients with severe chronic heart failure: importance of rest or inducible jugular venous distension. J Am Coll Cardiol 1993;22:968–974.

123. Badgett RG, Lucey CR, Mulrow CD. Can the clinical examination diagnose left-sided heart failure in adults? JAMA 1997;277:1712–1719.

124. Sola JE, Bender JS. Use of the pulmonary artery catheter to reduce operative complications. Surg Clin North Am 1993;73:253–263.

125. Berlauk JF, Abrams JH, Gilmour IJ, O'Connor SR, Knighton DR, Cerra FB. Preoperative optimization of cardiovascular hemodynamics improves outcome in peripheral vascular surgery. Ann Surg 1991;214:289–298.

126. Bender JS, Smith-Meek MA, Jones CE. Routine pulmonary artery catheterization does not reduce morbidity and mortality of elective

vascular surgery: results of a prospective, randomized trial. Ann Surg 1997 (in press).

127. Clinical competence in hemodynamic monitoring. A statement for physicians from the ACP/ACC/AHA Task Force on Clinical Privileges in Cardiology. J Am Coll Cardiol 1990;15:1460–1464.

128. Kannel WB. Cardioprotection and antihypertensive therapy: the key importance of addressing the associated coronary risk factors (the Framingham experience). Am J Cardiol 1996; 77:6B–11B.

129. Burt VL, Whelton P, Roccella EJ, et al. Prevalence of hypertension in the U.S. adult population: results from the Third National Health and Nutrition Examination Survey, 1988–1991. Hypertension 1995;25:305–313.

130. Goldman L, Caldera DL. Risks of general anesthesia and elective operation in the hypertensive patient. Anesthesiology 1979;50: 285–292.

131. Derbyshire DR, Smith G. Sympathoadrenal responses to anesthesia and surgery. Br J Anesth 1984;56:725–739.

132. Low JM, Harvey JT, Prys-Roberts C, Dagnino J. Studies of anesthesia in relation to hypertension. Br J Anesth 1986;58:471–477.

133. Bedford RF, Feinstein B. Hospital admission blood pressure: a predictor for hypertension following endotracheal intubation. Anesth Analg 1980;59:367–370.

134. Stamler J, Stamler R, Neaton JD. Blood pressure, systolic and diastolic, and cardiovascular risks. Arch Intern Med 1993;153:598–615.

135. Goldman L, Caldera DL, Southwick FS, et al. Cardiac risk factors and complications in noncardiac surgery. Medicine 1978;57:357–370.

136. Houston MC. Pathophysiology, clinical aspects, and treatment of hypertensive crises. Prog Cardiovasc Dis 1989;32:99–148.

137. Houston MC. Abrupt cessation of treatment in hypertension: consideration of clinical features, mechanisms, prevention and management of the discontinuation syndrome. Am Heart J 1981;102:415–430.

138. Johansson H, Brismar B, Hedenstierna G. Hypertensive crisis immediately after complete removal of phaeochromocytoma. Intensive Care Med 1986;12:56–57.

139. el-Ganzouri AR, Ivankovich AD, Braverman B, McCarthy R. Monoamine oxidase inhibitors: should they be discontinued preoperatively? Anesth Analg 1985;64:592–596.

140. Michaels I, Serrins M, Shier NQ, Barash PG. Anesthesia for cardiac surgery in patients receiving monoamine oxidase inhibitors. Anesth Analg 1984;63:1041–1044.

141. Lette J, Waters D, Bernier H, et al. Perioperative and long-term cardiac risk assessment: predictive value of 23 clinical descriptors, 7 multivariate scoring systems, and quantitative

dipyrimadole imaging in 360 patients. Ann Surg 1992;216:192–204.

142. Slogoff S, Keats AS. Does perioperative myocardial ischemia lead to postoperative myocardial infarction? Anesthesiology 1985;62: 107–114.

143. Slogoff S, Keats AS. Further observations on perioperative myocardial ischemia. Anesthesiology 1986;65:539–542.

144. Scheler S, Motz W, Vester J, Strauer BE. Transient myocardial ischemia in hypertensive heart disease. Am J Cardiol 1990;65: 51G–55G.

145. Harrison DG, Florentine MS, Brooks LA, Cooper SM, Marcus ML. The effect of hypertension and left ventricular hypertrophy on the lower range of coronary autoregulation. Circulation 1988;77:1108–1115.

146. Allman KG, Muir A, Howell SJ, Hemming AE, Sear JW, Foëx P. Resistant hypertension and preoperative silent myocardial ischaemia in surgical patients. Br J Anesthesia 1994;75: 574–578.

147. Shackelford DP, Hoffman MK, Kramer PR, Davies MF, Kaminski PF. Evaluation of preoperative cardiac risk index values in patients undergoing vaginal surgery. Am J Obstet Gynecol 1995;173:80–84.

148. Stone JG, Foëx P, Sear JW, Johnson LL, Khambatta HJ, Triner L. Myocardial ischemia in untreated hypertensive patients: effect of a single small oral dose of a beta-adrenergic blocking agent. Anesthesiol 1988;68:495–500.

149. Weiss SJ, Longnecker DE. Perioperative hypertension: an overview. Coronary Artery Dis 1993;4:401–406.

150. Brutsaert DL, Sys SU, Gillebert TC. Diastolic failure: pathophysiology and therapeutic implications. J Am Coll Cardiol 1993;22: 318–325.

151. Topol EJ, Traill TA, Fortuin NJ. Hypertensive hypertrophic cardiomyopathy of the elderly. N Engl J Med 1985;312:277–283.

152. Shapiro SM, Bersohn MM, Laks MM. In search of the Holy Grail: the study of diastolic ventricular function by the use of Doppler echocardiography. J Am Coll Cardiol 1991;17:1517–1519.

153. Thomas JD, Weyman AE. Echocardiographic Doppler evaluation of left ventricular diastolic function. Physics and physiology. Circulation 1991;84:977–990.

154. Nishimura RA, Housmans PR, Hatle LK, Tajik AJ. Assessment of diastolic function of the heart: background and current applications of Doppler echocardiography. Part II. Clinical studies. Mayo Clin Proc 1989;64:181–204.

155. Cuocolo A, Sax FL, Brush JE, Maron BJ, Bacharach SL, Bonow RO. Left ventricular hypertrophy and impaired diastolic filling in essential hypertension. Diastolic mechanisms

for systolic dysfunction during exercise. Circulation 1990;81:978–986.

156. Longnecker DE, Murphy FL, eds. Introduction to anesthesia. Philadelphia: WB Saunders, 1997.

157. Skydell JL, Machleder HI, Baker D, Busuttil RW, Moore WS. Incidence and mechanism of post-carotid endarterectomy hypertension. Arch Surg 1987;122:1153–1155.

158. Slotman GJ, Jed EH, Burchard KW. Adverse effects of hypothermia in postoperative patients. Am J Surg 1985;149:495–501.

159. Vaughan MS, Vaughan RW, Cork RC. Postoperative hypothermia in adults: relationship of age, anesthesia, and shivering to rewarming. Anesth Analg 1981;60:746–751.

160. Frank SM, Higgins MS, Breslow MJ, et al. The catecholamine, cortisol, and hemodynamic responses to mild perioperative hypothermia: a randomized clinical trial. Anesthesiology 1995; 82:83–93.

161. Frank SM, Higgins MS, Flesisher LA, Sitzmann JV, Raff H, Breslow MJ. Adrenergic, respiratory, and cardiovascular effects of core cooling in humans. Am J Physiol 1997;272: R557–R562.

162. Sessler DI. Perianesthetic thermoregulation and heat balance in humans. FASEB J 1993;7: 638–644.

163. Frank SM, Fleisher LA, Breslow MJ, et al. Perioperative maintenance of normothermia reduces the incidence of morbid cardiac events: a randomized clinical trial. JAMA 1997;277: 1127–1134.

164. Hulyalkar AR, Miller E Jr. Evaluation of the hypertensive patient. In: Rogers MC, Tinkler JH, Covino BG, Longnecker DE, eds. Principles and practice of anesthesiology. Mosby–Year Book, 1993;1:155–167.

165. Levi R. Therapies for perioperative hypertension: pharmacodynamic considerations. Acta Anaesthesiol Scand 1993;37:16–19.

166. Houston MC. Clonidine hydrochloride. South Med J 1982;75:713–721.

167. Coltart DJ, Mitchell NC, Stinson EB, et al. Investigation of the safe withdrawal period for propranolol in patients scheduled for open heart surgery. Br Heart J 1975;37:1228–1234.

168. Leaman DM, Levenson LW, Shiroff RA, et al. Persistence of biologic activity after disappearance of propranolol from the serum. J Thorac Cardiovasc Surg 1976;72:67–72.

169. Faulkner SL, Hopkins JT, Boerth RC, et al. Time required for complete recovery from chronic propranolol therapy. N Engl J Med 1973;289:607–609.

170. Viljoen JF, Estafanous FG, Kellner GA. Propranolol and cardiac surgery. J Thorac Cardiovasc Surg 1972;64:826–830.

171. Slogoff S, Keats AS, Ott E. Preoperative propranolol therapy and aortocoronary bypass operation. JAMA 1978;240:1487–1490.

172. Nattel S, Rangno RE, Van Loon G. Mechanism of propranolol withdrawal phenomena. Circulation 1979;59:1158–1164.

173. Goldman L. Noncardiac surgery in patients receiving propranolol. Case reports and a recommended approach. Arch Intern Med 1981; 141:193–196.

174. Goldman L. Cardiac risks and complications of noncardiac surgery. Ann Intern Med 1983;98: 504–513.

175. Pasternack PF, Imparato AM, Baumann FG, et al. The hemodynamics of ß-blockade in patients undergoing abdominal aortic aneurysm repair. Circulation 1987;76:III-1–III-7.

176. Leslie JB, Kalayjian RW, Sirgo MA, Plachetka JR, Watkins WD. Intravenous labetalol for treatment of postoperative hypertension. Anesthesiol 1987;67:413–416.

177. Grossman E, Messerli FH, Grodzicki T, Kowey P. Should a moratorium be placed on sublingual nifedipine capsules given for hypertensive emergencies and pseudoemergencies? JAMA 1996;276:1328–1331.

178. Breslow MJ, Jordan DA, Christopherson R, et al. Epidural morphine decreases postoperative hypertension by attenuating sympathetic nervous system hyperactivity. JAMA 1989;261: 3577–3581.

179. O'Keefe JH, Shub C, Rettke SR. Risk of noncardiac surgical procedures in patients with aortic stenosis. Mayo Clin Proc 1989;64:400–405.

180. Olson LJ, Subramanian R, Ackermann DM. Surgical pathology of the mitral valve: a study of 712 cases spanning 21 years. Mayo Clin Proc 1987;62:22–34.

181. Leavitt JI, Coats MH, Falk RH. Effects of exercise on transmitral gradient and pulmonary artery pressure in patients with mitral stenosis or a prosthetic mitral valve: a Doppler echocardiographic study. J Am Coll Cardiol 1991;17:1520–1526.

182. Passik CS, Ackermann DM, Pluth JR, Edwards WE. Temporal changes in the causes of aortic stenosis: a surgical pathologic study of 646 cases. Mayo Clin Proc 1987;62:119–123.

183. Otto CM, Pearlman AS, Kraft CD, Miyake-Hull CY, Burwash IG, Gardner CJ. Physiologic changes with maximal exercise in asymptomatic valvular aortic stenosis assessed by Doppler echocardiography. J Am Coll Cardiol 1992;20:1160–1167.

184. Deron SJ, Kotler MN. Noncardiac surgery in the cardiac patient. Am Heart J 1988;116: 831–838.

185. Otto CM, Mickel MC, Kennedy JW, et al. Three-year outcome after balloon aortic valvuloplasty: insights into prognosis of valvular aortic stenosis. Circulation 1994;89:642–650.

186. Nishimura RA, Holmes DR Jr, Reeder GS, et al. Doppler evaluation of results of percutaneous aortic balloon valvuloplasty in calcific aortic stenosis. Circulation 1988;78:791–799.

187. Levine MJ, Berman AD, Safian RD, Diver DJ, McKay RG. Palliation of valvular aortic stenosis by balloon valvuloplasty as preoperative preparation for noncardiac surgery. Am J Cardiol 1988;62:1309–1311.

188. Etchells E, Bell C, Robb K. Does this patient have an abnormal systolic murmur? JAMA 1997;277:564–571.

189. Currie PJ, Seward JB, Reeder GS, et al. Continuous-wave Doppler echocardiographic assessment of severity of calcific aortic stenosis: a simultaneous Doppler-catheter correlative study in 100 adult patients. Circulation 1985; 71:1162–1169.

190. Zoghbi WA, Farmer KL, Soto JG, Nelson JG, Quinones MA. Accurate noninvasive quantification of stenotic aortic valve area by Doppler echocardiography. Circulation 1986; 73:452–459.

191. Yeager M, Yock PG, Popp RL. Comparison of Doppler-derived pressure gradient to that determined at cardiac catheterization in adults with aortic valve stenosis: implications for management. Am J Cardiol 1986;57: 644–648.

192. Nakatani S, Masuyama T, Kodama K, Kitabatake A, Fujii K, Kamada T. Value and limitations of Doppler echocardiography in the quantification of stenotic mitral valve area: comparison of the pressure half-time and the continuity equation methods. Circulation 1988; 77:78–85.

193. Smith MD, Wisenbaugh T, Grayburn PA, Gurley JC, Spain MG, DeMaria AN. Value and limitations of Doppler pressure half-time in quantifying mitral stenosis: a comparison with micromanometer catheter recording. Am Heart J 1991;121:480–488.

194. Atwood JE, Kawanishi S, Myers J, Froelicher VF. Exercise testing in patients with aortic stenosis. Chest 1988;93:1083–1087.

195. Aronow WS, Harris CN. Treadmill exercise test in aortic stenosis and mitral stenosis. Chest 1975;68:507–509.

196. Linderholm H, Osterman G, Teien D. Detection of coronary artery disease by means of exercise ECG in patients with aortic stenosis. Acta Med Scand 1985;218:181–188.

197. Nylander E, Ekman I, Marklund T, Sinnerstad B, Karlsson E, Wranne B. Severe aortic stenosis in elderly patients. Br Heart J 1986;55: 480–487.

198. Samuels B, Kiat H, Friedman JD, Berman DS. Adenosine pharmacologic stress myocardial perfusion tomographic imaging in patients with significant aortic stenosis: diagnostic efficacy and comparison of clinical, hemodynamic and electrocardiographic variables with 100 age-matched control subjects. J Am Coll Cardiol 1995;25:99–106.

199. deFilippi CR, Willett DL, Brickner ME, et al. Usefulness of dobutamine echocardiography in distinguishing severe from nonsevere valvular aortic stenosis in patients with depressed left ventricular function and low transvalvular gradients. Am J Cardiol 1995; 75:191–194.

200. Isner JM. Acute catastrophic complications of balloon aortic valvuloplasty. J Am Coll Cardiol 1991;17:1436–1444.

201. Holmes DR, Nishimura RA, Reeder GS. In-hospital mortality after balloon aortic valvuloplasty: frequency and associated factors. J Am Coll Cardiol 1991;17:189–192.

202. Litvack F, Jakubowski AT, Buchbinder NA, Eigler N. Lack of sustained clinical improvement in an elderly population after percutaneous aortic valvuloplasty. Am J Cardiol 1988;62: 270–275.

203. Wilkins GT, Weyman AE, Abascal VM, Block PC, Palacios IF. Percutaneous mitral valvotomy: an analysis of echocardiographic variables related to outcome and the mechanism of dilatation. Br Heart J 1988;60:299–308.

204. Palacios IF, Tuzcu ME, Weyman AE, Newell JB, Block PC. Clinical follow-up of patients undergoing percutaneous mitral balloon valvotomy. Circulation 1995;91:671–676.

205. Vongpatanasin W, Hillis LD, Lange RA. Prosthetic heart valves. N Engl J Med 1996;335: 407–416.

206. Chesebro JH, Adams PC, Fuster V. Antithrombotic therapy in patients with valvular heart disease and prosthetic heart valves. J Am Coll Cardiol 1986;8:41B–56B.

207. Stein PD, Alpert JS, Copeland J, Dalen JE, Goldman S, Turpie AGG. Antithrombotic therapy in patients with mechanical and biological prosthetic heart valves. Chest 1992;102: 445S–455S.

208. Bärwolf CG, Acar J, Burckhardt D, et al. Ad Hoc Committee of the Working Group on Valvular Heart Disease, European Society of Cardiology. Guidelines for prevention of thromboembolic events in valvular heart disease. J Heart Valve Dis 1993;2:398–410.

209. Thompson RC, Liberthson RR, Lowenstein E. Perioperative anesthetic risk of noncardiac surgery in hypertrophic obstructive cardiomyopathy. JAMA 1985;254:2419–2421.

210. Loubser P, Suh K, Cohen S. Adverse effects of spinal anesthesia in a patient with idiopathic hypertrophic subaortic stenosis. Anesthesiology 1984;60:228–233.

12

Renal, Fluid, Electrolyte, and Acid-Base Disorders

Paul E. Turer and Gary R. Briefel

Disturbances of body fluid composition or renal function are commonly encountered in surgical patients by the consulting internist. The actual incidence of many electrolyte disorders and their effects on surgical morbidity, however, can only be estimated because of insufficient data. In general, renal-electrolyte disorders among surgical patients occur in complex settings and have significant morbidity associated with them.

Many times, fluid, electrolyte, and acid-base disturbances in surgical patients are multifactorial in origin. They are often as likely to arise from therapeutic maneuvers (e.g., nasogastric suction, fluid therapy) as from the underlying surgical problem. In addition, the body's metabolic and endocrinologic responses to surgery and trauma further predispose a patient to the development of fluid and electrolyte abnormalities.

Most of these disturbances of body fluid composition occur in patients with normal kidneys. However, the incidence of fluid and electrolyte problems increases as a patient's renal function declines. Even patients with mild renal impairment are likely to decompensate under the stress of surgery and trauma.

Acute renal failure (ARF) following surgery or trauma is one of the most difficult complications to manage, and it carries a high mortality rate. Although the morbidity of ARF has been modified by use of dialysis, the best hope of reducing the mortality of ARF lies in its prevention. Therefore, the recognition and treatment of factors predisposing to the development of ARF is paramount.

PREOPERATIVE EVALUATION AND TREATMENT OF PATIENTS WITH NORMAL RENAL FUNCTION

Epidemiology

Although most surgical patients have normal renal function and no significant disturbances of body fluid composition on hospital admission, it is important to be alert for the development of such abnormalities, which could complicate the postoperative course. Fluid, electrolyte, and acid-base disorders contribute to the risks that come with anesthesia, whereas development of ARF in the surgical setting is associated with a mortality rate of 50% or greater. The chances of developing renal-electrolyte disorders roughly depend on the underlying surgical illness and the nature of the operative procedure in patients with normal renal function preoperatively (see "High-risk Surgery" under "Special Considerations"). The incidence of such disturbances is also higher in elderly patients or in those with predisposing medical illnesses (e.g., preexisting renal insufficiency, diabetes, congestive heart failure, cirrhosis). The factors most clearly predisposing a patient to the development of postoperative renal failure are listed in Table 12.1.

Hou et al. (1) prospectively studied 2262 consecutive hospital admissions to the general medical and surgical services. The overall incidence of ARF in this group was 4.9%, but the incidence of ARF was even higher (14.4%) in those patients whose serum creatinine level on admission was greater than 1.2 mg/dL. Decreased renal perfusion, associated with both prerenal states and acute tubular necrosis (ATN), and postoperative ARF were the most common causes, occurring in 42 and 18%, respectively. Iatrogenic factors accounted for 55% of acquired renal insufficiencies, whereas no definite cause could be found in 8%.

Shusterman et al. (2) found a 2% incidence of ARF in a large teaching hospital. The odds ratio for the development of ARF in surgical patients was increased to 9.0, 3.0, 4.3, and 1.8 for those with volume depletion, aminoglycoside use, congestive heart failure, and exposure to radiocontrast, respectively. The risk of dying in all patients with ARF was increased sixfold compared to that of patients without renal failure.

Shires and Carrico (3) found the risk of ARF following elective surgery to be less than 1%. However, emergency or other high-risk surgical procedures (Table 12.2)

Table 12.1.   Risk Factors for Postoperative Renal Failure

1. Volume depletion
2. Hypotension
3. Sepsis
4. Nephrotoxins
   a. Drugs (aminoglycosides)
   b. Radiocontrast materials
   c. Hemoglobinuria
   d. Myoglobinuria
5. High-risk surgical procedures (see p. 176)
6. Preexisting renal insufficiency
7. Advanced age
8. Congestive heart failure
9. Obstructive jaundice

Table 12.2.   Incidence of Renal Insufficiency in Various Clinical Settings[a]

Clinical Setting	% Mild Acute Renal Failure (Scr <3 mg/dl)	% Severe Acute Renal Failure (Scr >3 mg/dl)
Elective surgery	1	<1
Admission to general medical/surgical service	4	1
Aminoglycoside administration	5–20	1–2
Open heart surgery	5–30	2–5
Abdominal aortic aneurysm resection		
Elective	5–10	2–5
Emergency	30–50	15–25
Severe trauma	10–20	1–5

[a]Adapted from Anderson and Schrier: Clinical spectrum of oliguric and nonoliguric acute renal failure, in Brenner BM, Stein JH (eds): Contemporary Issues in Nephrology: Acute Renal Failure. New York, Churchill Livingstone, 1980.

are associated with a much higher incidence of ARF (5–50%) and mortality (80–90%). For example, Green and Better (4) reported that the incidence of ARF was between 8 and 10% in a combined series of patients undergoing surgery for obstructive jaundice. These patients had a mortality rate of up to 80%, compared with the overall mortality rate of 16 to 18% in all surgical patients without obstructive jaundice.

Adequate maintenance of intravascular volume is essential in the prevention of ARF. In addition to resulting in prerenal azotemia, volume depletion appears to potentiate nephrotoxic insults of all types. Hypotension, whether resulting from fluid or blood losses, third spacing, sepsis, or myocardial dysfunction, is one of the most common causes of ATN in surgical patients. It is difficult, however, to correlate the degree and duration of hypotension with the development of ARF in any given patient. Hou et al. (1) documented hypotension in only 52% of the episodes of acute postoperative renal failure in their study.

Despite the presence of edema, patients with congestive heart failure, nephrotic syndrome, cirrhosis, and jaundice have decreased effective circulating volumes, and they may be excessively prone to hypotension from diuretics, sepsis, bleeding, and antihypertensive drugs. With or without hypotension or documented bacteremia, sepsis is considered to be a frequent cause of ARF in surgical patients. Intraabdominal infections with Gram-negative organisms are the most common cause of sepsis in these patients, and they often result in a nonoliguric renal failure. Visceral abscess of the lungs, abdomen, or sinuses has also been reported to cause ARF from an immune complex–mediated proliferative glomerulonephritis (5–7). Rather than producing direct nephrotoxicity, however, hyperbilirubinemia appears to predispose patients to the development of postoperative ARF by reducing peripheral vascular resistance, reducing cardiac performance, and inducing a diuresis that can result in volume depletion (4).

Nephrotoxic renal injury is another common cause of ARF in surgical patients. A wide variety of drugs have toxic effects on the kidney, ranging from impaired tubular functions to interstitial nephritis and ATN (8). Aminoglycoside antibiotics are some of the most frequent offenders, producing nephrotoxicity in 10 to 25% of patients even when the drug levels are within therapeutic concentrations (9). Radiocontrast materials also appear to be nephrotoxic, particularly in elderly patients (age, >60 years) and those with diabetes, preexisting renal disease, multiple myeloma, or volume depletion (10).

The precise incidence of radiocontrast-induced ARF is difficult to estimate from the literature. Overall, the incidence of reported renal dysfunction following radiocontrast administration is generally between 0 and 12%. Van Zee et al. (11) retrospectively reviewed the charts of 377 patients and found a greater than 1 mg/dL increase in the serum creatinine level following intravenous pyelography in 1.4, 9.2, and 39% of all cases when the initial levels were less than 1.5, 1.5 to 4.5, and greater than 4.5 mg/dL, respectively. In high-risk patients such as those without diabetes but with azotemia and an initial serum creatinine level greater then 4.5 mg/dL, 5 of 16 (31%) developed further renal dysfunction. In a study by Harkonen and Kjellstrand (12), exacerbation of renal failure occurred in 22 of 29 patients (76%) with diabetes with an initial serum creatinine level greater than 2 mg/dL. In another, prospective study, D'Elia et al. (13) found the incidence of ARF following nonrenal angiography to be 33% in patients with a baseline creatinine level greater than 1.5 mg/dL (mean, 2.3 mg/dL).

Newer, nonionic radiocontrast materials are quite expensive, and it was originally hoped they would be less nephrotoxic than ionic agents. Nonrandomized and retrospective studies have suggested a reduced incidence of ARF associated with the use of these agents, but a prospective, randomized study in 443 patients undergoing cardiac catheterization was unable to demonstrate any difference in the incidence of nephrotoxicity between patients receiving nonionic and those receiving ionic contrast agents (14–16). Clinically, radiocontrast-induced renal failure is often mild, and it is generally characterized by oliguria developing within the first 48 hours and lasting for an average of 2 to 4 days. The serum creatinine level usually peaks within 1 week of exposure and then returns to baseline in over 75% of cases.

Hemoglobinuria is more likely to occur following cardiopulmonary bypass surgery than after mismatched blood transfusions. Myoglobinuria, on the other hand, commonly occurs among surgical patients and should be considered in the clinical situations listed in Table 12.3.

The difficulty in successfully managing the complicated surgical patient arises from the fact that usually more than one of the risk factors discussed here are present.

Table 12.3.   Select Causes of Myoglobinuria in the Surgical Setting

1. Excessive muscular activity
   a. Seizures
   b. Agitated delirium, restraints
   c. High-voltage electric shock
2. Trauma
   a. Fallen weights, auto accident
   b. Compression by body in prolonged coma
3. Ischemic
   a. Arterial occlusion
   b. Compression and anterior tibial syndrome
4. Metabolic
   a. Hypokalemia
   b. Hypophosphatemia
5. Drugs
   a. Alcohol
   b. Narcotics (heroin)
   c. Succinylcholine
   d. Amphetamines
6. Infection (influenza)
7. Heat cramps, malignant hyperthermia, burns
8. Idiopathic

Evaluation

To use all of the available data most efficiently, a flow chart including sequential measurements of weight, blood pressure, intake and output, serum and urine chemistries, drugs, and other diagnostic or therapeutic interventions is recommended.

Patient History

The patient history helps the physician to recognize surgically unrelated disorders (e.g., diabetes, cirrhosis) or clinical manifestations of the present illness (e.g., vomiting, diarrhea) that predispose a patient to renal dysfunction or fluid and electrolyte abnormalities. The list of conditions leading to intravascular volume depletion is extensive (Table 12.4). The history should also include an inventory of all drugs, administered both in the past and in the present, that might have a bearing on renal-electrolyte problems (Table 12.5).

Physical Examination

The physical examination should emphasize clinical assessment of the extracellular and intravascular volume status. An orthostatic fall in blood pressure, nondistended neck veins, and resting tachycardia in the supine position when not resulting from other causes are associated with a significant (≥ 1 L) deficit in the intravascular volume. The "classical" signs of volume depletion (e.g., decreased

Table 12.4.   Factors Responsible for Volume Depletion

I. Decreased intake
   A. NPO during diagnostic procedures
   B. Defective thirst mechanism
   C. Lack of access to food/H_2O
   D. Anorexia
II. Excessive loss
   A. Gastrointestinal losses
      1. Vomiting
      2. Diarrhea
      3. Fistula or tube drainage
      4. Enemas (cleansing and barium), cathartics
      5. Bleeding
   B. Renal losses
      1. Diuretics
      2. Osmotic diuresis (radiocontrast dyes, high-protein tube feeding, mannitol, glycerol, glucose)
      3. Salt-wasting nephropathies
      4. Adrenal insufficiency
      5. Diabetes insipidus
         a. Central
         b. Nephrogenic
   C. Skin losses
      1. Excessive sweating
      2. Burns
      3. Extensive skin lesions
III. Third space sequestration
   A. Peritonitis
   B. Intestinal obstruction
   C. Pancreatitis
   D. Crush injuries
   E. Skeletal fractures
   F. Burns
   G. Sepsis
   H. Sites of surgical trauma including wounds (retroperitoneal)
   I. Bleeding
   J. Venous obstruction
      1. Mesenteric venous obstruction
      2. Acute ileofemoral thrombophlebitis

Table 12.5.   Drug-related Renal Syndromes Encountered in Surgical Patients

I. Renal dysfunction
  A. Acute renal failure
    Analgesics (aspirin, NSAIDs)
    Antibiotics (aminoglycosides, cepha-
      losporins, polymixin, tetracyclines,
      pentamidine, foscarnet)
    Antifungal agents (amphotericin B)
    Dextran
    Radiocontrast materials
    Anesthetics (methoxyflurange, enthrane)
  B. Interstitial nephritis
    Analgesics (aspirin, NSAIDs, phenacetin)
    Antibiotics (penicillins, cephalosporins,
      sulfonamides, rifampin, ciprofloxacin)
    Diuretics (furosemide, thiazide)
    allopurinol
    phenytoin
    captopril
    cyclosporin
    cisplatin
    nitrosureas (lomustine, carmustine)
    lithium
  C. Papillary necrosis
    Analgesics (aspirin, phenacetin)
  D. Obstructive uropathy
    Intrarenal: chemotherapy for hematologic
      malignancy-high-dose methotrexate
      (hyperuricuria), acyclovir, sulfadiazine,
      trimethoprim-sulfamethoxazole
    Extrarenal
    Methysergide
    Anticholinergics
    Morphine
    antihistamines
    alpha-adrenergic agonists
    diazepam
  E. Increased BUN (without change in GFR)
    Tetracyclines
    Glucocorticoids
  F. Increased creatinine (without change
    in GFR)
    Cimetidine
    Trimethoprim
    Probenecid
II. Fluid disorders
  A. Volume depletion
    Diuretics (thiazides, furosemide, mannitol)
    Cathartics
    Emetics
    Lactulose
  B. Nephrogenic diabetes insipidus
    Lithium
    Demeclocyline
    Methoxyflurane, enthrane

III. Electrolyte disorders
  A. Drug-induced hyponatremia
    Chlorpropramide
    Thiazides
    Vincristine
    Cyclophosphamide
  B. Hypernatremia
    Lactulose
  C. Hypokalemia
    Diuretics
    Gentamicin
    Carbenicillin
    Ticarcillin
  D. Hyperkalemia
    K^+-sparing diuretics
    NSAIDs
    ϵ-Aminocaproic acid
    Heparin
    ACE inhibitors
  E. Hypomagnesemia
    Gentamicin
    amphotericin B
    Cisplatin
    Cyclosporin
    diuretics
    foscarnet
    Pentamidine
IV. Acid-base disorders
  A. Renal tubular acidosis
    Amphotericin B
    Acetazolamide
  B. Metabolic alkalosis
    Carbenicillin
    Penicillin G
  C. Respiratory acidosis
    Sedatives
    Narcotics
    Barbiturates
    Muscle paralyzers
    Anesthetics
V. Electrolyte content of common drugs
  A. Sodium
    Ampicillin (3 mEq/gm)
    Penicillin G (1.7 mEq/million units)
    Cephalothin (2.5 mEq/gm)
    Carbenicillin (4.7 mEq/gm)
    Ticarcillin (5.2 mEq/gm)
    Kayexelate (65 mEq/16 gm)
    Fleets phosphosoda (24 mEq/15 ml)
  B. Potassium
    Penicillin G (1.7 mEq/million units)
    K phosphate (4.4 mEq/ml)
    Neutra phosphates (0.019 mEq/ml)
  C. Magnesium
    Cathartics
    Antacids

skin turgor, soft eyeballs, dry tongue) have minimal clinical value, because they only appear in advanced cases and may be misleading among patients who are elderly, cachectic, or breathing by mouth. When not resulting from local causes, peripheral and sacral edema always imply excess total body sodium and extracellular fluid volume. Intravascular volume, on the other hand, may be normal, increased, or decreased in patients with edema. Euvolemia is a diagnosis of exclusion, and it is made in the absence of evidence for volume overload or depletion (Fig. 12.1). The physical examination also detects evidence of urinary tract obstruction by percussing for a distended bladder, palpating for hydronephrotic kidneys, and performing rectal and pelvic examinations.

Reliance on any single measurement or observation in the patient history or physical examination, however, may be misleading when you are trying to assess volume status. In addition, orthopaedic patients in traction or surgical patients who are critically ill often present special problems in the assessment of intravascular volume, because their conditions preclude adequate testing for orthostasis.

Laboratory Evaluation

The minimal renal laboratory evaluation in a seemingly uncomplicated patient should include measurements of serum sodium, potassium, chloride, carbon dioxide content, urea nitrogen, creatinine, and glucose, as well as urinalysis with specific gravity. Urine output alone is not always a good reflection of renal function.

The key to preventing postoperative ARF is identifying, correcting, or avoiding the risk factors listed in Table 12.1. Assuring sufficient volume and tissue perfusion is of the utmost importance. In a stable patient not receiving diuretics and who is undergoing elective surgery, an hourly urine output of 40 to 50 mL generally reflects adequate volume status. If there is any doubt preoperatively about the patient's intravascular volume status, two coures of action are possible. In a young patient without significant medical problems and who is not obviously volume overloaded, a fluid challenge with normal saline, blood, or colloid may be attempted, and the patient's physical examination should be followed closely for signs of volume excess. In patients who are more severely ill, and particularly in those with edema, third-space losses, or underlying heart disease, determination of intravascular volume status is more difficult; use of a central line or, preferably, a Swan-Ganz catheter may be required. Preoperative fluid therapy should be individualized and may include the use of saline, blood, or albumin. Use of intraoperative mannitol or furosemide is discussed in the section on high-risk surgery.

Volume depletion (low-body sodium)	Interstitial depletion: poor skin turgor, dry skin and mucous membranes Intravascular depletion: orthostasis, azotemia, oliguria, flat neck veins, negative fluid balance, ↓ weight, $U_{Na} < 20$ meq/L
Hypervolemia (high-body sodium)	Interstitial excess: peripheral and sacral edema Intravascular excess: pulmonary congestion/edema, distended neck veins
Euvolemia (normal-body sodium)	Diagnosis of exclusion, i.e., absence of signs of volume overload or depletion

Figure 12.1. Clinical assessment of extracellular fluid volume.

When it is necessary to use radiocontrast materials diagnostically in preoperative patients, they should be well-hydrated and surgery deferred, if possible, until the dye has been cleared from the vascular system. Most dyes act as osmotic diuretics, so careful monitoring of the intravascular volume should be continued for up to 24 hours after radiography. Many nephrologists recommend use of low-ionic-strength agents in high-risk individuals, but it is probably more important to maintain good hydration and limit the dose of the dye. In patients who are particularly prone to developing ARF following use of radiocontrast material, the necessary information should be obtained by other means, if possible.

Use of nephrotoxic agents should be avoided or carefully controlled. Fluorinated anesthetic agents (e.g., methoxyflurane, enthrane) should not be used in patients with preexisting renal dysfunction. Minimizing the risk of antibiotic nephrotoxicity involves using the least toxic antibiotic that is consistent with the clinical situation and avoiding the use of other concomitant nephrotoxic agents. Serum drug levels should be monitored and drug dosage adjusted to the level of renal function. Serum creatinine levels should be monitored at least every 2 days during the course of nephrotoxic antibiotics and for at least 1 week afterward, because ATN may develop several days after the drugs have been discontinued. Patients with the greatest risk of aminoglycoside nephrotoxicity are those with preexisting renal disease, advanced age, or receiving prolonged courses (9–10 days) of therapy. Single daily-dose aminoglycosides have not been convincingly shown to reduce the incidence of nephrotoxicity, and loop diuretics, methoxyflurane, and, possibly, cephalosporins potentiate aminoglycoside nephrotoxicity.

Whenever possible, hypotension in preoperative patients should be corrected by treating the underlying source. When hypotension is refractory, dopamine in low to moderate dosages is preferable to more selective α-adrenergic agents, which further compromise renal blood flow. Adequate volume should be maintained during the intraoperative and the postoperative periods. In uncomplicated patients with normal renal function, monitoring the urine volume will suffice as a reflection of adequate hydration; more unstable patients may require monitoring with a Swan-Ganz catheter.

Urinary Tract Infections

Epidemiology

Up to 10% of hospitalized patients have a community-acquired urinary tract infection (UTI) on admission, whereas another 10% will develop a UTI during their hospitalization. Patients who are pregnant or who have diabetes or reduced host defenses are even more susceptible. The highest prevalence of UTIs is among patients with congenital renal diseases (57%), hydronephrosis or nephrolithiasis (85%), and indwelling open-drainage urinary catheters (98%) (17).

Between 70 and 80% of all hospital-acquired UTIs relate to urinary catheterization (18). Most of these patients are asymptomatic, and a proportion will clear their infections spontaneously on removal of the catheter.

Urinary tract infections account for 35 to 60% of all nosocomial infections (17). Of patients with Gram-negative sepsis, 20 to 30% have the urinary tract as the source. Sepsis is often associated with urologic abnormalities or follows instrumentation, and Gram-negative sepsis is also an important predisposing cause of ARF. The mortality rate of Gram-negative sepsis arising from the urinary tract is 15% (19).

Escherichia coli is still the most common infecting organism, even among hospitalized patients. The incidence of *Pseudomonas* sp., *Proteus* sp., *Klebsiella* sp., and other Gram-negative and Gram-positive UTIs is higher among hospitalized patients and those with urologic abnormalities.

Evaluation

Patient evaluation on hospital admission should include a routine urinalysis. If pyuria is found, a urine culture should be obtained. Pyuria may occur in the absence of infection or, occasionally, not be seen when an infected kidney is completely obstructed. The clean-catch method is the preferred means for obtaining a urine specimen, but many patients who are ill or immobile require straight catheterization.

Treatment

The following therapeutic guidelines should apply to most patients. Acute, uncomplicated infections or relapses in female patients should be treated. In elderly patients with frequent relapses who are asymptomatic, the risk of therapy often outweighs the benefits (20). Male or female patients with complicated infections (i.e., with foreign bodies such as stones, catheters, or anatomic abnormalities) should be treated only when blood or tissue invasion is suspected. Routine or prolonged treatment with broad-spectrum antibiotics in such cases only leads to the development of drug-resistant organisms.

When catheters are used, they should be left in place for the least amount of time possible. Strict antiseptic insertion and maintenance will help to reduce the infection rate, and closed-bag drainage (40% infection rate at 2 weeks) should be used. If indicated, 0.25% acetic acid or neosporin-polymixin irrigation can be used as a prophylactic measure against local infection, but this does not offer greater protection than a meticulously maintained, closed-drainage system.

It is rarely necessary to postpone nonurologic surgery because of an asymptomatic UTI. Treatment with antibiotics should be started preoperatively, and patients with bacteriuria who require instrumentation or urologic surgery should be treated to reduce the incidence of bacteremia following such procedures. Prophylactic therapy is also recommended before urologic surgery for patients with valvular heart disease or prosthetic devices. The long-term success of treatment for patients with anatomic abnormalities of the genitourinary tract depends on surgical correction of the defect.

Elective surgery may need to be postponed following symptomatic urinary infection. The length of this postponement can vary from a few days for uncomplicated lower-tract infections to 1 to 3 weeks after pyelonephritis with sepsis.

Postoperative Problems

Epidemiology

Metabolic and hormonal responses to trauma and surgery are intimately related to postoperative disorders of fluid and electrolyte balance (Table 12.6). Both the magnitude and character of the trauma as well as the preoperative condition of the patient will influence the response to surgical stress. Increased secretion of catecholamines, adrenocorticotropic hormone, aldosterone, and antidiuretic hormone (ADH) occur postoperatively and usually persist for 2 to 4 days in uncomplicated cases.

Release of ADH during the immediate postoperative period is unresponsive to the usual osmotic regulation, and volume depletion, morphine, and pain may further contribute to enhanced secretion. Excess secretion of ADH and aldosterone cause enhanced sodium and water reabsorption, resulting in oliguria. In uncomplicated cases, urinary electrolyte levels

Table 12.6. Metabolic Responses to Surgery and Trauma

Response	Effect
↑ Catecholamines	Hypertension, hyperglycemia, tachycardia
↑ ACTH-cortisol	Hyperglycemia, catabolism
↑ Aldosterone	Salt retention, K^+ wasting, alkalosis
↑ ADH	Water retention
Catabolism	Negative nitrogen balance, K^+ wasting
	↑ Endogenous water production

during this period show a low urinary sodium (U_{Na}) and increased urinary potassium (U_K) (70–90 mEq of K^+ per day), which may result in a negative potassium balance for 3 to 6 days postoperatively. Adequate preoperative and intraoperative volume replacement tends to minimize these changes.

Increased endogenous water production is the other major alteration seen postoperatively, and this might result in water intoxication if it is not considered when writing orders for fluids.

Evaluation and Treatment

See section on fluid and electrolyte disorders.

High-risk Surgery

Epidemiology

The incidence of ARF following most elective surgical procedures is 1% or less. Procedures that are associated with a higher risk of developing ARF, which is mainly ischemic (i.e., ATN), include cardiopulmonary bypass surgery; operations on the aorta and renal vessels, particularly aneurysectomy; and major gastrointestinal operations, especially when complicated by infection, hemorrhage, or biliary tract obstruction (21–28). Women undergoing surgery following third-trimester accidents such as abruptio placenta, elderly patients, and those with diabetes are also at high risk.

A prospective study of ARF following cardiac surgery at Stanford (29) showed that prolonged duration of cardiopulmonary bypass, preoperative left-ventricular dysfunction, and need for intra-aortic balloon pumping postoperatively were the best predictors of postoperative renal dysfunction (i.e., prerenal azotemia) and ARF. Additional risk factors included older age, a history of or active bacterial endocarditis, or prior cardiac surgery. Mean arterial pressure during cardiopulmonary bypass and the duration of aortic cross-clamping were not significantly different in the groups with renal dysfunc-

tion or ARF compared with the control group, which had a normal postoperative course. This study also found that postoperative depression of myocardial function, characterized by a low cardiac output and elevated pulmonary capillary wedge pressure accompanied by renal hypoperfusion (decreased glomerular filtration rate [GFR], fractional excretion of sodium [FE_{Na}] <1%), was present in all patients with postoperative renal dysfunction or ARF. However, hemodynamic function and GFR were similar in those with postoperative renal dysfunction (prerenal azotemia) and those with ARF. It was suggested that progression to ARF required the superimposition of additional renal insults, including sepsis, nephrotoxic antibiotics, hypotension, hemorrhage, prolonged low cardiac output, or withdrawal of mechanical or pharmacologic circulatory support.

Table 12.2 reviews the incidence of ARF following high-risk surgical procedures. The mortality rate for patients with postoperative ARF as a group is 50 to 70%. This rate is even greater, ranging between 60 and 98%, in the small subgroup of patients requiring dialysis.

Patients with acute rupture of an abdominal aortic aneurysm or who undergo suprarenal cross-clamping of the aorta are at high risk of ARF, which is usually ATN (30). However, there is also a group whose renal insufficiency is from atheroembolic disease, which develops more insidiously, is associated with peripheral manifestations such as livedo reticularis or embolic skin lesions, and is generally irreversible.

Patients undergoing surgery for the correction of obstructive jaundice have an increased risk of developing ARF as well. In addition to experiencing the effects of hyperbilirubinemia on the cardiovascular system, these patients are frequently septic.

The incidence of ARF, as defined by a 0.5 mg/dL increase in the serum creatinine level, was 18.9% in a large series of patients who were admitted to the Burn Center at the Johns Hopkins Bayview

Medical Center over a 3-year period (31). The mortality rate was 75% among those in whom renal failure developed after hospitalization even if they did not require renal replacement therapy. Among those who had renal insufficiency on hospital admission or when resolution occurred during the first week, mortality rates were not different from those of the general burn-patient population.

Evaluation

Evaluation in high-risk surgical candidates is similar to that outlined earlier for patients with normal renal function. Since the maintenance of intravascular volume assumes even greater significance in this group, we recommend use of a Swan-Ganz catheter. Even if the preoperative patient is judged on clinical grounds to be euvolemic, redistribution of volume or third-space losses during surgery as well as the effects of anesthesia on peripheral resistance will require continued readjustment of fluid intraoperatively.

When assessing the patient immediately postoperative, the development of a mannitol-induced or a furosemide-induced diuresis may be deceiving, because urine output and GFR are not always well correlated. Nonoliguric renal failure is common in these patients, and it will be missed without daily, careful monitoring of the serum creatinine level. In addition, if the patient is not monitored carefully, continued diuresis could lead to further volume depletion.

Treatment

Whenever possible, surgery should be delayed until the risk factors listed earlier have been controlled. Although primarily a surgical decision, intraoperative fluid management should also involve the consulting internist. The type and amount of fluids administered during surgery that are effective in preventing postoperative ARF, however, have not been established by rigorous studies.

Animal experiments indicate that volume expansion or mannitol-induced diuresis before the renal insult offers some protection. Mannitol and furosemide have also been used to reverse ARF immediately following the presumed renal injury, but with variable success (32–35). Whether there is a beneficial effect beyond that achieved through maintaining intravascular volume with saline, plasma, or blood is disputed (36–40). Since neither mannitol nor diuretics augment the intravascular volume, the primary form of both preoperative and intraoperative treatment should be the use of volume expanders.

EVALUATION AND TREATMENT OF THE SURGICAL PATIENT WITH ACUTE RENAL FAILURE

Epidemiology

More than 50% of the cases of ARF follow either surgery or trauma. The incidence of acute renal dysfunction ranges from 1% in the general surgical population to 25% in certain high-risk groups (Table 12.2). Dialysis is required in 30 to 80% of cases, and more often when patients are oliguric. The mortality rate averages between 50 and 70%, but it may exceed 90% following cardiopulmonary bypass surgery or the repair of ruptured aortic aneurysms.

Acute renal failure is a general term encompassing a wide variety of disorders that result in a rapid, but usually reversible, impairment of kidney function. For clinical purposes, an acute and progressive increase in blood urea nitrogen (BUN) or the serum creatinine level above the normal range (or the baseline value in patients with preexisting renal insufficiency) is sufficient for the diagnosis of ARF to be made. The quantity of urine is not always helpful, because only 50 to 70% of these patients are oliguric. Relying solely on urine output as a marker of renal function therefore may cause undue delay in making the diagnosis. Common examples of nonoliguric renal failure include

partial obstruction, hypercalcemic nephropathy, and aminoglycoside nephrotoxicity.

Oliguria is defined as a urine output of
less than 400 mL/day in a patient with
previously normal renal function. This
volume represents the minimum urine
output that is required to excrete the
average daily solute load. *Anuria* is defined as a urine volume of less than 50
mL/day. It should always suggest a possible obstruction, but other causes include
cortical necrosis, acute glomeruloncphri-
tis, and bilateral renal artery occlusion.
On occasion, ATN may be associated with
anuria, and alternating anuria and polyuria (especially with normal urinary sediment) may also indicate obstruction.

Dividing ARF into prerenal, postrenal,
and intrinsic categories is useful, because
it provides a framework for the diagnostic
classification. Postoperative oliguria, even
when associated with mild increments in
the serum creatinine level or urea nitrogen, often results from prerenal causes
and does not necessarily indicate kidney malfunction. Oliguria may result
from normal postoperative physiologic responses, such as increased ADH secretion
or, most commonly, depleted intravascular
volume. Diminished effective circulatory
volume may result from actual fluid losses
or relate to cardiac dysfunction.

Postrenal causes only account for a
minority of cases, but they should never be
overlooked as they are generally reversible. Bladder outlet obstruction is common
in the surgical patient who is often receiving narcotics or recovering from anesthesia. Obstruction should be suspected in
patients with a history of nephrolithiasis,
abdominal or pelvic surgery, rectal or
pelvic neoplasms, or prostatism (41, 42).
Rupture of the bladder may be seen
following pelvic fractures in up to 15% of
cases (43).

Although there are a variety of causes
for intrinsic ARF, the most common in
postoperative patients or in patients with
trauma is ATN. This is by no means the
only etiology, however, and others deserve

special mention. Acute drug-induced
nephrotoxicity is being recognized more
frequently, and acute interstitial nephritis
often develops following the use of drugs
such as penicillins (e.g., ampicillin, methicillin), nonsteroidal anti-inflammatory
agents, and diuretics. In addition to having ARF, patients with acute interstitial
nephritis may also have fever, rash, eosinophilia, or pyuria (with eosinophils).
Patients with bilateral renal artery stenosis treated with angiotensin-converting
enzyme (ACE) inhibitors may develop
a reversible form of renal insufficiency
because of the impaired autoregulation
of renal blood flow (44). Pyogenic visceral abscesses have also been associated
with ARF because of immune complex–
mediated glomerulonephritis (5–7), even
in patients without documented bacter-
cmia. Hematuria, hypertension, and pulmonary edema indicate the glomerular
nature of the lesion. In one study, cryoglobulins were frequently detected, although the serum complement level was
depressed in only 4 of 11 patients (35%).
Chronic renal failure or death is common
if the diagnosis or therapy is delayed, and
early treatment often results in complete
resolution. Cholesterol embolization to
the kidneys, arising either spontaneously
or, more commonly, following the insertion
of radiographic catheters or aortic surgery, may cause of renal failure in patients
with extensive atheromatous involvement
of the aorta. The presence of ischemic toes
or livido reticularis should suggest this
diagnosis.

Acute tubular necrosis, which is sometimes called "vasomotor nephropathy," is
the most common cause of intrinsic ARF
in surgical patients. The pathogenesis of
this disorder is complex, however, and is
not totally understood. Hemodynamic or
nephrotoxic insults are the usual initiating events (Table 12.7), and the maintaining factors are postulated to include persistent renal vasoconstriction, tubular
obstruction, decreased glomerular permeability, and leakage of filtrate back across
damaged tubules.

Table 12.7.   Causes of Acute Renal Failure

I. Prerenal
  A. Hypotension
  B. Volume depletion, including peripheral
    pooling 2° sepsis, acidosis
  C. Ineffective cardiac failure
    1. Congestive heart failure
    2. Tamponade
    3. Pulmonary embolism
    4. Cor pulmonale
II. Renal
  A. Toxins
    1. Exogenous: antibiotics, contrast media,
      anesthetics
    2. Endogenous: myoglobin and hemoglobin
  B. Arterial: emboli, thrombus, dissecting
    aneurysm, malignant hypertension
  C. Veins: thrombosis, vena caval obstruction
  D. Glomerulus: glomerulonephritis, vasculitis
  E. Tubule: ATN (ischemic and/or nephrotoxic)
  F. Interstitial: drug hypersensitivity,
    metabolic nephropathy, infection
III. Postrenal
  A. Urethral obstruction
  B. Bladder
    1. Outlet obstruction (BPH, bladder
      cancer, drugs)
    2. Ruptured bladder
  C. Bilateral urethral obstruction
    1. Intraureteral (uric acid, blood clots,
      pyogenic debris, stone, edema,
      necrotizing papillitis)
    2. Extraureteral
      a. Tumor: cervix, prostate, colon,
        endometriosis
      b. Periureteral fibrosis
      c. Accidental surgical ligature

The clinical course of ATN is generally divided into an oliguric and a diuretic phase. On average, the oliguric phase lasts between 10 and 14 days, with a range of a few hours to over 1 month. However, many patients never have a period of oliguria, or they have one of such short duration that it is missed. Complete clinical recovery occurs in most patients, even those with prolonged oliguria.

In the functionally anephric patient with uncomplicated ARF, the BUN usually increases by 20 to 40 mg/dL per day and the serum creatinine level by 1 mg/dL per day. In more seriously ill patients, hypercatabolism is reflected by: (a) increases of BUN greater than 40 mg/dL per day, or of the creatinine level greater than 1 mg/dL per day; (b) rapid onset of hyperkalemia; (c) severe metabolic acidosis; (d) a uric acid level greater than 15 mg/dL; and (e) hyperphosphatemia of 8 to 10 mg/dL or more, often in association with severe hypocalcemia.

Mortality during the oliguric phase relates to hyperkalemia, fluid overload, acidosis, bleeding, and infection (45–47). During the diuretic phase, the BUN and creatinine level may continue to rise for several days, despite increasing urine output. Once established, diuresis should proceed smoothly, with a gradual and persistent improvement in renal function. A second period of oliguria is associated with a poor prognosis, and the recovery phase generally last from 2 to 4 weeks.

The mortality rate for patients with postoperative or posttraumatic ARF approaches 60%. Cioffi et al. (48) analyzed the factors predicting unfavorable outcomes in 65 patients with postoperative ARF that required hemodialysis. They identified cardiac failure, multisystem organ failure, number of blood transfusions, type of surgery, patient age, severity of injury, creatinine level before first dialysis, and the interval from the onset of ARF to first dialysis as factors predicting higher mortality. Only the latter two factors can be modified by the clinician, however. Other investigators have found that preexisting renal dysfunction also correlates with increased mortality.

Complications related to the underlying surgical problems are the most important causes of death. In one autopsy series of postoperative ARF (49), the primary underlying disease or its extrarenal complications were considered to be the main cause of death in 92%. Sepsis occurs with a frequency of between 50 and 80% and accounts for approximately 33% of deaths. Gastrointestinal bleeding occurs in up to 40% of cases, with a mortality rate of approximately 25%, and infectious complications are particularly common in cases following trauma or major gastrointestinal operations. The most frequent sites of infection include the lungs, urine, wounds, peritoneum, intravenous sites, and the gastrointestinal tract. Other factors associated with a poor prognosis include advanced age, jaundice, and the requirement for mechanical ventilation. In some series, nonoliguric ARF is associated with a reduced need for dialysis and better prognosis. In surgical patients, however, nonoliguric renal failure carries a mortality rate of 40%.

Although most patients with ATN recover, from 40 to 50% have a reduced GFR and impaired ability to either concentrate or acidify their urine. Younger patients tend to have faster and more complete recoveries than elderly patients or those with preexisting mild renal insufficiency (50). In one large series, however, 10% of patients were left with severe, chronic renal failure (51).

Efforts to reduce the unacceptably high mortality in postoperative ARF center on three objectives: (a) reversal of early or established ARF, (b) more aggressive dialysis schedules, and (c) improved nutrition. Several pharmacologic maneuvers to restore GFR and correct the presumed pathophysiologic states resulting in ARF have been attempted, but none have unequivocally been shown to be of benefit. Of these various therapies, infusions of saline, mannitol, loop diuretics, and "renal-dose" dopamine are the most commonly used in the clinical setting, and when used judiciously, they are relatively safe. Complications tend to arise when these techniques are employed in an inappropriate setting or when the desire for diuresis leads to overly aggressive treatment. Both saline or mannitol infusions can result in pulmonary edema. In addition, too much mannitol can produce hyperosmolality and pseudohyponatremia, and both mannitol and loop diuretics can produce a vigorous diuresis, which can lead to worsening renal failure if not appropriately replaced. The combination of volume depletion and loop diuretics also can po-

tentiate the nephrotoxicity of other drugs. If any of these therapies is to have a chance of success, it must be used early in the course of ARF. Even when diuresis is achieved, however, it is not always associated with an improved GFR, but a larger urine output may make subsequent management easier. Whether these maneuvers in fact convert oliguric to nonoliguric renal failure requires further prospective studies (32). Brown et al. (33) have shown in a randomized, prospective study involving 58 surgical and trauma patients with ATN that high-dose furosemide (3 g/day) did not affect the duration of renal failure, number of dialyses, or the mortality rate.

If patients fail to respond to volume replacement and loop diuretics, then low-dose dopamine, administered at a rate of 2 to 3 μg/kg per minute, may increase urine output (52) and is almost universally given to patients with ARF. Despite the widespread practice of administering renal-dose dopamine, most data do not support its efficacy in either preventing or altering the course of established ARF (53, 54). Dopamine-induced increases in renal blood flow, GFR, and sodium excretion have been described best in euvolemic individuals with normal kidney function, and they cannot necessarily be extrapolated to critically ill patients with altered hemodynamic parameters. Although increased urine output may occur in some patients, it is also common that others have decreased output, presumably because of an increased sensitivity to its pressor effects. Even low-dose dopamine may increase myocardial oxygen consumption and result in vasoconstriction, leading to organ ischemia. Therefore, if low-dose dopamine is used, it is recommended that the duration be limited and the infusion stopped if prompt improvement in renal function does not occur.

Studies by Conger (55), Teschan et al. (56), Fischer et al. (57), as well as Kleinknecht and Graneval (58) suggest that early or "prophylactic" dialysis results in a lower mortality rate and decreased incidence of complications than occur with dialysis performed for specific uremic manifestations. In the study by Kleinknecht and Graneval, mortality in surgical patients with ARF was reduced from 54 to 42%, mortality from gastrointestinal bleeding fell from 17 to 6%, but the frequency of septic deaths was unaffected. Other studies using early and frequent dialysis have not shown a similar effect; nevertheless, it is generally conceded that aggressive dialysis facilitates the treatment of these patients.

Hypercatabolism, negative nitrogen balance, and weight loss contribute to the morbidity and mortality of postoperative and posttrauma patients with ARF.

Dudrick et al. (59) showed that an intravenous solution of hypertonic glucose and L-essential amino acids given to patients with postoperative renal failure reduces BUN and ameliorates hyperphosphatemia, hypercalcemia, and acidosis. In addition, dialysis requirements were simultaneously reduced. In a prospective, double-blind study, Abel et al. (60) gave "renal failure fluid" (i.e., hypertonic glucose and essential amino acids) to one group of patients with ARF and hypertonic glucose alone to another. Seventy-five percent of those receiving renal failure fluid survived, compared with only 56% of those receiving hypertonic glucose alone. The need for dialysis was not affected by hyperalimentation, nor was the incidence of pneumonia, sepsis, or gastrointestinal bleeding. In a similar study, Baek et al. (61) showed a reduction in the mortality rate from 70% in the glucose-treated group to 46% in the amino-acid-plus-glucose group. Although urea nitrogen levels were not reduced in this study, hyperkalemia occurred less frequently. In contrast, the renal group at Guy's Hospital was unable to reduce the mortality rate (62%) even with intensive dialysis combined with high-protein, high-calorie feedings (62). Since intravenous hyperalimentation is associated with a significant incidence of septic problems, volume overload, and iatrogenic electrolyte abnormalities, it should be reserved for those patients who are unable to take an oral diet.

Evaluation

The presence of ARF may be indicated by the development of oliguria or an actual rise in BUN or the creatinine level. The evaluation proceeds by excluding prerenal and postrenal causes, then matching the clinical and laboratory findings with the diagnosis of intrinsic renal disease.

Prerenal azotemia is evaluated through bedside determination of the intravascular volume status (described earlier), comparison of weights, input and outputs, Swan-Ganz or central venous monitoring, laboratory analysis of blood and urine chemistries, and, possibly, a diagnostic trial of volume expanders. Ultimately, prerenal azotemia is a retrospective diagnosis, whereby renal function should return to normal within 72 hours after the correction of volume depletion, hypotension, or congestive heart failure in a patient with previously normal renal function.

The possibility of bladder outlet obstruction is evaluated by physical examination, including a rectal and pelvic examination, and catheterization of the bladder (or by checking the patency of the catheter if one is already in place). Whenever the diagnosis of upper tract obstruction is being seriously considered, imaging studies are essential (discussed later).

Once prerenal and postrenal possibilities have been ruled out, a long list of causes for intrinsic ARF must then be considered. The diagnosis is often made by reviewing the patient's immediate past history and finding any factors predisposing to ARF. Unfortunately, surgical patients are frequently exposed to numerous nephrotoxic agents and events, and often, no single cause can be identified. Obviously, this should not detract from the diagnosis, because periods of hypotension may be minimal or missed entirely and exposure to nephrotoxins may have been brief but sufficient to cause harm.

Urinalysis, although at times very helpful, is usually nonspecific. It may be entirely normal or show fine, granular casts in prerenal azotemia. In obstructive uropathy, the findings may include hematuria, pyuria, or be normal. Hematuria with or without red-cell casts may also be seen in acute glomerulonephritis or vasculitis. Calcium oxalate crystals or urate crystals indicate methoxyflurane toxicity or uric acid nephropathy, respectively. Results of urinalysis in ATN may be normal, show a few red cells, or have the characteristic findings of many granular, pigmented casts associated with renal tubular epithelial cells. Pyuria with a high percentage of eosinophils is found in some cases of acute interstitial nephritis. When a urine test that is positive for blood by dipstick does not show red blood cells on microscopic examination, the diagnosis of myoglobinuria (or hemoglobinuria) should be strongly considered. The urine also often shows pigmented granular casts in myoglobinuric ARF.

The diagnosis of myoglobinuria can be more firmly established through blood analysis and the finding of a rapidly rising or markedly elevated creatinine, potassium, uric acid, phosphate, and creatinine phosphokinase levels. A definitive diagnosis depends on myoglobin beign present in the urine.

The specific technique of renal imaging to be used usually depends on the clinical circumstances. The simplest of these is the KUB, which might reveal kidney size, stones, or a distended bladder. Renal ultrasonography is the most commonly employed and least invasive method of visualizing the kidneys, and is usually reliable in ruling out the presence of obstruction without the need for radiocontrast materials. If hydronephrosis is detected by ultrasonography, one option is to proceed directly to percutaneous antegrade pyelography and placement of a nephrostomy tube. Computed tomography (CT), with or without contrast, or cystoscopy with retrograde urography would also be appropriate, but one needs to be

aware that patients with intraabdominal processes such as retroperitoneal fibrosis or pelvic cancers can present with minimal or no dilatation depicted on CT scans or ultrasounds (63). Intravenous urography is less commonly used because of the risk of radiocontrast-induced nephrotoxicity.

Chemical analysis of the urine may help in making the differential diagnosis of ARF, but it is most useful in differentiating prerenal azotemia from oliguric ATN (64, 65). Interpretation of these results presupposes previously normal renal function and that diuretics or other therapeutic maneuvers have not been recently administered. The most commonly obtained measurements include specific gravity, osmolality, urea, sodium, and creatinine concentrations. The urinary osmolality is more accurate than the specific gravity as an indication of urinary concentration, because urinary proteins or radiographic dyes do not interfere with its measurement.

In prerenal azotemia, one expects an elevated specific gravity (>1.015), a urinary osmolality greater than 500 mOsm/kg of H_2O, and a urinary sodium concentration less than 20 mEq/L. In oliguric ATN, the urine usually has an osmolality less than 350 mOsm/kg of H_2O, a specific gravity of 1.010, and a urinary sodium concentration of 40 mEq/L or greater. In those patients with oliguria whose urinary chemistries fall between these limits, the FE_{Na}[1] or the renal failure index (RFI)[2] are more reliable in differentiating prerenal causes from ATN (Table 12.8).

Formerly, an FE_{Na} or RFI of less than 1 was consistent with prerenal azotemia and of greaer than 1 with ATN. Today, many exceptions in both oliguric and nonoliguric ARF have been described with low FE_{Na} (<1%) (66) (Table 12.9). The FE_{Na} may may be elevated in patients receiving diuretics, those with chronic

---

[1]FE_{Na} = (U/P [Na])/(U/P [creatinine]) × 100%.
[2]RFI = (U[Na])/(U/P [creatinine]).

Table 12.8. Urinary Diagnostic Indices in Acute Renal Failure

	Prerenal Azotemia	Oliguria ARF	Non-oliguric ARF	Acute Obstruction	Acute Glomerulonephritis	Renal Vascular Occlusion
BUN/creatinine	>20:1	<20:1	<20:1	<20:1	<20:1	<20:1
(U/P) urea	>8	<3	<8	<12	>8	<8
(U/P) creatinine	>40	<20	<20	<20	>40	>20
(U/P)$_{Osm}$	>1.5	1–1.5	1–1.5	1–1.5	>1.2	1–1.5
U$_{Osm}$	>500	<350	<350	<400	>350	<350 (variable)
U$_{Na}$	<20	>40	>40[a]	>20	<20	<30
RFI	<1	>1	>1[a]	>1	<1	<1
FE$_{Na}$	<1	>1	>1[a]	>1	<1	<1
U/A	Normal	Renal tubular cells or casts, pigmented brown casts	Same as oliguric ARF	Normal or crystals or pyuria	Proteinuria RBC casts	Hematuria pyuria Proteinuria Cholesterol
Urine volume	<400 cc/day	<400 cc/day	>600 cc/day	Anuria or anuria-polyuria	<400 cc/day	Anuria-oliguria
Radiology	Not diagnostic	Not diagnostic, immediate dense, persistent nephrogram	Not diagnostic	Required for diagnosis. Delayed, but increasing nephrogram and delayed pyelogram evidence of obstruction		Renal scan or arteriogram or venogram for diagnosis
Sonography	Normal renal size	Normal renal size	Normal renal size	Dilated calyces		Normal renal size

[a]Tend to be lower on average than oliguric ARF.

Table 12.9.   Low Fractional Excretion of Sodium in ARF

1. Radiocontrast-induced ARF
2. Pigment nephropathy (myoglobin, hemoglobin)
3. Sepsis
4. Burns
5. Interstitial nephritis
6. Hepatorenal syndrome
7. Acute glomerulonephritis
8. Early obstructive uropathy
9. Nonoliguric ATN (10–15%)
10. Renal allograft rejection
11. Drugs (Captopril, nonsteroidal anti-inflammatory agents)
12. Postcardiac surgery

renal failure, or during postobstructive diuresis; therefore, it has less value in these situations.

Low urinary sodium concentrations may occur in ATN if there is a profound stimulus for sodium reabsorption, such as in terminal hepatic failure, shock, or severe cardiac failure. Nonoliguric renal failure is also associated with a lower urinary sodium concentration than in the oliguric form. In acute glomerulonephritis or vasculitis, the urinary sodium concentration and FE_{Na} also tend to be low. Urinary diagnostic indices in early, acute obstructive nephropathy may be similar to those in prerenal azotemia, but with time, they will resemble those in ATN. Urinary indices must be interpreted by considering the entire clinical picture. They are best used either to confirm a clinical impression or to question a diagnosis markedly different from that expected.

Treatment

Certain aspects of treatment differ depending on whether ARF occurs in the preoperative or the postoperative state (67). Preoperatively, nonurgent surgery should be postponed to allow time for establishing a diagnosis and assessing the effects of therapy. It is usually possible to arrive at a reasonable diagnosis within 24 to 48 hours.

Elective surgery should also be delayed

until the patient's renal function has returned to baseline. When surgery is more urgent, however, fluid and electrolyte disturbances should be managed as outlined in the section on fluid, electrolyte, and acid-base disorders. If renal function is severely compromised, dialysis may be necessary.

Since oliguria in surgical patients commonly occurs secondary to intravascular volume depletion, volume expansion should be considered if the signs of overload are absent. A Swan-Ganz catheter should be used when a fluid challenge is considered to be dangerous in the presence of cardiopulmonary diseases. A wedge pressure that continues to rise above optimal filling pressures (15–18 mm Hg) with no increment in cardiac or urine output indicates that volume depletion is not the cause of the oliguria. If the patient's clinical condition allows a fluid challenge without a Swan-Ganz catheter, 500 mL of normal saline may be given every 30 to 60 minutes while reassessing frequently for signs of fluid overload.

Once both prerenal and postrenal causes of ARF have been excluded and the likely diagnosis is ATN, therapy should be aimed at increasing urine output to make fluid management easier, shorten the duration of ATN, prevent the need for dialysis, and reduce mortality. Unfortunately, most studies that have systematically investigated the potential benefits of the pharmacologic agents purported to be useful in prophylaxis or treatment of established ATN have not demonstrated their efficacy (68).

With these caveats in mind, the usual recommendations for treating patients with ARF are: If euvolemia is achieved without improvement in urine output, then mannitol, a loop diuretic, or dopamine may be tried. Mannitol is given as 12.5 to 25.0 g over 10 minutes (50–100 mL of 25% solution). Furosemide may be given in increasing doses up to a maximum of 500 mg intravenously and bumetamide in increasing doses up to 12 mg intravenously. Continuous infusions of furosemide (20–160 mg/h) or bumetamide (1 mg/h) may be effective and possibly result in fewer toxic side effects than when these same drugs are administered as high-dose boluses. Continued administration of a loop diuretic when no effect is evident, however, is likely to result in ototoxicity, particularly if the patient is also receiving aminoglycoside antibiotics. Patients with ATN who respond to diuretics may have less severe ATN than those who do not respond (69). If urine output does not increase following the administration of loop diuretics, then dopamine may be infused at a rate of up to 3 μg/kg per min; if the patient's urine output still remains low, it is best to stop the diuretics or dopamine before toxicity becomes a problem. Calcium channel blockers and atrial natriuretic hormone are newer agents currently being investigated for their application in ATN (70).

Close attention must be paid when writing fluid orders, because in ARF, the kidney is unable to compensate. Daily fluid requirements should replace insensible losses ($\approx$ 400 mL/day) plus measurable losses (over the previous 24 hours) from the urine, gastrointestinal tract, wounds, and estimated third-space losses. Insensible water losses increase with fever (13% per each degree centigrade) and hyperventilation. Insensible losses through the lungs are nil in patients receiving mechanical ventilation, and hypercatabolic states result in increased endogenous water of oxidation, which tends to decrease net insensible losses.

Progressive weight gain is common in the first 36 to 48 hours following surgery, because fluids are administered to compensate for fluid sequestration into surgical third-spaces that accompany burns, inflammation, and soft-tissue trauma. Estimation of third-space requirements is based on hemodynamic measurements such as blood pressure and pulmonary wedge pressure. Fluid loss to surgical third-spaces is frequently rich in protein (30–50 g/L) and may need to be replaced by an infusion of albumin or Plasmanate. Resorption of third-space fluids should be anticipated after 36 to 48 hours and intravenous fluids reduced accordingly to prevent volume overload. Following this period, the semistarved, catabolic, postsurgical patient with ARF should be expected to lose 0.3 to 0.5 kg of body weight per day.

Excessive sodium intake during the oliguric period will lead to volume expansion and, possibly, to congestive heart failure or hypertension, whereas insufficient sodium replacement, particularly during the diuretic period, may result in hypotension and volume depletion. Daily sodium needs are assessed by following the daily weight and clinical determination of the intravascular volume. Although the exact electrolyte content of all available fluids is the best measure for accurately replacing fluid losses, Table 12.10

Table 12.10.   Composition of Gastrointestinal Fluids

	Na (mmol/l)	K (mmol/l)	Cl (mmol/l)	HCO$_3$ (mmol/l)	pH
Gastric Fluid	20–100	5–10	120–160	—	1–7
Bile	150–250	5–10	40–80	20–40	7–8
Pancreatic Fluid	120	5–10	10–60	80–120	7–8
Enteric Fluid	140	5	variable	variable	7–8

Reproduced with permission from Phillips SF, in Maxwell MH, Kleeman CR, Narins RG (eds): Clinical Disorders of Fluid and Electrolyte Metabolism, 4th ed. New York, McGraw-Hill, 1987.

can also be used to estimate gastrointestinal electrolyte losses. Once the volume has been replaced, it is general practice to begin water restriction to prevent dilutional hyponatremia. Replacement of the insensible losses in the euvolemic patient should be sufficient to maintain the intravascular volume.

Unless significant hypokalemia is present in the patient with oliguria, potassium intake should be restricted to approximately 20 mEq/day. Ongoing potassium losses, which can be quantitated, may be added to this amount, but special care should be taken to avoid hidden sources of potassium (e.g., antibiotics and certain forms of phosphate supplements). Other measures that may be taken to avoid hyperkalemia include prompt treatment of infection; debridement of necrotic tissue; providing nonprotein calories in the form of glucose or fat; drainage of accumulated blood; avoiding use of old, whole, banked blood; and cleaning out the gastrointestinal tract after bleeding. Frequent determinations of the serum potassium level are indicated in patients taking digoxin or those with internal bleeding or severe catabolic states. Patients who are prone to either hypokalemia or hyperkalemia should undergo frequent electrocardiographyc (ECG). When hyperalimentation is combined with diuretic therapy in ARF, hypokalemia may occur because of intracellular shifts of potassium.

Hypocalcemia is common and results from hyperphosphatemia, decreased renal production of the active form of vitamin D, and resistance to the skeletal effects of parathyroid hormone (PTH). Unless a patient becomes symptomatic or the ionized serum calcium level is less than 0.8 mmol/L (discussed later), calcium supplementation is not generally recommended for patients with ARF. Hypocalcemia can often be improved by controlling hyperphosphatemia through administration of phosphate binders such as calcium carbonate or aluminum hydroxide. Hypercalcemia may frequently occur during the diuretic phase of ATN secondary to rhabdomyolysis, and hyperuricemia, unless it is thought to be involved in producing the ARF or is present in a patient with gout, need not be treated.

Proper nutrition plays an important role in the treatment of postoperative patients with ARF. Protein-calorie malnutrition may lead to increased acidosis, azotemia, hyperphosphatemia, impaired wound healing, and decreased resistance to infection. Dialysis, particularly by the peritoneal route, may also result in further losses of amino acids, proteins, and water-soluble vitamins. In a noncatabolic patient with a functioning gastrointestinal tract, therapy should include moderate dietary-protein restriction, a high-calorie intake provided by carbohydrates and fats, and supplementation of essential amino acids. A packet of Amin Aid dissolved in 250 mL of water provides 680 kcal, which is the minimum adult requirement of amino acids, plus histidine. It can be given by mouth or nasogastric tube (starting at 20 mL/h, then increasing to 50–75 mL/h over the next 2–3 days). Since most essential amino acids are absorbed in the proximal intestine, Amin Aid can even be used in patients with enterocutaneous fistulas.

Hyperalimentation should be considered in severely stressed surgical patients, particularly following extensive trauma or when prolonged gastrointestinal dysfunction is anticipated. Although the benefits of nutritional therapy appear to be obvious, data conflict regarding what kind of amino acids should be used and whether they have any effect on patient recovery from ARF. The volume of fluid needed to administer the 30 to 50 kcal/kg per day that are required to prevent protein catabolism in postoperative surgical patients is often considerable. In these patients, however, it is probably better to combine aggressive hyperalimentation with early dialysis to avoid the debilitating effects of an unbalanced metabolism. Even so, an experienced hyperalimentation team is mandatory to avoid infections, hyperosmolality, and various disorders of electrolytes and mineral balance.

Use of early or prophylactic dialysis is recommended, although the data are somewhat conflicting. Even if early or prophylactic dialysis does not reduce mortality, it allows more leeway in the use of hyperalimentation or drug therapy. Dialysis may be performed on a daily or every-other day basis. A creatinine value that should not be exceeded has not been established; however, such a value would reasonably fall between 5 and 10 mg/dL.

It is difficult to define precise guidelines governing the timing for dialysis with respect to surgery in patients with preoperative ARF (71). When surgery is necessary before recovery of renal function can be achieved, it is recommended that the patient undergo dialysis if: *(a)* fluid, electrolyte, or acid-base disturbances are present and unresponsive to conservative management; *(b)* depressed mental status, uremic bleeding, or pericarditis are present; or *(c)* progression of renal insufficiency is such that dialysis would be likely within 24 hours after surgery. For any given level of serum creatinine, one would be more aggressive in performing dialysis preoperatively for patients with multiple metabolic derangements or who are about to undergo major surgery than for the patient with less extensive abnormalities. Patients with ARF who undergo dialysis with a "biocompatible" dialysis membrane made from synthetics such as polysulfone have faster recovery and fewer complications than patients who undergo dialysis with cellulose-derived membranes. In a recent prospective study, Hakim et al. (72) demonstrated improved outcomes with the use of biocompatible membranes compared to outcomes with conventional cellulose membranes. The beneficial effect of biocompatible membranes has been postulated to result from the absence of the alternate complement pathway activation that characterizes the use of cellulose-derived membranes. It is thought that repeated inflammatory responses to conventional dialysis with cellulose-derived membranes impairs patient recovery from ARF and has an adverse effect on the rate of mortality from sepsis.

Hypercatabolic patients with ARF secondary to multiple trauma or abdominal catastrophe should receive hemodialysis, because even continuous peritoneal dialysis is often unable to correct the severe metabolic disorders in such patients. In other words, hemodialysis is more efficient and therefore more effective than peritoneal dialysis in correcting metabolic abnormalities in these patient. Its disadvantages result from the need for anticoagulation, greater hemodynamic stresses, and requirement for vascular access. A peritoneal catheter may be placed during abdominal surgery if dialysis is anticipated in the immediate future (73). Peritoneal dialysis is simpler but may be complicated by atelectasis, pneumonia, hyperglycemia, and peritonitis. It is preferred in patients with an unstable cardiovascular status, however, and in those with head injuries or bleeding, because systemic heparinization is unnecessary. Antibiotics may be added to the dialysis solution in the presence of intra-abdominal infection. Recent abdominal surgery or the presence of vascular grafts are relative contraindications to peritoneal dialysis, but if needed, the catheter should be placed under direct vision rather than by the percutaneous route. Peritoneal lavage has not been shown to benefit patients with severe acute pancreatitis (74).

In the intensive care unit (ICU), continuous renal replacement therapy (CRRT) is becoming increasingly important role in the treatment of ARF (75). The main advantage of these techniques is their ability to correct fluid overload in patients who are hemodynamically unstable. However, by adding a diffusive dialysis component, the control of azotemia in severely catabolic patients also is possible. Maintaining hemodynamic stability is important not only to the technical success of CRRT but may be beneficial in recovery of renal function. In addition, Myers and Moran (76) have raised concerns that the hypotensive episodes frequently accompanying intermittent hemodialysis may delay patient recovery from ARF. They postulate that in the setting of lost renal blood flow autoregulation that characterizes ARF, hypotension will result in further ischemic insults to renal epithelium and delay recovery; thus, removal of inflammatory mediators by hemofiltration is another potential benefit of CRRT in sepsis and multiorgan failure.

To date, no prospective randomized trials have demonstrated continuous techniques as being superior to conventional intermittent techniques. In a historically controlled retrospective study involving 167 patients with ARF treated consecutively in one ICU between 1982 and 1991, Bellomo et al. (77) compared conventional dialysis with CRRT. The authors were unable to demonstrate an overall difference in patient survival between the two groups; however, by further characterizing these patients according to the severity of illness, they were able to show a significant difference in survival with CRRT among patients with an APACHE score of 24 to 29 or with two to four failing organs. There was no difference in survival among lesser or more seriously ill patients. Whether these improvements relate more to the use of biocompatible membranes in CRRT than to the mode of renal replacement therapy, however, remains to be proven.

Continuous renal replacement therapy is also very useful in patients with both liver disease and renal failure. Cerebral edema is a major cause of death in patients with fulminant hepatic failure, and rapid decreases in plasma osmolality or intravascular volume can exacerbate intracranial pressure. CRRT allows a more gradual change in plasma osmolality and intravascular volume, which would be beneficial in this situation. Biasioli et al. (78) reported that continuous venovenous hemofiltration (CVVH) resulted in the

improvement of congestive heart failure that was refractory to conventional therapy, and it may also be useful as a temporizing measure in patients waiting for a cardiac transplant. Hemofiltration may be better than intermittent hemodialysis at decreasing lung water in noncardiogenic pulmonary edema.

By continuously ultrafiltrating water, CRRT allows total parenteral nutrition to be given without restriction or concern of exacerbating volume overload. Total parenteral therapy has not been proven to definitely reduce mortality among patients with ARF patients, but it is still used commonly. At present, aggressive nutritional support aimed at maintaining positive nitrogen and caloric balance appears to be reasonable.

Continuous renal replacement therapy can be performed with or without (79, 80) the aid of a blood pump. If no blood pump is used, cannulation of the femoral artery with a large-bore catheter is necessary, and in this situation, the patient's own blood pressure is the driving force in the extracorporeal circuit. The femoral vein also is usually cannulated to allow a path for blood to return to the patient. In the absence of a preexisting coagulopathy, all patients receiving CRRT will require continuous infusions of heparin, with its attendant risk of bleeding. In patients already at high risk for bleeding or those with a coagulopathy, CRRT can be attempted without heparin. Some of the risks of arterial cannulation include vascular thrombosis, distal embolization of atherosclerotic placque, local or retroperitoneal hematoma, and infection. Because of the dangers of prolonged arterial cannulation, use of a simple blood pump to move blood through the extracorporeal circuit is becoming more common; although initially somewhat more demanding on the ICU nurses, this allows a dual-lumen hemodialysis catheter placed in the femoral, subclavian, or internal jugular vein to serve as a vascular access and avoids the risk associated with femoral artery catheterization. Such techniques using a blood pump are referred to as *venovenous*, because blood is both pumped out of and returned through a dual-lumen venous catheter.

Slow, continuous ultrafiltration is primarily indicated in fluid-overloaded patients without severe azotemia and who are resistant to diuretics. Ultrafiltration rates are usually less than 5 mL/min, and slow, continuous ultrafiltration is not adequate to correct azotemia. Continuous arteriovenous hemofiltration (CAVH) or CVVH typically result in ultrafiltration rates greater than 5 mL/min, and they may require up to 600 mL of replacement fluids to be infused per hour. In this situation, solute clearance is by convection only but still may control the level of azotemia if the patient is not severely catabolic. Continuous arteriovenous hemodialysis (CAVHD) or continuous venovenous hemodialysis (CVVHD) adds the element of solute removal via diffusion by infusing the peritoneal dialysis fluid through the hemofilter, typically at 1 L/h. Urea clearance rates average approximately 20 mL/min but can be greater if higher ultrafiltration rates or greater amounts of peritoneal dialysis fluid are infused through the hemofilter. However, with both CAVHD and CVVHD, ultrafiltration rates are generally less than 5 mL/min, and replacement fluid is typically not needed. Because of their higher rate of solute clearance, both techniques are suitable in severely catabolic patients to con-

Table 12.11.   Unbound Drug Fraction of Commonly Used Drugs

Antibiotics		Miscellaneous Drugs	
Drug	alpha	Drug	alpha
Amikacin	0.9	Bromide	1.0
Amphotericin B	0.1	Chlorodiazepoxide	0.05
Ampicillin	0.8	Cisplatin	0.1
Cefoperazone	0.1	Clofibrate	0.04
Cefotaxime	0.6	Cyclosporine	0.1
Cefoxitin	0.5	Diathybarbital	0.9
Ceftazidime	0.9	Diazepam	0.02
Ceftriaxone	0.1	Digitoxin	0.1
Cephapirin	0.6	Digoxin	0.8
Cilastatin	0.6	Famotidine	0.8
Ciprofloxacin	0.7	Glibenclamide	0.01
Clindamycin	0.4	Glutethimide	0.5
Doxycycline	0.2	Lidocaine	0.4
Erythromycin	0.3	Metamizole	0.4
Gentamicin	0.9	NAP	0.9
Imipenem	0.8	Nitrazepam	0.1
Metronidazole	0.8	Nomifensine	0.4
Mezlocillin	0.7	Oxazepam	0.1
Nafcillin	0.2	Phenobarbital	0.6
Netilmicin	0.9	Phenytoin	0.2
Oxacillin	0.05	Procainamide	0.9
Penicillin	0.5	Pyrithyldione	—
Streptomycin	0.6	Ranitidine	0.85
Sulfamethoxazole	0.6	Theophylline	0.85
Tobramycin	0.9		
Vancomycin	0.9		

Modified from Golper TA. Drug removal during continuous renal replacement therapies. Dial Transplant 22(4):185, 1993.

trol the level of azotemia and correct the volume overload. The nephrologist is best suited to decide which form of replacement therapy is best for an individual patient, but it is very important for the consulting internist to understand the implications of these therapeutic modalities.

Drug Therapy in Continuous Renal Replacement Therapy

Continuous renal replacement therapy is capable of providing significant daily clearance of urea (10–20 mL/min), which can result in substantial drug removal. Since CRRT is typically provided to patients who are critically ill, it is especially important to pay careful attention to proper administration to maintain therapeutic drug levels and avoid toxicity. Although significant amounts of vasopressors can be recovered in the ultrafiltrate, their rate of infusion typically exceeds their removal rate; thus, loss of pressors in the ultrafiltrate should not be a clinical concern.

The amount of drug removed by convection-based therapies (CAVH and CVVH) depends on the steady-state arterial concentrations (A), the fraction of the drug not bound to protein (α), and the ultrafiltration rate (UFR). It is expressed as follows:

Amount of drug removal $= A \times \alpha \times$ UFR

The blood sample for determining the arterial steady-state drug concentration should be drawn midway between the maintenance doses. The maintenance dose can also be determined by measuring drug concentration in the ultrafiltrate and multiplying this value by the daily ultrafiltrate volume. Table 12.11 lists the unbound-drug fraction of commonly used drugs to help calculate daily maintenance doses in patients receiving CAVH or CVVH.

Another method to estimate drug doses in CAVH or CVVH relies on the fact that each 10 L of ultrafiltrate per day corre-

Table 12.12. Approximate Drug Dosage in ARF treated by CAVHD/CVVHD

Cefuroxime	500 mg–700 mg per 24 hr
Ceftazidime	1 gm per 24 hr
Tobramycin	normal loading dose followed by 60–80 mg per 24 hr
Gentamicin	normal loading dose followed by 80–100 mg per 24 hr
Ciprofloxacin	200 mg per 8 hr
Vancomycin	1 gm per 24 hr

Modified from Sigler MH, Teehan BP. Continuous renal replacement therapy in Nissenson AR, Fine RN, Gentile DE (eds). Clinical Dialysis 3rd ed. Conn, Appleton and Lange, 1995.

sponds to a urea clearance of 7 mL/min. One can then follow the dosage guidelines in the *Physicians' Desk Reference* (PDR) for renal failure (assuming the patient had a GFR of 7 mL/min for each 10 L of ultrafiltrate).

In CAVHD and CVVHD, drug removal principally occurs by diffusion, although there is also a small element of convection. Again, the PDR can be used, estimating the GFR as 20 mL/min (assuming a dialysate flow of 1 L/h and ultrafiltrate rate of 4 mL/min) and following the dosage guidelines for chronic renal failure.

Table 12.12 lists the approximate dosage adjustments of antibiotics commonly used in ARF treated with CAVHD or CVVHD. In all patients who are critically ill, drug levels should be measured to verify the adequacy of dosing and to avoid toxicity. Strict attention to all other aspects of therapy, including the prevention and prompt treatment of infection, gastrointestinal bleeding, and appropriate tailoring of drug therapy, are also important.

EVALUATION AND TREATMENT OF PATIENTS WITH CHRONIC RENAL FAILURE

Epidemiology

Operations commonly performed in patients with renal failure include vascular access procedures, parathyroidectomy, pericardiectomy, nephrectomy, and renal transplantation. In patients with mild to moderate renal insufficiency, the most serious complication is the superimposition of ARF, although fluid and electrolyte disturbances are common. Patients with uremia have additional impairments of wound healing, hemostasis, and immunity. Nevertheless, even major surgery can be performed on patients undergoing hemodialysis with relative safety (81–83). The mortality rate in a series reported by Brenowitz et al. (84), encompassing 31 patients on hemodialysis undergoing 40 elective and 9 emergency operations, was 4%. Although intraoperative complications (e.g., such as bleeding) directly attributable to uremia were unusual, postoperative problems developed in more than 60%. Hemodialysis within 24 hours was required in 63%, mainly for treatment of hyperkalemia, the development of which appeared to relate to use of blood transfusions rather than to the preoperative potassium level. Fistula thrombosis, pneumonia (primarily with Gram-negative organisms), and wound infections were relatively common, and hypotensive episodes not related to fluid losses were also noted. Others have reported an increased incidence of wound dehiscence as well.

Evaluation

In patients with chronic renal failure of with an established cause, the diagnostic process should be directed at establishing the degree of impairment and documenting any uremic abnormalities (85–88). This evaluation should include a search for conditions that might aggravate existing renal failure, such as volume depletion or use of nephrotoxic drugs. When renal insufficiency is newly discovered, elective surgery should be postponed and the patient evaluated to establish the cause. The severity of renal impairment should be determined by the serum creatinine level and a timed creatinine clearance.

In general, serum electrolyte concentrations are only mildly affected, at least until late in the course of renal failure. Hyponatremia usually results from the administration of hypotonic fluids, and hyperkalemia often results from volume depletion, catabolic states, acidosis, use of ACE inhibitors, and excess potassium administration. Hyperkalemia should also suggest gastrointestinal bleeding or internal hemorrhage. Most patients with renal failure maintain a serum bicarbonate level of 15 mEq/L or greater; anything lower should suggest the presence of a superimposed acidosis. If hypermagnesemia is found, all medications should be examined for hidden sources of magnesium, such as that contained in many commonly used antacids.

Evaluation of the volume status in patients with azotemia is based on the physical examination, changes in body weight, urine output, or, possibly, invasive monitoring. These will usually provide sufficient information on the intravascular volume in patients with mild renal insufficiency. In more advanced cases, patients who might not tolerate fluid challenges, or those expected to have large volume losses or shifts during surgery, use of a Swan-Ganz catheter is appropriate. Since the usual criteria of volume depletion as applied to the urinary electrolytes presuppose normal kidney function, use of urinary indices such as sodium concentration, osmolality, or FE_{Na} have lesser value in patients with established renal disorders.

A generalized bleeding diathesis should not be attributed to uremia unless other commonly encountered causes, such as disseminated intravascular coagulation, can be ruled out. The finding of a normal bleeding time makes it unlikely that uremia is contributing to this problem.

Treatment

The most clearly defined risk in patients with abnormal kidney function is the development of superimposed ARF; therefore, a major focus preoperatively is to obtain optimal renal perfusion (89). Fluid therapy should be aimed at replenishing prior volume deficits as assessed by clinical and laboratory means, replacing ongoing losses, and providing daily metabolic needs. As renal function declines, it becomes more critical for the components of fluid therapy to reflect the actual losses. This is best accomplished by measuring the volume and electrolyte contents of urine and other body fluids being lost externally.

Many other details also require special attention in patients with chronic renal failure. Adequate nutrition is important in alleviating uremic symptoms and ensuring proper wound healing in the postoperative period. The type of dietary treatment chiefly depends on the degree of renal insufficiency; in general, only those patients with advanced renal insufficiency (creatinine clearance, <30 mL/min) have significant biochemical abnormalities or clinical manifestations warranting specific dietary therapy. Many patients with a diagnosis of renal disease are reflexively placed on "renal failure" diets, which are often interpreted to mean severe salt and protein restriction. Such a diet may lead to volume depletion and a negative protein balance, however. The role of protein restriction in preventing the progression of renal insufficiency is currently being investigated, but most patients with mild to moderate renal insufficiency do not require protein restriction to relieve their symptoms.

When protein restriction is necessary, essential amino acids or high-biologic-value proteins must be provided along with an adequate caloric intake (2000–3000 cal/day) in the form of carbohydrates and fats to prevent a negative nitrogen balance. Most often, patients on dialysis are not protein restricted. Those patients with moderate to advanced renal insufficiency do best on a 4- to 6-g salt diet unless they have edema, congestive heart failure, or hypertension, at which time either a loop diuretic (e.g., furosemide) can be added or salt intake restricted further.

Patients who cannot be fed should undergo hyperalimentation both before and after major surgery. For any given patients, prerenal azotemia indicates that the salt and volume restrictions are too severe.

Potassium restriction in stable patients is generally not necessary as long as the urine output is adequate. Care must be taken, however, to avoid use of potassium-sparing diuretics or potassium-containing drugs, such as most phosphate supplements, some penicillin preparations, and salt substitutes. ACE inhibitors may also cause hyperkalemia in patients with renal insufficiency. Most patients will not require water restriction unless hyponatremia develops, and keeping a patient NPO without an intravenous line in place may predispose to volume depletion in those with fixed salt losses.

Hypertension is often present in patients with renal failure, and it should be controlled throughout the surgical period. Oral medications should be continued up to the evening before the procedure. Short-acting drugs (e.g., parenteral hydralazine) may be required to maintain normotension until oral intake is resumed; patients with stable, minimal elevations of blood pressure may do well without parenteral supplementation. When related to volume overload, congestive heart failure should be treated with salt restriction, afterload reduction, or diuretics rather than with digitalis. If possible, volume overload should be corrected before surgery; however, some degree of edema is preferable to volume depletion.

While chronic anemia remains part of the uremic syndrome, widespread use of erythropoitein in patients undergoing dialysis has greatly diminished both its severity and the frequency of blood transfusion. Opinions still vary regarding acceptable preoperative hematocrit values, but factors to consider when assessing adequacy of the hematocrit in that setting include the presence of comorbid illnesses (e.g., coronary artery disease, congestive heart failure), magnitude of the surgical procedures, anticipated intraoperative blood loss, and the beneficial effect on platelet–vessel wall interactions when the hematocrit is 30% or greater. It appears to be reasonable to attempt achieving a 30% hematocrit in most patients preoperatively. It may be necessary to increase the patient's dose of erythropoietin to compensate for the increased resistance to this hormone that characterizes the postoperative state. Contraindications to transfusion include precipitation of volume overload or hyperkalemia. If possible, blood should be given in advance of the final preoperative dialysis to remove the excess potassium.

Use of prophylactic antibiotics is generally discouraged (84). In one study (83), their use did not prevent postoperative pneumonia, although the incidence of wound infections was slightly reduced. Prophylactic dialysis in patients with borderline renal function has not been shown to affect morbidity or mortality, and it should not be performed in the absence of specific indications (e.g., medically unresponsive fluid overload, uremia, pericarditis). One should anticipate, however, that the additional metabolic stress of surgery may require the use of postoperative dialysis. Therefore, surgery in these patients should be performed only in hospitals equipped for dialysis.

In the patients undergoing long-term dialysis, dialysis is generally performed again 24 hours before elective surgery to improve electrolyte balance and platelet function (90). Even a brief, 2- to 3-hour dialysis before emergency surgery is useful in correcting preoperative electrolyte disturbances. Dialysis can be performed using either regional heparinization (i.e., heparin is neutralized by the infusion of protamine after leaving the dialyzer) or "low-dose" heparin infusions. In most cases, patients with long-term Tenckhoff catheters for peritoneal dialysis may continue using their catheters postoperatively.

Intraoperative treatment should include careful infusion of potassium-free fluids and replacement of any fluid or blood loss. There is no convincing evidence that intraoperative mannitol or furosemide prevents postoperative ARF among patients with prior renal disease. Careful positioning of the fistula arm and avoidance of hypotension help to reduce the incidence of vascular access thrombosis. Frequent monitoring of the ECG and blood chemistries during prolonged operations is necessary for the early detection of electrolyte disturbances. Because of the prolonged effects of neuromuscular relaxants and central nervous system (CNS) depressants in patient with uremia, extubation should not be rushed and only performed with the anesthesiologist present. Postoperative reintubation is all too common but usually avoidable. During the immediate postoperative period, serum electrolyte levels should be obtained every 6 to 12 hours in patients who are seriously ill, and hourly urine outputs as well as daily weight should be recorded. Because even regional or minimal heparinization may increase the rate of hematoma formation, dialysis is usually delayed for at least 24 to 48 hours if possible. Administration of Kayexalate enemas (when not contraindicated) and careful administration of fluids often keeps patients in electrolyte balance.

In patients with uremia, sutures are often left in place for several additional days because of impaired wound healing. Respiratory therapy is an important part of postoperative treatment in reducing the incidence of pneumonia. Removal of indwelling Foley catheters and central or peripheral intravenous lines as soon as possible should help to reduce the incidence of infection.

Platelet dysfunction secondary to uremia often contributes to prolonged bleeding from the gastrointestinal tract or wound sites. Bleeding time is thought to be the best indicator of the adequacy of platelet function in patients with uremia, and severity of the anemia in chronic renal failure correlates with the prolongation of the bleeding time. Correction of the anemia to a hematocrit of 30% by either blood transfusion (91) or use of erythropoietin (92) improves platelet–vessel wall interaction and normalizes the bleeding time. When dialysis or raising the hematocrit to 30% or greater fails to completely correct a prolonged bleeding time, several drugs are useful (Table 12.13). Cryoprecipitate (93) or DDAVP (1-desamino-8-D-arginine vasopressin) are also capable of correcting an abnormal bleeding time. Cryoprecipitate is usually given intravenously, whereas DDAVP may be given either intravenously (94) or intranasally (95). Administration of cryoprecipitate carries a small risk of virus transmission, so it is best to start with DDAVP. However, the efficacy of DDAVP diminishes with repeated administration. The duration of action for both cryoprecipitate and DDAVP is typically less than a day, when a longer duration of action is required, intravenous administration of conjugated estrogens (96) is useful. These drugs may be used prophylactically in patients with uremia and prolonged bleeding times who are about to undergo procedures likely to be complicated by bleeding (e.g., surgery, organ biopsy). They are also useful in controlling active bleeding in patients with uremia.

Drug Therapy in Patients with Azotemia

Epidemiology

The frequency of adverse drug reactions is 25% in patients with azotemia, compared with 9% in patients with normal renal function (97). Side effects from drugs in patients with a reduced GFR can be divided into two groups: those adversely affecting kidney function, and those leading to systemic reactions. Drug nephrotoxicity can be induced by direct tubular damage (e.g., aminoglycoside antibiotics), interstitial nephritis (e.g., methicillin), glomerulonephritis (e.g., penicillamine), alterations in renal blood flow (e.g., ACE inhibitors, nonsteroidal antiinflammatories), or intrarenal crystal deposition (e.g., methoxyflurane) (8). Systemic effects may relate to abnormally high drug levels (e.g., penicillin-induced or cephalosporin-induced seizures) or increased sensitivity in uremia (e.g., CNS depression with narcotics).

Abnormalities of drug metabolism with renal failure include a prolonged half life of renally excreted drugs or active metabolites, alterations in bioavailability, volume of distribution, and protein binding. Decreased absorption of orally administered drugs may occur with nausea, vomiting, and by competition from phosphate-binding gels.

Significant edema or ascites in patients with renal failure will increase the apparent volume of distribution of highly water-soluble or highly protein-bound drugs. In such situations, subtherapeutic concentrations may result if drug levels are not monitored. Many acidic drugs have decreased protein binding in renal failure, which is thought to result from a combination of uremia-induced changes in the binding-site configuration and the accu-

Table 12.13.   Drugs Useful to Reduce the Bleeding Time in Uremia

Drug	Dose	Route	Onset of Action	Peak Effect	Duration of Effect
Cryoprecipitate	10 bags	iv	1 hr	4–12 hr	24–36 hr
DDAVP	0.3 micrograms/kg	iv	1 hr	2–4 hr	6–8 hr
DDAVP (intranasal)	3.0 micrograms/kg	intranasal	1 hr	2–4 hr	6–8 hr
Conjugated Estrogens	0.6 mg/kg daily for 5 days	iv	6 hr	5–7 days	21–30 days

mulation of undefined uremic toxins that compete with drugs for binding sites on albumin. As a result, there is an increase in the levels of unbound fraction of several acidic drugs. Serious toxicity may result even if the total plasma concentration of these drugs is in the therapeutic range, and it is important to measure both the total and the free plasma drug concentrations. Table 12.14 lists drugs commonly used in patients with renal failure patients that have decreased protein binding.

Evaluation

The internist is responsible for properly adjusting the dosage or frequency of renally excreted drugs in the presence of abnormal kidney function. Quantitation of both renal and hepatic function is crucial when selecting the proper drug dosage. Even if they have "normal" serum creatinine concentrations, elderly patients have an age-related decrease in the GFR; therefore, these patients should be treated as carefully as those with kidney failure.

Treatment

Methods of compensating for renal dysfunction include a reduction of drug dosage or a lengthening of the interval between administrations. In either situation, a normal loading dose should be given to achieve immediate effective levels. Monitoring should include measurement of blood levels (both peak and trough) and observing the patient carefully for side effects. Several excellent

reviews are available that provide complete information for prescribing most drugs in patients with renal insufficiency (98); this section only deals with those that are likely to be used perioperatively.

Nonnarcotic Analgesics Aspirin is generally avoided, because it aggravates platelet dysfunction. Nonsteroidal analgesics may be used, but a moderate reduction in their dosage may be required. However, nonsteroidal analgesics produce reversible decreases in the GFR, particularly in the presence of volume depletion, and have occasionally been implicated in the development of acute interstitial nephritis. Therefore, these drugs are best avoided in patients with renal insufficiency.

Narcotics   Most narcotics, including codeine, meperidine, morphine, and pentazocine, are hepatically metabolized. Doses of these drugs may need to be reduced, however, because patients with uremia tend to be sensitive to their depressant effects on the CNS. Prolonged use of meperidine has also been reported to cause twitching and seizures because of retained metabolites (99).

Barbiturates, Sedatives, and Hypnotics Short-acting, hepatically metabolized barbiturates such as pentobarbital are preferred over phenobarbital. Barbiturates are best avoided altogether, because they affect the metabolism and alter the protein binding of many drugs. Diazepam is a better alternative when sedation or tranquilization is necessary. Flurazepam is also an effective and relatively safe medication.

Anesthetics Most commonly used inhalational agents (e.g., cyclopropane, halothane) can be used for major surgery in patients with renal failure. Methoxyflurane and enthrane are nephrotoxic, however, and should not be used in patients with chronic renal failure. Succinylcholine may be used as a muscle relaxant, but it is known to cause an increase in the serum potassium level. Both intravenous and

Table 12.14.   Commonly Used Drugs in Renal Failure With Decreased Protein Binding

Phenytoin	Doxepin
Phenobarbital	Tamazepam
Theophylline	Penicillins
Furosemide	Sulfonamides
Oxazepam	Salicylates

spinal anesthesia should be used whenever deemed appropriate.

Diuretics Oral thiazide diuretics should not be used in moderate renal insufficiency (GFR, <30 mL/min), because they lose their effectiveness and also reduce the renal blood flow. Intravenous diuril is effective in patients with advanced renal failure, but potassium-sparing diuretics (e.g., spironolactone, triamterene, amiloride) are contraindicated in patients with chronic renal insufficiency because of their potassium-retaining effects. Loop diuretics are effective even in advanced renal insufficiency, although higher dosages are required. Use of prolonged, high-dose, and, particularly, intravenous furosemide may be complicated by the development of ototoxicity. Ethacrynic acid is also effective in advanced renal failure, but it has a higher incidence of ototoxicity than furosemide. Metolazone acts synergistically with the loop diuretics and is effective even in advanced renal failure.

Antihypertensives Most antihypertensive drugs are administered at the usual dosage. Intravenous nitroprusside can be used to control malignant hypertension in patients with mild renal failure, but the duration of such therapy should be brief (<12–24 hours). In addition, the levels of its toxic metabolite, thiocyanate, need to be monitored. Nitroprusside should be avoided in moderate to severe renal failure or in combined renal–hepatic diseases because of the risk of cyanide toxicity. β-Blockers such as propranolol may be used at the usual dose. The dosage of others however, such as atenolol and nadolol, should be reduced, because they are excreted by the kidney.

Cardiac Drugs The maintenance dose of digoxin should be reduced in patients with renal insufficiency, but the loading dose can remain unchanged. Since digoxin drug dosages in renal insufficiency are only approximated by nomograms, the drug levels need to be monitored, and

additional digoxin need not be administered following dialysis. Extra care must be taken in any patient receiving digitalis to maintain a normal potassium balance. Quinidine and lidocaine require no dose modifications in renal failure, and the active metabolite of procainamide, N-acetylprocainamide, accumulates in the setting of renal insufficiency. Therefore, levels of both the parent drug and its metabolite must be measured when assessing procainamide therapy. It is probably best to avoid use of procainamide altogether in patients with renal failure if an alternative antiarrhythmic drug is available.

Antibiotics Since excretion of penicillin G and most semisynthetic penicillins is by the kidney, large doses should be reduced in moderate to severe renal failure (100). An exception, however, is nafcillin, which does not require dose reduction because of hepatic metabolism. Significant amounts of sodium are given with large doses of sodium penicillin (1.7 mEq of Na^+ per 1 million U) and carbenicillin (4.7 mEq/g). Potassium penicillin G contains 1.7 mEq of K^+ per 1 million U.

Aminoglycosides are potentially nephrotoxic, and they can produce both vestibular and auditory problems as well. They are filtered by the glomerulus and concentrated in the proximal tubule. Early manifestations of aminoglycoside toxicity include concentrating defects, enzymuria, and proteinuria; there is some evidence that tobramycin may be less nephrotoxic than the other aminoglycosides (9). The use of single, daily-dose aminoglycoside therapy has become fashionable and may be as effective and less toxic than multiple-dose regimens (101).

Strict attention to adjusting dosages by means of nomograms and monitoring drug levels is essential in avoiding toxicity. The serum creatinine level should be measured every 1 to 2 days in patients receiving aminoglycosides. Urine volume alone is not a reliable index of renal function in these patients, because they often develop a nonoliguric form of ARF. It should also be noted that the onset of renal failure can be delayed for up to 1 week following discontinuation of the antibiotic.

Significant drug toxicity can occur even when drug levels are in the therapeutic range during renal insufficiency, volume depletion, metabolic acidosis, or when other nephrotoxic agents are being used simultaneously. Except for cephaloridine, most cephalosporins, including cefamandole and cefazolin, are not considered to be nephrotoxic. Drug dosage must be reduced in renal insufficiency for some of the second- and third-generation cephalosporins, however, because seizures may otherwise develop. Cephalosporins are thought to be nephrotoxic when used in conjunction with aminoglycosides, particularly in patients who are volume depleted.

Tetracycline derivatives should be avoided, because they increase BUN and potentiate acidosis. Neither chloramphenicol nor clindamycin require alteration of dosage in renal failure unless hepatic insufficiency coexists. Vancomycin can be used for staphylococcal infections in patients who are allergic to penicillin, but it requires a reduced dosage in this setting. With the older, cellulose-based dialyzers, a 1-g dose given intravenously lasts for approximately 7 days in patients without significant renal function. When patients undergo dialysis with the newer, more permeable, synthetic dialyzers, more frequent dosing is necessary and monitoring of vancomycin levels in the blood advisable.

Anticoagulants Both heparin and sodium warfarin (Coumadin) are given in the usual dosage. Both drugs, however, may potentiate uremic bleeding disorders.

Anticonvulsants Although the half-life of phenytoin (Dilantin) is decreased in renal failure, the usual dose tends to remain effective. This results both from accumulation of active metabolites and from reduced protein binding. It is recommended that divided doses of phenytoin be administered in patients with renal failure to avoid excessively high peak levels. Since the level of unbound (i.e., active) drug is higher relative to the total drug level, monitoring "free" phenytoin levels will help to avoid toxicity.

Antacids Surgical patients often receive large doses of antacids during therapy or prophylaxis for gastrointestinal bleeding. Since a patient's ability to excrete magnesium is impaired in renal insufficiency, use of magnesium-containing antacids is not recommended. Calcium carbonate may be used, but frequent monitoring of the serum phosphate level is necessary to avoid hypophosphatemia. The dose of cimetidine should be reduced to 300 mg given twice a day and that of ranitidine to 150 mg at bedtime in patients with significant renal insufficiency. Cimetidine has been reported to increase the serum creatinine level in patients with normal renal function, but this phenomenon does not appear to be progressive and reverses once therapy has been discontinued (102). There is also an increased incidence of CNS symptoms such as agitation, confusion, and coma in patients, particularly if they are elderly, with renal insufficiency who are receiving cimetidine.

TREATMENT OF RENAL TRANSPLANTATION DONORS AND RECIPIENTS
Epidemiology

In hospital centers that perform living-related donor kidney transplants, the consulting internist may be asked to aid in the medical evaluation of potential donors. The role of the "independent" internist is to examine the donor for any problems that would preclude the patient from this particular donation. There are three general categories of diseases that might adversely affect a person's ability to donate a kidney. In the first category are diseases that could damage the donor's remaining kidney (e.g., diabetes, hypertension, nephrolithiasis). In the second are diseases that might be transmitted to the transplant recipient (e.g., hepatitis B surface antigen–positive hepatitis, active syphilis, human-immunodeficiency-virus infection, malignancy). In the final group are diseases that increase the risk of surgery in general (e.g., coronary artery disease, pulmonary disease, liver diseases).

Evaluation of transplant recipients is generally the responsibility of the referring nephrologist and is beyond the scope of this chapter. However, a detailed review of the patient workup has been published by the Patient Care and Education Committee of the American Society of Transplant Physicians (103).

The incidence of renal abnormalities among family members (i.e., potential donors) of patients on dialysis appears to be increased. In a series of 209 potential donors (relatives of patients with hereditary renal diseases were excluded) reported by Spanos et al. (104), 10% had significant bacteriuria, 5% diastolic hypertension, 20% abnormal intravenous pyelograms, and 4% major abnormalities on renal arteriography. Of the original 209 potential donors, 40 (19%) were excluded based on one or more of these abnormalities.

Use of family members as donors for patients with hereditary forms of renal disease is controversial. Some centers simply restrict transplantation in such instances to cadaveric sources. Others, because the superior graft survival of living-related donor compared with that of cadaveric transplants (75 versus 50% 2-year graft survival, respectively), will evaluate and use family members as donors. Because of the shortage of transplantable kidneys, use of unrelated living donors is becoming more common, and it is also associated with improved graft survival compared to that with cadaveric kidneys (105).

Evaluation

Potential donors are selected after histocompatibility has been established and obvious physical or psychologic abnormalities have been excluded. The selected donor then is generally admitted for more extensive medical, psychologic, and urologic evaluation. Table 12.15 summarizes the donor evaluation.

When a living-related donor for a patient with hereditary renal disease is being considered, more extensive evaluations, including renal biopsy, are often necessary. For example, in Alport's disease, the earliest manifestations are seen in the glomerulus or tubules when examined by election microscopy. Milutinovic et al. (106) found that young siblings of patients with polycystic kidney disease may have a normal urogram, GFR, renal blood flow, ammonia production, and concentrating ability, yet have tubular dilatation seen in the renal biopsy specimen. As genetic markers become available, the evaluation of family donors will become more straightforward. Evaluation of the family members when a patient has diabetes is made more difficult by the complex nature of the genetic component; even HLA-identical siblings of such a patient may never develop glucose intolerance. If a relative is being considered in

Table 12.15. Living Related Transplant Donor Evaluation

1. Tissue typing
   ABO blood groups
   HLA typing, mixed lymphocyte culture,
   leukocyte cross-match (DR typing)
2. Psychological screening
3. History and physical
4. Repeat blood pressure determinations,
   urinalysis, urine culture
5. BUN, creatinine, creatinine clearance, IVP
6. Fasting blood sugar, liver functions, uric acid,
   calcium, phosphorus, CBC, prothrombin time,
   partial thromboplastin time, HAA, STS, HIV
7. Chest radiograph, ECG
8. Aortogram

this situation, the minimal evaluation of the potential donor should include a fasting glucose and oral glucose tolerance test. Some centers advocate the use of cortisone or intravenous glucose tolerance tests as well.

Treatment

A listing of postoperative complications in donors is provided by Table 12.16. Long-term follow-up of large numbers of donors has not revealed any change in life expectancy, and renal function returns to

Table 12.16. Postoperative Complications in Living Related Transplant Donors

	Boston[a] (N = 300)	Colorado[b] (N = 238)	Virginia[c] (N = 120)	Wisconsin[d] (N = 66)	Total (N = 724)
Group Characteristics	1954–1973	1964–1969	1966–1972	1966–1973	
Donor age (yr)	12–80	18–57	22–59	21–63	12–80
Percentage of potential donors rejected	23		66		
Overall complication rate (%)	28.3	47	21	34.8	33.8
Complications					
Wound infections	33	4	3		40 (5.5)
Pneumonia	5				5 (0.7%)
Atelectasis/fever/ pneumonia	29	33	5	2	69 (9.5%)
Pleural effusion		12		1	13 (1.8%)
Pneumothorax		26	3		29 (4%)
Pulmonary embolus				2	2 (0.3%)
Acute renal failure	1	1	1		3 (0.4%)
Gastric distention or intestinal ileus		4	3		7 (1.0%)
UGI bleed	1				1 (0.1%)
Hepatitis	2	4			6 (0.8%)
Serum	1				
Anesthesia-related	1	4			
Positive urine culture	39	24		15	78 (10.8%)
Persistent bacteriuria			3	2	5 (0.7%)
Transient hematuria		3			3 (0.4%)
Urinary retention		7			7 (1.0%)
Deep venous thrombosis		3		2	5 (0.7%)
Postaortogram thrombosis			1		1 (0.1%)
Phlebitis	3				3 (0.4%)
Transfusion requirement			3		3 (0.4%)
Transient hypertension	1	10			11 (1.5%)
Minor cardiac arrhythmias	3				3 (0.4%)
Psychiatric problems	21				21 (2.9%)
Transient nerve palsy		4			4 (0.5%)
Prolonged incisional pain		3			3 (0.4%)
Incisional hernia	1		3	2	6 (0.8%)
Mortality (in hospital)	0	0	1	1	2 (0.3%)
Myocardial infarct			1		
Pulmonary embolus				1	

[a]*Surg Gynecol Obstet* 139:894, 1974.
[b]*Arch Surg* 101:226, 1970.
[c]*J Urol* 110:158, 1973.
[d]*J Urol* 111:745, 1974.

between 70 and 80% of the preoperative level within a few months. There has been recent concern that the adaptive changes occurring in the remaining donor kidney (i.e., hyperfiltration) may eventually damage the organ. Several long-term series of donors examined to date, however, show only a slight increase in albuminuria and blood pressure, without significant decline in the GFR.

SURGERY IN RENAL TRANSPLANT RECIPIENTS

Epidemiology

Recipients of renal transplants are more likely to undergo surgery than patients in the general population. Most of their complications requiring surgical solutions derive from the transplant itself or from problems related to their prior uremic state. Surgical procedures directly related to the transplanted kidney include drainage of hematomas, lymphoceles, and wound abscesses, as well as urologic procedures such as the repair of leaking ureters or bladders. Procedures related to immunosuppression include operations to correct steroid-induced gastrointestinal bleeding and orthopaedic procedures for aseptic necrosis. Parathyroidectomy may be necessary for persistent hypercalcemia related to the prior development of secondary hyperparathyroidism. Since no direct comparisons between transplant recipients, patients with uremia, and "normal" individuals have been performed, the effect of renal transplant on surgical morbidity and mortality is unclear. It is evident, however, that transplant recipients are predisposed to unique complications arising from their prior uremic state or from transplant immunosuppression.

Combining the results from two series of renal transplant recipients in the United Kingdom and the United States, 106 of 280 patients required additional surgery (excluding transplant nephrectomy) (107, 108) (Table 12.17). In the U.S. series, 32% of the patients requiring ad-

Table 12.17. Surgical Experience in Two Groups of Renal Transplant Recipients

	Leapman et al. (United States) Numbers (%)	Bakkaloglu et al. (Britain) Numbers (%)
Transplant recipients	162	118
Transplants performed	202	132
Patients operated	67 (41)	39 (33)
Elective procedures	62 (60)	30 (46)
Emergency procedures	41 (40)	35 (54)
Mortality	20 (30)	0
Acute renal failure	1 (0.02)	0

ditional surgery underwent multiple procedures; most procedures related directly to the transplant itself or to the complications of immunosuppression. The U.K. group routinely treated their patients with 100 mg of hydrocortisone for 4 days, whereas the U.S. group did not augment the dose of steroids. Neither group reported complications attributable to hypoadrenalism, and only one patient in the combined series who already had severely compromised renal function showed any further deterioration. Although the U.K. group reported a 0% mortality rate, 20 patients died in the U.S. group, at an average of 2 months (range, 1 day to 1 year) following surgery. Most of the deaths related to sepsis, and urologic surgery tended to carry the poorest prognosis.

Treatment

Although many patients with successful transplants have "normal" levels of creatinine, it is unusual for the creatinine clearance to exceed 70 mL/min. Therefore, all precautions outlined in the treatment section of patients with chronic renal insufficiency should be observed. Tailoring drug dosages and maintaining adequate volume are particularly important. Antibiotics should be used only when specifically indicated based on Gram stain or culture results. Indwelling lines should be changed frequently, or removed if possible, and additional steroid may be required at the time of surgery to prevent the manifestations of adrenal insufficiency.

Fluid, Electrolyte, and Acid-Base Disturbances in Preoperative and Postoperative Patients

Fluid, electrolyte, and acid-base disturbances in surgical patients have several unique features compared with those seen in their medically treated counterparts. First, disturbances of body composition tend to be more complex and severe, largely resulting from the nature of the surgical disorders and their therapies (109). For example, burns, major trauma, and gastrointestinal disorders such as intestinal obstruction result in fluid, electrolyte, and acid-base problems that may be further complicated by use of potent diuretics, nasogastric suction, or bowel diversion. In addition, the postoperative state itself has the potential to induce changes in body fluid composition or renal function (110).

The second important consideration is the effect of body fluid disturbances on the proposed anesthesia and surgery. Since fluid and electrolyte disturbances often alter a patient's cardiovascular and neuromuscular function, they also increase the risk of intraoperative hypotension and life-threatening arrhythmias as well as increase the need for postoperative ventilatory assistance. Table 12.18 summarizes the clinical significance of fluid and electrolyte abnormalities in surgical patients, and it provides recommendations for their treatment with specific reference to preoperative patients.

Hyponatremia

Epidemiology

Hyponatremia is among the most commonly encountered electrolyte disturbances in surgical patients. The pathophysiology is relatively uncomplicated. It must either develop from an intake of water exceeding the ability of the kidney to excrete it or from the loss of salt from the body. Salt loss may lead to volume depletion, which stimulates thirst, ADH secretion, and increased proximal sodium reabsorption that in turn result in increased water intake and retention. Thus, as Figure 12.2 shows, water retention is usually the final common pathway leading to the development of hyponatremia, and it therefore follows that hypoosmolality, under most circumstances, does not occur without water intake. The water intake that results in hyponatremia is often low in absolute terms but is excessive relative to the volume of free water that can be excreted. Hidden sources of water in surgical patients include the increased water of oxidation in catabolic patients, dextrose and water used as a vehicle for drug administration (50–100 mL per dose), heparinized solutions used to maintain the patency of arterial lines and Swan-Ganz catheters, and decreased insensible water losses through the lungs in patients receiving mechanical ventilation.

Hyponatremia almost always occurs secondary to a physiologically induced impairment of renal dilution rather than as a primary disturbance in ADH secretion. Most conditions producing a low serum sodium level are associated with a low serum osmolality as well, and hypoosmolality results in the intracellular movement of water and cellular edema, which is responsible for the clinical manifestations of hyponatremia. Hyponatremia may occasionally be associated with a normal or an increased effective serum osmolality, and it is commonly referred to as "pseudohyponatremia." Pseudohyponatremia may be associated with either no fluid shifts (e.g., hyperproteinemia, hyperlipidemia) or intracellular dehydration (e.g., hyperglycemia, mannitol administration).

Effective serum osmolality may be calculated as follows:

Table 12.18.   Preoperative Disorders of Fluid, Electrolyte, and Acid-Base Balance and Their Management

Conditions	Clinical Significance	Recommendation
I. Volume disorders		
A. Hypovolemia	Predisposes to hypotension, renal failure	Restore volume to normal
B. Hypervolemia	Predisposes to intraoperative pulmonary edema with hypoxemia and acidosis	Restore volume to normal
II. Electrolyte disorders		
A. Sodium	Often associated with abnormalities of intravascular volume	Assess volume status and restore to normal
		Serum sodium concentration should be between 134–145 mEq/L prior to elective surgery, but may be between 130–150 mEq/L for emergency surgery
1. Hyponatremia	Produces cellular edema	Avoid hypotonic fluid administration
	Often associated with dilution or volume depletion	
2. Hypernatremia	Most have both water and salt depletion	Correct both water and salt depletion
B. Potassium	Associated with arrhythmias, muscle weakness, and ileus	Serum potassium should be between 3.5–5.0 mEq/L before elective surgery and 3.0–5.5 mEq/L for emergency surgery
1. Hypokalemia	Causes arrhythmias, potentiates digitalis toxicity	Oral replacement preferred
2. Hyperkalemia	Succinylcholine may further aggravate hyperkalemia in burn or trauma patients	Maintain ventilation intraopertively
		Monitor electrolytes and EKG
	Acidosis and transfusions may result in worsening of hyperkalemia	See text for discussion of management
C. Calcium		
1. Hypocalcemia	Produces tetany, seizures, and change in mental status	Postpone surgery if serum calcium is less than 7.5 mg/dl, even if patient is asymptomatic
	Rapid correction of acidosis may precipitate tetany	
	Potentiates neuromuscular effects of hyperkalemia	
2. Hypercalcemia	Frequently associated with volume depletion	May operate in asymptomatic patients with mild hypercalcemia (less than 12 mg/dl) if volume depletion and immobilization avoided
	Potentiates digitalis toxicity	
	Predisposes to pancreatitis, renal failure, nephrolithiasis, arrhythmia, and changes in mental status	Postpone surgery with calcium greater than 12 mg/dl

$$\text{Effective serum osmolality} = 2\,(Na^+) + glucose/18 + mannitol/18$$

The BUN is excluded from this calculation, because it does not cause osmotically induced water redistribution. The normal range for effective osmolality is between 280 and 290 mOsm per kg of H_2O. Serum osmolality may also be measured directly by freezing-point depression.

Serum osmolality is chiefly regulated by the hypothalamic-pituitary axis

Table 12.18. *(continued)*   **Preoperative Disorders of Fluid, Electrolyte, and Acid-Base Balance and Their Management**

Conditions	Clinical Significance	Recommendation
D. Phosphorus		
1. Hypophosphatemia	When severe (less than 1 mg/dl), may lead to respiratory failure, seizures, coma, cadiomyopathy, and increased affinity of hemoglobin for oxygen	Serum phosphorus of less than 1.5 mg/dl should be corrected preoperatively
2. Hyperphophatemia	Clinical manifestations secondary to hypocalcemia or mestastatic calcification	Not an indication by itself to postpone surgery
E. Magnesium		
1. Hypomagnesemia	Hypokalemia and hypocalcemia frequently coexist Potentiates digitalis toxicity Causes arrhythmia, seizures	Postpone surgery if serum magnesium less than 1 mEq/L
2. Hypermagnesemia	Causes depressed mental status, respiratory muscle paralysis, conduction disturbances	Postpone surgery if level exceeds 5 mEq/L
III. Acid-base disorders		
A. Metabolic acidosis	Severe acidosis results in decreased cardiac output, unresponsiveness to catecholamines, arrhythmias Reduced buffering capacity results in diminished ability to buffer further acid challenges Failure to maintain compensatory hyperventilation under anesthesia results in worsening acidosis, hyperkalemia, and arrhythmias Often associated with volume depletion	Correct acidosis if pH is less than 7.25 or bicarbonate is less than 16 mEq/L preoperatively Maintain appropriate degree of hyperventilation intraoperatively Correct volume abnormalities Follow serum potassium closely
B. Metabolic alkalosis	Frequently associated with volume depletion and hypokalemia May contribute to arrhythmias, shift of hemoglobin dissociation curve to left Hyperventilation causes severe alkalemia, arrhythmias, seizures Compensatory hypoventilation may interfere with weaning postoperative patients from mechanical ventilators	Correct volume depletion with normal saline Correct coexisting hypokalemia Avoid hyperventilation intraoperatively
C. Respiratory acidosis	Risk factor for postoperative respiratory failure Predisposes to hyperkalemia	Delay elective surgery until underlying cause corrected
D. Respiratory alkalosis	Results in lowered serum bicarbonate and diminishes body capacity to buffer acid challenge Associated with hypokalemia	Search for underlying cause

through the action of ADH on the kidney and by the control of thirst. The body defends itself against hypoosmolality by inhibiting thirst and ADH secretion, thereby decreasing water intake and producing dilute urine. For clinical purposes, maximally dilute urine has an osmolality of less than 100 mOsm per kg of H_2O. The expression "free-water clearance" represents the quantity of solute-free water

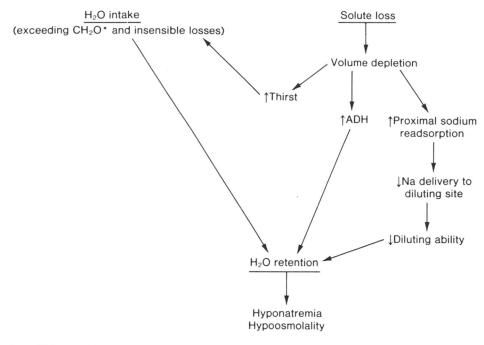

Figure 12.2. Pathophysiology of hyponatremia. C_{H_2O}, free-water clearance.

that is excreted during the process of urinary dilution.

Secretion of ADH is normally determined by changes in the serum osmolality, but several other important stimuli also affect its release. Chief among these nonosmotic stimuli is a perceived decrease in the circulatory volume, such as occurs with hemorrhage, isotonic fluid losses, congestive heart failure, or other edematous states. When hypovolemia is severe, the volume stimulus will predominate, resulting in persistent secretion of ADH despite a low serum osmolality. In additional, increased proximal sodium reabsorption because of volume depletion with decreased sodium delivery to the diluting sites impairs a patient's urinary dilution and also contributes to water retention. Emotion, pain, certain drugs (e.g., morphine, barbiturates, anesthetics), and the patient's metabolic response to surgery further enhance the stimulus of ADH secretion in the postoperative patient.

Hyponatremia can generally be maintained only if there is a defect in free-

Table 12.19.   Factors Diminishing Free H_2O Excretion

I. Decreased generation of free water at diluting site
   A. Decreased Na^+ and H_2O delivery to diluting site
      1. Renal failure ($\downarrow$ GFR)
      2. Effective volume depletion
   B. Decreased Na^+ and Cl^- reabsorption at diluting site
      1. Diuretics
II. Enhanced H_2O permeability of collecting ducts
   A. Presence of ADH
   B. Cortisol deficiency (primary or secondary)

water excretion, because the normal kidney can excrete 15 to 20 L of solute-free water per day. Free-water clearance is diminished by those conditions that lead to either decreased generation of free water at the diluting site in the ascending limb of Henle or to the enhanced permeability to water of the collecting ducts, as summarized in Table 12.19. Persistent secretion of ADH in response to nonosmotic stimuli is the most common cause for the diminished free-water clearance in patients with hyponatremia.

Administration of hypotonic fluids in the presence of nonosmotic-stimulated secretion of ADH is responsible for the hyponatremia that commonly occurs in postoperative patients. Chung et al. (111) prospectively studied 1088 operative procedures and found a 4.4% incidence of postoperative hyponatremia. Euvolemic hyponatremia was the most common cause of postoperative hyponatremia (42% of cases); edematous states (21%), hyperglycemia (21%), hypovolemia (8%), and renal failure (8%) accounted for the remainder. Postoperative hyponatremia was generally mild (P_{Na}, >125 mEq/L) and developed in the first 24 hours. Normovolemic hyponatremia usually resolved by the end of the first week, whereas patients with edema tended to remain hyponatremic for a longer period of time. Hyponatremia did not affect surgical mortality, but it may occasionally be associated with convulsions, respiratory arrest, and permanent brain damage after elective surgery (112). Most patients with this syndrome were females with the postoperative syndrome of inappropriate secretion of ADH (SIADH) who received excessive hypotonic fluids without frequent monitoring of electrolyte levels. Overall, the mortality rate of hospitalized patients who develop hyponatremia appears to be more closely associated with the underlying pathology than with the electrolyte disturbance per se (113).

Signs and Symptoms

The symptoms of hyponatremia are nonspecific and generally involve the CNS (e.g., disorientation, anorexia, nausea) or musculoskeletal system (e.g., cramps). Many patients remain asymptomatic. Physical findings are also nonspecific and may involve temperature regulation (e.g., hypothermia) or neurologic function (e.g., altered mental status, seizures, pathologic reflexes, Cheyne-Stokes respiration, pseudobulbar palsy, and, rarely, focal defi-

cits). The severity of neurologic symptoms depends on the absolute level of serum sodium as well as on the rate of change. Signs and symptoms are usually mild or absent when the serum sodium concentration is greater than 120 mEq/L, variably present between 110 and 120 mEq/L, and usually severe when less than 110 mEq/L. An acute fall in the serum sodium level produces more severe symptoms than occur with a gradual decline for any given serum sodium. A truly asymptomatic patient with very low serum sodium concentrations should indicate the possibility of pseudohyponatremia.

Diagnosis

Diagnosing the cause of hyponatremia is best approached by clinical assessment of the intravascular volume status, as previously described (114). Recall that the serum sodium concentration does not correlate with the total body sodium stores or with the volume of the intravascular or extracellular spaces. The patient history should be reviewed for any sources of solute or water loss or gain, intravenous therapy, and medications. Laboratory determinations of serum sodium, potassium, chloride, bicarbonate, urea nitrogen, creatinine, glucose, uric acid, osmolality, and the urinary sodium, creatinine (U_{Cr}), and osmolality (U_{Osm}) should be obtained before therapy is initiated. Once pseudohyponatremia has been excluded, correct determination of the volume status based on the complete clinical picture will limit the diagnostic considerations in each category, as listed in Table 12.20. When there is doubt regarding whether the patient is hypovolemic or euvolemic, a cautious fluid challenge with normal saline will usually clarify the situation. The approach to hyponatremia is summarized in Figure 12.3.

In surgical patients, certain electrolyte patterns will help to pinpoint the cause of hyponatremia. When metabolic acidosis is associated with a normal or low serum potassium levels, diarrhea or fistula drainage may be the source of electrolyte

Table 12.20.   Differential Diagnosis of Hyponatremia

I. Pseudohyponatremia
  A. Isotonic
    1. Hyperproteinemia
      a. Multiple myeloma
      b. Macroglobulinemia
    2. Hyperlipidemia
  B. Hypertonic
    1. Hyperglycemia
    2. Mannitol
    3. Glycerol
II. Hypovolemic hyponatremia
  A. Renal loss
    1. Diuretics[a]
    2. Adrenal insufficiency
    3. Salt-losing renal disease (medullary cystic disease, postobstructive diuresis, diuretic phase ATN)
    4. RTA with bicarbonaturia
  B. Extrarenal
    1. GI loss (vomiting, diarrhea) with hypotonic replacement[a]
    2. Third space (pancreatitis, burns, muscle trauma)[a]
    3. Skin (excess sweating with hypotonic replacement)
III. Euvolemic hyponatremia
  A. SIADH
  B. Psychogenic polydipsia
  C. Hypothyroidism
  D. Glucocorticoid deficiency
  E. Reset osmostat
  F. Drugs (thiazides, chlorpropamide, morphine, barbiturates, antipsychotics, acetaminophen, isoproteronol, indomethacin, cyclophosphamide)[a]
  G. Pain[a]
  H. Emotion
  I. Salt loss with hypotonic replacement resulting in euvolemia[a]
IV. Hypervolemic hyponatremia (edema)
  A. CHF[a]
  B. Cirrhosis[a]
  C. Nephrotic syndrome
  D. Renal failure[a]

[a]Common in surgical patients.

loss. A high bicarbonate level resulting from metabolic alkalosis and associated with a normal or low serum potassium level should indicate nasogastric suction or use of diuretics. A BUN less than 10 mg/dL is so infrequent in adults without liver disease or starvation that, when present in a patient with hyponatremia, it should indicate SIADH. The combination of hyponatremia and hypouricemia should also indicate SIADH, but psychogenic polydipsia or liver disease may also result from this combination. Extracellular volume depletion, on the other hand, can result in increased urate reabsorption and hyperuricemia. Determining the urinary sodium concentration (U_{na}) or FE_{Na} is useful in supplementing the clinical determination of intravascular volume, because the urinary sodium concentration is mainly determined by the effective circulating volume. Diagnostic use of urinary sodium is valid if renal tubular function is normal. Volume depletion with a low urinary sodium concentration suggests an extrarenal cause of hypovolemia, and a high urinary sodium concentration in a volume-depleted patient suggests renal salt loss as a cause. The urinary sodium concentration in patients with hyponatremia and who are euvolemic is variable and dependent on dietary salt intake. The urinary osmolality is only moderately helpful in the diagnosis of hyponatremia, because renal free-water excretion is impaired in most hyponatremic conditions. This diminished free-water excretion is associated with impairment in the ability of the kidneys to maximally dilute the urine (U_{Osm}, <100 mOsm per kg of H_2O). Urinary osmolality in most hyponatremic disorders will be hypertonic to plasma but may be isotonic or mildly hypotonic (U_{Osm}, 150–250 mOsm to kg of H_2O) and does not necessarily imply the presence of SIADH. Patients with psychogenic polydipsia or essential hyponatremia are the major exceptions, in which the urinary osmolality may be maximally dilute despite hyponatremia.

The syndrome of inappropriate ADH has five principle features: *(a)* hyponatremia with hypoosmolality; *(b)* urinary sodium concentration greater than 20 mEq/L; *(c)* absence of clinical evidence of volume depletion; *(d)* urinary osmolality less than maximally dilute; and *(e)* normal cardiac, renal, adrenal, and thyroid func-

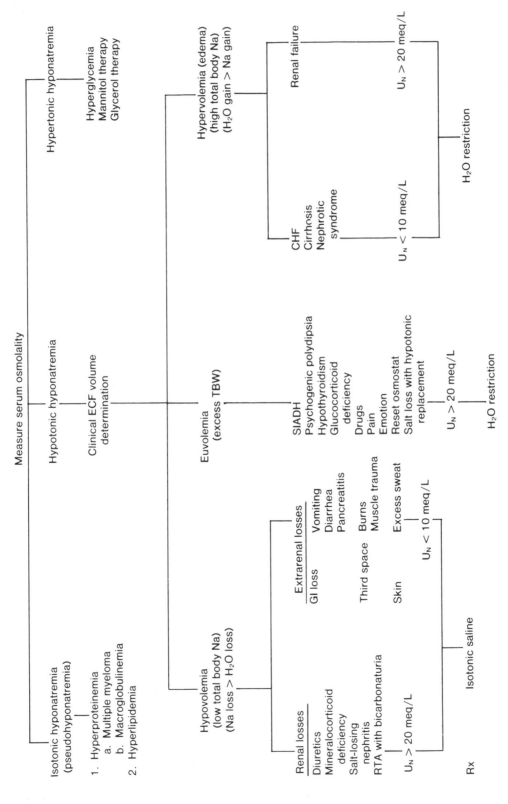

Figure 12.3.   Clinical approach to hyponatremia. *CHF*, congestive heart failure; *ECF*, extracellular fluid; *GI*, gastrointestinal; *RTA*, renal tubular acidosis; *TBW*, total body water.

tion. A water-load test (20 mL/kg given over 15–20 min) is not needed if all cardinal features are present. A normal person will excrete 80% or more of the ingested water within 4 hours and lower his or her urinary osmolality to less than 100 mOsm per kg of H_2O.

Patients with edema usually do not have serum sodium concentrations less than 125 mEq/L until end-stage hepatic or cardiac dysfunction occurs. Serum sodium values below this level in less severe disease may result from superimposed problems such as use of diuretics, vomiting, or compulsive drinking of water.

Treatment

Treatment of hyponatremia depends on the underlying cause, the level and duration of the disorder, and the presence or absence of symptoms. The study by Arieff et al. (115) reported a 50% mortality rate in acute hyponatremia of less than 12 hours, with only a 12% mortality rate in patients with chronic symptoms. No death in the chronic symptomatic group directly related to hyponatremia per se, and chronic asymptomatic hyponatremia was associated with a 0% mortality rate.

Treatment begins with correct assessment of the patient's volume status. The goal of therapy is to correct both the hyponatremia and any underlying causes.

Hypovolemic hyponatremia is treated with normal saline. In this situation, correction of the hyponatremia results from sodium retention and increased free-water excretion caused by decreased ADH secretion secondary to volume repletion.

Hyponatremia in patients with edema and congestive heart failure, cirrhosis, or nephrotic syndrome is treated with sodium and water restriction. Loop diuretics may sometimes be useful because of their ability to decrease urine-concentrating ability, thus resulting in increased free-water clearance.

Hyponatremia in euvolemic patients is treated with water restriction and the correction of underlying causes (e.g., hy-

pothyroidism, glucocorticoid deficiency, drugs, pain, conditions associated with SIADH). Patients with severe (serum sodium level, <110–115 mEq/L) or symptomatic (e.g., seizures, coma) hyponatremia should be treated with hypertonic saline and furosemide. The rationale behind use of hypertonic saline plus furosemide is to quantitatively replace diuretic-induced electrolyte losses (Na^+, K^+), which results in the net excretion of free water. Urinary and serum electrolyte levels should be monitored frequently (every 2 hours initially) to ensure proper corrections and prevent hypokalemia. Treatment is most safely performed in an ICU. The volume of excess free water that needs to be excreted to correct hyponatremia in a patient with SIADH is calculated as follows:

$$H_2O \text{ excess} = 0.6 \times \text{body weight [kg]} \times [1 - (P_{Na} \text{ actual}/140)]$$

The appropriate rate of correction depends on the patient's clinical condition, and the recommended rate for asymptomatic hyponatremia is slower than that for symptomatic hyponatremia. Current recommendations stem from a concern about the development of osmotic demyelination if the serum sodium level is corrected too rapidly. Clinical manifestations of this condition usually appear 2 to 6 days after correction of the hyponatremia, and they consist of paraparesis or quadraparesis, dysarthria, dysphagia, and altered mental state. Seizures are possible but less common. Characteristic demyelinating lesions can be seen on CT or magnetic resonance imaging but may take up to 4 weeks to be detectable. With symptomatic hyponatremia, which is most likely to develop in postoperative, premenopausal females receiving hypotonic fluids, or acute thiazide–induced hyponatremia, more aggressive therapy is indicated, because the risk of cerebral edema from persistent hyponatremia exceeds the risk of osmotic demyelination.

At present, correcting asymptomatic hyponatremia at a maximum rate of 0.5

mEq/L per hour appears to be prudent (116, 117). It is important to note that the total increase in serum sodium concentration should be less than 10 to 12 mEq/L in the first 24 hours, and less than 18 mEq/L over the first 48 hours, to minimize the risk of osmotic demyelination. Results of animal studies suggest that it is the daily rather than the hourly rate of correction that is the primary determinant of whether osmotic demyelination develops. More aggressive therapy is warranted in patients with symptomatic hyponatremia, who typically develop hyponatremia over 24 to 72 hours and present with neurologic abnormalities, including seizures resulting from cerebral edema. In this situation, the serum sodium concentration should be raised initally by 1.5 to 2.0 mEq/L per hour for the first 3 to 4 hours, or possible longer if the patient remains symptomatic. Even so, the total increase in serum sodium concentration should not exceed 12 mEq/L per hour in the first 24 hours (similar to that in asymptomatic hyponatremia). This can be followed by water restriction to allow evaporative and urinary losses to restore the sodium level to normal over the ensuing days.

Post-TURP Syndrome

Hyponatremia may also occur following transurethral resection of the prostate (post-TURP syndrome). It results from the systemic absorption of irrigating solution that has directly entered prostatic veins or has leaked into the retroperitoneal space through the perforated prostatic capsule. These irrigating solutions typically contain glycine, sorbitol, or mannitol. One prospective study involving 100 patients reported a 7% incidence of hyponatremia and one death (118). Measured osmolality, although variable, will usually be normal or modestly reduced because of the retained organic solute, so the diagnosis of post-TURP syndrome should be suspected on clinical grounds. Other supporting evidence includes an elevated osmolality gap, which is the difference between the measured and the calculated serum osmolality. Normally, this gap is between 5 and 10 but can exceed 30 to 60 mOsm per kg of H_2O. Hyperammonemia can also occur because of the accumulation of ammonia from glycine metabolism. A similar syndrome is being increasingly recognized with use of glycine-irrigant solutions during hysteroscopic endometrial ablation in women (119).

Asymptomatic patients with normal renal function require no treatment and will correct spontaneously by the movement of glycine and water into cells, renal excretion of excess fluid, and both metabolism and excretion of the excess solute. In symptomatic patients, however, the best therapy is less clear. Hypertonic saline may help if hypoosmolality exists. Hemodialysis may help to correct the hyponatremia and to remove both glycine and its toxic metabolites in patients with severe renal failure who cannot excrete the excess water and solute (120), and it may also help in patients with a relatively normal plasma osmolality and severe symptomatic hyponatremia (121).

Hypernatremia

Physiology

The incidence of hypernatremia in hospitalized patients is approximately 1%, and in one series, 20% of the cases were observed in the surgical setting, often in association with hypertonic intravenous fluids or hyperalimentation (122). Although the mortality rate in this group is increased by several times that of the general patient population, this is thought to be related to the underlying disease processes rather than to the hypernatremia itself. Hypernatremia most often develops as a result of excess water (i.e., hypotonic fluid) losses or inadequate water replacement of normal losses; only rarely does it develop primarily as a result of the gain of excess sodium. Excess water may be lost through the kidneys, gastrointestinal tract, or as insensible losses through the skin and lungs. The presence of a tracheostomy promotes pulmonary water loss of up to 1.0 to 1.5 L/day if continuous humidification is not used. Fever and burns also result in increased insensible water loss.

Most patients with hypernatremia have a combined water-and-sodium loss, with the loss of water exceeding that of sodium. The greater the degree of sodium loss, the more likely signs of volume depletion will be encountered. Such losses occur with an osmotic diuresis from glucose, mannitol, or urea, and a high-protein intake from tube feedings may result in an osmotic diuresis from urea production. In addition, excess sweating may result in hypotonic fluid losses. Loss of gastrointestinal secretions results in isotonic volume depletion, and hypernatremia results only if the water intake is less than normal. Iatrogenic hypernatremia associated with sodium depletion may occur in patients receiving diuretics if the water intake is inadequate.

Pure water loss from central or nephrogenic diabetes insipidus is not common in the general surgical setting. Approximately 50% of central diabetes insipidus cases are idiopathic, and the remainder result mostly from head trauma, hypoxic encephalopathy, hypophysectomy, and neoplasms. Acquired nephrogenic diabetes insipidus may occur with electrolyte abnormalities (e.g., hypercalcemia, hypokalemia) and with interstitial forms of renal disease. Certain drugs (e.g., lithium carbonate, demeclocycline, enthrane, methoxyflurane, amphotericin) may also produce nephrogenic diabetes insipidus.

Hypernatremia resulting from sodium excess is encountered much less frequently. The most common cause is the administration of sodium bicarbonate during cardiac arrests or during therapy for severe metabolic acidosis.

Hypernatremia is most likely to occur when the patient's access to water is limited. Commonly, this will occur in hospitalized patients who are debilitated or confined to bed by intravenous lines, catheters, or casts. In a series of patients who developed hypernatremia while hospitalized (123), most had a concentrating defect resulting from use of diuretics or an osmolar diuresis. Most also had increased insensible water losses or increased enteral water losses, and many had restricted access to water or inadequate intravenous replacement.

Hypernatremia is always associated with hyperosmolality and intracellular volume depletion. Intravascular volume, however, may be either high, low, or even normal. The degree of cellular shrinkage depends on the degree of hypernatremia as well as on the rate of its development. In chronic hypernatremic states, intracellular water loss is minimized by the creation of "idiogenic" osmoles, which tend to restore intracellular volume.

Signs and Symptoms

Hypernatremia is often asymptomatic, and it may be first detected with routine electrolyte studies. When present, symptoms result from intracellular dehydration and include thirst, muscle weakness, and neurologic symptoms such as lethargy, stupor, coma, and seizures. Symptoms relate both to the level and rate of change in the serum sodium concentration. Experimental studies in rabbits showed that neurologic symptoms developed when the plasma osmolality exceeded 350 mOsm per kg of H_2O. Signs of intravascular volume depletion resulting from pure water loss are not common unless the serum sodium concentration is greater than 170 mEq/L, because the intravascular volume sustains only 5 to 8% of any pure water loss. Combined water-and-salt losses will manifest themselves by hypotension at lower serum sodium levels.

Diagnosis

The diagnostic approach to hypernatremia is based on determination and interpretation of the urinary osmolality, as outlined in Figure 12.4. When the serum sodium concentration is increased (serum

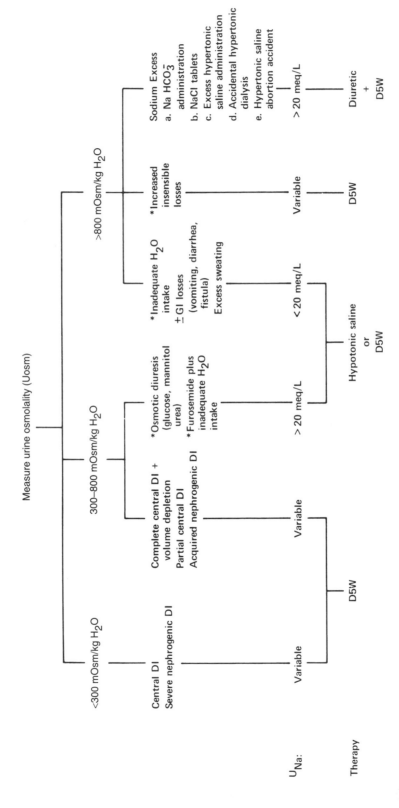

Figure 12.4. Clinical approach to hypernatremia. *DI*, diabetes insipidus; *GI*, gastrointestinal. *Common in surgical patients..

osmolality, >290 mOsm per kg of H_2O), the normal renal response should be a urinary osmolality of greater than 800 mOsm per kg of H_2O. A urinary osmolality less than this in a patient with hypernatremia represents a defect in ADH release or effect. Hypernatremia with a urinary osmolality greater than 800 mOsm per kg of H_2O suggests that sodium excess, increased insensible losses, or inadequate free-water intake is responsible for the hyperosmolar state.

Patients with central diabetes insipidus or severe nephrogenic diabetes insipidus usually have a urinary osmolality of less than 300 mOsm per kg of H_2O. When the urinary osmolality is between 300 and 800 mOsm per kg of H_2O, the most likely causes of hypernatremia are partial central diabetes insipidus, complete central diabetes insipidus with volume depletion, acquired nephrogenic diabetes insipidus, and osmotic diuresis. Osmotic diuresis can be verified through a timed urine collection with an osmolar excretion rate of greater than 60 mOsm/hr. When considering the diagnosis of diabetes insipidus, water restriction in conjunction with pitressin administration (i.e., water-deprivation test) will help to establish whether the defect is central or renal in origin. Water-deprivation tests should be delayed until after electrolyte abnormalities have been corrected and the patient is clinically stable.

Occasionally, osmotic diuresis may result in a urinary osmolality greater than 800 mOsm per kg of H_2O. Despite the urine having a high osmolality, an osmotic diuresis is characterized by a high urine output. Measuring the urinary glucose, urea, mannitol, or sodium concentration will determine which osmole is responsible for the process.

Treatment

Despite a high serum sodium concentration, patients with severe hypovolemia and hypernatremia should initially be treated with normal saline if they are hemodynamically unstable. This is followed by hypotonic saline or 5% dextrose in water (D5W). Hypernatremia resulting from pure water loss is treated with D5W, and hypernatremia associated with sodium excess is treated with diuretics and D5W. The free-water deficit should be estimated in all patients with the following equation:

$$H_2O \text{ deficit} = 0.6 \times \text{body weight [kg]} \times [1 - (140/\text{actual serum Na})]$$

While the optimal correction rate for hypernatremia has not been firmly established, overly rapid correction can lead to complications. These are more likely to occur after cerebral adaptation has restored the cell volume to normal (1–3 days). Rapid lowering of the serum sodium concentration after this period can result in cerebral edema, seizures, and permanent brain damage. Most reports on complications from the treatment of hypernatremia have involved children (124), but it is reasonable to extrapolate these results to adults. Therefore, the rate of correction in chronic hypernatremia should be limited to 0.5 mEq/L per hour. The total time to safely correct hypernatremia is given by the following equation:

$$\text{Correction time [hr]} = (\text{actual plasma sodium} - 140)/0.5$$

The rate of free-water administration, assuming a correction of 0.5 mEq/L per hour, is calculated by dividing the estimated water deficit by the correction time. It needs to be remembered, however, that the calculated water deficit estimates the net positive water balance that needs to be achieved to correct the hypernatremia. Thus, maintenance fluids and replacement of ongoing, abnormal losses must also be admistered simultaneously. It is also important that the calculated water deficit does not include any isosmotic fluid deficits that may additionally be present when sodium and water have been lost isosmotically, as with diarrhea. Initially, the plasma sodium concentration should be determined every 2 to 4 hours depending on the patient's symptoms. Acute symptomatic hypernatremia occurring less than 24 hours before cerebral cellular volume adaptation has occurred can probably be corrected more rapidly in relative safety. In this situation, the correction rate for the first 4 to 6 hours may be as high as 1 to 2 mEq/L per hour before eventually slowing to 0.5 mEq/L per hour.

Patients with complete central diabetes insipidus will also require ADH to be administered (see the section on endocrine disorders). Thiazide diuretics may be useful in chronically reducing the urine output of patients with nephrogenic diabetes insipidus by contracting the extracellular fluid volume.

Hypokalemia

Epidemiology

Among disorders of potassium balance in surgical patients with normal renal function, hypokalemia is seen more frequently than hyperkalemia. The most common conditions predisposing to hypokalemia in these patients include vomiting, nasogastric suction, inadequate potassium intake, and use of polystyrene sulfonate (Kayexalate), diuretics, and insulin.

Physiology

Potassium homeostasis represents a balance between intake, excretion (renal excretion accounts for 90% of potassium elimination from the body), and transcellular shifts. By itself, decreased intake is rarely the sole cause of potassium depletion, but it often contributes to the magnitude of the deficit. Tissue injury, acidosis, and catabolism result in the cellular release of potassium that may subsequently be excreted in the urine, and substantial amounts of potassium may be lost in the stool, with or without diarrhea.

Transcellular shifts affect potassium concentration but not the total body content. Alkalosis results in potassium movement into cells and acidosis in movement out of cells. Insulin, and possibly aldosterone, also cause potassium to shift into cells.

When hypokalemia results from extrarenal losses within 4 to 10 days, the renal excretion of potassium falls to less than 20 mEq/day, and the spot urinary potassium concentration should be less than 10 to 15 mEq/L. Renal potassium wasting (24-hour excretion, >20–30 mEq) occurs more often as a response to physiologic stimuli (e.g., alkalosis, hyperaldosteronism) or diuretic use than from primary kidney disease. Hypomagnesemia results in increased potassium excretion by an unknown mechanism, and it should be suspected in surgical patients with hypokalemia who are receiving gentamicin, hyperalimentation, or in those suffering from malabsorption.

Hypokalemia results in an increased resting cellular transmembrane potential (i.e., hyperpolarization) and decreased membrane excitability. This accounts for the clinical manifestations, which include muscle weakness and cardiac arrhythmias. The effect of any given decrease on the serum potassium level is augmented by the rapidity of the fall, hypercalcemia, and alkalosis.

It should be noted that the serum potassium and electrocardiographic findings correlate only roughly with the total body stores. A deficit of approximately 100 to 200 mEq will lower the serum potassium concentration from 4 to 3 mEq/L, and every fall of 1 mEq/L thereafter reflects another 200- to 400-mEq deficit. Continued loss in excess of 400 mEq produces relatively small changes in the serum potassium concentration because of the transcellular shift out of cells. Arterial pH and the resultant transcellular potassium shift must also be considered when estimating the deficit. Failure to estimate the true size of the deficit frequently leads to underreplacement and apparent "refractory" hypokalemia.

Signs and Symptoms

Signs and symptoms of hypokalemia may begin to appear when the serum potassium level is less than 3 mEq/L, but they do not occur with frequency until levels fall below 2.7 mEq/L. Symptomatic hypokalemia usually represents a total body deficit of at least 200 to 400 mEq. Skeletal muscle findings include cramps, tetany, weakness, and paralysis; muscle weakness usually affects the lower extremities first and then the trunk, upper extremities, and respiratory muscles. Rhabdomyolysis and myoglobinuria may rarely occur. Smooth muscle dysfunction results in paralytic ileus and symptoms of abdominal distention (e.g., nausea, vomiting, constipation). Chronic potassium depletion may result in hypotension, and renal abnormalities resulting from potassium depletion include: *(a)* decreased GFR, *(b)* nephrogenic diabetes insipidus, *(c)* increased ammonia production by renal tubules, *(d)* impaired urinary acidification, and *(e)* increased bicarbonate reabsorption. Encephalopathy may be precipitated by hypokalemia in patients with cirrhosis. ECG changes occurring with hypokalemia include flattened or inverted T waves, prominent U waves, and S-T changes.

Diagnosis

Table 12.21 lists the causes of hypokalemia. Often, the cause is obvious from the patient history. Important historical points include loss of gastrointestinal fluid (e.g., vomiting, diarrhea, fistula, nasogastric suction), drugs, and potassium intake (both oral and intravenous). The physical examination should emphasize clinical determination of the intravascular volume and blood pressure. If the diagnosis is not obvious after a careful patient history and physical examination, measurement of simultaneous serum and urinary potassium, serum sodium, bicarbonate, and creatinine levels, as well as of the arterial pH, is usually helpful. The approach to hypokalemia (Fig. 12.5) involves separat-

ing gastrointestinal from renal potassium losses. Measurement of arterial pH is helpful, because these losses are frequently associated with metabolic alkalosis or acidosis. Measurement of urinary chloride concentration (U_{Cl}) and urinary pH may also be useful in the evaluation of coexisting metabolic alkalosis or renal tubular acidosis (RTA), respectively.

Measurement of urinary potassium excretion helps to differentiate renal from gastrointestinal losses. However, diuretic therapy may confuse the interpretation of urinary potassium concentration regarding the site of potassium loss. Patients with diuretic-induced potassium deficiency will have a higher urinary potassium concentration while the diuretic agent is still acting, but they will have a low concentration once the diuretic effect has worn off. Since sodium depletion may limit urinary potassium excretion, a sodium intake (i.e., excretion) of 100 to 150 mEq/day is required to properly interpret urinary potassium concentrations; otherwise, a low urinary potassium concentration may be interpreted incorrectly as indicating extrarenal losses. Proper interpretation depends on correlating the urinary potassium concentration with 24-hour sodium excretion. Thus, hypokalemia with a low urinary potassium concentration (<10–15 mEq/L) suggests that: *(a)* the potassium deficiency most likely has been present for more than a few days, *(b)* the extrarenal potassium loss most likely is occurring from the gastrointestinal tract providing no diuretic agent has been administered recently, or *(c)* sodium depletion is limiting potassium excretion. Similarly, hypokalemia with a high urinary potassium concentration (>10–15 mEq/L) suggests renal potassium loss or that the potassium deficit has been present for less than 1 week.

Treatment

Potassium chloride is the usual preparation used to correct potassium deficits. The chloride is essential for any coexist-

Table 12.21.   Etiology of Hypokalemia

I. Decreased intake (oral, intravenous), prolonged administration of K$^+$-free fluids[a]

II. Transcellular shift into cells
    A. Alkalosis[a]
    B. Hypersecretion of insulin (hyperalimentation)[a]
    C. Treatment of megaloblastic anemia
    D. Hypokalemic periodic paralysis

III. Increased loss
    A. Renal
        1. Associated metabolic alkalosis
            a. Hyperaldosteronism
                (1) Primary
                (2) Secondary (renin mediated)
                    (a) Edematous states (CHF, cirrhosis, nephrotic syndrome)
                    (b) Non-edematous states (Bartter's syndrome, accelerated hypertension, renal vascular hypertension, renin-secreting tumor)
            b. Cushing's syndrome
                (1) Primary adrenal disease
                (2) Secondary to non-endocrine tumor
            c. Drugs
                (1) Diuretics (loop diuretics, thiazides)[a]
                (2) Antibiotics (penicillin, carbenicillin)
                (3) Licorice ingestion
                (4) Alkali loading
        2. Associated with metabolic acidosis
            a. Renal tubular acidosis
            b. Diabetic ketoacidosis
            c. Drugs (amphotericin B, outdated tetracyclines, acetazolamide)
        3. Normal acid-base status
            a. Osmotic diuretics (mannitol, glucose)
            b. Hypomagnesemia
            c. Gentamicin
            d. ? Acute myeloid leukemia
            e. Renal salt wasting
    B. Gastrointestinal losses
        1. Vomiting[a]
        2. Diarrhea[a]
        3. Villous adenoma
        4. Intestinal fistula or tube drainage[a]
        5. Laxative abuse
        6. Ureterosigmoidostomy
        7. Obstructed or long ileal loop[a]
    C. Skin (excess sweat)

[a]Common in surgical patients.

ing, chloride-sensitive metabolic alkalosis. Beside repairing the deficit, treatment of the underlying disorder should be initiated whenever possible to prevent further losses. Oral treatment is preferred in mild to moderate hypokalemia, with 80 to 120 mEq/day (20 mEq of K$^+$ = 15 mL of 10% KCl) administered in divided doses along with an addition amount to replace abnormal, ongoing losses. Intravenous therapy is indicated when a patient cannot take oral medications or severe hypokalemia is associated with serious arrhythmias (especially during therapy with digoxin), muscle weakness, respiratory paralysis, rhabdomyolysis, or diabetic ketoacidosis. It is best to keep intravenous replacement to less than 100 to 150 mEq/

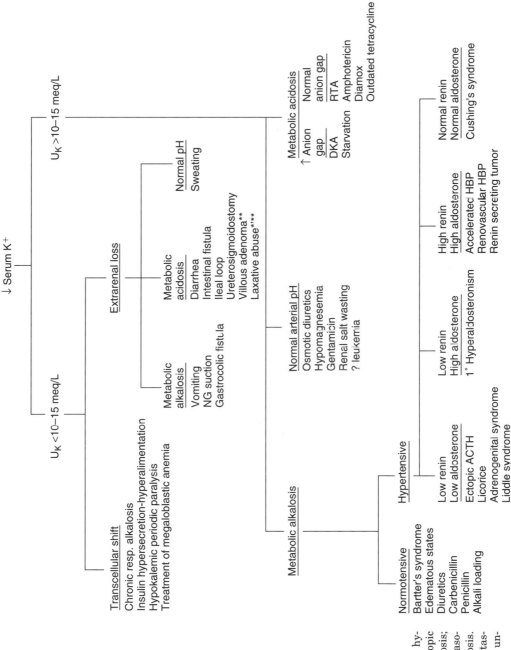

Figure 12.5. Clinical approach to hypokalemia. *ACTH*, adrenocorticotropic hormone; *DKA*, diabetic keotacidosis; *HBP*, high blood pressure; *NG*, nasogastric; *RTA*, renal tubular acidosis. *May have increased urinary potassium. **Actual acid-base status is unpredictable.

day (or 10 mEq/hr) unless life-threatening depletion is present or ongoing losses require larger amounts.

Concentrated potassium solutions are best administered through a large vein (e.g., the femoral vein). Although central veins are commonly used, such practice carries the danger of transiently high local serum potassium concentrations, leading to possible arrhythmias or cardiac arrest. Potassium solutions containing 200 mEq/L (20 mEq in 100 mL of isotonic saline) have been safely used to rapidly correct severe hypokalemia in patients manifesting life-threatening arrhythmias or paralysis (125). Up to 10 mEq of potassium may be administered intravenously per hour without monitoring; higher levels require continuous ECG monitoring and frequent determinations of the serum level. More than 20 mEq of potassium per hour intravenously is not recommended. The most difficult clinical situation is patients with RTA or urinary diversion procedures into the colon in which severe hypokalemia is associated with acidosis. In these patients, correction of the acidosis by vigorous bicarbonate therapy without potassium replacement results in life-threatening hypokalemia and respiratory paralysis. Therapy in these patients should include simultaneous administration of intravenous potassium and sodium bicarbonate.

Special Considerations

Hypokalemic metabolic alkalosis from vomiting or nasogastric suction commonly occurs in the surgical setting, and renal losses represent the major mechanism of potassium depletion in this situation. Factors contributing to kaliuresis include alkalosis, increased aldosterone secretion secondary to volume depletion, and increased nonreabsorbable anion (HCO_3^-) delivery to the distal tubule. Loss of potassium contained in gastric secretions (10 mEq/L) plays a minor role in the size of the deficit. When the total potassium deficit approaches 20% ($\approx$ 700 mEq), hy-

drogen ion is preferentially secreted despite alkalosis resulting in aciduria. Aciduria in a patient with metabolic alkalosis suggests severe potassium depletion.

Hyperkalemia

Epidemiology

Hyperkalemia in surgical patients occurs most commonly during ARF. It is similar to that occurring in medical patients except for two important considerations. First, hyperkalemia may be more difficult to control in catabolic, postoperative patients because of the increased endogenous potassium load originating from tissue breakdown, acidosis, resorption of blood from the gastrointestinal tract or hematomas, and multiple transfusions of stored whole blood. Second, use of potassium-exchange resins may not be possible in patients who have undergone bowel surgery. Even if sodium polystyrene sulfonate can be used, surgical patients appear to have an increased risk for intestinal necrosis (126). When this complication develops, the patient typically has severe abdominal pain, and surgery is frequently necessary. Two risk factors for intestinal necrosis have been identified: inceased duration of exchange-resin contact with the intestinal mucosa because of decreased colonic motility secondary to postoperative ileus, administration of narcotics, or both; and use of sorbitol, which may directly exacerbate the colonic inflammation. Shepard (127) has suggested that use of a cleansing enema after sodium polystyrene sulfonate enemas may prevent prolonged exchange-resin retention in the intestinal lumen.

Physiology

Renal potassium excretion represents the body's major defense against hyperkalemia; cellular uptake is of lesser importance. Sustained hyperkalemia rarely develops simply from increased intake, whether exogenous or endogenous, in patients with normal renal function, although abrupt increases in potassium intake through intravenous administration may lead to transient, potentially serious hyperkalemia. Impaired renal potassium excretion is essentially the only cause of chronic hyperkalemia.

Life-threatening hyperkalemia may develop within hours of the onset of acute oliguric renal failure in patients following surgery, with trauma, or with sepsis. Hyperkalemia in acute oliguric renal failure without these complications usually develops more slowly, however, appearing 4 to 5 days after onset. In noncatabolic, anephric patients, the serum potassium concentration should not increase by more than 0.5 mEq/L per day. Hyperkalemia may not develop in ARF if urine output is maintained.

Patients with chronic renal insufficiency in whom the serum creatinine level is less than 10 mg/dL or the GFR greater than 5 to 10 mL/min generally develop hyperkalemia only during excessive potassium intake (e.g., potassium-rich foods, salt substitutes), acidosis, volume depletion, or use of drugs that interfere with potassium excretion. These drugs include potassium-sparing diuretics, ACE inhibitors, heparin, or high-dose trimethoprim.

Signs and Symptoms

The signs and symptoms of hyperkalemia are mainly limited to muscle weakness and abnormalities of cardiac conduction. Paresthesia in the arms and legs is usually the first complaint. Muscle weakness may be seen with serum potassium concentrations greater than 8 mEq/L, beginning in the lower extremities and ascending to the muscles of the trunk and the upper extremities. Flaccid paralysis and respiratory arrest may occur.

In general, ECG findings parallel the severity of the hyperkalemia; however, cardiotoxic effects can occur without premonitory clinical signs. The cardiotoxic effects of hyperkalemia are enhanced by the presence of hypocalcemia, hyponatremia, acidosis, and a rapid rise in the levels

of potassium. Acute elevations will produce more marked effects at relatively lower serum potassium levels.

Diagnosis

The differential diagnosis of hyperkalemia is listed in Table 12.22, and the

Table 12.22.   Etiology of Hyperkalemia

I. Factitious
 A. Lab error[a]
 B. Pseudohyperkalemia: *in vitro* hemolysis, improper collection of blood, thrombocytosis, leukocytosis
II. Increased input[a]
 A. Exogenous (oral or IV): KCl, salt substitutes, K$^+$-containing medications, transfusions of old blood[a]
 B. Endogenous: hemolysis, GI bleeding, rhabdomyolysis[a]
III. Transcellular shift out of cells
 A. Acute acidosis[a]
 B. Drugs: succinylcholine, massive digoxin overdose, arginine HCl
 C. Insulin deficiency
 D. Cellular catabolism: trauma, burns, rhabdomyolysis[a]
 E. Hyperkalemic periodic paralysis
 F. Hyperosmolality (hyperosmotic mannitol or saline infusions)
IV. Decreased renal excretion
 A. Renal failure[a]
  1. Acute
  2. Chronic (GFR < 10 ml/min)
 B. Primary tubular defect in K$^+$ excretion (SLE, sickle cell disease, postrenal transplantation, amyloidosis)
 C. Impaired renin-angiotensin axis
  1. Primary hypoaldosteronism
  2. Addison's disease
  3. Primary hyporeninism
  4. Tubular unresponsiveness to aldosterone
  5. ACE inhibitors
 D. Volume depletion (inadequate Na delivery to distal tubule)[a]
 E. Drugs inhibiting

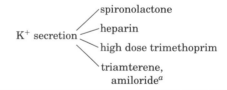

aCommon in surgical patients.

suggested clinical approach is outlined in Figure 12.6. The patient history should be reviewed for: (a) evidence of renal disease or diabetes mellitus, (b) endogenous or exogenous sources of potassium, and (c) drugs that interfere with potassium excretion or cause transcellular shifts of potassium out of cells. The physical examination emphasizes the determining the intravascular volume, searching for the stigmata of Addison's disease, and testing muscle strength. Laboratory determination of sodium, bicarbonate, and creatinine level as well as the arterial pH should be obtained.

If an unexpected elevation in the potassium level is found, a repeat sample should be immediately sent to rule out laboratory error and ECG performed. A false elevation in the serum potassium level may be seen with a hemolyzed blood specimen or when potassium is released from clotted blood that has a very high white-blood-cell count (>100,000/mL) or platelet count (>1,000,000/mL). These latter two, rare conditions can be excluded by checking the potassium concentration in heparinized blood; the difference in potassium concentrations between plasma and serum samples should be less than 0.5 mEq/L. Prolonged use of a tourniquet may also falsely elevate the serum potassium level. A potassium level of 7 mEq/L or greater with a normal ECG should indicate pseudohyperkalemia.

After eliminating these causes of false hyperkalemia, an arterial blood gas should be obtained to evaluate the contribution of acute metabolic or respiratory acidosis to the elevated potassium. Acute acidosis is associated with hyperkalemia.

The list of patient medications should be checked for potassium-containing drugs. In addition to the usual potassium supplements, drugs such as salt substitutes and phosphate supplements also contain large amounts of potassium. Diuretics with potassium-sparing effects should be sought as well, and ACE inhibitors can produce hyperkalemia by inhibiting the production of angiotensin. Impaired renal function should be sought next. Hyperkalemia out of proportion to the degree of renal dysfunction should suggest mineralocorticoid deficiency. Hyporeninemic-hypoaldosteronism occurs more often than Addison's disease and is commonly found in patients with diabetes or tubulointerstitial renal disease. Hyperchloremic metabolic acidosis may also be present in such patients, and this entity can be screened for by measuring stimulated plasma renin activity, aldosterone, and morning plasma cortisol levels.

Treatment

The aim of treatment is to correct both the hyperkalemia and its underlying cause. Significant ECG changes resulting from hyperkalemia indicate the need for immediate therapy, because the development of fatal cardiac toxicity is often unpredictable. The type of therapy depends on the absolute level of the serum potassium concentration, how rapidly it is rising, whether the source of potassium can be removed, and, most important, the type of ECG changes that are present and the patient's renal function.

In general, a serum potassium concentration between 5.5 and 6.5 mEq/L with only T-wave changes may be treated by potassium restriction and potassium exchange resins (Kayexalate). In postoperative patients, who are often catabolic, volume-depleted, hemorrhaging, or receiving blood transfusions, therapy may be started even sooner. Under these circumstances, treatment with these measures may begin if the potassium concentration is rising and reaches 5 mEq/L.

When the serum potassium concentration is between 6.5 and 7.0 mEq/L, treatment measures that shift potassium into cells should be initiated. Infusions of glucose and insulin will start to have an effect in 10 to 30 minutes, whereas administered sodium bicarbonate will have an onset of action in less than 1 hour. Sodium bicarbonate will be effective independent

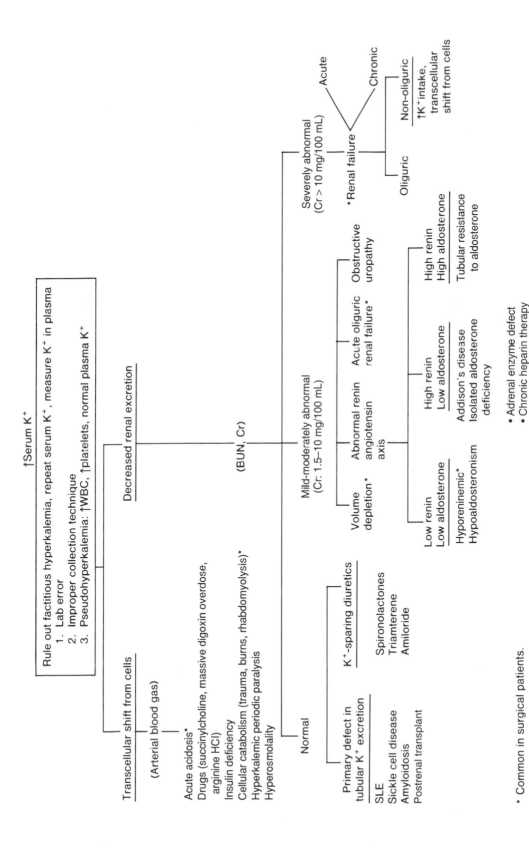

Figure 12.6.   Clinical approach to hyperkalemia. *SLE,* systemic lupus erythematosus; *WBC,* white blood cell.

Table 12.23.   **Treatment of Hyperkalemia**

Mechanism	Administration	Onset	Duration	Comments
I. Antagonism of cardiotoxic effects				
A. Calcium gluconate (10%)	1 amp (10 cc) IV over 2–3 min—may repeat q 5 min × 2 if EKG changes persistent or infusion: 2–3 amps in 1 L D5W	1–5 min	30 min	Contraindicated in patient on digoxin
B. Hypertonic saline (5%)	250 ml IV over 30–60 min	1 hr	1–2 hr	May cause volume overload
II. Enhanced K$^+$ entry into cells				
A. Glucose and insulin	500 ml D10W over 30 min plus 10 units regular insulin IV or 50 cc of D50 over 5–30 min plus insulin	30–60 min	2–4 hr	Use 1 unit reg. insulin per 5 gm glucose Use D50 when renal failure and volume overload a problem
B. Na HCO$_3$ (44.5 meq)	1 amp IV over 5 min may repeat q 5–10 min × 2 or 2 amps + 1000 cc D10 + 10 unit insulin infuses over 1–2 hr	30–60 min	1–2 hr	Especially useful when acidosis is present; subsequent doses determined by cause and severity of metabolic acidosis; can produce volume overload
C. Albuterol	20 mg inhaled over 10 min or 0.5 mg IV in 100 ml D5W over 15 min	30–60 min	2 hours	Shown to be useful in hemodialysis patients
III. K$^+$ removal from body				
A. K$^+$ exchange resins (sodium polystyrene sulfonate)	po: 20–50-gm resin + 20 cc 70% sorbitol may repeat q 4 hr for total 4–5 doses enema: 50–100 gm resin + 50 cc 70% sorbitol in 150–200 cc H$_2$O repeat enema q 2–4 hr as required	1–2 hr	4–6 hr	Sorbitol required to prevent constipation; enema must be retained for 30–60 min to be effective; each enema may decrease serum K$^+$ by 0.5–1 meq/L; side effects: Na$^+$ retention, nausea, constipation
B. Dialysis	Peritoneal dialysis; hemodialysis	Minutes after starting	Few hours after terminating dialysis	Useful for catabolic surgical/trauma patient when G.I. tract cannot be used to accept resins Hemo can remove more K$^+$ than peritoneal; 25–50 mEq K$^+$/hr *vs.* 10–15 mEq K$^+$/hr

of its effect on blood pH. Nebulized al-buterol, 20 mg inhaled over 10 minutes (or 0.5 mg intravenously over 15 min), reduces serum potassium levels in patients on hemodialysis within 30 minutes and has a duration of action of up to 2 hours (128).

Serum potassium concentrations greater than 7.0 mEq/L and ECG changes showing a loss of P waves or widening of the QRS complex requires immediate aggressive intervention. Calcium should be given intravenously and is immediately effective in reversing the electrophysiologic effects of hyperkalemia. Calcium administration should be immediately followed by infusions of glucose, insulin, and sodium bicarbonate.

No treatment that shifts potassium into cells reduces the total body potassium level; therefore, an attempt at removing potassium from the body should be initiated as soon as possible. Such removal can be achieved by using sodium exchange resins (Kayexalate) or dialysis. Loop diuretics generally have little value, particularly if renal function is impaired. Dialysis is rarely needed for the correction of hyperkalemia alone1, and it is typically used in patients with severely impaired renal function when volume overload and acidosis coexist. Peritoneal dialysis may not be efficient for potassium removal in severely catabolic patients; hemodialysis, which is much more effective, must then be used. Table 12.23 summarizes the various treatments of hyperkalemia.

Use of succinylcholine should be avoided in the presence of extensive third-degree burns, massive soft tissue injury, or certain neurologic diseases. These patients are exceptionally sensitive to the hyperkalemic effects of this drug.

Hypercalcemia

Epidemiology

Hypercalcemia occurs most frequently in surgical patients being prepared for parathyroidectomy or in patients with malignancy. Hypercalcemia can be wors-ened by immobilization and volume depletion, both of which are common in surgical patients.

Physiology

Calcium in the extracellular fluid is found in three forms: *(a)* ionized, ~50%; *(b)* protein bound, ~40%; and *(c)* nonionized and ultrafiltrable, ~10%. Only the ionized form is biologically active. Albumin is the major serum protein-binding calcium, and the total serum calcium level parallels the serum albumin level. For each change of 1 g per 100 mL in the serum albumin, there is a change of roughly 0.8 mg per 100 mL in the protein-bound calcium in the same direction.

Proper technique for drawing blood is important when measuring the serum calcium level. A tourniquet left on for 2 to 3 minutes may increase the total calcium level by 0.5 to 1.5 mg per 100 mL. This results from protein-free fluid leaving the capillaries, producing local hyperalbuminemia and increased total serum calcium.

Calcium excretion by the kidney on a normal intake averages between 250 and 300 mg per 24 hours. Calcium absorption parallels sodium reabsorption in the proximal tubule and loop of Henle, but not in the distal tubule. This is important clinically, because the conditions that promote renal sodium reabsorption (i.e., volume depletion) will also promote calcium reabsorption. Similarly, volume expansion will result in an increased renal excretion of both calcium and sodium. Both PTH and vitamin D result in decreased renal calcium excretion. Hypercalcemia related to malignancy can result from increased bone resorption, with subsequent release of calcium from bone, or from increased intestinal absorption of calcium. This can occur by three major mechanisms: *(a)* osteolytic metastases with release of local cytokines (e.g., tumor necrosis factor, interlukin-1, lymphotoxin), *(b)* production of PTH-related protein (PTHrP), or *(c)* production of calcitriol by the tumor.

Signs and Symptoms

The signs and symptoms of hypercalce-mia depend on the rapidity of onset, the prior general condition of the patient, and the underlying disease (e.g., renal CNS). Table 12.24 summarizes the various signs and symptoms.

Diagnosis

The differential diagnosis of hypercal-cemia is listed in Table 12.25. Malignancy (e.g., lung, breast, myeloma) and primary hyperparathyroidism account for most cases. Hypercalcemia of malignancy is generally more severe and its onset more rapid than primary hyperparathyroidism. Chronic hypercalcemia of several years' duration, without the appearance of new signs or symptoms, is more likely to result from primary hyperparathyroidism than from occult malignancy. Primary hyper-parathyroidism may coexist with malig-nancy, however, so the presence of a known malignancy during hypercalcemia does not necessarily imply a causal rela-

Table 12.25.   Differential Diagnosis of Hypercalcemia

I. Lab error[a]
II. Malignancy[a]
III. Primary hyperparathyroidism[a]
   A. Isolated
   B. Part of MEA syndrome
IV. Granulomatous disease
   A. Sarcoidosis
   B. Tuberculosis
V. Ingestions
   A. Milk alkali syndrome
   B. Thiazide diuretics
   C. Vitamins D, A
   D. Calcium supplements
   E. Ca^{2+}-containing antacids (Tums)
   F. Tamoxifen, estrogen, androgen (breast carcinoma)
   G. Lithium
VI. Hyperthyroidism
VII. Renal failure (acute, with rhabdomyolysis, chronic "tertiary" hyperparathyroidism)
VIII. Postrenal transplant
IX. Immobilization[a]
X. Adrenal insufficiency
XI. Hyperglobulinemia (normally ionized Ca^{2+})

[a]Common in surgical patients.

Table 12.24.   Signs and Symptoms of Hypercalcemia

A. General: somnolence, lethargy, weakness
B. Gastrointestinal: anorexia, nausea, vomiting, constipation, abdominal pain, peptic ulcer, pancreatitis
C. Renal: polydipsia, polyuria, nephrolithiasis, nephrocalcinosis, renal failure
D. Neurological: stupor, coma, psychotic behavior, visual abnormalities, hyporeflexia, myopathy, occasionally localizing signs, modest increase in CSF protein
E. Cardiac: shortened QT interval, loss of ST segment, and widening of T wave leads to prolonged QT interval with "cove-like" appearance, bradycardia, tachycardia, digitalis sensitivity, arrhythmias, hypertension
F. Skeletal: pain, fractures, skeletal deformities, loss of height
G. Miscellaneous: volume depletion, calcinosis, band keratopathy
H. Signs and symptoms of associated endocrinopa-thies: Zollinger-Ellison syndrome, pheochromo-cytoma, medullary cardinoma of thyroid, pituitary and adrenal tumors

tionship. Immobilization should be consid-ered as a cause in bedridden patients with a high rate of bone turnover (e.g., children, adolescents, those with Paget's disease).

The diagnostic approach to hypercalce-mia has changed over the last several years following the development of reli-able radioimmunoassays for PTH. Mea-surement of a patient's level of intact PTH has a 90 to 95% accuracy for hyper-parathyroidism. However, even in hyper-parathyroidism caused by hyperplasia or adenoma, secretion of PTH is not com-pletely autonomous and can be partially suppressed by elevations in the serum calcium levels. Hence, a normal level of PTH in a patient with hypercalcemia can still be considered as "inappropriate" and consistent with the diagnosis of hyper-parathyroidism. PTHrP is a 141–amino acid peptide that is immunologically dis-tinct from PTH; however, PTHrP can bind to the PTH receptor and thus mimic the action of PTH on bone resorption, stimulate distal renal calcium absorption, and inhibit proximal renal phosphate reabsorption. PTHrP is the most common cause of hypercalcemia in the setting of nonmetastatic solid tumors. Use of an assay measuring the amino terminal of PTHrP is preferred over the carboxy terminal assay in renal failure, because the carboxy assay can give elevated results because of reduced renal excretion and may not represent overproduction. Several studies have demonstrated a higher incidence of malignancy in patients with primary hyperparathyroidism and of primary hyperparathyroidism in patients with cancer (129, 130). If a patient with hypercalcemia and a solid tumor has elevated PTH and PTHrP levels, then coexisting primary hyperparathyroidism is probably also present (131).

Measurement of vitamin D metabolites can be useful when neither the PTH or the PTHrP level is elevated and there is no evidence of malignancy. Table 12.26 summarizes the use of these metabolites to diagnose disorders of calcium metabolism. Low levels of PTH and vitamin D metabolites, along with the absence of malignancy and elevated PTHrP, should indicate an unsuspected cause of increased bone resorption, such as thyrotoxicosis, immobilization, Paget's disease, or even milk-alkali syndrome. Milk-alkali syndrome occurs more commonly today because of the frequent use of calcium

carbonate to treat dyspepsia, osteoporosis, and to control hyperphosphatemia in patients with chronic renal failure. One recent study (132) showed that milk-alkali syndrome accounted for 12% of hypercalcemia cases in a hospitalized patient population.

The serum phosphate concentration may also sometimes be useful in suggesting a possible cause for hypercalcemia. Both hyperparathyroidism and humoral hypercalcemia of malignancy (PTHrP mediated) often present with hypophosphatemia. However, the plasma phosphate concentration is usually normal or elevated in vitamin D intoxication, granulomatous diseases, immobilization, thyrotoxicosis, metastatic bone disease, and milk-alkali syndrome. A suggested approach to the evaluation of patients with hypercalcemia is outlined in Table 12.27.

Treatment

Therapy for hypercalcemia involves general supportive measures, treatment of the hypercalcemia itself, and treatment of the underlying disorder. Serum calcium levels of 13 mg/dL or greater usually require immediate reduction, even without symptoms, to prevent soft-tissue calcification, renal failure, and disturbances of CNS function. Moderate hypercalcemia (serum calcium level, 11–13 mg/dL) without symptoms does not require immediate

Table 12.26.   Use of Serum Levels of Vitamin D Metabolites in Diagnosis of Disorders of Calcium Metabolism

	25 (OH) Vit D_3 (Calcidiol)	1.25 (OH) Vit D_3 (Calcitriol)
low	vit. D deficiency intestinal malabsorption nephrotic syndrome liver disease anticonvulsant therapy	reduced cholecalciferol intake or absorption renal failure hypoparathyroidism
high	cholecalciferol ingestion 25 (OH) cholecalciferol ingestion	calcitriol ingestion granulomatous diseases lymphoma primary hyperparathyroidism

Table 12.27.   Evaluation of Hypercalcemia

I. Initial evaluation
   A. History: ingestions (thiazides, vitamins D, A, Ca^{2+} supplements, Ca^{2+}-containing antacids (Tums), associated endocrinopathies, family history of hyperparathyroidism, childhood irradiation of head and neck, chronic hypercalcemia
   B. Physical exam: volume status, thyroid, evidence of malignancy, stigmata of Addison's disease, or hyperthyroidism
   C. Lab
      1. Blood
         a. Na^+, K^+, Cl^-, HCO_3^-
            1. Hypernatremia may be present in nephrogenic DI secondary to increased Ca^{2+}
            2. K^+ (Mg^{+2}) may be decreased in hypercalcemia of any cause
            3. HCO_3^- may be low in primary hyperparathyroidism secondary to renal HCO_3 loss; may be increased in cancer-related hypercalcemia not mediated by PTH; ? mechanism
         b. BUN/Cr: almost all hypercalcemic patients are volume-depleted; hypercalcemia may cause renal damage
         c. $CA^{2+}X2$: repeat to rule out lab error
         d. $PO_4^{-2}X2$
            1. May be low in primary hyperparathyroidism or humeral hypercalcemia of malignancy (PTHrP mediated)
            2. Suspect coexisting primary hyperparathyroidism when low in breast carcinoma
         e. Alkaline phosphatase
            1) May be hepatic or bone origin
            2) Elevated alkaline phosphatase from bone without evidence of osteitis fibrosa on x-rays of bone makes primary hyperparathyroidism less likely
         f. Albumin/globulin
            1) Required to properly interpret serum Ca^{2+}
            2) Initial step in detection of dysproteinemia
         g. Serum protein electrophoresis/immunoelectrophoresis
            1) Monoclonal spike of myeloma
            2) Diffuse hyperglobulinemia of sarcoid
            3) Increased $alpha_2$-, $beta_2$-globulins in hyperparathyroidism
         h. Intact PTH (RIA)
            1) Intact PTH assay is best assay in differential diagnosis of hypercalcemia when primary hyperparathyroidism is a consideration
            2) Increased PTH related protein (PTH_rP)-seen in 88% of solid tumors with hypercalcemia.
            3) Low or undetectable with hypercalcemia unrelated to PTH excess
         i. Vitamin D metabolites
            1) 25 (OH) Vit D_3-increased with ingestion of cholecalciferol and 25 (OH) cholecalciferol
            2) 1,25 (OH) Vit D_3-increased with calcitriol ingestion, granulomatous disease, lymphomas, primary hyperparathyroidism
         j. Angiotensin converting enzyme-increased in sarcoidosis
      2. Urine
         a. Urinalysis
            1) Hematuria may suggest hypernephroma, renal calculi
         b. 24-hr urinary Ca^{2+}
            1) Probably not required initially if no history of renal calculi
            2) Will be low in volume-depleted patients or patients with impaired renal function
            3) Disorders associated with hypercalcemia and relative hypocalciuria (Ca^{+2} excretion <100 mg/day)
               a) Milk alkali syndrome
               b) Thiazide diuretics
               c) Familial hypocalciuric hypercalcemia
         c. Urine protein electrophoresis/immunoelectrophoresis
            1) Monoclonal spike of myeloma

Table 12.27. *(continued)*   Evaluation of Hypercalcemia

3. X-rays
   a. Chest x-rays: may detect bronchogenic carcinoma, lymphoma, sarcoidosis, resorption of acro-
      mioclavicular joints (primary hyperparathyroidism)
   b. Flat plate of abdomen: nephrocalcinosis rare in cancer hypercalcemia and suggests primary
      hyperparathyroidism
   c. Skull: punched out lesions of myeloma, "salt and pepper" appearance of primary hyperpara-
      thyroidism
   d. Hands: subperiosteal reabsorption of primary hyperparathyroidism
   e. X-rays of abnormal areas on bone scan or symptomatic areas
4. Bone scan: looking for metastatic disease
5. ECG: look for changes due to hypercalcemia
II. Second order of evaluations
   A. Blood
      1. Thyroid function tests—hyperthyroidism
   B. X-rays
      1. IVP: hypernephroma
      2. No need to do GI series in absence of iron deficiency anemia, positive stools for occult blood or
         symptoms pointing to GI tract, since gastrointestinal malignancies are an uncommon cause of
         hypercalcemia
      3. CT of abdomen
   C. Biopsy
      1. Bone marrow aspirate and biopsy: myeloma, lymphoma, granuloma, metastatic tumor
      2. Abnormal tissue, including bone

reduction, and the aim in these patients is usually to lower the serum calcium level in 12 to 24 hours. The presence of coexisting hyperphosphatemia probably warrants prompt treatment at even lower elevations of serum calcium.

Hydration with normal saline (lactated Ringer's solution contains calcium) is the most important initial step in treating patients with hypercalcemia. Most patients are already volume-depleted secondary to vomiting, decreased intake, hypercalcemia-induced nephrogenic diabetes insipidus, and sodium diuresis. Only after the patient is well hydrated and an adequate urine output achieved should furosemide be given for its calciuretic effect. It is crucial to maintain intravascular volume by continuing infusions of normal saline up to 4 L/day for this method to work, because hypovolemia increases calcium absorption in the proximal tubule and decreases calcium excretion. Furosemide should be given intravenously in a dose of 40 to 80 mg and repeated as needed to maintain the urine output between 200 and 500 mL/h. Potassium and magnesium need to be replaced, because deficits of these electrolytes are commonly present in patients of hypercalcemia from any cause in addition to ongoing urinary losses resulting from the vigorous diuresis. Frequent monitoring (every 2 to 4 hours) of serum and urinary electrolyte levels will help to guide sodium, potassium, and magnesium replacement therapy. A CVP (central venous line) or a Swan-Ganz catheter is indicated in most of these patients to guide fluid therapy. Forced diuresis will not be successful in patients with significant intrinsic renal impairment.

Glucocorticoids may be effective in hypercalcemia secondary to myeloma, adrenal insufficiency, vitamin D intoxication, sarcoidosis, some malignancies (i.e., breast, lymphoma, myeloma), or tuberculosis. However, its onset of action is delayed by approximatly 48 to 96 hours. Calcitonin is particularly useful in treating hypercalcemia associated with Paget's disease, but patient tolerance may develop after hours or days. It is also less effective than mithramycin or phosphate in malignancy. Even so, because it is such a safe drug, little is lost by using it early, in addition to forced diuresis, in the treatment of severe hypercalcemia.

Biphosphonates inhibit the rate of bone resorption and appear to be one of the least toxic and most reliable forms of therapy for hypercalcemia. Pamidronate can be given as a single-dose (60 or 90 mg) infusion over 24 hours and repeated weekly if the response is inadequate (133).

Another agent that inhibits bone resorption is gallium nitrate, which is given at 200 mg/m^2 of body surface area in 1 L of normal saline given over 24 hours for 5 days. Because of potential nephrotoxicity, however, patients should be well hydrated, have frequent monitoring of renal function, and have their infusions stopped if the serum creatinine level exceeds 2.5 mg/dL.

Mithramycin, which acts by inhibiting the RNA synthesis that is necessary for PTH-induced bone resorption, may be given if significant hypercalcemia remains after hydration and other forms of therapy. The usual dose is 15 to 25 μg given over 4 to 6 hours, but side effects such as nephrotoxicity and hepatotoxicity limit the usefulness of this agent.

Intravenous phosphate should probably be reserved for situations in which other methods either fail or are contraindicated, because it may lead to soft-tissue calcification. However, in severe symptomatic hypercalcemia that does not respond to the measures described here, intravenous phosphate will predictably decrease the serum calcium level within minutes. The maximum decline may be delayed for as long as 5 days, however, and some hypocalcemic effect may persist for 5 to 15 days. It is not necessary to repeat the dose of phosphate within 24 hours, and generally no more than two doses is required. The serum calcium level should have reached its nadir and begun to rise before repeating the second dose. Significant hyperphosphatemia

(5–6 mg per 100 mL) contraindicates phosphate therapy, as does a rising creatinine level or oliguria. Complications (e.g., hypotension, hypocalcemia, ARF) from intravenous phosphate therapy have occurred with large doses given rapidly (100 mmol over 3–4 hours). Using a smaller dose over a longer period of time (50 mmol over 6–8 hours) and carefully monitoring the serum calcium and phosphorus levels should avoid these complications.

Oral phosphorus (1–3 g/day) may be used to treat chronic hypercalcemia. The lowest effective dose should be used to keep the serum phosphorus level less than 5.5 mg/dL to minimize soft-tissue calcification. All oral preparations can cause diarrhea, but hypotension or hypocalcemia does not occur with this route of administration.

Hemodialysis may occasionally be useful when diuresis either is not possible or is ineffective in patients with renal failure (134). The hypocalcemic effect is likely to be transient, however, and may sometimes be followed by rebound hypercalcemia.

Indomethacin (75–150 mg/day) may also be used for the treatment of chronic hypercalcemia resulting from cancer. Its effect relates to prostaglandin inhibition.

Table 12.28 summarizes drugs that are useful in the treatment of hypercalcemia.

Hypocalcemia

Epidemiology

Most patients in critical care settings will have decreased levels of total serum calcium, but the frequency of clinically significant decrements in the ionized calcium level that require immediate intervention is relatively low (135). Patients with sepsis often develop multifactorial hypocalcemia, and subtotal gastrectomy and gastrojejunostomy may lead to vitamin D deficiency, hypocalcemia, and osteomalacia as well. In addition, acute hypocalcemia is seen in patients with hemorrhagic pancreatitis.

Table 12.28. **Drugs Useful in Treatment of Hypercalcemia**

Drug	Dose	Administration Frequency	Route	Onset Hypocalcemic Effect	Complications	Contraindications
Furosemide and saline	40–200 mg	1–2 hr	IV push	Immediate	Hypovolemia; hypokalemia; hypomagnesemia	Impaired renal function; digoxin intoxication
Mithramycin	25 μg/kg	24–48 hr	IV push	24–48 hr	Hemorrhage; hepatocellular necrosis; azotemia, proteinuria	Thrombocytopenia; severe renal dysfunction; severe hepatic dysfunction
Phosphate (50 mmol/L)	1.5 gm	24 hr	IV over 6–8 hr	24 hr	Hypotension; hypocalcemia; soft tissue calcification	Hyperphosphatemia with severe renal impairment
Calcitonin	4–8 MRC U/kg	12 hr	IM, subcut	2–3 hr	None serious	None except allergy
	8 MRC U/kg	6 hr	IM, subcut	2–3 hr		
Steroids (hydrocortisone)	100–150 mg	12 hr	IV	48–96 hr	Hypokalemia; Na retention	GI bleeding; glucose intolerance
Prednisone	40–60 mg	24 hr	P.O.	48–96 hr	Hypokalemia; Na retention	GI bleeding, glucose intolerance
Pamidronate	60–90 mg	weekly	IV	24 hr	Fever and local pain	None
Gallium nitrate	200 mg/m^2	24 hrs	IV	2–5 d	Nephrotoxicity	$S_{CR} > 2.5$ mg/dl

Massive and rapid transfusions of citrate-containing blood (5–10 U) may result in hypocalcemia from calcium binding by citrate. This is more likely to occur during liver disease, in which the metabolism of citrate is reduced. Patients who receive massive doses of heparin after cardiopulmonary bypass surgery can also develop hypocalcemia from chelation. Patients with diffuse small bowel disorders and malabsorption may develop hypocalcemia as well.

Hypocalcemia following thyroidectomy is uncommon, but it may result in this setting from the inadvertent removal of the parathyroid glands, infarction of the parathyroid glands because of interference with their blood supply, or increased skeletal calcium uptake. Hypocalcemia in this situation usually develops within 24 hours following the procedure. Transient hypocalcemia frequently occurs after the removal of parathyroid adenomas because of atrophy of the remaining glands. Severe and persistent hypocalcemia (i.e., "hungry" bone syndrome) can be seen in patients with chronic uremia who undergo subtotal parathyroidectomy.

Gentamicin and other aminoglycosides may result in hypocalcemia secondary to excessive urinary losses of magnesium. Hypomagnesemia (<0.8 mEq/L) produces hypocalcemia by interfering with the release of PTH and its action on bone. Table 12.29 summarizes the causes of hypocalcemia.

Table 12.29.   Etiology of Hypocalcemia

I. Hypoalbuminemia (normal ionized Ca^{2+})[a]
   A. Malnutrition
   B. Hepatic cirrhosis
   C. Nephrotic syndrome
II. Hyperphosphatemia
   A. Renal failure (acute and chronic)[a]
   B. Oral or intravenous phosphate infusions
   C. Phosphate-containing enemas
   D. During therapy of leukemia
III. Hypoparathyroidism
   A. Idiopathic
   B. Surgical[a]
IV. Pseudohypoparathyroidism
V. Vitamin D deficiency
   A. Nutritional deficiency[a]
   B. Malabsorption from small bowel disease
VI. Magnesium deficiency[a]
VII. Acute pancreatitis[a]
VIII. Massive transfusion of citrated blood[a]
IX. Drugs
   A. Anticonvulsants (hydantoin,
      phenobarbitol)
   B. Gentamicin $-2°$ to renal Mg^{2+} loss
   C. Mithramycin
   D. Neomycin
   E. Glucocorticoids
   F. Glucagon
X. Neoplastic disorders
   A. Osteoblastic metastasis (breast, prostate)
XI. Renal tubular acidosis
XII. Healing phase of metabolic bone disease

[a]Common in surgical patients.

Signs and Symptoms

The important signs and symptoms of hypocalcemia relate to the cardiovascular and the neuromuscular systems; they depend on the level of serum calcium, its rate of development, and its duration. Cardiovascular manifestations of hypocalcemia include prolonged Q-T interval, hypotension, and arrhythmias. Neurologic manifestations include tetany, confusion, stridor, as well as Chvostek's and Trousseau's signs. Other causes of tetany besides hypocalcemia are both metabolic and respiratory alkalosis, hypomagnesemia, and acute hyperkalemia.

Diagnosis

In critically ill patients, the total serum calcium level is often abnormal, but clinically significant changes in the ionized calcium level are much less common. For example, a low total serum calcium often occurs in patients with hypoalbuminemia resulting from catabolism and malnutrition that accompany the postoperative state, but the ionized calcium may be high, low, or even normal. Unfortunately, multiple factors can affect the amount of free calcium relative to total calcium, particularly in acutely ill patients, so there is no simple and reliable way to estimate the ionized calcium level, which therefore should be measured directly. In general, symptoms do not occur unless the ionized calcium level falls to less than 0.8 mmol/L.

The patient history should emphasize: *(a)* previous surgery (e.g., thyroidectomy, parathyroidectomy, gastric, small intestinal resection), *(b)* blood transfusions, *(c)* drugs (e.g., anticonvulsants, phosphates, mithramycin, aminoglycosides), *(d)* symptoms suggesting malabsorption, *(e)* alcoholism (i.e., magnesium deficiency), and *(f)* renal failure. Initial blood chemistries should include calcium (total and ionized), phosphate, magnesium, albumin, BUN, creatinine, and PTH levels as well as arterial blood gases. Metastatic prostate cancer, in association with osteoblastic metastasis, is the most common cancer to produce hypocalcemia. Calcification of the basal ganglia on skull radiographs may be depicted in patients with hypocalcemia and idiopathic hypoparathyroidism. ECG may show a prolonged Q-T interval resulting from lengthening of the S-T segment.

The presence of hyperphosphatemia suggests renal insufficiency, hypoparathyroidism, or phosphate administration as the cause of hypocalcemia. Normal or low serum phosphorus levels suggest vitamin D deficiency or malabsorption. The serum phosphorus level in magnesium deficiency is variable, but the serum PTH concentration will be low in hypocalcemia resulting from hypoparathyroidism and high in vitamin D deficiency, malabsorption, renal failure, or pseudohypoparathyroidism. The PTH concentration may be low, high, or even normal in hypocalcemia resulting from magnesium deficiency.

Treatment

Symptomatic or severe hypocalcemia (ionized calcium level, <0.7 mmol/L) should be treated with intravenous calcium gluconate. Use of calcium gluconate is preferred over calcium chloride, which contains four times as much elemental calcium, because it may be less irritating if the solution undergoes extravasation. Calcium gluconate should be diluted with at least an equal volume of dextrose or normal saline to reduce any irritation that might be associated with parenteral administration.

Usually, two to three ampules of 10% calcium gluconate (1 amp = 10 mL = 5 mEq) in 100 mL of D5W administered over a 15-minute period are sufficient to alleviate the effects of symptomatic hypocalcemia. This should be followed by an intravenous calcium drip that is prepared by putting four to 6 ampules of 10% calcium gluconate in 1000 mL of D5W and titrating the rate to maintain a serum calcium level between 8.0 and 8.5 mg per 100 ml. Oral calcium supplements should be started when the clinical signs and symptoms have improved. The rate of calcium gluconate administration should not exceed 2 mL/min (200 mg of calcium gluconate = 0.92 mEq of calcium); the maximum rate should probably be slower (0.5 mL/min) if the patient is receiving digoxin. The serum calcium concentration needs to be monitored closely, and a total calcium gluconate dose of 2 g should not be exceeded without repeating the serum calcium measurement. Patients with hypocalcemia and simultaneous hypomagnesemia (<1.0 mg/dL) should receive magnesium replacement therapy (discussed later).

Asymptomatic and chronic hypocalcemia can be treated with oral calcium salts, various forms of vitamin D, or both. Several vitamin D preparations are available and used mainly for the treatment of chronic hypocalcemia. Calcitriol is the synthetically produced, active form of vitamin D (1,25-dihydroxycholecalciferol), and it is available both as an oral and an intravenous preparation. Both forms can be used in dosages ranging from 0.25 to 2.00 μg/day. Magnesium-containing antacids should not be used concomitantly with calcitriol, howeer, because of the danger of developing hypermagnesemia.

Patients already receiving calcium supplements and vitamin D preparations may require surgery, and those with chronic renal failure constitute the majority of such patients who are encountered clinically. Current vitamin D preparations have relatively long durations of action and can be safely discontinued perioperatively until the patient is able to resume oral intake. The duration of action for some common vitamin D preparations after therapy has ceased are: (a) vitamin D_2 (ergocalciferol), 6 to 18 weeks; (b) dihydrotachysterol, 1 to 3 weeks; (c) 25-hydroxy-D_3, 4 to 12 weeks; and (d) 1,25-dihydroxy-D_3, 3 to 7 days. Calcitriol is available as an intravenous injection (Calcijex), and it may be useful perioperatively in surgical patients with advanced renal failure.

Patients with renal insufficiency can have calcium supplements safely withheld for several days perioperatively while the serum calcium concentration is monitored and the serum phosphorus controlled. If a patient's condition will preclude oral intake or nasogastric administration for long periods of time, calcium may be given intravenously. Intravenous maintenance therapy with 200 to 400 mg of elemental calcium administered continuously over 24 hours should be sufficient in most patients who are stable. The serum calcium level should be measured at least once per day initially and intravenous calcium administered if the level falls to between 8.0 to 8.5 mg/dL.

Patients with PTH or vitamin D deficiency should receive intravenous maintenance calcium therapy throughout the intraoperative and the postoperative periods until oral intake can be resumed. There is usually no need for routine calcium administration in postoperative patients unless a specific indication exists.

Hypomagnesemia

Epidemiology

Hypomagnesemia occurs in up to 12% of hospitalized patients (136) and in up to 60 to 65% of patients in ICUs (137, 138). Hypomagnesemia should be suspected in surgical patients with malabsorption, small-bowel disease or resection, prolonged nasogastric suction, diarrhea, hyperalimentation, prolonged use of aminoglycosides, hypocalcemia, refractory hypokalemia, refractory arrhythmias, unexplained digoxin toxicity, or a history of alcoholism. Magnesium deficiency should always be considered in postoperative surgical patients exhibiting neuromuscular or CNS hyperactivity, especially if they also have a history of alcoholism. This is particularly true if the patient has a nonfunctioning gastrointestinal tract and has been on prolonged therapy with parenteral fluids; magnesium replacement should be routine in these patients. Transient hypomagnesemia on the day after an operation may occur, apparently as part of the metabolic response to surgery, and it does not necessarily indicate magnesium deficiency.

Physiology

Magnesium is predominantly an intracellular cation that is involved in various membrane and enzymatic functions. The serum magnesium concentration (1.5–2.0 mEq/L) does not correlate well with the total body content of magnesium. In fact, magnesium deficiency may be present despite a normal serum magnesium level.

Renal magnesium excretion is a major determinant of magnesium homeostasis in the body. A transport maximum (Tm) exists for magnesium near its normal serum concentration; therefore, small increases in serum magnesium concentration above the normal level quickly result in increased renal excretion. The kidney is also very efficient at conserving magnesium. In the presence of decreased intake or absorption resulting in magnesium deficiency, renal excretion will decrease to less than 1 mEq/day within 7 days. Thus, decreased intake alone is a rare cause of magnesium deficiency, but it may contribute to the magnitude of the deficiency when abnormal losses are occurring.

Hypokalemia and hypocalcemia frequently coexist with hypomagnesemia. Magnesium deficiency results in increased urinary potassium excretion by an unknown mechanism, and it also results in decreased PTH secretion and effect on bone.

Signs and Symptoms

Symptomatic hypomagnesemia usually corresponds to a serum magnesium concentration less than 1 mEq/L. The clinical manifestations of magnesium deficiency are somewhat difficult to define, however, because other electrolyte abnormalities (e.g., hypokalemia, hypocalcemia) frequently coexist. Most symptoms relate to neuromuscular function and altered mentation, and they are summarized in Table 12.30.

Diagnosis

The diagnosis of magnesium deficiency depends on an awareness of clinical conditions that are commonly associated with hypomagnesemia and recognition of their resultant symptoms, and the differential diagnosis of hypomagnesemia is listed in Table 12.31. A spot urinary magnesium level should be measured in all patients with hypomagnesemia when the cause is not obvious. Extrarenal causes are associated with a urinary magnesium excre-

Table 12.30.   Signs and Symptoms of Hypomagnesemia

General:	Anorexia, nausea, weakness, apathy
Neurologic:	Altered mentation (depression, irritability, psychosis), carpal pedal spasm, tetany, muscular fibrillation, vertigo, ataxia, tremor, Chvostek's sign, Trousseau's sign, hyperreflexia
ECG:	Prolonged QT interval, broadening and decreased amplitude of T waves, ST segment shortening, arrhythmias (supraventricular, ventricular)

tion less than 1 mEq/day provided that the deficiency is at least 1 week old. High renal excretion of magnesium in hypomagnesemia indicates that renal magnesium loss is at least partly responsible for the deficit.

Treatment

The preferred route of magnesium administration depends on the severity and clinical manifestations of the hypomagnesemia. Patients with severe hypomagnesemia and serious ventricular arrhythmias or tetany require intravenous administration; asymptomatic patients with lesser degrees of magnesium deficiency can be treated orally. When oral replacement is possible, it is best to use sustained-release preparations of oral magnesium (Slow Mag or Mag-Tab SR) to avoid an abrupt elevation in the serum magnesium concentration that will only result in increased magnesium excretion in the urine. Therapy for magnesium deficiency is empirical, because it is difficult to estimate the size of the deficit. The amount required for therapy is actually larger than the estimated deficit, because approximately one-half of the administered magnesium will be lost in the urine even during severe magnesium deficiency. Fifty-percent magnesium sulfate (1 g per 2 mL of $MgSO_4$ = 8 mEq of magnesium) is the preferred form for

parenteral therapy, and the dose and rate of administration depend on the clinical situation. For the initial treatment of severe deficiency, no more than 100 mEq of magnesium should generally be given in any 12-hour period, and the rate should be slowed to between 40 and 100 mEq/day once the symptoms subside. The rate of intravenous infusion should not exceed 1 mEq/min (0.3 mL of 50% $MgSO_4$ per min). There is little danger of overtreatment in

Table 12.31.   Etiology of Hypomagnesemia

I. Decreased intake
  A. Protein calorie malnutrition (kwashiorkor disease)
  B. Prolonged intravenous therapy without magnesium[a]
  C. Chronic alcoholism[a]
II. Increased loss
  A. Gastrointestinal
    1. Malabsorption
    2. Diarrhea
    3. Excessive use of cathartics
    4. Nasogastric suction[a]
    5. Intestinal or biliary fistula[a]
  B. Renal loss
    1. Diuretic therapy
    2. Diabetic ketoacidosis
    3. Drugs (aminoglycosides[a], cisplatin, cyclosporin, amphotericin B, pentamidine)
    4. Chronic ECF volume expansion: SIADH, hyperaldosteronism
    5. Chronic alcoholism
    6. Hypercalcemia
    7. RTA
    8. Hyperthyroidism
    9. Chronic renal failure with Mg^{2+} wasting
    10. Idiopathic renal Mg^{2+} wasting
    11. Diuretic phase of acute renal failure
    12. Bartter's syndrome
    13. Certain renal diseases (hydronephrosis, glomerulonephritis)
III. Miscellaneous
  A. Acute pancreatitis
  B. Multiple transfusions with citrated blood
  C. Severe burns
  D. Following parathyroidectomy
  E. Hypoparathyroidism
  F. Foscarnet therapy

[a]Common in surgical patients.

adults with normal renal function because of the large excretion capacity of the kidney; however, the dose should be decreased in patients with renal insufficiency.

Frequent monitoring of serum magnesium levels is mandatory. Magnesium should not be given to patients with renal insufficiency unless a deficit in the serum has been documented (Table 12.32). The patellar reflexes should be checked every several hours when magnesium is given parenterally, and administration should be stopped if these reflexes disappear. No more than 10 mL of 50% $MgSO_4$ is given intramuscularly at a time because of pain at the injection site. Less severe magnesium deficits can be replaced with 0.25 to 0.50 mEq of magnesium per kilogram per day until serum levels become normal. Magnesium can be give orally as either magnesium oxide, magnesium chloride (Slow Mag), or magnesium lactate (Mag Tab SR). Table 12.32 also includes appropriate doses for the oral repletion of magnesium deficiency, and at these doses, diarrhea is usually not a problem.

Prevention of hypomagnesemia is also important. Patients with gastrointestinal fluid losses or on prolonged intravenous therapy should receive from 10 to 15 mEq of magnesium per day to prevent depletion.

Hypermagnesemia

Epidemiology

Hypermagnesemia is essentially limited to patients with renal insufficiency who are receiving magnesium-containing antacids or cathartics. On surgical services, this occurs most commonly in patients with acute or chronic renal failure who are receiving magnesium antacids for gastrointestinal bleeding or through hyperalimentation fluids. Uncommon causes of hypermagnesemia include adrenal insufficiency, hypothyroidism, and hypothermia.

Signs and Symptoms

The signs and symptoms of hypermagnesemia result from the central and peripheral suppression of neuromuscular transmission. Changes in mental status (e.g., drowsiness, coma), decreased deeptendon reflexes, and muscle paralysis may occur. Reflexes are regularly lost with

Table 12.32.   Treatment of Severe Hypomagnesemia in Adults with Normal Renal Function

Preparation	Route	Dose
50% $MgSO_4$ (8.13 meq Mg^{2+}/gm $MgSO_4$)[a]	IV	Day 1: 12 ml (6 gm = 49 meq Mg^{2+}) in 1 liter of D_5W over 3 hr, followed by 10 ml (5 gm = 40 meq Mg^{2+}) in each of two 1-liter bottles of glucose-containing solution over remainder of the first 24 hr Days 2–5: 12 ml (49 meq Mg^{2+}) equally distributed in daily IV fluids
50% $MgSO_4$	IM	Day 1: 4 ml (2 gm = 16.3 meq Mg^{2+}) q2h × 3 doses, then q4h × 4 doses Day 2: 2 ml (8.13 meq Mg^{2+}) q4h × 6 doses Day 3–5: 2 ml (8.13 meq Mg^{2+}) q6h
MgO (magnesium oxide) (50 meq Mg^{2+}/gm MgO)	PO	250 (12.5 meq Mg^{2+}) to 500 mg (25 meq Mg^{2+}) q.i.d.
Mg chloride (5 meq Mg per tablet)	PO	6–8 tablets/day in divided dose
Mg lactate (7 meq Mg per table)	PO	6–8 tablets/day in divided dose

[a]One gram of hydrated magnesium sulfate ($MgSO_4$ $7H_2O$, MW = 246.5) contains 8.13 meq of elemental magnesium.

serum magnesium levels greater than 6 to 8 mEq/L, and respiratory paralysis may occur with serum magnesium concentrations greater than 10 mEq/L. Deep-tendon reflexes disappear before respiratory paralysis occurs. Hypotension and ECG changes (e.g., prolonged P-R and Q-T intervals, delayed atrioventricular and intraventricular conduction, sinus bradycardia, increased sensitivity to vagal stimuli) may also occur, and nausea, vomiting, and soft-tissue calcification sometimes occur as well. Hypermagnesemia should be suspected in lethargic patients with renal failure and unexplained hypotension with loss of deep-tendon reflexes.

Diagnosis

The diagnosis of hypermagnesemia should be suspected in patients with renal insufficiency who are receiving magnesium-containing compounds. It is confirmed by measuring the serum magnesium concentration.

Treatment

Prevention is the key to treatment in patients with renal insufficiency. A careful review of medications should verify that they are not receiving any antacids or cathartics that contain magnesium and are not taking any similar, nonprescription medications.

The initial step in therapy for magnesium intoxication involves stopping all forms of magnesium administration and providing calcium gluconate intravenously if the signs or symptoms of toxicity are present. Calcium antagonizes the effects of magnesium excess, including respiratory depression, hypotension, and cardiac arrhythmias, and it is the treatment of choice in life-threatening hypermagnesemia. Ten to twenty milliliters of 10% calcium gluconate slowly administered intravenously is usually effective. If not, or in patients with renal failure, dialysis can decrease the serum magnesium to safe levels in 4 to 6 hours. If renal function is adequate, hydration and furosemide may be tried to enhance magnesium excretion.

Hypophosphatemia

Epidemiology

Of the many causes of phosphorus depletion, few result in severe hypophosphatemia (<1 mg/dL) (139, 140). The most frequent situations that predispose to profound phosphorus depletion in surgical patients include hyperalimentation (without phosphorus supplementation), refeeding with protein-calorie malnutrition, and the recovery phase of severe burns. Hypophosphatemia rarely results from inadequate intake or decreased intestinal absorption, except in patients undergoing prolonged courses of phosphate-binding antacids (e.g., aluminum hydroxide) or with alcoholism. Prolonged respiratory alkalosis, diabetic ketoacidosis, and alcohol withdrawal are also associated with severe hypophosphatemia, and modest degrees of hypophosphatemia may be seen in patients following prolonged hypothermia (e.g., as used in open-heart surgery).

Physiology

Since several species of phosphorus are present in the serum (HPO_4^{-2}, $H_2PO_4^{-1}$) and are influenced by pH, the concentration is conventionally expressed in terms of elemental phosphorus (in mg) per 100 dL. The serum phosphorus concentration is not tightly controlled. It undergoes diurnal variation and may vary by 1 to 2 mg/dL over the course of a day. A fasting concentration must be obtained for proper interpretation.

Intestinal absorption of phosphorus is very efficient and varies inversely with the phosphorus content of the diet (normal range, 800–1500 mg/day). The daily phosphorus requirement is 600 to 1200 mg/day (20–40 mmol/day).

Most causes of acute hypophosphatemia are the result of phosphorus shifting into cells. Anything that stimulates glycolysis (e.g., acute respiratory alkalosis, glucose and insulin administration, epinephrine) shifts phosphorus intracellularly and may result in hypophosphatemia. Inhibition of glycolysis (i.e., acute acidosis) results in phosphorus leaving the intracellular compartment and hyperphosphatemia. Hyperalimentation without adequate phosphorus supplementation results in intracellular sequestration of phosphorus by rapidly dividing cells associated with normal total body stores. The anabolic/diuretic phase of recovery from burns or provision of a normal amount of calories to patients with protein-calorie malnutrition (i.e., nutritional recovery syndrome) results in the intracellular movement of phosphorus and hypophosphatemia. Patients with burns may also develop hypophosphatemia because of urinary losses when retained salt and water are mobilized during the diuretic phase.

Renal phosphorus excretion is the major determinant of phosphorus homeostasis. Volume expansion results in increased renal sodium and phosphate excretion, and metabolic acidosis, magnesium, and potassium depletion also result in increased renal phosphate excretion. Phosphorus depletion in diabetic ketoacidosis results from the combined effects of acidosis and osmotic diuresis, resulting in increased urinary phosphate loss. Phosphorus deficiency in hospitalized patients with alcoholism is multifactorial and relates partly to poor intake, magnesium deficiency, ketoacidosis, and glucose administration.

Signs and Symptoms

Severe hypophosphatemia (<1 mg/dL) can lead to: (a) muscle weakness with respiratory failure, or congestive cardiomyopathy; (b) neurologic dysfunction (e.g., apprehension, confusion, coma, seizures, paresthesia, ataxia, tremors); (c) hematologic disorders (e.g., hemolytic anemia, decreased phagocytosis, platelet dysfunction; and (d) rhabdomyolysis. The diverse consequences of severe hypophos-

phatemia reflect the important role of phosphorus in membrane structure and function. More moderate degrees (1.0–2.5 mg/dL) do not usually result in noticeable symptoms. Chronic hypophosphatemia in adults may result in osteomalacia.

Diagnosis

The differential diagnosis of hypophosphatemia is listed in Table 12.33. There should be a high index of suspicion for phosphate depletion in patients who are alcoholic, receiving hyperalimentation or other hypertonic glucose solutions, or on phosphate-binding antacids (e.g., for chronic renal failure, peptic ulcer disease, or prophylaxis against gastrointestinal bleeding). In addition to a serum phosphorus level, an arterial blood gas determination should be made to look for respiratory alkalosis, and a urinary phosphorus concentration should be obtained to help determine the site of phosphorus loss. A urinary phosphorus concentration greater than 4 mg/dL indicates renal losses, whereas a lower concentration indicates extrarenal losses.

Treatment

Like other predominately intracellular ions, serum phosphorus may not accu-

Table 12.33.   Etiology of Hyperphosphatemia

I. Administration of phosphate
   A. Oral: Laxatives containing PO_4, K^+ phosphate tablets
   B. Rectal: phosphate enemas
   C. Intravenous phosphate
II. Decreased renal phosphate excretion
   A. Renal failure[a]
      1. Acute
      2. Chronic (GFR <20–30 ml/min)
   B. Hypoparathyroidism
   C. Pseudohypoparathyroidism
III. Transcellular shift out of cells
   A. Acute acidosis
   B. Treatment of lymphoma/leukemia with chemotherapy
IV. Artifact: in vitro hemolysis

---

[a]Common cause in surgical patients.

Table 12.34. **Therapeutic Phosphorus Preparations**

| Preparation | Content | | | |
	Phosphate	Phosphorus	Sodium	Potassium
Oral				
Neutra phos capsule		250 mg/capsule	28.5 mEq/capsule	28.5 mEq/capsule
Neutra K phos capsule		250 mg/capsule	0 mEq/capsule	57 mEq/capsule
Phospho soda	4.2 mmol/ml	129 mg/ml	4.8 mEq/ml	0 mEq/ml
Parenteral				
K phosphate	3.0 mmol/ml	93 mg/ml	0 mEq/ml	4.4 mEq/ml
Na phosphate	3.0 mmol/ml	93 mg/ml	4.0 mEq/ml	0 mEq/ml
Neutral Na, K phosphate	0.1 mmol/ml	3.1 mg/ml	0.162 mEq/ml	0.019 mEq/ml

rately reflect the total body stores. In any patient with hypophosphatemia, neither the size of the deficit nor the response to phosphorus therapy can be predicted. Therapy is thus empirical and close monitoring of the serum phosphorus concentration required.

It is preferable to prescribe phosphorus therapy in millimoles of phosphate ion or in milligrams of elemental phosphorus (rather than mEq), because both are independent of pH (1 mg = 0.032 mmol). Tables 12.34 and 12.35 list suggested doses for phosphorus therapy and the available preparations (141).

Oral therapy may be used in mild to moderate hypophosphatemia (>1 mg/dL), with an initial daily dose of 1 to 2 g of elemental phosphorus. Milk, which contains 1 g of inorganic phosphorus per quart, is a good initial therapy. Oral therapy may produce diarrhea, but it is less likely than intravenous administration to result in hypocalcemia.

Intravenous phosphorus therapy is indicated in severe hypophosphatemia (<1 mg/dL), especially if seizures, coma, or respiratory muscle weakness is present. Parenteral therapy is required in patients who do not tolerate or absorb oral phosphate, but intravenous phosphorus therapy is potentially hazardous. Possible complications include: *(a)* hyperphospha-

Table 12.35. **Treatment of Severe Hypophosphatemia**[a]

Clinical Situation	Initial Dose[b]
Recent uncomplicated hypophosphatemia	2.5 mg of phosphorus/kg body weight (0.08 mmol/kg)
Prolonged multiple causes	5.0 mg phosphorus/kg body weight (0.16 mmol/kg)

[a]Adapted from Lentz RD, et al.: *Ann Intern Med* 89:941, 1978, with permission.

[b]Note:

1. All doses in severe hypophosphatemia should be given intravenously over a 6-hour period. Above doses are for patients with normal renal function.

2. The initial dose should be 25–50% higher if the patient is symptomatic; lower if the patient is hypercalcemic.

3. Maximum dose is 7.5 mg/kg (0.24 mmol/kg) (16.8 mmol = 525 mg for a 70-kg man) over 6 hr.

4. Major complications have been reported in the literature when doses of 50–100 mmol phosphate have been given intravenously in less than 3 hours.

5. Repeat serum phosphorus concentration and reassess clinical situation before repeating phosphorus dose.

6. Conversion factors:
  1 mmol phosphate = 31 mg elemental phosphorus
  0.032 mmol phosphate = 1 mg elemental phosphorus
  0.323 mmol phosphate/L = 1 mg/dl elemental phosphorus
  1 mmol phosphate/L = 3.1 mg/dl elemental phosphorus

temia, *(b)* hypocalcemia (calcium supplementation may be required if the patient is already hypocalcemic), *(c)* metastatic calcification, *(d)* hypotension, *(e)* hyperkalemia from potassium salts, and *(f)* dehydration and hypernatremia (from an osmotic diuresis caused by the hypertonic nature of parenteral phosphate solutions). Absolute contraindications to intravenous therapy include hypercalcemia (unless used for the treatment of severe hypercalcemia refractory to conservative measures) and conditions associated with a rising phosphorus level (e.g., oliguria, tissue necrosis). Parenteral phosphorus, 1 to 2 g/day initially, will correct most cases of severe hypophosphatemia. The serum phosphorus concentration should be monitored frequently and therapy started as soon as possible. Since patients who are likely to develop hypophosphatemia are also prone to hypokalemia, part of the potassium deficit may be replaced with potassium phosphate; maintenance phosphate requirements are 20 to 40 mmol/day.

Hyperphosphatemia

Epidemiology

Renal failure, whether acute or chronic, is the most common cause of hyperphos-

Table 12.36.   **Etiology of Hyperphosphatemia**

I. Administration of phosphate
  A. Oral: Laxatives containing PO_4, K^+
    phosphate tablets
  B. Rectal: phosphate enemas
  C. Intravenous phosphate
II. Decreased renal phosphate excretion
  A. Renal failure[a]
    1. Acute
    2. Chronic (GFR <20–30 ml/min)
  B. Hypoparathyroidism
  C. Pseudohypoparathyroidism
III. Transcellular shift out of cells
  A. Acute acidosis
  B. Treatment of lymphoma/leukemia with
    chemotherapy
IV. Artifact: in vitro hemolysis

[a]Common cause in surgical patients.

phatemia encountered in clinical practice (142). Very severe hyperphosphatemia (>10 mg/dL) may occur in myoglobinuric ARF associated with rhabdomyolysis and following chemotherapy for leukemia and lymphoma.

Signs and Symptoms

The clinical manifestations of hyperphosphatemia are secondary to hypocalcemia and extraskeletal calcification.

Diagnosis

The differential diagnosis of hyperphosphatemia is listed in Table 12.36.

Treatment

Decreasing the intestinal absorption of phosphate is the major means of treating hyperphosphatemia. It is achieved by administering aluminum salts (e.g., aluminum hydroxide, aluminum carbonate), which bind the phosphate in the gut and thus prevent absorption.

ACID-BASE DISORDERS

Epidemiology

Acid-base disturbances are common in surgical patients. Various circumstances, either related to the illness requiring surgery or to therapy, may contribute to the development of a primary disturbance in the acid-base balance or alter the expected compensation. Table 12.37 summarizes the factors that lead to production of or affect the response to acid-base disorders in the surgical setting. Because of the complex nature of these problems in surgical patients, a few principles of acid-base physiology deserve mention.

Physiology

The acidity of blood may be expressed in terms of either the hydrogen ion concentration $[H^+]$ or the pH. It follows from the Henderson equation:

$$[H^+] = 24 \times P_{CO_2}/[HCO_3^-]$$

Table 12.37. Conditions Affecting Acid-Base Balance and Factors Contributing to Development of Acid-Base Disorders in Surgical Patients

Primary Acid-Base Disorders	Contributing Factors
Respiratory alkalosis	Overventilation
	Hypoxemia
	Sepsis
	Pain
	Apprehension
	Neurologic damage
	Liver disease
	Pulmonary embolism
Metabolic alkalosis	Vomiting
	NG suction
	Massive blood transfusions
	Excess HCO_3 administration
	Steroids
Respiratory acidosis	Drugs (preanesthetic medication, muscle paralyzing drugs)
	Pneumothorax
	Flail chest
Metabolic acidosis	Loss of alkaline GI fluids (biliary, small bowel, pancreas)
	Hypotension (hemorrhage, sepsis)
	Renal failure
	Vasopressor usage without adequate volume repletion
	Starvation ketosis
	Hyperalimentation

Factors Contributing to Impaired Compensation to Acid-Base Disorders in Surgical Patients

Conditions	Interferes With
Thoracic-abdominal operations	Respiratory compensation for metabolic acidosis
Peritonitis	″
COPD	″
CHF	″
Drugs (respiratory depressants)	″
Volume depletion	Renal HCO_3^- excretion for correction of metabolic alkalosis
K$^+$ depletion	
Renal failure	
Hypercapnea	″
Renal failure	Metabolic compensation for respiratory acidosis

that [H$^+$] is determined by the ratio of P_{CO_2}/[HCO_3^-] and not by their absolute values alone. This equation may be used to calculate [H$^+$], [HCO_3^-], or P_{CO_2} when the values for any two of these three are known. The [pH$^+$] may also be calculated from the Henderson-Haselbach equation:

$$pH = 6.1 + \log{[HCO_3^-]}/0.03 \times P_{CO_2}$$

If the measured [H$^+$], pH, P_{CO_2}, and [HCO_3^-] fail to satisfy the Henderson-Haselbach equation, there is either a laboratory error or the serum electrolytes and arterial blood gas samples were not drawn simultaneously.

Acid-base homeostasis is maintained by three mechanisms: *(a)* body fluid and tissue buffers, *(b)* respiratory excretion or retention of carbon dioxide, and *(c)* renal HCO_3 absorption or excretion. The bicarbonate system is the most clinically important buffer of the extracellular fluid (ECF). Chemical buffering via the bicarbonate system occurs instantaneously; intracellular buffering with intracellular–extracellular shifts takes 2 to 4 hours to occur. Respiratory compensation for primary metabolic disturbances in acid-base balance begins within minutes, but it may take 12 to 24 hours for maximum compensation to be achieved. If the acidosis develops slowly, full compensatory hyperventilation develops simultaneously. Renal compensation requires up to 5 days but is usually 90% complete within 3 days.

Acid-base disorders are categorized as either simple or mixed. Simple disorders are defined as the presence of one primary disorder coupled with its appropriate amount of compensation. Mixed disorders are defined as the presence of two or more primary acid-base disorders.

Before discussing the four simple disorders, it is important to note that you cannot diagnose an acid-base disorder by examining the [HCO_3^-] level or the P_{CO_2} alone. The pH, P_{CO_2}, and [HCO_3^-] level must be combined with the clinical picture to correctly interpret any set of arterial blood gases. Any increase or decrease in

[HCO$_3^-$] or Pco$_2$ may be part of the primary disorder or its compensation (Table 12.38) (143).

Simple Metabolic Acidosis

Epidemiology

The common causes of metabolic acidosis in surgical patients are those associated with a high anion gap, and they include lactic acidosis, ketoacidosis, and uremic acidosis. Lactic acidosis is usually associated with poor tissue perfusion secondary to low cardiac output, hypotension, or sepsis. The common causes of normal anion gap acidosis in surgical patients are loss of bicarbonate from the gastrointestinal tract, early renal failure (creatinine level, 3–8 mg/dL), and ureteral diversion (particularly when accompanied by obstruction).

Morbidity will more likely be attributable to the underlying disease (i.e., sepsis) than to the acidosis itself. However, severe acidosis may be harmful in itself, because it results in direct myocardial depression, unresponsiveness to the effects of catecholamines in maintaining vascular tone, and decreased threshold for ventricular fibrillation. These manifestations are thought to appear as the pH falls to less than 7.1 or 7.2. Patients who are elderly or with cardiovascular disease are more likely than young patients to suffer the consequences of acidosis.

Table 12.38. Etiology of Abnormal HCO$_3^-$ or pCO$_2$ Concentrations

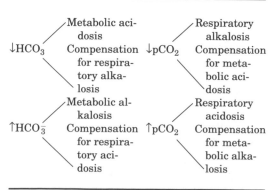

Diagnosis

The first step in determining the cause of a metabolic acidosis is calculation of the serum anion gap (AG). The anion gap is defined as the difference between the serum sodium concentration and the sum of the serum Cl$^-$ and HCO$_3^-$ concentrations:

$$AG = Na^+ - (HCO_3^- + Cl^-)$$

The anion gap normally ranges between 3 and 11 mEq/L when measured using the newer autoanalyzers, which give a higher reading for the serum chloride concentration and explain why the normal value of the anion gap is lower now than in the past (144). Since albumin accounts for most of this gap, hypoalbuminemia will lower the measured value. A useful rule of thumb is that for each reduction of 1 g/dL in the serum albumin concentration, the anion gap will decrease by 2.5 mEq/L (145). It is important to know, if possible, what a patient's baseline anion gap is; otherwise, a low baseline value may mask the presence of a high anion gap acidosis. All cases of metabolic acidosis can be divided into one of two types (Table 12.39): high anion gap metabolic acidosis, and normal anion gap (i.e., hyperchloremic) metabolic acidosis. The normal anion gap metabolic acidoses may be further subdivided into two groups according to the serum potassium concentration: normal to high, and low.

Gabow et al. (146) reported that the anion gap is most useful when its value exceeds 25 mEq/L. In this situation, lactic acidosis, ketoacidosis, renal failure, or certain ingestions are usually present and easily identifiable. Ketoacidosis is easily diagnosed by the finding of ketones in the blood. However, the nitroprusside reaction (Acetest) detects only acetoacetate and not beta-hydroxybutyrate, and it may produce a false-negative result in clinical situations of tissue hypoxia in which beta-hydroxybutyrate predominates. Typical uremic acidosis (i.e., anion gap) is seen

Table 12.39. Etiology of Metabolic Acidosis

High Anion Gap	Normal Anion Gap
1. Ketoacidosis[a]	Normal to high potassium type
a. Diabetic	1. Early renal failure (Cr = 6–8 mg/100 ml)[a]
b. Alcoholic	2. Obstructive uropathy[a]
c. Starvation	3. Hypoaldosteronism
2. Lactic acidosis[a]	a. Hyporeninemia
3. Renal failure[a]	b. Renal aldosterone resistance
4. Ingestions	4. Dilutional acidosis
a. Salicylate	5. Acidifying agents (HCl, NH_4Cl, arginine HCl,
b. Methanol	lysine HCl, $CaCl_2$)
c. Ethylene glycol	6. Sulfur toxicity
d. Paraldehyde	7. Recovery stage of diabetic ketoacidosis
	Low potassium type
	1. GI HCO_3^- loss[a]
	a. Diarrhea
	b. Pancreatic, biliary, small bowel drainage, or external fistula
	c. Cholestyramine
	2. Renal tubular acidosis
	a. Proximal
	b. Distal
	3. Carbonic anhydrase inhibitors
	a. Acetazolamide (Diamox)
	b. Mafenide (Sulfamylon)
	4. Posthypocapnic metabolic acidosis
	5. Ureteral diversions[a]
	a. Ureterosigmoidostomy
	b. Ileal ureter
	c. Obstructed ileal bladder

[a]Common in surgical patients.

only in advanced renal failure (creatinine clearance, <25 mL/min). Lactic acidosis is usually a diagnosis of exclusion in the appropriate clinical setting, but may be confirmed by an elevated serum lactate level.

Although one might initially believe that the increase in the anion gap (ΔAG) would match the decrease in the serum HCO_3 (ΔHCO_3) in a high anion gap acidosis, this is usually not the case. There are several explainations why the ratio of ΔAG:ΔHCO_3 ratio is usually 1.0 to 2.0 in uncomplicated high anion gap acidosis. First, anions responsible for the increased anion gap remain mostly in the extracellular space, whereas more that 50% of the H^+ produced by the metabolic acidosis will be buffered intracellularly, by bone, and thus will not contribute to lowering the serum HCO_3 (i.e., different volumes of distribution for anions and H^+). Second, excretion of anions in the urine (e.g., ketonuria), D-lactate, and hippuric acid (i.e., metabolism of toluene) also can explain this ratio. Excretion of the anion that is responsible for the elevated anion gap can convert a high anion gap acidosis to a normal anion gap acidosis. This urinary loss of anions will be of lesser quantitative importance in patients with preexisting renal failure or severe volume depletion. The ΔAG:ΔHCO_3 ratio will be useful in evaluating high anion gap metabolic acidosis only if the baseline anion gap is known and the anions that accumulate in the body derive from the acids causing the acidemia (147). Figure 12.7 summarizes interpretation of the ΔAG:ΔHCO_3 ratio.

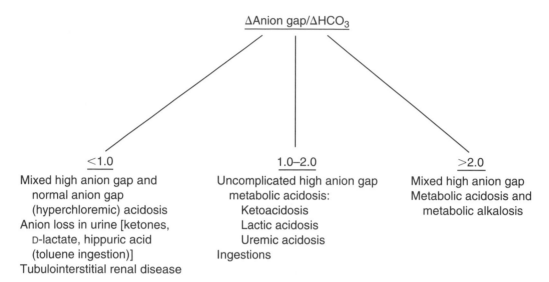

ΔAnion gap/ΔHCO$_3$

<1.0

Mixed high anion gap and
   normal anion gap
   (hyperchloremic) acidosis
Anion loss in urine [ketones,
   D-lactate, hippuric acid
   (toluene ingestion)]
Tubulointerstitial renal disease

1.0–2.0

Uncomplicated high anion gap
   metabolic acidosis:
   Ketoacidosis
   Lactic acidosis
   Uremic acidosis
Ingestions

>2.0

Mixed high anion gap
Metabolic acidosis and
   metabolic alkalosis

Figure 12.7.   Use of ΔAG/ΔHCO$_3$ ratio in the diagnosis of high-anion-gap metabolic acidosis.

Measurement of the urinary anion gap and the urinary osmolality gap is sometimes useful in evaluating normal anion gap metabolic acidosis by estimating the urinary ammonium excretion, which will allow differentiation of a renal from an extrarenal acidosis. The normal kidney responds to extrarenal acidosis by increasing NH_4Cl excretion up to 200 mEq/day. Significant ammonium in the urine indicates an extrarenal acidosis, whereas low ammonium excretion indicates a renal acidosis. The urinary anion gap is calculated by the following equation:

$$\text{Urinary AG} = \text{Urinary } (Na^+ + K^+ - Cl^-)$$

The urinary anion gap will usually be from −20 to −50 mEq/L in an extrarenal acidosis, signifying that the kidney is responding appropriately by excreting hydrogen ions as NH_4Cl. This gap will generally be positive in a renal acidosis. The cause of normal anion gap acidosis will usually be apparent from the clinical situation and the analysis of serum electrolytes, glucose, BUN, creatinine, blood, and urine pH. However, severe hypokalemia and metabolic acidosis from diarrhea may sometimes resemble a distal RTA because of a urinary pH greater than 5.5.

Hypokalemia stimulates renal ammonia production independent of the extracellular pH, thus raising the urinary pH to greater than 5.5 and indicating a distal RTA. For the urinary anion gap to be a valid measure of ammonium excretion, the patient must not be significantly volume depleted. If the urinary sodium concentration is less than 25 mEq/L because of volume depletion, then proximal reabsorption of NaCl will limit the kidney's ability excrete NH_4Cl, and the laboratory findings will resemble those of a distal RTA, with a urinary pH of greater than 5.5. In fact, the decreased net acid secretion that is induced by volume depletion plays an important role in the development of metabolic acidosis with diarrhea. Increased excretion of unmeasured anions will also interfere with use of the urinary anion gap to measure ammonium excretion, and excretion of the Na^+ and K^+ salts of unmeasured urinary anions will produce a positive urinary anion gap even though ammonium excretion is greatly increased. In this situation, the calculated urinary osmolality gap can be used as a measure of ammonium excretion. Any gap between the measured and the calculated urinary osmolality is mainly comprised of ammonium salts. The following equation is used to calculate the urinary osmolality:

Calculated urinary osmolality = $2 \times$ [$Na^+ + K^+$] + BUN/2.8 + glucose/18.

The glucose term can be ignored if the urine dipstick test is negative for glucose. Subtracting the calculated urinary osmolality from the measured urinary osmolality gives the urinary osmolality gap. Dividing the urinary osmolality gap by 2 to adjust for the accompanying anions will estimate the urinary ammonium excretion. Figure 12.8 summarizes use of both the urinary anion gap and urinary osmolality gap in evaluating difficult cases of normal anion gap metabolic acidosis.

Treatment

To be successful in either lactic acidosis or ketoacidosis, therapy must be directed at the underlying cause (i.e., improving tissue perfusion or the administration of insulin). Often, this will result in normalization of the pH without additional (i.e., bicarbonate) therapy.

Guidelines for the use of sodium bicarbonate in severe metabolic acidosis include: (a) a serum pH less than 7.1 (or 7.2 in patients with heart disease), (b) a serum bicarbonate less than 12 mEq/L, or (c) presence of a maximum ventilatory response ($Pco_2 \leq 15$ mm Hg). The initial aim of therapy is to increase the serum bicarbonate concentration by approximately 4 to 6 mEq/L over the first several hours and to 14 to 16 mEq/L by 24 hours. Elderly patients with Gram-negative sepsis, shock, arrhythmias, and a pH of 7.2 should probably receive bicarbonate. Young patients with diabetes and a pH of 7.1 but without hypotension may not require bicarbonate, because treatment with insulin should rapidly improve the acidosis and their cardiovascular systems are more stable.

The serum bicarbonate concentration should be raised to between 16 and 18 mEq/L in patients with metabolic acidosis who have lung disease or are about to receive anesthesia. These patients are more prone to having impaired respiratory compensation.

The approximate total amount of bicarbonate needed to achieve a desired serum bicarbonate level can be estimated by the following formula:

Bicarbonate deficit = weight [kg] $\times 0.5$ [(HCO_3^- desired) – (HCO_3^- measured)]

The actual required amount will vary widely, however, because of large differences in the volume of bicarbonate distribution. The actual amount tends to be greater when acidosis is severe or ongoing and when bicarbonate continues to be lost. Therefore, there is no substitute for the frequent measurement of pH and bicarbonate concentration.

Bicarbonate therapy should never be considered lightly. Potential complications include hypokalemia, decreased ionized calcium with tetany, volume overload, hypernatremia, and cerebral acidosis. "Overshoot" alkalosis may occur when the change in bicarbonate level is more rapid than the change in Pco_2 or when lactate or the salts of ketoacids are remetabolized to bicarbonate. Volume overload may impair the respiratory compensatory response and result in a lower pH. Diuretics or dialysis may occasionally be needed to handle the excess sodium load resulting from bicarbonate therapy.

In patients with severe acidosis from renal failure and with hypocalcemia, it may be necessary to provide intravenous calcium (20–30 mL of 10% calcium gluconate) to avoid precipitating tetany or convulsions. When severe acidosis and hypokalemia coexist, a large potassium deficit is usually also present; in this situation, the pH and the potassium deficiency must be corrected simultaneously.

D-Lactic acidosis is an uncommon form of lactic acidosis that may occur in patients who have undergone jejunoileal bypass or suffer from small-bowel syndrome as a result of prior small-bowel surgical resection or disease (148). This

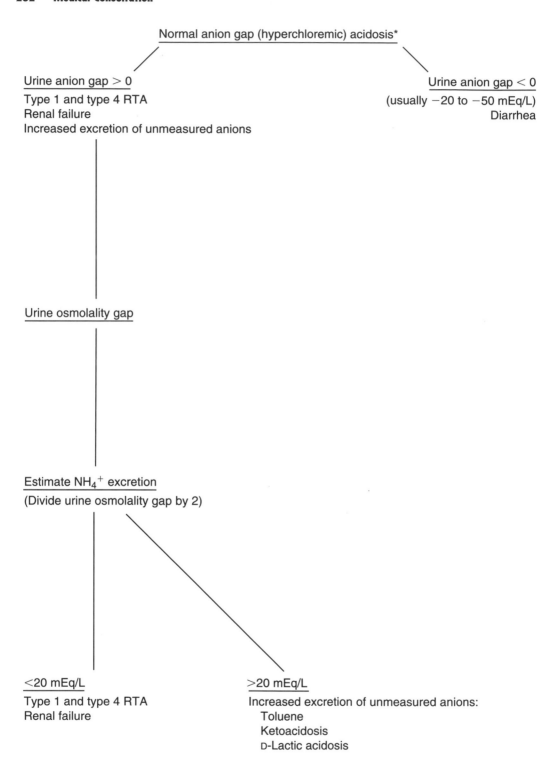

Normal anion gap (hyperchloremic) acidosis*

Urine anion gap > 0
Type 1 and type 4 RTA
Renal failure
Increased excretion of unmeasured anions

Urine anion gap < 0
(usually −20 to −50 mEq/L)
Diarrhea

Urine osmolality gap

Estimate NH_4^+ excretion
(Divide urine osmolality gap by 2)

<20 mEq/L
Type 1 and type 4 RTA
Renal failure

>20 mEq/L
Increased excretion of unmeasured anions:
    Toluene
    Ketoacidosis
    D-Lactic acidosis

*U_{Na} should be >25 mEq/L to assure NH_4Cl excretion is not limited by NaCl absorption in proximal tubule in response to volume depletion.

Figure 12.8.   Use of urinary anion gap and urinary osmolality gap in the evaluation of normal-anion-gap metabolic acidosis. *RTA*, renal tubular acidosis.

will result in an increased delivery of glucose and starch to the colon secondary to a limited absorption of these substrates in the small intestine. If bacterial overgrowth with Gram-positive anaerobes (e.g., lactobacilli) has also occurred, the colonic bacteria are capable of converting dietary carbohydrate into D-lactate rather than into the normal, physiologically occuring L-lactate. Characteristic neurologic findings in D-lactic acidosis include confusion, slurred speech, memory loss, and cerebellar ataxia. The diagnosis should be suspected in patients with a history of small-bowel disease who develop unexplained high anion gap metabolic acidosis associated with neurologic manifestations after the ingestion of a carbohydrate-rich meal. However, if the D-lactate is rapidly excreted in the urine, a normal anion gap acidosis can be seen. Treatment consists of administering sodium bicarbonate to correct the acidosis and oral antibiotics (e.g., vancomycin, flagyl) to reduce the number of D-lactate–producing organisms. A low-carbohydrate diet or the use of starch polmyers should also be provided to decrease carbohydrate delivery to the colon (149).

Simple Metabolic Alkalosis

Epidemiology

In surgical patients, metabolic alkalosis most commonly develops from gastric losses of hydrogen through vomiting or gastric suction (150). Alkalosis resulting from potassium depletion, use of diuretics, or posthypoventilation syndrome is common as well. Because many of these patients are also volume depleted, which leads to the renal retention of bicarbonate, the metabolic alkalosis will tend to persist.

Surgical patients who are critically ill are commonly alkalotic (metabolic, respiratory, or both), and the mortality rate has been shown to increase with a pH greater than 7.55 (Table 12.40) (151). Metabolic alkalosis also results in hypoventilation, which may interfere with weaning a pa-

Table 12.40. Acid-Base Disorders in Critically Ill Patients[a]

Frequency of Acid-Base Disorders in Critically Ill Patients

	N = 105 Surgical Patients (Lyons)	N = 1415 Surgical Patients (Wilson)	N = 8209 ABG Determinations in an ICU (Mazzara)
Alkalosis	64%	12.5%	69%
Respiratory	57%	11.0%	46%
Metabolic	13%	1.5%	23%
Acidosis			21.5%
Respiratory			13.4%
Metabolic			8.1%
Normal			8.6%

Mortality Related to pCO_2 or pH in Critically Ill Alkalotic Patients

Mazzara		Wilson[b]	
pCO_2 (mm Hg)	Mortality (%)	pH	Mortality (%)
15	88	7.55–7.56	41
20–25	77	7.57–7.59	47
25–30	73	7.60–7.64	65
35–45	29	7.65–7.7	80

[a]Sources: Mazzara JT, Ayres SM, Grace WJ: Extreme hypocapnea in the critically ill. *Am J Med* 56:450–456, 1974; Wilson RF, et al.: Severe alkalosis in critically ill surgical patients. *Arch Surg* 105:197–203, 1972; Lyons JH, Moore FD: Posttraumatic alkalosis: Incidence and pathophysiology of alkalosis in surgery. *Surgery* 60:93–106, 1966.
[b]Wilson did not find mortality related to pCO_2.

tient from mechanical ventilation. Correction in patients with mixed respiratory acidosis and metabolic alkalosis improves arterial blood gases and clinical symptoms.

Physiology

Metabolic alkalosis can be divided into two types: chloride responsive and chloride resistant. Most chloride-responsive forms are associated with intravascular volume depletion and a low spot urinary

Table 12.41. Etiology of Metabolic Alkalosis

Chloride-Responsive ($U_{Cl} < 10$–20 mEq/L)	Chloride-Resistant ($U_{Cl} > 10$–20 mEq/L)

1. Gastrointestinal causes
  a. Gastric losses (vomiting, nasogastric suction)[a]
  b. Cl^--losing diarrhea (villous adenoma of colon, congenital Cl^--losing diarrhea)
2. Diuretic administration (late)[a]
3. Posthypercapneic metabolic alkalosis[a]
4. Antibiotics (carbenicillin, penicillin)
	1. Hyperaldosteronism
	2. Cushing's syndrome
	3. Bartter's syndrome
	4. Licorice ingestion
	5. Severe K^+ depletion
	6. Excessively rapid HCO_3^- administration (especially in renal failure)
	7. Drugs
	  a. Diuretics (early)
	  b. Exogenous glucocorticoid or mineralocorticoid
	  c. Carbenoxalone

[a]Common in surgical patients.

chloride concentration (U_{cl}, >10–20 mEq/L). The urinary chloride concentration is more useful than the urinary sodium concentration in assessing the effective circulating volume in metabolic alkalosis, because sodium may be lost in the urine despite volume depletion if bicarbonaturia is present. The urinary chloride concentration may be high despite intravascular volume depletion in three conditions: *(a)* renal insufficiency, *(b)* severe hypokalemia (potassium level, <2 mEq/L), and *(c)* acute hypercapnea. Chloride-sensitive metabolic alkalosis can be corrected with chloride administered as either KCl, NaCl, or both.

Chloride-resistant metabolic alkalosis is associated with a high urinary chloride level (U_{cl}, >10–20 mEq/L). Most are rare, however, and result from some form of mineralocorticoid excess. Chloride administration in this group has no effect, because these patients are not chloride (i.e., volume) depleted. Table 12.41 lists the differential diagnosis of metabolic alkalosis.

Signs and Symptoms

Severe alkalosis can result in mental confusion, seizures, or coma. The oxyhemoglobin dissociation curve shifts to the left, and this results in impaired oxygen release from hemoglobin. Arrhythmias are much more common in patients with alkalosis, who may also have coexisting hypokalemia or hypomagnesemia and may be receiving digoxin.

Diagnosis

Patient history and bedside determination of the intravascular volume are the keys to diagnosing the cause of metabolic alkalosis. If the cause is not obvious from the history and physical examination, then surreptitious vomiting, ingestion of diuretics, and mineralocorticoid excess should be suspected. Measurement of the urinary chloride concentration will help in these cases.

Treatment

Definitive treatment of any metabolic alkalosis involves correcting the underlying cause. Increased renal bicarbonate excretion can be achieved by correcting those conditions responsible for maintaining the metabolic alkalosis (e.g., decreased extracellular fluid volume, potassium deficiency, hypercapnea) by elevating the renal bicarbonate threshold. An increase in urinary chloride excretion to between

60 and 100 mEq/day indicates adequate replacement of chloride stores. If the effective circulating volume cannot be improved (e.g., edematous states), acetazolamide (250–500 mg two to four times a day) may help in improving pulmonary function in patients who are hypoventilating as a response to metabolic alkalosis. The combination of metabolic alkalosis (e.g., from nasogastric suction) and postoperative renal failure represents a special problem when the alkalosis is severe. Volume replacement and the administration of NaCl and KCl do not reverse the alkalosis, because the kidney cannot excrete the excess bicarbonate. In this situation, administration of dilute (0.1 N) hydrochloric acid or dialysis with a high chloride–low acetate bath (152, 153) can be an effective treatment. Use of ammonium HCl and arginine HCl are less desirable in patients with renal failure because of the increased nitrogen load. Dilute (0.1 N) HCl contains 100 mEq of hydrogen ions per liter, and it must be administered through a central line to avoid its sclerosing effects. The dose of dilute HCl may be estimated as follows:

$$\text{Acid required [mEq]} = \text{weight [kg]} \times 0.5 \times [\text{HCO}_3^- \text{ initial} - \text{HCO}_3^- \text{ desired}]$$

From this formula, it follows that approximately 5 mEq of acid per kg is required to reduce the serum bicarbonate concentration by 10 mEq/L. This decrease in bicarbonate should be accomplished over 12 to 24 hours. If the amount of gastric drainage is large, the ongoing hydrogen ion loss can be estimated by applying the electroneutrality principle to the gastric contents:

$$\text{Ongoing gastric H}^+ \text{ loss [mEq/L]} = \text{Cl}^+ - (\text{Na}^+ + \text{K}^+)$$

This ongoing acid loss should be added to the calculated acid deficit when correcting severe metabolic alkalosis. H_2-blockers or proton-pump inhibitors, which reduce gastric acid secretion, can also be used to minimize the loss of hydrogen ions.

Severe, chloride-resistant metabolic alkalosis can be treated with large doses of potassium or acidifying agents. Definitive treatment, however, depends on correcting the underlying disorder.

Simple Respiratory Acidosis

Epidemiology

Acute respiratory acidosis is not an uncommon problem in the postoperative period, and severe chronic obstructive pulmonary disease is a definite risk factor for its development. Factors contributing to postoperative hypoventilation include pain from abdominal incisions and abdominal distention that limit diaphragmatic excursion, flail chest, atelectasis, pleural effusions, pneumonia, airway obstruction, and drugs (e.g., sedatives, anesthetics, muscle paralyzers).

Diagnosis

Postoperative restlessness, hypertension, and tachycardia may result from respiratory acidosis, hypoxia, or pain, and they should be evaluated with an arterial blood gas measurement. Table 12.42 summarizes the causes of respiratory acidosis.

Treatment

Treatment involves improving pulmonary ventilation by clearing secretions, use of bronchodilators and corticosteroids, and, possibly, intubation.

Simple Respiratory Alkalosis

Epidemiology

Apprehension, pain, and overventilation contribute to the development of respiratory alkalosis, and unexplained respiratory alkalosis may be an important first clue to the presence of sepsis in surgical patients. On surgical services, acute respiratory alkalosis is also seen following head trauma, pneumothorax, overventilation by a mechanical respirator, and with pulmonary embolism.

Signs and Symptoms

Hypocapnea leads to cerebral vasoconstriction, and it may further compromise cerebral blood flow in patients with cerebrovascular disease. Cardiac arrhythmias may also develop with severe respiratory alkalosis, especially the patient has hypokalemia and is receiving digoxin. Table 12.43 summarizes the causes of respiratory alkalosis.

Treatment

The primary mode of treatment involves correction of the underlying disorder. On occasion, reducing the respiration rate by pharmacologic (e.g., sedation,

Table 12.42.   Causes of Respiratory Acidosis

1. Respiratory center depression
   a. Drugs (general anesthesia, narcotics, sedatives)[a]
   b. CNS lesions (trauma, medullary tumor, vertebral artery occlusion)
   c. Pickwickian syndrome
   d. Increased intracranial pressure
   e. Oxygen therapy in chronic hypercapnea[a]
2. Neuromuscular disorders
   a. Neuropathies (poliomyelitis, Guillain-Barre syndrome, botulism, spinal cord injury)
   b. Myopathies (myasthenia gravis, muscular dystrophy, hypo- and hyperkalemic paralysis)
3. Thoracic cage disorders
   a. Kyphoscoliosis
   b. Flail chest[a]
   c. Alkylosing spondylitis
   d. Pneumothorax[a]
   e. Scleroderma
4. Airway obstruction
   a. Aspiration
   b. Foreign body
   c. Laryngeal edema
5. Pulmonary disease
   a. COPD[a]
   b. Pulmonary edema
   c. Pneumonia
   d. Severe bronchospasm

[a]Common in surgical patients.

Table 12.43.   Causes of Respiratory Alkalosis

1. Hypoxemia[a]
2. Anxiety[a]
3. Drugs (hormones)
   a. Salicylates
   b. Progesterone (pregnancy)
   c. Epinephrine
4. CNS disorders
   a. Subarachnoid hemorrhage
   b. Meningitis, encephalitis
   c. Head trauma
   d. Cerebrovascular accident
   e. Brain tumor
5. Pulmonary disorders
   a. Pneumothorax[a]
   b. Pulmonary emboli[a]
   c. Early restrictive disorders
   d. Pneumonia[a]
   e. Pulmonary hypertension
   f. Congestive heart failure[a]
6. Hypermetabolic states
   a. Fever[a]
   b. Thyrotoxicosis
   c. Anemia
   d. Delirium tremens
7. Miscellaneous
   a. Gram-negative septicemia[a]
   b. Endotoxemia[a]
   c. Ventilator-induced[a]
   d. Liver disease
   e. Sudden recovery from metabolic acidosis[a]
   f. Severe burns[a]

[a]Common in surgical patients.

muscle paralyzers) or mechanical (e.g., increasing dead space) means may be necessary.

Mixed Acid-Base Disorders

Epidemiology

A mixed acid-base disorder should be suspected when arterial blood gas and electrolyte analyses reveal either an inadequate or an excessive degree of compensation. Often, it will be clinically obvious that several individual processes are occurring simultaneously and combining to produce more than one primary acid-base disturbance. For instance, a patient who might be septic (e.g., respiratory alkalosis, metabolic acidosis) following surgery for an abdominal abscess and who has a nasogastric tube (i.e., metabolic alkalosis) and is on a respirator (e.g., respiratory acidosis or alkalosis) has several separate processes, each of which is capable of producing abnormalities in acid-base homeostasis. The final pH in this patient would depend on the relative severity of each individual disorder.

Physiology

Before one can properly approach mixed disorders, it is necessary to understand the normal patterns of compensating for primary acid-base disturbances. This topic is well reviewed elsewhere (154, 155), and the expected compensation for each primary acid-base disorder can be derived from the acid-base map con-structed by Goldberg (156) (Fig. 12.9) or from the equations in Table 12.44.

The more severe the primary acid-base disturbances, the less likely the pH will be normal and the more likely a normal pH indicates a mixed acid-base disorder. Compensation does not usually return the pH to normal. In mild disorders, however, it may possibly return the pH to the normal range but not to the initial value.

What appears to be an "inappropriate" degree of compensation may actually be the effect of a separate primary disorder. Even apparently appropriate compensation may represent the chance occurrence of dual or triple acid-base disorders. The duration of the acid-base disorder must be known to interpret how appropriate the compensatory mechanisms are. Other-

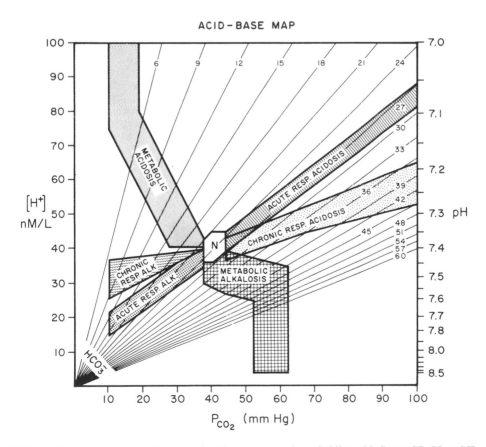

Figure 12.9. Acid-base nomogram. (Reprinted with permission from Goldberg M, Green SB, Moss ML, et al. Computer-based instruction and diagnosis of acid-base disorders: a systematic approach. JAMA 1973; 223:269.)

Table 12.44.   Compensation for Acid-Base Disorders

Metabolic acidosis	$pCO_2 = 1.5\ [HCO_3^-] + 8 \pm 2$ $pCO_2 \downarrow$ by 1–1.3 per mEq/L $\downarrow HCO_3^-$	Measured $pCO_2 >$ expected pCO_2: superimposed primary respiratory acidosis or insufficient time for complete resp. compensation (acidosis <24 hr) Measured $pCO_2 <$ expected pCO_2: superimposed primary respiratory alkalosis or delayed ventilatory adjustment to sudden increase in plasma HCO_3^-
Metabolic alkalosis	$pCO_2 \uparrow$ by 0.5–0.7 mm Hg per mEq/L $\uparrow HCO_3^-$	Measured $pCO_2 >$ expected pCO_2: suggests superimposed primary respiratory acidosis (resp. compensation may be absent in mild metabolic alkalosis HCO_3^- <37 mEq/L) Measured $pCO_2 <$ expected pCO_2: suggests superimposed primary respiratory alkalosis
Acute respiratory acidosis	$HCO_3^- \uparrow$ by 1 mEq/L for every 10 mm Hg rise in pCO_2, not increasing more than total of 3–4 mEq/L or exceeding a $HCO_3^- = 30$ mEq/L $\Delta H^+ = 0.8\ \Delta pCO_2{}^a$	$HCO_3^- >$30 mEq/L suggests superimposed primary metabolic alkalosis $HCO_3^- <$24 mEq/L suggests superimposed primary metabolic acidosis $\Delta H^+ \neq 0.8\ \Delta pCO_2$ suggests superimposed metabolic disorder or laboratory error
Chronic respiratory acidosis	$\Delta HCO_3^- = 0.4\ \Delta pCO_2 \pm 3$ $\Delta H^+ = 0.33\ \Delta pCO_2$	Measured $HCO_3^- >$ expected HCO_3^- suggests superimposed primary metabolic alkalosis Measured $HCO_3^- <$ expected HCO_3^- suggests superimposed primary metabolic acidosis $\Delta H^+ \neq 0.33\ \Delta pCO_2$ suggests superimposed metabolic disorder or laboratory error
Acute respiratory alkalosis	$\Delta HCO_3^- = 0.2\ \Delta pCO_2 \pm 2.5$ (HCO_3^- usually not <18 mEq/L) $\Delta H^+ = 0.8\ \Delta pCO_2$	Measured $HCO_3^- >$ expected HCO_3^- suggests superimposed primary metabolic alkalosis $HCO_3^- <$18 mEq/L suggests superimposed primary metabolic acidosis $\Delta H^+ \neq 0.8\ \Delta pCO_2$ suggests superimposed metabolic disorder or laboratory error
Chronic respiratory alkalosis	$\Delta HCO_3^- = 0.5\ \Delta pCO_2 \pm 2.5$ (HCO_3^- usually not <15 mEq/L) $\Delta H^+ = 0.17\ \Delta pCO_2$	Measured $HCO_3^- >$ expected HCO_3^- suggests superimposed primary metabolic alkalosis $HCO_3^- <$15 mEq/L suggests superimposed primary metabolic acidosis $\Delta H^+ \neq 0.17\ \Delta pCO_2$ suggests superimposed metabolic disorder or laboratory error

$^a\Delta$, change from normal.

wise, insufficient compensation will be attributed incorrectly to a complicating primary disorder rather than to insufficient time to reach a new steady state of acid-base balance with maximal compensation.

Values falling within the confidence bands for a simple acid-base disorder do not prove that a simple disorder exists, only that the data are consistent with a single disturbance. If a point falls outside a band, a mixed disorder is indicated. Since there are always several possible explanations for any point on the acid-base map, the correct interpretation can be made only by using the available clinical information. Table 12.44 lists the possible explanations when actual compensatory responses differ from the expected or the calculated responses.

Diagnosis

A systematic approach to the diagnosis of both simple and mixed acid-base disorders is outlined in Table 12.45 and is largely self-explanatory. The patient history and physical examination search for conditions associated with disorders of the acid-base balance. The indicated laboratory data confirm the presence of an acid-base disorder and help in establishing its cause. Finally, to decide if a mixed acid-base disorder is present, the expected compensation for any primary acid-base disorder must be compared with the actual compensation. It cannot be overemphasized, however, that only by incorporating the actual clinical picture, including the estimated duration of the acid-base disturbance, can the arterial blood gas measurements be interpreted correctly. The common causes of mixed acid-base disorders are summarized in Table 12.46.

Treatment

The treatment of mixed and simple acid-base disorders is similar. The aim is to restore the pH toward normal and to identify and correct all underlying conditions. If the pH is severely abnormal in a patient with mixed metabolic acidosis and metabolic alkalosis, the predominant disorder should be treated first.

Table 12.45. **Diagnostic Approach to Acid-Base Disturbances**

I. History
   A. Clinical diagnoses capable of producing acid-base disorders (COPD, renal failure, diabetes mellitus)
   B. Drugs
      1. Diuretics
      2. Steroids
      3. Acidifying/alkalinizing agents
      4. Respiratory stimulants/depressants
      5. Antibiotics
         a. Aminoglycosides (renal failure, neuromuscular blockade)
         b. Carbenicillin (metabolic alkalosis)
      6. Toxins (aspirin, methanol, ethylene glycol, paraldehyde)
   C. Therapeutic maneuvers
      1. Mechanical ventilation
      2. Sodium restriction
II. Physical examination
   A. Vital signs: Kussmaul respiration, hypotension → metabolic acidosis
   B. Fundus: papilledema (CO_2 retention, methanol)
   C. Cyanosis, COPD → respiratory acidosis
   D. Nasogastric tube → metabolic alkalosis
   E. Fever → respiratory alkalosis

Table 12.45. *(continued)*   Diagnostic Approach to Acid-Base Disturbances

III. Laboratory
   A. Routine electrolytes
      1. Na^+
      2. K^+
      3. Cl^-
      4. HCO_3^-
      5. Calculate anion gap: $AG = Na^+ - (Cl + HCO_3^-)$
         a. Look for value of anion gap before acid-base disorder developed or factors that may decrease its size (i.e., hypoalbuminemia)
      6. Calculate $\Delta AG/\Delta HCO_3$
   B. Arterial blood gases
   C. Supplementary data
      1. Blood
         a. Glucose
         b. BUN, creatinine
         c. Osmolality
         d. Serum ketones
         e. Toxicology screen (methanol, ethylene glycol, paraldehyde, salicylate)
         f. Lactate level
      2. Urinalysis: glucose/ketones, oxylate (ethylene glycol)
      3. Pulmonary function tests
      4. Blood cultures
      5. Calculate urine anion gap: $Na^+ + K^+ - Cl$
      6. Calculate urine osmolality gap
IV. Synthesize data
   A. Rule out lab error
   B. Arterial blood gases different from expected
      1. ? Miss something
      2. ? Overemphasis of some process in history
   C. Calculate expected compensation for any primary acid-base disorder present

---

Table 12.46.   Examples of Mixed Acid-Base Disorders

   I. Respiratory acidosis + metabolic acidosis
      A. COPD (chronic respiratory acidosis) + septic shock[a]
      B. COPD + severe acute hypoxia (pO_2 <30 mm Hg)[a]
      C. Cardiopulmonary arrest[a]
      D. Acute respiratory failure + renal failure[a]
      E. Pulmonary edema[a]
      F. Metabolic acidosis with inadequate respiratory compensation due to pulmonary disease (COPD, pleural effusion), CHF, severe hypokalemia, severe PO_4 depletion[a]
  II. Respiratory acidosis plus metabolic alkalosis
      A. COPD + diuretics/Na restriction/glucocorticoids
      B. ARDS + nasogastric suction[a]
 III. Respiratory alkalosis plus metabolic acidosis
      A. Septic shock[a]
      B. Liver disease[a]
         1. Hepatorenal syndrome
         2. Cirrhosis + alcoholic ketoacidosis or RTA
      C. Salicylate intoxication
      D. Severe burns treated with Sulfamylon[a]
      E. Recovery phase of severe metabolic acidosis
      F. Hemodialysis (high mass transfer of acetate)

Table 12.46. (continued)   Examples of Mixed Acid-Base Disorders

IV. Respiratory alkalosis plus metabolic alkalosis
   A. CHF + diuretics[a]
   B. Posthypercapneic metabolic alkalosis[a]
   C. Cirrhosis + vomiting[a]
   D. Pregnancy + vomiting/diuretics
   E. Excessive HCO_3^- therapy in metabolic acidosis with persistence of compensatory hyperventilation[a]
   F. Sepsis + massive transfusions or nasogastric suction[a]
   G. Severe hypoxemia + metabolic alkalosis
V. Acute and chronic respiratory acidosis: COPD with exacerbation (infection, O_2 therapy, sedatives)[a]
VI. Metabolic acidosis plus metabolic alkalosis
   A. Diarrhea + vomiting/nasogastric suction
   B. Renal failure + vomiting/nasogastric suction
   C. Ketoacidosis + vomiting/nasogastric suction
   D. Organic (lactate, ketones) acidosis + "overshoot" metabolic alkalosis from excessive HCO_3^- therapy[a]
VII. Mixed metabolic acidosis
   A. Mixed hyperchloremic and high-anion gap metabolic acidosis
   B. Mixed high-anion gap acidosis
   C. Mixed hyperchloremic acidosis
VIII. Triple disorder
   A. Metabolic acidosis + metabolic alkalosis + respiratory acidosis
   B. Metabolic acidosis + metabolic alkalosis + respiratory alkalosis

[a]Common in surgical patients.

REFERENCES

1. Hou SH, Bushinsky DA, Wish JB, et al. Hospital acquired renal insufficiency: a prospective study. Am J Med 1983;74:243–248.
2. Shusterman N, Strom BL, Thomas MG, et al. Risk factors and outcome of hospital-acquired acute renal failure: clinical epidemiologic study. Am J Med 1987;83:65.
3. Shires GT, Carrico CJ. Renal responses. Philadelphia: WB Saunders, 1972.
4. Green J, Better OI. Systemic hypotension and renal failure in obstructive jaundice—mechanistic and therapeutic aspects. J Am Soc Neprol 1995;5:1853–1
5. Beaufils M, Morel-Maroger L, Sraer JD, et al. Acute renal failure of glomerular origin during visceral abscesses. N Engl J Med 1976;295:185.
6. Zappacosta AR, Ashby FL. Gram-negative sepsis with acute renal failure. Occurrence from acute glomerulonephritis. JAMA 1977;238:1389.
7. Spector DA, Millan J, Zauber N, et al. Glomerulonephritis and staphylococcal aureus infections. Clin Nephrol 1980;14:256.
8. Bennett WM, Plamp C, Porter GA. Drug-related syndromes in clinical nephrology. Ann Intern Med 1977;87:982.
9. Smith CR, Lipsky JJ, Laskin OL, et al. Double-blind comparison of the nephrotoxicity and auditory toxicity of gentamicin and tobramycin. N Engl J Med 1980;320:1106.
10. Byrd L, Sherman RL. Radiocontrast-induced acute renal failure: a clinical and physiologic review. Medicine 1979;58:270.
11. Van Zee BE, Hoy WE, Talley TE, et al. Renal injury associated with intravenous pyelography in nondiabetic and diabetic patients. Ann Intern Med 1978;89:51.
12. Harkonen S, Kjellstrand DM. Exacerbation of diabetic renal failure following intravenous pyelography. Am J Med 1979;63:939.
13. D'Elia JA, Gleason RE, Alday M, et al. Nephrotoxicity from angiographic contrast material: a prospective study. Am J Med 1983;72:719.
14. Lautin EM, Freeman NJ, Shoenfeld AH, et al. Radiocontrast-associated renal dysfunction: a comparison of lower-osmolality and conventional high-osmolality contrast media. AJR 1991;157:59–65.
15. Barrett BJ, Calisle EJ. Metaanalysis of the relative nephrotoxicity of high- and low-osmolality iodinated contrast media. Radiology 1993;188:171–178.
16. Schwab SJ, Hlatky MA, Pieper KS, et al. Contrast nephrotoxicity: a randomized controlled trial of nonionic and ionic radiographic contrast agent. N Engl J Med 1989;320:149.
17. Kunin CM. Detection, prevention, and manage-

ment of urinary tract infections. 3rd ed. Philadelphia: Lea and Febiger, 1979.

18. Schaberg DR, Haley RW, Highsmith AK, et al. Nosocomial bacteriuria: a prospective study of case clustering and antimicrobial resistance. Ann Intern Med 1980;93:420.

19. McHenry MC, Hawk WA, Straffon RA. Gram-negative bacillemia. Urol Clin North Am 1976; 3:333.

20. Nicolle LE, Mayhew WJ, Bryan L. A prospective randomized comparison of therapy and no therapy for asymptomatic bacteriuria in institutionalized elderly women. Am J Med 1987; 83:27.

21. Anderson RJ, Schrier RW. Clinical spectrum of oliguric and nonoliguric acute renal failure. In: Brenner BM, Stein JH, eds. Contemporary issues in nephrology: acute renal failure. New York: Churchill Livingstone, 1980.

22. Abel RM, Buckley MJ, Austen WG, et al. Etiology, incidence, and prognosis of renal failure following cardiac operations. J Thorac Cardiovasc Surg 1976;71:323.

23. Abbott WM. Renal failure complicating vascular surgery. In: Bernhard VM, Towne JB, eds. Complications in vascular surgery. New York: Grune & Stratton, 1980.

24. Bhat JG, Gluck MC, Lowenstein V, et al. Renal failure after open heart surgery. Ann Intern Med 1976;84:677.

25. Casali R, Simmons RL, Najarian JS, et al. Acute renal insufficiency complicating major cardiovascular surgery. Ann Surg 1975; 181:370.

26. McLeish KR, Luft FC, Kleit SA. Factors affecting prognosis in acute renal failure following cardiac operations. Surg Gynecol Obstet 1977; 145:28.

27. Tilney NL, Bailey GL, Morgan AP. Sequential system failure after rupture of abdominal aortic aneurysm. Ann Surg 1973;178:117.

28. Dawson JL. Renal failure in obstructive jaundice: clinical aspects. Postgrad Med J 1975; 51:510.

29. Hilberman M, Myers BD, Carrie BJ, et al. Acute renal failure following cardiac surgery. J Thorac Cardiovasc Surg 1970;77:880.

30. Berisa F, Beamon M, Adu D, et al. Prognostic factors in acute renal failure following aortic aneurysm surgery. Q J Med 1990;76:689–698.

31. Rossiter K, Kulaylat N, Anderson J: Acute renal failure, burns, and death: patterns and probabilities in the burn center (1991–1993) [abstract]. J Am Soc Nephrology 1995;6:474.

32. Anderson RJ, Linas SL, Berns AS, et al. Nonoliguric acute renal failure. N Engl J Med 1977;296:1134.

33. Brown CB, Ogg CS, Cameron JS. High dose furosemide in acute renal failure: a controlled trial. Clin Nephrol 1981;15:90.

34. Levinsky NG, Bernard DB, Johnston PA. Enhancement of recovery of acute renal failure: effects of mannitol and diuretics. In: Brenner BM, Stein JH, eds. Contemporary issues in nephrology. New York: Churchill Livingstone, 1980.

35. Tiller DJ, Mudge GH. Pharmacologic agents used in the management of acute renal failure. Kidney Int 1980;18:700.

36. Thompson JE, Vollman RW, Austin DJ, et al. Prevention of hypotensive and renal complications of aortic surgery using balanced salt solution. Ann Surg 1968;167:767.

37. Barry KG, Mazze RI, Schwartz FD. Prevention of surgical oliguria and renal hemodynamic suppression by sustained hydration. N Engl J Med 1964;270:1371.

38. Bismuth H, Kuntziger H, Corlette MD. Cholangitis with acute renal failure: priorities in therapeutics. Ann Surg 1975;181:881.

39. Shin B, Mackenzie CF, McAsland TC, et al. Postoperative renal failure in trauma patients. Anesthesiology 1979;51:218.

40. Polk HC, Vargas A. The prevention of postoperative renal failure. South Med J 1970;63: 1068.

41. Rastogi SP, Reid IS. Bilateral ureteral obstruction following aortic bypass surgery. Clin Nephrol 1980;14:250.

42. Hinman F. Postoperative overdistention of the bladder. Surg Gynecol Obstet 1976;142:901.

43. Mazze RI. Critical care of the patient with acute renal failure. Anesthesiology 1977; 47:138.

44. Coulie P, DePlaen JF, Van Ypersele de Strihou C. Captopril induced acute reversible renal failure. Nephron 1983;35:108.

45. Baek SM, Makabali GG, Shoemaker WC. Clinical determinants of survival from postoperative renal failure. Surg Gynecol Obstet 1975; 140:685.

46. Milligan SL, Luft FC, McMurray SD, Kleit SA. Intra-abdominal infection and acute renal failure. Arch Surg 1978;113:467.

47. Polk HC, Shields CL. Remote organ failure: a sign of occult intra-abdominal infection. Surgery 1977;81:310.

48. Cioffi WG, Ashikaga T, Gamelli RL: Probability of surviving postoperative acute renal failure. Development of a prognostic index. Ann Surg 1984;200:205.

49. Kornhall S. Acute renal failure in surgical disease with special regard to neglected complications. A retrospective study of 298 cases treated during the period 1960–1968. Acta Chir Scand (Suppl) 1971;419:3.

50. Hall JW, Johnson WJ, Maher FI, et al. Immediate and long-term prognosis in acute renal failure. Ann Intern Med 1970;73:515.

51. Merino GE, Buselmeier TJ, Kjellstrand CM. Post-operative chronic renal failure: a new syndrome? Ann Surg 1975;182:37.

52. Grazioni G, Cantaluppi A, Casati S, et al. Dopamine and furosemide in oliguric acute renal failure. Nephron 1984;37:39.

53. Chertow GM, Sayegh MH, Allgren RL, et al. Is the administration of dopamine associated with favorable outcomes in acute renal failure. Am J Med 1996;101:49–53.

54. Denton MD, Chertow GM, Brady HR. Renaldose dopamine for the treatment of acute renal failure: scientific rationale, experimental studies and clinical trials. Kidney Int 1996;49:4–14.

55. Conger JD. A controlled evaluation of prophylactic dialysis in posttraumatic acute renal failure. J Trauma 1975;15:1056.

56. Teschan PE, Baxter CR, O'Brien TF, et al. Prophylactic hemodialysis in the treatment of acute renal failure. Ann Intern Med 1960; 53:992.

57. Fischer RP, Griffen WO, Reiser M, et al. Early dialysis in the treatment of acute renal failure. Surg Gynecol Obstet 1966;123:1019.

58. Kleinknecht D, Graneval D. Preventive hemodialysis in acute renal failure. Its effect on mortality and morbidity. In: Friedman EA, Eliahou HE, eds. Proceedings conference on acute renal failure. DHEW Publications No. (NIH) 74-608. New York: National Institutes of Health, 1973:165.

59. Dudrick SJ, Steiger E, Long JM. Renal failure in surgical patients. Treatment with intravenous essential amino acids and hypotonic glucose. Surgery 1970:68:180.

60. Abel RM, Beck CH, Abbott WM, et al. Improved survival from acute renal failure after treatment with intravenous essential L-amino acids and glucose. Results of a prospective, doubleblind study. N Engl J Med 1973;288:695.

61. Baek SM, Makabali GC, Bryan-Brown CW, et al. The influence of parenteral nutrition on the course of acute renal failure. Surg Gynecol Obstet 1975;141:405.

62. Brown CB, Cameron JS, Ogg CS, et al. Established acute renal failure following surgical operations. In: Friedman EA, Eliahou HE, eds. Proceedings conference on acute renal failure. DHEW Publications No. (NIH) 74-608. New York: National Institutes of Health, 1973:187.

63. Spital A, Valvo JR, Segal AJ. Nondilated obstructive uropathy. Urology 1988;l21:478–482.

64. Miller TR, Anderson RJ, Linas SL, et al. Urinary diagnostic indices in acute renal failure. A prospective study. Ann Intern Med 1978;89:47.

65. Miller PD, Krebs RA, Neal BJ, et al. Polyuric prerenal failure. Arch Intern Med 1980;140: 907.

66. Zarich Z, Fang L, Diamond JR. Fractional excretion of sodium. Exceptions to its diagnostic value. Arch Intern Med 1985;145:108.

67. Knochel JP. Acute renal failure. Semin Nephrol 1981;1:5.

68. Conger J. Interventions in clinical acute renal failure: what are the data? Am J Kidney Dis 1995;26:565–576.

69. Levinsky NG, Bernard DB, Johnston PA. Mannitol and loop diuretics in acute renal failure. In: Brenner BM, Lazarus JM, ed. Acute renal failure. Philadelphia: WB Saunders, 1983: 712–722.

70. Alkhunazi AM, Schrier RW. Management of acute renal failure: new perspectives. Am J Kidney Dis 1996;28:315–328.

71. Champion H, Long W, Smith H, et al. Indications for early hemodialysis in multiple trauma. Lancet 1974;i:1125.

72. Hakim RM, Wingard RL, Parker RA. Effect of the dialysis membrane in the treatment of patients with acute renal failure. N Engl J Med 1994;331:1338.

73. Tzamaloukas AH, Garella S, Chazan JA. Peritoneal dialysis for acute renal failure after major abdominal surgery. Arch Surg 1973; 106:639.

74. Mayer AD, McMahon MJ, et al. Controlled clinical trial of peritoneal lavage for the treatment of severe acute pancreatitis. N Engl J Med 1985;312:399.

75. Bell C, Smithies M. Selection of patients for continuous renal replacement therapy. Semin Dialysis 1996;9:125.

76. Myers DB, Moran SM. Hemodynamically mediated acute renal failure [review]. N Engl J Med 1986;314:97.

77. Bellomo R, Mansfield D, Rumble S, Shapiro J, Parkin G, Boyce N. Acute renal failure in critical illness. Conventional dialysis versus acute continuous hemodiafiltration. ASAIO J 1992;38:M654.

78. Biasioli S, Barbaresi F, Barbiero M, et al. Intermittent venovenous hemofiltration as a chronic treatment for refractory and intractable heart failure. ASAIO J 1992;138:M658.

79. Bosch JP. Continuous arteriovenous hemofiltration (CAVH): operational characteristics and clinical use. Nephrol Lett 1986;3:15.

80. Bartlett RH, Mault JR, Dechert RE, et al. Continuous arteriovenous hemofiltration: improved survival in surgical acute renal failure? Surgery 1986;100:400.

81. Francis GS, Sharma B, Collins AJ, et al. Coronary-artery surgery in patients with endstage renal disease. Ann Intern Med 1980; 92:499.

82. Lansing AM, Leb DE, Berman LB. Cardiovascular surgery in end-stage renal failure. JAMA 1968;204:134.

83. Haimov M, Glabman S, Schupak E, et al. General surgery in patients on maintenance hemodialysis. Ann Surg 1974;179:863.

84. Brenowitz JB, Williams CD, Edwards WS. Major surgery in patients with chronic renal failure. Am J Surg 1977;134:765.

85. Burke GE, Gulyassy PF. Surgery in patients with renal disease and related electrolyte disorders. Med Clin North Am 1979;63:1191.

86. Dornfeld L, Narins RG. Pre- and postoperative renal failure. Urol Clin North Am 1976;3:363.

87. Egan JD. How to evaluate the surgical patient with renal disease. Geriatrics 1977;32:46.

88. Herrin JT. Preparation of the renal patient for surgery. Int Anesthiol Clin 1975;13:183.

89. Tasker PR, MacGregor GA, DeWardener HE. Prophylactic use of intravenous saline in patients with chronic renal failure undergoing major surgery. Lancet 1974;ii:911.

90. Silberman H. Renal failure and the surgeon. Surg Gynecol Obstet 1977;144:775.

91. Livio M, Gotti E, Marchesi D, et al. Uraemic bleeding: the role of anemia and beneficial effect of red cell transfusions. Lancet 1982;ii:1031.

92. Vigano G, Benigni A, Mendogini D, et al. Recombinant human erythropoietin shortens the uraemic bleeding time without causing intravascular haemostatic activation. Thromb Res 1990;7:171.

93. Janson PA, Jubilerer SJ, Weinstein MJ, et al. Treatment of the bleeding tendency in uremia with cryoprecipitate. N Engl J Med 1980;303:1318.

94. Mannucci PM, Remuzzi G, Posineri R, et al. Deamino-8-D-arginine vasopressin shortens the bleeding time in uraemia. N Engl J Med 1983;308:8.

95. Shapiro MD, Kelleher SP. Intranasal deamino-8-D-arginine vasopressin shortens the bleeding time in uremia. Am J Nephrol 1984;4:260.

96. Liu YK, Kosfeld R, Marcum SG. Treatment of uremic bleeding with conjugated estrogens. Lancet 1984;ii:887.

97. Smith JW, Seidl LG, Cluff LE. Studies on the epidemiology of adverse drug reactions: V. Clinical factors influencing susceptibility. Ann Intern Med 1966;65:629.

98. Bennett WM, Aronoff GR, Golper TA, et al. Drug prescribing in renal failure: dosing guidelines for adults. 2nd ed. Philadelphia: American College of Physicians, 1991.

99. Inturrisi CE. Disposition of narcotics in patients with renal failure. Am J Med 1977;62:528.

100. Bryan CS, Stone WJ. "Comparably massive" penicillin G therapy in renal failure. Ann Intern Med 1975;82:189.

101. Hatala R, Dinh T, Cook DJ. Once-daily aminoglycoside dosing in immunocompetent adults: a meta-analysis. Ann Intern Med 1996;124:717–725.

102. Finkelstein W, Isselbacher K. Cimetidine. N Engl J Med 1978;299:992.

103. Kasiske BL, Ramos EL, Gaston RS, et al. The evaluation of renal transplant candidates: clinical practice guidelines. J Am Soc Nephrol 1995;6:1–34.

104. Spanos PK, Simmons RL, Lampe E, et al. Complications of related kidney donation. Surgery 1974;76:741.

105. Terasaki PI, Cecka JM, Gjertson DW, et al. High survival rates of kidney transplants from spousal and living unrelated donors. N Engl J Med 1995;333:333–336.

106. Milutinovic J, Agodoa LCY, Cutler RE, et al. Autosomal dominant polycystic kidney disease. Early diagnosis and consideration of pathogenesis. Am J Clin Pathol 1980;73:740.

107. Bakkaloglu M, Hamilton NH, Macpherson SG, Briggs JD. Morbidity and mortality in renal transplant patients after incidental surgery. Br J Surg 1978;65:228.

108. Leapman SB, Vidne BA, Butt KM, et al. Elective and emergency surgery in renal transplant patients. Ann Surg 1976;183:266.

109. Brown RS, Epstein FH. Fluid and electrolyte disorders in urologic patients. Urol Clin North Am 1976;3:267.

110. Orloff MJ, Hutchin P. Fluid and electrolyte response to trauma and surgery. In: Kleeman CR, Maxwell MH, eds. Clinical disorders of fluid and electrolyte metabolism. New York: McGraw-Hill, 1972.

111. Chung HM, Kluge R, Schrier RW, et al. Postoperative hyponatremia. A prospective study. Arch Intern Med 1986;146:333.

112. Arieff AI. Hyponatremia, convulsions, respiratory arrest, and permanent brain damage after elective surgery in healthy women. N Engl J Med 1986;314:1529.

113. Baran D, Hutchinson TA. The outcome of hyponatremia in a general hospital population. Clin Nephrol 1984;22:72–76.

114. Berl T, Anderson RJ, McDonald KM, Schrier RW. Clinical disorders of water metabolism. Kidney Int 1976;10:117.

115. Arieff AI, Llach F, Massry SG. Neurological manifestations and morbidity of hyponatremia: correlation with brain water and electrolytes. Medicine 1976;55:121.

116. Karp BI, Laurenco R. Pontine and extrapontine myelinolysis: a neurologic disorder following rapid correction of hyponatremia. Medicine 1993;72:359.

117. Sterns RH, Cappuccio JD, et al. Neurologic sequelae after treatment of severe hyponatremia: a multicenter perspective. J Am Soc Nephrol 1994;4:1522.

118. Rhymer JC, Bell TJ, et al. Hyponatremia following transurethral resection of the prostate. Br J Urol 1985;57:450.

119. Gonzalez R, Brensilver JM, et al. Posthysteroscopic hyponatremia. Am J Kidney Dis 1994;23:735.

120. Campbell HT, Fincher ME, et al. Severe hy-

ponatremia with severe hypoosmolality following transurethral resection of the prostate (TURP) in end-stage renal disease. Am J Kidney Dis 1988;12:152.

121. Agarwal R, Emmett M. The post-transurethral resection of prostate syndrome: therapeutic proposals. Am J Kidney Dis 1994;24:108.

122. Snyder N, Feigal DW, Arieff AI. Hypernatremia in elderly patients. Ann Intern Med 1987;107: 309–319.

123. Palevsky PM, Bhagrath R, Greenberg A. Hypernatremia in hospitalized patients. Ann Intern Med 1996;124:197–203.

124. Blum D, Brasseur, et al. Safe oral rehydration of hypertonic dehydration. J Pediatr Gastroenterol Nutr 1986;5:232.

125. Kruse JA, Carlson RW. Rapid correction of hypokalemia using concentrated intravenous potassium chloride infusions. Arch Intern Med 1990;150:613.

126. Gerstman BB, Kirkman R, Platt R. Intestinal necrosis associated with post-operative orally administered sodium polystyrene sulfonate in sorbitol. Am J Kidney Dis 1992;20:159.

127. Shepard KV. Cleansing enemas after sodium polystyrene sulfonate enemas [letter]. Ann Intern Med 1990;112:711.

128. Allon, M, Dunlay R, Copkney C. Nebulized albuterol for acute hyperkalemia in patients on hemodialysis. Ann Intern Med 1989;110: 426–429.

129. Farr HW, Fahey TJ Jr, Nash AG, et al. Primary hyperparathyroidism and cancer. Am J Surg 1973;126:539.

130. Skrabanek P, McPartlin J, Powell D. Tumor hypercalcemia and "ectopic hyperparathyroidism." Medicine (Baltimore) 1980;59:262.

131. Ratcliffe WA, Hutchesson CJ, et al. Role of assays of parathyroid hormone-related protein in investigation of hypercalcemia. Lancet 1992; 339:164.

132. Beall DP, Scofield RH. Milk-alkali syndrome associated with calcium carbonate consumption. Report of seven patients with PTH levels and an estimate of prevalence among patients hospitalized with hypercalcemia. Medicine 1995;74:89.

133. Mundy GR, Wilkinson R, Heath DA. Comparative study of available therapy for hypercalcemia of malignancy. Am J Med 1983;74:421.

134. Cardella CJ, Birkin BL, Roscoe M, et al. Role of dialysis in the treatment of severe hypercalcemia: report of two cases successfully treated with hemodialysis and review of the literature. Clin Nephrol 1979;12:285.

135. Suleiman MY, Zaloga GP. How—and when—to manage ionized hypocalcemia in critically ill patients. J Crit Illness 1993;8:372–390.

136. Wong ET, Rude RK, Singer FR. A high prevalence of hypomagnesemia in hospitalized patients. Am J Clin Pathol 1983;79:348.

137. Ryzen E. Magnesium homeostasis in critically ill patients. Magnesium 1989;8:201.

138. Chernow B, Bamberger S, Stoiko N, et al. Hypomagnesemia in patients in post-operative intensive care. Chest 1989;95:391.

139. Knochel JP. The pathophysiology and clinical characteristics of severe hypophosphatemia. Arch Intern Med 1977;137:203.

140. Juan D, Elrazak M. Hypophosphatemia in hospitalized patients. JAMA 1979;242:163.

141. Lentz RD, Brown DM, Kjellstrand CM. Treatment of severe hypophosphatemia. Ann Intern Med 1978;89:941.

142. Slatopolsky E, Rutherford WE, Rosenbaum R, et al. Hyperphosphatemia. Clin Nephrol 1977; 7:138.

143. Carroll HJ, Oh MS. Water, electrolyte, and acid-base metabolism: diagnosis and management. Philadelphia: JB Lippincott, 1978.

144. Winter SD, Pearson R, Gabow PA, et al. The fall of the serum anion gap. Arch Intern Med 1990;150:311.

145. Gabow PA. Disorders associated with an altered anion gap. Kidney Int 1985;27:472.

146. Gabow PA, Kaehny WD, Fennessey PV, et al. Diagnostic importance of an increased anion gap. N Engl J Med 1980;303:854.

147. Rose DB. Clinical physiology of acid-base and electrolyte disorders. 4th ed. New York: McGraw-Hill, 1994:540–603.

148. Oh MS, Uribarri J, Carroll HJ. A cause of unusual organic acidosis in humans, not bacteria. Am J Kidney Dis 1988;11:80.

149. Mayne AJ, Dandy DJ, et al. Dietary management of D-lactic acidosis in short bowel syndrome. Arch Dis Child 1990;65:229.

150. Lyons JH, Moore FD: Posttraumatic alkalosis: incidence and pathophysiology of alkalosis in surgery. Surgery 1966;60:93.

151. Wilson RF, Gibson D, Percinel AK, et al. Severe alkalosis in critically ill surgical patients. Arch Surg 1972;105:197.

152. Shavelle HS, Parke R. Postoperative metabolic alkalosis and acute renal failure: rationale for the use of hydrochloric acid. Surgery 1975; 78:439.

153. Swartz RD, Rubin JE, Brown RS, et al. Correction of postoperative metabolic alkalosis and renal failure by hemodialysis. Ann Intern Med 1977;86:52.

154. McCurdy DK. Mixed metabolic and respiratory acid base disorders. Chest 1972;62:355.

155. Narins RG, Emmett M. Simple and mixed acid base disorders: a practical approach. Medicine 1980;59:161.

156. Goldberg M, Green SB, Moss ML, et al. Computer-based instruction and diagnosis of acid base disorders: a systematic approach. JAMA 1973;223:269.

13
Gastroenterology

Gerald A. Hofkin[1]

Disorders of the digestive system may affect the outcome of surgical procedures. This chapter emphasizes the preoperative assessment of patients with hepatic and peptic ulcer disease and the treatment of postsurgical complications related to the digestive system.

NUTRITION

Significant nutritional deficiencies may result from disorders of the intestinal tract. Impairment of wound healing and immune competence may result from protein malnutrition, and there may be depletion of the intravascular volume, electrolyte imbalance, protein loss, and catabolism. Evaluation of the patient's nutritional status and treatment of his or her nutritional deficiencies are described in Chapter 6.

LIVER DISEASE

Underlying liver disease may predispose a patient to greater surgical risk for deterioration of liver function. The advice of the consulting internist must be based on consideration of the pathophysiology and cause of the disease, the functional capacity of the liver, and the urgency of the surgery.

Pathophysiology

In general, liver disease can be divided into hepatocellular and cholestatic categories. In a1dvanced liver disease, there is a hyperdynamic cardiovascular state. Reduced responses to catecholamines exist, and both ascites and edema are prone to occur as these patients are in a sodium-avid state. Alcoholic cardiomyopathy may be present in patients who have abused ethanol over long periods of time. Renal blood flow is well preserved, and electrolyte abnormalities relate to increased aldosterone effect and diuretic therapy. Because of reduced hepatic blood flow, the metabolism of both exogenous and endogenous compounds and drugs is impaired, resulting in a decreased affinity of hemoglobin for oxygen because of changes in the red blood cell. Because of intrapulmonary shunts and possible hypoventilation, hypoxia may develop. In addition, pancytopenia may result from hypersplenism, and anemia may result from nutritional protein-calorie deficiencies, hemolysis, or gastrointestinal bleeding. Abnormalities of coagulation are not infrequent. Because of damage to the synthetic and metabolic responsiveness of hepatic cells, glucose intolerance also develops in these patients.

In cholestatic liver disease, which may result from either intrahepatic or extrahepatic causes, the cardiovascular changes are less pronounced than in hepatocellular disease. A prolonged prothrombin time is the most common co-

---

[1]Harold Tucker contributed to this chapter in the first and second edition of this book.

297

agulation abnormality found, resulting from a deficiency of vitamin K–dependent factors (2).

There is a dual supply of blood to the liver. The portal vein provides 75% of the oxygen for nutrient-rich blood, and the hepatic artery, which is oxygen rich, provides 25%. In addition, the liver is a blood reservoir that is capable of delivering 500 mL of blood into the circulation. α-Adrenergic control is the main regulator of hepatic portal flow. Since the sensitivity to catecholamines may be decreased in liver disease, the response to hypovolemia or hemorrhage may be impaired, and this response may be further inhibited through suppression of the sympathetic nervous system by anesthetics. The hepatocytes subserve the functions of storage, secretion, synthesis, metabolism, and detoxification.

Incidence of Complications

Although it is generally well accepted that severe liver disease poses special risks for surgical patients, the actual frequency of adverse outcomes from surgery is not well documented in the literature. Several reports have described hepatic deterioration following surgery in patients with acute hepatitis. Harville and Summerskill (3) reported a 9.5% operative mortality rate in patients with acute viral hepatitis (0% in patients with drug-induced hepatitis) and a 12% incidence of serious complications. These data suggests that the risk of surgery is significantly increased during acute viral hepatitis.

Increased mortality and morbidity rates may also occur in the setting of alcoholic hepatitis. The incidence of complications for nonshunt surgery in these patients is unknown.

Surgery in patients with cirrhosis has been accepted as carrying a high risk. Little literature is available, however, to document this increased risk, to quantify the magnitude of the risk, or to determine which factors identify subgroups of high-risk patients (4, 5).

Gallbladder surgery in the presence of cirrhosis carries a total mortality risk of over 20%. The risk rises to between 30 and 83% if the prothrombin time is prolonged. Not all of these deaths relate to the liver disease; liver disease–specific mortality figures are not available. The Child's classification, or the factors making up this index, seem to be predictive of mortality (Table 13.1) (6), similar to more extensive studies for mortality from portasystemic shunts (Table 13.2) (7).

Identification of High-risk Patients

Both the severity and the activity of liver disease are major determinants of the surgical risk in patients with hepatic dysfunction. Elevated levels of the transaminases, now named aspartate aminotransferase (AST), formerly known as serum glutamic-oxaloacetic transaminase (SGOT), and alanine aminotransferase (ALT), formerly known as serum glutamic-pyruvic transaminase (SGPT), indicate some degree of inflammatory activity in the liver. They are not useful as prognostic indicators, however, and they do not reflect severity of the hepatic pathology. Hypoalbuminemia, which is a reflection of impaired hepatic synthetic function, may indicate chronic liver disease and is an indicator of increased surgical risk.

Routine measurements of AST or ALT levels in asymptomatic patients without a history of liver disease is generally not indicated as a screening test because of

Table 13.1. Risk of Biliary Surgery in Cirrhosis: Preliminary Data on Child's Classification

Child's Classification[a]	Mortality (%)
A	13
B	25
C	50

Data from Cryer HM, Howard DA, Garrison RN. Liver cirrhosis and biliary surgery: assessment of risk. South Med J 1985; 78:138–141.
[a]See Table 13.2 for an explanation of this classification.

Table 13.2.   Classification of Hepatic Function and Surgical Risk for Portasystemic Shunt

	Child's Classification		
	A	B	C
Albumin (gm/100 mL)	>3.5	3.0–3.5	<3.0
Bilirubin	<2.0	2.0–3.0	>3.0
Ascites	None	Easily controlled	Poorly controlled
Encephalopathy	None	Minimal	Moderate to severe
Nutrition	Excellent	Good	"Wasted" to poor
Operative mortality[a]	0–1%	9–10%	>50%

Adapted from Child CG III. Portal hypertension. Philadelphia: WB Saunders, 1974; 82.
[a]Mortality rate for portasystemic shunting.

their low specificity (1). The prevalence of hepatitis in asymptomatic patients is also low at 0.25 per 1000. Transaminase, alkaline phosphatase, and bilirubin levels should be obtained for those patients in whom history, physical examination, or routine screening tests suggest either liver disease or risk factors for liver disease, including alcohol or drug abuse and other high-risk behaviors.

A useful classification of patients with liver disease combines both clinical and biochemical parameters (Table 13.2). Measurements of the serum bilirubin, albumin, and prothrombin time in conjunction with assessment of the patient's nutritional status, degree of ascites, and degree of encephalopathy are used to categorize patients, and with this classification, the surgical risk can be evaluated for different patients. Class C patients with obvious evidence of severe liver disease have the worst risk, with 53% operative mortality, while class A patients tolerate surgery well.

Differentiation between fatty liver and alcoholic hepatitis as well as determining the presence of active hepatitis (either acute or chronic) is best made by liver biopsy, not by various biochemical tests. Steatosis, or fat accumulation in the liver, disappears rapidly, usually within several weeks, once the patient abstains from alcohol and begins consuming a nutritious diet. Therefore, the finding of excessive fat

in the liver may warrant delaying surgery for several weeks to allow the liver function to improve. The presence of Mallory's bodies in liver biopsy specimens suggests a higher risk. Finally, cirrhosis can be readily detected in liver biopsy specimens, even when the biochemical parameters are only minimally abnormal or even normal (8).

For patients with newly discovered hepatomegaly or abnormal liver function tests, further investigation into the nature of the hepatic disease is indicated before surgery. Analysis of the results of liver function tests generally dictates the direction of the evaluation. Abnormalities of liver function tests can be divided into hepatocellular (e.g., hepatitis) and cholestatic patterns. Hepatocellular disease is characterized predominantly by elevations of the ALT and AST levels. Cholestatic liver disease is associated predominantly with elevation of the alkaline phosphatase level but either no or low elevations of the ALT and AST levels.

Hepatitis, either infectious or drug induced, is generally characterized by markedly abnormal transaminase levels, with only mild elevation of alkaline phosphatase. The family of known hepatitis viruses includes hepatitis A, B, C, delta, E, G, and GB, but the most common concerns are hepatitis A, B, and C. Further identification of the offending agent should be determined by measuring hepatitis B surface antigen (HBsAg), hepatitis B core antibody (HBcAb), hepatitis B surface antibody (HBsAb), hepatitis A antibody, and hepatitis C antibody, as well as by obtaining a detailed patient history of exposure to potential hepatotoxins (including alcohol and medications).

In patients with disproportionately high levels of alkaline phosphatase in relation to the transaminase levels, cholestatic liver disease should be suspected. Intrahepatic and extrahepatic causes of cholestasis may be differentiated by clues in the patient history and physical examination, but generally not by analysis of the chemistry values. Recent use of drugs that are known to induce cholestasis (e.g., phenothiazines, estrogen compounds) or the presence of a palpable gallbladder are helpful distinguishing features for intrahepatic and extrahepatic disease, respectively. A dilated biliary tract depicted by ultrasonography or computed tomography (CT) of the abdomen is a clear indication of extrahepatic disease (e.g., stones or tumor). Further preoperative delineation of the cause of extrahepatic obstruction can be obtained through endoscopic or transhepatic cholangiography. The overall accuracy of ultrasonography in distinguishing intrahepatic and extrahepatic cholestasis is 90% (9). The cause of intrahepatic cholestasis should be corrected before elective, non–biliary tract surgery as the morbidity and mortality rates of surgery in such patients may be increased. In patients with extrahepatic obstruction, mortality and morbidity for biliary tract surgery increases with increasing elevations of the bilirubin, particularly with levels greater than 20 mg per 100 mL (10).

Nonalcoholic fatty liver is a common cause of elevated liver enzyme levels, which often occur in asymptomatic patients when routine biochemistries are done during a periodic health maintenance or preoperative evaluation. The usual pattern elevated levels of AST and ALT with minimal or no elevations of alkaline phosphatase, but other patterns may occur. Either ultrasonography or CT may depict fatty liver, and use of these modalities has reduced the need for liver biopsy. The clinical and laboratory findings are usually not distinguishable from those of alcoholic fatty liver, except for a patient history or other findings of alcohol ingestion. Other causes of liver disease must be excluded.

Common, treatable complications of liver disease, which increase the risk of surgery, should be sought preoperatively in all patients with liver disease. These complications include encephalopathy, ascites, infection, electrolyte disturbance, gastrointestinal bleeding, infection, malnutrition, abnormal clotting factors and platelets, anemia, and decreased renal function. Medications should be reviewed to identify those that are hepatotoxic, will worsen liver function, or produce complications such as bleeding and encephalopathy; these especially include aspirin, sedatives, and pain medications.

In summary, patients undergoing anesthesia and surgery should be screened for liver disease by a careful patient history and physical examination. When evidence suggests the presence of liver disease, further evaluation is needed. In patients with significant liver disease, either acute or chronic, the morbidity and mortality rates from surgery appear to be increased. Hepatic deterioration commonly occurs in such patients postoperatively for a variety of reasons, including ischemic injury to the liver secondary to the effects of anesthesia on liver blood flow. Recognizing the severity of liver disease preoperatively is essential in predicting the risk of surgical procedures and preventing postoperative complications. Poor prognostic features include: *(a)* ascites, *(b)* encephalopathy, *(c)* poor nutritional status, *(d)* hypoalbuminemia, *(e)* hyperbilirubinemia, *(f)* prolonged prothrombin time, and *(g)* alcoholic hyaline on liver biopsy specimens.

Coagulation Defects

The prothrombin time is often prolonged in patients with severe liver disease, reflecting low levels of the clotting factors I, II, V, VII, IX, X, XI, and XII, whose production depends on normal liver function (11, 12). Thrombocytopenia because of hypersplenism, folate deficiency, and alcoholism is also common. These abnormalities need be identified and corrected before surgery.

In patients with a prolonged prothrombin time, parenteral vitamin K_1, 10 to 20 mg/day for 3 consecutive days, should be administered. This dose will generally correct the prothrombin time if coagulation defect results from obstructive jaundice or malabsorption. However, in advanced parenchymal liver disease with severe depression of the clotting factors, the prothrombin time may remain prolonged; in such cases, fresh-frozen plasma should be given preoperatively to correct the coagulation abnormality and continued through the operative and postoperative periods to prevent bleeding.

Platelet transfusions are rarely needed, because very low platelet counts are unusual and the platelets function normally. Thrombocytopenia may be caused by primary bone marrow suppression secondary to alcohol exposure or folate deficiency, or it may be caused by hypersplenism resulting from the portal hypertension. When hypersplenism is the cause, platelet transfusions have little value and will be rapidly consumed by the spleen.

Effect of Liver Disease on Renal Function

The incidence of postoperative renal failure may be increased in patients with marked hyperbilirubinemia. This complication occurs more often than in the anicteric population and is most common in those with obstructive jaundice. Various causes have been suggested, including hypoxia, decreased renal blood flow, possible toxic effects from bilirubin, and excess endotoxin produced from the patient's own bowel flora (10).

Diuretic-induced hypovolemia may result in hypotension during surgery, with its consequent deleterious effect on the liver. Similarly, hypokalemia may result from a brisk diuresis and precipitate hepatic encephalopathy. Other measures that have been recommended to prevent postoperative renal failure in patients with hyperbilirubinemia include volume repletion before surgery, selection of anesthetic agents with the least vasoconstrictive effect on renal blood flow, preoperative antibiotics to reduce bowel flora capable of producing endotoxins, and use of dopamine to dilate the splanchnic circulation (13). The efficacy of these various measures in preventing postoperative renal failure, however, has not been established.

Treatment

Patients with known liver disease should be prepared for surgery with attention paid to the possibility of specific postoperative complications. The risks of surgery should be well understood by the patient, his or her family, and the surgeon. The anesthesiologist should be well aware of the patient's hepatic disease, and any electrolyte abnormalities and coagulation defects should be corrected preoperatively. Ascites should be well controlled, and both infection and gastrointestinal bleeding should be sought and stabilized as effectively as the time before surgery allows. Nutritional support will be required in some cases of malnutrition. In addition, the patient's mental status should be documented preoperatively so that any changes occurring postoperatively can be readily identified. Care should be taken to maintain an adequate intravascular volume to minimize intraoperative hepatic ischemia while, at the same time, not excessively increasing portal pressure. Defining the patient's hepatic status preoperatively with attention paid to potential postoperative complications is the best way to handle these challenging patients.

The decision to proceed with, postpone, or cancel surgery depends on the type of liver disease and the urgency of the surgery; severity of the liver disease has a significant but less important impact on the surgical decision. In general, all but emergency, immediately lifesaving surgery should be postponed in the presence of acute viral or alcoholic hepatitis. Surgery should be postponed for drug hepatitis as well. There is no information regarding the optimal waiting time for elective surgery following acute hepatitis. However, general clinical guidelines suggest waiting for at least 6 weeks from the time that all clinical and laboratory parameters of hepatitis have normalized, although some authorities suggest waiting for up to 6 months. The decision in individual cases must also consider both the type and severity of the hepatitis and the urgency of the surgery.

Surgery needs to be carefully considered in the setting of cirrhosis. Patients in Child's class A with cirrhosis and no ascites, bilirubin concentration less than 2 mg per 100 mL, normal albumin level, no encephalopathy, and good nutrition seem to be at lower risk. A normal prothrombin time, stable rather than deteriorating cirrhosis, and lack of superimposed acute liver disease also appear to lower risk, although the latter two clinical factors have not been confirmed statistically.

There are no firm data on the risk of deteriorating liver function, major complications, or death in patients with no known liver disease but mildly elevated liver enzyme levels that are found unexpectedly during preoperative laboratory testing. Evaluation can often find a cause in patients with substantial elevations of liver enzymes (i.e., two or three times normal levels), but often no, or only an uncertain, etiology can be found in patients with small elevations.

Repeating the liver enzyme measurements is the first step in evaluating mild, unexpected abnormalities of liver function. Other tests that should be done include a full set of liver enzymes (i.e., AST, ALT, alkaline phosphatase), prothrombin time, and albumin level (if not done as part of the original blood testing).

Often, the results of repeat testing will be normal, either because of laboratory error or, more commonly, the way that normal values are set. Normal values for most screening batteries are based on the 95th percentile; therefore, 1 in 20 normal patients will be screened as abnormal. If the remainder of the patient history, physical examination, and laboratory tests point against the presence of liver disease, this is often as far as the evaluation needs to be taken.

If the repeat liver enzyme levels remain elevated, the enzymes should be evaluated as for patients with liver disease (described earlier) and the surgery postponed. If laboratory testing does not discover a cause of the liver dysfunction, possibilities to be considered are hidden alcoholism (a very common cause), medications (especially over the counter, such as aspirin), drug abuse, and a mild viral illness. If no cause can be found, as is often the case, the surgery might be postponed until the situation is clarified. However, if the elevations are only a few points, the surgery is minor, and only local or regional anesthesia will be used, surgery may not need to be postponed.

In patients with severe liver disease, efforts should be made to correct coagulopathy and electrolyte abnormalities as well as to control infection, encephalopathy, and ascites. The prothrombin time should be maintained within 3 seconds of the control value. Vitamin K, 10 mg parenterally, or fresh-frozen plasma should be used for this purpose. When present, hypokalemia and hyponatremia usually result from use of diuretics.

If possible, massive ascites should be reduced. A diagnostic paracentesis should be done when the patient presents for the first time, and several key tests need to be performed on the ascitic fluid:

1. *Ascitic fluid albumin*: Use of the serum–ascites albumin concentration gradient has replaced the total protein content to classify the cause of the ascites (14). The serum–ascites

albumin gradient is superior to the exudate–transudate concept in the differential diagnosis of ascites. This gradient is calculated by subtracting the ascitic fluid albumin concentration from the serum albumin concentration. Values greater than 1.1 g/dL indicate that cirrhosis is the cause of ascites; values less than 1.1 g/dL suggest causes such as carcinomatosis, tuberculosis, pancreatic ascites, heart failure, nephrotic syndrome, constrictive pericarditis, or Budd-Chiari syndrome.

2. *Cell count and cultures*: More than 250 polymorphonuclear cells per milliliter of ascitic fluid indicates bacterial peritonitis.

3. *Cytology*: In the presence of malignant ascites, cytology will give a positive result in at least 60% of cases.

In the treatment of patients with normal renal function who are excreting at least 30 mEq of sodium in the urine per day, salt restriction will produce a response. Unless the serum sodium concentration is less than 120 mEq/L, however, fluid restriction has no additional benefit. In patients with chronic ascites and excretion of less than 10 mEq of sodium per liter of urine, diuretic therapy is required. A weight loss of approximately 0.5 kg/day avoids potential electrolyte problems. Spironolactone is used in a starting dose of 100 mg/day and can be increased stepwise to 400 mg/day depending on the patient response; it usually takes several days after initiating therapy for the effect of a drug to be seen. Patients must be monitored for azotemia and hyperkalemia. Furosemide is used to enhance the effect of spironolactone, is usually started at 40 mg/day, and can be increased to 160 mg/day. Thiazide diuretics should be avoided because of the risk of triggering hepatic encephalopathy. Nonsteroidal anti-inflammatory drugs (NSAIDs) should not be used because of the danger of inducing water retention.

Massive ascites that does not respond to adequate therapy will respond to large-volume paracentesis of up to 6 L with the administration of 40 g of albumin intravenously, which is a safe and effective treatment. Although quite effective in relieving ascites, peritoneovenous shunts are associated with complications of disseminated intravascular coagulation and sepsis. Transjugular intrahepatic portosystemic shunts (TIPS), which is the side-to-side portacaval shunt created by interventional radiologists, successfully controls ascites, although there may be an initial delay before the full natriuretic response is evident. Occlusion of TIPS can occur as well. Encephalopathy is the most frequent and troublesome complication of this procedure.

Special Considerations

HBsAg Carriers

Patients who are chronic carriers of HBsAg pose the special problem of infecting surgical personnel and contaminating hospital equipment. Such patients may be entirely asymptomatic, with normal liver function, or they may suffer from chronic hepatitis. For asymptomatic carriers without evidence of liver disease, there is no increased risk from surgery, nor is there any evidence of activation of the virus by anesthesia (15).

Effects of Anesthesia

In general, inhalation agents decrease hepatic blood flow. There may also be hepatotoxicity. Halothane is well recognized as causing severe hepatic dysfunction, with an incidence of approximately 1 in 6000, and the toxic mechanism is probably immunogenic. Furthermore, its effect on both synthetic and excretory function and hepatic oxygen supply and blood flow are greater than those of other inhalation agents. Risk is increased in women and those who have had multiple exposures to the medication, in the presence of obesity, and in middle-aged patients.

Enflurane and isoflurane are safe to use in patients with liver disease. Nitrous oxide has no hepatotoxicity (16), and although intravenous anesthetics and opiates do not significantly affect hepatic function, dosing adjustments may be needed. For example, the half-life of lidocaine is increased by approximately 300% and that of benzodiazepines by 100% in liver disease. In patients with decreased serum albumin levels, the dosage of drugs bound to albumin (e.g., pentothal) must be reduced. Atracurium and vecuronium, which are muscle relaxants, may be used in liver disease.

In patients with decompensated disease, it is a good practice to reduce the initial dose by 50%. Then, modify subsequent doses based on patient tolerance.

Effects of Surgery on the Liver

Minor surgical procedures are unlikely to cause changes in the intestinal blood flow. However, exploratory laparotomy does reduce blood flow to the intestines and the liver related to both endocrine and paracrine activation. The greatest reduction in hepatic blood flow occurs with upper abdominal surgery, and biliary tract surgery is most likely to result in elevation of the so-called "liver function tests." Factors that may also affect hepatic blood flow include hypotension, hypoxia, sepsis, congestive failure, and hemorrhage.

Surgical Risk with Liver Disease

Patients with acute viral hepatitis and who undergo laparotomy have a reported 10% mortality rate and 12% morbidity rate. These rates related to the extent of surgery. The approach to patients with subclinical hepatitis, however, is more difficult. In general, if the transaminase levels are greater than 3 times the normal value for the performing laboratory, surgery should be postponed. Another indicator of high risk is prolongation of the prothrombin time, the activated partial thromboplastin time, or both. Also of interest, drug-induced hepatitis has a lesser adverse impact on surgical risk.

Patients with chronic hepatitis must be evaluated based on their liver function. Few studies on the question of surgical risk in chronic hepatitis have been published, but asymptomatic patients with good synthetic capacity are at no significantly increased risk.

The type of alcoholic liver disease also influences the surgical risk. Severity of the liver dysfunction may be underestimated by the transaminase levels, because these levels frequently are only mildly abnormal. An indication of the reserve capacity of the liver is found by measuring the prothrombin time, and the histologic finding of alcoholic hyaline indicates a worse outcome from surgery. Patients with an alcoholic fatty liver without evidence of significant liver dysfunction do not present an increased surgical risk; however, acute alcoholic hepatitis is associated with a high mortality. Such patients should have their surgery postponed until there has been clinical improvement, biochemical improvement, and abstinence for 3 months.

Whether resulting from alcohol, viral disease, or immunologic disease, cirrhosis has an increased rate of postoperative mortality. Risk factors include Child's class B and C, which take into the account the presence of ascites, albumin level, bilirubin level, and coagulopathy. Abdominal surgery and preoperative infection are associated with poor outcome.

Laboratory clues to the diagnosis of alcoholic liver disease include reduction of the γ-glutamyl transpeptidase (GGT) when the patient is hospitalized and unable to obtain alcohol as well as a ratio of AST to ALT of greater than 2:1. This ratio occurs because alcoholic liver damage produces leakage of mitochondrial AST. The Child's class C patient has obvious evidence of severe liver disease, with a 53% risk of operative mortality.

The value of measuring the serum ammonia level is limited, because factors other than hepatic function also influence this level. Therefore, the serum ammonia level alone should not be used as a measure of liver function. In the presence of an elevated alkaline phosphatase level, GGT will differentiate its origin from that found in bone. Together with the clinical findings, laboratory studies form the basis of the Child-Pugh classification of liver disease. This classification correlates well with clinical prognosis.

Postoperative Treatment

Postoperative treatment of patients with known liver disease is similar to preoperative treatment, with close monitoring and correction of any abnormalities of coagulation, electrolytes, and fluid balance. Monitoring for and correction of hepatic encephalopathy and infection are also necessary.

When liver dysfunction occurs postoperatively in patients who had no liver disease preoperative, a search for the cause is necessary. In the immediate postoperative period, the number of conditions that may cause liver dysfunction are limited. They include exacerbation of subclinical chronic hepatitis, drug-induced hepatitis, anesthesia-induced hepatitis, blood transfusions, infection, and intraoperative hepatic hypoxia. In addition, acute viral hepatitis that was not clinically expressed preoperatively can manifest itself postoperatively.

The first manifestation of postoperative liver dysfunction may be jaundice. This can occur because of the increased bilirubin load from hemolysis, hematomas, or blood transfusions, or it can occur secondary to hepatocellular injury because of hypoxia or drugs and extrahepatic biliary obstruction. The first step is to assess what fraction of the total bilirubin is direct reacting. If the predominance of the bilirubin is indirect reacting, then hemolysis is the most common cause. The presence of predominantly direct-reacting bilirubin with elevated levels of alkaline phosphatase and GGT indicates a biliary cause, either intrahepatic or extrahepatic.

The next study should be ultrasonography of the gallbladder and liver with a search for dilated ducts. Ultrasonography is the preferred imaging modality for studying the biliary tract and ductal dilatation; abdominal CT is the preferred imaging modality for visualization of the pancreas.

The treatment of postoperative jaundice is supportive and specific only for the treatment of any complications. The treatment of ascites has already been discussed.

Treatment of bleeding esophageal varices has undergone significant changes since the last edition of this book. Infusion of Octreotide is effective in the treatment of acute variceal hemorrhage. This involves an IV loading dose of a 50-μg bolus of Octreotide that is followed by a continuous infusion of 50 μg/h for 48 hours (17). Sclerotherapy and, more recently, variceal banding have become the interventional techniques of choice for the treatment of variceal bleeding. Use of nadolol, 80 mg/day, adjusting to the heart rate was decreased by 25% or less than 55 beats per minute, and oral isosorbide, added progressively to a dose of 40 mg twice a day, significantly decreased the likelihood of variceal rebleeding following sclerotherapy (18). TIPS is a highly effective technique for the treatment of acute variceal hemorrhage that is unresponsive to endoscopic sclerotherapy, and because aspiration pneumonia is the major cause of mortality during bleeding esophageal varices, early intubation for airway protection is essential in these patients (19). The use of vasopressin as an infusion for the treatment of variceal bleeding is no longer advocated, however, because of the high incidence of serious reactions to this drug in the arterial vasculature throughout the body. In addition, controlled studies have failed to demonstrate a benefit from the use of vasopressin intravenously. As a result of the pharmacologic approaches as well as the endoscopic techniques described, use of open surgical portacaval shunts is exceedingly rare at present.

Both the intraoperative, operative, and postoperative care of patients with liver disease involves protection of the caregivers from exposure to any potentially infectious agents. Therefore, patients with active hepatitis A, HbsAg, or HBcAb without the presence of HbsAb, and all patients with hepatitis C, should be identified (even with use of universal precautions within the hospital and doctors' offices).

Intercurrent Liver Disease and Pregnancy

Viral hepatitis, biliary tract disease, toxic hepatitis, nonviral hepatic infections, and Budd-Chiari syndrome may occur during pregnancy. Viral hepatitis is the most common cause of jaundice in women of childbearing age. Of all cases of jaundice during pregnancy, approximately 40% relate to viral hepatitis, with the exception of epidemic non-A, non-B hepatitis, in which the presentation, course, and treatment are similar in women who are pregnant and in women who are not. Prematurity, but not congenital malformation, can be attributed to viral hepatitis. Hepatitis B is far less contagious than hepatitis A, but with hepatitis B, there is the potential of transmission to the fetus during delivery. These infants will not become HBsAg positive for at least a month or two after birth, however, and this lag time provides the rationale for prophylaxis by combined administration of hepatitis B immune globulin and hepatitis B virus vaccine.

Epidemic non-A, non-B hepatitis is now thought to result from hepatitis E, which is an RNA virus frequent in Southeast Asia, Africa, and Mexico. The morbidity and mortality rates of this viral disease are much higher in pregnant women than in any other group. The clinical treatment of acute viral hepatitis is conservative, and as breastfeeding does not lead to transmission of the infection, it may be continued. Unnecessary obstetric procedures such as amniocentesis should be avoided (20, 21).

Biliary tract disease is one of the most frequently encountered surgical diseases during pregnancy, and the clinical presentation varies little from that seen in nonpregnant women. Ultrasonography is the imaging modality of choice. Initial treatment should consist of intravenous fluids, nasogastric suction, and parenteral antibiotics if there is an indication of sepsis. Medical therapy is often successful, and cholecystectomy may be deferred until after delivery. Endoscopic retrograde cholangiopancreatography (ERCP) with papillotomy and stone extraction is possible, particularly in those patients with pancreatitis, and it may be preferable to surgery. Bile acid–dissolution therapy in pregnant women is not indicated, however, because these substances cross the placenta. Use of ERCP has virtually eliminated the use of extracorporeal biliary lithotripsy.

Budd-Chiari syndrome (i.e., obstruction of hepatic venous outflow because of hepatic vein thrombosis with onset during pregnancy) is uncommon. Since its natural history is progressive in relentless hepatic failure and ascites, various therapies have been attempted, including thrombolytic therapy, percutaneous transluminal angioplasty, and surgical therapies, including side-to-side portacaval shunting and thrombectomy (22).

Nonviral Hepatic Infections

The most common parasitic infection that involves the liver in temperate climates is amebiasis. Women are more susceptible than men to hepatic abscess, and pregnant women represent an even greater risk. Metronidazole and emetine are used in the treatment of amebiasis. Women must be counseled about the teratogenic effects of these drugs, but this therapy is almost always successful.

Preexisting Liver Disease in Pregnancy

Women with cirrhosis do not easily become pregnant, and those who conceive have a high incidence of fetal wastage. The complications of portal hypertension and cirrhosis (i.e., cholestasis, ascites, and variceal bleeding) are all exacerbated during pregnancy. Cooperation between the internist, gastroenterologist, obstetrician, and surgeon is essential when caring for the pregnant woman with cirrhosis. Treatment of the complications of cirrhosis is basically similar to that in nonpregnant women.

Autoimmune chronic liver disease in the absence of significant portal hypertension is not particularly detrimental in women who are pregnant. Prompt recognition and treatment of the hepatic complications of pregnancy have reduced the fatality rate, and improved therapy for chronic liver disease as well as successful orthotopic liver transplantation have also improved the prospects of pregnant women with chronic liver disease.

PANCREATITIS

Epidemiology

It has long been a dictum that surgery should be avoided in the presence of acute pancreatitis. Factors associated with acute pancreatitis that may increase the surgical risk include preoperative hypovolemia and electrolyte disturbance; technical factors in dealing with peripancreatic tissues that are inflamed, edematous, and highly vascular; potential for introducing infection into the inflamed pancreatic tissue, thus producing an infected pseudocyst or pancreatic abscess; increased renal and pulmonary complications; and postoperative exacerbation of pancreatitis. Following surgery, it may be difficult to distinguish the consequences of the surgical procedure from the complications of ongoing pancreatitis. Thus, in most patients of acute pancreatitis, surgical exploration should be avoided.

Evaluation

Because of the variable clinical presentations of acute pancreatitis, it may be difficult to establish the diagnosis or distinguish this condition from other disorders that require surgical therapy. While acute abdominal pain and hyperamylasemia are the most characteristic features of acute pancreatitis, other conditions, including cholecystitis, choledocholithiasis, penetrating peptic ulcer, and intestinal infarction, may present in a similar fashion. In these conditions, use of ultrasonography and CT of the abdomen may be helpful; in others, only serial observations of the clinical course over several hours or days may permit definitive differentiation among these clinical entities.

The laboratory diagnosis of acute pancreatitis is based on the detection of hyperamylasemia greater than three times the upper limits of normal. The lipase level, which has a delayed rise from and prolonged fall to normal, may be more specific; it tends to be less than three times the upper limit of normal in conditions such as perforated ulcer, mesenteric ischemia, and renal failure (23). In the setting of abdominal pain, a significantly elevated lipase level indicates acute pancreatitis until proven otherwise (23). The magnitude of the rise in serum amylase does not correlate with the severity of attack, and prolonged hyperamylasemia does not indicate developing complications. The amylase:creatinine clearance ratio is only useful for diagnosing asymptomatic macroamylasemia; therefore, this ratio has no value in diagnosing acute pancreatitis. With the technologic advancements in noninvasive imaging techniques, improved diagnosis is now possible quite early in the course of the disease. Ultrasonography is the most sensitive (67%) and specific (100%) method of biliary tree evaluation (24).

Computed tomography with contrast is the imaging method of choice for evaluating the pancreas in moderately severe to severe disease. The scan, however, may be normal in up to one-third of patients with mild disease.

Clinical severity of the disease during the first 48 hours may be determined by criteria combining clinical and laboratory data. The original criteria, created by Ranson et al., has been modified by physicians in Glasgow, producing the so-called "modified Glasgow criteria" (25):

Age > 55 years
White-blood-cell count > 15×10^3 cells/mL
Glucose > 180 mg/dL
Blood urea nitrogen > 45 mg/dL
Lactic dehydrogenase > 600 U/L
Albumin < 3.3 g/dL
Calcium < 8 mg/dL
Oxygen partial pressure < 60 mm Hg

Among patients with fewer than three of these factors during the first 48 hours, the mortality rate is very low. As the number of risk factors increases, however, the mortality and morbidity rates also increase. The acute physiology and chronic health evaluation (i.e., APACHE) grading score done on admission has been demonstrated to predict survival; if the score is less than eight during the first 48 hours, survival is assured (26).

Treatment

The role of surgery in the treatment of pancreatitis has become more limited with the availability of ERCP and interventional radiologic procedures. Surgical exploration may still be required for an impacted common duct stone, drainage of an abscess or pseudocyst, or for other conditions such as an infarcted bowel or perforated viscus. The timing of cholecystectomy and the role of common bile duct exploration in patients with gallstone-induced pancreatitis remains controversial. Nevertheless, cholecystectomy is the standard therapy for biliary pancreatitis. It has been accepted that surgery should be postponed for up to 6 weeks following an acute attack for the effects of pancreatic inflammation to subside. There is some evidence that the optimal time to operate is during the same hospitalization, usually 5 to 7 days after resolution of the acute pancreatic inflammation (27).

Patient with mild pancreatitis can be treated by stopping oral intake and using both intravenous hydration and parenteral analgesics on a regular schedule. In the presence of vomiting, use of nasogastric suction is helpful; otherwise, nasogastric tubes do not hasten patient recovery. The degree of recovery is based on the clinical status of the patient rather than on the level of lipase or amylase. If the patient is afebrile with evidence of bowel function, all feedings can be resumed despite abnormalities in these enzyme levels. Convincing evidence that a fat-restricted diet is especially helpful to patients with acute pancreatitis is lacking, but use of other medications, including H_2-receptor antagonists, anticholinergics, and pancreatic enzyme replacement, in the treatment of mild pancreatitis have shown no efficacy unless there was an underlying condition known to benefit from such medications.

If possible, removal of factors that may have precipitated the attack, such as alcohol, toxins, and gallstones, is advisable. In severe acute pancreatitis, complications can rapidly develop that affect the cardiovascular, pulmonary, and renal systems, and treatment in an intensive care unit may be needed. The specific therapy prescribed will be dictated by which systems have been affected. In this setting and in the presence of fever, antibiotic therapy is beneficial.

POSTOPERATIVE PANCREATITIS
Epidemiology

The most common cause of postoperative pancreatitis at present is ERCP. The mechanism of this injury includes rupture of ducts during the injection of contrast material, reactions of the ductal system to the contrast material, as well as other factors that may remain unidentified. The severity of post-ERCP pancreatitis can range from mild abdominal pain with elevated amylase levels lasting 24 hours to a prolonged course lasting several

weeks and requiring use of total parenteral nutrition. Common bile duct exploration, sphincteroplasty, distal gastrectomy, and splenectomy are the surgical
operations most frequently associated
with postoperative pancreatitis. The condition is thought to result from injury to
the gland or from an obstructed flow of
pancreatic juices. Cardiopulmonary bypass and cardiac transplantation have
been associated with pancreatitis, and it is
thought that hypoperfusion or emboli may
be the mechanism responsible (28). Acute
pancreatitis has been observed following
inguinal hernia repair, parathyroidectomy, and thyroidectomy. The mechanism
by which the pancreatitis is induced following these surgeries, however, is unknown (29).

Treatment

Treatment includes careful attention to
intravascular volume, electrolyte balance,
and relief of pain. In this regard, analgesics should be prescribed on a scheduled
rather than an "as-needed" basis. Total
parenteral nutrition should be employed
in patients who are moderately to severely
ill, but the use of nasogastric suction is not
recommended unless vomiting is present.
Intravenous antibiotics may be helpful as
well. Other therapies, such as H_2-receptor
antagonists, atropine, glucagon, somatostatin, indomethacin, aprotinin, fresh-
frozen plasma, and peritoneal lavage,
have been tried in pancreatitis, but little
objective evidence supports their use.

PEPTIC ULCER DISEASE

Epidemiology

Peptic ulcer disease is quite common.
However, the literature contains little
information concerning the effect of existing peptic ulcer disease on the outcome of
nonulcer surgery.

A group of patients at high risk for
ulcers that may be clinically silent at the
time include elderly patients who are
taking NSAIDs. A significant number of
patients with peptic ulcer disease may
remain asymptomatic until a complication
such as hemorrhage or perforation occurs.
Theoretically, patients with a history of
ulcer disease might be more likely to
develop exacerbations during the perioperative period. There is little evidence to
suggest an increased risk of new peptic
ulcers forming perioperatively, however,
and there is no evidence for an increased
risk of stress ulcerations in patients with
a previous history of peptic ulcer disease.

Risk factors for peptic ulcer disease
include smoking tobacco, use of NSAIDs,
and a family history of peptic ulcer disease. Identification of the relationship of
Helicobacter pylori to peptic ulcer disease
has been one of the outstanding medical
discoveries in the past decade (30). Testing
for *H. pylori* is indicated if ulcer disease is
present; it has been estimated that over
95% of duodenal ulcers and over 60% of
gastric ulcers are associated with this
bacteria. Available tests for this organism
include a nonradioactive urea breath test,
a serologic test for antibodies, and endoscopic biopsy staining for the bacteria.

Features in the patient history suggesting exacerbation of the ulcer condition
include: (a) change in the pain–food relief
pattern, (b) change in the daily pattern of
pain, (c) nocturnal pain, (d) radiation of
the pain to the back, and (e) vomiting.
Food typically relieves the pain of duodenal ulcers, but for patients with gastric
ulcers, the pain may not have a clear
relationship to meals or may even be
exacerbated by eating. Vomiting and
weight loss may occur in such patients. On
physical examination, epigastric tenderness may be elicited, and the stool may be
positive for occult blood.

The diagnosis of peptic ulcer disease
can be confirmed by barium contrast radiography or by endoscopy. With these
techniques, not only ulcers but gastritis
and gastric erosions can be identified.
Nevertheless, barium studies are less sensitive and specific than endoscopy. Upper
endoscopy is generally well tolerated, and

in the preoperative setting, if documentation of an ulcer crater would alter plans for surgery, endoscopy is the diagnostic test of choice. For patients with active ulcer disease, elective surgery is generally deferred until the ulcer has healed. The major concern is the risk of precipitating either hemorrhage or perforation in the postoperative period, because gastric acid output is increased. The mucosal resistance of the stomach may be diminished during periods of hypotension and hypoxia that occur during surgery. Nevertheless, the incidence of postoperative ulcer-related complications is poorly documented in the literature. It would appear to be prudent, however, to delay elective surgery until healing has occurred. Healing, rather than simple relief of symptoms, is necessary, because the presence of ulcer pain correlates poorly with the presence of an ulcer crater, particularly in patients older than 65 years of age.

Patients with active ulcer disease should be treated intensively for 4 weeks or so before surgery. If patients are on NSAIDs, these should be stopped if possible. Tobacco is interdicted as well. The H_2-receptor antagonists cimetidine, ranitidine, famotidine, and nizatidine are equally effective and usually well tolerated. The proton-pump inhibitors omperzole and lansoprazole can also be used and may offer an advantage in the rapidity with which healing of ulcers occurs. Sucralfate is also effective, acting topically and with little systemic absorption. Antacids may be used on an "as-needed" basis by the patient to control symptoms.

Eradication of *H. pylori* holds the promise of preventing recurrence of ulcer disease, and several different regimens have been developed. Most involve simultaneous administration of from two to four drugs for 2 weeks, followed by an H_2-receptor antagonist in therapeutic doses for another 2 to 4 weeks. The proton-pump inhibitors omeprazole or lansoprazole combined with clarithromycin is a two-drug regimen that is effective in approximately 80% of cases. Another regimen

that involves three drugs, but only in tablet form, is marketed under the trade name of Tritec. This regimen includes a tablet containing both ranitidine and bismuth citrate, and it is taken with a course of clarithromycin. Clarithromycin resistance is a problem, and in such cases, a four-drug regimen that includes bismuth subsalicylate, tetracycline, metronidazole, and a proton-pump inhibitor for 2 weeks has been successful. With the development of treatment for *H. pylori*, use of low-dose, long-term H_2-receptor antagonists to prevent ulcer recurrence has become less frequent. When such maintenance therapy is used, the H_2-receptor antagonist is given as a single dose at bedtime (e.g., cimetidine, 400 mg; ranitidine, 150 mg; famotidine, 20 mg).

If *H. pylori* is present, treatment for gastric ulcers is similar to that for duodenal ulcers. In patients receiving NSAIDs, these drugs should be stopped. No NSAID is completely safe, and no dosage of an NSAID is completely safe. If, however, the NSAID cannot be discontinued, then use of a proton-pump inhibitor is protective against both gastric and duodenal ulcer development in this setting. Use of misoprostol, a prostaglandin analogue, helps to reduce the effects of NSAIDs on the mucosa of the stomach and duodenum. Because of the small but real possibility of a gastric ulcer representing a malignancy, all gastric ulcers should be followed to complete healing, and large ulcers may require up to 12 weeks of therapy for this to occur.

Stress Ulcers

Epidemiology

Acute stress ulcers or erosions may present with postoperative gastrointestinal hemorrhage. These lesions represent disruptions in the gastric or duodenal mucosa that are rapid in onset and occur in the setting of severe physical stress. Retrospective endoscopic studies in high-risk patients with trauma or burns have identified discreet mucosal changes that occur within the first 24 to 72 hours in over 75% of these patients (31).

Significant bleeding occurs infrequently from the superficial lesions. Clinically ill patients in an intensive care unit and who have respiratory failure or sepsis have an extremely high incidence of stress ulcers.

The pathophysiology of stress ulcer formation is uncertain. Ischemic injury, disruption of the mucosal barrier, and impaired energy metabolism of the gastric mucosal cells have all been suggested.

Evaluation

Clinically, stress ulcers usually present with painless bleeding, either slow and occult or massive. Endoscopy provides the best method for establishing the correct diagnosis. During endoscopy, multiple superficial lesions may be seen, and these occur most often in the proximal portion of the stomach. Barium studies have little diagnostic value in this setting. At times, elective angiography may be helpful.

Treatment

Primary therapy should aim at preventing the formation of stress ulcers in those critically ill patients with the highest incidence of such ulcers. Prophylactic therapy may include antacids, sucralfate, or an H_2-receptor antagonist. In a study of patients on mechanical ventilation (32), the mortality rate was not significantly different among these three therapies; however, patients who received sucralfate had a lower median gastric pH and significantly less frequent gastric bacterial colonization.

It is recommended that critically ill patients with sepsis or on respirators be given some form of stress prophylaxis. If a nasogastric tube is in place, administration of sucralfate appears to be most appropriate; when no nasogastric tube is present, intravenous administration of an H_2-antagonist in sufficient quantity to maintain an intragastric pH greater than 4 is recommended. Once bleeding has occurred from stress ulcers, supportive therapy is needed. Raising the intragastric pH to 7 by antacids is not superior to standard therapy. Nevertheless, this measure should be tried to stem the bleeding. Other therapies with varying efficacy include the intravenous infusion of octreotide or vasopressin. Selective intra-arterial infusion of vasopressin after angiography is able to control acute gastric mucosal hemorrhage (33). Complications of vasopressin administration include myocardial, mesenteric, and systemic vasoconstriction as well as water overload from its antidiuretic effect. Intravenous vasopressin for mucosal hemorrhage may be initiated before angiography, but its effect on mucosal hemorrhage has not been well studied. Surgery for stress ulceration carries a high mortality rate and requires extensive gastric resection; such surgery is reserved for bleeding that is refractory to medical or endoscopic therapy.

Gastroesophageal Reflux

Gastroesophageal reflux may be exacerbated by surgery as a result of the abdominal distention associated with an ileus and prolonged nasogastric intubation. If the patient has a preoperative history of significant reflux, the head of the bed should be elevated to at least 30 at all times and the nasogastric tube removed as soon as possible. Intravenous H_2-receptor antagonists can be used to decrease both the acidity and the volume of gastric contents. Metoclopramide can be given intravenously at a dose of 10 mg every 6 hours to promote gastric emptying and improve the lower esophageal sphincter tone. An alternative intravenous medication is low-dose erythromycin, such as 200 mg intravenously every 6 hours; erythromycin is effective because of its motilin-like activity. When the patient is able to take all feeding, Cisapride, 10 to 20 mg four times a day, may be used as a promotility agent. Drugs that reduce the lower esophageal sphincter tone, such as anticholinergics and antidepressants, should be avoided if possible.

COMPLICATIONS FROM SURGERY

There is little evidence that extraintestinal surgery is associated with any increased risk, such as for exacerbation of ulcerative colitis or Crohn's disease in patients with inflammatory bowel disease. Stressful events may produce increased symptoms in some patients, but this reaction is highly variable and unpredictable—even in the same patient. When exacerbations of the disease do result, specific therapies should be instituted. There are scant data to support prophylactic increases in the dosage of steroids or other therapeutic agents before surgery, but patients who have been on all mesalamine preparations or sulfasalazine before surgery may need alternative medications in the postoperative period until they are able to resume their oral medications. An increased steroid dose may be needed in these particular patients, or the concomitant use of parenteral antibiotics, such as intravenous metronidazole, may be needed. Those patients with inflammatory bowel disease and receiving long-term steroid therapy will require an increased steroid dosage for stress during the immediate operative and postoperative periods.

Jaundice

Epidemiology and Pathophysiology

Jaundice is an infrequent complication of surgery. The incidence varies with the type of surgery, occurrence of intraoperative hypotension, use of various drugs, and the patient's underlying preoperative liver function. Severe jaundice develops in approximately 2% of patients with shock (34), and jaundice develops in 25% of patients undergoing cardiopulmonary bypass surgery (35). Cytomegalovirus hepatitis may develop after cardiac surgery as well. Delayed-onset jaundice following surgery most often results from posttransfusion hepatitis (PTH) caused by hepatitis C.

Three pathophysiologic mechanisms are responsible for postoperative jaundice: *(a)* overproduction of bilirubin, *(b)* hepatocellular dysfunction, and *(c)* extrahepatic obstruction (Table 13.3). In some cases, clear delineation of the specific cause may be impossible, but an understanding of the underlying mechanism allows a rational approach to such patients. The mechanism of jaundice is suggested by the relative elevation in the level of unconjugated (i.e., indirect) and conjugated (i.e., direct) bilirubin, as well as by the relative rise in the serum transaminase and alkaline phosphatase levels.

Hemolysis and reabsorption of blood results in an overproduction of bilirubin pigment, which causes an indirect component, jaundice. Associated with hemolysis are an elevated reticulocyte count and

Table 13.3.   Classification of Postoperative Jaundice

I. Increased pigment load
   A. Hemolysis
   B. Transfusions
   C. Resorption of hematomas or hemoperitoneum
II. Impaired hepatocellular function
   A. Hepatitislike picture
      1. Viral hepatitis
      2. Drug- and anesthetic-induced hepatitis
      3. Ischemia
      4. Sepsis
      5. Post-pump syndrome
   B. Cholestatic picture
      1. "Benign" intrahepatic cholestasis
      2. Drug-induced cholestasis
      3. Sepsis
   C. Fatty liver and cirrhosis following intestinal bypass surgery
   D. Hepatic resection
   E. Hepatic transplantation and rejection
III. Extrahepatic obstruction
   A. Choledocholithiasis
   B. Bile duct injury
   C. Pancreatitis
   D. Cholecystitis

Adapted from LaMont J, Isselbacher K. Postoperative jaundice. N Engl J Med 1973; 288:305–307.

lactate dehydrogenase level and a depressed haptoglobin level.

When the jaundice is predominantly direct reacting, differentiation must be made between hepatic parenchymal disease and extrahepatic obstruction. Hepatocellular dysfunction can present as a hepatitislike pattern or as cholestasis. The picture of hepatocellular cholestasis can mimic that occurring with extrahepatic biliary obstruction in the biochemistry studies.

Bilirubin Pigment Overproduction

The liver is responsible for handling approximately 300 mg of bilirubin, formed from the breakdown of hemoglobin resulting from the destruction of senescent erythrocytes. A small portion of the bilirubin comes from immature cells in the spleen and bone marrow, and a smaller portion is formed in the liver from heme proteins such as myoglobin and cytochromes. When liver function is impaired or the erythrocyte breakdown is rapid and massive, the hepatic capacity can be overwhelmed, and jaundice ensues. Hypoxia, hypotension, and sepsis impair the liver's ability to handle bilirubin. Excessive pigment load that can overwhelm the liver reserve comes from massive hemolysis, resorption of hematomas or hemoperitoneum, and transfusion of stored red blood cells.

Jaundice from postoperative hemolysis is commonly caused by blood transfusions, sickle cell anemia, and glucose-6-phosphate dehydrogenase. Drugs such as aspirin, sulfonamides, sulfones, and nitrofurans can reduce hemolysis in these patients. Hemolytic episodes in patients with sickle cell anemia may be precipitated by hypoxia or infection at the time of surgery.

In patients with preexisting liver disease, blood transfusion may result in jaundice. In addition, prolonged cardiopulmonary bypass contributes to decreased erythrocyte survival during cardiac surgery.

Resorption of blood from hematomas, gastrointestinal bleeding, or intraperitoneal bleeding causes excessive production of bilirubin. However, jaundice in these situations usually occurs only when parenchymal liver disease is also present (36).

Hepatocellular Dysfunction

The most common cause of postoperative jaundice is hepatocellular dysfunction. Medications, hypoxia, decreased liver blood flow, and sepsis may cause injury to the liver during surgery, and either a hepatitic or a cholestatic picture may result. A few conditions may produce a mixed picture.

Hepatitislike Pattern

Hepatocellular inflammation can result from anesthetic compounds, drugs, infections, and ischemia. The clinical, biochemical, and histologic presentation for these various conditions may be similar.

Halothane-induced liver injury is infrequent but serious. A similar hepatitislike pattern has been reported for enflurane, but this is rare. The National Halothane Study found an incidence of fatal liver injury secondary to halothane of 1 per 36,000. The cause of the liver damage is believed to be a hypersensitivity reaction (37). Repeated exposures, particularly within a short interval, and obesity appear to be major risk factors for severe liver injury, and a history of multiple exposures can be found in 75 to 90% of patients (38).

Clinically, halothane hepatitis presents with fever and leukocytosis occurring 2 to 3 days after surgery. Jaundice usually occurs within 3 to 10 days. Jaundice occurring more than 3 weeks after surgery is rarely the result of exposure to halothane.

Marked elevations in the bilirubin level (>10 mg per 100 mL) and prolongation of the prothrombin time are the most reliable biochemical indicators of a poor prognosis. Eosinophilia may occur, but its absence does not exclude halothane as a cause for the liver injury.

The histologic picture is one of acute hepatocellular necrosis. Fatty infiltration and eosinophils are occasionally found. In severe cases, massive necrosis may be seen, and cirrhosis may occur following repeated exposures (39).

In most cases, complete recovery occurs; however, the mortality rate is approximately 20%, with a wide range in the severity of acute illness. Chronic hepatitis is generally not a consequence of an isolated episode of halothane hepatitis. In patients with a history of halothane hepatitis, repeated use of this anesthetic agent is contraindicated; however, there is no evidence of increased risk from halothane in patients with preexisting liver injury. Treatment is supportive. Corticosteroids are of no value.

Methyoxyflurane hepatitis may be caused by a halogenated anesthetic agent that is structurally related to halothane. Its clinical picture is similar to that of halothane-induced hepatitis. Cross-sensitivity to halothane has been reported (31), and nonoliguric renal failure may occur in combination with hepatic injury or as a separate entity (40).

Drugs that are commonly administered in the perioperative period are also capable of causing liver damage. Drug-induced hepatitis may present with a hepatitislike pattern, a cholestatic pattern, or a mixed reaction (Table 13.4). Isoniazid, methyldopa, and tetracycline are examples of drugs that may produce a hepatitislike pattern, and careful scrutiny of the medication chart is necessary to identify exposure to potential hepatic toxins. With removal of the offending agent, the hepatitis rapidly resolves. Rechallenge is generally unnecessary, and it may even be hazardous. Liver biopsy generally is not revealing, because the specimen rarely demonstrates any features that are specific for drug-induced injury. The finding of peripheral eosinophilia or excessive eosinophilic infiltration in the portal area or in the hepatic parenchyma strongly suggests drug-induced hepatitis.

Ischemic hepatitis is an infrequent cause of postoperative jaundice, but it may play a significant role in hepatic deterioration postoperatively among patients with preexisting, severe liver disease. Patients with cirrhosis or active hepatitis tolerate hypotension poorly, and in patients with a normal hepatic architecture,

Table 13.4. **Drug-Induced Liver Injury**

Histologic Classification	Hepatocellular Necrosis	Cholestasis	Mixed (Hepatocellular Necrosis and Cholestasis)	Fat
Biochemical features				
SGOT, SGPT	↑↑ (often >10-fold)	↑	↑	Slightly ↑
Alkaline phosphatase	↑ (<3-fold)	↑↑ (>4-fold)	↑	Normal to ↑ slightly
Examples	Halothane, enflurane, methoxyflurane Isoniazid, Dilantin (phenytoin) Tetracycline, methyldopa	Chlorpromazine Oral contraceptives Erythromycin estolate Amitriptyline Chlorpropamide Anabolic steroids	Sulfonamides Phenylbutazone Thiouracil	Tetracycline Methotrexate

significant hepatic injury usually occurs only after prolonged hypotension, as in shock secondary to trauma or following a cardiac arrest. In such patients, marked elevations in transaminase levels and jaundice occur in the first week postoperatively. Transaminase values may range from a hundred to several thousand units, and the bilirubin level may rise to 20 mg per 100 mL. Other factors, such as transfusions, infections, and passive congestion of the liver from heart failure, may also play a role in promoting hepatic injury. In most cases, complete resolution occurs, often with rapid falls in the markedly elevated transaminase levels. The mortality rate is highest in patients with preceding hepatic disease, especially chronic, passive congestion of the liver resulting from congestive heart failure.

Posttransfusion hepatitis is another cause of hepatocyte damage and jaundice in postoperative patients. Unlike halothane hepatitis, which occurs within 2 weeks of exposure, PTH is usually not evident for up to 5 to 12 weeks following exposure. Because many patients undergoing major surgery receive blood, this diagnosis must be recognized as a potential late complication.

The major cause of PTH in the United States is hepatitis C virus. The prevalence of antibodies to hepatitis C virus among blood donors is 0.3%. Previously, hepatitis B virus was believed to be the main cause of PTH, but with routine screening of blood for hepatitis B over the past several years, it has now become an infrequent cause. At present, the incidence of PTH in hospitalized patients is similar to that of hepatitis among patients who do not receive blood transfusions (41).

Hepatitis A virus does not appear to play a role in PTH. The incubation period, generally 3 to 4 weeks, is too short for the observed incubation period of most PTH. Furthermore, hepatitis A is not associated with a chronic carrier state and does not progress to chronic liver disease, which are two features that characterize PTH. Nevertheless, there is the potential for transmission of hepatitis A by blood transfusion (42).

Evidence suggests the existence of more than one causative agent for PTH that is not hepatitis A or hepatitis B virus, hence the general term *non-A, non-B hepatitis*. The hepatitis C virus has been identified as the major virus in this group. Earlier indications of a non-A, non-B hepatitis unrelated to the hepatitis C virus have been found to be less convincing than they originally seemed (43). The virus is found in intravenous drug users, health care workers, persons of low socioeconomic status, and patients on hemodialysis.

The incubation period for transfusion-associated hepatitis C is 5 to 12 weeks, which is intermediate between that for type A and type B hepatitis. Only approximately 25% of these patients have jaundice. Clinically, the course of non-A, non-B hepatitis resembles more closely that of type B hepatitis, and overall, it appears to be less severe of an illness than hepatitis B. Hepatitis C RNA is detectable 1 to 2 weeks after infection. Transaminase levels rise, often up to 15 times their normal value, at 7 to 8 weeks. In those who recover completely, hepatitis C RNA is lost. Most patients will still have raised levels of transaminase at 1 year, and most of these persons will develop chronic hepatitis. Morphologically, the chronic hepatitis appears, using the older descriptive terminology, as either "chronic active" or "chronic persistent" hepatitis. Cirrhosis has also been noted in approximately 20% of patients with chronic disease, and hepatocellular carcinoma can complicate hepatitis C virus–related cirrhosis, usually after approximately 20 years (44). There is no evidence to support the use of steroids or immunosuppressive therapy for chronic non-A, non-B hepatitis. The only approved treatment for hepatitis C is interferon-α in a dose of 3 million U three times a week for at least 3 months. At that time, the level of hepatitis C RNA should have fallen. If so, therapy for another 3 months is recommended; if not, therapy should be discontinued. The overall success rate is only approximately 25%, however, and studies are in progress using other antiviral agents, such as ribavirin, with interferon (45).

Among the other viral agents that may cause PTH, only cytomegalovirus has been shown to be of definite clinical importance, particularly when the recipient of the blood transfusion is immunocompromised.

Extrahepatic Obstruction

Biliary duct obstruction may occur postoperatively from a variety of causes and may result in jaundice. This complication is significant, because endoscopic or surgical intervention may be required. Retained common duct stones may present with jaundice and an elevated alkaline phosphatase level; they must be differentiated from intrahepatic cholestasis syndromes. Most often, pain and fever are associated with the extrahepatic blockage, but retained stones should also be suspected in patients with persistent, painless jaundice following cholecystectomy. Imaging of the biliary tree is often necessary for the diagnosis to be made. The initial study may be abdominal ultrasonography, but cholangiography is frequently necessary and may be performed endoscopically (i.e., ERCP), either through a T-tube drain if the common duct has already been explored or by transhepatic cholangiography depending on the availability of facilities and the skill of the medical personnel. Intravenous cholangiography may be attempted if the bilirubin concentration is less than 2 mg per 100 mL. Should retained common duct stones be found, removal is generally indicated, which can be achieved by endoscopic sphincterotomy, reoperation, or through the T-tube (if still present).

Bile duct injury may inadvertently occur following upper abdominal surgery, common duct exploration, or cholecystectomy. Failure to properly identify the common bile duct intraoperatively can result in resection or ligation of the duct, which many times goes unrecognized during surgery. Jaundice often occurs within 1 week postoperatively, and it may be associated with cholangitis, bile peritonitis, and abscess formation. Prompt surgical repair is necessary to avoid further hepatic damage. Once injured, the bile duct may become strictured, thus leading to intermittent cholangitis, jaundice, and biliary cirrhosis if uncorrected.

Postoperative pancreatitis or cholecystitis may also cause postoperative jaundice or abnormal liver function tests. In 20 to 30% of patients with postoperative pancreatitis, jaundice occurs secondary to partial bile duct obstruction by the edematous pancreas. Postoperative cholecystitis is an unusual occurrence, but it may present with right upper quadrant pain and mild hyperbilirubinemia. The pathogenesis of both pancreatitis and cholecystitis in postoperative patients is unclear. High mortality has been reported with both complications.

Cholestatic Jaundice (Cholestasis)

Postoperative hepatic dysfunction may also present with a cholestatic picture that is characterized by markedly elevated alkaline phosphatase levels and hyperbilirubinemia. This pattern may occur as part of a benign intrahepatic cholestasis syndrome, secondary to drugs, or in association with sepsis.

Benign postoperative intrahepatic cholestasis is a syndrome occurring in postoperative patients that is characterized by transient cholestatic jaundice. The incidence of this complication is uncertain, but it generally occurs in one out of every several hundred general surgical patients. Schmid et al. (46) described 11 patients with postoperative cholestasis that occurred in one hospital during an 8-month interval. Typically, patients had undergone a major operative procedure and required multiple transfusions of blood. Jaundice was often noted on the first or second postoperative day but may have been delayed up to 10 days following surgery. The hyperbilirubinemia generally peaked about 1 week postoperatively, with values of 15 to 40 mg per 100 mL. The alkaline phosphatase was also abnormal, often with markedly elevated values. Transaminase levels were minimally abnormal. Hepatosplenomegaly and hepatic encephalopathy are not features of this condition, but liver biopsy specimens revealed characteristic changes of cholestasis, with bile canalicular dilatation, biliary casts, and bile staining of hepatocytes. Necrosis of liver cells and a prominent inflammatory infiltrate are not usually seen. These features reflect the cholestatic process; however, they are not specific for this postoperative syndrome as they may be found in drug-induced cholestasis as well.

The cause of this condition is unclear. Common features include hypotension, hypoxemia, and multiple blood transfusions. However, as discussed, these conditions generally do not produce a cholestatic pattern; more often, they cause hepatocellular necrosis.

The prognosis of this condition is good. Generally, jaundice subsides within 2 to 3 weeks. Resolution is complete, and chronic liver disease is not associated with this postoperative syndrome. Benign, transient cholestasis, however, must be differentiated from more serious causes of jaundice and, in particular, extrahepatic causes of jaundice (e.g., stones or common bile duct injury). Clinically, these conditions may be difficult to distinguish, especially during the first week, when bilirubin levels are rising. Hepatomegaly, abdominal pain, and fever suggest common bile duct obstruction rather than the syndrome of benign postoperative cholestasis. Ultrasonography usually clarifies the situation, but in doubtful cases, cholangiography, either ERCP or percutaneous transhepatic cholangiography, may be needed to differentiate these conditions.

Drug-induced cholestasis is another type of liver injury that must be considered in postoperative patients. A chole-static pattern may be seen following the use of various drugs such as chlorpromazine, erythromycin, anabolic steroids, oral hypoglycemic agents, and antithyroid medications. In general, drug-induced cholestatic injury is less likely to produce hepatic failure; therefore, it has a better prognosis than the acute hepatitislike syndrome. Rarely, however, a chronic cholestatic picture resembling biliary cirrhosis has been reported to develop following acute injury by drugs.

Sepsis has been associated with a cholestatic picture as well. Pneumococcal pneumonia and bacteremia with Gram-negative organisms are the infections most commonly associated with development of jaundice. The hepatic dysfunction is usually mild, with abnormalities of liver function tests usually occurring 5 to 12 days after the onset of infection (47). Other factors capable of causing liver damage, such as drugs and hypotension, are also often present. The mechanism for this type of injury associated with sepsis is unknown.

Treatment of Postoperative Hepatic Dysfunction

Postoperative hepatic dysfunction is most often mild, with complete resolution occurring in most patients. In a small percentage, however, the hepatic injury is extensive, and hepatic failure may occur. In patients with preexisting liver diseases, even mild damage may result in a marked deterioration in hepatic function, and in general, patients with a hepatitislike pattern of injury have higher morbidity and mortality rates than those who develop a cholestatic pattern postoperatively. In patients who develop hepatic coma, the mortality rate is greater than 80% (48).

Fulminant hepatic failure may occur as a complication of viral hepatitis or from exposure to hepatotoxic agents. The clinical course is one of rapid deterioration in mental status, often progressing from agitation to deep coma within several days. Serum transaminase levels are usually markedly elevated, bilirubin values rise progressively, and the prothrombin time becomes markedly prolonged. In patients with preexisting liver disease, hepatic failure may occur more insidiously, but mental status still deteriorates progressively and liver function tests worsen.

Therapy is largely supportive. Early identification of patients with severe liver injury and intensive effort to prevent potential complications are important. Therapy should be instituted to reduce blood ammonia levels and to prevent infection, bleeding, and electrolyte abnormalities. Drugs that may exacerbate encephalopathy, either by inducing further liver damage or deterioration in mental status, should be discontinued.

Oral protein intake should be reduced to no more than 50 g/day. Gastrointestinal bleeding should be treated aggressively, and colonic contents, including blood, should be evacuated with enemas and laxatives. Lactulose or sorbitol should be given to decrease the absorption and production of ammonia.

In addition to treating the encephalopathy, other complications should be prevented. Hypoglycemia may occur because of depleted glycogen stores and failure of gluconeogenesis within the liver, and its resultant symptoms may be confused with those of the hepatic encephalopathy. Monitoring of serum glucose levels and appropriate administration of glucose are essential. Gastrointestinal bleeding may occur from stress ulcers as often as from variceal hemorrhage in this setting, and prophylactic use of H_2-antagonists or proton-pump inhibitors are indicated. Finally, sepsis should always be suspected.

Ascites may develop in the face of hepatic dysfunction, but other potential causes in the postoperative setting must be ruled out as well. These include infections, either resulting from perforation of a viscus with peritonitis or spontaneous bacterial peritonitis; venous occlusion; pancreatic duct disruption; and metastatic disease. A diagnostic paracentesis should be done when the patient presents with ascites, and four key tests need to be performed on the ascitic fluid:

1. *Ascitic fluid albumin:* The serum–ascites albumin concentration gradient has replaced total protein content to classify the cause of the ascites (14, 49). This gradient is calculated by subtracting the ascitic fluid albumin concentration from the serum albumin concentration. Values greater than 1.1 g/dL indicate that cirrhosis is the cause of ascites; values less than 1.1 g/dL suggest causes such as carcinomatosis, tuberculosis, pancreatic ascites, heart failure, nephrotic syndrome, constrictive pericarditis, or Budd-Chiari syndrome.
2. *Cell count and cultures:* More than 250 polymorphonuclear cells per milliliter of ascitic fluid indicates bacterial peritonitis.
3. *Cytology:* The fluid should be collected for cytologic examination and placed in transport media at the bedside.

Variceal hemorrhage is a serious complication of postoperative hepatic dysfunction. Documentation that the bleeding results from varices is essential, because other causes of postoperative gastrointestinal bleeding require different therapies. Restoration of blood volume, correction of coagulation defects, and prevention of hepatic encephalopathy are all essential features in the treatment of these patients, and injection sclerotherapy or endoscopic variceal banding is the preferred method to arrest acute variceal bleeding. In addition, vasopressin could be infused intravenously to decrease portal pressure and control the variceal hemorrhage; the required dose usually ranges from 0.2 to 0.4 U/min following a bolus injection. Because of the arterial vasoconstrictor effect of vasopressin, concomitant use of a nitroglycerin medication, such as tridil intravenously, is indicated (50). Alternatively, octreotide, usually given as a 50-μg bolus intravenously and followed by 50 μ/h as a continuous infusion, may be used (51). For patients in whom vasopressin infusion fails, balloon tamponade may be beneficial. Use of this tube assembly requires greater expertise in placing the tube and maintaining its proper position; thus, endotracheal intubation is recommended in this situation to minimize the risk of aspiration (52). Use of this tube is a temporizing measure, however. The newest technique to control variceal hemorrhage that does not respond to endoscopic techniques has been given the acronym *TIPS*, which stands for *trans-jugular intrahepatic portosystemic shunt.* This interventional radiologic technique consists of inserting a stent through the jugular vein into the hepatic vein and then forcing it into a branch of the portal vein. The technique has a very good success rate (53), and its main complications are the development of portal encephalopathy and occlusion. The development and success of these methods of dealing with this life-threatening complication has replaced the use of emergency portacaval shunting.

Postoperative Cholecystitis

Acute cholecystitis, which is an infrequent postoperative complication, often presents as a diagnostic dilemma. The acute attack may develop following any form of surgery. It may occur within several days of the initial operation but it more often is delayed for up to 4 weeks postoperatively.

Clinically, the patient presents with fever, right upper quadrant pain, and tenderness. Mild liver enzyme abnormalities may occur with mild hyperbilirubinemia, and with this presentation in a postoperative setting, the condition is easily confused with a subhepatic abscess or with hepatic dysfunction. Radionuclear biliary scanning may demonstrate occlusion of the cystic duct, but both false-positive and false-negative scans frequently occur in this setting. In some patients, surgical exploration is needed before the diagnosis can be established,

because many of the usual preoperative tests may be either normal or difficult to perform. Pathologically, acute cholecystitis is found, but stones are absent in as many as 50% of patients. Common bile duct obstruction is generally not observed. The mechanism for this acalculous cholecystitis is unclear, but a similar phenomenon has been observed in patients with trauma. Gangrene of the gallbladder occurs in one-third of patients, and the mortality rate is reported to be as high as 20% (54).

Postcholecystectomy Syndrome

Pathophysiology and Epidemiology

The term *postcholecystectomy syndrome* has been applied to a heterogeneous group of disorders and symptoms that are present following cholecystectomy. The term is confusing, because it implies a causal relationship between the cholecystectomy and the symptoms that, in fact, does not exist in most cases. Indeed, in many cases, the symptoms are present before the operation and often are used as the indication for cholecystectomy. Categorizing such patients as having the postcholecystectomy syndrome only confuses the issue and obscures the correct diagnosis. Most often, patients with biliary dyskinesia present with recurrent biliarylike colic, often postprandially. Nausea and vomiting are common, and dyspeptic symptoms include vague abdominal discomfort following a meal, food intolerance, and gaseousness. Alteration in bowel habits are also reported, with both diarrhea and constipation occurring. Fever, chills, and jaundice are generally absent. The condition is more common in females between 20 to 50 years of age, and most patients with the syndrome have a thin-walled, unscarred gallbladder at the time of surgery.

The causes for postcholecystectomy syndrome are varied, and they include: *(a)* biliary tract disease, such as retained common duct stones, common bile duct strictures, stenosis of the sphincter of

Oddi, and cystic duct remnant; *(b)* extra-biliary tract disease, such as irritable bowel syndrome, gastritis, gastroesophageal reflux, peptic ulcer disease, and pancreatitis; and *(c)* functional disorders, such as biliary dyskinesia. Retained stones occur in approximately 40% of patients with postcholecystectomy syndrome following cholecystectomy. In more than 50% of patients, no demonstrable organic pathology can be found; motor abnormality of the extrahepatic biliary ductal system is then suspected (i.e., the so-called "biliary dyskinesia").

The cystic duct remnant has often been blamed for persistent syndromes following cholecystectomy. However, a remnant can be identified in many asymptomatic patients; thus, its causal relationship in symptomatic patients is unclear.

In some cases, the symptoms of irritable bowel syndrome are exacerbated following cholecystectomy. Irritable bowel syndrome may be characterized by intermittent and sometimes severe pain, and it may be overlooked in a patient with gallstones.

Evaluation

Currently, the diagnosis is generally made by exclusion of the other causes of postcholecystectomy syndrome. Careful evaluation of the biliary tract must be performed to rule out small stones or strictures, and liver function studies should be normal, even during an attack of pain. Other disorders, such as gastroesophageal reflux and the irritable bowel syndrome, are to be ruled out, as noted earlier. Endoscopic manometry of the sphincter of Oddi has demonstrated an altered pattern of abnormalities in patients with postcholecystectomy syndrome (55).

Postgastrectomy Syndromes

Postgastrectomy syndromes are uncommon but frustrating for both the patient and physician.

Postcibal Problems

Postcibal problems include abdominal pain, bilious vomiting, early satiety, and the dumping syndrome. The most common complaints include early satiety, postprandial vomiting, and epigastric pain. It has been suggested that postcibal complications relate to abnormal emptying of the fluid gastric contents into the small intestine. The onset of symptoms usually occurs within the first 30 minutes following a meal. Experimentally, distention of the proximal small bowel may reproduce many of these same symptoms, and vagotomy inhibits the fundic relaxation that occurs with the swallowing of food. Thus, as the stomach fails to distend, liquids in particular are emptied more rapidly into the small bowel, resulting in distention of the intestine as well as rapid delivery of hypertonic contents.

These complaints may be associated with vasomotor phenomena such as light-headedness, diaphoresis, and postural hypotension, the combination of which is termed the *dumping syndrome*. The effects of various hormones (e.g., serotonin, gastric inhibitory peptide) are thought to induce these vasomotor phenomena, and release of these hormones may be induced by intestinal distention, the influx of hypertonic solutions into the jejunum, or both.

Therapy for this condition is directed toward slowing the gastric emptying and avoiding hypertonic solutions and over-distention of the intestine. Frequent small feedings that are high in protein and low in carbohydrate have been recommended, and it important that liquids, which may accelerate gastric emptying, be avoided while eating a solid meal. Lying down after a meal may be beneficial as well, because it slows gastric emptying and may reduce the intensity of vasomotor symptoms.

The epigastric pain and vomiting may result from a variety of disorders. These include distention of the stomach or small bowel, afferent loop obstruction, gastric outlet obstruction, recurrent ulcerations, and reflux gastritis.

Partial afferent loop obstruction is an unusual complication that results in postprandial abdominal pain and bilious vomiting. The pain occurs with distention of the afferent limb by pancreatic and biliary secretions, which are stimulated following a meal. The vomiting is typically bilious and contains little, if any, food. The diagnosis is made by radiographic demonstration of a dilated, afferent limb that is slow to empty, and endoscopy may either document the inability to pass the endoscope into the afferent loop or demonstrate the retention of copious volumes of biliary secretions within the obstructed limb. When the diagnosis is established, surgical revision is necessary.

Gastric outlet obstruction, on the other hand, is generally associated with vomiting large amounts of retained or undigested food. Barium studies will typically demonstrate the gastric obstruction with retention of the barium. Causes for such obstruction include scarring or surgical deformity at the anastomosis as well as recurrent ulcerations, which may be documented by upper endoscopy.

Anastomotic ulcers must always be considered as a cause for postprandial pain and vomiting. These ulcers generally occur around the intestinal side of the anastomosis, and they most commonly present with epigastric pain. Air-contrast barium studies and endoscopy are both able to detect these lesions.

Bile gastritis (also termed *alkaline gastritis* or *reflux gastritis*) is a poorly defined entity that may cause abdominal pain and bilious vomiting. The correlation between severity of the symptoms and severity of both the gross and microscopic appearance of the gastritis is poor. When the gastritis is endoscopically and histologically severe and no other cause is evident, the diagnosis of bile gastritis is usually made.

Therapy for this condition is extremely difficult. No medical therapy has proven value or efficacy, and binding the bile

with cholestyramine has proved to have only a transient benefit. Use of proton-pump inhibitors may offer somewhat more benefit, however, and surgical diversion of the bile flow away from the stomach appears to be the most successful approach to ameliorating the patient's symptoms. Formation of a Roux-en-Y anastomosis has achieved very good results in a number of reports, but conversion of a vagotomy and pyloroplasty to a Billroth II or of a Billroth II to a Billroth I has been of little value.

Diarrhea

Chronic diarrhea is common following surgery for ulcers, occurring in 10 to 40% of patients. It appears to be a less common complication following parietal cell vagotomy. A prospective Veterans Administration study demonstrated no difference in the incidence of diarrhea at 2 and 5 years postoperatively (56). Causes for this type of diarrhea include: (a) rapid intestinal transit, (b) rapid gastric emptying, (c) lactose intolerance, (d) increase in fecal bile acid, (e) malabsorption, (f) gastrocolic fistula, (g) Zollinger-Ellison syndrome, and (h) inadvertent gastroileal anastomosis.

The evaluation of patients with postgastrectomy diarrhea follows the same guidelines as the evaluation of patients with chronic diarrhea. Significantly, one must differentiate the problems of absorption from those related to mechanical and motility factors. Thus, fecal collections for volume and fat content are important, with a fecal fat excretion of greater than 10 to 12% indicating significant malabsorption. Barium studies should also be performed to review the anatomy and to provide a crude estimate of the motility pattern.

Many of these patients respond to the empiric use of the bile salt–binding resin cholestyramine. Lactose intolerance is a common cause of diarrhea in the postgastrectomy setting, and patients with borderline levels of the intestinal enzyme lactase may become symptomatic with the rapid delivery of a lactose load. Thus, lactose-restricted diets are often advocated.

Significant malabsorption rarely occurs in the postgastrectomy state. Causes for malabsorption include poor mixing of food with pancreatic and biliary secretions, rapid transit, bacterial overgrowth in the afferent loop, and latent celiac disease being unmasked by ulcer surgery. When greater than 12% of ingested fat is excreted in the stool, evaluation for these causes should be performed. A blood test for antiendomysium antibodies has reduced the need for small-bowel biopsy to rule out celiac disease (57), and a hydrogen breath test may be useful in documenting bacterial overgrowth.

In still other patients, rapid transit will be seen on the barium study, and some patients will also complain of a prominent postprandial urge to defecate. In such patients, antidiarrheal medications such as diphenoxylate or loperamide may be useful.

Weight Loss

Weight loss is a significant problem following surgery for ulcers. A 10% reduction in preoperative body weight may occur after any standard ulcer operation. Often, these patients avoid eating because of postprandial symptoms, resulting in a reduction of their caloric intake. Encouraging these patients to consume small feedings, and even to supplement their intake with high-caloric additives, may be helpful.

Anemia

The gradual development of mild anemia (hemoglobin values, 10–12 g/mL) is common following surgery for ulcers, and it appears to occur somewhat more frequently after gastrojejunostomy than after other operations. Most frequently, this anemia results from iron deficiency. Iron absorption is commonly decreased in these patients because of bypass of the duodenum. In addition, reflux gastritis and stomal ulcerations may cause bleeding, thus accounting for the iron deficiency.

A macrocytic anemia may develop because of vitamin B_{12} or folate deficiency. Vitamin B_{12} deficiency develops in fewer than 10% of patients after gastrectomy, resulting from either loss of intrinsic factor secretion by the stomach or from bacterial overgrowth. Folic acid deficiency may also develop in the setting of bacterial overgrowth. This anemia is generally mild, and in patients with severe anemia or precipitous falls in the hemoglobin level, other causes should be considered.

Postoperative Recurrent Ulcer

Recurrent ulceration following surgery for ulcers is an infrequent but significant problem. The incidence of these anastomotic or marginal ulcers varies with the type of ulcer surgery that is performed, with a recurrence rate of less than 1% after vagotomy and gastric resection and from 6 to 8% after vagotomy plus pyloroplasty. These recurrent ulcers are most common on the intestinal side of the anastomosis.

Clinically, these ulcers present with abdominal pain, bleeding, and, often, weight loss. The pain from these ulcers may not be relieved by meals, vomiting and weight loss are common, and bleeding occurs in two-thirds of patients. Occasionally, the recurrent ulcer may penetrate into the colon, thus forming a gastrojejunal-colonic fistula, which can present dramatically with feculent vomiting.

The diagnosis is best made by endoscopy or an air-contrast, upper gastrointestinal series. A conventional barium study may miss these lesions in 50% of cases.

The most common cause for recurrent ulcerations is an inadequate initial surgery, either incomplete vagotomy or inadequate gastric resection. Other causes include retained antrum, ulcerogenic drugs, and Zollinger-Ellison syndrome.

Thus, an evaluation of these patients should include several fasting serum gastrin determinations to rule out Zollinger-Ellison syndrome and retained antrum. In both of these conditions, the gastrin level is markedly elevated, and they can be differentiated by performing a secretin stimulation test. After injection of the secretin, basal gastrin levels decline over the first 30 to 45 minutes in normal patients and in those with retained antrum. However, in patients with Zollinger-Ellison syndrome, gastrin levels paradoxically rise.

A gastric analysis is technically difficult to perform in patients after gastrectomy, because there is often mixing of gastric secretions with bile. The insulin-hypoglycemia gastric analysis (i.e., the Hollander test) carries too greater a risk of nervous system injury to be recommended.

Both medical and surgical therapy are useful in the treatment of recurrent ulcers. H_2-antagonists and proton-pump inhibitors are effective in the healing of these postoperative recurrences, but for patients in whom medical therapy fails or who develop a serious complication (e.g., bleeding, fistula formation) from the recurrence, surgical therapy is required. In general, a repeat vagotomy with more extensive gastric resection is required, with lesser operations resulting in a high frequency of second recurrence. In some patients with an initial adequate gastric resection, only a repeat abdominal or even a thoracic vagotomy may be needed.

parenteral nutrition, and the occurrence of abdominal distention was a particularly ominous sign.

Treatment includes discontinuation of antibiotic therapy, if possible, or changing the antibiotic regime, as well as replacement of fluid and electrolytes. Specific antibiotic therapy is indicated. Although *C. difficile* is highly sensitive to vancomycin, use of this antibiotic should be restricted to the most seriously ill patients because of the increasing prevalence of vancomycin resistance in general. The dose of vancomycin is 125 mg orally four times a day to 1 g orally three to four times a day for 10 days. Metronidazole is effective in oral doses of 250 mg four times daily for 10 days. For patients who are seriously ill, metronidazole may be given intravenously (60).

Although bacitracin is effective, it has a very unpleasant taste, and *C. difficile* resistance is not a rare occurrence. Use of cholestyramine is an option in mild or moderately severe cases, and specific antimicrobial therapy is more effective in severe cases. Cholestyramine binds vancomycin.

Use of antiperistaltic agents is to be discouraged, because they lead to intestinal stasis, toxin retention, and complications, particularly in older patients. Use of biotherapeutic agents in the prevention and treatment of intestinal infections has been reported, and the most effective agent in the treatment of *C. difficile* colitis is *Saccharomyces boulardii* (61). *Lactobacillus* sp. give more variable results.

POSTOPERATIVE DIARRHEA

Postoperative diarrhea can be a troublesome and a dangerous occurrence. One study (59) reported a mortality rate of 8% in patients with antibiotic-associated diarrhea, which most commonly results from the *Clostridium difficile* toxin. Risk factors for increased mortality that were identified included the use of multiple antibiotics, steroids, laxatives, and total

TREATMENT OF "OSTOMATES"

Proper treatment of the ostomate, which is the preferred term for a patient with an ostomy, begins with preoperative preparation of both the patient and his or her family. During this period, the patient should be encouraged to express both fears and concerns about being an ostomate. Certain aspects should be emphasized to the patient, including: (a) modern appliances are easy to use and keep the patient clean; *(b)* no one will be able to detect that the patient is wearing an appliance under his or her clothing; *(c)* there will be no problem with foul odor; *(d)* physical activity, including swimming, sports, and dancing, are not limited by an ostomy; and *(e)* sexual function depends on the results of the surgery but may remain normal.

A nurse who is specially trained in the management of ostomies and the treatment of ostomates (i.e., an enterostomal therapist) should visit the patient preoperatively. The therapist will mark the proper location for the ostomy depending on the patient's posture, skin crease lines, and location of the incision. The therapist is also helpful in providing information and counseling to the patient. In addition, a visit from a member of the local chapter of the United Ostomy Association is very helpful in allowing the patient to overcome any misconceptions about life with an ostomy.

Ileostomy

An ileostomy and a colostomy have differing features. Conventional ileostomies require that the patient continuously wear an appliance or pouch to retain the frequent discharge of ileal effluent. This pouch adheres to the skin by an adhesive that provides a water tight seal, and it can be emptied into a toilet by unclipping the bottom end of the pouch several times per day. The ileal discharge is watery and odorless. In some patients, a continent ileostomy is performed by creating a reservoir pouch in the abdomen from loops of the small bowel, thus allowing the patient to be free of an outer appliance. The patient can drain this intestinal pouch several times a day by inserting a catheter through a nipplelike opening in the abdominal wall and into the pouch. The choice of which type of ileostomy to perform depends on the patient's illness (e.g., Crohn's disease of the ileum is a contraindication), the experience of the surgeon, and the desires of the patient.

Colostomy

Most permanent colostomies are sigmoid colostomies (following the resection of a rectal carcinoma). As only the rectum is removed, the patient's preoperative bowel function will generally persist following surgery. Thus, patients who are "regular by the clock" in their bowel habits will continue that same pattern even with a colostomy, and they can develop control of the evacuation by use of irrigation enemas. As a result, some "colostomates" will need to wear only a small gauze pad instead of a pouch, whereas others will prefer the security of the pouch. Similarly, those patients who had erratic bowel habits preoperatively will continue to have unpredictable bowel movements through the ostomy. In these patients, continence between irrigations is very difficult, and the appliance will generally need to be worn.

When the colostomy is performed proximal to the splenic flexure, the discharge is looser and contains a greater liquid content. This type of colostomy is generally only temporary, such as to relieve obstructions or to permit healing of a diverticular abscess. This type of colostomy is less desirable as well, because evacuation is very frequent and cannot be controlled by irrigation. In addition, the discharge is malodorous because of colonic bacterial action. These ostomies are often placed above the belt line, thus making them difficult to wear an appliance. In short, a permanent ileostomy is preferable to this type of "wet" colostomy.

While in the hospital, both patients and their families should learn about management of the ostomy and the appliance and become comfortable with its use. The physician should also feel comfortable with inspecting the stoma periodically and being sure that patients are managing the appliance properly. At times, skin breakdown may be a problem, and hypersensitivity to adhesives or the pouch may also occur. Skin problems occur more frequently among the ileostomates. Skin irritation can be treated with a cortisone spray and an antifungal powder, and ointments and creams are both to be avoided as they interfere with adhesion of the appliance.

Occasionally, odor is a problem. This is more often the case in colostomates than in ileostomates. Dietary factors may be important, and certain foods such as onions, eggs, and oils should be eliminated in such cases. Malabsorption from small-bowel disease may also produce malodorous discharge. A variety of deodorants are available and can be placed into the pouch, and proper cleansing and drying of the appliance between uses is important in preventing colonization with odor-forming bacteria. The sudden onset of problems with excessive gas or odor should suggest the possibility of partial bowel obstruction.

Leakage rarely occurs with modern appliances under usual circumstances. Significant weight gain postoperatively or pregnancy, however, may alter the abdominal configuration, thus necessitating a refit of the appliance. The stoma can be expected to retract during the first few months postoperatively, and monitoring the amount of stomal protrusion is important. A stoma that is flush with the abdominal wall will create problems with leakage and frequently result in skin breakdown.

Significant problems related to the stoma include obstruction, prolapse, and retraction. Crampy abdominal pains, distention, vomiting, and diarrheal discharge suggest an obstruction, which may result from volvulus, herniation, or adhesions. Herniation can be suspected from the presence of a large parastomal bulge. The stoma may retract, or loops of bowel may prolapse through the stomal opening in the abdominal wall. These problems occur more frequently with ileostomies, and they usually require surgical consultation and correction.

Sexual dysfunction may occur secondary to neurologic impairment, depression with loss of libido, inhibition because of the stoma, and, occasionally, because of rejection by the spouse. Impotence is common after colostomies for rectal carcinoma, occurring in up to 50% of such patients; impotence following ileostomy is unusual. The physician should inquire about these potential problems. Supportive therapy, involvement in a local ostomy chapter, and, when appropriate, psychiatric therapy can all be very beneficial to the ostomate in coping with these problems. Newer surgical techniques, including ileoanal pull-through for patients with total colectomy and rectal mucosectomy for patients undergoing left-sided hemicolectomy for reanastomosis of the bowel, avoid many of these problems.

REFERENCES

1. Schemel WH. Unexpected hepatic dysfunction found in multiple laboratory screening. Anesth Analg 1976;55:810–812.
2. Conn M. Preoperative evaluation of the patient with liver disease. Mt Sinai J Med 1991;58:75–80.
3. Harville DD, Summerskill WH. Surgery in acute hepatitis. Causes and effects. JAMA 1963;184:261–275.
4. Friedman LS, Maddrey WC. Surgery in the patient with liver disease. Med Clin North Am 1987;71:453–476.
5. Aranha GV, Greenlee HB. Intra-abdominal surgery in patients with advanced cirrhosis. Arch Surg 1986;121:275–277.
6. Cryer HM, Howard DA, Garrison RN. Liver cirrhosis and biliary surgery: assessment of risk. South Med J 1985;78:138–141.
7. Resnick RH, Iber FL, Ishihara AM, Chalmers TC, Zimmerman H. A controlled study of the therapeutic portacaval shunt. Gastroenterolgy 1974;67:843–857.
8. Abdi W, Millan J, Mezey E. Sampling variability on percutaneous liver biopsy. Arch Intern Med 1979;139:667–669.
9. Malini S, Sabel J. Ultrasonography in obstructive jaundice. Radiology 1977;123:429–433.
10. Baum M, Sterling G, Dawson JL. Further study into obstructive jaundice and ischemic renal damage. BMJ 1969;2:229–231.
11. Strunin L. Preoperative assessment of the patient with liver dysfunction. Br J Anaesth 1978;50:25–31.
12. Robbins JA, Mushlin A. Preoperative evaluation of the healthy patient. Med Clin North Am 1979;63:1145–1156.
13. Siefkin AD, Bolt RJ. Preoperative evaluation of

the patient with gastrointestinal or liver disease. Med Clin North Am 1979;63:1309–1320.

14. Runyon BA, Montana A, Akriviadis EA, et al. The serum-ascites albumin gradient is superior to the exudate-transudate concept in the differential diagnosis of ascites. Ann Intern Med 1992;117:215–220.

15. Dykes MH. Is halothane hepatitis chronic active hepatitis? Anesthesiology 1975;46:233–235.

16. Gelman S. Anesthesia and the liver. In: Barash PG, Cullen BF, Stoetting RK, eds. Clinical anesthesia. Philadephia: JB Lippincott, 1989.

17. Sung JJY, Chung SCS, Ylai CW, et al. Octreotide infusion or emergency sclerotherapy for variceal hemorrhage. Lancet 1993;342:637–641.

18. Villanueva C, Balanzo J, Novella MT, et al. Nadolol plus isosorbide mononitrate compared with sclerotherapy for the prevention of variceal bleeding. N Engl J Med 1996;334:1624–1629.

19. Sanyal AJ, Freedman AM, Luketic VA, et al. Transjugular intrahepatic portosystemic shunts for patients with active variceal hemorrhage unresponsive to sclerotherapy. Gastroenterology 1996;111:138–146.

20. Rustgi VF, Hoofnagle JH. Viral hepatitis during pregnancy. Semin Liver Dis 1987;7:40–46.

21. Bjorkman DJ, Burt RW, Tolman KG. Primary care of women with gastrointestinal disorders. Clin Obstet Gynecol 1988;31:974–988.

22. Maddrey WC. Hepatic vein thrombosis (Budd-Chiari syndrome): possible association with the use of oral contraceptive. Semin Liver Dis 1987;7:32–39.

23. Gumaste V, Dave P, Sereny G. Serum lipase: a better test to diagnose acute alcoholic pancreatitis. Am J Med 1992;92:239–242.

24. Malini S, Sabel J. Ultrasonography in obstructive jaundice. Radiology 1977;123:429–432.

25. Blamey SL, Imrie W, O'Neil J, et al. Prognostic factors in acute pancreatitis. Gut 1984;25:1340–1346.

26. Wilson D, Heath DI, Imrie CW. Prediction of outcome in acute pancreatitis: a comparative study of APACHE-II, clinical assessment and multiple factor scoring systems. Br J Surg 1990;77:1260–1264.

27. Kelly TR. Gallstone pancreatitis: the timing of surgery. Surgery 1980;88:345–350.

28. Rattner DW, Gu ZY, Vlahades GJ, Warshaw AL. Hyperamylasemia after cardiac surgery: incidence, significance and management. Ann Surg 1989;209:279–283.

29. White TT, Morgan A, Hopton D. Postoperative pancreatitis: a study of 70 cases. Am J Surg 1970;120:132–137.

30. Peterson WL. *Helicobacter pylori* in peptic ulcer disease. N Engl J Med 1991;324:1043–1048.

31. Craja A, McAllnany JC, Pruitt BA Jr. Acute gastroduodenal disease after thermal injury: an endoscopic evaluation of incidence and natural history. N Engl J Med 1974;291:925–929.

32. Prod'hom G, Leuenberger P, Koerfer J, et al. Nosocomial pneumonia in mechanically ventilated patients receiving antacid, ranitidine or sucralfate as prophylaxis for stress ulcer. Ann Intern Med 1994;120:653–662.

33. Athanasoulis C, Baum S, Waltman AC, et al. Control of acute gastric hemorrhage with intra-arterial infusion of posterior pituitary extract. N Engl J Med 1974;290:597–603.

34. Nunes G, Blaisdell FW, Margaretten W. Mechanism of hepatic dysfunction following shock and trauma. Arch Surg 1970;100:646–656.

35. Chu C, Chang C-H, Liaw Y-F, et al. Jaundice after open heart surgery: a prospective study. Thorax 1994;39:52–56.

36. Kantrowitz PA, Jones WA, Greenberger NJ, Isselbacher KJ. Severe postoperative hyperbilirubinemia simulating obstructive jaundice. N Engl J Med 1967;276:590–598.

37. Klatskin G, Kimberg D. Recurrent hepatitis attributable to halothane sensitization in anesthetist. N Engl J Med 1969;280:515–522.

38. Summary of the National Halothane Survey. Possible association between halothane anesthesia and postoperative hepatitis. JAMA 1966;197:775–788.

39. Trey C, Lipworth L, Chalmers TC, et al. Fulminant hepatic failure. N Engl J Med 1968;279:798–801.

40. Joshi PH, Conn H. The syndrome of methoxyflourane-associated hepatitis. Ann Intern Med 1974;80:395–401.

41. Bianco C. Hepatitis testing. Immunol Invest 1995;24:155–161.

42. Lemon SM. The natural history of hepatitis A: the potential for transmission by transfusion of blood or blood products. Vox Sang 1994;67(Suppl 4):19–23.

43. Alter HJ, Bradley DW. Non-A, non-B hepatitis unrelated to the hepatitis C virus (non-ABC). Semin Liver Dis 1995;15:110–120.

44. Sherlock S. Chronic hepatitis C. Dis Mon 1994;40:117–196.

45. Lai MY, Kao JH, Yang PM, et al. Long-term efficacy of ribavirin plus interferon alfa in the treatment of chronic hepatitis C. Gastroenterology 1996;111:1307–1312.

46. Schmid M, Hefti ML Gattiker R, et al. Benign postoperative intrahepatic cholestasis. N Engl J Med 1965;272:545–550.

47. LaMont JT, Isselbacher K. Postoperative jaundice. N Engl J Med 1973;288:305–307.

48. Scharschmidt BF. Approach to management of fulminant hepatic failure. Med Clin North Am 1975;59:927–935.

49. Sherlock S. Alcoholic liver disease. Lancet 1995;345:227–234.

50. Teres J, Planas R, Panes J, et al. Vasopressin/nitroglycerin infusion vs esophageal tamponade

in the treatment of acute variceal bleeding. Hepatology 1990;11:964–968.

51. Sung JJY, Chung SCS, Lai CW, et al. Octreotide infusion or emergency sclerotherapy for variceal hemorrhage. Lancet 1993;342:637–641.

52. Boyce HW Jr. Modifications of the Sengstaken-Blakemore balloon tube. N Engl J Med 1962; 267:195–196.

53. Sanyal AJ, Freedman AM, Luketic VA, et al. Transjugular intra-hepatic portosystemic shunts for patients with active variceal hemorrhage to sclerotherapy. Gastroenterology 1996; 111:138–146.

54. Ottinger LW. Acute cholecystitis as a postoperative complication. Ann Surg 1976;184: 162–165.

55. Rolny P, Geenen JE, Hogan WJ. Postcholecystectomy patient with "objective signs" of partial bile outflow obstruction: clinical characteristic, sphincter of Oddi manometry findings, and results of therapy. Gastrointest Endosc 1993;39:778–781.

56. Postlethwait RW. Five-year follow-up results of operations for duodenal ulcer. Surg Gynecol Obstet 1973;137:387–392.

57. Valdimarsson T, Franzel L, Grodzinsky E, et al. Is small bowel biopsy necessary in adults with suspected celiac disease and IgA anti-endomysium antibodies? 100% positive predictive value for celiac disease in adults. Dig Dis Sci 1996;41:83–87.

58. Steinberg W, Tenner S. Medical progress: acute pancreatitis. N Engl J Med 1994;330:1998–1209.

59. Prendergast TM, Marini CP, D'Angelo AJ, et al. Surgical patient with pseudomembranous colitis: factors affecting prognosis. Surgery 1994; 116:768–774.

60. Fekety R, Shah AB. Diagnosis and treatment of *Clostridium difficile* colitis. JAMA 1993;269: 71–75.

61. Elmer GW, Surawicz CM, McFarland LV. Biotherapeutic agents: a neglected modality for the treatment and prevention of selected intestinal and vaginal infections. JAMA 1996;275: 870–876.

14

Endocrine Disorders

Thomas J. McGlynn, Jr. and Richard J. Simons

DIABETES MELLITUS

Epidemiology

With careful management, the perioperative morbidity of surgical patients with diabetes approaches 2%, or that of other patients. Preoperative assessment and perioperative management should focus on controlling glycemia, renal and cardiovascular function, wound healing, and consequences of neuropathies and other end-organ damage (1). Cardiovascular complications account for 30% and infections 20% of perioperative morbidity.

Pathophysiology

Surgery increases the release of glucagon, growth hormone, catecholamine, and cortisol, which produces a state of relative and absolute insulin deficiency (2). The degree to which insulin-mediated anabolic and anticatabolic effects are decreased depends on the type of surgery, underlying illnesses, and the type of diabetes (3). Increased liver glucose production and decreased peripheral disposal foster hyperglycemia, and lipolysis produces ketosis and increases in protein catabolism. Basal insulin requirements (0.5–1.0 U/h) rise to from 1.0 to 2.0 U/h for uncomplicated surgery and 1.5 to 5.0 U/h for coronary artery bypass surgery with the added stresses of hypothermia and pump perfusion. Without regular insulin supplements during the perioperative period, patients with insulin-dependent diabetes mellitus begin to develop ketosis and hyperglycemia within 4 to 6 hours of their last insulin dose. Ketosis and dehydration resulting from hyperglycemia are the major risks of insulin-dependent diabetes mellitus, and dehydration secondary to a hyperglycemia-induced osmotic diuresis presents the greatest clinical risk in non–insulin-dependent diabetes mellitus.

Most perioperative complications are determined by the patient's overall physiologic state. In vitro white-cell dysfunction increases with glucose levels greater than 250 mg/dL. Antecedent microvascular and macrovascular disease, increased platelet aggregation, poor tissue oxygenation, lowered red-cell 2,3-diphosphoglycerate levels, granulocyte chemotaxis, phagocytosis, and lymphocyte responsiveness, along with altered urinary acidification, are either proven or suspected factors that predispose a patient to infectious and vascular complications.

Preoperative Assessment

Elective surgery provides the opportunity to enhance control of glycemia (4, 5). Measurements of preoperative random blood glucose, serum glycosylated hemoglobin, creatinine, urinalysis, and electrolytes provide essential baseline information. Patients who are poorly controlled (fasting blood sugar, >240 mg/dL; glycosylated hemoglobin, >10%) and require more urgent surgery should be admitted, if possible, for metabolic control 24 hours in advance of surgery. During the hospital stay, a diabetes nurse specialist and dietitian should assess the patient's motivation, knowledge, self-monitoring, interpretation skills, dietary compliance, exercise, and weight control measures.

Long-term hypertension should be optimally controlled (<140/80 mm Hg) to slow progression of renal and retinal complications, although the short-term preoperative goals may not be as strict. Angiotensin-converting enzyme inhibitors provide an advantage for patients with nephropathy (6, 7), and despite side effects, thiazides (for hyperglycemia) and β-blockers (for decreased cardiac response to hypoglycemia) can be used in select cases (8). Cardiac evaluation includes careful assessment for ischemic heart disease and congestive heart failure through interview, physical examination, standard electrocardiography and chest radiography. Before transplant or other major vascular surgery, dynamic testing or cardiac catheterization should be considered in those with long-standing diabetes (9).

Hyperkalemia, hyperchloremia, and a reduced bicarbonate level indicate low-renin hypoaldosteronism. Nonsteroidal anti-inflammatory drugs, potassium supplements, and volume contraction can induce clinically significant hyperkalemia and acidosis, and they can aggravate renal insufficiency in these patients. Pyuria suggests infection, and culture should be taken. Bacteriuria should be treated with antibiotics based on patients sensitivities. Unnecessary urinary catheters should be avoided.

Hospitalization offers a chance to assess the potential for lower extremity complications. Examine the patient's feet for ischemic changes: ulceration, erythema, inflammation, calluses, drying, cracking, and abnormalities of toe nails (10). A lanolin-based lotion should be used for dry skin, and dermatophytes should be treated with topical agents applied to entire foot. (A review of diabetic ulcers and infection is provided in Chapter 18.)

Intermediate Metabolism

Although controlled trials are currently lacking, most experienced authors recommend a perioperative target glucose level of 120 to 180 mg/dL. No prospective study has established a precise target range and regimen that will produce fewer complications, lower cost, and other favorable outcomes. The key to successful management is close monitoring of laboratory parameters. Effective monitoring for patients with well-controlled non–insulin-dependent diabetes mellitus who are undergoing uncomplicated, brief surgery (i.e., less than 2 hours) consists of nurse-supervised, before-meal bedside assessments (Autolet and glucose monitor or Chem Strip Bg) twice a day. For all other patients, bedside monitoring is conducted before every meal, and a 4-hour, postprandial evening assessment is performed.

Clinicians achieve favorable results with different strategies for patients controlled by diet or oral agent, who are insulin-dependent, well controlled or poorly controlled, and with ketoacidosis or hyperosmolar complications. Table 14.1 summarizes several popular strategies.

The pancreas normally secretes 0.5 to 1.0 U of insulin per hour, or 12 to 24 U/day. This amount maintains the balance between glucose production and peripheral use, so that an average of 2.0 mg/kg per minute, or 8.4 g/h, is metabolized by a 70-kg patient. An infusion of 5% glucose and water at 100 mL/h provides 5 g of glucose per hour, or 120 g over 24 hours, which covers most daily metabolic requirements (approximately 120–240 g/day).

The stress of surgery can increase hourly insulin requirements by two- to threefold. However, clinical experience has demonstrated that a continuous infusion of 1.0 to 2.0 U of insulin per hour maintains balanced glucose production and use (i.e., blood glucose levels between

Table 14.1.   Perioperative Management of Diabetes Mellitus

Optimum control: Glucose range 120 to 180 mg/dl, glycohemoglobin 7 to 9.9%, average fasting glucose <180 mg/dl.

Baseline data: Examination focuses on end organ damage (hypertension, cardiac, peripheral vascular, neuropathic, retinal, gastrointestinal, infectious and renal). Urinalysis (microscopic and microalbuminuria), electrolytes, BUN, creatinine, fasting glucose, glycosylated hemoglobin, EKG.

Monitoring: Bedside, nurse supervised: before each meal and 10-11 P.M. blood glucose.

Indications for insulin therapy: All IDDM patients, all NIDDM insulin-taking patients, surgery longer than 2 hours, sub-optimal glucose control.

Continuous intravenous insulin: For all IDDM patients and poorly controlled NIDDM patients, mix 50 U regular insulin 500 cc of 0.45% saline. Run 50 cc through tubing to saturate receptors. Piggyback insulin line to fluid maintenance line. Intravenous fluid containing 5% Dextrose is infused at 100 cc/hr at all times. Continue hourly bed side monitoring during surgery and until optimally controlled. *Infusion rate for insulin:* For plasma glucose 81-100 mg/dl-0.5 U/hour. Increase or decrease amount by 0.5 U/hr for each 50 mg/dl increase or decrease in plasma glucose above 100 mg/dl. (To estimate infusion dose: Required dose (U/hr.) = blood glucose/100). If blood glucose is less than 80 mg/dl, discontinue infusion and give 25 ml of 50% D & W. Insulin needs can be increased 2 to 5 fold in the presence of factors such as: obesity, infection, bypass or transplant surgery, steroids, etc.

Sliding scale subcutaneous insulin: For well controlled (average fasting glucose <180 mg/dl) NIDDM patients, undergoing a short (<2 hour) procedure that does not invade a body cavity. The patient can take usual evening oral hypoglycemic or insulin dose on the evening before surgery. Hold AM oral agent and Lente or NPH insulin. Administer subcutaneous insulin on sliding scale every 6 hours until eating. Amount based on blood glucose: <120 mg/dl-0 U regular insulin, 120-160-4 U, 161-200-6 U, 201-240-8 U, 240 300 10 U, >300 mg/dl initiate insulin drip until tight control is achieved. If eating full meals on the evening after surgery, give half of usual evening dose of NPH or Lente, restart usual dose of insulin in AM. Continue 5% D&W (100 cc/hour) until patient is eating full meals. Monitor q 2-4 hours through surgery and immediate recovery.

Ketoacidosis: Loading dose 10 units IV (repeat once if needed) then maintain at rate of 2-5 Units per hour. Infuse 5% Dextrose IV (100 cc/hour) once glucose falls to 200 mg/dL. Continue fluid replacement and insulin at 0.5-1 U/hour until HCO_3 returns to >20 meq/dL, monitor glucose closely to avoid hypoglycemia.

Hyperosmolar states: Loading dose: 0 to 5 units IV then give 1-3 units per hour as a continuous piggyback infusion. Insulin requirements are small. Aggressive fluids as per text. Most important part of therapy is fluid replacement.

120–180 mg/dL) during most major but uncomplicated surgeries. On average, 0.5 U of insulin per hour reduces the blood glucose level to approximately 50 mg/dL.

The popularity of Insulin infusions continues to increase because of their advantages over older sliding scale and bolus strategies. They are simple to use, provide immediate control throughout therapy, and are less labor-intensive for the nursing staff. The biologic half-life of intravenous insulin is 8 minutes and the metabolic effect 20 minutes. To prepare the solution, mix 50 U of regular insulin in 500 mL of 0.45% saline to provide 1 U per 10 mL of infused fluid. The insulin receptors of intravenous tubing are satu-

rated by running 50 mL of the solution through the tubing before starting the infusion. With a continuous insulin infusion, the plasma glucose level rarely falls by more than the predictable 50 mg/dL each hour. The exceptions are during the first 2 hours of treatment for ketoacidosis and hyperosmolar states, when fluid compartment expansion can induce an hourly fall in glucose that is two- to threefold greater.

Perioperative Management

Patients with diabetes controlled through diet are simply monitored and placed on an individualized American

Diabetes Association diet. Patients who require only **oral sulfonurea hypoglycemics** usually do well with discontinuation of oral hypoglycemics 24 hours in advance of surgery, or 48 hours for glyburide and chlorpropamide. Well-controlled patients who normally receive an evening dose are given their oral hypoglycemic the evening before surgery. Patients begin to fast at midnight and receive 5% dextrose in water (D & W) at 50 to 75 mL/h beginning on the morning of surgery. Sulfonurea hypoglycemics are reinstituted once the patient begins eating again on the following morning or on the evening of surgery according to the patient's prehospitalization schedule. Bedside monitoring is conducted four times a day until control is established and the patient is eating.

Metformin (Glucophage) therapy is temporarily suspended for any surgery that involves restriction of oral intake or fluid until unrestricted intake resumes and renal function has been evaluated as normal. Biguanide therapy carries an increased risk of lactic acidosis in the presence of infection, hypoxia, altered tissue or renal perfusion (including transient alterations), and contrast agents; therefore it should be discontinued for major surgical procedures.

Well-controlled patients who require insulin and are undergoing brief, uncomplicated surgery can be given subcutaneous regular insulin (Table 14.1), but the total daily dose is decreased by one-third to one-half of their total daily units. When an uncomplicated course is anticipated, some physicians give a small dose of an intermediate-acting insulin (e.g., 30–50% of usual AM NPH or Lente insulin). Begin 5% D & W at 100 mL/hour by 8 AM on the day of surgery. Supplemental sliding-scale regular insulin can be administered as needed based on the results of bedside monitoring.

For **patients who require insulin but are poorly controlled** or who will undergo **prolonged, complicated surgery**, continuous infusions are preferred.

This approach provides a highly efficient method in restoring patients with ketoacidosis, hyperosmolar states, and poor control to a euglycemic state over 24 hours (11). Table 14.1 outlines these strategies.

Ketoacidosis

Patients with ketoacidosis present with tachypnea, nausea, vomiting, gastric dilatation, and polyuria. A few develop abdominal distention, pain, and guarding. The diagnosis of pancreatitis and acute abdomen need to be established with care in the presence of acute ketoacidosis or profound hyperglycemia. Patients with severe ketoacidosis occasionally appear to have an acute abdomen; such patients are young (usually less than 40 years), have profound acidosis (bicarbonate, <10), and nausea and vomiting that usually precede the abdominal pain. The white blood cell count is often elevated. Abdominal pain persisting for longer than a few hours into the treatment of ketoacidosis indicates an underlying, acute abdominal cause. Serum amylase can be elevated in 60% of patients with ketoacidosis because of salivary amylase activity and an enhanced amylase:creatinine ratio. Serum amylase can rise to over 1000 Samoji units several hours after therapy has been initiated and in the absence of pancreatitis (10, 12).

A serum bicarbonate of less than 20 mEq/dL with an increased anion gap can reflect ketones of ketoacidosis, lactate of lactic acidosis, or increased phosphates and sulfates from renal insufficiency. Levels of serum creatinine, electrolytes, lactate, and ketone should be measured to sort out the difficult anion-gap acidosis. Venous serum bicarbonate or arterial pH levels every 2 hours provide equally valid measures of the patient's acidosis provided that bicarbonate is not given.

Rapid replacement of insulin, fluids (i.e., free water), and electrolytes are essential (12), and continuous infusion of insulin is indicated. Give 10 U of regular insulin as an intravenous bolus to saturate the available insulin receptors in the presence of insulin resistance. A continuous infusion is maintained according to the algorithm in Table 14.1. Intermittent intramuscular insulin every 2 hours is also effective, but it also has no advantage. Subcutaneous insulin is absorbed erratically and is less effective overall.

Patients with ketoacidosis and hyperosmolar states are de facto hypovolemic and require volume expansion to downregulate catecholamine release, replace electrolytes, and enhance renal perfusion. Intravenous fluids are initiated aggressively, with normal saline infused at a rate of 500 to 1000 ML for the first and, perhaps, second hour. A common management error is underreplacement of fluids. On average, patients with ketoacidosis require volume expansion of 4 to 6 L, and patients with hyperosmolar states 6 to 8 L, over 24 hours.

For these reasons, initial infusion rates should be aggressive and modified only in the presence of prior clinical cardiovascular disease and the appearance of clinical signs and symptoms indicating the patient's inability to tolerate fluid replacement. After the first hour or 1 to 2 L of fluid, the rate can be reduced and the amount of saline (e.g., one-half or one-quarter normal saline, 5% D&W) tailored to clinical circumstances. Requirements for fluid replacement vary according to the clinical circumstances. Average requirements provide rough target volumes: 4 to 6 L fluids in first 24 hours for diabetic ketoacidosis, and 6 to 8 L for hyperosmolar states.

Electrolytes should be monitored every 2 hours, and hypokalemia can be anticipated as insulin improves the entry of glucose into cells. If the serum potassium level is greater than 4.0 mEq at the onset of therapy, replacement can be deferred until the level falls. Twenty milliequivalents of KCl can be added to each liter of fluid once urine flow is established. Hyponatremia (i.e., sodium and free-water depleted) and hypernatremia (i.e., free-water depleted and excess of sodium) provide some guidance on the choice of fluid replacement therapies. Each 100 mg of glucose displaces 2 mEq of plasma sodium. A patient with a glucose level of 600 mg/dL and sodium level of 135 mEq/dL is severely free-water depleted, and he or she will require a small volume of saline and a large volume of D&W. A patient with a glucose level of 600 mg/dL and a sodium level of 123 mEq/dL will require a larger volume of saline to replace the lost sodium.

Replacement of bicarbonate is not required in most patients, even in the presence of severe acidosis. One to two ampules of $NaHCO_3$ (44 mEq of HCO_3 per ampule) can contribute to recovery when given to clinically unstable patients with a pH of 7.0 or lower. Phosphate can be given as K_2PO_4 if the patient exhibits cardiac insufficiency and fails to respond or stabilize with initial therapy, although in practice, this is rarely done. The serum PO_4 status does not accurately predict tissue PO_4 status.

Cerebral disequilibrium is a rare, late complication that presents as progressive stupor, coma, areflexia, and death when glucose levels are decreasing and bicarbonate levels increasing. The syndrome appears to be produced by cerebral edema that is precipitated by overly aggressive bicarbonate therapy or electrolyte replacement and persistent cerebral acidosis. Treatment consists of 8 mg of dexamethasone intravenously and osmotic diuresis (e.g., mannitol).

Hyperosmolar States

Hyperosmolar states occur most commonly among patients with type II diabetes and those who require oral hypoglycemic agents. Medications such as diazoxide, corticosteroids, immunosuppressive agents, diuretics, dilantin, β-blockers, and other factors such as parenteral hyperalimentation, cerebrovascular accidents, pancreatitis, and so on can precipitate progressive hyperglycemia with associated dehydration but without ketoacidosis. Clinical presentation is often insidious, over 10 to 12 days, and early clinical signs can be nonspecific, such as irritability, nausea, vomiting, polydypsia, polyuria, and decreased activities of daily living, only to progress to obtundation and coma. Therapy emphasizes large quantities (average, 6–8 L) of free-water replacement, often beginning with 0.45% normal saline followed by 5% D&W. Insulin requirements can be quite small and are often only 1 to 3 U/h.

HYPERTHYROIDISM

Epidemiology

The risk of surgery in the patients with untreated hyperthyroidism is substantial. The major concern is precipitation of "thyroid storm," which is a life-threatening clinical syndrome characterized by hypermetabolism, adrenergic excess, or both. In the past, the most common precipitant of thyroid storm was surgery (i.e., thyroidectomy for Graves' disease in an inadequately prepared patient) (13). A spectrum of both major and minor surgical and obstetric procedures can precipitate thyroid storm, including dental extraction, abdominal surgery, childbirth, and cesarean section. With the advent of more sensitive assays for thyroid hormone, efficacious antithyroid drugs, and improved preparation of patients before surgery, perioperative thyrotoxic storm should be a rare occurrence today.

Preoperative Assessment

The best treatment of surgically induced thyroid storm is prevention through preoperative recognition of hyperthyroidism. Symptoms of thyroid hormone excess—palpitations, heat intolerance, weight loss without anorexia, diarrhea, tremor, dyspnea, menstrual irregularity or amenorrhea, and muscular weakness—should be sought. Older patients may not present with the classic symptoms or

signs of hyperthyroidism, which often presents in the elderly with monosystemic features, the cardiovascular, neuromuscular, and gastrointestinal systems predominating. Thus, patients may present with new-onset atrial fibrillation, worsening congestive heart failure, or angina pectoris. In one study (14), two-thirds of elderly patients with hyperthyroidism presented with symptoms of heart failure, arrhythmia, or angina. Other patients may present with fatigue, muscle weakness, and emotional lability. Occasionally, elderly patients are labeled as senile, depressed, or psychotic when hyperthyroidism is the actual culprit.

A special variant of hyperthyroidism is "apathetic hyperthyroidism," a phrase coined nearly a half-century ago to describe those elderly patients who present with blunted affect and who appear to be depressed, lethargic, and apathetic (15). The usual hyperkinesis is replaced by nonactivation. These patients generally do not have eye signs or flushing and have minimal thyroid enlargement. Weight loss is usually marked. Thus, this form of hyperthyroidism is more likely to be missed in a preoperative evaluation.

Because the clinical features of hyperthyroidism may be subtle and masked by an underlying medical illness, the diagnosis is established by thyroid function tests. A major breakthrough in such testing occurred in the early 1980s with the application of monoclonal antibody technology to thyroid-stimulating hormone (TSH) testing, which led to the development of immunometric assays. These newer, "sensitive" TSH assays measure very low concentrations of TSH (0.001 mIU/L) depending on the assay used. Measurement of the serum TSH level and an appropriate estimate of free thyroxine (T_4) should be performed for all patients in whom hyperthyroidism is suspected. Patients with hyperthyroidism usually demonstrate TSH suppression to levels less than 0.1 mIU/L and elevated concentrations of free T_4 or free triiodothyronine (T_3) (16). In addition, the consulting internist should be aware of other factors that can suppress TSH to the subnormal range, including thyroid hormone overreplacement, effects of medication (e.g., dopamine and dopamine agonists, glucocorticoids, somatostatin), pregnancy, hypothalamic-pituitary failure, and nonthyroidal illness.

Causes of thyrotoxicosis include Graves' disease, toxic or multinodular goiter, and thyroiditis. A radionuclide scan will show increased uptake of iodine in overproduction hyperthyroidism (e.g., Graves' disease). In patients with thyroiditis, hyperthyroidism results from unregulated, inflammation-induced release of stored T_4 and T_3; thus, radioiodine uptake into the thyroid is low. Treatment with an antithyroid drug or radioiodine is contraindicated in patients with thyroiditis.

The three major classes of pharmacologic agents used in the treatment of hyperthyroidism include thioamides (i.e., propylthiouracil, methimazole), iodides, and β-adrenergic antagonists. Thioamides block thyroid peroxidase and thus inhibit biosynthesis of thyroid hormone. This inhibitory effect may be seen within 1 hour of administering these agents, and both drugs have weak immunosuppressive effects. Agranulocytosis is the most feared complication but occurs in less than 0.2 % of patients; routine blood counts do not predict this complication. The half-life of propylthiouracil is 1 to 2 hours, whereas that of methimazole is 4 to 8 hours. The usual starting dose of propylthiouracil is 300 mg/day in three divided doses. Methimazole can be given as a single daily dose and is generally started at 10 to 20 mg/day. Dosage should be titrated to achieve and then maintain biochemical and clinical euthyroidism.

Iodide is a potent and prompt inhibitor of thyroid hormone release. It is the most effective agent for lowering thyroid hormone acutely, which is useful in patients who need rapid correction of the hyperthyroid state. Because iodide interferes with the synthesis of thyroid hormone and reduces the vascularity of an overactive thyroid gland, it is an ideal agent for the preoperative preparation of patients with hyperthyroidism. Its dose and route of administration are discussed later.

β-Adrenergic blocking agents are usually employed in the treatment of thyrotoxicosis. The time-honored β-blocker propranolol is effective in abolishing many hyperdynamic signs and symptoms of thyrotoxicosis. It is postulated that patients with hyperthyroidism exhibit an extreme sensitivity to the action of catecholamines.

For elective surgery, and even minor procedures, the patient should be rendered euthyroid before the operation. Propylthiouracil has been the mainstay of therapy; however, methimazole can be given as a single daily dose and is associated with a lower rate of major toxicity (17). Although euthyroid levels of thyroid hormone can sometimes be achieved in 2 to 3 weeks, surgery is usually postponed by 1 to 3 months to ensure the effects of hyperthyroidism have been reversed.

If a patient with untreated or only partially treated hyperthyoidism requires emergency surgery, treat with propranolol and iodides before the induction of anesthesia. Intravenous preparations of both propranolol and iodide can be used (discussed later). These patients require careful postoperative care in terms of their fluid and hemodynamic status. Antithyroid drugs should be initiated as soon as the patient is able to take oral or nasogastric fluids. With appropriate preoperative evaluation and care, thyroid storm will be averted in most patients. However, the internist who consults with the surgeon should be prepared to treat this condition, because it can arise unexpectedly following any surgical procedure.

Definitive therapeutic options for the patient with hyperthyroidism include antithyroid medications, thyroid surgery, and radioactive iodine. Treatment decisions are individualized and based on age, concomitant medical illness, and patient preference. Discussion of the pros and cons of each therapeutic modality is beyond the scope of this book, but there are excellent reviews of this subject (17).

Thyroid Storm

Thyroid storm is severe hyperthyroidism characterized by high fever, agitation, and weakness. Additional manifestations may include tremor, overt psychosis, obtundation and coma, high-output congestive heart failure, tachyarrhythmias, diarrhea, vomiting, and jaundice. Criteria for the diagnosis vary, because there is no defined point at which severe thyrotoxicosis becomes thyroid storm. Clinical manifestations of thyroid storm are outlined in Table 14.2, and measurement of T_4, T_3, and TSH levels is necessary to confirm the diagnosis. The diagnosis itself is made on clinical evaluation, however, and a delay in therapy while awaiting laboratory confirmation may result in further clinical compromise and even death.

Surgery frequently precipitates thyroid storm, and recognition by the consultant demands immediate action (Table 14.3). Therapy has five goals: (a) identification and treatment of the precipitating cause,

Table 14.2. **Clinical Features of Thyroid Storm**

General	Neurological
Agitation	Tremor
Fever	Restlessness
Sweating, heat intolerance	Psychosis
	Hyperreflexia
	Coma

Cardiovascular	Gastrointestinal
Palpitations	Vomiting
Tachyarrhythmias	Diarrhea
Congestive heart failure	Jaundice

Eyes
Stare
Proptosis

(b) blockade of thyroid hormone production, (c) blockade of the release of thyroid hormone, (d) blockade of excess β-adrenergic stimulation, and (e) general supportive measures.

General supportive measures include the replacement of fluid and electrolytes and the control of hyperthermia. Aspirin should be avoided, because it may further increase the patient's metabolic rate by displacing thyroid hormone from its binding proteins. Hypothermic blankets, fans, and ice packs may be used to control fever.

Most authorities recommend use of glucocorticoids, because there may be a relatively inadequate adrenal reserve (18). Hydrocortisone, 300 mg/day in divided doses, is usually sufficient. Congestive heart failure may require use of oxygen and diuretics, and antibiotics should be administered for established infection.

Antithyroid drugs should be administered as quickly as possible. Propylthiouracil, 900 to 1200 mg as a loading dose and then 100 mg every 6 hours by mouth or nasogastric tube, is preferred in light of its ability to inhibit extrathyroidal conversion of T_4 to T_3. Administration of iodide should be delayed for at least 1 to 2 hours after propylthiouracil has been administered to avoid any thyroidal accumulation of iodide that could later be used to synthesize more thyroid hormone. Iodide is given orally in the form of a Lugol's solution, at a dose of up to 30 drops per day. Alternatively, sodium iodide, 1 to 2 g slow push intravenously, can be given. The iodide is usually continued for 7 to 10 days.

A β-adrenergic blocking agent should be given to all patients with thyroid storm unless there is an absolute contraindication. Propranolol, 2 to 5 mg every 4 hours intravenously or 320 to 480 mg/day by mouth, is the preferred drug, having a peripheral inhibitory effect on the conversion of T_4 to T_3. β-Blockers quickly control the cardiac and psychomotor manifestations of thyrotoxicosis, and fever, restlessness, and tremor usually respond promptly.

Table 14.3. Management of Thyroid Storm

I. Treatment of precipitating cause (sepsis, diabetes, etc.)
II. Blockade of thyroid hormone production
    1. Propylthiouracil (600-1000 mg p.o. or by nasogastric tube as loading dose, then 100-300 mg every 9 hours)
III. Blockage of thyroid hormone release
    1. Lugol's solution (30 drops/day p.o.) or sodium iodide (1 gm intravenously every 8-12 hr). Note: Iodide should be started after propylthiouracil and continued for 7-10 days.
IV. Beta-Adrenergic blockade
    1. Propranolol (initially, 20-40 mg p.o. every 6 hr or 2-10 mg by slow intravenous infusion every 6 hr). Note: Dosage should be titrated to achieve a resting pulse <90.
V. General supportive measures
    1. Hydrocortisone (200-500 mg daily parenterally).
    2. Control fever with fans, hypothermic blankets, or acetaminophen. Avoid aspirin.
    3. Fluid and electrolyte replacement.

Even with the therapeutic modalities mentioned here and summarized in Table 14.3, thyroid storm still carries significant morbidity and mortality. Prevention through early recognition of impending thyroid storm remains the most important aspect of treatment.

HYPOTHYROIDISM

Surgical Risk

Surgery in patients with untreated hypothyroidism carries the risk of several potential complications. These patients may manifest extreme sensitivity to sedatives and anesthetic agents, thus resulting in prolonged unconsciousness following the administration of seemingly normal doses. Induction of anesthesia in patients with hypothyroidism has also resulted in hypotension, cardiac arrest, and myxedema coma. Other risks of anesthesia and surgery include hypoventilation, cardiopulmonary arrest, hyponatremia, and precipitation of congestive heart failure.

Patients with hypothyroidism have a reduced maximal breathing capacity, diminished carbon monoxide diffusion capacity, and reduced hypoxic ventilatory drive. Alveolar hypoventilation is especially common in obese patients with this condition. These abnormalities in pulmonary function can be corrected with thyroid-hormone replacement therapy.

Left ventricular dysfunction has been documented in patients with severe hypothyroidism. Also, electrocardiographic abnormalities, including flat or inverted T waves, sinus bradycardia, and low voltage, are common. Occasionally, the presenting manifestation is congestive heart failure associated with bradycardia and with pericardial and pleural effusion. Such effusions are not hemodynamically significant, however. Tamponade rarely occurs, and they resolve with thyroid-hormone replacement therapy. However, in the stressed patient with hypothyroidism, congestive heart failure may develop rapidly and respond poorly to conventional therapy.

Patients with hypothyroidism have an impaired ability to excrete free water. This abnormality, which is corrected by giving replacement doses of thyroid hormone, is probably caused by inappropriate secretion of antidiuretic hormone (ADH). Such patients are at risk for significant iatrogenic hyponatremia.

Several studies have attempted to better define the surgical risk for patients with untreated hypothyroidism. Ladenson et al. (19) performed a retrospective, controlled analysis that compared the relative frequencies of perioperative complications in those with hypothyroidism and in control patients undergoing surgery with general anesthesia. Most in the hypothyroid group were judged to have mild or moderate hypothyroidism (serum T_4 level, $2.4 \pm 1.2 \, \mu g/mL$ [mean $\pm$ SD]). The hypothyroid group had a statistically greater incidence of intraoperative hypotension, heart failure, and gastrointestinal as well as neuropsychiatric complications. There were no differences in perioperative blood loss, length of hospitalization, or prevalence of perioperative arrhythmia, hypothermia, hyponatremia, delayed anesthetic recovery, abnormal tissue integrity, impaired wound healing, pulmonary complications, or death. Drucker and Burrrow (20) compared 10 patients with untreated mild to moderate hypothyroidism undergoing cardiac surgery with cardiopulmonary bypass to a control group of 30 patients, and they found no difference in the number of postoperative complications or the length of hospitalization. Furthermore, no problems were encountered with discontinuation of cardiopulmonary bypass or reversal of hypothyroidism. Caution should be exercised, however, in extrapolating these results to patients with severe or profound hypothyroidism.

Preoperative Evaluation and Diagnosis

The diagnosis of hypothyroidism can be easily missed. Clinical onset is usually insidious, and the manifestations are protean. Associated signs and symptoms are often ascribed to debilitation caused by illness and aging. Common complaints include lethargy, weakness, dyspnea, fatigue, cold intolerance, and weight gain with little or no change in appetite. Distension, flatulence, and constipation dominate the gastrointestinal complaints, whereas arthritis and carpal tunnel syndrome are the most common musculoskeletal problems. Neuropsychiatric manifestations include memory loss, dementia, cerebellar ataxia, and myxedema

coma. Bradycardia, hypothermia, brittle hair, dry skin, and slow relaxation of deep-tendon reflexes are common physical findings, and laboratory clues include a normocytic or macrocytic anemia, hypercholesterolemia, elevated levels of muscle enzymes (e.g., creatine phosphokinase), and hyponatremia.

The diagnosis is confirmed by thyroid function tests. A low serum T_4 (or free T_4) level in combination with an elevated TSH level is diagnostic of primary hypothyroidism. The common clinical entity of a mildly elevated TSH (usually < 20 mIU/L) with normal levels of thyroid hormone and a lack of clinical symptoms typical of hypothyroidism is defined as "subclinical hypothyroidism." This may be evidence of early thyroid failure, or it may represent a possible "resetting" of the pituitary-thyroid axis as many patients with these findings remain stable for prolonged periods of time (21).

The clinician must be aware that in moderately to severely ill patients, serum total or free T_4 levels may not accurately reflect thyroid status. Despite a low T_4 level, most of these patients are thought to be clinically euthyroid and constitute the **"euthyroid sick syndrome."** A classic study (22) supports the theory that the low T_4 state of severe illness at least partially relates to suppression of thyrotropin secretion. The TSH concentration in such patients may be low or high depending on the clinical circumstance. During a nonthyroidal illness, TSH levels typically remain in the normal to low-normal range until the recovery phase, when a transient, mild (<20 mIU/L) elevation of TSH may be seen in the absence of medications known to suppress TSH release (i.e., dopamine, glucocorticoid therapy) (23). At present, most authorities do not recommend thyroid replacement in patients with the euthyroid sick syndrome.

Primary hypothyroidism often results from thyroid surgery or treatment with radioactive iodine. The most common spontaneous form of hypothyroidism is Hashimoto's thyroiditis, which is characterized by circulating antithyroid antibodies and a firm, rubbery thyroid gland. Medications also known to cause hypothyroidism include lithium, iodide, and amiodarone.

Primary and secondary hypothyroidism can be differentiated by measuring the TSH level, which is elevated in primary hypothyroidism and normal or low in secondary hypothyroidism. In a patient with low T_4 and normal or low TSH levels, it is necessary to evaluate other pituitary functions, including gonadotropins, prolactin, and cortisol. Sparse or absent pubic and axillary hair, absence of a palpable thyroid gland, and thin, finely wrinkled, pale skin suggest secondary hypothyroidism.

Perioperative Management

Because of the multiple abnormal physiologic responses already discussed, the risk of surgery can be considerable in patients with severe hypothyroidism. Therefore, in those with moderate to severe hypothyroidism, elective surgery should be postponed until the patient is treated with thyroid hormone and rendered clinically euthyroid. Optimal replacement may require 2 to 3 months to be achieved, especially in older patients or those with suspected cardiac disease, because rapid replacement can precipitate angina and even myocardial infarction. Patients with subclinical or mild hypothyroidism may be cleared for elective surgery; however, close follow-up in the postoperative period, with anticipatory planning for the potential complications discussed earlier, is essential.

If an untreated or inadequately treated patient with hypothyroidism requires emergency surgery, the anesthesiologist must be informed. Lower anesthetic doses are usually required, and recovery from anesthesia will generally be prolonged. Assisted ventilation will probably be required not only during the anesthesia itself but also for up to 2 or 3 days postoperatively. Indiscriminate use of sedatives and narcotics in these patients should be avoided. **Sudden respiratory arrest** has been reported in postoperative patients with hypothyroidism. In addition, because these patients have an impaired ability to handle a free-water load, particular attention must be devoted to fluid and electrolyte management to prevent hyponatremia and congestive heart failure from overhydration.

The ultimate expression of severe hypothyroidism is myxedema coma. Although it can occur at any age, it is most common in elderly women with hypothyroidism who develop myxedema coma during the winter months after some stressful event, with pneumonia leading the list. Other precipitating factors include cold or alcohol exposure, gastrointestinal bleeding, myocardial infarction, injuries, and, of course, surgery. These individuals have a long antecedent history of symptoms suggesting hypothyroidism, and their physical examination will provide corroborative findings. Most will be hypothermic, and in fact, a normal body temperature suggests an intercurrent infection. Other physical findings to be sought include puffy eyelids, loss of the outer one-third of eyebrows, alopecia, thickened nails, bradycardia with soft heart sounds, and muscle weakness.

Myxedema coma is usually associated with hypoventilation and carbon dioxide retention, with a variable degree of respiratory acidosis. Carbon dioxide narcosis is reported to be the predominant factor in at least one-third of patients. Hypoglycemia can occur in both primary and secondary hypothyroidism, although it is more common in the latter. Hyponatremia, cerebral hypoxia from decreased cardiac output and decreased cerebral perfusion, hypothermia, intercurrent infection, and thyroid hormone deficiency itself can contribute to this neurologic state.

Myxedema coma is a medical emergency, and therapy must begin promptly, before laboratory confirmation of the hypothyroid state is obtained. General guidelines for the treatment of myxedema coma are outlined in Table 14.4. Replacement of thyroid hormone is the single most specific aspect of therapy. In the past, there was a tendency to administer T_4 in small doses because of fear over precipitating coronary ischemia. However, it has been suggested that therapeutic failures in myxedema coma may have been secondary to the inadequate administration of T_4. The current recommendation is to administer 500 μg of T_4 as a slow bolus infusion, followed by an appropriate maintenance dose given either intravenously or orally (18). This approach rapidly normalizes the levels of circulating thyroid hormone, so that by 24 hours, the TSH level has decreased and the serum T_4 level is within the normal range.

A number of other general principles regarding the treatment of these patients should be emphasized. Although most of these individuals are hypothermic, attempts at rewarming should be discouraged, because this inappropriately increases body metabolism and oxygen consumption. Since the laboratory distinction between primary and secondary hypothyroidism could require several days, patients should be given **parenteral glucocorticoids.** Also, even in myxedema resulting from primary hypothyroidism, the adrenocorticotropin hormone (ACTH) response to stress is impaired.

If a patient is hypotensive, the blood pressure usually responds to thyroid hormone and volume replacement. Vasopressors should be used with caution, however, because serious cardiac arrhythmias may occur when they are given with large doses of thyroid hormone. In addition, doses of digitalis should be reduced, because even normal levels of digoxin can be associated with digitalis intoxication.

ADRENAL INSUFFICIENCY
Epidemiology

Acute perioperative adrenal insufficiency occurs in less than 0.001% of all surgical patients, and recognizing adrenal insufficiency in the perioperative period presents special challenges to the consulting internist. The most commonly addressed issue is ACTH suppression resulting from exogenous corticosteroids and the need for perioperative corticosteroid prophylaxis.

Pathophysiology

Adrenocorticotropin hormone stimulates glucocorticoid (i.e., cortisol) and catecholamine (e.g., epinephrine, norepinephrine) secretion, whereas mineralocorticoid secretion (i.e., aldosterone) is controlled primarily by the angiotensin-renin mechanism. Secretion of ACTH is regulated by cortisol levels, stress, circadian rhythm, and corticotropin-releasing hormone (CRH) from the hypothalamus.

Table 14.4.   Treatment of Myxedema Coma

I. General supportive measures
  1. Maintain a patent airway and adequate ventilation.
  2. Rewarming hypothermic patients is unnecessary.
  3. Careful monitoring of fluid and electrolytes to prevent volume overload and hyponatremia.
  4. Hydrocortisone (100 mg q 8 hr) for at least a week. The dose can be tapered in the second week.
II. Treatment of metabolic complications
  1. Hypoglycemia
  2. Hyponatremia
III. Treatment of precipitating cause
  1. Careful evaluation for a source of infection or other intercurrent medical illness.
IV. Thyroid hormone replacement
  1. Thyroxine (500-1000 μg) by slow intravenous infusion followed by 50-100 μg per day.

Hypothalamic-pituitary-adrenal (HPA) suppression is influenced by the type of corticosteroid used as well as the dose, route, and duration of therapy (24). Long-acting agents with 48-hour duration of action (e.g., betamethasone, dexamethasone, triamcinolone) suppress HPA feedback and provide no chance for recovery between daily doses. Cortisol, cortisone, prednisone, prednisolone, and methyl-prednisolone with a shorter duration of action (24–36 hours) in small, once-daily (AM) doses permit HPA recovery and function between doses. Large doses as well as daily AM and PM doses effectively suppress HPA function.

Pituitary response (i.e., ACTH secretion) to fluctuations in glucocorticoid level deteriorates within weeks of initiating continuous exogenous corticoids. With continued steroid administration, adrenal hyporesponsiveness to ACTH follows over several more weeks to months. Recovery of function occurs in reverse order, over weeks to months depending on the degree and duration of HPA suppression. The adrenal stress response of patients receiving high doses of exogenous corticoids for 1 week can be inadequate.

Primary adrenal insufficiency involves adrenal gland dysfunction. Secondary insufficiency results from pituitary insufficiency, and tertiary insufficiency results from the lack of normal CRH secretion (25). Mineralocorticoids (primarily aldosterone) are secreted by the zona glomerulosa of the cortex and foster both sodium reabsorption and potassium excretion by the renal tubules. Mineralocorticoid function is preserved in secondary and tertiary adrenal insufficiency. The adrenal cortex secretes glucocorticoids, cortisol, and androgens through ACTH stimulation, whereas the medulla secretes catecholamines (e.g., epinephrine, norepinephrine) in response to ACTH and stress.

Clinical Presentation

Most patients with primary adrenal insufficiency present with hyponatremia from relative ADH excess in secondary and tertiary insufficiency. Patients with secondary and tertiary insufficiency do not exhibit hyperkalemia from loss of aldosterone and, in general, exhibit less severe clinical manifestations of volume and sodium depletion (i.e., prerenal azotemia) because their mineralocorticoid function is preserved. They require less fluid and sodium replacement compared to patients with primary adrenal insufficiency, who require 3 to 4 L of fluids on average to replace renal fluid and sodium losses. The core treatment of secondary and tertiary insufficiency is volume support and prompt intravenous administration of a soluble corticosteroid (e.g., cortisol).

Patients with primary adrenal insufficiency have lost mineralocorticoid, glucocorticoid, and stress response (i.e., catecholamine) hormones. They are sodium and volume depleted because of the absent mineralocorticoid effect, and they also lack vascular tone because of the absent glucocorticoid effect. Treatment requires the aggressive replacement of glucocorticoid, mineralocorticoid (as fludrocortisone), volume, and sodium.

The effective consulting internist considers adrenal insufficiency whenever unexplained but compatible findings are present (26). Insufficiency can be partial, complete, acute, emergent, or evolve over months to years after an adrenal or pituitary insult. Causes include infectious (e.g., tuberculosis, acquired immunodeficiency syndrome) or metastatic diseases (e.g., lung cancer), hemorrhage, immune disorders, and drugs (e.g., aminoglutethimide). On surgical services and in the postoperative setting, symptoms resulting from adrenal insufficiency can be erroneously attributed to other conditions. Patients with adrenal insufficiency can present with any combination of fever, hypotension, abdominal pain, nausea, vomiting, polyuria, fatigue, myalgias, anorexia, weakness, weight loss, psychiatric symptoms, delirium, and so on. Less than one-half of these patients present with the classic constellation of symptoms and findings: hyponatremia, hyperkalemia, acidosis, eosinophilia, hypoglycemia, and prerenal azotemia. The challenge is to consider the diagnosis.

Diagnosis

Once adrenal insufficiency becomes a consideration, the diagnostic evaluation is straightforward on surgical consultation services (27). During acute stress, a random screening cortisol level of 20 μg/dL in the presence of hypotension, fever, and so on makes the diagnosis of insufficiency very unlikely. In the same setting, a level of 5 μg/dL or less provides presumptive evidence of insufficiency, and a level of 10 μg/dL or less makes the diagnosis likely. To confirm adrenal competency, administer 250 μg/dL of ACTH (Cortrosyn) intramuscularly or intravenously, and measure the serum cortisol level at baseline, 30 minutes, and 1 hour. Any serum cortisol level of 20 μ/dL (550 mmol/L) or greater indicates that the HPA axis and adrenal response to acute stress are intact. If primary insufficiency is suspected, measure the aldosterone level as well; it does not rise above 4 ng/mL in primary insufficiency. Tests that clarify the cause of primary and secondary insufficiency (e.g., prolonged ACTH stimulation, insulin tolerance, metapyrone, CRH stimulation tests, computed tomography [CT]) are not necessary during the acute perioperative period.

Treatment

An acute crisis is treated with cortisone sodium succinate, 100 mg given intravenously immediately and then 100 mg again every 6 to 8 hours until vital signs, fluid, and electrolytes are stable. If a rapid Cortrosyn stimulation test is to be done, administer dexamethasone (3–4 mg intravenously), which will not interfere with the cortisol assay. Fluid replacement is guided by clinical parameters, laboratory findings, and the type of insufficiency. Fluid therapy begins with rapid intravascular compartment expansion using normal saline during the first hour at a rate of 500 to 1000 mL/h. Individual clinical circumstances determine the rate, volume, and type of any subsequent fluid replacement. Monitor electrolytes and creatinine hourly, and anticipate late hypokalemia. Add potassium supplements (20 mEq to each liter of intravenous fluid) as needed.

Once the patient is stable, switch to maintenance therapy of oral cortisone, 25 mg in the morning and 12.5 mg in the evening, for glucocorticoid replacement (equivalent to 7.5 mg of prednisone daily). In primary adrenal insufficiency, mineralocorticoid supplements may be necessary (e.g., fludrocortisone, 0.1–0.2 mg daily by mouth), especially when less than 50 mg of hydrocortisone daily is prescribed. Before discharge, educate patients about the signs and symptoms of adrenal insufficiency, use of an emergency steroid kit (e.g., hydrocortisone Mix-o-vial), and prescribe a "medic-alert" bracelet.

Perioperative Prophylactic Steroids

During severe stress, maximum adrenal secretion is equivalent to 300 to 400 mg of cortisone daily. After major surgery, increased endogenous secretion of adrenal hormones is sustained for 3 days but then returns quickly to normal (over 24 hours for minor surgery). Therefore, stress dose coverage can be safely administered on the day of major surgery and the first two postoperative days, and then it can be abruptly discontinued. Table 14.5 identifies patients who are at risk and summarizes an approach to treatment; when uncertain about the meaning of compatible symptoms or the need for prophylaxis, always treat as recommended. There is no documentation of patients being harmed when physicians provide exogenous steroids, which patients would have produced endogenously during acute stress, for a few days.

Table 14.5.   Corticosteroids and Adrenal Insufficiency

Candidates for Prophylaxis: (Prednisone or Equivalent)

- >20 mg Prednisone (or equivalent) daily for one week, within one year
- 7.5 to 10 mg Prednisone daily for one month within one year
- 5 mg of Prednisone daily for one year or longer
- Repetitive doses of intramuscular or "depot" corticosteroids within one year
- All steroid regimens within a year which were longer than one week duration and dosing was more than once daily or the dose was given other than in the A.M. or the agent was not short acting.

Prophylaxis Options

1. Cortrosyn stimulation test prior to surgery (250 μg IV, serum level of 20 ug after)
2. Monitor closely and treat immediately for adrenal insufficiency if any compatible symptoms evolve.
3. Minor stressful procedure: 50-100 mg hydrocortisone on the morning of (dilatation and curettage, hand surgery, etc.)
   Major surgery: 100 mg soluble intravenous corticosteroid (hydrocortisone sodium succinate) every 8 hours for 3 days. Can be discontinued abruptly without taper once stress is completely resolved.

Treatment of Adrenal Crisis

Baseline electrolytes, creatinine; monitor vital signs, input, output, etc.
Immediate intravenous cortisone hemisuccinate, 100 mg
Repeat cortisone dose every 6 hours until clinical and laboratory parameters are stable.
Rapid fluid compartment expansion; begin with 500-1000 cc of 5% D (cover hypoglycemia) and normal saline (replenish sodium) for the first 4 hours. Additional fluids as needed. Primary insufficient patients often require 3-4 liters.
Anticipate and monitor for late hypokalemia; add 20 meq of potassium to each liter of fluid as appropriate.

SELECTIVE ALDOSTERONE DEFICIENCY

Epidemiology and Pathophysiology

Selective aldosterone deficiency is an infrequent but potentially lethal disorder in patients with renal insufficiency (70%) resulting from many causes (28, 29), but most frequently among patients with diabetes mellitus (50% of cases). It can be the underlying cause of significant hyperkalemia in elderly patients who use nonsteroidal anti-inflammatory drugs (30) and in others receive angiotensin-converting enzyme inhibitors (31). Electrolyte abnormalities alert the consulting internist to this disorder. Hyperkalemia, hyperchloremia, and metabolic acidosis are present in one-half of these patients. Most (75%) are asymptomatic, but a minority present with weakness or arrhythmias. In the presence of volume contraction, deteriorating renal function, potassium replacement, or use of spironolactone, clinically significant hyperkalemia and acidosis can evolve over several hours.

The syndrome is characterized by low stimulated-renin and plasma-aldosterone values as well as decreased fractional potassium and ammonium excretion. However, the patient's ability to acidify urine is preserved. A recent clinical study (32) suggests that atrial natriuretic peptide contributes to the pathogenesis of this syndrome. A similar syndrome, hyperkalemic distal renal tubular acidosis, is associated with obstructive uropathy, amiloride or hydrochloride therapy, and sickle cell disease (33). These patients have impaired distal tubular function and the inability to excrete hydrogen and potassium or to lower their urinary pH below 5.5 in the presence of acidosis and hyperkalemia. Lead nephropathy and obstructive uropathy can produce a combined syndrome as well (34).

Diagnosis

Recognition of the disorder coupled with prudent adjustments in patient care are usually adequate; a definitive diagnostic evaluation is rarely done. Other potential causes of hyperkalemia may be identified by the patient interview, such as salt substitutes, potassium-sparing diuretics, and potassium supplements. Clinical events associated with hyperkalemia are also identified through the patient assessment: gastrointestinal bleeding, hemolysis, catabolic states, crush injuries, pseudohyperkalemia, leukocytosis, or thrombocytosis. The latter three are excluded by a normal peripheral blood smear, CBC, and differential as well as a simultaneous measure of serum and plasma potassium, which should agree within 0.2 mEq/dL.

Other commonly available tests can also help (Table 14.6). Severely dehydrated patients can develop hyperkalemia if their urinary sodium excretion falls below 10 to 20 mEq/day. Chronic renal failure produces hyperkalemia if the glomerular filtration rate falls below 10 to 15 mL/min. Measurements of serum creatinine and, occasionally, urinary sodium levels are therefore in order. The acidosis of selective aldosteronism is a non–anion-gap acidosis.

A normal Cortrosyn stimulation test eliminates Addison's disease, which is another cause of hyperkalemic, hyperchloremic metabolic acidosis. The experienced consulting internist knows that an occasional patient with diabetes and chronic azotemia who is recovering from ketoacidosis may not achieve a normal bicarbonate level despite ample therapy, because recovery reveals an underlying electrolyte pattern of selective aldosterone deficiency. Additional tests including basal and stimulated (furosemide-induced volume

Table 14.6. Selective Aldosterone Deficiency

Presentation

Hyperkalemia, hyperchloremia, acidosis
Most commonly among diabetics with renal insufficiency, those using prostaglandin or ACE inhibitors and Addison's disease

Diagnostic Strategy

CBC, peripheral smear, platelet count, electrolytes, creatinine, BUN. Occasionally the Cortrosyn stimulation test and simultaneous serum and plasma measures of potassium help.

Treatment

Avoid volume contraction and dehydration, potassium supplements or sparing diuretics, ACE inhibitors and nonsteroidal anti-inflammatory agents. Monitor electrolytes closely if agents listed above are essential to therapy. If potassium is <5.6 meq/dl conservative measures (above) usually suffice.
Potassium wasting diuretics, sodium-potassium exchange resins for more severe cases.
Fludrocortisone acetate (Florinef) 0.1-0.2 mg orally for most severe cases.

contraction) renin levels, ACTH level, or angiotensin infusions to demonstrate subnormal aldosterone responses as well as an evaluation of urine acidification capabilities can confirm the diagnosis. In practice, however, they are rarely needed.

Treatment

Many patients are elderly and vulnerable to complications. If the potassium level does not exceed 5.6 mEq/dL, then avoidance of precipitating situations (i.e., volume contraction), potassium supplements, or offending drugs (e.g., nonsteroidal anti-inflammatory and angiotensin-converting enzyme inhibitors) is adequate. Administration of potassium-wasting diuretics, anion resin exchange, or bicarbonate can also correct the hyperkalemia and acidosis. Fludrocortisone acetate (Florinef), 0.1 to 0.2 mg daily, is reserved for severe cases.

PRIMARY HYPERALDOSTERONISM

Epidemiology

In 1955, Conn (35) described a patient with hypertension, hypokalemia, and neuromuscular symptoms who was found to have an aldosterone-producing adenoma of the adrenal cortex. Removal of the tumor reversed the clinical and biochemical abnormalities. Since the original description of primary hyperaldosteronism, this disorder has been studied extensively, and debate still rages as to the most appropriate diagnostic evaluation. Primary hyperaldosteronism is an uncommon cause of hypertension, however, with a prevalence among unselected patients with hypertension of less than 1%. Despite its rarity, the consulting internist must be familiar with this disorder, because it represents one of the potentially curable forms of hypertension. Effective consultation in this area requires consideration of the following questions: Which patients should be evaluated for primary hyperaldosteronism? What are the appropriate screening tests? How should patients be

evaluated definitively for this syndrome? And, finally, how should patients with suspected primary hyperaldosteronism be treated during the perioperative period?

Diagnosis

The consulting internist should consider this entity in all patients with hypertension and spontaneous hypokalemia. The hypertension may be mild, moderate, or severe, and symptoms reflect the hypokalemia and include muscle weakness, polyuria, nocturia, paresthesia, tetany, and muscle paralysis. Headache is often a predominant feature. It should be remembered, however, that approximately 20% of patients with primary hyperaldosteronism have serum potassium values greater then 3.5 mEq/L (36). Patients who develop moderately severe hypokalemia (serum potassium concentration, <3.0 mEq/L) or have difficulty maintaining normal serum potassium values despite supplementation during therapy with diuretics also should be investigated for hyperaldosteronism. Hyperaldosteronism should also be considered in patients with refractory hypertension when no other, secondary cause is obvious.

The diagnosis is relatively simple in patients with hypertension receiving no diuretics and who have significant hypokalemia (serum potassium, <3.0 mEq/L) with inappropriate kaliuresis (24-hour urinary potassium, >30 mEq), plasma renin activity less than 1 ng/mL, and elevated plasma or urinary aldosterone values. However, the results of these diagnostic screening tests are often ambiguous or equivocal because of the effects of antihypertensive medications (e.g., β-blockers, angiotensin-converting enzyme inhibitors, diuretics) as well as the inherent variability of plasma aldosterone levels, even in the presence of a tumor. The literature contains many seemingly different methods to assess primary hyperaldosteronism. Despite the subtle differences among the various protocols, all are designed to bring out the two biochemical hallmarks of hyperaldosteronism: patients with this disorder fail to increase their plasma renin activity in response to a variety of stimuli (e.g., furosemide, sodium depletion, upright posture), and they fail to suppress their plasma or urinary aldosterone level in response to salt loading or mineralocorticoid administration.

Before proceeding with the diagnostic evaluation, all antihypertensive agents should be discontinued for at least 2 weeks, and the serum potassium level should be normalized by oral supplements. According to Bravo (37), the best test for primary hyperaldosteronism is measurement of the 24-hour urinary level aldosterone during salt loading. This can be accomplished in the ambulatory setting by adding 10 to 12 g of sodium chloride to the patient's daily intake for 3 to 5 days before measuring the 24-hour urinary sodium and aldosterone levels. A 24-hour urinary sodium of at least 250 mEq is evidence of adequate sodium repletion. A 24-hour urinary aldosterone excretion rate of greater than 14 μg per 24 hours distinguishes most patients with primary hyperaldosteronism from those with essential hypertension. Weinberger and Fineberg (38), however, argue that a single plasma aldosterone:plasma renin activity ratio (PA/PRA) provides a simple, sensitive, and specific test for primary hyperaldosteronism. In their study, use of a PA/PRA ratio of more than 30 and a plasma aldosterone value greater than 20 μg/dL as criteria had a sensitivity of 90%, specificity of 91%, positive predictive value of 69%, and negative predictive value of 98%.

Once the biochemical diagnosis of primary hyperaldosteronism has been established, it is important to determine which of the two principal forms is present. Not only is the pathogenesis of each distinct, the treatment is different as well. Adrenal surgery is indicated for patients with adrenal tumor, whereas medical therapy with spironolactone is the treatment of choice for bilateral adrenal hyperplasia or idiopathic hyperaldosteronism. CT of the adrenal glands is the initial step in localization because of this modality's noninvasive nature and overall sensitivity for detecting adenomas. In a patient with biochemical criteria for primary aldosteronism whose CT scan of the adrenal gland is normal, additional evaluation is required, because a subgroup of these patients will be cured by unilateral adrenalectomy. A positive postural stimulation test (i.e., plasma renin activity does not increase with upright posture), elevated urinary excretion rates of 18-methyl oxygenated cortisol metabolites, and lateralization of aldosterone secretion suggest an adenoma and a favorable response to surgery (39).

Treatment

Medical therapy with spironolactone or amiloride is the treatment of choice for patients with adrenal hyperplasia or with adenoma who are poor candidates for surgery. In most patients with adenoma, surgical adrenalectomy results in cure or improvement of the hypertension and reversal of the biochemical abnormalities. Patients undergoing surgery should receive antihypertensive therapy and potassium supplementation for at least 8 to 10 weeks, and it is important to remember that these patients have a significant deficit of total body potassium that must be corrected preoperatively to avoid the risk of arrhythmias during anesthesia. Antihypertensive agents are continued until the day of surgery, and glucocorticoid administration is not necessary. Finally, after removal of an aldosterone-producing adenoma, selective hypoaldosteronism develops in most patients (40). Potassium values should be monitored closely, and if required, supplementation must be given cautiously. Usually, there is sufficient activity to prevent hyperkalemia. Most patients do not require treatment with fludrocortisone.

PHEOCHROMOCYTOMA

Pheochromocytoma is a rare tumor. Most physicians will only encounter one or two patients with this disorder in their careers. Nonetheless, the consulting internist must be familiar with this entity, because it carries the potential for a fatal outcome if the diagnosis is missed as well as the potential for cure if proper diagnosis and surgical treatment are achieved.

Most patients with pheochromocytoma have hypertension, which may be either sustained, sustained with paroxysms, or purely paroxysmal. The classic triad of symptoms is headache, diaphoresis, and palpitations. In fact, the absence of all of three components of this triad makes this diagnosis unlikely (41). Other symptoms include chest pain, nervousness, weakness, and nausea. Paroxysms of these and other symptoms are frequently present in these patients, and hypermetabolism, weight loss, mild glucose intolerance, and orthostatic hypertension are also common. The astute clinician will at least consider this disorder in patients with less esoteric diagnoses, such as labile hypertension, panic disorder, thyrotoxicosis, and functional bowel disease. However, it should be noted that recent advances in diagnostic technology (e.g., new catecholamine assays, CT) may be changing the clinical presentation of patients with pheochromocytoma. In other words, more patients may present "asymptomatically" with an incidental adrenal mass depicted on a CT scan.

Diagnosis

Once the diagnosis is suspected, it must be established through biochemical methods. Controversy abounds as to the best test in diagnosing pheochromocytoma. Measurements of the levels of urinary catecholamine metabolites or free catecholamines are the standard initial laboratory tests. Measurement of 24-hour metanephrine excretion has a sensitivity of 80 to 85% and a specificity in excess of 90% (42). Because of the practical problems with 24-hour urine collections, assays of plasma catecholamines have also been developed and used in patients suspected of pheochromocytoma; reported sensitivities have ranged from 67 to 94% (41). One recent study (43) suggests that tests for plasma metanephrines are more sensitive than tests for plasma catecholamines or urinary metanephrines. Our preference for initial screening is a 24-hour urine collection for metanephrines and free catecholamines, but it is important to recognize that certain medications may interfere with urinary assays, which may make these tests less reliable.

Most patients with pheochromocytoma have plasma catecholamine levels greater than 2000 pg/mL (44). Patients with essential hypertension, anxiety states, or congestive heart failure may have plasma catecholamine levels between 1000 and 2000 pg/mL; for these patients further testing is necessary. The clonidine suppression test uses the ability of clonidine, a centrally acting α-adrenergic agonist, to suppress the release of neurogenically mediated catecholamine (45). The test is based on the premise that increases in plasma catecholamine levels among normal individuals are mediated through activation of the sympathetic nervous system, but in patients with pheochromocytoma, the excess plasma catecholamines originate from the tumor, bypassing normal storage and release mechanisms. The clonidine suppression test should be performed in a standard fashion, as originally described by Bravo et al. (45). Blood for baseline catecholamine levels should be drawn at least 30 minutes after an indwelling venous catheter is placed. Oral clonidine, 0.3 mg, is then administered and blood sampled at 1-, 2-, and 3-hour intervals. A normal response is a total plasma catecholamine level of 500 pg/mL or less. Using this criteria, the clonidine suppression test is 92% accurate in diagnosing pheochromocytoma (46).

Once there is biochemical evidence for pheochromocytoma, the next question is the location of the tumor. Although CT has been widely used for tumor localization, T2-weighted magnetic resonance imaging (MRI) may be a more sensitive study (47). If the MRI is negative, the methyl-iodo-benzyl guanidine (MIBG) scanning test may be helpful. This radiolabeled guanethidine analogue is concentrated by pheochromocytomas, and because MIBG localizes to areas of abnormal adrenergic function, it may be useful in localizing very small lesions as well as extra-adrenal tumors.

Preoperative Management

Surgery offers the potential for cure in most patients with pheochromocytoma, and the consulting internist's task is to ensure the patient has been properly prepared. All patients undergoing exploratory surgery for a pheochromocytoma or needing urgent, unrelated surgery when a pheochromocytoma is present should be treated with adrenergic-blocking agents. The α-blocking agent of choice is phenoxybenzamine, which has a long duration of action and thus can be given as a single daily dose. The starting dose is 10 mg, which is increased to achieve the desired blood pressure; a dose of 40 to 60 mg/day is usually required. Orthostatic hypotension and tachycardia suggest overdosage. Phenoxybenzamine should be given several days before surgery to ensure the patient has adequate α-blockade. Phentolamine is a rapidly acting α-blocker and available for intravenous administration. Its major use is in the management of hypertensive crisis. This agent is particularly helpful to the anesthesiologist intraoperatively, because manipulation of the tumor by the surgeon can trigger catecholamine release and excessive elevations in blood pressure.

Propranolol, a β-blocking agent, is useful in controlling tachycardia, and intravenous propranolol is of great utility intraoperatively for the treatment of multiple tachyarrhythmias. It must be emphasized that propranolol should not be administered until α-blockade is established to avoid a paradoxical rise in blood pressure mediated by unopposed α-vasoconstricting effects. Although β-blockade is often necessary to control tachycardia, one must also be aware of possible hypotension caused by the removal of α-mediated vasoconstriction combined with an inability to mount a reflex tachycardia. Volume replacement is the initial therapy for such hypotension, but β-agonists are sometimes also necessary to restore the blood pressure.

SYNDROME OF INAPPROPRIATE ANTIDIURETIC HORMONE
Epidemiology and Pathophysiology

From 1 to 4% of all hospitalized patients develop hyponatremia. The most common cause among euvolemic patients is the syndrome of inappropriate antidiuretic hormone (SIADH) (48). A variety of stimuli and circumstances can result in excess the ADH effect through one of three mechanisms: (a) production of excess ADH or ADH-like substance by nonhypothalamic tissue (i.e., tumors), (b) excess central nervous system production and release (i.e., head trauma), or (c) excess ADH effect on renal tubules (i.e., drugs). The end result is hyponatremia and a low serum osmolality.

Thirst and ADH are the major regulators of volume homeostasis. Serum osmolality is the primary stimulus, but blood pressure, volume, and, less commonly, hypoxia, hypercarbia, nausea, pregnancy, hypertension, mechanical ventilation, and some drugs can increase ADH secretion. The ADH effect on the renal tubules leads to free-water retention. In the presence of normal ADH secretion and functional kidneys, patients with low serum osmolalities (i.e., hyponatremia) stop secreting ADH, immediately decrease their urine osmolality to less than 100 mOsm/kg, and increase their urine production to greater than 10 mL/min. Maximum ADH secretion produces a urine flow of less than 1 mL/min and a urine osmolality of 800 mOsm/kg when serum osmolality is 295 mOsm/kg (sodium, 145 mmol/L).

SIADH is a normovolemic or slightly volume-expanded condition. Two criteria establish the diagnosis: an "inappropriately high" urine osmolality (>100 mOsm/kg) that is not maximally dilute in the presence of a low serum osmolality (<280 mOsm/kg; serum sodium, <135 mmol/L), and the absence of clinical disorders that normally produce excess ADH excretion or effect. The patient's clinical circumstances suggest the diagnosis. A few simple tests can exclude other disorders.

If clinical circumstances indicate SIADH but the urine sample is maximally dilute, repeat the urine osmolality measurements as serum sodium is restored toward the normal level. Patients with SIADH from the resetting of their osmostat can achieve maximal urinary dilution, because they can suppress their ADH secretion if their water intake is high enough. Therefore, a correct diagnosis can be made with repeat urine and serum osmolality measurements if the urinary concentration increases (101–150 mOsm/kg) before the patient is normonatremic.

Clinical Presentation and Diagnosis

The rate at which patients develop hyponatremia determines their symptoms. The clinical symptoms of confusion, lethargy, headache, nausea, vomiting, and anorexia correlate loosely with the level of hyponatremia. Early cerebral edema occurs with relatively rapid development of serum sodium levels from 120 to 125 mEq/dL along with mild symptoms. As the serum sodium decreases to 110 mEq/dL or less, seizures, decreased deep-tendon reflexes, lower extremity clonus, positive Babinski's signs, weakness, hyperventilation, coma, and death evolve. Rapid development of hyponatremia produces symptoms at higher serum sodium levels.

Table 14.7 identifies six categories of

disorders that are associated with SIADH as well as an approach to assessment. Clinical assessments identify patients with hypovolemia (e.g., diarrhea, vomiting, hypotension, dehydration) and edematous states or conditions in which "effective intravascular hypovolemia" is common (e.g., congestive heart failure, cirrhosis, nephrosis, renal failure). The diagnosis is often straightforward after neurosurgery and in other clinical situations (49, 50). Urine and serum osmolality measurements frequently suffice diagnostically.

TSH and Cortrosyn stimulation tests help to exclude causes of "appropriate" ADH excess. When volume status is unclear, a high plasma renin level, which is usually suppressed in SIADH, supports the diagnosis of hypovolemia. Patients who are elderly or have hypoaldosteronism can have a low renin level even in the presence of hypovolemia. Two other easily available tests can also support the correct diagnosis, but their results need to be interpreted according to the individual clinical circumstances. First, the serum creatinine and uric acid levels are not elevated in SIADH, and second, the urine sodium level is usually greater than 20 mEq/L. Urinary sodium is usually less than 20 mEq/dL in edematous and hypovolemic states; it is also low during recovery from SIADH. Use of diuretics, salt-losing nephropathy, and adrenal insufficiency are three hypovolemic, hyponatremic states that are associated with a high urinary sodium (>20 mEq/L).

The water-loading test is rarely needed. Before testing, the patient's serum sodium level must be 125 mEq/dL; after testing, fluids may need to be restricted for 24 hours to avoid water intoxication. Patients are given 20 mL of water per kilogram of body weight over 20 minutes, and hourly urine samples are measured and tested for osmolality over the next 5 hours. Normal patients excrete 80% of the water load at 5 hours, and the urine osmolality falls to less than 100 mOsm/kg (specific gravity, 1.005). Patients with

Table 14.7.   Syndrome of Inappropriate Antidiuretic Hormone

Differential: (Disorders Where ADH Excess is Expected):

Adrenal insufficiency (Cortrosyn stimulation), hypothyroid (TSH), reset osmoreceptor states (congestive heart failure, renal disease, psychogenic water drinker, cirrhosis)

Associated Conditions (Causes of SIADH):

Malignancy: Adeno and oat cell carcinoma of lung, thymoma, pancreatic, duodenal or prostate cancer
CNS: Aneurysm, hemorrhage and cerebral vascular disease, encephalitis, Guillain-Barré, malformations, paroxysmal cerebral dysrhythmia, trauma, tuberculosis, tumors, neurosurgery, spine surgery.
Pulmonary: Aspergillosis, pneumonia and chronic lung infections, tuberculosis, asthma, pneumothorax, acute respiratory failure, adult respiratory distress syndrome
Metabolic and Endocrine: Myxedema and porphyria
Drugs: Vincristine, cyclophosphamide, other antineoplastics, chlorpropamide, tolbutamide, phenformin, amitriptyline, barbiturates, carbamazepine, fluphenazine, thiothixene, thioridazine, acetaminophen, clofibrate, isoproterenol, morphine, monoamine oxidase inhibitors, oxytocin.
Miscellaneous: Idiopathic, post commisurotomy dilutional syndrome, pain, stress, post surgery and operative distress spinal surgery, mechanical ventilation, nausea.

Diagnostic Strategy:

Hyponatremia (<135 mmol/L, 280 mOsm/kg) identified; review clinical circumstances
Urine osmolality (>100 mOsm/kg) in presence of hypotonic serum (<280 mOsm/kg)
Creatinine, urine sodium, TSH or T4, cortisol and Cortrosyn tests as appropriate
Above efforts usually suffice—water loading and other tests are rarely done.

Treatment of SIADH:

Determined by severity of symptoms and rapidity of hyponatremia
Restrict fluids (500-1000 cc/24 hours), discontinue offending drugs
Demeclocycline (900-1200 mg p.o. daily)
Diuresis (IV Furosemide); IV electrolyte replacement as normal or 3% saline
Risk of pontine myelinolysis is increased by correcting sodium more than 0.5 mmol/L/hour.
Raising serum sodium acutely above 120-125 meq/dl is unnecessary and potentially dangerous.
To estimate sodium replacement:
$0.6 \times$ body weight [kgs] $\times$ (125 − measured serum Na[mmol/L]) = required sodium in mmol

SIADH excrete less than 40% of the water load and fail to fully dilute their urine.

Treatment

Clinical symptoms, severity, rapidity of onset, and chronicity dictate therapy. Fluid restriction (both dietary and discretionary intake) to 500 to 1000 mL daily and withdrawal of offending drugs are the first, and usually successful, conservative options. Demeclocycline, 900 to 1200 mg/ day, antagonizes ADH over several days and provides effective long-term therapy. Chronic SIADH can be well tolerated by patients, and slow correction of sodium levels over several days is in order. Rapid corrections when levels are greater than 120 to 125 mEq/dL are unnecessary and potentially dangerous. Symptoms are uncommon at sodium levels greater than 120 mEq/dL, even in the presence of acute hyponatremia.

When symptoms are severe, rapid diuresis with intravenous furosemide (40 mg) in conjunction with intravenous replacement of measured urine sodium and potassium losses should be initiated. Replacement fluids are either isotonic saline or, if necessary, 3% saline (i.e., for severe symptoms such as seizures). An infusion of 3% saline at a rate of 0.1 mL/g per minute raises the serum sodium level to 10 mEq/dL over 2 hours. A target correction rate of 0.5 mEq/h avoids the risks of neurologic complications (e.g., central pontine myelinolysis) because of overly rapid correction. Young women with acute, severe hyponatremia appear have a greater risk of respiratory arrest, neurologic complications, and death. A correction rate of 1 to 2 mmol/h is prudent in this group until the serum sodium is 125 mmol/L. Adjust the rate of saline infusion to replace urine output and closely monitor urine volume, serum, and urine electrolytes along with the patient's clinical status. Restrict the patient's fluid intake to complete correction of the serum sodium level from 125 mEq/dL to normal over several days.

DIABETES INSIPIDUS

Epidemiology

Polyuria most often raises the possibility of diabetes insipidus among patients after pituitary surgery (5–20% transsphenoidal surgery) or who have facial and head trauma, brain tumors, central nervous system granulomatous disease, aneurysms, or infections. Diabetes insipidus also occurs uncommonly among those with chest wounds and hypotension, drug overdose, hypoxic encephalopathy, electrical burns, brain death, or deep coma (51). The diagnosis is supported by the presence of hypernatremia and a 4- to 6-L daily diuresis.

Pathophysiology

In the postoperative and acute trauma settings, central diabetes insipidus is a dynamic process. It is characterized by rapidly changing urine output and electrolyte patterns over several hours to days as central regulatory centers evolve through an injury. After neurosurgery, onset is usually within 24 hours, and following an injury, cerebral edema evolves after 12 to 24 hours and peaks at 48 to 72 hours. Patients with profound nervous system damage exhibit immediate and permanent polyuria. If the injury is not severe or is transient following pituitary surgery, polyuria persists for approximately 7 days and resolves. When hypothalamic structures are more severely compromised, early polyuria (i.e., onset over 4–8 days after insult) is followed by a brief period (i.e., 1–2 weeks) of normal urine volumes and, occasionally, an SIADH pattern as stores of ADH are depleted. This is followed by the persistent polyuria of a permanent deficiency. A partial defect in some patients is revealed during the period of cerebral edema and presents as a relatively distinct clinical pattern. Polyuria develops over 2 to 3 days after surgery and is followed by small, gradual decreases in urine volume over several days (52).

ADH insufficiency is characterized by polyuria, thirst, polydipsia, and, ultimately, dehydration. Increasing osmolality stimulates carotid, atrial, and aortic osmoreceptors, and it is the primary determinant of ADH secretion. Pain, stress, emotions, and certain drugs (e.g., clofibrate, carbamazepine) can also trigger the release of vasopressin (i.e., ADH) by supraoptic and paraventricular nuclei. ADH activation of cyclic AMP within the medullary nephrons allows water transported across tubular cells to reenter the systemic circulation, thereby conserving total body water and increasing the urine concentration.

Diagnosis

The diagnostic challenge is to distinguish the postoperative diuresis of diabetes insipidus from that of other causes.

These include iatrogenic fluid overload, solute excretion (e.g., glucose, urea, mannitol), adrenal insufficiency, posturinary obstruction, hypercalcemia, hypokalemia, acute renal failure, and drugs such as lithium (in therapeutic range), methoxyflurane, enflurane, narcotic antagonists, and demeclocycline.

Assessment begins with a comprehensive fluid and electrolyte flow sheet that includes weight, renal and extrarenal output, and parenteral and oral intake. Measure several simultaneous urine and serum osmolalities (Table 14.8). Iatrogenic fluid overload and the associated diuresis are characterized by low urine osmolality but low serum osmolality. Solute-induced diuresis (e.g., mannitol, glucose) produces urine osmolalities of 250 to 350 mOsm/kg (specific gravity, 1.009–1.035), but the serum sodium and osmolality are near normal.

Four findings characterize diabetes insipidus: *(a)* diuresis of 30 mL/kg over 24 hours (2–10 L/day), *(b)* low urine specific gravity (1.001–1.005) and urine osmolality (<200 mOsm/kg or <200 mmol/kg), *(c)* normal or elevated serum osmolality and sodium levels, and *(d)* complaints of thirst if the patient is alert and oriented. Two caveats apply here. First, incomplete loss of ADH permits significant urine concentration, which can be associated with urine osmolalities of 290 to 600 mOsm/kg. Second, patients with unrecognized complete loss of ADH who develop profound volume contraction can also develop a urine specific gravity of 1.010 and slightly greater urine osmolality (300 mOsm/kg) through renal compensatory mechanisms.

After neurosurgery, a serum sodium level of 143 mmol/L and 24-hour diuresis of 3 L with hypotonic urine allow a presumptive diagnosis of diabetes insipi-

---

Table 14.8.   Diabetes Insipidus

Presentation

Brain trauma or surgery patients primary group
Low urine specific gravity (1.001-1.005), diuresis >2 liters/day
Drugs which cause nephrogenic diabetes insipidus

Diagnosis

Low urine osmolality (50-200 mOsm/kg) in presence of high serum osmolality
Urine osmolality <200 mOsm/kg after water deprivation and positive pitressin response = central DI
Urine osmolality <200 mOsm/kg after water deprivation and negative response to pitressin =
  nephrogenic DI

Treatment

Central DI: Fluid replacement, aqueous pitressin and then Desmopressin
Nephrogenic diabetes insipidus: thiazide diuretic and indomethacin
To estimate osmolality:

$$2 \times (\text{Na} + \text{K meq/L}) + \frac{\text{blood glucose (mg/dl)}}{18} + \frac{\text{BUN (mg/dl)}}{2.8} = \text{Serum osmolality}$$

To estimate total body water deficit:
$0.6 \times \text{Body weight } (1 - 140/[\text{Na}+]) = \text{body weight deficit}$

---

dus to be made. A 4- to 18-hour water-deprivation test with pitressin administration confirms the diagnosis in less obvious situations. When the clinical circumstances are stable (i.e., euvolemic), the patient should be weighed and the blood pressure, pulse, and urine osmolality recorded. If the patient has a large daily diuresis (6–10 L/day) before scheduled surgery, begin at 6 AM and measure the urine osmolality each hour until three consecutive hourly osmolalities increase by less than 30 mOsm/kg compared with the previous reading. For patients with less than a 6-L daily diuresis, begin fluid restriction at midnight and hourly monitoring at 6 AM.

Once three stable urine osmolality measurements are obtained, adequate dehydration is confirmed by a serum osmolality of 288 mOsm/kg or greater. Patients often lose 1 to 2 kg, and losses that approach 5% of baseline body weight should be replaced. Give 5 U of subcutaneous aqueous pitressin, and measure a final urine osmolality 1 hour later.

When a patient is sufficiently water deprived, the body's normal response is to decrease urine output to 0.5 mL/min and increase osmolality to a level two to four times greater than that of plasma, often to 800 mOsm/kg (specific gravity, ≥1.020). The absolute level of urine concentration is nondiagnostic, because maximal concentration depends on the renal medullary tonicity and the presence of ADH. Patients with diabetes insipidus rarely achieve a urine osmolality of 200 mOsm/kg (specific gravity, 1.001–1.005). After the administration of 5 U of subcutaneous pitressin, patients with partial central diabetes insipidus increase their urine osmolality by at least 9%, whereas normal patients do not. Those patients with complete ADH deficiency increase their urine osmolality by as much as 50%. Patients with chronic fluid overload (e.g., psychogenic water drinkers) or who are severely debilitated usually cannot achieve the same pitressin response. Pa-

tients with nephrogenic diabetes insipidus, chronic hyperkalemia, or renal disease alter their urine osmolality little after dehydration and pitressin challenge (53).

Treatment

Weight and vital signs should be monitored and urine output measured every 1 to 6 hours depending on the volume of diuresis. Replace urine losses with 5% D & W. Patients with hypernatremia who have sodium levels of 165 mEq/dL are at risk for permanent neurologic damage and require prompt, aggressive intravenous therapy. Such patients with a marked diuresis suffer some loss of sodium and may require some fluid replacement as 0.5 N or normal saline (1–2 L).

Initial administration of 5 to 10 U of aqueous pitressin either intramuscularly or subcutaneously (duration of action, 4–6 hours) avoids the risk of water intoxication (4). Doses can be repeated when two consecutive, hourly urine samples reveal an osmolality of 200 mOsm/kg. If the patient is unresponsive to subcutaneous pitressin, an intravenous infusion (1.0 U/h) should be tried. After several days of aqueous pitressin, switch to desmopressin (duration of action, 8–24 hours), administered once or twice daily through nasal insufflations (2.5–40 μg daily). Patients adjust to use of a rhinyl catheter that is calibrated to progressive doses of 5, 10, and 20 μg by first controlling nocturnal diuresis (5–10 μg) and then titrating a morning dose that will be required to control daytime urine volumes (same as or double the evening dose to begin). Pitressin tannate in oil injections provides 24 to 48 hours of control as well as an effective alternative strategy. Lysine nasal vasopressin is a synthetic peptide, but it requires insufflation three to eight times daily. Chlorpropamide, 250 to 500 mg daily, potentiates endogenous vasopressin and can treat very mild cases of partial diabetes insipidus, in which patients with only 2- to 6-L daily diuresis may require no treatment as long as the patient has access to ample water replacement.

Paradoxically, nephrogenic diabetes insipidus can be treated with thiazide diuretics, which induce a negative salt balance and decreased sodium delivery to the loop of Henle. This in turn results in decreased extracellular fluid and urine flow. The addition of indomethacin, which also inhibits the delivery of solute to distal tubules but through prostaglandin inhibition, can add to the control of urine volumes (52, 53).

PITUITARY INSUFFICIENCY

Epidemiology and Clinical Manifestations

The partial to complete deficiency of any one of six anterior pituitary hormones produces a spectrum of clinical manifestations (54). Acute panhypopituitarism on surgical services is uncommon, but it does occur following severe head trauma, pituitary apoplexy associated with anticoagulation or radiation therapy for pituitary tumors, following pituitary surgery, or in patients with pituitary adenomas or parasellar diseases (55). Autopsy studies of patients with severe head trauma have revealed pituitary hemorrhage in 40 to 50%, but pituitary insufficiency is a rare sequela. When pituitary insufficiency is present, the manifestations can be subtle to obvious, transient to progressive and permanent, or evolve over weeks to years after intracranial events (56). A few patients also develop acute panhypopituitarism only to gradually recover function over months to years.

Transient or permanent diabetes insipidus during an intracranial event identifies those patients who are likely to evolve some degree of pituitary insufficiency. The most common symptoms are those of hypogonadism. The classic finding in complete panhypopituitarism is loss of production in the following order: gonadotropins (i.e., luteinizing hormone, follicle-stimulating hormone), growth hormone, TSH, and ACTH. Prolactin deficiency is uncommon except with pituitary infarction, and manifestations of hypoadrenalism or hypothyroidism can predominate. Dysfunction is suggested in the appropriate setting by acute or slowly progressive stupor, easy fatigue, somnolence, cold intolerance, hypotension, hyponatremia, coarse and dry skin, or any combination of these and other endocrine hormone–related symptoms and signs. Acute pituitary apoplexy presents with severe headache, meningismus, changes in vision, extraocular muscle dysfunction, syncope, manifestations of acute adrenal insufficiency, and evidence of bleeding on analyses of spinal fluid.

Diagnosis and Treatment

A low T_4 level, abnormal Cortrosyn stimulation test, or presence of hyponatremia can provide initial clues to the diagnosis. Primary insufficiency is confirmed by demonstration of a lack of growth hormone release following hypoglycemia, a failure of TSH release after thyrotropin-releasing factor infusion, ACTH deficiency, and deficient secretion of luteinizing hormone and follicle-stimulating hormone. This approach is not required to screen for panhypopituitarism or care for patients in the surgical setting. A functional assessment following the rapid sequential administration of four hypothalamic-releasing hormones is available (Table 14.9) (57). Details of a complete pituitary evaluation, however, are beyond the scope of this text.

Replacement therapy involves coverage for ACTH, TSH, and gonadotropin deficiency, in that order. Vascular collapse can follow within hours to days because of adrenal insufficiency. Other deficiencies also manifest and require replacement therapy over several weeks. The insulin requirements of patients with diabetes may fall dramatically in the acute setting because of the loss of adrenal hormones. Table 14.9 summarizes an approach to diagnosis and treatment in this setting.

Table 14.9.   Diagnosis and Treatment of Pituitary Dysfunction

Presentation:

Head trauma, surgery or intracranial disease and any symptoms and signs associated with gonad, thyroid, adrenal, or growth hormone deficiency.

Diagnosis Through Screening:

ACTH deficiency: Inadequate Cortrosyn stimulation test, low A.M. or "during stress" cortisol.
Thyroid deficiency: Serum TSH low, T4 low
Gonadal deficiency: Serum FSH and LH low. For men, draw three serum samples 20 minutes apart and average results. Menstruating women not on contraceptives do not need an FSH or LH level. Random prolactin levels usually preserved and are not helpful.
Combined anterior pituitary test (4): Screen for suspected pituitary dysfunction (post pituitary surgery and radiation). Obtain baseline hormone levels at 8 A.M.: cortisol, T4, T3, resin uptake, estradiol, testosterone and IGR I. Give IV over 20 seconds: LHRH, 100 μg; TRH, 200 μg; CRH, 1 μg/kg body weight; and GHRH 1 μg/kg body weight. Measure serum ACTH, TSH, LH, FSH, GH and prolactin 30 minutes before, at the time of injection and 15, 30, 60, 90 and 120 minutes after injection. Interpret results in the light of baseline hormone measurements. Consult reference 4, Pituitary.
Growth hormone deficiency: Growth hormone response to hypoglycemia is low. Check 8 A.M. cortisol before testing. With physician in attendance and prepared to treat severe hypoglycemic symptoms give regular insulin 0.15 U/kg body weight IV and measure serum GH in 45–60 minutes. Treat hypoglycemia if necessary. Contraindications include: seizure disorder, ischemic heart disease, adrenal insufficiency (8 A.M. serum cortisol of less than 5 μg/dl). Test should be done by an experienced consultant.

Replacement Therapy:

ACTH deficiency: Anticipate deficiency and provide stress dose replacement before surgical intervention or diagnostic procedures. Administer Dexamethasone (treat brain edema as well as adrenal insufficiency) 4 mg IV every 4 to 6 hours, taper rapidly over 5–7 days post-surgery. Upon discharge prescribe preassembled syringe of dexamethasone (4 m/ml) or hydrocortisone sodium succinate, 100 mg (Solu Cortef Mix-O-Vial) and educate about use in the event of symptoms of acute crisis. If daily replacement is required long-term: Oral cortisone 25 mg in A.M. and 12.5 mg in P.M. or Prednisone 7.5 mg daily (5 mg in A.M. and 2.5 mg in P.M.) to begin.
Thyroid deficiency: 8–10 days after pituitary ablation early symptoms begin to evolve. Give adrenal replacement first to avoid adrenal crisis. Thyroxin (synthroid) 0.1–0.2 mg daily, orally. Preoperative replacement needed only if hypothyroid before surgery.
Gonadal deficiency: Testosterone deficiency is treated after discharge. Testosterone ethanate or cypionate 200 mg I.M. every 2 to 3 weeks. Cyclic daily oral conjugated estrogens (0.625–1.25 mg Premarin, 20–50 μg ethynil estradiol days 1 through 25) in conjunction with 5-10 mg medroxy-progesterone acetate on days 21-25 will produce menstruation.
Growth hormone, prolactin: Not replaced in adults.
Antidiuretic hormone: See Diabetes Insipidus section.

HYPERPARATHYROIDISM AND HYPERCALCEMIA

Hyperparathyroidism

Primary hyperparathyroidism was once considered to be a rare disease characterized by bone disease, renal calculi, and a variety of gastrointestinal complaints. With the advent of inexpensive, routine serum multiple-chemical analysis now available to the clinician, many more cases of previously unrecognized asymptomatic hyperparathyroidism have been diagnosed. It is currently estimated that 0.2% of patients in an outpatient or a hospital facility will have primary hyperparathyroidism (58). Approximately 100,000 new cases develop each year in the United States. Accordingly, the consulting internist must be familiar with this disease to correctly diagnose and treat patients with primary hyperparathyroidism.

The following discussion addresses two major questions. First, how is the diagnosis of hyperparathyroidism established? Second, which patients should be referred for surgery, and which should be treated medically?

Diagnosis

The presenting clinical features of primary hyperparathyroidism are varied. Patients may be relatively asymptomatic, or they may come to clinical attention because of nephrolithiasis, gastrointestinal complaints, or fatigue. Severe bone disease (i.e., osteitis fibrosa cystica) with loss of stature and weakness rarely occurs today. Other clinical manifestations include myopathy, pseudogout, hypertension, and anemia.

The biochemical hallmark of hyperparathyroidism is hypercalcemia. Most patients have sustained elevations in their serum calcium level, but it is important to remember that total serum calcium concentrations may be misleading in patients with decreased serum albumin levels. This problem can be resolved with use of the ionized serum calcium level. Other biochemical abnormalities in these patients may include a low phosphorus, high chloride, low bicarbonate, and high alkaline phosphatase level.

The development of highly sensitive, two-site immunoradiometric assays has made it possible to measure the level of intact parathyroid hormone (PTH), and this represents a major advance in diagnosis. Most patients with hyperparathy-roidism have elevated baseline plasma levels of intact PTH. An elevated serum calcium level with an elevated intact PTH level is generally sufficient biochemical evidence to make the diagnosis. Intact PTH concentrations are low in nonpara-thyroid hypercalcemia, including the humoral hypercalcemia of malignancy. Borderline levels of intact PTH may be found in patients with familial hypocalciuric hypercalcemia, which can be diagnosed by measurements of serum and urinary calcium concentrations.

A small percentage of patients with primary hyperparathyroidism have high-normal or minimal elevations of intact PTH. One shortcoming of intact PTH assays is the overlap of values among healthy patients and those with hyperparathyroidism. In patients who are strongly suspected of hyperparathyroidism but have normal intact PTH levels, a calcium-loading test may be a valuable diagnostic tool (59).

Treatment

Once the diagnosis of primary hyper-parathyroidism is established, the next step is to decide if the patient can be followed medically or be referred to a surgeon for parathyroidectomy. Indications for surgical treatment are: (a) markedly elevated serum calcium concentration, (b) previous episode of life-threatening hypercalcemia, (c) reduced creatinine clearance (i.e., 30% of age-matched normal persons), (d) kidney stones, (e) markedly elevated 24-hour urine calcium excretion (i.e., >400 mg), and (f) bone mass of more than 2 SD less than those of age-, gender-, and race-matched controls. A National Institutes of Health consensus conference recommended nonoperative surveillance for patients without symptoms, with a serum calcium level less than 12 mg/dL, and without renal calcification or radiographically evident bone disease (60). Other authorities, however, advocate a more liberal approach when selecting patients for surgery based on the safety and benefits of parathyroidectomy in light of the natural progression of mild, "asymptomatic" hyperparathyroidism (61, 62).

For the patient undergoing parathyroid surgery, careful observation is essential. Serum calcium and phosphorus measurements should be obtained daily, and the consulting internist must be aware of the transient hypocalcemia that usually occurs on the third or fourth day following the surgery. If the serum calcium concentration does not drop below 7 mg/dL and the patient's symptoms are mild, supplemental calcium is probably not indicated. The serum calcium level usually returns to normal within a week's time, but if symptoms become severe (e.g., muscle cramping, numbness, twitching) or hypocalcemia persists, intermittent calcium should be given (i.e., 10 mL of a calcium gluconate solution over 5 to 10 minutes). Occasionally, oral calcium and vitamin D are necessary in patients with persistent hypocalcemia.

Hypercalcemia

Occasionally, an internist may be asked to see a patient scheduled for elective surgery who was found to have hypercalcemia on routine preoperative testing. In this situation, the consulting internist must address the following questions: What is the cause of the hypercalcemia? What are the implications for patient care? What risk does hypercalcemia impose on the patient?

Hypercalcemia most often results from primary hyperparathyroidism or malignancy. In the ambulatory setting, hyperparathyroidism accounts for 50 to 60% of these cases. In contrast, malignancy is responsible for approximately 65% of cases among hospitalized patients. The cancers that are associated with hypercalcemia most frequently include lung, breast, head and neck, urogenital, and multiple myeloma. Other causes include familial hypocalciuric hypercalcemia, hy-

perthyroidism, Paget's disease, thiazide diuretic, vitamin D excess, milk alkali syndrome, sarcoidosis and other granulomatous diseases, and immobilization. In most cases, a careful patient history and physical examination, routine laboratory testing, chest radiography, and renal ultrasonography will reveal the cause. Attention to the breast examination in women and the prostate examination in men is essential. The laboratory distinction between primary hyperparathyroidism and humoral hypercalcemia of malignancy is facilitated by the serum immunoradiometric intact PTH assay, in which patients with humoral hypercalcemia of malignancy have consistently low or low-normal levels and patients with primary hyperparathyroidism have high or high-normal levels. If a malignancy is uncovered or strongly suspected, it is usually prudent to postpone or cancel elective surgery until the patient's overall prognosis is better defined and the impact of this diagnosis on the surgical condition has been considered.

Mild hypercalcemia (i.e., calcium <12 mg/dL) poses no special perioperative problems for patients with normal renal and cardiovascular function. Because hypercalcemia can lead to hypovolemia, however, restoration of normal intravascular fluid and electrolyte status is required. The electrocardiography should be examined for signs of hypercalcemia (i.e., short P-R and Q-T interval). For patients with more marked hypercalcemia (i.e., calcium >12 mg/dL) or symptomatic hypercalcemia, surgery should be postponed until the serum calcium level has been lowered by the methods outlined in Chapter 11 (renal and acid-base disorders).

REFERENCES

1. Nathan DM. Long-term complications of diabetes mellitus. N Engl J Med 1993;328:1676–1685.
2. Gavin LA. Perioperative management of the diabetic patient. Endocrinol Metab Clin North Am 1992;21:457–475.
3. Raucou-Aime M, Lugrin D, Boussofara M, et al. Intraoperative glycaemic control in non-insulin-

dependent and insulin-dependent diabetes. Br J Anaesth 1994;73:443–449.

4. The Diabetes Control and Complications Trial Research Group. The effect of intensive treatment of diabetes on the development and progression of long-term complications in insulin-dependent diabetes mellitus. N Engl J Med 1993;329:977–986.

5. American Diabetes Association. Detection and management of lipid disorders in diabetes. Diabetes Care 1993;14:839–855.

6. Mathiesen ER, Hommel E, Giese J, et al. Efficacy of captopril in postponing nephropathy in normotensive insulin dependent diabetic patients with microalbuminuria. BMJ 1991;303:81–87.

7. Ravid M, Savin H, Jutrin I, et al. Long-term stabilizing effect of angiotensin-converting enzyme inhibition on plasma creatinine and on proteinuria in normotensive type II diabetic patients. Ann Intern Med 1993;118:577–581.

8. Weidmann P, Boehlen LM, de Courten. Pathogenesis and treatment of hypertension associated with diabetes mellitus. Am Heart J 1993;125:1498–1513.

9. Manske CL, Wang Y, Rector T, et al. Coronary revascularization in insulin-dependent diabetic patients with chronic renal failure. Lancet 1992;340:998–1002.

10. Gibbons GW, Habershaw GM. Diabetic foot infections: anatomy and surgery. Infect Dis Clin North Am 1995;9:131–142.

11. Saperstein MD. Diabetic keoacidosis and hyperosmolar coma. Endocrinol Metab Clin North Am 1992;21:415–432.

12. Grayson ML. Diabetic foot infections: antimicrobial therapy. Infect Dis Clin North Am 1995;9:143–161.

13. McArthur JW, Rawson RW, Means JH, et al. Thyrotoxic crisis. JAMA 1947;134:868–874.

14. Davis PJ, Davis FB. Hyperthyroidism in patients over the age of 60 years. Medicine 1974;53:161–181.

15. Lahey FH. Non-activated (apathetic) type of hyperthyroidism. N Engl J Med 1931;204:747–748.

16. Franklyn JA, Black EG, Betteridge J, et al. Comparison of second and third generation methods for measurement of serum thyrotropin in patients with overt hyperthyroidism, patients receiving thyroxine therapy, and those with non-thyroidal illness. J Clin Endocrinol Metab 1994;78:1368–1371.

17. Franklyn JA. The management of hyperthyroidism. N Engl J Med 1994;330:1731–1738.

18. Gavin LA: Thyroid crises. Med Clin North Am 1991;75:179–193.

19. Ladenson PW, Levin AA, Ridgeway EC, et al. Complications of surgery in the hypothyroid patients. Am J Med 1984;77:261–266.

20. Drucker DJ, Burrow GN. Cardiovascular surgery in the hypothyroid patient. Arch Intern Med 1985;145:1585.

21. Kabadi UM. "Subclinical hypothyroidism"—natural course of the syndrome during a prolonged follow-up study. Arch Intern Med 1993;153:957–961.

22. Wehmann RE, Gregerman RI, Burns WH, et al. Suppression of thyrotropin in the low-thyroxine state of severe non-thyroidal illness. N Engl J Med 1985;312:546–552.

23. Hamblin PS, Dyer SA, Mohr VS, et al. Relationship between thyrotropin and thyroxine changes during recovery from severe hypothyroxinemia of critical illness. J Clin Endocrinol Metab 1986;62:717–722.

24. Schlaghecke E, Kornely E, Santen RT, Ridderkamp P. The effect of long-term glucocorticoid therapy on pituitary-adrenal responses to exogenous corticotropin-releasing hormone. N Engl J Med 1992;326:226–230.

25. Werbel SS, Ober KP. Acute adrenal insufficiency. Endocrinol Metab Clin North Am 1993;22:303–328.

26. Boulanger BR, Gann DS. Management of the trauma victim with pre-existing endocrine disease. Crit Care Clin 1994;10:537–554.

27. Dickstein G, Shechner C, Nicholson WE, et al. Adrenocorticotropin stimulation test: effects of basal cortisol level, time of day, and suggested new sensitive low dose test. J Clin Endocrinol Metab 1991;72:773–778.

28. Shaked Y, Blau O, Shpiberg O, Samra Y. Hyporeninemic hypoaldosteronism asssociated with multiple myeloma: 11 years of follow-up. Clin Nephrol 1993;40:79–82.

29. Etzel JV, Brocavich JM, Torre M. Endocrine complications associated with human immunodeficiency virus infection. Clinical Pharmacy 1992;11:705–713.

30. Murray MD, Brater DC. Renal toxicity of the nonsteroidal anti-inflammatory drugs. Annu Rev Pharmacol Toxicol 1993;33:435–465.

31. Uchida K, Sadahide A, Shigeru N, et al. Reversible hyperkalemia during antihypertensive therapy in a hypertensive diabetic patient with latent hypoaldosteronism and mild renal failure. South Med J 1994;87:1153–1155.

32. Clark BA, Brown RS, Epstein FH. Effect of atrial natriuretic peptide on potassium-stimulated aldosterone secretion: potential relevance to hypoaldosteronism in man. J Clin Endocrinol Metab 1992;75:399–403.

33. Kokko JP. Primary acquired hypoaldosteronism. Kidney Int 1985;27:690–702.

34. Ashouri O. Hyperkalemic distal renal tubular acidosis and selective alsosterone deficiency. Arch Intern Med 1985;145:1306–1307.

35. Conn JW. Primary aldosteronism: a new clinical syndrome. J Lab Clin Med 1955;45:3–7.

36. Bravo EL, Taraz RC, Dustan HP, et al. The

changing clinical spectrum of primary hyperaldosteronism. Am J Med 1983;4:641–651.

37. Bravo EL. Primary aldosteronism: issues in
diagnosis and management. Endocrinol Metab
Clin North Am 1994;23:271–283.

38. Weinberger MH, Fineberg NS. The diagnosis of
primary aldosteronism and separation of two
major subtypes. Arch Intern Med 1993;153:
2125–2129.

39. Blumenfeld JD, Sealey JE, Schlussel Y, et al.
Diagnosis and treatment of primary hyperaldosteronism. Ann Intern Med 1994;121:877–885.

40. Bravo EL, Tarazi RC, Dustan HP. Selective
hypoaldosteronism despite prolonged pre- and
postoperative hyperreninemia in primary hyperaldosteronism. J Clin Endocrinol Metab 1975;
41:611–617.

41. Stein PP, Black HR. A simplified diagnostic
approach to pheochromocytoma. A review of the
literature and report of one institution's experience. Medicine 1991;70:46–66.

42. Krakoff LR. Management of the hypertensive
patient. New York: Churchill Livingstone,
1995:75–86.

43. Lenders JW, Keiser HR, Goldstein DS, et al.
Plasma metanephrines in the diagnosis of pheochromocytoma. Ann Intern Med 1995;123:
101–109.

44. Bravo E, Tarazi R, Gifford R, Stewart B. Circulating and urinary catecholamines in pheochromocytoma. Diagnostic and pathophysiologic implications. N Engl J Med 1979;301:682–686.

45. Bravo EL, Tarazi RC, Fouad FM, et al. Clonidine
suppression test: a useful aid in the diagnosis of
pheochromocytoma. N Engl J Med 1981;305:
623–626.

46. Sjoberg JF, Simcic KJ, Kidd GS. The clonidine
suppression test for pheochromocytoma. A review of its utility and pitfalls. Arch Intern Med
1992;152:1193–1197.

47. Peplinski GR, Norton JA. The predictive value of
diagnostic tests for pheochromocytoma. Surgery
1994;116:1101–1110.

48. Kovacs AU. Syndrome of inappropriate antidi-
uresis. Endocrinol Metab Clin North Am 1992;
4:859–875.

49. Callewart CC, Menchew JT, Kanim LE, et al.
Hyponatremia and the syndrome of inappropriate antidiuretic hormone secretion in adult
spinal surgery. Spine 1994;19:1674–1679.

50. Olson BR, Rubino D, Gumowski J, et al. Isolated

hyponatremia after transpheniodal pituitary
surgery. J Clin Endocrinol Metab 1995;80:
85–91.

51. Urquhart CK, Craft PD, Nehlowe MM. Transient diabetes insipidus following electrical
burns in two patients. South Med J 1994;87:
412–413.

52. Johnson MA, Ogorman J, Golembiewski GH, et
al. Nephrogenic diabetes insipidus secondary to
lithium therapy in the postoperative patient: a
case report. Am Surg 1994;60:836–839.

53. Seckl JR, Dunger DB. Diabetes insipidus: current treatment recommendations. Drugs 1992;
44:216–224.

54. Rolih CA, Ober KP. The endocrine response to
critical illness. Med Clin North Am 1995;79:
211–214.

55. Vance ML. Hypopituitarism. N Engl J Med
1994;330:1651–1662.

56. Constine LS, Woolf PD, Cann D, et al.
Hypothalamic-pituitary dysfunction after radiation for brain tumors. N Engl J Med 1993;328:
87–94.

57. Sheldon WR Jr, DeBold CR, Evans WS, et al.
Rapid sequential intravenous administration of
four hypothalamic releasing hormones as a
combined anterior pituitary function test in
normal subjects. J Clin Endocrinol Metab 1885;
60:623–630.

58. Heath H, Hodgson SF, Kennedy MA. Primary
hyperparathyroidism: incidence, morbidity and
potential impact in a community. J Clin Endocrinol Metab 1976;41:415–425.

59. Monchik JM, Lamberton RP, Roth U. Role of the
oral calcium-loading test with measurement of
intact parathyroid hormone in the diagnosis of
symptomatic subtle primary hyperparathyroidism. Surgery 1992;112:1103–1110.

60. NIH Consensus Development Conference Panel.
Diagnosis and management of asymptomatic
primary hyperparathyroidism: consensus development conference statement. Ann Intern Med
1991;114:593–597.

61. Clark OH, Wilkes W, Siperstein AE, Duh QY.
Diagnosis and management of asymptomatic
hyperparathyroidism: safety, efficacy, and deficiencies of our knowledge. J Bone Min Res
1991;6(Suppl 2):S135–1342.

62. Harrison BJ, Wheeler MH. Asymptomatic primary hyperparathyroidism. World J Surg 1991;
15:724–729.

15

Hematology

James O. Ballard and Robert A. Gordon

Timely recognition and treatment of hematologic disorders are essential for an optimal surgical outcome. Some abnormalities of the blood, blood-forming organs, and hemostatic system are not routinely encountered by the general internist and therefore may require a hematologist. However, the consulting internist can assess and manage many hematologic problems that arise during the preoperative and the postoperative periods. This chapter provides an overview of the more common disorders, and it highlights those of special interest in surgical patients.

THE PREOPERATIVE PATIENT WITH ANEMIA

When evaluating a patient with anemia in the preoperative setting, the major goals are to determine the underlying cause of the anemia, to estimate its physiologic significance in the operative setting, and to assess the need for blood transfusion.

Diagnostic Activities

Both acute and chronic blood loss are leading causes of anemia. The patient should first be questioned about overt, traumatic blood loss or gastrointestinal bleeding in the form of melena, hematochezia, and hematemesis. Women should be asked to describe the extent of blood loss both with menses and during prior pregnancies. It should be remem-

bered that regular phlebotomy for voluntary blood donation may also lead to the gradual onset of iron deficiency anemia.

Additional historical data of importance include prior history of anemia, requirement for blood transfusion, jaundice, any current medications, ethanol consumption, dietary habits, and renal, hepatic, endocrine, and rheumatologic diseases. A family history of anemia, cholelithiasis at a young age, or splenectomy indicate the possibility of a congenital hemolytic process.

A review of the complete blood count, including indices by automated cell counter, reticulocyte count, peripheral smear, and stool occult blood testing, can be quickly accomplished. The anemia can then be classified as either microcytic, macrocytic, or normocytic, thus narrowing the diagnostic possibilities (Table 15.1). A reticulocyte count should be obtained, because it reflects the production rate of the erythroid bone marrow.

The reticulocyte count more accurately indicates the marrow capacity for red blood cell (RBC) production when it is corrected for the degree of anemia and the premature release of reticulocytes from the stressed bone marrow. This corrected reticulocyte count is expressed as the reticulocyte production index (RPI), which is calculated as follows:

$$\text{RPI} = \text{Observed reticulocyte count (\%)} \times \text{Patient's hematocrit/45}$$

Table 15.1.   Causes of Anemia Classified by RBC Indices and Peripheral Blood Smear

---

Microcytic (MCV, <80 fL)
    Iron deficiency
    Thalassemia (beta, alpha)
    Anemia of chronic disease
    Sideroblastic anemia
Macrocytic (MCV, >100 fL)
    Folic acid deficiency
    Vitamin B_{12} deficiency
    Liver disease
    Alcoholism
    Drugs
    Hypothyroidism
    Myelodysplastic syndromes
    Reticulocytosis (marked)
Normocytic (MCV, 80–100 fL)
    Hypoproliferative (RPI, <2)
    Anemia of chronic disease
    Chronic renal failure
    Bone marrow failure (hypoplasia, infiltration)
    Early iron deficiency
    Hypothyroidism
    Hypopituitarism
    Combined deficiency states (iron, vitamin B_{12},
        folate)
    Acute hemorrhage (RPI, >3)
    Hemolytic anemia (RPI, >3)
        Drugs
        Autoimmune
        Tranfusion reaction
        Microangiopathic (e.g., DIC, cancer, TTP,
            vasculitis, prosthetic surfaces)
        Congenital
            Hemoglobinopathy
            Hereditary membrane defects (e.g.,
                hereditary spherocytosis)
            RBC enzyme deficiency (e.g., G-6-PD)
            Other congenital abnormalities
        Hypersplenism

MCV, mean corpuscular volume; *TTP,* thrombotic thrombocytopenic purpura.

If increased numbers of bluish (i.e., polychromatophilic) RBCs are seen on the peripheral blood smear, the RPI is divided by 2.

An RPI of greater than 3% is found with hemolysis, acute blood loss, or erythroid response to the replacement of a deficient hematinic (e.g., iron, vitamin B_{12}, folate). An RPI of 2% or less indicates inadequate erythroid production because of erythroid hypoplasia, ineffective RBC maturation, or marrow replacement. In the absence of acute blood loss or recent repletion of iron, vitamin B_{12}, or folate stores, an RPI of greater than 3% indicates hemolytic anemia. Both direct and indirect Coombs' tests should then be performed to exclude immune hemolysis, because compatible units of blood may be difficult to find and transfusion could be hazardous in this situation.

Clues to the underlying cause of anemia are frequently apparent on the peripheral blood smear. In addition to the hemoglobin content of RBCs, abnormalities such as red cell spherocytosis or fragmentation may suggest specific forms of hemolytic anemia. Leukocyte and platelet abnormalities on the peripheral blood smear may lead to diagnosis of an unsuspected leukemic disorder even when the total white blood cell count is within the normal limits.

After classification of the anemia by indices, RPI, and peripheral blood smear, patient serum should be obtained for ferritin, iron, total iron-binding capacity, vitamin B_{12}, and folate determinations before transfusion, because transfused blood will alter these values and confound diagnostic efforts. The RBC folate level provides a more reliable estimate of tissue folate reserves over the preceding 2 to 3 months and, unlike the serum folate level, is not affected by acute changes in dietary intake. When emergency surgery is required, there is little time for a specific diagnosis or treatment, because improvement of the hemoglobin and hematocrit following therapy with iron, vitamin B_{12}, folic acid, or recombinant human erythropoietin requires days to weeks. Thus, preoperative correction of anemia by replacing a deficient hematinic is only practical in candidates for elective surgery.

Assessing the Need for Blood Transfusion

Reliable data correlating the hemoglobin level and patient risk during general anesthesia and surgery are sparse. For many years, surgeons and anesthesiologists used a hemoglobin of 10 g/dL and a hematocrit of 30% as the values below which preoperative RBC transfusion was indicated (1).

Experience with renal transplantation and patients with religious prohibitions against blood transfusion, however, has shown that some types of surgery can be safely performed at hemoglobin levels as low as 6 to 7 g/dL when a compensated intravascular volume exists. In a study involving 125 patients who refused blood transfusion (2), the surgical mortality rate was 7% for those with hemoglobin values greater than 10 g/dL but 62% for those with values less than 6 g/dL. When intraoperative blood loss did not exceed 500 mL, the mortality rate was 8%; when intraoperative blood loss exceeded 2000 mL, the mortality rate was 43%. In addition, a study of a small number of patients at high risk for myocardial ischemia (3) suggested an association between lower postoperative hematocrit levels and the occurrence of myocardial infarction and other cardiac abnormalities during arterial bypass procedures. The decision to transfuse blood should be based on the clinical condition of the patient and the expected blood loss during the specific surgical procedure.

Factors favoring transfusion are continuing acute blood loss, underlying cardiopulmonary disease, and the need for major procedures with significant anticipated blood loss that require general anesthesia. Patients with continued bleeding should be transfused promptly, because the hematocrit may not adequately reflect the degree of blood loss as volume depletion and hemoconcentration are also usually present. Cardiopulmonary compromise with dyspnea, angina, or congestive heart failure is also an indication for transfusion if these symptoms are attributable to the anemia. The National Institutes of Health Consensus Development Conference on perioperative RBC transfusion (4) concluded

No single measure can replace good clinical judgement as the basis for decisions regarding perioperative transfusion. However, current experience suggests that otherwise healthy patients with hemoglobin values of 10 g/dL or greater rarely require perioperative transfusion, whereas those with hemoglobin values of less than 7 g/dL will frequently require RBC transfusion.

Transfusions for elective surgery should be completed at least 24 hours before the procedure. Transfusion of packed RBCs into a patient with chronic anemia further increases the total circulating blood volume, and heart failure may occur if the transfusion is given too rapidly. Also, banked blood that is used for transfusions may have abnormal oxygen dissociation characteristics. For example, storage of blood depletes the level of 2,3-diphosphoglycerate (2,3-DPG), causing a significant displacement of the oxyhemoglobin dissociation curve to the left and preventing oxygen unloading to the tissues. Transfused RBCs will regenerate 2,3-DPG, but with multiple-unit transfusions, an adequate level may not be restored for 24 hours or more.

Autologous Blood Transfusion

Blood transfusion carries a significant potential risk of disease transmission. Donor units are uniformly tested for hepatitis B, hepatitis C, human immunodeficiency virus (HIV-1), and human T-cell leukemia virus, type 1 (HTLV-I), thus making homologous blood transfusion a safer procedure than in the past. Nonetheless, the patient's need for a blood transfusion should be clearly documented by the physician on the medical record, and a growing number of institutions now require informed consent from the patient before a transfusion.

Except for potential bacterial contamination of autologous units, there is no risk for the transmission of infectious diseases (e.g., hepatitis, syphilis, cytomegalovirus, HIV-1, HTLV-I) with autologous transfusion. This mode of transfusion also avoids the risk of alloimmunization to erythrocyte, leukocyte, platelet, or protein antigens. Preoperative donation of autologous blood is appropriate for all patients requiring an elective surgical procedure in which blood transfusion will likely be necessary. Autologous transfusion is particularly valuable for patients with rare blood types, a history of previous transfusion reactions, and whose religious beliefs prohibit homologous transfusions. It can be used effectively in patients undergoing cardiopulmonary bypass and in pregnancy for women in whom increased blood loss is anticipated with delivery. In this latter situation, donations can begin after the 13th week of gestation, with most occurring in the third trimester.

Autologous blood can be stored for up to approximately 35 to 42 days depending on the anticoagulant used. Except in unusual circumstances, phlebotomy can be performed in most patients with a hemoglobin of 11 g/dL or greater. No more than 450 ± 45 mL or 12% of the estimated blood volume, whichever is less, should be withdrawn at a single donation. The usual schedule is 1 U donated per week, with the last phlebotomy performed 72 hours before surgery. Iron supplementation should begin at least 1 week before the first donation and continue for 2 to 3 months after the last. This is especially important for female donors.

Despite its advantages, however, autologous transfusion has recently come under closer scrutiny. Because many donated autologous units are not transfused, the expense of collecting, processing, and storing these discarded units must be weighed against the potential health benefit of this method. In an era when the transmission of infection by homologous transfusion has been dramatically reduced, the role of autologous transfusion is somewhat less certain.

In a recent study using a decision-analysis model (5), the cost of preoperative autologous transfusion for several common surgical procedures at a large university medical center was compared with the expected health benefit. The authors concluded that the increased safety afforded by autologous transfusion may not justify the increased cost associated with this method.

Alternative methods of providing autologous blood have also been developed. During intraoperative isovolemic hemodilution, blood is removed immediately after the induction of anesthesia and is followed by reexpansion with intravenous fluids and subsequent return of autologous blood to the patient during the surgical procedure. This is simpler and less costly than preoperative autologous collection. In addition, intraoperative blood salvage involves the collection of shed blood during surgery with centrifugation and washing of the RBCs before returning them to the patient (6).

With the availability of recombinant human erythropoietin, anemias of underproduction, such as anemia associated with renal failure, chronic diseases, HIV infection, and myelosuppressive chemotherapy, can sometimes be ameliorated or reversed without a blood transfusion. Use of recombinant human erythropoietin also decreases the need for perioperative homologous blood transfusion for elective hip replacement (7, 8).

POSTOPERATIVE ANEMIAS

Diagnostic Activities

Evaluation of the cause of postoperative anemia should begin with a search for anemias that existed preoperatively or were acquired because of the patient's underlying disease. Stools should be tested for occult blood, because gastrointestinal bleeding from stress ulceration is not uncommon postoperatively. The operative report should be reviewed for estimated blood loss, and the intake and output records should be examined. If the postoperative fall in hematocrit is greater than would be expected from the estimated blood loss at surgery, causes of anemia other than operative blood loss should be considered. A useful clinical axiom is that **1 U of blood lost or transfused (i.e., 250–350 mL of packed RBCs) correlates with approximately three percentage points of hematocrit** (assuming a stable intravascular volume).

A review of the complete blood count, including indices, RPI, and peripheral blood smear, should help to classify the anemia into one of the three major categories: microcytic, macrocytic, or normocytic (Table 15.2). Direct and indirect Coombs' test, lactate dehydrogenase, and bilirubin should be obtained to help exclude hemolysis.

Most postoperative anemias are normocytic and normochromic, and they are generally multifactorial. Common causes are underestimation of the surgical blood

loss or continued bleeding, occult gastrointestinal bleeding, dilutional anemia because of excess fluid administration, repeated drawing of blood for diagnostic tests, and anemia from chronic disease and inflammation. In patients who had borderline iron stores preoperatively, a significant anemia is more likely to have occurred from blood loss at surgery.

Dilutional anemia is often overlooked. Overhydration during surgery and the postoperative period can cause significant dilution of the RBC mass, and fluid intake and output as well as preoperative and postoperative weights should be compared.

Drawing blood for diagnostic studies is a significant cause of anemia in hospitalized patients, and it has been termed **nosocomial anemia.** One study of patients in coronary and pulmonary care units (9) recorded a mean blood loss of approximately 55 mL/day. It was estimated that the hematocrit value may decrease by 6% during a hospitalization period averaging 21 days. The authors concluded that for most seriously ill adults who are hospitalized for 3 to 4 weeks, an average of 500 to 1000 mL of blood will be drawn for diagnostic studies. In patients with nosocomial anemia, an observed reticulocyte count of 2 to 4% is common. However, patients with preexisting medical illnesses or iron deficiency may not be able to increase RBC production to compensate for blood loss from both surgery and frequent diagnostic blood studies.

Anemia associated with chronic disease may complicate disorders such as chronic infection and inflammation, cancer, and collagen vascular diseases. Current research suggests that the anemia of chronic disease results from the marrow-suppressing effects of cytokines such as tumor necrosis factor and certain interleukins. These humoral substances appear to impair utilization of iron by the developing RBC precursors. This type of anemia develops slowly, and by itself, it should not produce a rapid fall in hematocrit. Postoperatively, however, the de-

Table 15.2. Anemias in the Postoperative Period

Most Common
Normocytic (MCV, 80–100 fL)
  Surgical blood loss
  Active bleeding (surgical site, GI ulceration)
  Dilutional anemia
  Nosocomial anemia
  Acute inflammation/chronic disease
  Renal insufficiency
  Drug-induced bone marrow suppression
  Hemolysis
    Drugs
    Bacterial sepsis (e.g., *Clostridium* sp.)
    Delayed transfusion reaction
    Underlying immunologic disorder
Less Common
Macrocytic (MCV, >100 fL)
  Folic acid deficiency
  Drugs
  Liver disease
  Reticulocytosis (marked)
Microcytic (MCV, <80 fL)
  Anemia of chronic disease
  Iron deficiency from chronic blood loss

GI, gastrointestinal; MCV, mean corpuscular volume.

crease in marrow erythroid response caused by anemia of chronic disease may contribute to the failure of compensation for blood loss from operative bleeding and blood drawing. In the anemia of chronic disease, both the serum iron and the total iron-binding capacity are reduced, whereas the serum ferritin level and bone marrow iron stores are normal to increased.

Postoperative renal insufficiency will also contribute to decreased RBC production because of a reduced erythropoietin response to anemia. Patients with renal failure demonstrate a mildly shortened RBC survival as well. When anemia results primarily from renal failure, treatment with recombinant human erythropoietin (50–150 U/kg subcutaneously three times a week) will reverse or significantly ameliorate the anemia.

If thrombocytopenia, neutropenia, or both accompany anemia, marrow suppression because of drugs should be excluded. In unexplained anemias, all medications should be reviewed, including any drugs used preoperatively. Bone marrow aspiration and biopsy may be necessary to establish the diagnosis of marrow hypoplasia.

Hemolysis is a less common cause of postoperative anemia, but it should be sought after blood loss and marrow underproduction have been excluded. Helpful clues are splenomegaly and an elevated, unexplained preoperative reticulocyte count. A mild preoperative hemolytic anemia may go unnoticed if the reticulocyte response is adequate to maintain the hematocrit near normal. If a preoperative reticulocyte count is unavailable, a peripheral smear from blood drawn before surgery can be examined for bluish, macrocytic erythrocytes, which is an indication of reticulocytosis.

Causes of postoperative hemolysis include:

1. *Drug-induced hemolysis*: Penicillin, methyldopa, and quinidine are the prototypes of drug-induced immune hemolytic anemia, but several other agents have also been implicated. Oxidant, drug-induced hemolysis should be considered in patients of African and Mediterranean descent who have been diagnosed with or are at risk for glucose-6-phosphate dehydrogenase (G-6-PD) deficiency. Drugs that are frequently implicated as causing hemolysis in patients with G-6-PD deficiency include sulfa drugs, antimalarials, and nitrofurantoin.

2. *Hemolysis resulting from sepsis*: Some degree of hemolysis can be seen in sepsis and severe infection. Routine tests for hemolysis (e.g., Coombs' test) are usually negative, and disseminated intravascular coagulation (DIC) may also be present. Severe intravascular hemolysis may accompany sepsis resulting from *Clostridium* sp. Hemolysis resulting from red cell G-6-PD deficiency may be exacerbated by infection and sepsis.

3. *Hemolysis following transfusions*: Acute, severe transfusion reactions are easily recognized, but a delayed transfusion reaction with less severe hemolysis resulting from "minor" antibodies may be missed (see "Delayed Transfusion Reactions").

4. *Hemolysis related to the underlying disease*: Lymphoma, collagen vascular disease, and malignancies (especially lymphoproliferative diseases) may be associated with hemolytic anemia.

Macrocytic anemias are uncommon postoperatively. A brisk, postoperative reticulocytosis from blood loss or hemolysis should be excluded first as a cause for macrocytosis. Drugs that have been implicated in producing macrocytosis (without necessarily causing anemia) include trimethoprim, triamterene, hydantoin, zidovudine, and various chemotherapeutic agents. Macrocytosis may also signal liver disease or folate deficiency in patients with prolonged hospitalization and poor nutrition. Folate deficiency may manifest earlier, however, if the patient was malnourished at the time of admission.

Microcytic anemias rarely occur postoperatively; they require considerable time to develop. However, patients with a prolonged preoperative or postoperative course may develop the anemia of chronic disease, which can occasionally produce mild microcytosis.

THE TRANSFUSED PATIENT

A variety of clinical problems can arise because of blood transfusion. The physician should be aware that the clinical signs and symptoms of reactions to a blood transfusion are numerous, and they include anxiety, shortness of breath, chest pain, rigors, fever, hypotension, pulmonary edema, wheezing, and skin rashes. When evaluating a patient with a suspected transfusion reaction, he or she should be **questioned about previous blood transfusions.** In women, the number of pregnancies and any associated complications should be noted in particular.

Transfusion reactions are discussed here in the temporal sequence in which they usually arise, not by the traditional classification based on immunologic and nonimmunologic mechanisms.

Immediate Reactions

Hypersensitivity Skin Reactions

Hypersensitivity skin reactions are characterized by urticaria, pruritus, or blotchy erythema. They usually begin within minutes of starting the transfusion. It is generally agreed that they result from sensitization to plasma proteins such as immunoglobulin subtypes. They can occur with the transfusion of fresh-frozen plasma and cyroprecipitate as well as with RBCs. Hypersensitivity skin reactions are usually responsive to antihistamines, and they can be avoided, or at least minimized, by pretreatment with these medications.

Acute Hemolytic Transfusion Reactions

The incidence of hemolytic reactions is estimated at 1 in 6000 transfusions, and that of fatal hemolytic reactions at 1 in 100,000. Of greatest concern are those resulting from ABO incompatibility. Rhesus blood group (Rh) isoantibodies are a less common cause. Clerical error during blood collection, such as incorrect labeling of blood samples and administering blood to the wrong patient, are the most frequent causes of an acute hemolytic transfusion reaction.

Clinical manifestations of this type of reaction result from two factors: (a) acute antigen–antibody reaction with release of cytokines and subsequent activation of the complement, coagulation, and the kallikrein systems; and (b) intravascular RBC destruction by isoantibodies. Clinical findings during these reactions include apprehension, facial flushing, chest or lumbar pain, chills, tachypnea, tachycardia, and nausea. These symptoms may be followed by signs of shock, acute oliguric renal failure, and diffuse bleeding. In a comatose or anesthetized patient, the first sign may be coagulopathy manifested by bleeding from mucus membranes, the operative site, or hemoglobinuria.

When an acute hemolytic transfusion reaction is suspected, the transfusion must be stopped immediately. Careful attention should be paid to the blood pressure, urine output, and clinical evidence of bleeding. Laboratory findings include hemoglobinemia, hemoglobinuria, and a transiently positive direct antiglobulin (i.e., Coombs') test. Since DIC may occur, coagulation studies, including prothrombin time (PT), activated partial thromboplastin time (aPTT), platelet count, fibrinogen and fibrin degradation products, or D-dimer assay, should be performed. The supernatant plasma of a centrifuged blood sample should be examined for pinkish discoloration, which indicates free hemoglobin and rapidly confirms the diagnosis of intravascular hemolysis.

Therapy for patients with acute hemolytic transfusion reactions is the treatment of cardiovascular collapse, acute tubular necrosis, and DIC. Intravenous fluids should be infused as soon as the reaction is suspected, and vasopressor medications are indicated if hypotension supervenes. The urine output should be maintained at greater than 100 mL/h. Low-dose dopamine can be used to maintain adequate renal perfusion, and mannitol or furosemide should be used to maintain urine output only after appropriate resuscitation of fluid volume. Shock is the most life-threatening complication of an acute hemolytic transfusion reaction, and diuretics can contribute to hypoperfusion if they are given indiscreetly. Use of heparin for DIC depends on the clinical situation (see "Disseminated Intravascular Coagulation").

Anaphylactic Reactions

Anaphylactic reactions are rare complications of transfusions. They are seen in patients with immunoglobulin A (IgA) deficiency, occur soon after beginning the transfusion, and are characterized by hypotension, bronchospasm, cyanosis, and abdominal, back, or chest pain. The incidence of IgA deficiency in the general population has been estimated to vary between 1 in 600 and 1 in 800, but reactions because of IgA deficiency occur at a rate of less than 1 reaction per 20,000 U of blood products transfused. Anti-IgA antibodies in the recipient are responsible for the reaction, and a prior history of transfusion or pregnancy is not required. Therapy is the same as that for anaphylaxis from any cause (i.e., intravenous fluids, pressors, oxygen, steroids, and epinephrine). Once IgA deficiency has been diagnosed, the patient should receive only washed RBCs or blood components from IgA-deficient donors.

Acute Noncardiac Pulmonary Edema

Acute noncardiac pulmonary edema, which is also termed *transfusion-related*

acute lung injury, is characterized by the abrupt onset of chills, fever, tachycardia, nonproductive cough, and dyspnea. Chest radiography depicts bilateral perihilar and lower-lung-field infiltrates without cardiac enlargement or pulmonary vascular engorgement. This transfusion reaction occurs primarily because of HLA antigen–antibody interactions from passively transfused HLA antibodies in the recipient's plasma that react with the recipient's own leukocytes, or it may occur because of alloimmunization to HLA antigens on transfused leukocytes. The antigen–antibody interaction activates granulocytes, causing them to migrate into the interstitial space between the alveolar epithelium and the capillary endothelium, which in turn causes a capillary leak syndrome and noncardiogenic pulmonary edema. Therapy consists of epinephrine and steroids as well as the traditional measures for treating pulmonary edema.

Intermediate Reactions

Febrile Transfusion Reactions

Febrile transfusion reactions are characterized by flulike complaints such as malaise, fatigue, fever, myalgia, and headache. Onset varies from within several minutes of beginning the transfusion to, more commonly, 1 to 2 hours after the transfusion has ended. The symptoms can persist for several hours. **These reactions occur in patients with a history of prior transfusion or pregnancy.** Febrile reactions may not occur with each transfusion, however, and they are dependent on individual donors.

Febrile transfusion reactions result from antileukocyte and antiplatelet antibodies. These reactions can be prevented, or at least lessened in severity, by pretreatment with acetaminophen and, when this is ineffective, by transfusing leukocyte-depleted blood. Washed or frozen-thawed RBCs have almost no contaminating leukocytes, but they are more expensive to prepare. Commercially available leukocyte filters effectively reduce the leukocyte count in RBC units and platelet concentrates by more than 99% and prevent most nonhemolytic febrile transfusion reactions.

Leukocyte-depleted blood should be ordered when a patient receiving multiple transfusions develops febrile transfusion reactions despite premedication. Treatment is otherwise symptomatic, using aspirin or acetaminophen, 650 mg by mouth. In a patient with frequent or unusually severe reactions, hydrocortisone, 50 to 100 mg intravenously before the transfusion, may be effective. Meperidine, 25 to 50 mg by slow intravenous bolus, will usually reduce the severity of rigors associated with the reaction. A hemolytic transfusion reaction and bacterial sepsis should be excluded with appropriate laboratory studies and blood cultures depending on the patient's transfusion history and the physician's clinical judgment.

Volume Overload

Volume overload is a common and often misdiagnosed complication in elderly patients with renal or cardiac insufficiency and chronic anemia. Patients may develop clinical manifestations varying from dyspnea to overt pulmonary edema. Onset may be delayed by up to 24 hours after the transfusion. The risk of volume overload can be avoided through awareness of the potential problem in elderly individuals, slow transfusion of packed RBCs (<2 mL/min), and judicious use of diuretics. Small doses of intravenous furosemide (e.g., 20 mg) between transfused units may also help to prevent volume overload in such patients.

Delayed Transfusion Reactions

Delayed hemolytic transfusion reactions are well recognized by blood-bank personnel but often missed by physicians. The hallmark of such a reaction is **an unexplained decrease in the hematocrit 2 to 21 days after a transfusion.** The recipient has always been sensitized to blood-group antigens by previous transfusion or pregnancy, but at the time of the current transfusion, antibody titers are below the level that screening agglutination reactions can detect. The transfusion initiates an anamnestic response, and alloantibodies directed against the donor RBCs are then produced, causing hemolysis.

Most delayed hemolytic transfusion reactions cause low-grade fever, decreased hemoglobin level and hematocrit, elevated corrected reticulocyte count, and a mildly elevated indirect bilirubin level. In one study (10), fever was the most common sign of an ongoing hemolytic process, occurring in 78% of those affected. Although it is uncommon, these reactions can be serious, with patients developing oliguric renal failure and death. When investigated early, the direct antiglobulin test is positive and one or more RBCs antibodies usually detected; however, the direct Coombs' test becomes negative once the donor RBCs have been cleared by the recipient's reticuloendothelial system. Therefore, a positive direct Coombs' test is helpful, but a negative direct Coombs' test does not exclude the diagnosis of a delayed hemolytic transfusion reaction. In contrast, the **indirect Coombs' test** remains positive for weeks following the reaction. Delayed hemolytic reactions may also lead to the mistaken diagnosis of autoimmune hemolytic anemia.

The **triad of anemia, fever, and recent blood transfusion** should alert clinicians to the possibility of a delayed hemolytic reaction. Because the serum alloantibody titer may become undetectable with time, it is advisable to provide these patients with a warning device (e.g., a wristband or wallet card) listing the type of RBC antigen(s) to avoid if a transfusion becomes necessary again.

Massive Transfusions

A massive transfusion is defined as the replacement of one or more blood volumes within 24 hours. In a 70-kg individual, the blood volume is approximately 75 mL/kg, or approximately 10 U of whole blood. In the past, numerous electrolyte, coagulation, and other complications have been attributed to the transfusion of large quantities of banked blood, and Table 15.3 lists the potential problems that have been seen in some patients receiving massive transfusion. It is likely, however, that some of these complications result from the circumstances responsible for the massive transfusion being needed in the first place (e.g., trauma, surgery, massive hemorrhage) (11).

After 24 hours of storage, the platelet count of the blood is nil. Diffuse bleeding accompanying massive transfusion may result from thrombocytopenia, and the administration of platelet concentrates to maintain a platelet count of 50,000 cells/μL is indicated in this setting. Levels of factors V and VIII decrease in stored blood but remain at hemostatic levels in patients receiving massive transfusion unless DIC is also present (11). Both PT and aPTT prolongations should be treated with fresh-frozen plasma (i.e., contains all clotting factors) and cryoprecipitate (i.e., contains fibrinogen and factor VIII coagulant activity). Microparticles that are present in stored blood should be removed by in-line, 20- to 40-micron filters to prevent microembolization, which may lead to the adult respiratory distress syndrome in massively transfused patients. Surgical patients who continue to bleed after normalization or significant improvement in platelet count, PT, and aPTT should be considered for surgical reexploration.

The clinical efficacy of an algorithm to guide component replacement, such as recommendations to transfuse a certain quantity of fresh-frozen plasma for a defined quantity of RBCs, has not been established by clinical studies. The presence or absence of diffuse bleeding and abnormalities of platelet count, PT, aPTT, and fibrinogen still currently serve as a guide to blood component replacement.

Table 15.3. Problems Associated with Massive Blood Transfusion

Dilutional thrombocytopenia
Coagulation factor deficiency (especially factors V and VIII)
Citrate toxicity (paresthesias, hypocalcemia, alkalosis)
Hypothermia
Hyperkalemia and hypokalemia
Respiratory distress syndrome
Ammonia toxicity (if liver disease coexists)

SPECIAL OPERATIVE CONSIDERATIONS IN PATIENTS WITH ERYTHROCYTE ABNORMALITIES

Sickle-cell Hemoglobinopathies

The common sickle cell–hemoglobin disorders include homozygous sickle-cell disease (Hgb SS), sickle-cell trait (Hgb AS), sickle cell–hemoglobin C disease (Hgb SC), and sickle cell–β-thalassemia. Except for Hgb AS, all of these disorders are characterized by some degree of recurrent microvascular occlusion under conditions predisposing to reduced tissue oxygenation. The sickle-cell prep or the more rapid dithionite tube test are the available tests that screen for hemoglobins that sickle. A positive screening test should be followed by hemoglobin electrophoresis to confirm the presence of hemoglobin S and evaluate for combined hemoglobinopathies.

Patients with a sickling disorder other than Hgb AS present challenging diagnostic problems. For example, sickling in mesenteric and intestinal vessels can produce an abdominal crisis that mimics the acute surgical abdomen, with abdominal pain (frequently in the right upper quadrant), leukocytosis, fever, and jaundice. Cholelithiasis and cholecystitis are common sequelae of the bilirubin stones that result from chronic hemolytic anemia, and surgical intervention may be required in these circumstances. However, hepatic infarction, intrahepatic cholestasis, and hepatitis should also be considered in the differential diagnosis of abdominal pain and jaundice in these patients.

Preoperative Treatment

Hemoglobin AS (i.e., sickle trait) does not increase the incidence of anesthetic and surgical complications. However, patients with other forms of sickle cell hemoglobinopathies are at significant risk for acute episodes of sickling and tissue infarction if they are stressed by hypoxia, infection, dehydration, and acidosis.

Hemoglobin values for patients with the more severe sickling disorders usually vary between 5.5 and 10.0 g/dL. A preoperative corrected reticulocyte count and serum bilirubin level will help to assess the status of bone marrow RBC production and the rate of hemolysis. Patients with congenital hemolytic anemias are predisposed to aplastic crises resulting from infection by parvovirus B19 or folic acid deficiency. During an aplastic crisis, the reticulocyte count drops to less than 1%, and the erythroid bone marrow can no longer sustain its compensation for the chronic hemolytic anemia. Elective procedures should be performed when the hemoglobin is at its optimum value for the individual patient. If possible, surgical procedures should be deferred until any infection and metabolic, fluid, or electrolyte abnormalities are corrected. In addition, the general condition of the patient is equally as important as the absolute preoperative hemoglobin level.

Prophylactic packed RBC transfusions are frequently given before major surgical procedures to reduce a patient's hemoglobin S concentration and suppress bone marrow production of hemoglobin S–containing RBCs. Although RBC transfusions could theoretically increase the viscosity of the blood and accentuate vascular occlusive crises, many clinicians favor preoperative transfusions to protect against inadvertent hypoxia during general anesthesia.

Levels of hemoglobin S may be reduced by manual or automated exchange transfusion with the general goal of lowering the hemoglobin S concentration to 40% or less. Exchange transfusion eliminates the potential problem of increasing blood viscosity that comes with simple transfusion. Use of agents such as low-molecular-weight dextran or urea during surgery has no clinical value. Alkalinization with sodium bicarbonate should be used if the patient is acidemic.

The cytotoxic drug, hydroxyurea, has recently been shown to increase fetal hemoglobin levels in over 50% of treated patients with sickle cell anemia. In general, patients who demonstrate this increase in fetal hemoglobin experience a decrease in the frequency of sickle cell crisis and fewer episodes of acute chest syndrome. Presumably this favorable response is explained by the fact that intracellular fetal hemoglobin does not participate in intracellular sickle hemoglobin polymerization. Patients receiving this drug should be carefully monitored for bone marrow suppression by physicians familiar with the use and side effects of hydroxyurea (12).

The choice of anesthetic agent appears to be less important than the quality of anesthetic management. The main objectives of **anesthetic management in the perioperative period** include: (a) provision of adequate oxygenation and ventilation, (b) avoidance of hypothermia, and (c) maintenance of adequate circulating volume and cardiac output (13).

Postoperative Treatment

Patients with sickle cell hemoglobinopathy are subject to many potential postoperative problems, including a well-recognized increase in the incidence of pulmonary complications. Attention also has recently focused on the acute chest syndrome (14), which is characterized by pulmonary sequestration of sickled erythrocytes, hypoxia, and bilateral pulmonary infiltrates seen on chest radiographs. Treatment of this serious complication includes partial or total RBC exchange transfusion with maintenance of hemoglobin S levels at less than 30%, careful attention to volume status, treatment of infection, and, if necessary, ventilatory support.

Bone marrow–fat embolism arising from areas of marrow infarction may cause pulmonary infarction and infiltrates as well as fat embolism of the eye, brain, and kidneys. Marrow fat embolism may also complicate pregnancy and delivery. In addition, patients with sickling disorders are prone to pneumonia, which can occur related to their susceptibility to bacterial infection, particularly with *Streptococcus pneumoniae*. Prevention of pulmonary atelectasis with incentive spirometry (15), maintenance of adequate arterial oxygen levels, and prompt treatment of infection are important principles of treatment.

Since preexisting heart disease and impaired renal function with hyposthenuria are common, meticulous attention to fluid intake, output, and daily weight are important observations in the postoperative treatment of patients with sickling disorders. Worsening postoperative anemia without blood loss or a positive direct Coombs' test should raise the suspicion of hemolysis resulting from coexisting G-6-PD–enzyme deficiency, which is not uncommon among black patients.

Immune Hemolytic Anemias

Diagnostic Activities

Immune hemolytic anemias can be classified based on whether the antibody causing the increased RBC destruction is maximally active at body temperature (i.e., warm reactive) or at lower temperatures (i.e., cold reactive). In addition, it is important to establish whether immune hemolysis results from an underlying disease process or drug or, by exclusion, is idiopathic in origin (16). When an autoimmune hemolytic anemia is diagnosed, the secondary causes to be considered include drugs, lymphoproliferative disorders, various cancers, collagen vascular diseases (e.g., systemic lupus erythematosus), infections (e.g., viral infections, *Mycoplasma pneumoniae* infection, subacute bacterial endocarditis), and delayed hemolytic transfusion reaction. If an underlying disease cannot be found, the diagnosis is idiopathic autoimmune hemolytic anemia (Table 15.4).

Surgical patients not infrequently receive multiple medications in the postoperative period. Penicillin and other β-lactam antibiotics are recognized as causes of immune hemolytic anemia. The usual clinical setting is a patient who has received large doses of these agents for 10 days or longer. Renal insufficiency causing high serum drug levels may be present as well. The drug becomes firmly bound to the red cell membrane and elicits an immunoglobulin G (IgG)-antibody response. Other drugs that are associated with hemolytic anemia include quinidine, procainamide, captopril, and methyldopa; drugs that are less frequently associated include antimycobacterials, nonsteroidal anti-inflammatory agents, and anticonvulsants. Drugs such as cephalosporins and methyldopa may cause a positive direct Coombs' test in the absence of active clinical hemolysis. In addition to the usual laboratory indicators of hemolysis (i.e., elevated RPI, serum indirect bilirubin, and serum lactate dehydrogenase), a positive direct or indirect Coombs' test, or both, establishes the diagnosis of immune hemolytic anemia.

Table 15.4. Causes of Immune Hemolytic Anemia

Warm Antibody
Drugs
Lymphoproliferative disorders (CLL, lymphoma)
Collagen vascular diseases
Carcinoma (rare)
Delayed transfusion reaction
Idiopathic
Cold Antibody
Infection (mycoplasma, Epstein-Barr virus)
Lymphoproliferative disorders
Chronic cold agglutinin disease

Treatment of Warm Autoimmune Hemolytic Anemia

Patients with severe warm antibody–induced hemolytic anemia can present with hypoxia and heart failure, and general cardiovascular support is of great importance. **Blood transfusions should be avoided whenever possible**, because they may accelerate hemolysis. However, blood transfusions may be necessary to reverse circulatory failure or hypoxemia resulting from severe anemia. Even so, finding totally compatible units of blood for these patients is frequently impossible, because the autoantibody coating the patient's erythrocytes confounds cross-matching. If a transfusion is imperative, a blood bank that has experience with these problems should be consulted to select the **least-incompatible units** of blood (17). Although the autoantibody may cause the transfused RBCs to be eliminated rapidly, relatively small amounts of RBCs may provide sufficient oxygen-carrying capacity to alleviate cardiopulmonary or central nervous system symptoms until corticosteroid treatment is effective. Transfusion to a predetermined hematocrit should not be the goal; rather, the least amount of transfused RBCs that is necessary to alleviate symptoms should be the goal. Blood should be transfused very slowly, with close monitoring for evidence of an acute intravascular hemolytic reaction (see "Acute Hemolytic Transfusion Reactions"), in which case the transfusion should be immediately discontinued.

Corticosteroids are the initial treatment of warm antibody–type autoimmune hemolytic disease. Prednisone or methylprednisolone should be given, 1 to 2 mg/kg daily in divided doses, or hydrocortisone, 100 to 200 mg intravenously every 6 hours, can be given initially. High-dose corticosteroids should be used until the hematocrit stabilizes at an acceptable value, after which their dosage can be reduced gradually. Folic acid, 1 mg daily by mouth, should be given empirically. If autoimmune hemolytic anemia is associated with a known disease process, therapy for that disease may ameliorate the anemia.

Maintenance corticosteroid therapy should be given in the lowest dosage possible to relieve the symptoms of anemia and achieve an acceptable, stable hematocrit value. **Splenectomy may be indicated in patients not responding to high doses of corticosteroids** or when these agents cannot be successfully withdrawn. Immunosuppressant drugs (e.g., cyclophosphamide, vincristine, azathioprine) should generally be reserved for patients with severe anemia that is unresponsive to steroids and splenectomy.

If splenectomy is necessary for steroid-dependent autoimmune hemolytic anemia, the procedure can be performed with a low risk of morbidity and mortality in patients with anemia that has been first stabilized with corticosteroids. Complications are significantly increased in patients with severe anemia that is unresponsive to medical therapy or who are severely ill from an underlying disease. Perioperative treatment includes continuing higher doses of corticosteroids, maintaining adequate oxygenation, and judicious transfusion of the least-incompatible packed RBCs for unacceptably low hematocrits.

Hemolytic anemia caused by drugs or drug metabolites usually resolves within a few days of discontinuing the drug. The exception is hemolytic anemia caused by α-methyldopa, which may persist for months following discontinuation of this agent. Corticosteroid therapy usually has little value in treating drug-induced hemolytic states, but it may be beneficial if the hemolysis is prolonged. Blood transfusion can usually be employed, if necessary, to correct severe anemia in this setting.

Evaluation and Treatment of Cold Autoimmune Diseases

Cold autoimmune diseases are a relatively uncommon group of immunologic disorders. They are characterized by the abnormal production of cold-reactive immunoglobulins, usually of the immunoglobulin M (IgM) class. These autoantibodies may be of low titer and little clinical consequence, or they may cause RBC agglutination, vaso-occlusive phenomena, and hemolytic anemia.

Polyclonal cold autoantibodies may be produced in various infections, such as influenza, mumps, infectious mononucleosis, and acute **mycoplasma pneumonia.** Monoclonal cold agglutinins are most often associated with lymphoproliferative disorders or chronic cold agglutinin disease (Table 15.4). Perioperative problems in patients with cold autoantibodies are obstruction of the microcirculation, active immune hemolysis, or both. Gangrene of the acral tissues (e.g., fingers, toes, earlobes) also can occur. When these patients undergo systemic hypothermia, acute renal failure because of immune complex glomerulonephritis is a potential complication, and use of iced potassium cardioplegic solution during cardiac surgery may cause intracoronary hemagglutination with coronary thrombosis, subendocardial ischemia, and, possibly, myocardial infarction.

Cryoglobulinemia is a multisystem disorder in which abnormal cold-reactive immunoglobulins do not cause hemolysis but, instead, form immune complexes, fix complement, and precipitate in the peripheral circulation with cold exposure. This syndrome can be idiopathic (i.e., essential) in origin or secondary to autoimmune disorders or plasma cell dyscrasias. Vascular occlusion, leukocytoclastic vasculitis, and crescentic glomerulonephritis are frequent sequelae of this syndrome.

In the preoperative evaluation of cold autoimmune disorders, it is important to **determine the critical temperature of the cold antibodies** (i.e., the temperature above which activity as agglutinins or precipitins ceases). This can be done in vitro by noting the highest environmental or water-bath temperature at which hemagglutination persists (18).

Preoperative recognition and treatment of the underlying condition associated with cold agglutinins will prevent or decrease the intraoperative risk. Corticosteroids and splenectomy have little benefit in cold agglutinin disease, but long-term treatment with alkylating agents (e.g., chlorambucil, cyclophosphamide) has been effective in some patients with idiopathic cold agglutinin disease. Chemotherapy for an associated plasma cell dyscrasia or lymphoma may control the disease process and reduce titers of cold autoantibodies. When cold agglutinins are caused by an infectious process, elective surgery should be postponed until the infection resolves, either naturally or with specific therapy. Preoperative plasmapheresis performed under warmed environmental temperatures can be used to rapidly reduce high antibody titers of patients with clinically important cold agglutinins or cryoglobulins in whom surgical hypothermia will be induced.

Perioperative treatment is directed at **warming the patient** above the critical temperature of activity for the cold autoantibodies. Intraoperative monitoring of temperature and maintenance of the critical temperature are essential. Intravenous fluids should be given at normal body temperature, and if a transfusion is necessary, RBCs should be washed to eliminate plasma complement and then given through a blood warmer. For several days following the surgery, evidence of continuing hemolysis should be sought with serial hemoglobin, hematocrit, and serum as well as urine free hemoglobin determinations.

Erythrocytosis

Erythrocytosis is defined as an increase in the number of circulating RBCs above the normal range for individuals of the same sex, as reflected by the hemoglobin level and hematocrit. **The hematocrit should be considered as elevated**

when it is greater than 54% in men
and 48% in women. In approaching an
elevated hematocrit, the consulting internist should have several strategies in
mind: to determine the cause of the erythrocytosis, to determine whether the patient is symptomatic from hyperviscosity,
and to appreciate the potential risks of
hemorrhage and thrombosis in patients
with untreated erythrocytosis.

An elevated hemoglobin level and hematocrit represent either a relative or an
absolute increase in RBC mass. **Relative
erythrocytosis** occurs when there is a
loss or contraction of plasma volume,
which may occur because of loss into the
interstitial tissues or a third space; extracellular losses from persistent vomiting,
diarrhea, or severe diaphoresis; inadequate fluid intake; or aggressive diuretic
therapy. A mild, stable erythrocytosis with
an unexplained contraction of plasma
volume is termed *stress polycythemia*, or
Gaisböck's syndrome. This condition is
seen most frequently in overweight, hypertensive males, and it is accompanied
by an excess rate of cardiovascular morbidity and mortality.

The first step in evaluating erythrocytosis is to document an absolute increase
in erythrocytes by measuring the RBC
mass. If this mass as measured by the ^{51}Cr
method is elevated (in men, >36 mL/kg; in
women, >32 mL/kg), then three categories
of **absolute erythrocytosis** should be
considered:

1. An appropriate absolute erythrocytosis secondary to systemic hypoxemia,
   increased carboxyhemoglobin levels,
   or a hemoglobinopathy in which the
   hemoglobin molecule has a high
   oxygen affinity.
2. An inappropriate absolute erythrocytosis secondary to increases in erythropoietin secretion secondary to renal diseases or tumors.
3. An inappropriate absolute erythrocytosis resulting from polycythemia vera,
   which represents an autonomous,
   clonal myeloproliferative disorder.

An elevated serum erythropoietin level is
evidence against the diagnosis of polycythemia vera; however, a normal serum
erythropoietin level does not exclude secondary erythrocytosis.

Clinical and laboratory information
help to differentiate the types of erythrocytosis that result from an absolute increase in the RBC mass. In patients with
increased RBC mass, normal arterial oxygen saturation (>92%), and splenomegaly,
the diagnosis of polycythemia vera can be
made with confidence. However, in the
absence of palpable splenomegaly, which
is present in approximately 25% of patients with polycythemia vera at presentation, two of the following abnormalities
are required: *(a)* thrombocytosis with a
platelet count greater than 400,000 cells/
μL, *(b)* leukocytosis with a white blood cell
count greater than 12,000 cells/μL without fever or infection, *(c)* elevated leukocyte alkaline phosphatase score, and *(d)*
increased serum vitamin B_{12} level or
unbound vitamin B_{12}–binding capacity.
Other findings that support a diagnosis of
polycythemia vera are an elevated baso-
phil and eosinophil count, abnormal platelet morphology, and elevated uric acid
level.

If absolute erythrocytosis is present
and the criteria for polycythemia vera
cannot be met, one must then determine
whether the patient has an **appropriate
or inappropriate secondary erythrocytosis**. Hypoxemia is a common cause of
appropriate increase in the RBC mass,
and it occurs because of pulmonary disease, cardiac disease with right-to-left
shunts, alveolar hypoventilation, and
residence at high altitudes. These patients have an arterial oxygen saturation
of less than 92%. If the arterial oxygen
saturation is normal, however, then abnormal hemoglobin function or ectopic
production of erythropoietin should be
sought.

The most common cause of secondary
erythrocytosis from abnormal hemoglobin
function is the presence of carboxyhemoglobin from heavy cigarette smoking.

Patients with **smoker's erythrocytosis** have an elevated carboxyhemoglobin level, and the oxyhemoglobin dissociation curve is shifted to the left, with a lower P_{50} (i.e., the partial pressure of oxygen at which hemoglobin is 50% saturated) (19). Rare congenital hemoglobinopathies may also cause erythrocytosis with a leftward shift in the P_{50}.

If an appropriate cause for erythrocytosis cannot be found, the patient does not smoke, and the P_{50} is normal, one needs to consider an inappropriate elaboration of erythropoietin. Renal lesions, particularly adenocarcinoma and polycystic kidney disease, are the most frequent causes of inappropriate secondary erythrocytosis. Hepatic adenomas, uterine tumors, and pheochromocytoma are other, rarer causes.

The pathophysiologic consequences of true erythrocytosis include hyperviscosity, hypervolemia, and decreased systemic oxygen transport. As the hematocrit increases above 45%, the viscosity of blood increases exponentially (Fig. 15.1), and this increase in viscosity is responsible for many of the signs and symptoms of polycythemia vera. Complaints of altered circulation such as dizziness, headache, vertigo, tinnitus, and visual alterations, including scotomata and double or blurred vision, should be sought. Cerebral blood flow is significantly lowered in patients with hematocrits between 47 and 53% when compared to patients with hematocrits between 36 and 46%. Reduction of hematocrit to the lower range by phlebotomy increases the cerebral blood flow by a mean of 50% (20).

Thrombotic manifestations are particularly common in polycythemia vera, but they can also occur from any of the causes of absolute erythrocytosis. Paradoxically, hemorrhage is a common problem in polycythemia vera. Hemorrhage from mucous membranes can be attributed to blood vessel distention and intrinsic platelet dysfunction. The nose and gastrointestinal tract are the most common sites of bleeding in patients with erythrocytosis.

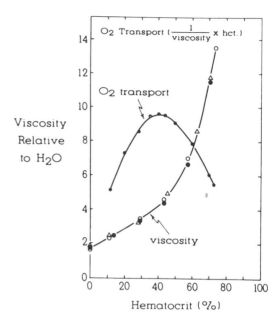

Figure 15.1. Oxygen transport as calculated from blood oxygen-carrying capacity (hematocrit) and blood flow (reciprocal of viscosity). (Reprinted with permission from Erslev AJ, Gabuzda TG (eds). Pathophysiology of blood. 2nd ed. Philadelphia: WB Saunders, 1979:35.)

Hyperviscosity results in sluggish flow of blood and decreased transport of oxygen to tissues. The optimal hematocrit for oxygen transport is between 40 and 45% (Fig. 15.1). An increased blood viscosity also elevates the pulmonary arterial pressure. If erythrocytosis occurs because of hypoxemia, the combined elevation of pulmonary vascular resistance and pulmonary arterial pressure contributes to the development or worsening of cor pulmonale.

Treatment of erythrocytosis is dependent on its cause. **Patients with polycythemia vera and a hematocrit greater than 45% should undergo phlebotomy,** and phlebotomy is especially important in patients with polycythemia vera who must undergo surgery. The intraoperative and postoperative morbidity and mortality rate are four to five times greater in those who have not undergone phlebotomy compared with those who have (21). Much of this increased risk results from thrombosis and hemorrhage. In addition, patients who have had effective, consistent, long-term control of their polycythemia vera are at less risk of complications from surgery than are those who have had short-term control.

In an emergency situation, the RBC mass can be reduced quickly by phlebotomy with a suitable plasma replacement to prevent the vascular instability that is associated with an overly rapid reduction in the total blood volume. **If a patient with polycythemia vera has significant thrombocytosis (platelet counts, >600,000 cells/µL), elective surgery is contraindicated.** If emergency surgery is required, the platelet count should be reduced quickly (see "Thrombocytosis"). If the surgery is not an emergency, the platelet count can be reduced by a cytoreductive agent such as hydroxyurea, and the surgery can then be performed after lowering of the platelet count and the RBC mass.

WHITE BLOOD CELL DISORDERS
Neutrophilia

An absolute neutrophil count of greater than 10,000 cells/µL is above the normal range (1800–7700 cells/µL). Certain pharmacologic agents, including corticosteroids, epinephrine, lithium carbonate, and granulocyte-colony stimulating factor (G-CSF), are associated with neutrophilia, and acute or chronic bacterial infection is the most common cause. At times, the response to infection and chronic inflammation or malignancy causes a striking neutrophilia, which is termed the **granulocytic leukemoid reaction**. Common causes of this neutrophilic response are sickle cell anemia, trauma, burns, pregnancy, myocardial infarction, electric shock, invasive malignancy, tuberculosis, and bacterial abscess. The consulting internist's principal objective in evaluating preoperative neutrophilia is to exclude drugs and simple infection as causes and then to differentiate a myeloproliferative disorder such as CGL from a leukemoid reaction.

The clinical complex of neutrophilia, granulocytic cells of all stages of maturation on peripheral blood smear, and splenomegaly suggest the diagnosis of CGL. In contrast, the elevated white blood cell count in a leukemoid reaction results primarily from an increase in polymorphonuclear leukocytes, with a mild increase in bands and metamyelocytes. Finding myelocytes, promyelocytes, and a rare myeloblast on the peripheral blood smear would be more suggestive of CGL or another myeloproliferative disease (e.g., myelofibrosis). Leukocyte alkaline phosphatase is present in low levels or is absent in CGL, but it is usually present at elevated levels in leukemoid reactions or myeloproliferative disorders other than CGL.

The Philadelphia chromosome, which represents a balanced translocation between chromosomes 9 and 22 (t9;22), can be demonstrated in the peripheral blood or bone marrow cells of almost all patients with CGL. **Presence of the t9;22 translocation differentiates CGL from the granulocytic leukemoid reaction.** The translocation is also absent in other chronic myeloproliferative disorders, such as polycythemia vera, myelofibrosis, and thrombocythemia. The (t9;22) translocation can now be detected in peripheral blood or bone marrow cells by a DNA probe that is sensitive to the *bcr/abl* transcript using a polymerase chain reaction assay.

Operating on patients in the **chronic phase** of CGL, when their white blood counts are less than 50,000 cells/µL, is not problematic as long as the RBC and platelet counts are normal. However, absolute blast cell counts greater than 80,000 cells/µL in association with the **blast crisis phase** of CGL or in acute myelogenous leukemia and acute lymphoblastic leukemia may predispose the patient to **leukostasis,** which refers to the vascular sludging of poorly deformable, immature leukocytes. The consequence of leukostasis is obstruction of cerebral and pulmonary capillaries, which can lead to cerebral hemorrhage and hypoxemia. The granulocytes of patients with chronic phase CGL have normal phagocytic and microbicidal function; in contrast, a predisposition to infection is seen when CGL accelerates into blast crisis and in patients with de novo acute leukemia. Patients with myeloproliferative disorders frequently have an elevated serum uric acid level, so adequate hydration, urine alkalinization, and allopurinol therapy may prevent postoperative gout and uric acid nephropathy.

The diagnostic approach to **postoperative neutrophilia** is usually straightforward: infection and drug effect (see the pharmacologic agents listed earlier) should be excluded as causes. A transient postoperative elevation in the neutrophil count may occur because the stress of surgery, but in this form of neutrophilia, the white blood cell count usually does not exceed 15,000 to 30,000 cells/μL. Transient neutrophilia is also anticipated following splenectomy.

Neutropenia

The term *neutropenia* refers to an absolute neutrophil count of less than 2000 cells/μL. Commonly encountered causes are listed in Table 15.5. An absolute neutrophil count of less than 1500 cells/μL is abnormal, and the cause of such a count should be elucidated before any surgery is undertaken. As the absolute neutrophil count falls to less than 1000 cells/μL, the risk of infection rises, but serious spontaneous infection usually is not encountered until the absolute neutrophil count is less than 500 cells/μL. In addition to the neutrophil count, the risk of infection also relates to the primary disease causing the neutropenia.

Neutropenia due to drugs should be considered in both pre- and post-operative settings. Drugs which can be associated with isolated neutropenia are listed in Table 15.6. However, it is more common

Table 15.5. Common Causes of Neutropenia

Drugs (see Table 15.6)
Benign neutropenia (ethnic/racial differences)
Infection
   Viral (EBV, influenza, HIV, others)
   Nonviral (TB, typhoid, rickettsia, brucella)
   Overwhelming bacterial sepsis
Vitamin B_{12} or folate deficiency
Autoimmune disorders
   Seropositive rheumatoid arthritis
   Systemic lupus erythematosus
   Hashimoto's thyroiditis
Hypersplenism
Bone-marrow stem cell disorder (aplasia, myelodysplasia, acute leukemia)
Hairy-cell leukemia

EBV, Epstein-Barr virus; *TB,* tuberculosis.

that drugs cause pancytopenia with a reduction in all hematopoietic elements (see "Pancytopenia"). Autoimmune disorders such as rheumatoid arthritis and systemic lupus erythematosus, lymphoid neoplasms, and acute infections (especially viral) may be associated with neutropenia and should also be considered in the differential diagnosis.

Patients with "pseudoneutropenia" have an increased proportion of neutrophils that are marginated on the capillary endothelium. This phenomenon occurs in some black patients and, occasionally, in Yemenite Jews. Affected individuals

Table 15.6. Drugs Associated with Isolated Neutropenia

Analgesic/anti-inflammatory drugs
   Indomethacin, gold, ibuprofen, phenylbutazone, penicillamine
Antibiotics
   Sulfa drugs, semisynthetic penicillins, cephalosporins, chloramphenicol, vancomycin, antituberculosis agents
Phenothiazines
Anticonvulsants
Antithyroid agents
Cardiovascular agents
   Procainamide, captopril, aprindine
H_2-blockers
   Cimetidine, ranitidine

rarely develop serious infection even with absolute neutrophil counts of 500 cells/μL. In contrast, similar reductions in the neutrophil count among patients with congenital agranulocytosis (i.e., Kostmann's syndrome), neutropenia caused by diseases of the bone marrow stem cells (e.g., acute leukemia, myelodysplasia, aplastic anemia), or bone marrow infiltrative disorders predispose to a significant risk of bacterial infection.

A record of prior neutrophil counts and a patient history targeted at determining both the number and severity of previous bacterial infections will allow the consulting internist to decide the clinical significance of neutropenia. A bone marrow examination may be necessary to determine if the neutropenia is caused by underproduction, ineffective production, or a bone marrow infiltrative disorder. If anemia and thrombocytopenia are also present, the differential diagnosis is that of pancytopenia (see "Pancytopenia").

Elective surgery should be postponed in patients with an absolute neutrophil count less than 1000 cells/μL if the process causing the neutropenia is expected to resolve over time. If the neutropenia is irreversible, however, a clinical decision regarding the urgency of surgery must be made. If the surgery is essential, broad-spectrum, prophylactic antibiotics should be given immediately both preoperatively and postoperatively. Except in neonates with life-threatening infections, granulocyte transfusions are no longer recommended because of the inability to obtain a sufficient yield of donor granulocytes to elevate recipient's blood neutrophil count to an effective, antimicrobicidal level. Transfusions of granulocyte also carry the risk of life-threatening side effects, particularly when random, unmatched granulocytes are transfused.

Use of recombinant G-CSF shortens the duration of neutropenia following myelosuppressive chemotherapy. G-CSF also is effective in the treatment of neutropenia resulting from congenital agranulocytosis, cyclic neutropenia, and hairy-cell leuke-

mia (22). Other recombinant human growth factors, such as granulocyte-monocyte colony-stimulating factor, are currently undergoing clinical trials.

Patients with absolute neutrophil counts less than 1000 cells/μL should be placed in reverse isolation postoperatively until wound healing is satisfactory. Anyone having physical contact with the patient should practice meticulous infection-control procedures, such as washing hands before and after contact with the patient. Any postoperative fever should be presumed to represent infection. Broad-spectrum antibiotics should be instituted immediately after cultures are obtained in the febrile patient with neutropenia.

Lymphocytosis

Lymphocytosis is defined as an absolute lymphocyte count greater than 4000 cells/μL. The causes of lymphocytosis in adult surgical patients are limited, and the principal differential diagnosis is between viral infections (e.g., infectious mononucleosis, viral hepatitis, cytomegalovirus) and chronic lymphocytic leukemia (CLL). The peripheral blood smear of patients with viral infections frequently shows a mild lymphocytosis that is accompanied by the transient appearance of reactive, "atypical" lymphocytes with increased amounts of clear, bluish cytoplasm. **An absolute lymphocytosis of 15,000 cells/μL or greater that persists for several months is required for the diagnosis of CLL.** The peripheral blood smear of patients with CLL usually shows morphologically normal-appearing small- and medium-sized lymphocytes and smudged cells.

Marked lymphocytosis resulting from CLL is not, by itself, a contraindication to surgery. A lymphocyte count of 100,000 to 200,000 cells/μL does not usually result in vascular sludging, because small lymphocytes are readily deformable in the microcirculation. When anemia, thrombocytopenia, or both accompany CLL, a reticulocyte count and bone marrow examination will help to determine if these cytopenias result from autoimmune hemolytic anemia, immunologic thrombocytopenia, or marrow replacement with lymphocytes. Quantitative immunoglobulin levels should also be measured, because patients with CLL may have hypogammaglobulinemia, thus predisposing them to recurrent bacterial infections. If such infections recur in severe hypogammaglobulinemia, intravenous IgG can be given together with appropriate antibiotics.

Lymphocytopenia

Lymphocytopenia is present when the absolute lymphocyte count falls to less than 1500 cells/μL. It is often associated with an altered host immune response, and the importance of chronic lymphocytopenia is the underlying disorder, which may predispose to or be associated with infection. Important causes include malignancies, malnourishment, infection with HIV-1 and the acquired immunodeficiency syndrome, corticosteroid therapy, and autoimmune diseases such as systemic lupus erythematosus.

Pancytopenia

When blood concentrations of neutrophils, platelets, and RBCS are all reduced, a broad differential diagnosis must be considered (Table 15.7). Pancytopenia accompanied by normal or macrocytic RBC morphology may result from drug effects, aplastic anemia, myelodysplastic syndrome, megaloblastic anemia from vitamin B_{12} or folic acid deficiency, and, occasionally, collagen vascular disorders. Pharmacologic agents that are classically associated with pancytopenia include chloramphenicol, phenylbutazone and its derivatives, sulfonamides, gold salts, quinacrine, mephenytoin, trimethadione, and cancer chemotherapeutic agents.

Pancytopenia accompanied by peripheral blood smear findings of nucleated RBCs, immature leukocytes, and tear-

Table 15.7. Differential Diagnosis of Pancytopenia

With Normal or Macrocytic RBCs
Drugs
Aplastic anemia
Myelodysplastic syndrome
Vitamin B_{12} or folate deficiency
Collagen vascular disorders
With Leukoerythroblastic Peripheral Blood Smear[a]
Metastatic cancer
Myelofibrosis
Leukemia
Granulomatous infections (tuberculosis, fungi)
With Marked Splenomegaly
Chronic liver disease (cirrhosis)
Lymphoma
Hairy-cell leukemia
Myelofibrosis

[a]*Leukoerythroblastic* refers to a peripheral blood smear that contains nucleated RBCs, teardrop RBCs, and immature granulocytes.

drop erythrocytes (i.e., "leukoerythroblastic" smear), with or without splenomegaly, indicate pathologic processes that are replacing the bone marrow and causing extramedullary hematopoiesis (e.g., metastatic carcinoma, myelofibrosis, leukemia, granulomatous infections). When splenomegaly is marked, conditions such as hypersplenism caused by chronic liver disease, lymphoma, hairy-cell leukemia, and myelofibrosis should be considered. A bone marrow aspirate and bone marrow core biopsy are frequently helpful in evaluating patients with pancytopenia.

EVALUATION AND TREATMENT OF HEMOSTASIS IN SURGICAL PATIENTS

Evaluation of the Hemostatic System

A thorough patient history incorporating certain key questions (Table 15.8) is the single most valuable screening technique in evaluating patients for bleeding disorders and ensuring adequate hemostasis during surgery (23). Although preoperative laboratory tests to exclude abnormalities of platelets and coagulation factor deficiency are readily available and reasonably sensitive, the results of these **tests of hemostasis must be interpreted in light of the patient history.** On the other hand, if the patient is a poor historian or minimizes his or her symptoms, laboratory testing assumes a greater importance in estimating the operative risk. In addition, an abnormal coagulation test result may be the first evidence of a mild, congenital coagulation factor deficiency or platelet disorder in patients who have escaped prior surgical challenge or significant trauma.

A careful screening history and tests of hemostasis are especially indicated when patients are scheduled for major surgical procedures that are associated with higher risks of operative bleeding. Examples are radical surgery for prostate cancer and cardiac surgery during which the pump-oxygenator is used. The same degree of caution is also warranted in patients undergoing ophthalmologic and neurologic surgery, because even small amounts of bleeding could be detrimental.

When the history is positive for prior excessive bleeding, determining the age of onset will help to define whether the disorder is congenital or acquired. Next, the pattern of the bleeding episodes should be established. For example, a history of bleeding predominantly from the skin and mucosal surfaces (i.e., oral, nasal, gastrointestinal and genitourinary tracts) that is spontaneous or occurs immediately after minimal trauma indicates a quantitative or qualitative platelet deficiency. In contrast, coagulation factor deficiency is more likely to manifest as bleeding into the muscles and joints, and it may be delayed in onset for several hours following trauma.

Questions regarding chronic medical illnesses (especially renal, liver, and autoimmune diseases) as well as a detailed listing of medications are of obvious importance. The patient may not realize that over-the-counter medications contain aspirin or nonsteroidal anti-inflammatory drugs.

Finally, the family history, obtained from either the patient or his or her relatives, is an essential part of the preoperative evaluation. However, a negative family history does not exclude a congenital bleeding disorder.

The physical examination may provide clues that help to determine the cause of abnormal bleeding. Petechiae (i.e., small, pinpoint capillary hemorrhages), which are seen most frequently on the feet and legs, are commonly present in thrombocytopenia or platelet dysfunction. Ecchymoses greater than 4 cm in diameter, hematomas, hemarthroses, and chronic flexion contractures of joints suggest coagulation factor deficiency. Purpura (i.e., irregularly shaped, purple macular lesions with clearly defined margins) may have the same significance as petechiae;

Table 15.8. Key Questions for Evaluating Hemostasis

I. Do you bruise easily without good reason? Have you bled excessively after minor trauma to your tongue, cheek, or lip? If so, how old were you when this began?

II. Have you had teeth extracted? If so, which ones? How long did you bleed after the extraction? Did the bleeding start again a day or so later? Did you need stitches to control the bleeding?

III. What operations have you had? Was bleeding after surgery or childbirth hard to stop? Were transfusions necessary? How well did your wounds heal?

IV. Have you had general medical illnesses? Which ones, and how were/are they being treated? Have you had kidney, liver, or joint diseases?

V. What medicines do you take? Do you use over-the-counter drugs for colds, allergy, headaches, arthritis, backache, menstrual pain, or other types of pain?

VI. Have any blood relatives experienced prolonged or excessive bleeding?

Modified from Rappaport SI. Preoperative hemostatic evaluation: which tests, if any? Blood 1983;61:229–231.

however, purpura is quite common on the dorsal surfaces of the arms and hands of otherwise healthy elderly individuals (i.e., senile purpura). It is also not unusual to find purpura on the extremities of patients receiving long-term corticosteroid therapy, and in these patients, it does not indicate a defect in hemostasis. Palpable purpuric lesions in patients with a generalized illness should suggest the diagnosis of vasculitis. Generalized oozing from mucosal surfaces and venipuncture sites occurs in hemostatic disorders affecting both platelets and coagulation factors (e.g., DIC).

When the screening history or physical examination are abnormal, an accurate history is unobtainable, or the patient is scheduled to undergo a surgical procedure involving highly vascular areas, a platelet

Table 15.9. Preoperative Testing to Identify Bleeding Disorders in Patients Undergoing High-risk Surgery

I.   Platelet count by automated counter
II. Template bleeding time
III. Prothrombin time (extrinsic pathway)
IV. Partial thromboplastin time (intrinsic pathway)

count, template bleeding time, PT, and aPTT should be obtained (Table 15.9). These tests permit identification of the area of the hemostatic system that may be affected and indicate the need for other, more specific tests to determine the precise nature of the defect. Figure 15.2 depicts an approach to the initial laboratory screening for defects in hemostasis.

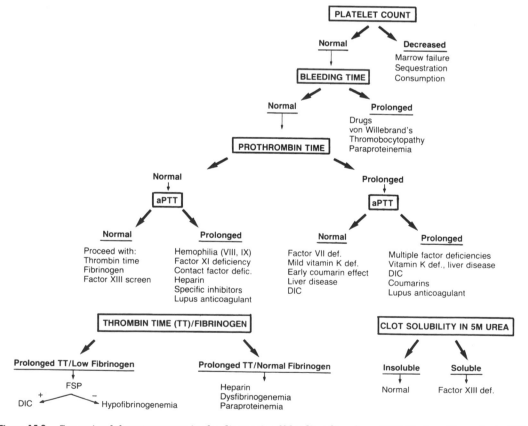

Figure 15.2. Screening laboratory tests in the diagnosis of bleeding disorders. *FSP*, fibrin split products; *TT*, thrombin time. (Modified from Edwards RL, Rickles FR. The evaluation of the patient with a bleeding disorder. In: Lichtman MA, ed. Hematology and oncology. New York: Grune & Stratton, 1980:208.)

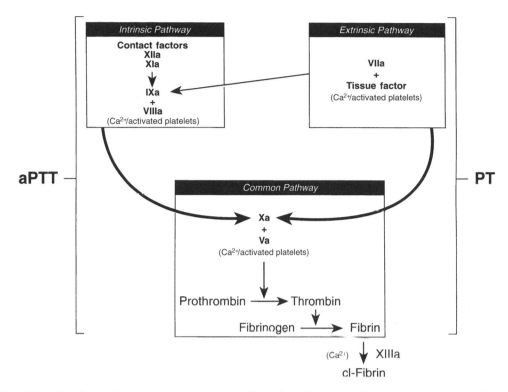

Figure 15.3. Blood coagulation occurs as a series of interdependent steps that terminate in formation of a fibrin clot. The intrinsic pathway, as measured by the aPTT, is initiated when blood contacts a negatively charged surface. The extrinsic system, as measured by the PT, is triggered by the release of tissue factor at the site of injury. Both systems lead to the formation of complexes of activated clotting factors [IXa + VIIIa] and [VIIa + tissue factor], which assemble on activated platelet membranes. Each of these complexes are able to activate factor X to Xa. The platelet-bound complex of factors Xa, Va, and Ca++ converts prothrombin into thrombin. Thrombin leaves the platelet surface and converts fibrinogen to fibrin, which is cross-linked (cl) by factor XIIIa. Products of the initial stages of coagulation—factors XIa (intrinsic) and VIIa (extrinsic)—both can activate factor IX.

The platelet count and bleeding time are considered together in diagnosing platelet disorders. If the platelet count is normal but the template bleeding time is longer than 10 minutes, platelet dysfunction should be suspected. This dysfunction is commonly caused by drugs such as aspirin, but it also may result from von Willebrand's disease, renal insufficiency, liver disease, or congenital thrombocytopathy. When the patient has no history of prior medications, further testing, including platelet aggregation studies, may be indicated. Platelet-related problems can be excluded as the cause of a predisposition to bleeding if both the platelet count and the bleeding time are normal.

A prolonged template bleeding time helps to diagnose a platelet-related cause of bleeding or von Willebrand's disease. However, comprehensive reviews of large numbers of clinical studies examining predictive value have concluded that **the preoperative template bleeding time does not adequately predict the degree of bleeding risk** that is associated with invasive procedures and surgery (24, 25). The clinical usefulness of this test appears to be limited to diagnosis of a platelet-related cause of bleeding in patients with a history of a bleeding tendency.

The PT, which measures the extrinsic coagulation pathway and those clotting factors that are common to both the intrinsic and the extrinsic systems (Fig. 15.3), is the next test in the screening sequence. If the PT is prolonged and the aPTT normal, there is a defect in the extrinsic pathway. This may be caused by a deficiency of factor VII, which is rare, or by an acquired coagulopathy, including an early, mild, combined defect in the vitamin K–dependent clotting factors (i.e., II, VII, IX, and X) resulting from vitamin K deficiency, liver disease, or the early effect of coumarin anticoagulants. Factor VII has the shortest half-life of all the coagulation factors ($\approx$ 5 hours), which explains an isolated, prolonged PT early in the course of these clinical situations.

If both the PT and the aPTT are prolonged, single or multiple deficiencies of common pathway factors are present. Causes for these deficiencies include severe vitamin K deficiency, liver disease, coumarin anticoagulation, congenital factor X or V deficiency, and, rarely, prothrombin (i.e., factor II) deficiency.

When the aPTT is prolonged and the PT normal, there is a defect in the intrinsic pathway (Fig. 15.3). The physician should first confirm that an isolated prolongation of the aPTT is not the result of heparin in the specimen or laboratory error by **repeating the test on a carefully collected blood sample.** Heparin contamination of blood drawn from an indwelling catheter is a frequent cause of aPTT elevation in hospitalized patients.

An isolated, marked prolongation of the aPTT in patients without a history of abnormal bleeding despite previous surgery or trauma indicates a deficiency of factor XII or one of the contact factors, such as prekallikrein or high-molecular-weight kininogen. Patients with any one of these three congenital deficiencies can be operated on safely without clotting factor replacement. In patients with abnormal bleeding, an isolated, prolonged aPTT will usually be caused by hemophilia (i.e., factor VIII or IX deficiency) or by factor XI deficiency. When both the aPTT and the template bleeding time are prolonged, von Willebrand's disease is the most likely diagnosis (Table 15.10).

The thrombin time and fibrinogen level should be evaluated in conjunction with each other. These tests monitor the final stage of clot formation, in which fibrinogen is converted to fibrin. The thrombin time and fibrinogen level should be normal in all the specific disorders mentioned thus far. If the fibrinogen level is low and the thrombin time prolonged, a test for fibrin split products or D-dimer should also be obtained. The D-dimer test is a more sensitive assay for the breakdown of cross-linked fibrin, which occurs in DIC, and the test is not confounded by the presence of

Table 15.10. Diagnosis of Common Bleeding Disorders

Disorder	Platelet Count	Bleeding Time	PT	aPTT	Fibrinogen	Fibrinogen Degradation Products
Hemophilia A (factor VIII deficiency)	N	N	N	A	N	–
Hemophilia B (factor IX deficiency)	N	N	N	A	N	–
von Willebrand's disease	N or A	A	N	N or A	N	
Vitamin K deficiency	N	N	A	A	N	–
Coumarin excess	N	N	A	A	N	–
Liver disease	N or A	N or A	A	A	N or A	+ or –
DIC	A	N or A	A	N or A	A	+

A, abnormal; *N,* normal; +, present; –, absent.

fibrinogen fragments. The combination of elevated levels of fibrin degradation products or D-dimers, decreased fibrinogen level, and a low platelet count is a good indicator of ongoing DIC. In the absence of fibrin degradation products or D-dimer, hypofibrinogenemia from decreased synthesis should be suspected. If the fibrinogen level is normal or high and the thrombin time prolonged, heparin contamination of the specimen or an abnormal fibrinogen (i.e., dysfibrinogenemia) should be considered.

If these tests are normal in a patient with a history of bleeding, wound dehiscence, or exaggerated scar formation, factor XIII deficiency should be sought by determining if the fibrin clot is soluble in 5-M urea. Factor XIII deficiency results in a non–cross linked clot that readily dissolves in this solution, and this represents the only screening test for the disorder. Factor XIII deficiency is usually congenital; however, inhibitors to factor XIII may be acquired after long-term exposure to certain drugs (e.g., isoniazid, phenytoin).

A major consideration in evaluating the cause of an abnormal screening coagulation test is the need to **establish whether the abnormality reflects a decreased level of clotting factor(s) or presence of a circulating coagulation inhibitor.** The latter is a substance (frequently an immunoglobulin) that circulates in plasma and interferes with the normal function of one or more clotting factors. Inhibitors may produce bleeding as severe as that in congenital coagulation factor deficiencies, or they may interfere only with the in vitro clotting test without causing actual clinical bleeding (e.g., lupuslike anticoagulant). The presence of an inhibitor can usually be demonstrated by repeating the abnormal clotting test (e.g., PT, aPTT, thrombin time) on a mixture of equal parts of the patient's plasma and normal plasma. A clinically significant coagulation inhibitor in the patient's plasma will prolong the aPTT of the normal plasma, and the aPTT of the mixture will remain prolonged. In con-

Table 15.11.   Screening Test for Coagulation Inhibitors

I.   Perform aPTT on:
     Patient (Pt) plasma
     Normal (Nl) plasma
II. Mix and incubate at 37° C for 1 hour:
     1 part Pt plasma + 1 part Nl plasma
III. Repeat aPTT on the mixture:
     aPTT corrects completely = clotting factor
       deficiency
     aPTT fails to correct = coagulation inhibitor

trast, if the initial test is abnormal because of a deficiency in one or more of the coagulation factors, addition of normal plasma will provide approximately 50% of the missing factor(s) and correct the test (Table 15.11). Heparin, even in small quantities, prolongs the thrombin time, and the addition of normal plasma will not correct the thrombin times of patients receiving heparin as the drug remains in the mixture.

Preoperative Planning for Surgery in Patients with Coagulation Factor Disorders

Before any patient with a coagulation factor disorder is taken to surgery, the following questions must be addressed:

1. Has the diagnosis been firmly established? Does the patient have more than one hemostatic defect?
2. Is there an associated platelet deficiency or qualitative platelet defect?
3. Is there evidence of a coagulation factor inhibitor?
4. Can the blood bank provide adequate clotting factor replacement for the entire preoperative and postoperative periods?
5. Which therapy would pose the least risk for transmission of viral infections?
6. Is a hematology consultant available? Is a specialized coagulation laboratory available? In what institution can the patient best be treated?

A **care plan** that details both the frequency and amounts of clotting factor support as well as the timing of coagulation testing should be developed before surgery and circulated to everyone involved in the patient's care. **Intramuscular injections, antiplatelet medications, and anticoagulants must be avoided** in patients with coagulation factor disorders, and clotting factor replacement should precede invasive procedures and vigorous physical therapy.

Treatment of Congenital Coagulation Factor Disorders

The most common congenital clotting disorders are hemophilia A (i.e., factor VIII:C deficiency), hemophilia B (i.e., factor IX deficiency), and von Willebrand's disease (i.e., combined deficiency of factors VIII:vWF and VIII:C). Rare deficiency states that also require replacement therapy for surgery include deficiencies of factors XI, VII, X, V, XIII, prothrombin, and fibrinogen.

Patients with **hemophilia** resulting from either deficiency of congenital factor VIII clotting factor activity (VIII:C) or factor IX deficiency demonstrate an isolated prolongation of the aPTT, unless the deficiency is very mild (plasma factor level, >30%), in which case the aPTT is frequently normal. Occasionally, the diagnosis of hemophilia is first made because of postoperative hemorrhage in patients with mild hemophilia who have had no prior surgical challenge.

Circulating inhibitors to factor VIII:C develop in approximately 15% of patients with severe factor VIII deficiency; inhibitors are less common in patients with factor IX deficiency. A **test for a coagulation factor inhibitor** should be performed before surgery and at intervals during the postoperative period of factor replacement, because an inhibitor may first appear during prolonged factor replacement therapy following surgery. Elective surgery is contraindicated in patients with hemophilia and an inhibitor or with a history of an inhibitor, especially if the antibody has been shown to be of the high-titer, easily stimulated type. If emergency surgery is required, the procedure should ideally be performed at a center providing specialized resources for the treatment of such patients.

In the absence of a factor VIII:C inhibitor, factor VIII replacement is accomplished by use of third-generation, high-purity factor VIII concentrate (i.e., monoclonal antibody–purified and heat-treated or detergent/solvent-treated to inactivate HIV and the hepatitis C virus), recombinant human factor VIII concentrate, or single-donor cryoprecipitate. Heat-treated prothrombin complex concentrates and monoclonal antibody–purified (i.e., "pure") factor IX concentrates are sources of factor IX for the treatment of factor IX deficiency (Table 15.12).

Both factor VIII and factor IX concentrates are prepared from the pooled plasma of thousands of donors. Earlier products carried an unacceptably high risk of transmitting viral infections, but high-purity clotting factor concentrates of both factors now are widely available. These third-generation concentrates have essentially eliminated the risk of HIV-1 transmission, and they have greatly reduced the risk of hepatitis. Use of recombinant human factor VIII concentrate should be considered for patients with hemophilia A who have not been previously transfused (26).

The plasma half-life of transfused clotting factor is 8 to 12 hours for factor VIII and 18 to 24 hours for factor IX. Calculation of the dosage and planning of treatment schedules should be done in collaboration with the hematology consultant and take into account the patient's plasma volume ($\approx$40 mL/kg), the percentage of normal clotting factor desired to control or prevent bleeding, half-life of the transfused factor, and the concentration of clotting factor in the replacement product. In vivo recovery and survival of a test dose should be determined before surgery, and these studies should be repeated at regular intervals during prolonged periods of postoperative replacement therapy.

Patients with hemophilia and moderate or mild factor VIII deficiency may show a twofold (or higher) rise above baseline factor VIII levels 30 minutes following the intravenous infusion of desmopressin acetate (DDAVP; Stimate). The maximum increase occurs immediately at the end of the infusion, and it persists for 6 to 12 hours (27). Theoretically, tachyphylaxis

Table 15.12.   Blood Component Therapy of Common Coagulation Disorders[a]

Disorder	Deficient Factor(s)	Component	Dosage	
			Initial Dose	Maintenance
Congenital				
Hemophilia A	VIII:C	Third-generation AHF[b]	40–50 U/kg	10–20 U/kg per 12 h
		Recombinant AHF[c]	40–50 U/kg	10–20 U/kg per 12 h
		Cryoprecipitate[d]	—	—
		DDAVP[e]	0.3 µg/kg IV	May repeat q 12 h
Hemophilia B	IX	Heat-treated PCC[f]	50–75 U/kg	20–40 U/kg per 12–24 h
		"Pure" IX[g]	50–75 U/kg	20–40 U/kg per 12–24 h
von Willebrand's disease	VIII:C and VIII:vWF	Cryoprecipitate[d]	—	—
		Int-purity AHF[h]	30–80 U/kg	—
		DDAVP[e]	0.3 µg/kg IV	May repeat q 12 h
Acquired				
Vitamin K deficiency	II, VII, IX, X	Plasma (FFP)	10–20 mL/kg	10 mL/kg q 6–12 h
Coumarin excess		Heat-treated PCC[f]	20–40 U/kg	—
Liver disease	II, VII, IX, X, V (and I if severe)	Plasma (FFP)	10–20 mL/kg	10 mL/kg q 6–12 h
DIC	Platelets	Platelet concentrates[i]	0.1 U/kg	—
	V, VIII	Plasma (FFP)	10–20 mL/kg	—
	Fibrinogen	Cryoprecipitate[d]	2 bags per 10 kg	—

FFP, fresh-frozen plasma.

[a]Component dosage varies depending on severity of the deficiency, severity of bleeding, and clinical response to treatment. The preoperative and postoperative treatment of patients with bleeding disorders requires close supervision by a specialist who has training in these disorders.

[b]Third-generation (high-purity) AHF = human factor VIII coagulant activity prepared by monoclonal antibody purification or solvent/detergent.

[c]Recombinant AHF = human factor VIII coagulant activity prepared by recombinant DNA technology. Not derived from pooled plasmas.

[d]Cryoprecipitate of plasma contains approximately 80–100 U of factor VIII per bag and 100–250 mg of fibrinogen per bag. Single-donor cryoprecipitate reduces the risk of viral transmission.

[e]Used for minor procedures only, rise in factor VIII:C is short-lived, tachyphylaxis may occur with repeated doses, and preoperative trial with factor VIII levels postinfusion must be performed to ensure adequate response.

[f]Prothrombin complex (II, VII, IX, and X) concentrate prepared from pooled plasmas and heated to destroy viral agents.

[g]"Pure" IX = factor IX concentrate prepared by monoclonal purification of pooled plasmas; preferred for extended periods of postoperative support beause of reduced risk of thrombotic complications.

[h]Intermediate-purity FVIII concentrate (Humate-P) is a heat-treated, pooled plasma product. It contains both factor VIII coagulant and vWF activity.

[i]The initial dose is 6 to 8 U of pooled platelet concentrates for an adult patient; response to transfusion is assessed by repeating a platelet count 1 hour postinfusion.

may occur when repeated doses of DDAVP are given within a 24-hour period; however, patients generally show continued responsiveness with repeated dosing. This form of therapy is feasible only for minor surgical procedures and dental extractions, but it spares patients with moderate or mild hemophilia from exposure to plasma components and their potential for transmitting viral infections. A test infusion of DDAVP with measurement of both preinfusion and postinfusion factor VIII levels should be completed at least 7 days before minor surgery to confirm a rise in the factor VIII level. A special, high-potency formulation of DDAVP is now available for nasal administration in mild and moderately affected patients with factor VIII deficiency and von Willebrand's disease who require minor surgical procedures (28).

Von Willebrand's disease, which is the most common congenital coagulopathy, produces a combined deficiency of factor VIII clotting activity (factor VIII:C) and the factor VIII von Willebrand factor (factor VIII:vWF), which is necessary for normal platelet adhesion to the vascular subendothelium. Thus, a mildly prolonged aPTT and a prolonged template bleeding time are both usually characteristic of this disorder. Three principal types of von Willebrand's disease are recognized. In type I, an autosomal dominant disorder, levels of factor VIII:C (as measured by an assay based on the aPTT) and factor V:vWF (as measured by the ristocetin-induced platelet agglutination assay) are decreased to the same extent. Type II is inherited in the same fashion and results in a dysfunctional factor VIII:vWF, but factor VIII:C in these patients may be normal. SDS-agarose electrophoretic analysis of plasma from patients with type II disease using Western blot technology reveals a loss of higher and intermediate VIII:vWF multimers (i.e., type IIa) or a selective absence of higher-molecular-weight multimers (i.e., type IIb). Type III is inherited as an autosomal recessive disorder and results in a marked reduc-

tion or absence of both VIII:C and VIII:vWF levels, causing a severe bleeding disorder.

The control of surgical bleeding in patients with von Willebrand's disease generally depends more on achieving normal factor VIII clotting factor activity than on correcting the prolonged bleeding time (29). On the other hand, arrest of bleeding from mucosal surfaces appears to require at least temporary elevation of the factor VIII:vWF concentration and accompanying correction of the bleeding time.

Patients with von Willebrand's disease may respond to **intravenous infusion or nasal administration of DDAVP** with an increase in factor VIII clotting factor activity, with or without a rise in factor VIII:vWF activity. If a test infusion of DDAVP confirms an adequate rise in factor VIII levels, this drug can be used for transient augmentation of factor VIII in preparation for minor surgery. Patients with other forms of the disease (i.e., type III) may show no response, however, or may develop severe thrombocytopenia (i.e., type IIb). Therefore, therapy with DDAVP should generally be reserved for the treatment of types I and IIa.

Plasma products will usually be necessary to provide adequate factor VIII support for **major surgery** in patients with von Willebrand's disease. Fresh-frozen plasma or cryoprecipitate of fresh-frozen plasma contain both factor VIII clotting factor and factor VIII:vWF activities. Cryoprecipitate is enriched with the higher-molecular-weight forms of factor VIII:vWF. It is transfused as a pool of the cryoprecipitate from several donors, and it thus carries the risk of virus transmission. Standard purified and heat-treated factor VIII concentrates that are used in the treatment of hemophilia A generally lack sufficient quantities of higher-molecular-weight von Willebrand factor to be effective in the treatment of von Willebrand's disease. However, a limited number of commercial, intermediate-purity, virus-inactivated factor VIII concentrates that contain higher concentrations of factor

VIII:vWF are undergoing clinical trials in patients with von Willebrand's disease who require replacement therapy because of major surgery.

Treatment of Acquired Coagulation Factor Disorders

An acquired coagulopathy may be discovered during preoperative evaluation. If so, the goal should be to make the correct diagnosis and, if possible, to reverse the abnormality before surgery. More commonly, however, an acquired clotting factor deficiency may develop postoperatively, especially if surgery or recovery are prolonged and complicated by hypotension, infection, poor nutrition, or the need for massive transfusion of blood. Acquired coagulopathies usually involve deficiencies of more than one clotting factor, and the correct diagnosis is suggested by the clinical setting combined with the pattern of screening laboratory test results (Table 15.10).

Vitamin K deficiency is quite common, particularly in very ill patients postoperatively (30). Body stores of vitamin K are limited, and a deficiency state can develop as quickly as 1 to 3 weeks in the following situations: *(a)* prolonged, inadequate oral intake of food in combination with antibiotic therapy, especially when the gut flora responsible for the synthesis of vitamin K_2 have been eliminated; *(b)* malabsorption of vitamin K; and *(c)* therapy with oral anticoagulants.

Vitamin K is fat soluble, and conditions such as celiac disease, biliary tract obstruction, pancreatitis, regional enteritis, and cholestyramine therapy can result in deficiency. Broad-spectrum antibiotics, especially neomycin and certain cephalosporins such as cefotetan, cefamandole, and cefoperazone, can promptly interfere with the normal synthesis of vitamin K–dependent clotting factors (i.e., factors II, VII, IX and X). Early in the course of vitamin K deficiency, only the PT is prolonged, but over time, the aPTT also becomes abnormal.

Treatment of this coagulopathy depends on the urgency of the clinical situation. If bleeding is absent or surgery is elective, vitamin K_1 can be given subcutaneously or intramuscularly in doses of 10 to 20 mg. Intravenous administration should be avoided if possible because of occasional anaphylactoid reactions; if vitamin K_1 must be given intravenously, it should be diluted with saline or dextrose and given at a rate not to exceed 1 mg/min. Correction of the abnormal clotting tests following therapy with vitamin K_1 requires approximately 10 to 12 hours. Response to therapy should always be confirmed by repeating the PT. If the PT is not satisfactorily shortened within 24 hours, the dose may be repeated, but this failure usually indicates hepatocellular disease or concomitant, non-vitamin K–dependent coagulation factor deficiencies.

In patients with vitamin K deficiency who have serious bleeding or in those who require urgent surgery, fresh-frozen plasma, 10 to 20 mL/kg, will immediately replace the vitamin K–dependent clotting factors (Table 15.12), and 20 mg of vitamin K_1 should be given concurrently. Fresh-frozen plasma will also rapidly reverse the anticoagulant effect of coumarin drugs and is the treatment of choice when emergency surgery is required in patients receiving long-term warfarin therapy. Vitamin K_1 should be given prophylactically at a dose of 10 mg at least once per week during antibiotic therapy with some second- and third-generation cephalosporins that are known to cause vitamin K carboxylase antagonism.

Patients taking **coumarin drugs** for antithrombotic prophylaxis and who will undergo elective surgery require a specific preoperative treatment plan. Warfarin or dicumarol should be discontinued 4 days before surgery, and prophylactic subcutaneous heparin should be substituted. A preoperative PT is obtained to assure that the PT international normalized ratio (INR) has returned to the normal or near-normal range. On postoperative day

1, oral anticoagulants can be resumed. A loading warfarin dose of 10 mg/day for 2 days, followed by resumption of the patient's preoperative dose, will usually reestablish adequate prophylactic anticoagulation within 4 to 5 days, at which time the use of heparin can be discontinued. However, each patient will require variable loading and maintenance doses of warfarin. When new medications have been introduced or liver disease has developed postoperatively, the patient's warfarin requirements may change dramatically. Vitamin K_1, administered to temporarily reverse the warfarin effect, may render the patient transiently refractory to warfarin anticoagulation.

A common dilemma is the need to perform outpatient dental surgery on patients who require long-term warfarin therapy. Mandibular anesthetic blocks and dental extractions pose a risk of soft-tissue bleeding extending into the retropharyngeal space in anticoagulated patients. If possible, dental procedures should be postponed during the early phases of warfarin therapy, when continuous, effective antithrombotic prophylaxis is essential. Patients at high risk of developing recurrent thromboembolism, such as those with prosthetic heart valves, require uninterrupted anticoagulation, and they are best treated as inpatients with intravenous or subcutaneous adjusted-dose heparin until adequate warfarin anticoagulation can be reestablished after the dental procedure. When the risk of recurrent thrombosis is less (e.g., during the chronic maintenance phase of anticoagulation following a deepvenous thrombosis), warfarin can usually be discontinued safely 4 days before and resumed at the original dose on the day of the procedure.

Liver disease is one of the most common causes of acquired coagulation disorders. Individuals with advanced, chronic liver disease pose complex problems as far as treatment, because multiple abnormalities contribute to their hemostatic defects (31). There is defective synthesis of factors II (i.e., prothrombin), V, VII, IX, and X. In severe liver disease, there is deficient and, rarely, defective synthesis of fibrinogen. These patients may also be thrombocytopenic, particularly when portal hypertension leads to splenomegaly and splenic pooling of platelets. Compounding these deficiencies is increased fibrinolytic activity, because the liver is the site of antiplasmin synthesis and clearance of plasminogen activators. The individual contributions of these factors differs in each patient; however, inadequate synthesis of coagulation factor is usually the most important defect in chronic liver disease. In these patients, both a prolonged PT and aPTT are common, and in patients with end-stage liver disease, the plasma fibrinogen level may also be low and the thrombin time prolonged.

Either preoperatively or before procedures such as liver biopsy, these patients should receive infusions of fresh-frozen plasma to restore their coagulation factors to normal. Vitamin K_1 therapy is usually ineffective, because the liver cannot produce the vitamin K-dependent factors. Even so, vitamin K_1 should be administered as vitamin K deficiency resulting from malabsorption or inadequate intake may accompany liver disease. Infusion of prothrombin complex concentrates should be avoided, because these may precipitate intravascular clotting in this setting. Both thrombocytopenia and a qualitative platelet abnormality may be present as well, necessitating the transfusion of platelets in addition to fresh-frozen plasma if the platelet count is less than 80,000 cells/μL. Unfortunately, complete correction of the coagulation and platelet abnormalities that are associated with liver disease is not always possible.

Disseminated intravascular coagulation results in the consumption of coagulation factors following the intravascular activation of coagulation during a serious, underlying illness. This disorder should be thought of both as a syndrome and as a complication of a number of clinical disorders. Common clinical conditions triggering DIC are listed in Table 15.13.

The clinical manifestations of DIC are variable. They may present acutely with generalized bleeding from multiple sites and organ damage from ischemia. In the chronic and subacute forms, patients may have minimal or no spontaneous bleeding but a significant risk of bleeding from minor challenges such as arterial punctures. The diagnosis of DIC is confirmed by demonstrating the consumption of prothrombin, factor V, factor VIII, fibrinogen, and platelets. The abnormalities of coagulation factors and platelets are reflected by a prolonged PT, partial thromboplastin time, and thrombin time, as well as by the presence of thrombocytopenia and fibrin degradation products or D-dimer (Table 15.10).

Not all coagulation factors that are consumed during the coagulation process are depressed below their normal limits in patients with DIC. The initial clotting factor concentrations and their rates of

regeneration vary from individual to individual. Since fibrinogen is an acute phase reactant, it may be elevated before the onset of intravascular coagulation. Although it is being consumed, the level may be in the normal range; therefore, only a relative decrease in fibrinogen is seen. This may also be true for platelets, factor V, and factor VIII. Thus, the PT, aPTT, and platelet count may be normal early in the course of DIC, especially if the only clinical manifestation of the syndrome is thrombosis. However, fibrin degradation products or D-dimer should be present and the thrombin time prolonged in the early stages.

Treatment of patients with intravascular coagulation begins with the identification and correction of the underlying cause. Intravascular coagulation associated with placental separation or fetal death should be treated by removal of the uterine contents. In patients with septicemia, appropriate antibiotic therapy is the initial requirement. Every effort should be made to reverse shock with replacement of fluids and maintenance of adequate blood pressure to prevent vasoconstriction, venous stasis, acidosis, and hypoxemia. Even with meticulous attention to the appropriate medical problems, however, the underlying disorder causing the intravascular coagulation cannot be reversed in some patients.

The **initial treatment of patients with DIC** is based primarily on whether intravascular coagulation is occurring with bleeding, thrombosis, or both. If bleeding is the major problem, the appropriate clotting factors should be replaced. If thromboembolic phenomena dominate, heparin therapy may be indicated, but studies confirming its value are lacking. Fortunately, the need for heparin is rare. If simultaneous bleeding and clotting are present, the use of heparin requires a careful strategy. Heparin will inhibit intravascular clotting and permit improvement of the clotting factor levels. However, bleeding is frequently exacerbated by heparin alone. Thus, it is imperative to

Table 15.13. Conditions Triggering Disseminated Intravascular Coagulation

Acute Disorder
Gram-negative bacteremia
Gram-positive bacteremia
Hypotension
Obstetrical emergencies
    Abruptio placenta
    Amniotic fluid embolism
    Toxemia
    Burns and severe trauma
Heat stroke
Acute hemolytic transfusion reaction
Acute leukemia (especially promyelocytic)
Rocky Mountain spotted fever
Snake (pit viper) envenomation
Chronic / Subacute Disorder
Mucin-producing adenocarinomas
Large arteriovenous malformations
Obstetrical problems
    Toxemia
    Retained dead fetus
Hepatic failure
Tumor lysis syndrome

administer platelets initially if the platelet count is less than 20,000 to 50,000 cells/μL; to replace clotting factors II, V, and VIII; and to supplement fibrinogen if the level is less than 150 mg/dL.

A reasonable initial dosage for platelets in adults is 8 to 10 U. Consumable factors can be replaced with fresh-frozen plasma (i.e., prothrombin and factor V) and cryoprecipitate (i.e., fibrinogen and factor VIII). Fresh-frozen plasma can be given at 10 mL/kg. The dosage of cryoprecipitate to restore the fibrinogen and factor VIII to adequate levels is empiric; an initial trial of 0.1 bags/kg should be given to adults. If necessary, both fresh-frozen plasma and cryoprecipitate can be repeated every 12 to 24 hours, as indicated by serial aPTT and fibrinogen levels.

After the fibrinogen level and platelet count have been restored to acceptable levels, a continuous intravenous infusion of heparin, 10 U/kg per hour, can be initiated if thrombosis has been documented. Loading doses of heparin should be avoided if bleeding is apparent. In addition, significantly smaller doses should be used in severe thrombocytopenia (platelet count, ≤20,000 cell/μL), because heparinization in this circumstance significantly increases the risk of hemorrhage.

The best index of hemostatic effectiveness is cessation or reduction of bleeding. **The most sensitive laboratory indicator of patient response to heparinization is a rise in the fibrinogen level.** In patients who respond, the fibrinogen level returns toward normal within 24 to 48 hours, and the platelet count rises (but more slowly). A reduction in fibrin degradation products or the D-dimer concentration may be delayed but provides evidence that intravascular fibrinolysis has been interrupted. Other coagulation test abnormalities slowly revert to normal and are less helpful in following the intravascular clotting process.

Use of the fibrinolytic inhibitor ε-aminocaproic acid (EACA) is rarely indicated in the treatment of intravascular coagulation. This drug should be considered when there is excessive fibrinolytic activity following prostatectomy or in patients with prostate carcinoma. Also, combined therapy with heparin and EACA may be indicated in patients with acute promyelocytic leukemia. In these situations, adequate heparinization must be accomplished before EACA is used, because when used alone, it can produce a disastrous thrombotic tendency.

Massive transfusion syndrome was discussed previously (see "The Transfused Patient").

Circulating anticoagulants develop in many clinical settings, including hemophiliacs receiving clotting factor replacement, some postpartum women, patients with autoimmune disorders and drug reactions, and, occasionally, in otherwise healthy, elderly patients who have no apparent underlying disease (32). Presence of a circulating anticoagulant is indicated by failure to correct the abnormal clotting test when repeated on a mixture of the patient's plasma and normal plasma. Inhibitors to all clotting factors have been described; however, those directed against factor VIII and the lupuslike anticoagulant are most common. Patients with **factor VIII inhibitor** usually have **severe hemorrhagic tendency**, and control of bleeding in these patients is very difficult. Elective surgery is contraindicated in patients with coagulation factor inhibitors, and specialized laboratory investigations and therapeutic maneuvers are required.

On the other hand, bleeding tendency is not present in patients with the lupuslike anticoagulant unless thrombocytopenia or low levels of prothrombin are also present. Surgery can be performed in the absence of these deficiencies without fear of excessive bleeding. This IgG or IgM antibody interferes with in vitro, phospholipid-dependent clotting tests and prolongs the partial thromboplastin time and, occasionally, the PT. Paradoxically, however, it is associated with an increased risk of thrombosis (see "Antiphospholipid Antibody Syndrome").

HYPERCOAGULABLE STATES

The term *hypercoagulable state* refers to a number of conditions that may predispose an individual to inappropriate and excessive thrombosis (33, 34). This enhanced tendency to form blood clots may be acquired during an illness that causes alterations in coagulation factors, platelet function, blood vessels, or properties of blood flow. Alternatively, it may result from a congenital deficiency of some naturally occurring coagulation factor inhibitor or of fibrinolytic proteins that normally limit the extent of thrombus formation following vascular injury (Table 15.14).

Diagnostic Approach

The **preoperative assessment of thromboembolic risk begins with the patient history,** which should identify any factors that are associated with in-

Table 15.14. Risk Factors for Thromboembolism

Secondary Risk
Advancing age
Obesity
Immobilization
Postoperative state
Prior thromboembolism
Venous stasis (congestive heart failure,
    cardiomyopathy, venous insufficiency)
Malignancy
Oral contraceptives
Hyperviscosity
Paroxysmal nocturnal hemoglobinuria
Nephrotic syndrome
Myeloproliferative disorders
Inflammatory bowel disease
Diabetes mellitus
Artificial surfaces (prosthetic valves and grafts)
Antiphospholipid antibody syndrome
Primary Risk (Thrombophilia)
Antithrombin III deficiency
Protein C deficiency
Activated protein C resistance
Protein S deficiency
Dysfibrinogenemia
Fibrinolytic disorders
Homocystinuria

Modified from Schafer AI. The hypercoagulable states. Ann Intern Med 1985; 102:814–828.

creased thrombotic tendency in the postoperative period. These include advanced age, obesity, repeated thromboembolism, venous insufficiency, estrogen therapy, pregnancy, malignancy, and medical illnesses such as valvular heart disease and congestive heart failure. Even in the absence of any clearly defined, predisposing factors, patients undergoing surgery such as orthopaedic, abdominal, urologic, gynecologic, and neurosurgical procedures have an increased risk of developing deep-venous thrombosis and pulmonary embolism.

Certain historical findings suggest the possibility of a hypercoagulable state caused by an inherited deficiency or abnormality of a naturally occurring anticoagulant or secondary to an acquired antiphospholipid antibody. These include: *(a)* family history of repeated thrombosis, especially if occurring at a young age; *(b)* history of recurrent thrombosis without precipitating factor; *(c)* history of multiple spontaneous abortions; *(d)* history of thrombosis occurring in adolescence or early adulthood; *(e)* history of clot formation in unusual anatomic locations (e.g., mesenteric or hepatic veins); and *(f)* history of a resistance to heparin anticoagulation. Evaluating these primary conditions requires access to a laboratory that can perform assays for antithrombin III, proteins C and S, antiphospholipid antibody, and activated protein C resistance. Rarely, studies to exclude abnormalities in the fibrinolytic system or abnormal fibrinogens may also be necessary.

The clinical expression and mode of inheritance for antithrombin III deficiency, which is the major physiologic antagonist of thrombin and other activated serine protease clotting factors, is the prototype of the primary hypercoagulable states. Typically, a quantitative or qualitative abnormality in the antithrombin III molecule is inherited in an autosomal dominant fashion. Patients not uncommonly develop venous thrombosis, pulmonary embolism, or both in adolescence or young adulthood, and they may present with thrombosis in unusual anatomic locations. Most symptomatic heterozygotes have antithrombin III levels that are 30 to 50% of normal, and the severity of disease expression may vary considerably within affected families. Patients with a congenital deficiency of protein C, which inactivates the activated coagulation factors VIII and V, or of protein S, which is a cofactor for protein C, have a clinical presentation and mode of inheritance similar to those of antithrombin III deficiency. Both proteins C and S are vitamin K–dependent proteins.

The most common inherited cause of thrombophilia is **activated protein C resistance**. Patients with this disorder have inherited a mutation of the factor V molecule that renders it resistant to the inhibitory action of activated protein C (35). For many patients, it appears that more than one mechanism may be involved in a predisposition to thrombosis. For example, a congenital deficiency of protein C or other clot-limiting proteins may be recognized first in pregnancy or the postoperative setting when factors favoring venous stasis are also present.

Antiphospholipid Antibody Syndrome

Antiphospholipid-protein antibodies (36) may appear during infection (including infection with HIV-1); systemic lupus erythematosus or other autoimmune diseases; malignancies; therapy with drugs such as phenothiazines, quinidine, procainamide, and hydralazine; and in patients with no apparent underlying disease. They are frequently discovered when a plasma sample from an asymptomatic patient is found to have a prolonged aPTT before surgery or in patients with thrombosis or other clinical symptoms of the antiphospholipid antibody syndrome.

These antibodies interact with negatively charged phospholipids, and they are detected by phospholipid-dependent coagulation assays (e.g., kaolin clotting time, aPTT, platelet neutralization assay,

Russell's viper venom), in which case they are termed *lupuslike anticoagulants*, or the solid-phase enzyme-linked immunoadsorbent assay using cardiolipin as the antigen (i.e., "anticardiolipin antibodies"). Approximately 90% of plasma samples demonstrating lupuslike anticoagulant activity will also demonstrate anticardiolipin antibody activity. Those patients with clinical thrombosis usually have moderate to highly positive IgG anticardiolipins, with or without IgM antibodies, whereas those with isolated IgM antibodies are usually asymptomatic. Other accompanying serologic abnormalities include VDRL positivity and, occasionally, antibodies to double-stranded DNA and low-titer antinuclear antibodies (36).

Thrombosis is uncommon when antiphospholipid-protein antibody formation is associated with drugs, solid tumors, or infection. The term *antiphospholipid antibody syndrome* refers to patients who have clinical symptoms in association with the presence of these antibodies, because many apparently normal individuals possess low-titer antibodies to phospholipid. To establish the diagnosis of antiphospholipid antibody syndrome, the patient with plasma containing these antibodies must have demonstrated: *(a)* venous or arterial thrombosis, including gangrene, myocardial infarction, and stroke; *(b)* recurrent pregnancy loss; or *(c)* thrombocytopenia. Vasculitis, rash (including livedo reticularis), arthralgias, migraine headache, transient ischemic attacks, amaurosis fugax, nonbacterial endocarditis, and Coombs' test–positive hemolytic anemia may also be present.

The finding of antiphospholipid-protein antibodies before surgery carries no risk of hemorrhage, but it should alert physicians to a substantial risk of perioperative thrombosis, especially in patients with a history of prior thrombosis in association with high-titer, IgG antiphospholipid-protein antibodies. Perioperative heparin prophylaxis and long-term oral anticoagulation with warfarin are recommended for this latter group of patients. Recent studies support the recommendation that these patients should be maintained on warfarin in doses that are sufficient to achieve an INR of 3.0 or greater (37).

Risk Reduction and Treatment

Before elective surgery, an attempt should be made to eliminate any reversible cause of hypercoagulability. For example, oral contraceptives should be discontinued several weeks before the procedure, and the treatment of congestive heart failure and other edematous states should be maximized. Hyperviscosity from increased RBC mass (i.e., erythrocytosis), extreme thrombocytosis, or increased serum paraprotein concentrations (i.e., macroglobulinemia and other plasma cell dyscrasias) should be corrected with phlebotomy, cytapheresis, or plasmapheresis.

Available data support the use of **prophylactic subcutaneous heparin,** 5000 U subcutaneously every 8 or 12 hours, in patients at high risk for thrombosis who are to undergo general surgical, urologic, or gynecologic procedures. Therapy begins 2 hours before surgery and continues at least until the patient is ambulatory. The aPTT usually remains normal during low-dose subcutaneous heparin therapy.

Prophylactic heparin may increase the risk of bleeding and hematoma formation at the operative site, but the risk of life-threatening bleeding complications is minimal. Low-dose heparin has not been shown to provide effective prophylaxis in orthopaedic patients, and it is considered to be contraindicated in those undergoing neurosurgical operations for intracranial or spinal lesions. For orthopaedic patients, low-dose warfarin or adjusted-dose heparin may provide adequate prophylaxis. Physical measures such as pneumatic gradient compression stockings, early ambulation, and physical therapy are important general antithrombotic adjuncts for surgical patients and should not be overlooked. Currently ongoing clinical trials (37) are testing the efficacy and safety of low-molecular-weight heparin as antithrombotic prophylaxis for surgery.

Perioperative treatment of patients with a hypercoagulable state, such as antithrombin III deficiency, protein C or S deficiency, activated protein C resistance, or the lupuslike anticoagulant, should be carried out in collaboration with a specialist familiar with these fairly uncommon disorders. As with all surgical patients, risk factors such as obesity, pregnancy, immobilization, and estrogen-containing medication will further increase the potential for thrombosis in these individuals.

Prophylactic replacement of antithrombin III with fresh-frozen plasma or commercially available antithrombin III concentrate, with or without low-dose heparin therapy, can be used in surgical patients with a congenital deficiency of this naturally occurring inhibitor. Fresh-frozen plasma and commercially available heat-treated prothrombin complex concentrates are potential sources of proteins C and S; however, prothrombin complex concentrate carries some risk of transmitting viral hepatitis and, occasionally, has itself been associated with thrombotic manifestations. Symptomatic patients with a congenital deficiency of antithrombin III and of proteins C and S usually require long-term prophylactic anticoagulation with warfarin directed at maintaining a prothrombin time INR of 2.0 to 2.5. For symptomatic patients with the antiphospholipid antibody syndrome who require long-term warfarin anticoagulation, a target INR of approximately 3.0 is recommended (38).

The lupuslike anticoagulant may disappear during treatment of the underlying condition or with corticosteroid therapy. As mentioned, if emergency surgery is required, heparin prophylaxis is indicated. Measures such as early ambulation and pneumatic compression stockings are also essential for preventing thromboembolism in these patients.

TREATMENT OF PLATELET DISORDERS IN SURGICAL PATIENTS

Preoperative Diagnostic Studies

Platelets arrest bleeding from small vessels by forming a plug at the site of vascular damage within 2 to 10 minutes of injury. To succeed, the platelets must circulate at a minimum concentration of 50,000 to 100,000 cells/μL. They must also adhere to exposed subendothelial collagen, release their granule contents, bind clotting factors to their phospholipid membranes, and form aggregates to seal the edges of the wound. Fibrin then forms at the site of the platelet seal, thus strengthening the plug.

Some authors have proposed that a bleeding time be obtained for all surgical candidates as part of the preoperative screening for hemostatic defects. In a retrospective study at a single institution, Barber et al. (39) found that 110 of 1941 routine preoperative bleeding times were prolonged. However, in approximately 75% of these patients, the abnormality could have been predicted because of a recorded history of recent ingestion of aspirin or nonsteroidal anti-inflammatory drugs, azotemia, or thrombocytopenia. Furthermore, as mentioned, the template bleeding time appears to have little clinical value in predicting the likelihood of bleeding with surgery and invasive procedures (24, 25).

Thrombocytopenia

As the platelet count decreases to less than 100,000 cells/μL, there is a proportional increase in the template bleeding time as well as an increase in the potential risk of bleeding. It is unusual for bleeding to occur with surgery or trauma when the platelet count is greater than 50,000 cells/μL unless platelet dysfunction is also present. Both spontaneous and induced bleeding are more likely to occur when the platelet count is between 10,000 and 20,000 cells/μL. It is not only the absolute number of platelets that must be consid-

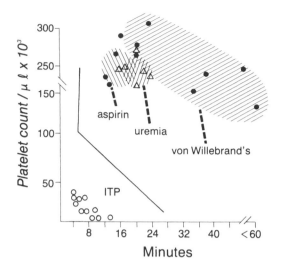

Figure 15.4. Relationship of template bleeding time to platelet count. *ITP*, idiopathic thrombocytopenic pupura. (Modified from Harker LA. Hemostasis manual. 2nd ed. Philadelphia: FA Davis, 1974:9.)

ered, however, but also the underlying process causing the thrombocytopenia, the presence or absence of other hemostatic defects, the duration of thrombocytopenia, and any coexisting qualitative platelet abnormalities. For example, life-threatening bleeding is unusual in patients with autoimmune thrombocytopenia who appear to have platelets with increased hemostatic potency. Not infrequently, such patients have normal template bleeding times, even when the platelet count is less than 10,000 cells/μL (Fig. 15.4).

Usually, minor procedures involving easily visualized surgical sites at which direct pressure can be applied can be safely performed when the platelet count is only moderately reduced (platelet count, >50,000 cells/μL). Below this count, however, hemorrhage is more likely, and major elective procedures should be deferred until a higher platelet count can be achieved. Before emergency surgery, every attempt should be made to obtain a minimum platelet count of 80,000 cells/μL.

Thrombocytopenia in adult patients is usually acquired by one of four mechanisms: *(a)* decreased or ineffective platelet production, *(b)* increased platelet destruction, *(c)* abnormal platelet distribution, and *(d)* platelet dilution. Specific causes for each mechanism are shown in Table 15.15.

Decreased platelet production occurs with systemic infection (especially viral), vitamin B_{12} and folate deficiencies, various drugs, chemotherapy, and bone marrow involvement by fibrosis, infection, or malignancy. It may be a component of bone marrow aplasia, affecting all cell lines; less commonly, it can be an isolated deficiency of platelet production. Drugs that may specifically inhibit platelet production include ethanol, thiazides, and anticonvulsants. A bone marrow aspirate showing severely reduced or absent megakaryocytes confirms this mechanism.

Treatment or prevention of serious hemorrhage is achieved by use of platelet concentrates. Usually, 6 to 8 U of platelets are infused, and platelet counts are obtained at 1 and 12 hours postinfusion to estimate platelet recovery and survival. When patients have been alloimmunized by prior transfusions or pregnancies, random donor platelets may be ineffective; platelets obtained from relatives, random single donors, or donors more closely matched for the recipient's HLA antigens may be required. Whenever family-donor blood products are used, these should be irradiated to prevent transfusion-induced graft-versus-host disease.

Increased platelet destruction is the most common mechanism of acquired thrombocytopenia seen in a general clinical practice. Severe thrombocytopenia with a bone marrow aspirate showing abundant megakaryocytes and no other abnormality is consistent with platelet destruction in the peripheral circulation. Drug-associated immune thrombocytopenia occurs with some of the most commonly prescribed medications (Table 15.15).

Thrombocytopenia associated with heparin therapy can occur in as many as 10% of patients receiving this drug and results from drug-dependent antibody formation. In patients who have previously received heparin, thrombocytopenia may develop as early as 2 days after therapy has been initiated, but the average time of onset for previously unexposed patients is 7 to 10 days. These patients not only have an increased risk for bleeding but, paradoxically, may develop fatal arterial or, less commonly, venous **thrombosis**. Patients receiving heparin should be monitored for thrombocytopenia with platelet counts every 2 to 3 days. If a falling platelet count is documented, heparin must be discontinued in favor of other methods for anticoagulation (40); warfarin or ancrod therapy are usually substituted for heparin, depending on the clinical situation. Although thrombocytopenia may be less likely to develop in patients receiving low-molecular-weight heparin (41), low-molecular-weight heparin should not be substituted for high-molecular-weight

Table 15.15. Causes of Thrombocytopenia

Decreased or Ineffective Production
Drugs (e.g., ethanol, thiazides, anticonvulsants)
Viral infection (e.g., HIV-1, rubella, influenza)
Vitamin B_{12} and folic acid deficiency
Hematopoietic stem cell disorders (e.g., aplastic anemia, PNH, leukemia)
Myelophthisis (e.g., metastatic cancer)
Chemotherapy
Ionizing radiation
Increased Peripheral Destruction
Drug-immune thrombocytopenia (e.g., heparin, quinidine, quinine, gold, sulfa drugs, penicillins)
Autoimmune thrombocytopenia (e.g., ITP, SLE, CLL, lymphoma)
Immune complex–mediated thrombocytopenia (e.g., bacterial sepsis, HIV-1, endocarditis, IV drug abuse, posttransfusion purpura)
DIC
Mechanical (e.g., prosthetic surfaces)
Abnormal Platelet Distribution or Dilution
Hypersplenism
Massive transfusion syndrome

ITP, idiopathic thrombocytopenic purpura; *PNH,* paroxysmal nocturnal hemoglobinuria; *SLE,* systemic lupus erythematosus.

forms if thrombocytopenia develops. Clinical trials are now being conducted to assess the efficacy of hirudin, a new anticoagulant enzyme with specific antithrombin activity. When available, this drug should be of great benefit to patients with heparin-associated thrombocytopenia.

Autoimmune thrombocytopenic purpura is a form of destructive thrombocytopenia resulting from the spontaneous development of an IgG antibody that is directed against the host's platelets. It is frequently idiopathic in nature (e.g., autoimmune thrombocytopenia) but may be secondary to other diseases, such as lymphoid malignancies and systemic autoimmune disorders. Initial treatment involves several weeks of high-dose oral corticosteroids (equivalent of prednisone, 1–2 mg/kg). Most adult patients with autoimmune thrombocytopenia will fail to achieve a lasting remission when steroid doses are tapered, however, and **splenectomy is frequently necessary.** A significant improvement in the platelet count during corticosteroid treatment seems to predict the ability to achieve a complete remission with splenectomy. Because of potential adrenal suppression from chronic steroid use and to maintain the highest possible platelet count, corticosteroids should be continued throughout the preoperative and early postoperative periods.

Patients with autoimmune thrombocytopenia who fail to respond to corticosteroids require splenectomy at a time when they are severely thrombocytopenic and generally unresponsive to platelet transfusion. Usually, intraoperative and postoperative bleeding are surprisingly mild, and once the splenic pedicle is clamped, the platelet count frequently rises spontaneously. If thrombocytopenia persists and bleeding occurs, platelet transfusion and steroid therapy may be somewhat more effective after splenectomy.

Three patterns of response to splenectomy are recognized. Approximately 70 to 75% of patients achieve a complete remission, and their platelet counts rise sharply in the first 1 to 2 weeks after surgery. Another 20% experience improvement in platelet counts to a hemostatically safe, although not normal, level. The remaining 5 to 10% remain severely thrombocytopenic and require other treatment modalities for refractory autoimmune thrombocytopenia, including danazol, high-dose intravenous gamma globulin (IgG), or immunosuppressive agents (42).

Other forms of destructive thrombocytopenia include immune complex–mediated thrombocytopenia associated with sepsis (43), bacterial endocarditis, intravenous drug abuse, posttransfusion purpura, and acquired immunodeficiency syndrome. Thrombin-induced platelet consumption occurs in DIC (see "Treatment of Acquired Coagulation Factor Disorders"). The constellation of intravascular platelet consumption, hemolytic anemia, fever, renal dysfunction, and central nervous system abnormalities is diagnostic of **thrombotic thrombocytopenic purpura**. Recognizing this syndrome is important, because treatment with plasma exchange combined with plasma or cryosupernatant infusions is usually life-saving (44).

Abnormal platelet distribution and platelet dilution commonly occur with hypersplenism and the massive transfusion syndrome, respectively (see "Splenomegaly: Preoperative and Postoperative Treatment" and "Massive Transfusion Syndrome").

Qualitative Platelet Dysfunction

A prolonged bleeding time with a normal or near-normal platelet count indicates abnormal platelet function. The patient history will often detect these functional platelet disorders preoperatively and help to suggest whether they are congenital or acquired.

Patients with **congenital platelet dysfunction** have a longstanding history of bruising and mucosal bleeding, which may be exacerbated by antiplatelet medications such as aspirin and nonsteroidal anti-inflammatory drugs. These drugs are an important cause of acquired platelet dysfunction, and a history of their use within 1 to 2 weeks of the preoperative evaluation should be sought. Von Willebrand's disease is a hereditary disorder in which platelets do not adhere to the vascular subendothelium. This abnormality is not intrinsic to the platelet; it is caused by a deficiency of plasma factor VIII:vWF, which is corrected through plasma-derived products or DDAVP. Hereditary defects of intrinsic platelet function are relatively common causes of mild bleeding disorders, and the family history is often positive for mucosal or skin bleeding and menorrhagia. These patients should be evaluated preoperatively with platelet aggregation studies and testing to exclude von Willebrand's disease.

Except for the well-defined platelet dysfunction that is associated with Glanzmann's thrombasthenia and Bernard-Soulier syndrome, the congenital, qualitative platelet disorders are poorly characterized. Platelet aggregation testing helps to diagnose these disorders, and a defect in platelet granule release is the most common type of congenital dysfunction. If a platelet release–type defect is confirmed by platelet aggregation testing, preoperative therapy with corticosteroids (e.g., prednisone, 30 mg/d for 5–7 days) will occasionally correct the bleeding time to normal or near-normal. If corticosteroids are ineffective, DDAVP may be beneficial, and platelet transfusions are indicated if excessive bleeding occurs during surgery. As in the treatment of all hemostatic disorders, close communication between the consulting internist and surgeon is important to ensure the patient's safety.

Acquired platelet dysfunction (Table 15.16) occurs most commonly with use of aspirin and other nonsteroidal anti-inflammatory drugs that inhibit platelet cyclooxygenase, a key enzyme that is required for platelet thromboxane A_2 production and subsequent platelet

Table 15.16. Causes of Acquired Platelet Dysfunction

Drugs
    Aspirin and other nonsteroidal anti-inflammatory agents, dipyridamole, semisynthetic penicillins, clofibrate, dextran, hydroxychloroquine)
Uremia
Hepatic cirrhosis
Ethanol
Paraproteins
    Myeloma, macroglobulinemia
Cardiopulmonary bypass
Fibrin degradation products
    DIC, fibrinolytic therapy
Hematopoietic stem cell disorders
    Leukemia, myeloproliferative diseases, myelodysplastic syndromes

aggregation. Duration of the antiplatelet effect varies among these agents. Aspirin irreversibly acetylates cyclooxygenase, resulting in an antiplatelet effect lasting for up to 1 week; other nonsteroidal drugs have antiplatelet effects lasting for less than 24 hours. Penicillins, especially semisynthetics, can cause a dose-related prolongation of the bleeding time, and they may produce a bleeding diathesis, especially in patients with renal insufficiency. The antiplatelet effect persists for as long as 4 to 5 days after these drugs are stopped. Thus, medications associated with platelet dysfunction should be discontinued at least 1 week before elective surgery (45). Serious bleeding caused by drug-induced platelet dysfunction should be treated with platelet transfusion.

Acquired defects in platelet function can accompany several types of systemic illnesses. The hemorrhagic tendency that is associated with uremia appears to parallel the progressive loss of renal function, and it may relate to failure of the kidney to clear metabolic products. Partial or complete correction of the bleeding tendency in uremia has been reported following both peritoneal dialysis and hemodialysis, cryoprecipitate infusion, intravenous DDAVP, and estrogen therapy. The shortening of the bleeding time is transient after DDAVP infusion, lasting only for approximately 6 hours (46). Cryoprecipitate, 10 bags infused over 30 minutes, may also shorten the bleeding time (47); the period of maximum shortening occurs between 1 and 12 hours after infusion and usually returns to pretreatment levels by 24 hours. Of greatest interest is the observation that prolonged bleeding times in patients with renal insufficiency may normalize following correction of their anemia with recombinant human erythropoietin therapy. Clearly, responses to these treatments vary from patient to patient.

Platelet dysfunction also occurs in paraproteinemic states (e.g., multiple myeloma), myeloproliferative diseases, DIC, and hepatic cirrhosis. Response to platelet transfusion may be less than optimum in these conditions, and treatment of the primary disease is an important aspect of care. Alkylating agents may correct the qualitative platelet abnormality in myeloproliferative syndromes, and DDAVP may shorten the bleeding time in patients with cirrhosis (48). Plasmapheresis will remove paraproteins and correct a prolonged bleeding time resulting from these abnormal immunoglobulins.

The results of several studies have implicated acquired platelet defects as the major hemostatic abnormality in CPB surgery (see "Hemostatic Problems in Cardiac Surgery").

Thrombocytosis

A platelet count in excess of 400,000 cells/μL is encountered in many clinical circumstances. The relevant question is whether the thrombocytosis reflects a primary marrow disorder (i.e., a myeloproliferative disorder) or is secondary to an underlying disease (i.e., secondary or reactive thrombocytosis). A clear-cut distinction may be difficult, but because of the prognostic implications, this differentiation is important.

Secondary thrombocytosis occurs in various clinical conditions, including ma-

lignancy, infections, rheumatoid arthritis, other collagen vascular disorders, iron deficiency anemia, inflammatory bowel disease, and following splenectomy. The platelets in these disorders function normally, and these patients are usually not at an increased risk for thromboembolic phenomenon, even with platelet counts greater than 1,000,000 cells/μL.

Platelets in patients with primary thrombocytosis secondary to myeloproliferative disorders (e.g., polycythemia vera, essential thrombocythemia, CGL, myelofibrosis) can be hyperaggregable, hypoactive, or normal. Thrombocytosis places these patients at a substantial risk for either thromboembolic phenomena, including vascular graft occlusion, or bleeding (49).

The preoperative approach to patients with thrombocytosis resulting from a myeloproliferative disorder depends on the platelet count and the urgency of surgery. A platelet count in excess of 1,000,000 cells/μL should be reduced before surgery. Hydroxyurea or busulfan will reduce the number of platelets over several weeks to months. Combined therapy with alkylating agents and automated plateletpheresis (50) will also reduce the platelet count, usually within 3 to 5 days of treatment. If emergency surgery is required, plateletpheresis should be instituted immediately, and hydroxyurea can be given concomitantly to reduce the production of platelets. **For patients with chronic myeloproliferative disorders such as thrombocythemia, polycythemia vera, myelofibrosis, and CGL who require surgery, it is important to reduce the platelet count to less than 600,000 cells/μL, because life-threatening thromboembolic phenomena or hemorrhage can occur in the perioperative setting.** Thrombosis of vascular grafts is also common in patients with uncontrolled thrombocytosis associated with a myeloproliferative disorder.

SPECIAL HEMATOLOGIC TREATMENT ISSUES IN SURGICAL PATIENTS

Hemostatic Problems in Cardiac Surgery

The patient who has undergone CPB surgery not infrequently acquires multiple hemostatic defects. The consulting internist is often called to evaluate these patients postoperatively because of bleeding.

Diagnostic Activities

Postoperative bleeding most commonly occurs from an open vessel, which may necessitate surgical exploration and suturing. Occasionally, however, excessive bleeding occurs both at the operative site and systemically. CPB produces thrombocytopenia, altered platelet function, decreased coagulation factors, and activation of the fibrinolytic system.

After the initiation of CPB, there is a prompt decrease in all clotting factors, antithrombin III, platelets, and plasminogen resulting from the hemodilution effect of priming the pump with crystalloid solution. By the end of the procedure, levels of most of these factors remain low, approximating 50% of their baseline values; for unknown reasons, the level of factor V may decrease markedly, to less than 20% of baseline. Since a 30% level of most coagulation proteins is adequate for hemostasis, it is difficult to attribute the bleeding that occurs in these patients to a coagulation factor deficiency. A decreased factor V level is the exception and may occasionally contribute to bleeding. Measurement of the PT and aPTT will help to determine the extent of factor deficiencies; if these screening tests are prolonged, fresh-frozen plasma can be used for clotting factor replacement. The levels of all coagulation factors return to the their baseline values by 48 hours after the procedure.

Anticoagulation with heparin is necessary during CPB, and although its use is indispensable, heparin has given rise to abnormal bleeding both during and after the surgical procedure. The causes of such hemorrhage have been traced to excessive heparin during surgery, failure of administered protamine sulfate to neutralize the heparin at the end of surgery, and heparin rebound. Heparin "rebound" refers to reappearance of the anticoagulated state and bleeding tendency after adequate neutralization of the heparin has been accomplished. A prolonged activated clotting time suggests excessive heparinization.

When patients are placed on the pump oxygenator, the platelet count decreases, and this decrease persists for 48 to 96 hours postoperatively. However, it is unusual for the platelet count to decrease to less than 80,000 cells/μL, and bleeding from thrombocytopenia as the sole mechanism is uncommon. In addition to mild or moderate thrombocytopenia, the bleeding time is often prolonged with a near-normal platelet count, which is diagnostic of a qualitative platelet defect. Thus, **loss of platelet function is the most significant hematologic consequence of CPB and is usually the main contributor to bleeding in the immediate postoperative period.** Platelet dysfunction gradually improves over a 2- to 3-day period after surgery as increasing numbers of fully functional platelets are released from the bone marrow. Mechanisms that have been proposed to explain this loss of platelet function include an alteration in platelet glycoprotein membrane receptors, which normally mediate platelet adhesion and aggregation, and the release and depletion of platelet alpha granules, causing defective aggregation. Transfusion of 6 to 8 U of platelet concentrates should reverse the platelet dysfunction associated with CPB.

Prophylaxis and Treatment

Prophylactic treatment to prevent bleeding in patients undergoing CPB has increased in importance. Salzman et al. (51), in a randomized, prospective, double-blind study, found that intravenous administration of DDAVP, 0.3 μg/kg, significantly reduced blood loss both during and in the first 24 hours after CPB in **complicated cardiac operations** (i.e., valve replacement, repeat coronary artery bypass graft). Patients undergoing uncomplicated coronary artery bypass graft surgery were not included in this study. Two additional randomized, placebo-controlled studies (52, 53) did not confirm that DDAVP decreased the total operative blood loss with coronary artery bypass graft surgery; however, one of the studies did show significant shortening of the bleeding time and reduced intraoperative blood loss. A double-blind, randomized trial in patients undergoing insertion of Harrington spinal fusion rods found a significant decrease in operative bleeding among patients treated with DDAVP compared to untreated controls (54).

Use of aprotinin, which inhibits the fibrinolytic enzyme plasmin, significantly reduces blood loss in patients undergoing cardiac bypass (55). It was also shown to decrease the need for autologous transfusion in patients undergoing coronary artery bypass graft surgery (56). In this latter study, patients treated with aprotinin were less likely than controls to have a prolonged bleeding time during bypass. Aprotinin may help to preserve platelet function by preventing plasmin degradation of platelet glycoprotein membrane receptors.

Every attempt to identify the specific hemostatic defect (or defects) should be made if bleeding occurs after CPB, and therapy should be tailored to the specific defect. Available **therapeutic modalities** include use of platelet concentrates, DDAVP, cryoprecipitate, and fresh-frozen plasma. Administration of platelet concentrates is usually the first step to control bleeding if the PT, aPTT, and platelet count are normal and the template bleeding time prolonged. DDAVP has not been used as extensively once bleeding has occurred with CPB, but this agent may be beneficial in slowing established bleeding.

In the less common situation of bleeding that cannot be attributed to platelet dysfunction, fresh-frozen plasma to replace factor V and cryoprecipitate to supplement factor VIII and fibrinogen can be given empirically. If bleeding fails to be controlled after a reasonable attempt with multiple agents, **reoperation to explore for an open vessel is strongly recommended.**

Preoperative and Postoperative Treatment of Splenomegaly

The preoperative treatment of patients with marked splenomegaly requires an understanding of the hemodynamic and hematologic changes that occur with progressive splenic enlargement (57). With marked splenic enlargement, from whatever cause, the flow of blood through the organ increases from a normal value of 5% to as much as 50% of the cardiac output. With massive splenomegaly, the splenic blood volume may increase such that the organ contains as much as 25% of the total blood volume. Blood flow through the portal system increases dramatically; at the same time, blood is shunted away from other intravascular spaces, including the renal circulation. This stimulates the renin-angiotensin-aldosterone system, causing retention of both sodium and water. Patients with a massively enlarged spleen characteristically show evidence of high cardiac output and wide pulse pressure on physical examination. Care must be taken to avoid further volume expansion from vigorous hydration or rapid transfusion. Following surgical removal of the spleen, the expanded intravascular volume slowly returns to normal over several months.

Hypersplenism is the increased sequestration of the formed elements in blood that occurs as the splenic blood pool enlarges. Anemia, neutropenia, or thrombocytopenia may exist in any combination. The bone marrow compensates for the peripheral cytopenias by increasing its basal rate of blood cell production. The anemia that occurs with splenomegaly is a result of both hemodilution from the expanded blood volume and increased RBC trapping in the spleen.

The thrombocytopenia that occurs with hypersplenism is usually moderate in severity, with platelet counts between 30,000 to 50,000 cells/μL. The markedly enlarged spleen may sequester as much as 90% of the total body pool of platelets. Transfused platelets are rapidly removed from the circulation in hypersplenic states; however, if bleeding is present, platelet transfusions should be given as the bleeding may respond even though a platelet increment cannot be achieved. When significant thrombocytopenia is present before splenectomy, the blood bank should be requested to have 10 to 20 U of platelet concentrates available for emergency use if excessive operative bleeding develops. Platelet transfusion will be more effective in raising the platelet count once the surgeon has clamped the splenic pedicle.

Following splenectomy for any cause, the platelet count commonly rises to greater than 600,000 cells/μL, and it often exceeds 1,000,000 cells/μL. **Postsplenectomy thrombocytosis** usually resolves within weeks to a few months after surgery; however, marked elevations in the platelet count may persist indefinitely in patients with underlying myeloproliferative disorders (e.g., chronic myelogenous leukemia, polycythemia vera, agnogenic myeloid metaplasia, essential thrombocythemia) and those with acquired idiopathic sideroblastic anemia.

Thrombocytosis following splenectomy may be of such magnitude that the physician considers antithrombotic therapy as prophylaxis against thromboembolism. One study, however, suggests that the incidence of thrombotic complications in patients with platelet counts of greater than 1,000,000 cells/μL is not significantly different from that in patients with normal platelet counts as long as those with myeloproliferative disorders are excluded (58). Therefore, the value of routine use of aspirin or anticoagulants to prevent postsplenectomy thrombosis in patients without underlying myeloproliferative disorders cannot be substantiated. Furthermore, use of antiplatelet drugs may enhance bleeding in patients with myeloproliferative disorders (see "Treatment of Platelet Disorders in Surgical Patients").

When splenectomy is performed in patients with myeloproliferative diseases, there is a heightened risk of thrombosis risk, because these individuals produce large numbers of qualitatively abnormal platelets. Myelosuppressive therapy should be given preoperatively to normalize both the platelet count and function. Even when this is done, however, postoperative thrombocytosis may still occur.

Asplenic adult patients are predisposed to fulminant sepsis resulting primarily from encapsulated bacteria such as *Streptococcus pneumoniae, Haemophilus influenzae,* and meningococcus (59). The risk appears to be greater for infants and young children, and the underlying cause necessitating removal of the spleen is also an important determinant. The incidence appears to be greatest in splenectomized patients with thalassemia or malignant hematologic disorders, and the risk is greatest within 2 to 3 years of splenectomy but continues at a lower probability for several years thereafter. Rates of mortality from postsplenectomy sepsis are high, and prophylactic immunization with pneumococcal vaccine before splenectomy is important in attempting to prevent this complication. Splenectomized patients should be counseled that fever may signal a life-threatening infection and should be reported to their physician immediately.

Therapeutic Apheresis

Removal of selected cellular components in the blood or plasma can be performed efficiently with automated cell centrifugation or the newer technique of hemofiltration. The latter technique uses membranes that selectively remove un-

Table 15.17.   Accepted Indications for Therapeutic Apheresis

Standard Therapy
Plasma exchange
    Thrombotic thrombocytopenic purpura
    Cryoglobulinemia
    Coagulation factor inhibitor
    Posttransfusion purpura
      Cold agglutinin hemolysis
    Myasthenia gravis
    Goodpasture's syndrome
    Guillain-Barré syndrome
    Homozygous familial hypercholesterolemia
    Refsum's disease
Cytapheresis
    Sickle-cell disorders
    Leukemia and hyperleukocytosis
    Symptomatic thrombocythemia
Adjunctive Therapy
Chronic cold agglutinin disease
Chronic inflammatory demyelinating
    polyneuropathy
Autoimmune thrombocytopenia
Rapidly progressive glomuerlonephritis
Systemic vasculitis
Hemolytic-uremic syndrome
Cutaneous T-cell lymphoma
Hairy-cell leukemia

desired plasma components by ultrafiltration while retaining albumin and clotting factors.

For some medical conditions, use of apheresis has been established as the standard and, in some cases, the primary therapy in controlling disease manifestations or complications. For others, it may play an adjunctive role. Plasma exchange has assumed a primary role in the treatment of thrombotic thrombocytopenic purpura (44), and preoperative cytapheresis for extreme thrombocytosis, hyperleukocytosis in myeloproliferative diseases, and in sickling disorders can help to prepare patients for emergency surgery. Other specific indications for therapeutic apheresis are listed in Table 15.17.

REFERENCES

1. Stehling L, Simon TL. The red cell transfusion trigger. Arch Pathol Lab Med 1994;118:429–434.
2. Carson JL, Spence RK, Poses RM, Bonavita G. Severity of anaemia and operative mortality and morbidity. Lancet 1988;i:727–729.
3. Nelson AH, Fleisher LA, Rosenbaum SH. Relationship between postoperative anemia and cardiac morbidity in high-risk vascular patients in the intensive care unit. Crit Care Med 1993;21:860–866.
4. Consensus Conference. Perioperative red blood cell transfusion. JAMA 1988;260:2700–2703.
5. Etchason J, Petz L, Keller E, et al. The cost effectiveness of preoperative autologous blood donation. N Engl J Med 1995;332:719–724.
6. Welch HG, Meehan KR, Goodnough LT. Prudent strategies for elective red blood cell transfusion. Ann Intern Med 1992;116:403–406.
7. Biesma DH, Marx JJ, Kraaijenhagen RJ, et al. Lower homologous blood requirement in autologous blood donors after treatment with recombinant human erythropoietin. Lancet 1994;344:367–370.
8. Canadian Orthopedic Perioperative Erythropoietin Study Group. Effectiveness of perioperative recombinant human erythropoietin in elective hip replacement. Lancet 1993;341:1227–1232.
9. Eyster E, Bernene J. Nosocomial anemia. JAMA 1973;223:73–74.
10. Pineda A, Taswell H, Brzica S. Delayed hemolytic transfusion reaction: an immunologic hazard of blood transfusion. Transfusion 1978;18:1–7.
11. Pisciotti PT, ed. Blood transfusion therapy: a physician handbook. 4th ed. Bethesda, MD: American Association of Blood Banks, 1993:60.
12. Rodgers GP. Recent approaches to the treatment of sickle cell disease. JAMA 1991;265:2097–2101.
13. Searle J. Anaesthesia in sickle cell states. Anaesthesia 1973;28:48–58.
14. Davies SC, Luce PJ, Win AA. Acute chest syndrome in sickle cell disease. Lancet 1984;i:36–38.
15. Bellet PS, Kalinyak KA, Shukla R, et al. Incentive spirometry to prevent acute pulmonary complications in sickle cell diseases. N Engl J Med 1995;333:699–702.
16. Pirofsky B. Immune hemolytic disease: the autoimmune hemolytic anemias. Clin Haematol 1975;4:167–180.
17. Petz LD. Autoimmune hemolytic anemia: transfusion in special situations. Hum Pathol 1983;14:251–255.
18. Diaz JH, Cooper ES, Ochsner JL. Cold hemagglutination pathophysiology: evaluation and management of patients undergoing cardiac surgery with induced hypothermia. Arch Intern Med 1984;144:1639–1641.
19. Smith JR, Landaw SA. Smoker's polycythemia. N Engl J Med 1978;298:6–10.
20. Thomas D, Marshall J, Du Boulay GH, et al.

Cerebral blood-flow in polycythemia. Lancet 1977;ii:161–163.

21. Wasserman L, Gilbert H. Surgery in polycythemia vera. N Engl J Med 1963;269:1226–1230.

22. Gabrilove J. The development of granulocyte colony stimulating factor in its various clinical applications. Blood 1992;80:1382–1385.

23. Rapaport SI. Preoperative hemostatic evaluation: which tests, if any? Blood 1983;61:229–231.

24. Rodgers RPC, Levin J. A critical reappraisal of the bleeding time. Semin Thromb Hemost 1990;16:1–20.

25. Lind SE. The bleeding time does not predict surgical bleeding. Blood 1991;77:2547–2552.

26. Lusher JM, Arkin S, Abildgaard CF, et al. Recombinant factor VIII for the treatment of previously untreated patients with hemophilia A. N Engl J Med 1993;328:453–459.

27. Bolan CD, Alving BM. Pharmacologic agents in the management of bleeding disorders. Transfusion 1990;30:541–551.

28. Rose EH, Aledort LM. Nasal spray desmopressin (DDAVP) for mild hemophilia A and von Willebrand disease. Ann Intern Med 1991;114:563–568.

29. Mannucci PM. Desmopressin (DDAVP) for treatment of disorders of hemostasis. Prog Hemost Thromb 1986;8:19–45.

30. Ansell JE, Kumar R, Deykin D. The spectrum of vitamin K deficiency. JAMA 1977;238:40–42.

31. Lechner K, Niessney H, Thaler E. Coagulation abnormalities in liver disease. Semin Thromb Hemost 1977;4:40–56.

32. Green D, Lechner K. A survey of 215 nonhemophilic patients with inhibitors to factor VIII. Thromb Haemost 1981;45:200–203.

33. Nachman RL, Silverstein R. Hypercoagulable states. Ann Intern Med 1993;119:819–827.

34. Schafer AI. Hypercoagulable states: molecular genetics to clinical practice. Lancet 1994;344:1739–1742.

35. Svensson PJ, Dahlback, B. Resistance to activated protein C as a basis for venous thrombosis. N Engl J Med 1994;330:517–522.

36. Triplett DA. Protean clinical presentation of antiphospholipid antibodies (APA). Thromb Haemost 1995;74:329–337.

37. Ten Cate JW, Koopman MMW, Prins MH, Buller HR. Treatment of venous thromboembolism. Thromb Haemost 1995;74:197–203.

38. Green D, Hirsh J, Heit J, et al. Low molecular weight heparin: a critical analysis of clinical trials. Pharmacol Rev 1994;46:89–109.

39. Barber A, Green D, Galluzzo T, et al. The bleeding time as a preoperative screening test. Am J Med 1985;78:761–764.

40. Warkintin TE, Kelton JG. Heparin-induced thrombocytopenia. Annu Rev Med 1989;40:31–44.

41. Warkintin TE, Levine MN, Hirsh J. Heparin-induced thrombocytopenia in patients treated with low-molecular-weight heparin or unfractionated heparin. N Engl J Med 1995;332:1330–1335.

42. Berchtold P, McMillan R. Therapy of chronic idiopathic thrombocytopenic purpura in adults. Blood 1989;74:2309–2317.

43. Poskitt TR, Poskitt PK. Thrombocytopenia of sepsis. The role of circulating IgG-containing immune complexes. Arch Intern Med 1985;145:891–894.

44. Rock GA, Shumak KH, Buskard NA, et al. Comparison of plasma exchange with plasma infusion in the treatment of thrombotic thrombocytopenic purpura. Canadian Apheresis Study Group. N Engl J Med 1991;325:393–397.

45. Davies D, Steward D. Unexpected excessive bleeding during operation: role of acetylsalicyclic acid. Can Anaesth Soc J 1977;24:452–458.

46. Mannucci PM, Remuzzi G, Pusineri F, et al. Deamino-8-arginine vasopressin shortens the bleeding time in uremia. N Engl J Med 1983;308:8–12.

47. Janson P, Jubelirer S, Weinstein M, et al. Treatment of the bleeding tendency in uremia with cryoprecipitate. N Engl J Med 1980;303:1318–1322.

48. Mannucci PM, Vicante V, Vianello L, et al. Controlled trial of desmopressin in liver cirrhosis and other conditions associated with a prolonged bleeding time. Blood 1986;67:1148–1153.

49. Schafer AI. Bleeding and thrombosis in the myeloproliferative disorders. Blood 1984;64:1–12.

50. Taft E, Babcock R, Scharfman W, et al. Plateletpheresis in the management of thrombocytosis. Blood 1977;50:927–933.

51. Salzman EW, Weinstein MJ, Weintraub RM, et al. Treatment with desmopressin acetate to reduce blood loss after cardiac surgery: a double-blind randomized trial. N Engl J Med 1986;314:1402–1406.

52. Seear M, Wadsworth L, Sheps S, et al. The effect of desmopressin acetate (DDAVP) on postoperative blood loss after open heart surgery in children [abstract]. Blood 1987;70:380A.

53. Rocha E, Llorens R, Paramo JA, et al. Does desmopressin acetate reduce blood loss after surgery in patients on cardiopulmonary bypass? Circulation 1988;77:1319–1323.

54. Kobrinsky NL, Letts RM, Patel LR, et al. 1-Desamino-8-D-arginine vasopressin (desmopressin) decreases operative blood loss in patients having Harrington rod spinal fusion surgery. A randomized, double-blinded, controlled trial. Ann Intern Med 1987;107:446–450.

55. Royston D, Bidstrup BP, Taylor KM, Sapsford

RN. Effect of aprotinin on need for blood transfusion after repeat open-heart surgery. Lancet 1987;ii:1289–1291.

56. Bidstrup BP, Royson D, Sapsford RN, Taylor KM. Reduction in blood loss and blood use after cardiopulmonary bypass in high dose aprotinin (Trasylol). J Thorac Cardiovasc Surg 1989;97: 364–372.

57. Hess C, Ayers C, Sandusky W, et al. Mechanism of dilutional anemia in massive splenomegaly. Blood 1976;47:629–644.

58. Boxer M, Braun J, Ellman L. Thromboembolic risk of postsplenectomy thrombocytosis. Arch Surg 1978;113:808–809.

59. Krivit WM. Overwhelming postsplenectomy infection. Am J Hematol 1977;2:193–201.

16
Oncology

Robert A. Gordon

The consulting internist deals with numerous medical and surgical situations involving patients with cancer. Although certain aspects of oncology are specialized, the internist is frequently involved in the preoperative and postoperative decisions involving these patients, and he or she is often consulted regarding complications of both the treatment and disease. The internist is commonly involved in the care of the terminally ill patients with cancer as well.

Therefore, the internist should know the natural history of the common cancers and be prepared to make decisions concerning the diagnostic, therapeutic, and supportive care issues of these patients. Since the care of patients with cancer often involves a multidisciplinary approach, the internist should also understand the importance of a good working relationship with their surgical and radiologic colleagues.

Many of the hematologic, metabolic, and infectious problems in patients with cancer are covered in other chapters. This chapter emphasizes the principles of performing perioperative consultation on these patients and discusses the treatment of specific complications caused by metastatic cancer. A pragmatic approach to the control of commonly encountered complaints is presented as well.

Surgical patients with cancer can be classified into two general groups:

1. Patients who require surgery that is unrelated to their cancer. This incidental surgery may be necessary whether the patient is undergoing active therapy or not and whether the cancer is present or in remission.
2. Patients with recently diagnosed cancer and who require therapeutic cancer surgery.

INCIDENTAL SURGERY IN PATIENTS WITH CANCER

General Considerations

Patients with cancer undergoing active chemotherapy, radiation therapy, or both and who develop an acute surgical problem may have complex metabolic, infectious, and hematologic abnormalities. The internist must perform a complete history and physical examination, and he or she must carefully evaluate the laboratory and radiologic data.

The internist should focus on the patient's nutritional and hydration status, because therapy for cancer may result in cachexia, dehydration, and a catabolic state, which will result in delayed wound healing and additional risk for infection. Examination of the mouth may detect mucositis, which is assumed to involve the mucosa of the entire gastrointestinal tract. Early institution of hyperalimentation may prevent certain postoperative metabolic problems.

A careful review of the patient's present medications is also important, because glucocorticoids may be a component of the chemotherapy regimen or a prescribed treatment for some complication. Appropriate glucocorticoid replacement therapy may be necessary to prevent adrenal insufficiency during the postoperative period.

Meticulous attention to laboratory abnormalities may prevent serious postoperative complications. Electrolyte abnormalities (i.e., hypokalemia, hypomagnesemia, hypophosphatemia) commonly occur in patients undergoing therapy for cancer. Neutropenia, thrombocytopenia, or both may be present preoperatively, but if not, they should be anticipated when chemotherapy has been recently administered. Granulocyte colony-stimulating factor (Neupogen) may be given for neutropenia to hasten granulocyte recovery. Broad-spectrum antibiotic coverage is essential for febrile patients.

Patients with cancer (especially metastatic cancer) are hypercoagulable. Prophylactic heparin should be given preoperatively if there is no contraindication.

The internist should appreciate that chemotherapy given in the remote past can result in end-organ impairment of the heart, lungs, kidneys, and intestinal tract. The stresses imposed by surgery may result in demands on body organs that have inadequate reserve function.

Clearly, a knowledgeable estimate of the patient's prognosis as it relates to his or her cancer is important. If the cancer is potentially curable, aggressive medical and surgical treatment is indicated, and correction of the underlying, acute problem is most critical (Table 16.1).

Specific Problems

Gastrointestinal Tract

Acute **abdominal pain in patients with neutropenia** following chemotherapy is a common reason for combined medical and surgical treatment. Localized abdominal pain is more likely than generalized abdominal pain to result from a surgically correctable condition. Surgery should be avoided unless the pain is accompanied by specific signs or radiologic findings. Patients with neutropenia undergoing operations tolerate these procedures well if aggressive supportive care is administered and the granulocyte recovery is rapid. Prolonged neutropenia following surgery, however, portends a poor outcome. Broad-spectrum antibiotic therapy with specific coverage of Gram-negative enteric and anaerobic organisms is essential, and granulocyte colony-stimulating factor (Neupogen) should be administered to hasten granulocyte recovery.

Bowel obstruction in patients with cancer, especially those who have had

---

Table 16.1.   Evaluation of Surgical Patients with Cancer

Incidental Surgery
Carefully evaluate metabolic, infectious, and hematologic abnormalities associated with cancer and
    treatment.
Anticipate or prevent problems related to previous or current cancer therapy. Consider remote effects
    of chemotherapy and radiation therapy on organ systems.

Therapeutic Surgery
Evaluate the extent of the cancer preoperatively (stage and anticipate intraoperative therapy).
Understand the changing role for initial chemotherapy and therapy before or in place of surgery
    (neoadjuvant therapy).
Recognize the benefit and limitations of postoperative adjuvant therapy for specific cancers.
Appreciate the indications for "second look" surgery.
Consider the resectability of a single or a few metastases.

previous surgery for gastrointestinal and gynecologic malignancies, is not uncommon. One study that evaluated 95 patients with cancer and bowel obstruction, of which 57 patients underwent surgery, found that 27% of the 57 patients had either a benign cause or a new primary tumor as the cause of the obstruction (1). However, the remaining 73% had recurrent or metastatic cancer. The authors concluded that patient performance status before entering the hospital was the most important predictor of successful outcome of the bowel obstruction, and they point out that **early surgical intervention** is indicated in patients with a good performance status. In contrast, patients with poor performance status, who are clearly terminal and who have extensive visceral metastases, have little chance of benefitting from operative intervention.

Judicious use of prophylactic antibiotics and the early institution of parenteral nutrition will minimize the risk of postoperative complications. **Adynamic ileus** is common in patients with cancer who take opioid drugs or antidepressants that have anticholinergic properties, and it can be difficult to differentiate from a partial colonic obstruction. Medical treatment with bowel rest, intravenous fluids, correction of electrolyte abnormalities, intubation of the stomach or small intestine for decompression, placement of a rectal tube, colonic enemas, cathartics, and avoidance of drugs that depress intestinal motility will often restore bowel function. Decompressive colonoscopy may be beneficial to patients when all other measures fail, and if mechanical obstruction is documented, early surgery is indicated.

Perirectal infections are relatively common in patients with neutropenia and are associated with a high mortality rate. The usual physical findings of fluctuance and erythema are uncommon because of the neutropenia, however, but fever, pain, and induration are present. One study of perirectal infections in patients with acute leukemia and severe neutropenia found that early surgical incision and debride-

ment was associated with rapid relief from pain, excellent healing, and improved survival (2).

Remote Organ Toxicity Caused by Cancer Therapy

When surgery is indicated in patients previously treated with chemotherapy, radiation therapy, or both, several potential complications from the remote effects of such treatment on organ systems may result. These complications are usually preventable and require special consideration.

Lungs

Bleomycin has major toxicity on the lung, and it can cause chronic pneumonitis that progresses to pulmonary fibrosis. It is important to identify any associated risk factors that will increase the incidence of pulmonary toxicity in patients undergoing general anesthesia. These risk factors include:

1. Cumulative dose of bleomycin (the incidence of pulmonary fibrosis increases significantly after a total dose of 400 U).
2. Age older than 70 years.
3. Prior or concomitant thoracic radiation therapy.
4. Concurrent use of cyclophosphamide or doxorubicin (Adriamycin).
5. Administration by intravenous bolus technique, which causes more toxicity than constant infusion.
6. Exposure to high-dose oxygen.
7. Preexisting lung disease, especially emphysema.

Administration of **high oxygen concentration** in patients previously treated with bleomycin deserves special emphasis. There appears to be a synergistic effect between prior use of bleomycin and a high-oxygen concentration during anesthesia. This synergistic effect is toxic to lung tissue, and it can cause progressive pulmonary fibrosis. Since many patients who receive bleomycin are young, have been cured of their malignancy (e.g., testicular cancer, Hodgkin's disease, lymphoma), and may require incidental surgery in the future, this should not be overlooked. It is recommended that the **inspiratory oxygen concentration not exceed 40%** at any time either during or after the surgery, and the internist should ensure that the surgeon and anesthesiologist are aware of the patient's history of chemotherapy before the procedure. Also, since bleomycin will frequently decrease the lung volumes and cause a diffusion abnormality, careful pulmonary evaluation, including spirometry, DLCO, and arterial blood gas before major surgery, is indicated (3).

Mitomycin is an additional chemotherapeutic drug that will increase the risk of pulmonary toxicity when a patient is exposed to a high oxygen concentration. The same guidelines as recommended for bleomycin apply to patients who have received mitomycin as well.

Heart

Doxorubicin (Adriamycin) is one of the most commonly used anticancer drugs and is active against many malignancies. An important toxicity, however, is a cumulative, **dose-dependent cardiomyopathy**, which can result in congestive heart failure. The frequency of this cardiomyopathy ranges from only a few to over 50% depending on the population treated and the specific techniques used to study cardiac function.

Risk factors for doxorubicin-induced cardiomyopathy (4) include:

1. Cumulative dose (significant increase in risk when the dose is 450 mg/m^2 or greater).
2. Dose schedule (lower incidence when a weekly or an infusion schedule is used compared with "standard" bolus, every-3-week schedule).
3. Age older than 40 years.
4. Mediastinal radiation therapy.

5. Previous underlying cardiac disease.
6. Concurrent use of cyclophosphamide (possible risk factor).

At least one-third of all patients with doxorubicin-induced cardiomyopathy are asymptomatic, and left ventricular dysfunction is only abnormal in this group when evaluated by an exercise radionuclide ventriculography gated scan (5). These patients should be identified before major surgery so that appropriate cardiac monitoring can be employed. The left ventricular dysfunction lasts for years, but it tends to be stable, nonprogressive, and is not a contraindication to necessary surgery.

Mediastinal radiation therapy is standard treatment for a number of malignancies, including Hodgkin's disease, lung cancer, both nonsmall-cell and limited small-cell carcinoma. Despite use of techniques that limit the dose of radiation to the heart, a small percentage of patients will eventually suffer radiation-induced heart disease. This problem is best studied in Hodgkin's disease because of its high rate of curability. Constrictive pericarditis is the cardiac problem most commonly induced by radiation, but severe coronary artery disease, valvular injury, and conduction system abnormalities have all been reported. These radiation-induced abnormalities are often occult. However, because these patients are now surviving longer after therapy, cardiac abnormalities may be seen with increasing frequency (6). A careful cardiac evaluation should be performed in patients with a prior history of mediastinal irradiation before they undergo any major surgical procedure.

Kidneys

Cisplatin (Platinol) commonly causes a subclinical reduction in kidney function that appears to be **irreversible.** Even when the blood urea nitrogen and creatinine level are normal or only minimally elevated, a marked decrease in the creatinine clearance rate can be documented (7).

Hypomagnesemia occurs in a substantial number of patients who have received cisplatin. This results from the renal wasting of magnesium caused by a toxic effect of cisplatin on the renal tubules (8). Cisplatin also may cause hypocalcemia and hypokalemia.

Several recommendations can be made regarding surgery in patients who have received cisplatin. Adequate hydration and a urinary output of 100 mL/h both during and after surgery may prevent additional renal injury, and mannitol, 25 to 50 g, should be used to ensure diuresis during surgery. Avoidance of nephrotoxic drugs, especially aminoglycoside antibiotics, is recommended as well.

Magnesium, calcium, and potassium measurements should be a part of the preoperative evaluation. Appropriate replacement is indicated for low levels.

Intestine

Radiation injury to the small intestine and colon is a significant complication of radiation therapy for pelvic and abdominal malignancies. The incidence of such injury has been estimated to approach 10%, and this complication usually occurs several years after radiation therapy. The most common presenting signs and symptoms relate to bowel obstruction, although fistula formation, ulceration, or perforation also occur.

Several important **principles regarding treatment** of radiation enteropathy (9) include:

1. Early diagnosis and surgical intervention are critical.
2. Total parenteral nutrition should be given both before and after definitive surgery.
3. Broad-spectrum antibiotic coverage is necessary. Nonabsorbable antibiotics should be given either orally or through a long intestinal tube preop-

eratively, and parenteral antibiotics, which cover bowel flora, should be given preoperatively and for at least 3 to 5 days postoperatively.

Preoperative consideration of the effects of previous therapy for cancer on organ systems may prevent significant postoperative complications.

THERAPEUTIC SURGERY IN PATIENTS WITH CANCER

Patients with cancer undergo therapeutic surgery for many reasons during the course of their illness. The first step after establishing the diagnosis is to critically and effectively stage the cancer. In addition to other factors that are specific to the individual cancer, the stage will determine the patient's prognosis and direct treatment. Early in therapy, surgery is often indicated to remove a localized cancer for potential care. Local or regionally advanced cancers may be treated initially with chemotherapy, radiation therapy, or both to make surgery possible in the future (i.e., neoadjuvant therapy). "Second-look" surgery may be recommended to evaluate a therapeutic effect or to debulk a tumor. On occasion, surgery may also be performed on selected patients with a single or a few metastases (Table 16.1).

Initial Treatment Of Specific Cancers

Each specific cancer should be thought of as a unique disease with its own natural history and patterns of spread. The major treatment modalities include surgery, chemotherapy, and radiation therapy, and they can be employed in a variety of sequences and combinations that are specific to the individual cancer. Organ preservation and quality of life are important considerations when deciding on specific therapy.

This section deals with the staging studies and therapeutic options for specific cancers. These cancers have been selected for discussion because of the frequency with which the internist is involved in their treatment.

Breast Cancer

Breast cancer is the most common malignancy in women, and it accounts for almost one-third of all new cancers in women and one-fifth of deaths from cancer in women. The internist is often asked to consult on many aspects of the care of women with this cancer. The internist should be able to advise women of the surgical options for newly diagnosed breast cancer, and it is important for the internist to have a working knowledge of the risk factors that predict eventual recurrence and to understand the role of adjuvant systemic therapy.

Staging Studies When evaluating asymptomatic women with clinical **stage I or II breast cancer** (see "Appendix"), there is no benefit to obtaining a brain or a liver scan. Metastases to these organs are extremely uncommon on initial presentation.

Although bone scanning has been considered to be a routine procedure before definitive surgery for breast cancer, objec-

Table 16.2. Five-Year Relapse Rate Correlated to Size of Primary and Axillary Node Involvement

	Size of Primary Tumor (cm)		
Axillary lymph node status	<2	2–5	>5
	5-Year Relapse Rate (%)		
Negative nodes	8–13	19–24	19–27
Positive nodes	37–50	50–64	65–79

Modified from Harris JR, Morrow M, Bonadonna G. Cancer of the breast. In: Devita VT, Hellman S, Rosenberg SA, eds. *Cancer. Principles and practice of oncology.* 4th ed. Philadelphia: JB Lippincott, 1993; 1276.

Table 16.3. Ten-Year Survival and Survival Without Recurrence Relative to Histologic Node Status at Radical Mastectomy[a]

	10-Year Survival (%)	
Node status	Overall	Without Recurrence
All patients	60	47
Nodes negative	82	72
Nodes positive	40	25
1–3 nodes	54	34
>4 nodes	26	16

Reprinted with permission from Valagussa P, Bonadonna G, Veronesi U. Patterns of relapse and survival following radical mastectomy. Cancer 1978; 41:1170–1178.
[a]No adjuvant systemic therapy given.

tive data do not support its use in early breast cancer (stage I or II) (10). The risk of metastases at presentation and recurrent disease is best determined by the size of the primary tumor, the presence or absence of metastases in the axillary lymph nodes, and the number of lymph nodes involved (Tables 16.2 and 16.3). It is unusual ($\approx$1%) for women with a primary tumor smaller than 2 cm in size and negative axillary lymph nodes to have a "truly" positive bone scan. When the primary tumor is between 2 and 5 cm and axillary lymph nodes are positive, the incidence of positive bone scans is approximately 5%, and less than one-half of these patients with positive scans will have proven bony metastases. The extra cost, time, and anxiety of additional tests such as skeletal radiography, bone biopsy, and computed tomography (CT) or magnetic resonance imaging (MRI) required to clarify spurious findings on bone scans is significant. Bone scans need not be part of the routine workup for patients who are free of musculoskeletal complaints and who have normal blood chemistry profiles before their initial treatment of truly early breast cancer. Imaging studies of the liver (i.e., ultrasonography or CT) are not necessary if the liver function tests and physical examination are normal. On the other hand, women with stage II and many positive lymph nodes or stage III (local-regional advanced) breast cancer have a greater likelihood of metastases, which would alter treatment, and a bone scan and liver imaging study are indicated.

Surgical Options Conservative surgery for early stage breast cancer (stages I and II) is an acceptable alternative to mastectomy in selected women. Although breast cancer appears clinically to be localized, hematogenous micrometastases frequently occur, resulting in ultimate relapse and proving that breast cancer is a systemic disease.

A randomized study of more than 1800 women with stages I and II breast tumors 4 cm or small in size compared total mastectomy to lumpectomy both with and without breast irradiation (12). Through an average 12 years of follow-up, similar distant disease-free and overall survival rates were found (12). The cumulative incidence of tumor recurrence in the ipsilateral breast was 35% in those treated with lumpectomy alone and 10% in those treated with lumpectomy and breast irradiation.

More women elect conservative surgery as their primary therapy for breast cancer now than in the past. The patient must understand that an **axillary lymph node dissection is necessary** for staging the disease. The optimal axillary staging procedure is controversial, but an adequate sample should include at least 10 level-one lymph nodes. **Adjuvant radiation therapy to the ipsilateral breast** is an integral part of therapy, because local recurrence rates are unacceptably high if irradiation is not given.

It is important for the consulting internist to understand the indications and contraindications for conservative breast surgery, because this type of surgery is not indicated in all women. Patient selection for breast-conserving treatment involves assessment of whether the primary tumor can be successfully **removed with an acceptable cosmetic result**, estimation of local recurrence after breast-conserving surgery, and understanding the patient's desires and expectations. Before any treatments are discussed with the patient, mammograms of both breasts must be obtained. These mammograms are critical in evaluating the size and location of the primary tumor, the presence and extent of microcalcifications, the presence or absence of multicentric disease, and the status of the contralateral breast. Consultation between the internist, surgeon, radiologist, and radiation therapist is often necessary.

In 1992, the American College of Radiology, American College of Surgeons, College of American Pathologists, and the Society of Surgical Oncology published standards for breast-conservation treatment (13). Both absolute and relative contraindications were determined (Table 16.4); although there is little debate regarding absolute contraindications, the relative contraindications deserve comment. Tumor size is not an absolute contraindication to breast-conservation treatment, but there is little published

Table 16.4. Absolute and Relative Contraindications to Breast-Conserving Treatment

Absolute Contraindications
First or second trimester of pregnancy
Two or more gross tumors in separate quadrants of the breast
Diffuse, indeterminate or malignant-appearing microcalcifications
History of therapeutic irradiation of the breast region

Relative Contraindications
Large tumor size in small breast
History of collagen vascular (connective-tissue) disease
Large breast size
Tumor location beneath the nipple

Reprinted with permission from Winchester DP, Cox JD. Standards for breast-conservation treatment. *CA* 1992;42:3;134–162.

experience on treating patients with tumor larger than 4 or 5 cm. Excision of a large tumor in a small breast may result in an unacceptable cosmetic outcome. An extremely large breast is not a contraindication to breast preservation provided that the available radiation-therapy technical resources are adequate to immobilize the breast and obtain dose homogeneity. Tumor location in the breast may be a consideration in the choice of local treatment, and in patients with a tumor directly beneath the nipple, adequate resection involves removal of the nipple areola complex. Whether this is preferable to mastectomy, however, needs to be assessed by the patient and her physician. The patient will be left with a sensate breast and a breast mound, and nipple reconstruction can be performed after radiation therapy has been completed. Finally, a history of collagen vascular disease is a relative contraindication to breast-conservation treatment, because the experience of radiation therapists indicates that patients with lupus and scleroderma develop severe fibrotic reactions to irradiation.

Several conservative surgical techniques are available, including wide local excision (i.e., lumpectomy) or quadrantectomy. Whichever technique is used, it is crucial that all of the tumor be removed and that the resected margins be tumor-free. Lumpectomy generally gives a better cosmetic result, but the technique is not always feasible.

Ductal carcinoma in situ (DCIS) may be found with or without invasive carcinoma. When it occurs with invasive carcinoma, clear surgical margins should be obtained, and an extensive intraductal component coexisting with invasive carcinoma is an indication for total mastectomy. Patients with DCIS alone should have breast surgery similar to that performed in patients with invasive cancer (i.e., total removal of the primary tumor with clear resected margins). If this goal is not possible, mastectomy should be performed. Axillary lymph node dissection is

not indicated in patients with DCIS without an invasive component. Breast irradiation after lumpectomy decreases the occurrence rate of second ipsilateral breast cancers, whether recurrent DCIS or invasive cancer (14).

Locally advanced breast cancer and inflammatory breast cancer (stages IIIA and IIIB) should be treated with combined modalities. After a tissue diagnosis has been established, patients should initially be treated with induction systemic chemotherapy (15). Subsequent treatment is aimed at local and regional control with a combination of radiation therapy and mastectomy. Adjuvant chemotherapy is given after local and regional control has been established (16).

Adjuvant Systemic Therapy   The rationale of adjuvant systemic therapy for breast cancer is that subclinical micrometastases occur in certain women long before the cancer is detected. There is excellent evidence that systemic adjuvant therapy alters the natural history of invasive breast cancer. Unfortunately, the magnitude of the overall treatment benefit is modest, despite statistical significance.

Several factors define the prognosis of patients who should, or should not, receive any form of adjuvant systemic therapy. The most important prognostic factor is the status of the axillary lymph nodes. Breast cancer metastases to axillary lymph nodes place women at high risk for the eventual development of clinically detectable metastases (Table 16.3). In the absence of any lymph node involvement, tumor size, hormone-receptor status, histologic grade, and patient age or menopausal status are the important prognostic factors (17, 18). Other prognostic factors are either controversial or still investigational in their ability to predict recurrence.

The Early Breast Cancer Trialists' Collaborative Group, an international group of experts, has performed the most comprehensive **meta-analysis** of the available randomized, adjuvant trials. In all,

133 trials involved more than 74,000 women. More than two-thirds of these women were node-positive, but 31% were node-negative (19).

The 10-year results of the meta-analysis are described in Table 16.5. Postoperative adjuvant combination **chemotherapy in premenopausal women with lymph node involvement** prolonged the disease-free interval and reduced the annual "odds of death" by approximately 25% in women with cancer that would otherwise recur. Use of combination chemotherapy in postmenopausal women with lymph node involvement remains controversial, but it is recommended in those who are younger or have estrogen receptor–negative tumors. Although the Early Breast Cancer Trialists' Group recommends tamoxifen as adjuvant systemic therapy in postmenopausal women with lymph node involvement and have estrogen receptor–rich tumors, re-

cent data suggest that many of these postmenopausal women will benefit from the addition of chemotherapy to tamoxifen. Table 16.6 lists the treatment recommendations for women with lymph node–positive breast cancer.

Adjuvant treatment for patients with lymph node–negative breast cancer varies substantially depending on the definition of their risk (Table 16.7). For patients considered to be at high risk, treatment is similar to that for patients with lymph node–positive disease. These high-risk patients with lymph node–negative cancer do not have a good prognosis, with 30 to 40% experiencing recurrence and death from metastatic breast cancer over a 10-year interval (20). Several studies have shown the efficacy of treating patients with **lymph node–negative, estrogen receptor–negative** breast cancer with adjuvant chemotherapy (21, 22). A significant benefit in overall disease-free sur-

Table 16.5. Ten-Year Results of Treatments Included in the Early Breast Cancer Trialists' Collaborative Group Meta-analysis

	Patients	Typical Reduction in Annual Odds (% ± SD)[a]	
		Recurrence or Prior Death	Death from Any Cause
Patients Younger Than 50 Years			
Tamoxifen	8,578	12 ± 4	6 ± 5
Tam alone vs. nil	2,216	27 ± 7	17 ± 10
Tam + Ctx vs. Ctx	6,362	7 ± 4	3 ± 5
Polychemotherapy	3,363	36 ± 5	25 ± 5
Ctx alone vs. nil	2,976	37 ± 5	27 ± 6
Ctx + Tam vs. Tam	386	32 ± 16	−6 ± 23
Ovarian ablation	1,817	26 ± 6	25 ± 7
Ablation vs. nil	878	30 ± 9	28 ± 9
Abl-x + Ctx vs. Ctx	939	21 ± 9	19 ± 11
Patients 50 Years and Older			
Tamoxifen	21,262	29 ± 2	20 ± 2
Tam alone vs. nil	13,114	30 ± 2	19 ± 3
Tam + Ctx vs. Ctx	8,148	28 ± 3	20 ± 4
Polychemotherapy	7,677	23 ± 33	12 ± 4
Ctx alone vs. nil	3,745	22 ± 4	14 ± 5
Ctx + Tam vs. Tam	3,932	26 ± 5	10 ± 7

Reprinted with permission from Early Breast Cancer Trialists' Collaborative Group. Systemic treatment of early breast cancer by hormonal, cytotoxic, or immune therapy. Lancet 1992;339:1–15.
Abl-x, ablation; *Ctx,* chemotherapy; *Tam,* tamoxifen.
[a]The annual odds of death is the probability of dying during a given year divided by the probability of surviving the year.

Table 16.6. Adjuvant Treatment for Patients with Lymph Node–Positive Cancer

Patient Group	Treatment[a]
Premenopausal	
Positive ER status	**Chemotx** ± Tamoxifen[b]
	Ovarian ablation ± Tamoxifen[b]
	GnRH[b]
	Chemotx ± ovarian abl-x + Tamoxifen[b]
Negative ER status	**Chemotx**
Postmenopausal	
Positive ER status	**Tamoxifen** ± Chemotx[b]
Negative ER status	**Chemotx** ± Tamoxifen[b]
Elderly	**Tamoxifen**; if ER negative then chemotx ± Tamoxifen[b]

Reprinted with permission from Goldhirsch A, Wood WC, Senn HJ, et al. Meeting highlights: international consensus panel on the treatment of primary breast cancer. J Natl Cancer Inst 1995;87:1441–1445.

abl-x, ablation; *ER,* estrogen receptor; *GnRH,* gonadotropin-releasing hormone analogue.

[a]**Bold entries are treatments accepted for routine use.**

[b]Treatments still being tested in randomized clinical trials.

vival was demonstrated at 8 years in the National Surgical Adjuvant Breast and Bowel Project (NSABP) B-13, in which 760 patients were randomized between systemic chemotherapy with methotrexate, 5-fluorouracil (5-FU), and leucovorin and no systemic therapy (74 vs. 59%, respectively), and a survival advantage was evident in woman 50 years and older (89 vs. 80%). NSABP B-19 randomized 1095 lymph node–negative patients to receive Cytoxan (cyclophosphamide), methotrexate, and 5-FU (CMF) or methotrexate, 5-FU, and leucovorin. A median follow-up of 5 years revealed a disease-free survival advantage (82 vs. 73%, respectively) and a borderline survival advantage (88 vs. 85%, respectively) to those who received

CMF. The survival benefit was greater in women 49 years and younger (89 vs. 84%).

Patients who are classified as "good risk" are treated with endocrine therapy, usually with tamoxifen. For those with minimal-risk or low-risk disease, the decision to treat with tamoxifen depends on a cost–benefit analysis and consideration of the potential reduction in the incidence of contralateral breast cancer. A randomized, double-blind, placebo-controlled trial of postoperative therapy with tamoxifen in 2644 patients with **lymph node–negative, estrogen receptor–positive** breast cancer revealed significant prolongation of disease-free survival among both premenopausal and postmenopausal women treated with tamoxifen. Use of tamoxifen reduced the recurrence rate at both local and distant sites, and it decreased the incidence of tumor recurrence after lumpectomy and breast irradiation. No survival advantage was observed, however, during a 4-year follow-up period (23). Table 16.8 summarizes the adjuvant treatment of women with lymph node–negative breast cancer (24).

Table 16.7. Definition of Risk Categories for Patients with Lymph Node–Negative Breast Cancer

Factor/risk	Minimal-low[a]	Good	High[b]
Tumor size (cm)	<1	1-2	>2
Estrogen-receptor status	+	+	−
Grade	1	1–2	2–3
Age (y)[c]	>35		

Reprinted with permission from Goldhirsch A, Wood WC, Senn HJ, et al. Meeting highlights: international consensus panel on the treatment of primary breast cancer. J Natl Cancer Inst 1995;87:1441–1445.

[a]Risk for patients with all listed factors.

[b]Risk for patients with at least one listed factor.

[c]Patients who develop breast cancer at a young age are considered to be at high risk of relapse, although an exact age threshold for this increased risk has not been defined.

Table 16.8.   Adjuvant Treatment for Patients with Lymph Node–Negative Breast Cancer[a]

Patient Group	Minimal-low	Good	High
Premenopausal			
Positive ER status	No tx vs. Tam[b]	**Tamoxifen** Oophor-x[b] Chemotx[b] GnRH[b]	**Chemotx** ± Tam[b] Oophor-x[b] GnRH[b]
Negative ER status	Not applicable	Not applicable	**Chemotx**
Postmenopausal			
Positive ER status	No tx vs. Tam[b]	**Tamoxifen**	**Tamoxifen** ± Chemotx[b]
Negative ER status	Not applicable	Not applicable	**Chemotx** ± Tam[b]
Elderly	No tx vs. Tam[b]	**Tamoxifen**	**Tamoxifen** Chemo ± tx[b]

Reprinted with permission from Goldhirsch A, Wood WC, Senn HJ, et al. Meeting highlights: international consensus panel on the treatment of primary breast cancer. J Natl Cancer Inst 1995;87:1441–1445.
Chemotx, chemotherapy; *ER*, estrogen receptor; *GnRH*, gonadotropin-releasing hormone; *Oophor-x*, oophorectomy; *Tam*, tamoxifen; *tx*, treatment.
[a]**Bold entries are treatments accepted for routine use.**
[b]Treatments still being tested in randomized clinical trials.

Despite encouraging improvements in the disease-free survival and overall survival of women with various subsets of breast cancer treated with adjuvant chemotherapy or hormonal therapy, the ideal therapy for these patients is yet to be achieved. Patients with newly diagnosed breast cancer should be encouraged to participate in ongoing clinical trials.

Colorectal Cancer

Colorectal cancer is the second most common cause of cancer-related death in the United States. Colon and rectal cancers should be staged using the TNM classification; however, several other staging systems are also commonly used, (e.g., the Duke's and modified Astler-Coller), which confounds analysis of the literature (see "Appendix"). Prognosis correlates closely to the stage and relates to the depth of tumor penetration into the bowel wall, presence and number of regional lymph node involvement, and distant metastases.

The same TNM staging system is used for both colon and rectal cancer; however, these cancers have a somewhat different natural history and treatment. The primary determinant of recurrence patterns in colorectal cancer is the location of the primary tumor in relation to the peritoneal reflection. Tumors at or below the peritoneal reflection (i.e., rectal cancer) are more likely to recur in the pelvis; tumors above the peritoneal reflection (i.e., colon cancer) have a higher incidence of failure within the abdominal cavity. Both colon and rectal cancer can spread systemically. The different patterns of recurrence explain the different recommendations for postoperative adjuvant treatment.

Staging Studies and Surgical Considerations Colorectal cancer is a malignancy that usually requires surgery regardless of its stage, and the detection of metastases need not preclude tumor resection in patients with tumor-related symptoms such as bleeding or obstruction. A thorough evaluation for metastatic disease should include a complete physical examination, chest radiography, liver chemistries, CT of the abdomen and pelvis, and plasma carcinoembryonic antigen (CEA) level. When possible, colonoscopy of the entire large bowel should be performed to identify synchronous neoplasms or polyps. Preoperative liver imaging by CT is useful in surgical planning and provides a baseline for subsequent comparison (25). This cancer rarely metastasizes to bone on presentation, so a routine bone scan is not indicated.

In patients with colorectal cancer and abnormal liver function tests, evaluation for liver metastases is important before surgery. CT or ultrasonography of the liver will show better delineation of liver metastases than radionuclide scans. If limited liver metastases are depicted, then surgical resection of these lesions should be considered. Patients with unresectable liver metastases could be candidates for an implantable Infusaid pump for continuous-infusion chemotherapy through the hepatic artery. It is important to identify these patients preoperatively, and arteriography in this period may be necessary to evaluate the vascular supply to the liver. Although whether treatment of liver metastases by the Infusaid pump prolongs life is controversial, there is good evidence that response rates in the liver are very high and that such treatment does change the natural history of colorectal carcinoma with metastases to the liver. If these patients are carefully selected, prolonged life and good palliation are possible (26).

Adjuvant Therapy Adjuvant systemic therapy for patients with **stage III (i.e., lymph node–positive) colon cancer** is now considered to be standard postoperative treatment. In a randomized study with a median follow-up of 6.5 years, Moertel et al. (27) divided 929 patients with surgically staged, lymph node–positive colon cancer in three groups. These groups included observation alone, treatment with levamisole (an antihelminth with im-

munomodulating properties), and treatment with levamisole plus 5-FU. Levamisole plus 5-FU reduced the recurrence rate by 40% ($P < 0001$) and the death rate by 33% ($P = .0007$). Treatment with levamisole alone did not have a statistically significant, beneficial effect on either the recurrence or the death rate. Levamisole plus 5-FU regimen produces toxicity, however, which, although usually mild and tolerable, can be troublesome.

Studies using 5-FU plus leucovorin for the adjuvant treatment of stage III colon cancer report results similar to those obtained with 5-FU and levamisole.

There is little evidence that patients with stage II (i.e., lymph node–negative) colon cancer benefit from adjuvant systemic therapy. However, depending on the prognostic characteristics of the individual cancer, the option should be discussed with the patient.

Adjuvant therapy of rectal cancer is directed at preventing both local and systemic recurrences. As mentioned, patients with rectal cancer who have undergone total surgical resection have a higher likelihood of developing pelvic recurrence compared to patients with colon cancer. Numerous trials have demonstrated significant reduction in the likelihood of pelvic recurrence after radiation therapy, but such treatment alone has not been demonstrated to prolong survival.

The superiority of postoperative therapy with combined chemotherapy and radiation has been confirmed in patients with **stage II (T3, N0, M0) and stage III (lymph node–positive) rectal cancer** (28). A randomized study of 240 patients with stages II and III rectal carcinoma compared radiation therapy alone to combined radiation and chemotherapy (5-FU and methyl-CCNU) (29). After a median follow-up of more than 7 years, the combined-modality therapy was statistically superior, having reduced the overall probability of recurrence by 34%, the local recurrence rate by 46%, the distant recurrence rate by 37%, and the mortality rate by 29%. However, methyl-CCNU is a leukemogen, and it is not commercially available. A subsequent study randomized 210 patients to receive radiation therapy and either 5-FU and methyl-CCNU or to receive 5-FU alone (30), and these results showed no difference in the survival or recurrence rates. The authors concluded that methyl-CCNU is not an essential component of effective postoperative combined-modality therapy for adjuvant rectal cancer.

Despite data showing the combination of 5-FU and radiation as effective therapy for rectal cancer, the optimal method of administering 5-FU is still under investigation. A coordinated effort of multiple cooperative groups evaluated 660 patients with stages II and III rectal cancer to determine whether the efficacy of chemotherapy with 5-FU can be improved with administration by protracted venous infusion throughout the duration of radiation therapy. Patients also received methyl-CCNU plus 5-FU or 5-FU alone both before and after irradiation. With a median follow-up of almost 4 years, patients who received 5-FU through protracted venous infusion had significantly increased time to relapse and improved survival. This study also confirmed previous data that patients who received methyl-CCNU plus 5-FU received no added benefit compared with those patients who received 5-FU alone (31).

Preoperative treatment of rectal cancer offers several potential advantages. First, preoperative treatment increases downstaging and resectability rates (32, 33). Second, preoperative therapy increases the likelihood that a sphincter-preserving procedure can be performed (34).

Many trials using preoperative radiation therapy have been performed in patients with clinically resectable rectal cancer. Both randomized and nonrandomized studies have shown that preoperative irradiation can decrease tumor volume and allow patients to successfully undergo a low-anterior resection with coloanal

anastomosis and sphincter preservation. However, even the randomized studies in this area have been criticized for their design.

Use of preoperative combined-modality therapy with radiation and chemotherapy (5-FU and leucovorin) has had encouraging preliminary results. Such therapy has been used to treat both resectable and unresectable rectal cancer, and it has been shown to convert unresectable to resectable rectal cancer. In a small study of patients with resectable rectal cancer (34), patients who received 5-FU with leucovorin and concurrent irradiation had a higher complete-response rate (20 vs. 6%) and a lower incidence of positive nodes (30 vs. 53%) compared with those patients who received radiation therapy alone. Well-designed trials evaluating preoperative combined-modality treatment of rectal cancer are currently in progress.

Nonsmall-cell Lung Cancer

Nonsmall-cell lung cancer (NSCLC) is the most frequent cause of cancer and the most common cause of cancer-related death. The three most common histologic types include adenocarcinoma, squamous or epidermoid carcinoma, and large-cell (or large-cell anaplastic) carcinoma. The internist is called on to evaluate patients with lung cancer in many situations, including to determine the stage, to evaluate the patient for resectability and operability, and to decide on appropriate palliative care.

Staging Evaluation The internist must understand the staging of NSCLC to determine the best therapeutic approach. In 1992, the **TNM classification for NSCLC** was changed to reflect important differences in prognosis and therapy (see "Appendix"). Stages I and II include localized tumors for which complete resection is the treatment of choice. Stage III includes patients with locally advanced disease and is divided into stages IIIA and IIIB based on extent of the primary tumor, extent of nodal involvement, and presence of pleural effusion. Stage IIIA NSCLC is a heterogeneous disease, and its therapy is varied (discussed later). Stage IV consists of patients with metastatic disease who are candidates for palliative treatment.

Patients with NSCLC must be critically staged both anatomically and physiologically, and the importance of a complete history and physical examination cannot be overstated. The history should focus on the patient's performance status and presence of weight loss. Both of these historical factors have important prognostic significance, because patients with low performance status and weight loss greater than 10% rarely respond to any specific therapy.

Computed tomography of the chest and abdomen is essential to determine the stage of cancer. Specifically, CT is important to evaluate the mediastinal lymph nodes and tumor extension into the pleural surfaces, diaphragm, chest wall, and vessels, and to detect occult abdominal disease, with the liver and adrenal glands being common sites for metastases (35). Bone and brain metastases are relatively common in patients with NSCLC. Such metastases are usually symptomatic, however, and routine radionuclide bone scans and brain CT scans are not necessarily indicated in patients who are asymptomatic and who are clinical stage I or II. If a bone scan is performed, plain radiography of any suspicious bony metastases should also be performed.

Whether all patients with NSCLC who are considered to be curable by surgery should have preoperative histologic evaluation of their mediastinal lymph nodes is controversial. Important therapeutic decisions are based on size of the mediastinal lymph nodes on CT scans. These lymph nodes are considered to be abnormal when they are larger than 1.5 cm and normal when smaller than 1 cm; nodes between these limits are considered to be indeterminate. The problem is that a small percentage of mediastinal lymph nodes smaller than 1 cm on CT scans harbor metastases and a small percentage larger

than 1.5 cm are not involved with metastases. Therefore, patients being considered for curative surgery should undergo mediastinoscopy for right-sided tumors and lateral mediastinotomy for left-sided tumors. Some surgeons proceed directly to thoracotomy after a "negative" mediastinoscopy, whereas others perform thoracotomy at a latter time.

The **physiologic staging** of patients with NSCLC is imperative, because many have significant cardiopulmonary disease and it is necessary to determine their ability to withstand surgery as well as to predict their postresection pulmonary function. Pulmonary function tests should be performed, and a forced expiratory volume at 1 second (FEV_1) of greater than 2 L and the absence of an elevated arterial carbon dioxide tension ($Paco_2$) indicate the patient will most likely tolerate pneumonectomy. Patients with an FEV_1 of between 2 and 1 L require additional evaluation and judgment. These patients require split pulmonary function tests by radionuclide ventilation–perfusion lung scanning. Using this technique, it is possible to predict the postresection pulmonary function, and a predicted FEV_1 of greater than 800 to 1000 mL is most likely adequate to proceed with surgery and afford the patient a decent quality of life after the resection. Major contraindications to surgery include uncontrolled major arrhythmias, maximum breathing capacity less than 40% of that predicted, an FEV_1 of less than 1 L, carbon dioxide retention, and severe pulmonary hypertension.

Before surgery, the consulting internist should attempt to maximally improve pulmonary function with medical therapy. Use of inhaled β-agonists, a short course of steroids, and smoking cessation may prevent postoperative pulmonary complications.

Therapy for Localized Nonsmall-cell Lung Cancer Resection is the most effective treatment for stages I and II NSCLC. Five-year survival is unaffected by traditional adjuvant treatment, including radiation therapy, chemotherapy, or a combination of both. Five-year survival for stage II NSCLC is approximately 50%. Radiation therapy can decrease the local recurrence rate, but it has no effect on survival. Newer chemotherapeutic regimens have yet to be tested in patients with stage II NSCLC and a high risk of systemic recurrence.

Stage III NSCLC is a heterogeneous group, and treatment remains under investigation. However, there is good evidence that a combined-modality approach can prolong life in selected patients heretofore destined to have a poor outcome (36). As mentioned, stage III NSCLC is now divided into stage IIIA and stage IIIB. Stage IIIA includes a particularly heterogeneous group of patients (see "Appendix"); T3, N0 or N1 disease includes tumors that directly invade the chest wall or diaphragm either without lymph node involvement or with ipsilateral hilar node involvement. (Superior sulcus tumors are included in this group.) Such situations are surgically resectable, and patients may achieve 5-year survival rates of 30 to 50%. However, patients with N2 disease (ipsilateral mediastinal lymph node involvement) have a poor 5-year survival rate of approximately 15% for those who are treated surgically. It is the group of good-performance patients with stage IIIA and N2 status that benefit the most from a combined-modality approach with neoadjuvant chemotherapy with either radiation therapy alone, surgery alone, or the combination or radiation therapy and surgery.

Results from numerous studies (37–42) have shown that induction chemotherapy with or without concurrent irradiation followed by surgery is feasible, and pathologic complete responses have been documented in up to 20% of patients treated in this manner. Improvements in both median survival and 2-year and 3-year survival rates have also been confirmed. Selected patients with "minimal" stage IIIB cancer have been treated with this neoadjuvant approach as well; results have been similar to those in stage IIIA patients. Patients with stage IIIA or IIIB NSCLC and good performance status should be offered treatment with induction chemotherapy. Such newer regimens have been effective in a fair percentage of patients, whereas radiation therapy has been of little value in improving the poor survival in these groups of patients. When feasible, patients with stage IIIA or IIIB cancer should enter into well-designed clinical trials.

Most patients with stage IIIB, N3 or T4 are considered to be inoperable. These patients are treated with palliative intent (see the previous discussion of "minimal" stage IIIB cancer).

Small-cell Carcinoma of the Lung

Small-cell carcinoma of the lung is considered to be incurable surgically. It is a systemic disease, and initial chemotherapy is indicated. Initial response rates are high, but long-term survival beyond 2 years is very uncommon. Rarely, small-cell carcinoma of the lung may present as a solitary pulmonary nodule, in which case surgery is usually performed to remove the cancer.

Prostate Cancer

During the past decade, the incidence of prostate cancer has increased by over 300%, and it is now the most commonly diagnosed cancer in men. The frequent practice of ordering a prostate-specific antigen (PSA) to detect such cancer in an earlier stage is the major reason for this increased incidence. In addition, prostate cancer, which has always been considered to be a cancer of older men, is being diagnosed more often today in men between 55 and 65 years of age. Furthermore, before 1989, most cases were either locally advanced or metastatic at diagnosis; in 1995, the exact opposite became true, in that most cases were locally confined at diagnosis. For these reasons, the internist is becoming more involved in the care of these patients and needs to understand the rationale for staging, natural history, therapeutic options, and long-term complications of treatment.

Staging Considerations and Selection of Patients for Specific Therapy The selection of patients with prostate cancer for specific treatments depends on the extent of tumor at diagnosis, the patient's age, and any other medical illnesses. The histologic grade of the cancer and PSA levels affect the prognosis and are also important factors in making therapeutic decisions.

When the cancer is confined to the prostate gland, the disease is considered to be curable and usually treated by radical prostatectomy or radiation therapy. Surgery is considered to be a better therapeutic option in patients who are younger than 70 years old, free of significant medical problems, and predicted to have longevity. Patients with locally advanced cancer are considered to be incurable, and standard treatment is radiation or, if asymptomatic, watchful waiting. However, preliminary results of a randomized clinical trial have shown that immediate hormonal therapy with goserilin (Zoladex), a luteinizing hormone–releasing hormone analogue, started on the first day of radiation therapy and continued for 3 years improves local control, reduces the incidence of metastases, and prolongs survival compared with patients who receive radiation therapy alone (43). If the cancer is metastatic to distant organs, current therapies will not cure it, and treatment should be aimed at palliation. Therefore, it is critical in patients with documented prostate cancer to determine if the cancer is localized and to decide on the optimal treatment.

Detection of asymptomatic metastatic disease in prostate cancer is facilitated by the results of staging studies in conjunction with the pathologic grade of the tumor. The radionuclide bone scan is used to determine metastases to bone, which is the most common site of distant tumor spread. There is evidence that the PSA level can, with a detailed patient history, reliably predict the results of radionuclide bone scans in newly diagnosed patients. In one study of 852 patients (44), only 2 (0.23%), who had a PSA level of less than 20 μg/L, in the absence of bone pain had a truly positive bone scan.

The degree of differentiation of the cancer is an important predictor for capsular penetration, seminal vesicle invasion, or regional lymph node metastases. There is marked variability in tumor differentiation from one microscopic field to another in biopsy specimens of prostate cancer. Many pathologists will report the range of differentiation in a specimen, using a score from well differentiated (score, 1 or 2) to poorly differentiated (score, 4 or 5); **the sum of the total score from the most well-differentiated to the most poorly differentiated area is called the Gleason score.** This score correlates directly with the prognosis, and it should be considered when making any therapeutic decision. If the prostate cancer is considered to be localized, the Gleason score is favorable, and the patient is considered to be a good surgical candidate (i.e., good health and, ideally, younger than 70 years of age), then radical prostatectomy is considered to be the optimal therapy.

Prostatectomy can be performed by either the retropubic or the perineal approach. The retropubic approach is most often used. Before the procedure, pelvic lymph node dissection should be performed to stage the cancer, and this can be accomplished either by an open surgical technique or by laparoscopy. Pelvic lymph node dissection is not therapeutic, and it spares patients with involved pelvic nodes the morbidity of prostatectomy, because if metastases are present, the patient is considered to be incurable and the surgical procedure terminated.

Surgical Complications It is important for the internist to have a detailed understanding of the **morbid events associated with total prostatectomy.** Despite the significant recent decline in perioperative morbidity from radical prostatectomy, this surgery is associated with important quality-of-life issues and, as with any operation, a rare death. Varying percentages for morbid events following radical prostatectomy have been reported in the literature, and the results of these studies are difficult to compare. Differences in their outcomes depend on at least some of the following factors: *(a)* national studies versus case series, *(b)* varying surgical expertise among reporting centers, *(c)* selection factors (especially age), *(d)* publication bias of favorable series, and *(e)* different methods of collecting information from patients.

One study performed at a reputable institution evaluated the morbidity of 1000 consecutive patients with clinically localized prostate cancer treated with bilateral pelvic lymph node dissection and radical prostatectomy between 1989 and 1992 (45). The assessment of their surgical complications are shown in Table 16.9, and it is important to understand that their results are as good as any reported. A national review of 10,600 radical prostatectomies determined that 30-day mortality and cardiovascular morbidity rates were 2 and 8%, respectively. The most common complication, vesical neck contracture, has been reported to occur in up to 22% of patients treated with radical prostatectomy.

The continence status of these 1000 patients was assessed 1 year after radical prostatectomy. Results of their functional assessment were:

1. Dry (i.e., no pads), 79%.
2. Rare incontinent episodes (i.e., one pad or less per day), 16%.
3. Stress incontinence (i.e., more than one pad per day), 4%.
4. Totally incontinent, 0.8%.
5. Incontinent preoperatively, 0.4%.
6. Required artificial genitourinary sphincter, 0.6%.

The literature indicates that urinary incontinence is a quality-of-life issue in

Table 16.9. Morbidity Assessment of Contemporary Radical Retropubic Prostatectomy in 1000 Consecutive Patients

Complication	Morbidity (n [%])
Intraoperative	
Hospital mortality	0
Mean blood loss (mL)	844
Hospital transfusion requirement	217 (22)
Rectal injury	6 (0.6)
Early	
Myocardial infarction	7 (0.7)
Pulmonary embolism	6 (0.6)
Deep-vein thrombophlebitis	8 (0.8)
Sepsis	2 (0.5)
Wound infection	9 (0.9)
Late / Post-discharge events	
Vesical neck contracture	87 (8.7)
Pulmonary embolism	1 (0.1)
Deep-vein thrombosis	5 (0.5)
Pelvic abscess	1 (0.1)
Pelvic lymphocele	1 (0.1)

Reprinted with permission from Lerner SE, Blute ML, Lieber MM, et al. Morbidity of contemporary radical retropubic prostatectomy for localized prostate cancer. Oncology 1995;9(5):379–386.

approximately 5 to 10% of patients undergoing radical prostatectomy. Erectile dysfunction is another complication of retropubic prostatectomy and an important quality-of-life issue for many men. Several factors correlate with the likelihood of erectile dysfunction, including the patient's age, whether neurovascular bundles were preserved at surgery, and preoperative potency. Preservation of potency with the nerve-sparing technique of radical prostatectomy depends on tumor stage and patient age, but the operation appears to induce at least a partial defect in nearly all patients (46).

Esophageal Cancer

Esophageal cancer is relatively uncommon and has a poor prognosis. The 5-year survival rate is approximately 5%, and the internist may be involved in selecting which patients are operable and in the palliative care of inoperable and terminal patients with complicated morbid problems. Although squamous cell carcinoma was previously the most common histologic type by far, adenocarcinoma now accounts for between 30 and 50% of all newly diagnosed esophageal cancers. Adenocarcinoma of the esophagus occurs in the distal esophagus and in areas affected by Barrett's syndrome, a premalignant condition that is associated with chronic reflux esophagitis.

Staging esophageal cancer is critical in determining the limited group of patients for whom surgical cure is possible. Radiography of the esophagus and endoscopy have usually been performed before tissue diagnosis is made. CT of the chest and abdomen is necessary for preoperative staging, and CT has a sensitivity and specificity of approximately 90% in depicting mediastinal invasion. Several reports have stated that endoscopic ultrasonography is superior to CT in staging patients with stages I and II esophageal cancer (tumor limited to the esophagus). The transducer, however, cannot be passed through many tumors, thus limiting the ability of endoscopic ultrasonography to completely stage the patient. The use of endoscopic ultrasonography in staging patients with esophageal cancer requires greater experience.

The therapeutic options for localized esophageal cancer are currently under investigation. If careful imaging studies show that cancer is limited to the esophagus, surgical resection is considered to be the standard treatment. However, because fewer than 20% of patients who undergo esophagectomy remain alive at 5 years, alternative treatments should be considered. Several studies have evaluated concurrent therapy with chemotherapy (5-FU and cisplatin) and radiation therapy as the primary treatment for patients with localized esophageal cancer. Although follow-up has been limited thus far, the available data from these studies suggest that combined therapy results in better local control, fewer distant metastases, and improved overall survival compared with radiation therapy alone (47). A randomized, controlled study also compared multimodality therapy consisting of concurrent chemotherapy (5-FU and cisplatin) and radiation therapy followed by surgical resection to surgery alone in patients with esophageal adenocarcinoma (48). Patients who received multimodality therapy had a 3-year survival rate of 32%, compared with 6% in the patients who had surgery alone; this survival advantage was statistically significant. Twenty-five percent of patients who underwent surgery after multimodality therapy also had a complete response determined pathologically.

Patients with incurable esophageal cancer can have a miserable existence, and **palliative care to improve the quality of life** is an important part of their management. **Dysphagia, malnutrition, and tracheoesophageal fistulas** are common issues. **Palliation of dysphagia** that occurs after primary therapy can be managed in several ways (49):

1. Simple dilatation can temporarily relieve obstruction, but repeated dilatations are necessary.
2. Endoscopic laser fulguration of an obstructing tumor can be effective but requires appropriate equipment and expertise.
3. A self-expanding stent can be placed endoscopically in almost all patients, alleviating dysphagia in most and preventing tumor ingrowth.

The **surgical placement of a gastrostomy or jejunostomy** for feeding and hydration is another important palliative approach to patients with esophageal cancer who cannot eat or drink because of obstruction or treatment-related mucositis. A **tracheoesophageal fistula** can be difficult to palliate; surgical correction is usually neither possible nor indicated. Intubation of the esophagus with a plastic prosthesis can occlude the fistula, restore the natural lumens, and prevent aspiration pneumonia. These prostheses can migrate, however, and tumor can grow either over or under the stent.

Bladder Cancer

The internist may be called on to render an opinion regarding therapeutic options in patients with bladder cancer, which should be thought of as either superficial, invasive, or metastatic. Superficial bladder cancer is treated by the urologist with local therapy, including transurethral endoscopic resection with or without intravesical immunotherapy (bacille Calmette-Guérin [BCG] vaccine) or intravesical chemotherapy. Patients with metastatic bladder cancer are treated by the medical oncologist with palliative intent. However, patients with transitional-cell bladder cancer that invades muscle or perivesical fat can have important therapeutic options. The classic standard therapy is considered to be radical cystectomy. Preoperative radiation therapy followed by cystectomy has been widely employed, but the only prospective, randomized trial reported to date failed to show any survival advantage for this approach compared with radical cystectomy alone. This therapy also gives inadequate results, with a 5-year survival rate of approximately 50%, and most patients with invasive bladder cancer experience recurrence with systemic disease. Several studies have evaluated the administration of chemotherapy before cystectomy or in conjunction with radiation therapy; the rationale for this combined therapy being to improve local tumor control, prevent distant metastases, and allow for bladder preservation (50–52). One particular chemotherapeutic regimen, M-VAC (methotrexate, vinblastine, Adriamycin, cisplatin), produced a complete pathologic response in approximately 20% of patients treated before radical cystectomy (51). Another combined-modality approach used the MCV regimen (methotrexate,

cisplatin, and vinblastine) followed by concurrent radiotherapy and cisplatin, and this **combined-modality therapy resulted in bladder preservation in most patients with invasive bladder cancer.** The overall survival rate was similar to that reported with aggressive surgical approaches (52). Long-term survival and quality-of-life assessments, however, require longer follow-up periods, and these encouraging reports require additional confirmatory trials.

Pancreatic Cancer

Pancreatic adenocarcinoma accounts for only 2 to 3% of all cancers, but it is the fifth-leading cause of cancer-related death in the United States. The reason for its poor prognosis is that symptoms are often nonspecific, so disease is often far advanced before a diagnosis is established. Approximately two-thirds of pancreatic cancers arise in the head area. Many of these patients will present with obstructive jaundice, which can represent an early sign of the disease, and it is this subset of patients in which the most progress has been made and about which the internist should have knowledge of the diagnostic and therapeutic options. This section only discusses treatment of adenocarcinoma of the head of the pancreas, because carcinoma of the body and tail are usually nonresectable and far advanced.

Diagnosis and Staging (Considerations for Resectability) Several diagnostic studies can be performed when a patient presents with obstructive jaundice and is suspected of having a periampullary carcinoma. CT of the abdomen, ultrasonography of the biliary tract, endoscopic retrograde cholangiopancreatography (ERCP), or percutaneous cholangiography are all appropriate diagnostic procedures. The goal, however, is to obtain the most information with the fewest tests performed. CT of the abdomen should be the initial diagnostic study, because it gives the most information concerning cause of the obstructive jaundice and extent of the tumor (i.e., stage). If the CT scan depicts a tumor that is potentially resectable, further staging with visceral angiography is indicated. Visceral angiography is an important study in patients with pancreatic cancer. If the study is normal, it demonstrates that the tumor is likely to be resectable. Encasement of the celiac axis or superior mesenteric artery significantly decreases, but does not completely exclude, the chances of resection, but if major vessel occlusion is present, the patient should be palliated nonoperatively and not be explored as these tumors are unresectable. The exception is the patient who is operated on with palliative intent to relieve or prevent duodenal or biliary tract obstruction (see section on treatment of biliary tract obstruction).

Preoperative percutaneous biopsy of the tumor should be reserved for patients who are not operative candidates. A definitive tissue diagnosis can be made at the time of laparotomy.

Treatment Pancreaticoduodenectomy or Whipple operation is the only potentially curative treatment for a patient with carcinoma of the head of the pancreas. The major centers with experience in performing this procedure report a low mortality rate (<2%). This operation can be performed safely in virtually any age group (including many patients older than 80 years) as long as reasonable preoperative screening is done. However, postoperative morbidity can be substantial. The most common postoperative complication is delayed gastric emptying, and one author with extensive experience in pancreaticoduodenectomy has reported that approximately one-third of all patients undergoing this procedure will experience vomiting that keeps the patient hospitalized for 2 to 3 weeks after surgery (53). The vomiting results from delayed gastric emptying or gastric atony. Motilin, a gastrointestinal hormone that is produced primarily in the duodenum, stimulates gastric peristalsis. Since the duodenum is removed during a pancreaticoduodenec-

tomy, the loss of motilin is believed to cause the gastric atony. Administration of parenteral erythromycin, an antibiotic that is a motilin agonist, can improve gastric emptying and alleviate vomiting; however, upper endoscopy may be required to ensure the anastomosis is patent. The second most common complication following pancreaticoduodenectomy is postoperative pancreatic cutaneous fistula, which occurs in 10 to 20% of patients. This complication used to be responsible for most of the deaths following the Whipple operation. However, now that pancreatic anastomoses can be well drained with closed-suction drains, most fistulas close spontaneously, although extended hospitalization may be required.

A patient with pancreatic cancer at a stage allowing for pancreaticoduodenectomy has a finite chance for long-term survival. Twenty years ago, patients rarely survived 5 years following pancreaticoduodenectomy for carcinoma of the head of the pancreas. A study of 195 patients from a single institution undergoing pancreaticoduodenectomy for such carcinoma reported an actuarial 5-year survival rate of 26% (53). Although selection bias influences these results, prolonged survival following pancreaticoduodenectomy for this carcinoma is now possible. The important prognostic indicators for long-term survival included tumor size, blood vessel invasion seen microscopically, and lymph node status. Among patients who were lymph node negative at the time of surgery, 5-year survival was greater than 40%; among patients who were lymph node positive, 5-year survival fell to 8%.

After successful pancreaticoduodenectomy for carcinoma of the head of the pancreas, patients should receive adjuvant therapy with postoperative radiotherapy and 5-FU. In a prospective, randomized study performed by the Gastrointestinal Study Group, those patients receiving no adjuvant therapy following pancreaticoduodenectomy had a median survival of 11 months;

median survival doubled with the addition of postoperative radiotherapy and 5-FU (54).

Despite careful preoperative screening, too many patients are found to be unresectable at the time of laparotomy. Surgical palliation can be performed safely and effectively, however. A prophylactic gastrojejunostomy usually will eliminate gastric outlet obstruction from duodenal involvement with tumor, and hepaticojejunstomy can effectively eliminate subsequent jaundice.

Head and Neck Cancer

Cancers of the head and neck are uncommon malignancies involving the upper aerodigestive tract, paranasal sinuses, and salivary glands. Approximately 90% of all head and neck cancers are squamous cell carcinomas, but in the salivary glands, cancers are usually adenocarcinomas.

Head and neck malignancies are usually the domain of surgical subspecialists; however, the internist should understand some important principles of the diagnosis and treatment of early head and neck cancer. Signs and symptoms of a primary head and neck neoplasm can be obvious, but they may prove to be very illusive. Not infrequently, the initial presentation is a mass in the neck. If so, and if a primary lesion cannot be visualized, CT imaging should be performed along with a nasolaryngoscopic examination under general anesthesia. **Incisional or excisional biopsy of such a mass should not be performed initially. Fine-needle aspiration of the neck mass should be performed if a primary lesion cannot be detected. If a diagnosis still cannot be established at this point, then— and only then—should incisional or excisional biopsy of the neck mass be performed.** If open biopsy is initially performed, the neck is violated, and there is the potential for spread of the cancer.

The choice of treatment should depend on histology, size and location of the primary tumor, and status of the cervical lymph nodes. In early stage disease, surgery is often the preferred treatment, but radiation therapy can be equally effective (55). In more advanced-stage cancers, however, combined-modality therapy is superior to single-modality treatment. The role of neoadjuvant chemotherapy in advanced-stage head and neck cancer remains investigational, but a **meta-analysis of randomized, controlled studies indicates that chemotherapy (cisplatin alone or combined with 5-FU) given synchronously with radiation therapy confers a modest survival advantage** (56). The role of surgery following combined-modality therapy has yet to be clearly defined; decisions regarding surgery must be individualized for each patient. The combination of chemotherapy and radiation therapy is particularly important when organ preservation is feasible, and such therapy preserves the larynx in some patients with advanced laryngeal cancer.

Anal Carcinoma

Anal carcinoma is an uncommon malignancy that was previously treated with surgery, often requiring an anteroposterior resection and colostomy. Even with surgery, however, systemic recurrences and death were still common. At present, initial chemotherapy with mitomycin and 5-FU, given by a continuous, 4-day infusion and simultaneously with radiation therapy, has essentially eliminated the need for surgery. Cure rates today are high (57).

"Second Look" Surgery

"Second look" surgery to evaluate the effectiveness of chemotherapy and remove local recurrent cancer for potential cure is only valuable in a few, selected patients. These include patients with ovarian carcinoma and with colorectal carcinoma.

Patient reponses to chemotherapy of advanced **ovarian carcinoma** are impressive. Unfortunately, cure is uncommon, and these patients often have residual carcinoma at second look surgery. Preoperative CT evaluation has limited value, because CT usually does not visualize small residual ovarian carcinoma (58). The tumor marker CA-125 is useful in determining the efficacy of therapy and the development of progressive disease, but its sensitivity is low in patients with small-volume tumors. Extensive surgical debulking of residual carcinoma with bowel resection, if necessary, can prolong life and palliate symptoms; however, overall survival rates are not influenced (59).

Second look surgery in patients with **colorectal carcinoma** can be palliative and, rarely, even curative. An **increasing CEA level** on follow-up often indicates the need to evaluate for recurrence. Second look surgery in this situation, even when residual carcinoma is not found by noninvasive studies, is indicated in good-risk patients. Resection of a local recurrence or of liver metastases can prolong life and, potentially, be curative (60–62).

Resection of a Single or Few Metastases

An isolated metastasis, or several metastases, in an important organ should be considered for surgical resection. Depending on the solid-tumor histology, number of metastases, and the disease-free interval, prolonged survival and even cure can be anticipated. Metastases from certain solid tumors should receive higher consideration for surgical resection, and these are discussed here by the organ of metastases.

Pulmonary Metastases The lung is a common site of metastases for many cancers, including osteogenic and soft-tissue sarcomas, melanoma, nonseminomatous germ-cell tumors of the testes, as well as head and neck, colorectal, renal, endometrial, cervical, and breast carcinomas. Although lung metastases usually represent only one site of extensive spread, there are important exceptions.

Osteogenic and soft-tissue sarcomas frequently metastasize to the lungs, and these pulmonary metastases are often exclusive from other sites (i.e., metastasizing only to the lungs). In these patients, surgical resection prolongs survival and may even be curative (63).

Patient selection is important, and patients should meet the following criteria:

1. The primary site must be controlled.
2. The patient must be a good surgical candidate.
3. No extrapulmonary metastases may be present.
4. The tumor doubling time should be calculated as longer than 20 days.
5. The disease-free interval should be longer than 12 months.
6. Less than five nodules should be depicted on preoperative chest CT scans.
7. Adequate lung functioning should remain after potential resection.

A median sternotomy approach is recommended so that both lungs can be explored.

A pulmonary nodule occurring in a patient with a previous diagnosis of head and neck cancer represent an important situation, because these patients have a second primary lung cancer at least as often as metastases from their primary head and neck cancer. Since preoperative radiologic differentiation of metastases versus a primary lung cancer is inaccurate, surgery should be considered. Patients who are good surgical candidates, show no evidence of distant metastases or mediastinal involvement, and have had disease-free interval of at least 1 year, should undergo thoracotomy (64).

Pulmonary metastases from all other primary cancer sites are less well studied. Individual judgment is necessary.

Liver Metastases It is unknown whether resection of a solitary or a few liver metastases has any palliative or curative benefit. However, if liver resection is contemplated, it should be considered a curative, not a palliative, procedure.

Only two groups of adult patients should be considered for resection of their liver metastases. The first includes highly selected patients with primary colon and rectal cancers and localized liver metastases as their only manifestation of recurrent or persistent disease. The second, and even more unusual, group includes those patients with endocrine tumors (e.g., carcinoid or islet-cell tumors) and who have disabling symptoms from liver metastases. These malignancies are usually slow-growing, and surgical resection may benefit these patients if widespread metastases are not evident.

Liver resection for patients with metastases from other common sites, such as the pancreas, stomach, lung, breast, and melanoma, is not justified.

Brain Metastases Use of combination chemotherapy to control systemic cancer has led to an increased incidence of brain metastases, because most chemotherapeutic agents cannot cross the blood–brain barrier. Brain metastases may be the only site of recurring cancer. Lung and breast are the most common primary malignancies to metastasize to the brain, but melanoma, renal cell, and those of unknown histologies occur with important frequency.

Dexamethasone, 10 mg intravenously and followed by 4 mg every 6 hours orally or intravenously, should be the initial treatment of patients with brain metastases and neurologic deficit. This therapy usually results in dramatic and rapid improvement of the neurologic deficit if cerebral edema is present. Anticonvulsant therapy should be given to patients with seizures and to patients who undergo surgical resection of a metastasis. Use of prophylactic anticonvulsant therapy should be considered in patients with multiple brain metastases.

Most brain metastases are treated with radiation therapy. However, some patients benefit from resection followed by radiation therapy (65). These patients have the following characteristics:

1. They are ambulatory.
2. The brain metastasis is solitary (or, rarely, a few) and is localized to the cerebrum, especially in an area in which resection will not cause significant neurologic deficit.
3. The primary site of cancer is controlled.
4. There is no evidence of metastatic disease outside the brain.

Whole-brain irradiation should be performed after the surgical resection. Stereotactic radiosurgery is a newer technology that is relatively safe and reasonably effective in small intracranial metastases, and it may be preferable to surgery in appropriately selected patients (66).

Treatment of Complications Caused by Metastases

There are special considerations in the treatment of the complications caused by metastases, and these require that the consulting internist and surgeon to work closely together.

Superior Vena Cava Syndrome Superior vena cava (SVC) syndrome may be acute, but it is more often a subacute syndrome usually resulting from a malignant tumor. The most common causes include lymphomas, Hodgkin's disease, and bronchogenic carcinomas (both small-cell and nonsmall-cell types). Less common causes include thymic, testicular, and other metastatic tumors.

Treatment and prognosis are very different among these malignancies. A **definitive histologic diagnosis should be established before therapy** begins.

The previous idea that the SVC syndrome was an acute emergency and invasive diagnostic procedures were dangerous has been proven to be wrong. On the contrary, SVC syndrome usually presents with subacute symptoms, and invasive diagnostic procedures (i.e., mediastinoscopy, bronchoscopy or even thoracotomy) can be safely performed (67). A patient who presents with life-threatening symptoms in whom a tissue diagnosis should be deferred before therapy is unusual.

Chemotherapy is the initial treatment for SVC syndrome caused by small-cell lung carcinoma and diffuse large-cell lymphoma, and it is highly effective in alleviating symptoms rapidly. Radiation therapy is the initial therapy for NSCLC. Chemotherapy, radiation therapy, or both may be the initial therapy for Hodgkin's disease, depending on the clinical circumstances.

Malignant Pleural Effusion Many different malignancies can cause a pleural effusion, and treatment of malignant effusions will vary according to the specific cancer involved. Pleural effusions from lymphomas, germ-cell cancer, small-cell lung cancer, and breast cancer usually respond to systemic chemotherapy or, in the case of breast cancer, hormonal therapy. However, many common malignancies that cause pleural effusions, such as colon, pancreatic, and NSCLC, do not respond to systemic therapy (68).

It should be remembered that not all effusions in patients with cancer are malignant. Other causes, particularly congestive heart failure and infection, should be considered. A diagnostic thoracentesis should be performed early in the investigation; following thoracentesis for malignant effusion, there is usually a rapid reaccumulation of fluid.

A malignant pleural effusion requires treatment when the patient has respiratory symptoms. The therapeutic options available include:

1. Tube thoracostomy combined with sclerosis produced by intrapleural bleomycin or doxycycline (tetracycline is no longer available in this preparation).
2. Video-assisted thoracoscopy (VAT) with insufflation of talc into the pleural space.
3. Pleural stripping (in a rare, selected patient).

4. Pleuroperitoneal shunt placement (shunts frequently become occluded).

Tube thoracostomy or VAT with pleurodesis are the most common and pragmatic options. The effectiveness of these procedures depends entirely on the underlying lung to expand. If a bronchus is occluded by intrinsic or extrinsic tumor or the effusion is loculated, these procedures will not control the patient's symptoms.

The literature reports that tube thoracostomy with pleurodesis will control 50 to 70% of malignant pleural effusions; VAT with pleurodesis performed under general anesthesia will control approximately 90% of effusions (69). These success rates are possible only provided that the underlying lung can be reexpanded. In addition, the VAT procedure is limited to those physicians with the appropriate expertise and available technology.

Tube thoracostomy combined with sclerosis is performed by placing a large-bore chest tube into the pleural cavity with closed-tube suction drainage followed by instillation of a sclerosing agent into the pleural cavity. A successful outcome is more likely if thoracostomy drainage is continued for at least 48 to 72 hours, or until complete drainage has been achieved. Complete drainage may not be possible, however. Drainage limited to between 50 and 100 mL/day may have to be acceptable. Many sclerosing agents have been used, but the obliteration of the pleural space, not the particular agent used, determines the effectiveness of therapy. Doxycycline and bleomycin are the most commonly used agents. The liquid preparation of tetracycline is no longer available, but similar efficacy has been shown for doxycycline (69). A randomized trial comparing bleomycin and tetracycline has shown a slight superiority of bleomycin in preventing recurrence, but the cost of this agent compared with doxycycline is prohibitive (70). The dose of doxycycline is 500 mg in 50 mL of volume, and the dose of bleomycin is 60 U. Routine use of 2% lidocaine, 10 mL injected into the pleural cavity 15 minutes before sclerosis, will often eliminate associated pleuritic pain. To ensure patient comfort, parenteral administration of a narcotic 1 hour before instillation of the sclerosing therapy is recommended. Following instillation, the chest tube is clamped for 4 to 6 hours, and the patient instructed to change positions frequently to distribute the sclerosing agent throughout the pleural cavity. The tube can then be unclamped and reattached to drainage. If no significant drainage occurs during the subsequent 12 to 24 hours, the tube can be removed.

Neoplastic Pericardial Effusion Pericardial involvement in patients with cancer can occur either from contiguous extension by an adjacent cancer in the lung or mediastinum or from metastases of a distant primary cancer. Lung cancer, breast cancer, leukemia, and both Hodgkin's and non-Hodgkin's lymphoma account for more than three-fourths of cases involving the pericardium. Radiation-induced pericardial injury may manifest as acute pericarditis, either during the treatment itself or weeks to months after its completion, or as chronic pericarditis, occurring several months to many years after treatment. The importance of differentiating (and treating) radiation-induced pericarditis from progressive malignant disease with pericardial metastases in a patient who may be cured of their cancer is obvious (71).

Echocardiography is the easiest and most sensitive method to detect a pericardial effusion, and it may detect impending cardiac tamponade as well. Total electrical alternans on electrocardiography, involving both the atrial and ventricular complexes, is virtually pathognomonic of cardiac tamponade. Approximately three-fourths of documented malignant pericardial effusions will have a positive cytology. Therefore, negative cytology may not differentiate cancer from radiation as the cause of pericardial effusion, and there are no other characteristics of the effusion that will help in differentiation.

Treatment of pericardial effusion depends on the clinical setting. Cardiac tamponade is an emergency situation, and pericardiocentesis should be performed immediately, preferably under electrocardiographic monitoring. The effusion usually recurs within 1 to 2 days after the initial pericardiocentesis. Therefore, additional therapy will be required, and planning should be based on the cause of the effusion, the type of the effusion (i.e., effusive or constrictive), and the patient's medical condition and long-term prognosis.

If therapy is aimed at short-term palliation because of extensive metastatic disease, a transcutaneous catheter can be placed into the pericardial space to drain the effusion. Tetracycline, 500 mg in 20 mL of normal saline solution, can be subsequently instilled through the catheter to sclerose the pericardial surfaces and obliterate the pericardial space (72). This method is efficacious in preventing recurrent pericardial tamponade, and additional radiation therapy or chemotherapy can be given, depending on the sensitivity of the cancer.

In patients with a malignant pericardial effusion and good prognosis, prolonged palliation can be obtained by surgical placement of a pleuropericardial window. This procedure is well tolerated, but the window may eventually close because of adhesions. In addition, this procedure may be difficult technically if the tumor encases the heart and pericardium.

Pericardectomy is the treatment of choice for radiation-induced pericardial effusion causing cardiac tamponade. This surgical procedure is more extensive, requires a thoracotomy, and has significant associated morbidity and mortality. It rarely is justified in patients with malignant pericardial effusion and a limited life span.

Malignant Ascites A common and difficult problem is malignant ascites that is refractory to systemic anticancer therapy. Use of spironolactone, a low-salt diet, and repeated paracentesis are the mainstays of treatment, but they are often ineffective. Intraperitoneal administration of radioactive elements is not available to most patients, and many chemotherapeutic agents have been instilled intraabdominally but have resulted in limited success and frequent morbidity (73).

Use of **peritoneovenous shunting** in the palliative treatment of intractable, malignant ascites should be considered for carefully selected patients. The main problem is clotting of the shunt, which renders it nonfunctional. Patients with positive cytology, high ascitic-fluid protein content, and bloody ascites have frequent clotting of these shunts; peritoneovenous shunting is best avoided in these patients. These contraindications are relative, however. Absolute contraindications include recent or concurrent infection, liver failure, loculated intraperitoneal fluid, and preoperative coagulopathy (74).

Complications of peritoneovenous shunting include disseminated intravascular coagulation, which is usually subclinical and does not require treatment; pulmonary edema, which can occur in the immediate postoperative period from large volumes of peritoneal fluid shunted into the systemic circulation; and infection. A Tenckhoff catheter can be surgically placed into the peritoneal cavity in selected patients who require frequent paracentesis to palliate the symptoms of recurrent ascites.

Malignant Biliary Obstruction Biliary obstruction results from many types of cancer. However, therapy of the obstruction depends on the site of obstruction and the type of cancer involved.

Surgical resection of the primary tumor for cure is the first approach, but this is often impossible. Nonoperative techniques for palliation of obstructive jaundice include either placement of a stent internally by ERCP or transhepatically for percutaneous biliary drainage. Surgery for the sole purpose of biliary tract decompression is not recommended.

Indications for biliary tract drainage are jaundice associated with any of the following: (a) cholangitis, (b) sepsis, (c) pruritis, and (d) intractable nausea and vomiting. Cancer causing low obstruction within the common bile duct, such as unresected cancer of the pancreas or periampullary cancer, is usually palliated through the endoscopic route. High obstruction at the ductal confluence, which may result from cholangiocarcinoma, gallbladder carcinoma, or adenopathy in the porta hepatis, may be unreachable by the endoscopist; the percutaneous route may be more approachable.

There is no advantage to either the endoscopic or the percutaneous approach with regard to patient survival, and the choice of technique is often based on the available local expertise. However, there is a growing consensus among specialists with experience in both techniques that endoscopy should be the primary approach and the percutaneous technique a secondary therapy. In one randomized study, the success rate of endoscopic stents in relieving jaundice was higher and the complication rate lower than with the percutaneous technique (75). Endoscopically placed stents also require no maintenance, and they provide greater patient comfort and quality of life compared with percutaneously placed stents using external catheters, which require emptying of the drainage bag, skin care, catheter exchanges every 2 to 3 months, as well as a constant reminder to patients of their cancer (76).

When either percutaneous or endoscopic stents are compared with surgical bypass, the success rates in relieving jaundice are similar (≈90%). The incidence of major complications, 30-day mortality, and number of days in hospital, however, are all lower in the nonsurgical group. In addition, costs are significantly lower with the nonoperative approach.

Complications from both percutaneous and endoscopic stent placement are comparable in incidence, and they include stent occlusion or migration, sepsis, abscess, and hemobilia. Stent occlusion is a significant problem. The advent of expandable, metallic stents (placed either endoscopically or transhepatically) has reduced the rate of stent occlusion, but occlusion secondary to tumor ingrowth through the mesh or tumor overgrowth remains a problem.

One significant advantage of percutaneous placement is that it allows for implantation of radioactive seeds through the catheter for local radiation therapy of the tumor.

External-beam irradiation to radiosensitive tumors or metastatic porta hepatis lymph nodes may occasionally be palliative as well.

Ureteral Obstruction Bilateral complete obstruction of the ureters is a life-threatening condition, and the most common primary tumors causing ureteral obstruction occur in the cervix, ovary, bladder, prostate, and rectum. The diagnosis of upper tract obstruction is best made with renal ultrasonography. The intravenous administration of contrast medium should be avoided in patients with azotemia, because this may result in further renal damage.

Percutaneous nephrostomy with antegrade pyelography will determine both the site and nature of the obstruction and provide drainage for the obstructed kidney. A percutaneous nephrostomy will provide temporary relief of obstruction. It should not be considered a permanent form of drainage, however, because of the difficulty in maintaining the tubes and patient discomfort.

Permanent indwelling ureteral stents can be positioned by retrograde ureteral catheterization over a guide wire, and they are well tolerated by the patient. Permanent surgical urinary diversion techniques may be indicated, depending on the clinical circumstances.

Treatment of Pathologic and Impending Pathologic Long-bone Fractures Bone metastases are common in patients with cancer, and more than three-fourths of adult patients who develop bone metastases have common malignancies, including breast, lung, and prostate carcinomas. Involvement of the proximal femur accounts for more than one-half of all pathologic long-bone fractures and causes significant morbidity because of immobilization. Metastases distal to the elbow or knees are uncommon, except in preterminal patients, and accounted for only 10% of pathologic fractures in one series (76).

A pathologic fracture of a long bone should not be interpreted as a terminal event in most patients with cancer. In fact, directed treatment of the fracture can result in a markedly improved quality of life for many patients, especially those with breast or prostate cancers. Prosthetic replacement or internal fixation of proximal femoral pathologic fractures is the best approach to ensure early ambulation and relief of pain, and the selection of patients for such surgery is an important decision. Harrington (76) recommended that the **following criteria be met before this surgery**: *(a)* a life expectancy of at least 2 months, and a general patient's condition such that major surgery can be tolerated; *(b)* the procedure must be expected to expedite mobilization of the patient or to facilitate general care; and *(c)* the quality of bone both proximal and distal to the fracture must be adequate to support metallic fixation or secure the prosthetic seating.

Harrington developed a technique in which the diseased bone and tumor tissue is replaced by methylmethacrylate supplemented by metal internal fixation devices or prostheses, resulting in a structural capacity able to withstand the stresses of early weight-bearing. In his experience, 94% of 400 patients who were ambulatory before their pathologic fractures regained the ability to walk postoperatively, and pain relief was rated as excellent or good in 85% and poor in only 2% (76).

Some metastatic bone lesions, particularly those from renal, pancreas, and colon cancer, tend to be highly vascular, and blood loss at the time of attempted fixation or even biopsy may become prohibitive. If such situations can be anticipated preoperatively, arterial embolization of the bone tumor site may be attempted.

Prophylactic fixation of an impending fracture of the femur should be performed in high-risk patients. Criteria to assess this risk include: *(a)* primarily lytic lesion, *(b)* size of 2.5 cm or larger, *(c)* cortical involvement, *(d)* lytic lesion involving more than 50% of the diameter of the femur, and *(e)* persistent pain despite radiation therapy.

Complications that relate specifically to operative fixation or prosthetic replacement of malignant pathologic fractures include infection, thromboemboli, local tumor seeding, and delayed wound healing. The complication rate is acceptable, however, particularly considering the physiologic fragility of these patients.

Radiation therapy should be administered at the involved area after internal fixation or prosthetic replacement. Radiation therapy can usually be initiated safely 10 to 14 days following surgery. The prognosis for union of a pathologic fracture depends on rigid fixation and the tumor cell type. Fractures secondary to metastatic breast or prostate carcinoma, myeloma, or lymphoma unite far more frequently than those secondary to malignant tumors of the lung, kidney, or the gastrointestinal tract. Fortunately, metastatic breast cancer is the most common cause for pathologic fracture of long bones, and internal fixation followed by irradiation results in good local tumor control and fracture union in most patients (77).

Spinal Cord Compression Spinal cord compression is a relatively common complication of cancer that metastasizes to the vertebral column, and it often causes severe disability. Early diagnosis requires a high index of suspicion. Therapy must be instituted rapidly to prevent morbidity.

Spinal cord compression by an epidural tumor is **almost always preceded by back pain.** Typically, the pain has been present for weeks to months and is located over the spinal column, with or without radicular radiation (78). Motor weakness, autonomic dysfunction, sensory loss, and ataxia are late signs and often indicate irreversible neurologic impairment.

Plain radiography of the spine usually depicts vertebral involvement. Despite the increased sensitivity of bone scans in detecting bone metastases, their predictive value in spinal cord compression is inferior to that of plain radiographs. MRI provides the most important information regarding vertebral destruction and tumor involvement near the spinal cord and spinal nerves, and it has replaced myelography in evaluating patients for suspect spinal cord compression.

A patient with cancer, back pain, and a plain radiograph depicting vertebral involvement should undergo MRI even if the neurologic examination is normal. Using this approach, a high incidence of epidural spinal metastases will be found, and the institution of appropriate therapy will usually prevent neurologic morbidity.

The appropriate treatment for epidural spinal cord compression is controversial. It depends on the primary cancer, level of the block, rapidity of onset, and the patient's overall clinical condition and prognosis. Treatment options include surgery or radiation therapy, either alone or in combination. No single therapy has been proven to be superior. Early diagnosis and patient selection are the critical factors in predicting a successful outcome.

Patients with lymphoma or myeloma who develop spinal cord compression are usually treated with radiation therapy alone, because these tumors are highly radiosensitive and tumor shrinkage rapidly occurs. Other cancers with favorable histologies include those of breast and prostate. Patient survival and ability to walk after radiation therapy are better in those with favorable tumor histology compared to those with poor tumor histology (i.e., lung cancer). Radiation therapy without operation provides good symptomatic relief in most patients with metastatic spinal cord compression (79). **Indications for an aggressive surgical approach** include relapse after radiation therapy, neurologic deterioration during radiation therapy, or the absence of histologic diagnosis of the tumor.

Dexamethasone should be used when the diagnosis of spinal cord compression is established. The optimal dosage has not been determined but ranges from 16 to 100 mg/day. Dexamethasone at 100 mg/day has been shown to be oncolytic in some patients. Patient tolerance is initially acceptable at this level, but the dose should be rapidly tapered after 3 days.

Malignant Hypercalcemia Hypercalcemia is a common metabolic disorder, occurring in approximately 10% of all patients with cancer. The patient with cancer and hypercalcemia can be a difficult treatment problem, and the consulting internist should be aware of the spectrum of symptoms and understand the therapeutic options. Carcinomas of the breast, lung, head and neck, kidney, and certain hematologic malignancies (particularly multiple myeloma and lymphoma) are most frequently associated with hypercalcemia. However, hypercalcemia occurs more frequently in some malignancies (e.g., squamous cell carcinomas of the lung, head and neck, and esophagus) than in others.

The fundamental cause of cancer-induced hypercalcemia is increased bone resorption with calcium mobilization into the extracellular fluid and, secondarily, inadequate renal clearance of calcium. Two types of cancer-induced hypercalcemia have been described: osteolysis by primary or metastatic tumor infiltrating bone, and humoral hypercalcemia of malignancy mediated by circulating factors that are secreted by malignant cells and without evidence of bony disease. Circulating factors that have been implicated with humoral hypercalcemia of malignancy include parathyroid hormone–like protein, known as *parathyroid hormone–related protein or peptide (PTHrP)*; transforming growth factor–α and –β; interleukin-1 and interleukin-6, formerly referred to as *osteoclast-activating factor;* tumor necrosis factor–α and –β; and prostaglandin E_2 (80, 81).

Symptoms associated with hypercalcemia are characteristically nonspecific and can be easily attributed to chronic or terminal illness. Some patients have no symptoms, but those with corrected total serum calcium concentrations greater than 14 mg/dL (>7.0 mEq/L or 3.5 mmol/L) are generally symptomatic. Clinical manifestations are closely related to the rapidity of hypercalcemia onset and may include neurologic symptoms (e.g., fatigue, apathy, depression, confusion, obtundation, restlessness), cardiovascular abnormalities (e.g., hypertension, electrocardiographic changes, arrhythmias, digitalis toxicity), renal symptoms (e.g., polyuria, nocturia, polydipsia), and gastrointestinal complaints (e.g., anorexia, nausea, abdominal pain, constipation, abdominal distention).

Treatment of Hypercalcemia Treatment is typically based on severity of the hypercalcemia. Immediate, aggressive hypocalcemic treatment is warranted in patients with a corrected total serum calcium concentration greater than 14 mg/dL (>7 mEq/L or 3.5 mmol/L). In patients with a total corrected serum calcium concentration between 12 and 14 mg/dL (6–7 mEq/L or 3.0–.5 mmol/L), clinical manifestations should guide therapy and the urgency of its implementation. Aggressive treatment is not generally indicated in patients with mild hypercalcemia (corrected total serum calcium concentration, <12 mg/dL [<6 mEq/L or 3.0 mmol/L]) unless coexistent central nervous system symptoms are present. Response to treatment is indicated by resolution of the symptoms attributable to hypercalcemia and diminishing serum calcium concentrations.

Symptomatic treatment for hypercalcemia focuses first on correcting dehydration and enhancing the renal excretion of calcium, followed by specific hypocalcemic treatment with agents that inhibit bone resorption. Definitive treatment is that which effectively treats the malignant disease underlying the hypercalcemia.

Mild Hypercalcemia Patients who are asymptomatic or only minimally symptomatic and who have corrected total serum calcium concentrations less than 12 mg/dL (<6 mEq/L or <3.0 mmol/L) are considered to have mild hypercalcemia. Hydration, either alone or followed by loop diuretics, is an option for asymptomatic patients with tumors that are likely to respond to antineoplastic treatment (e.g., lymphoma, breast cancer, ovarian cancer, head and neck carcinoma, multiple myeloma) if such treatment is about to be implemented. In symptomatic patients, or when the tumor response is expected to occur slowly, hypocalcemic therapy should be implemented to treat symptoms and stabilize their metabolic states.

Moderate to Severe Hypercalcemia Patients who are symptomatic and have corrected total serum calcium concentrations of 12 mg/dL or greater (≥6 mEq/L or ≥3 mmol/L) are considered to have moderate to severe hypercalcemia, and rehydration is the essential first step in their treatment. Although few patients achieve normocalcemia with use of hydration alone, replenishing extracellular fluid, restoring intravascular volume, and saline diuresis are fundamental to initial therapy. Adequate rehydration may require 3 to 6 L of 0.9% sodium chloride within the first 24 hours to restore fluid volume. Restoring a normal extracellular fluid volume will increase daily urinary excretion of calcium, but rehydration is a temporizing intervention. Loop diuretics should be administered only after hydration has been is established.

For patients with severe symptomatic hypercalcemia, salmon calcitonin should be given for its rapid, although short-lived, effect. Pamidronate is the bisphosphonate of choice, and because its onset of action is delayed for 1 to 2 days, it should also be administered.

Additional ancillary interventions should be directed toward control of nausea and vomiting, encouragement of mobility, attention to febrile episodes, and minimal use of sedatives.

Specific Drug Therapy

Loop diuretics (e.g., furosemide, bumetanide, ethacrynic acid) induce calciuresis by inhibiting calcium reabsorption in the ascending limb of the loop of Henle, but they should not be administered until volume expansion has been achieved. Otherwise, loop diuretics can exacerbate fluid loss, further reducing calcium clearance. Moderate doses of furosemide, 20 to 40 mg every 12 hours, increase saline-induced urinary excretion of calcium and are useful in preventing or managing fluid overload in adequately rehydrated patients. Aggressive treatment with furosemide, 80 to 100 mg every 2 to 4 hours, is problematic, because it requires concurrent administration of large volumes of saline to prevent intravascular dehydration. In turn, this requires intensive hemodynamic monitoring to avoid volume overload and cardiac decompensation, as well as frequent measurements of serial urinary output and serum electrolyte levels to prevent life-threatening hypophosphatemia, hypokalemia, and hypomagnesemia.

Salmon calcitonin is a potent hypocalcemic hormone. It is given at 4 IU/kg, initially subcutaneously and then either subcutaneously or intramuscularly every 12 hours. Both the dose and the schedule may be escalated after 1 or 2 days to 8 IU/kg every 12 hours and, finally, to 8 IU/kg every 6 hours if the response at lower doses is unsatisfactory. Unfortunately, tachyphylaxis commonly occurs. Also, with repeated use, calcitonin's beneficial hypocalcemic effect wanes, even at the upper recommended limits of dose and schedule; therefore, its calcium-lowering effect persists for only a few days. There is evidence to suggest that the effect of calcitonin on bone resorption may be prolonged by concomitant glucocorticoid administration, and that it may hasten the onset and duration of hypocalcemic response when combined with bisphosphonates. Calcitonin is usually well-tolerated. Adverse effects, however, include mild nausea, transient and cramping abdominal pain, and cutaneous flushing. Calcitonin is most useful within the first 24 to 36 hours of treatment for severe hypercalcemia, and it should be used in conjunction with more potent, slower-acting agents.

Bisphosphonates are the most effective pharmacologic alternative for controlling hypercalcemia. They bind to hydroxyapatite in calcified bone, rendering it resistant to hydrolytic dissolution by phosphatases and thereby inhibiting both normal and abnormal bone resorption. At present, only etidronate and pamidronate are approved in the United States for the treatment of malignant hypercalcemia. Compared with etidronate, which requires daily administration for 3 or more days, pamidronate is administered once over 4 to 24 hours in a dose of 60 to 90 mg. Regarding serum calcium reduction and duration of hypocalcemic response, pamidronate, 60 mg given intravenously as a single dose over 24 hours, is more effective than etidronate, 7.5 mg/kg per day administered over 2 hours as a daily intravenous infusion for 3 consecutive days.

Different pamidronate dosages and schedules may be indicated by the severity of the hypercalcemia. In moderate hypercalcemia, 60 mg is as effective as 90 mg. For serum calcium levels of 13.5 mg/dL or greater, 90 mg administered over 4 hours is both safe and somewhat more effective than 60 mg.

The effects of pamidronate are apparent within 3 to 4 days, with maximal effects occurring within 7 to 10 days, after treatment has commenced. The duration of effect may persist for 7 to 30 days. Adverse effects include transient, low-grade temperature elevations (1–2°C), which typically occur within 24 to 36 hours of administration and persist for as long as 2 days in up to 20% of patients; the incidence of temperature elevation, nausea, anorexia, dyspepsia, and vomiting may be increased by rapid administration. New-onset hypophosphatemia and hypomagnesemia may occur, and preexisting abnormalities in these same electrolytes may be exacerbated by treatment. The serum calcium level may drop below the normal range, and hypocalcemia, which is typically asymptomatic, may result. Renal failure has been reported only after rapid injection of etidronate; however, rapid administration should be avoided with all bisphosphonates.

Plicamycin (also referred to as *mithramycin*) is an inhibitor of RNA synthesis by osteoclasts. It inhibits bone resorption in vitro and is clinically effective in the presence or absence of bone metastases. Onset of response occurs within 12 hours of a single intravenous dose of 25 to 30 μg/kg, either as a short 30-minute or longer infusion. Maximum response, however, does not occur until approximately 48 hours after administration, and the effect may persist for 3 to 7 days (or more) after administration. Repeated doses may be given to maintain the hypocalcemic effect. Thrombocytopenia, hepatotoxicity, and renal insufficiency are important adverse effects, and for the most part, bisphosphonate therapy has replaced the need for plicamycin except in the most severe conditions.

Glucocorticoids are effective hypocalcemic agents primarily in steroid-responsive tumors (e.g., lymphoma, myeloma). They increase the urinary excretion of calcium and inhibit the vitamin D–mediated gastrointestinal absorption of calcium. However, the response is typically slow; 1 to 2 weeks may elapse before serum calcium concentrations decrease.

Gallium nitrate is a newer agent that is effective in the treatment of hypercalcemia caused by malignancy. The disadvantage of gallium is that it must be given

Table 16.10. Commonly Prescribed Analgesic Drugs for Patients with Cancer

Drug (Formulation)	Route	Usual Starting Dose and Interval	Dose Equianalgesic to Morphine, 10 mg IM	Comments
Step 1[a]		Nonopioids ± Adjuvant[b]		
Acetaminophen	PO	650–1000 mg q 4–6 h		OTC; available in tabs and liquid
Ibuprofen	PO	400–800 mg q 6–8 h		
NSIADs		Numerous drugs available by prescription		
Step 2[a]		Opioids + Nonopioids ± Adjuvant[b]		
Codeine	PO	30–60 mg q 3–4 h	200 mg	Usually combined with nonopioids (ASA or acetaminophen)
Hydrocodone (Lorcet, Lortabs, Vicodin)	PO	10 mg q 3–4 h	30 mg	
Oxycodone	PO	5–10 mg q 3–4 h	30 mg	Available in tabs and liquid
Tabs (immediate release) (Percocet, Tylox, Roxicodone)				
Oxycontin Tabs (sustained release)	PO	10–20 mg q 12 h	30 mg	Available in 10-, 20-, and 40-mg tabs
Step 3[a]		Opioids ± Nonopioids ± Adjuvant[b]		
Morphine				
Tabs (immediate release) (MSIR)		15–30 mg q 3–4 h	30 mg (repeated dosing) 60 mg (single or intermittent dosing)	
Liquid (Roxanol, MSIR)	[20 mg/mL]	0.5–1.5 ml q 3–4 h		30- and 120-mL bottles
Tabs (sustained release) (MS Contin)		60–120 mg q 12 h	30 mg	15, 30, 60, 100, and 200-mg tabs
(Oramorph)	IV or SQ (single dose)	0.1 mg/kg q 3–4 h	10 mg	30, 60, and 100-mg tabs
	Continuous IV infusion	(Total 24-h dose of oral and/or parenteral opioids; determine appropriate equianalgesic dose and then divide by 24 to obtain hourly rate)		
Rectal (Roxanol)		Same as oral dose		5, 10, 20, and 30-mg suppository
Hydromorphone (Dilaudid)				
Tabs		2–4 mg q 3–6 h	7.5 mg	Available in 1, 2, 3, 4, and 8-mg tabs
Liquid (1 mg/mL)	IV, SC	Same as tabs		
	Rectal	0.015 mg/kg q 3–4 h	1.5 mg	
		3 mg q 3–6 h	N/A	
Fentanyl (Duragesic)	Transdermal	Use after pain controlled on morphine q 48–72 h	100 μg = MS 2 mg/hr	Patches available in 25, 50, 75, and 100 μg Slow onset (12 h)

ASA, aspirin; *N/A,* not applicable; *NSAIDs,* nonsteroidal anti-inflammatory drugs; *OTC,* over the counter.
[a]World Health Organization three-step analgesic ladder, which portrays a progression in the doses and types of analgesic drugs for effective pain management.
[b]Adjuvant drug therapy includes corticosteroids, antidepressants, anticonvulsants, and psychostimulants.

over a 5-day infusion, and it should not be used in patients with a serum creatinine concentration greater than 2.5 mg/dL.

Control of Symptoms in Patients with Cancer

The internist is often asked to help surgical colleagues palliate symptoms in patients with cancer, and the principles of symptom control are best suited to application by the internist. These principles include expertise in eliciting a careful patient history in a compassionate manner, determining the significance of a patient's symptoms, and skillfully prescribing treatments to alleviate these symptoms. The internist should be familiar with medications for the treatment of common symptoms in terminally ill patients with cancer, and the flexible routes of administration for these medications are also important to understand. Common symptoms the internist will encounter during consultations for palliative treatment of patients with cancer include pain, nausea, vomiting, constipation, cough, and dyspnea.

Effective treatment of **cancer pain** requires an understanding of the patho-physiology of pain, the ability to identify and evaluate pain syndromes, and a familiarity with proven therapeutic modalities. This section deals with pharmacotherapy for pain.

Opioid therapy is the mainstay of treatment, and practical aspects of such therapy include selection of both the drug and the route, dose titration, and treatment of side effects. Several opioids with flexible drug formulations are described in Table 16.10. Knowing how to prescribe a few drugs well in this situation is more effective than knowing how to prescribe many drugs. Table 16.10 is organized by the World Health Organization three-step analgesic ladder, which portrays a progression in the doses and types of analgesic drugs for effective treatment of pain (82). The internist should also understand the value of adjuvant drug therapy (83) (Table 16.11).

Constipation is a common and distressing symptom in patients with cancer, and use of opioids without adequate doses of laxatives is the most common cause of constipation in these patients. Other important causes include spinal cord compression, bowel obstruction from tumor, adhesions, or impacted stool and meta-

Table 16.11. Adjuvant Analgesic Drugs

Drug (Formulation)	Route	Usual Starting Dose and Interval	Comments
Corticosteroids	PO		May decrease pain associated with CNS and spinal cord tumors and bone pain. May increase appetite. Many side effects
(*Dexamethasone*)		4–8 mg q 6–8 h	
(*Prednisone*)		10–20 mg q 6–8 h	
Antidepressants	PO		Useful for neuropathic pain. Onset of analgesic effect may take 1–2 weeks. Side effects: dry mouth, hypotension, constipation, urinary retention
(*Amitriptyline*)		10–25 mg t.i.d. or HS	
(*Doxepin*)		10–25 mg t.i.d. or HS	
(*Trazodone*)		50 mg t.i.d.	
Anticonvulsants	PO		Useful for neuropathic pain
(*Phenytoin*)		300 mg daily	
(*Carbamazepine*)		200 mg b.i.d.	
Psychostimulants	PO		Improves opioid analgesia
(*Dextroamphetamine*)		5–10 mg daily to t.i.d.	Decreases sedation
(*Methylphenidate*)		10 mg daily to t.i.d.	

CNS, central nervous system; *HS*, bedtime.

Table 16.12.   Commonly Prescribed Drugs for Nausea, Vomiting, and Dyspepsia

Drug (Formulation)	Dose (mg)	Route	Interval (h)	Considerations
Prochlorperazine (*Compazine*)				Extrapyramidal reactions, sedation, hypotension, anticholinergic effect
Tablet	5 & 10	PO	4–8	
Spansule	10 & 15	PO	12	
Suppository	25	Rectal	12	
Syrup[a]	5–10	PO	4–8	
Parenteral	5–10	IM, IV	4–8	
Triethylperazine (*Torecan*)				Same as prochlorperazine
Tablet	10	PO	8	
Suppository	10	Rectal	8	
Chlorpromazine	10–50	PO	4–6	Usually more side effects than Prochlorperazine. Available in syrup and suppository
Lorazepam (*Ativan*)	0.5–1.0	PO/SL	4–8	Sedation, amnesia, confusion
Metoclopramide (*Reglan*)	10–20	PO	6–8	Extrapyramidal reactions, sedation, diarrhea; contraindicated with GI obstruction
	10–40	IV	6–8	
Haloperidol	1–2	PO	4–6	Dystonia, hypotension, sedation; may be effective if opioid-induced
Droperidol	0.5–2.0	IV	4	Same as haloperidol
Dexamethasone	4–8	PO	6–12	Hyperglycemia, euphoria, insomnia, dyspepsia; may be effective if resistant to other antiemetics
	10–20	IV		
Metodiphenex		Rectal	4–6	Combination metoclopramide, diphenhydramine, dexamethasone in suppository form; helpful in refractory cases
Dronabinol (*Marinol*)	2.5–10.0	PO	3–4	Dysphoria, ataxia, confusion, dry mouth
Promethazine (*Phenergan*)	25–50	PO	4–6	Drowsiness, dry mouth
	25 mg per 5 mL			
	12.5–50	Rectal	4–6	
Hydroxyzine	25–50 mg	PO	6–8	Drowiness, dry mouth; may potentiate opioids; anxiolytic
	25 mg per 5 mL			
	50–100	IM	6–8	
H$_2$-receptor antagonists (*Cimetidine, Ranitidine, Famotidine*)		PO		Use for GI irritation, especially from NSAIDs
		IV		
Omeprazole (Prilosec)	20 mg	PO	Daily	For GI irritation, hyperacidity
Sulcrafate (*Carafate*) (tabs, suspension)	1 gm	PO	6	For GI irritation
Antacids				For GI irritation
Ondansetron (*Zofran*)	8–32 mg	IV	Daily	Headache, constipation
	8 mg	PO	8–12	To be used for the prevention and treatment of chemotherapy induced nausea and vomiting
Granisetron (*Kytril*)	40 μg/kg	IV	Daily	
	1 mg	PO	Daily	

GI, gastrointestinal; *NSAIDs*, nonsteroidal anti-inflammatory drugs.
[a]5 mg per 5 mL.

Table 16.13.   Commonly Prescribed Laxatives

Type of Laxative	Trade Name	Route of Administration and Dose	Schedule	Onset of Action	Type of Stool Formed
Bulk-forming					
Psyllium	Metamucil, many others	Oral (1–2 tsp in 8 oz of fluid)	q.i.d.-t.i.d.	12–24 h (up to 3 days)	Soft
Polycarbophil	FiberCon, Mitrolan	Oral (1–2 tabs in 8 oz of fluid)	1–2 tabs q.i.d.-q.i.d.	1–3 days	Soft
Stool Softener or Emollient					
Docusate				24–48 h (up to 3–5 days)	Soft
Sodium	Colace	Oral 50–100 mg	q.i.d.-t.i.d.		
Calcium	Surfak	Oral 50 and 240 mg	q.i.d.-t.i.d.		
Lubricant					
Mineral oil		PO	15–45 mL	6–8 h q.i.d.	Soft
		Rectal	30–60 mL	5–15 min q.i.d.	
Peristalsis Stimulants					
Casanthranol		Oral (30 mg)	Daily	6–12 h	Soft-semisolid
Sennosides	Senokot	8.6-mg tab or 5 mL of syrup q.i.d.	q.i.d.-b.i.d.	6–12 h	Soft or formed
Bisacodyl		Oral (5 mg)	2 tabs/h	6–12 h	Soft or formed
		Rectal (10 mg)		15–60 min	
Cascara sagrada		5 mL	Daily	6–12 h	Soft
Phenolphthalein		Oral (65 mg) 10–20 mL	q.i.d.-b.i.d.	6–12 h	Semifluid
Castor oil		15–60 mL	Daily	1–6 h	Watery
Danthron	Modane	37.5–75.0 mg	1–2 tab q.i.d.-b.i.d.	6–8 h	Soft-semifluid
Hyperosmotic					
Magnesium hydroxide	MOM	15–40 mL	q.i.d.-b.i.d.	3–6 h	Soft-formed
Magnesium citrate		Oral (8–10 oz)	Daily	3–6 h	Watery
Lactulose		Oral (30–60 mL)	q.i.d.	24–48 h	Soft
Sodium phosphates		Oral (15–30 mL)	q.i.d.	½–3 h	
	Fleet	Enema (60–120 mL)	PRN	2–5 min	Soft-formed
Polyethylene glycol		Oral	8 oz q15 min	1–4 h	Watery
Glycerine		Rectal	PRN	¼–1 h	Soft
Combinations					
Sennosides and docusate	Senokot-S		1–2 tabs q.i.d.-t.i.d.		
Casanthranol and docusate	Pericolace		1–2 tabs q.i.d.-t.i.d.		
Danthron and docusate	Doxidan		1–2 tabs q.i.d.-t.i.d.		

bolic abnormalities (specifically, hypokalemia and hypercalcemia). Commonly prescribed laxatives, their route of administration, and their mode and onset of action are described in Table 16.12.

Nausea and vomiting are also frequent symptoms in patients with cancer. Nausea and vomiting are commonly induced by medications such as opiates, nonsteroidal anti-inflammatory drugs,

Table 16.14.   Cough in the Patient with Cancer

Pharmacologic Options
Bronchodilators
    Inhaled β2-agonists (nebulized or inhaler)
    Anticholinergic inhaler (ipratropium bromide)
    Theophylline compounds
Corticosteroids (dexamethasone or prednisone)
Antitussives
    Dextromethorphan
    Bensonatate (Tessalon perles, 100 mg q.i.d.)
    Hydrocodone (Hycodan [with homatropine],
        Tussionex [with chlorpheniramine])
Opioids (codeine, morphine)
Atropine (to decrease secretions)
Mucolytics
    Guaifenesen
    Potassium iodide (saturated solution of
        potassium iodide)
Antibiotics
Nebulized lidocaine
Nebulized morphine (Astromorph)

Nonpharmacologic Options
Aspiration of oropharynx
Humidification of air (vaporizer)
Drainage of pleural effusion
Radiotherapy to cancer
Chest physiotheray (to improve clearance of
    secretions in patient with copious pulmonary
    secretions)

---

of a productive cough include acute and chronic bronchitis, pneumonia, and aspiration. A dry cough commonly occurs from bronchospasm (from any cause), pleural effusion, or an endobronchial or obstructing cancer. Both pharmacologic and non-pharmacologic treatments are described in Table 16.14.

Dyspnea is another common symptom in patients with cancer and can range in severity from mild to severe. Treatable causes in these patients include anemia, cardiac failure, pleural effusion, pericardial effusion, bronchospasm, pulmonary infection, atelectasis, ascites, and pulmonary emboli. Treatment of patients with preterminal dyspnea can be difficult and is described in Table 16.15.

Pelvic Exenteration

See Chapter 22.

Radical Neck Surgery

See Chapter 22.

---

and steroids. Intra-abdominal cancer resulting in obstruction and peritonitis can also cause nausea and vomiting. Metabolic consequences of cancer such as hypercalcemia and uremia may produce symptoms of nausea and vomiting. In addition, disorders that are unrelated to the specific cancer (e.g., esophagitis, gastritis, peptic ulcer disease, anxiety, depression) should not be overlooked as treatable causes. Commonly prescribed medications for nausea, vomiting, and dyspepsia are described in Table 16.13. A trial of different combinations and routes of administration can improve refractory symptoms.

Cough can be a disturbing symptom and result in anorexia, nausea and vomiting, insomnia, musculoskeletal pain, syncope, and exhaustion. Common causes

Table 16.15.   Treatment of Preterminal Dyspnea

For Respiratory Panic:
Calmly educate patient about breathing control
Trial of lorazepam, 0.5–1.0 mg intravenously

*For Shortness of Breath Associated with
    Tachypnea:*
Give morphine sulfate IV or SQ
Oxygen therapy
Trial of corticosteroids

For Air Hunger:
Give morphine sulfate IV, titrate to symptoms
Give lorazepam IV, titrate to symptoms

*For Shortness of Breath Associated with Excess
    Secretions:*
Oropharyngeal suctioning
Atropine, 0.4–0.6 mg SQ q 2–4 h

Appendix
Staging Systems of Common Cancers

Breast Cancer—TNM Classification

Primary Tumor (T)
T1: Tumor 2 cm or smaller in greatest dimension
T2: Tumor 2–5 cm in greatest dimension
T3: Tumor larger than 5 cm in greatest dimension
T4: Tumor of any size with direct extension to the chest wall or skin (including inflammatory carcinoma)

Regional Lymph Nodes (N)
N0: No regional lymph node metastasis
N1: Metastasis to movable ipsilateral axillary lymph node(s)
N2: Metastasis to ipsilateral axillary lymph node(s) fixed to one another or to other structures
N3: Metastasis to ipsilateral internal mammary lymph node(s)

Distant Metastases (M)
M0: No evidence of distant metastases
M1: Distant metastases (includes metastases to ipsilateral supraclavicular lymph node[s])

Group Stage
Stage I: T1, N0, M0
Stage IIA: T1, N1, M0
T2, N0, M0
Stage IIB: T2, N1, M0
T3, N0, M0
Stage IIIA: T0–3, N2, M0
T3 N1 M0
Stage IIIB: Any T, N3, M0
T4, Any N, M0
Stage IV: Any T, Any N, M1

Colorectal Cancer—TNM Classification

Primary Tumor (T)
T1: Tumor invades submucosa
T2: Tumor invades muscularis propria
T3: Tumor invades through the muscularis propria into the subserosa or into the nonperitonealized pericolic or perirectal tissues
T4: Tumor directly invades other organs or structures, perforates the visceral peritoneum, or both

Regional Lymph Nodes (N)
N0: No regional lymph node metastasis
N1: Metastasis in 1 to 3 pericolic lymph nodes
N2: Metastasis in 4 or more pericolic lymph nodes
N3: Metastasis in any lymph node along the course of a named vascular trunk, metastasis to apical node(s), or both.

Distant Metastasis (M)
M0: No distant metastasis
M1: Distant metastasis

Group Stage
Stage I: T1, N0, M0
T2, N0, M0
(Stage I may be equivalent to Dukes' A or Modified Astler-Coller [MAC] A or B1. Tumor is limited to bowel wall [i.e., mucosa, muscularis mucosae, submucosa, and muscularis propria].)
Stage II: T3, N0, M0
T4, N0, M0
(Stage II may be equivalent to Dukes' B or MAC B2 or B3. Tumor has spread to extramural tissue.)

Stage III: Any T, N1, M0
Any T, N2, M0
Any T, N3, M0
(Stage III may be equivalent to Dukes' C
or MAC C1–C3. Regional nodes are in-
volved.)
Stage IV: Any T, any N, M1
(Stage IV may be equivalent to Dukes' D
or MAC.)

Colorectal Cancer—Astler-Coller (Modified Duke's) Staging

A: Limited to mucosa; nodes are negative
B1: Extension through mucosa but still
within bowel wall; nodes are negative
B2: Extension through entire bowel
wall; nodes are negative
C1: Limited to bowel wall; nodes are
positive
C2: Extension through entire bowel
wall; nodes are positive

Treatment decisions are often made in
reference to the older Dukes or the MAC
classification schema. Stages should preferably be defined by the TNM classification.

Prostate Cancer—TNM Classification

Primary Tumor (T)
T1: Clinically inapparent tumor not palpable or visible by imaging
T1a: Tumor an incidental histologic
finding in 5% or less of tissue
specimens resected
T1b: Tumor an incidental histologic
finding in more than 5% of tissue
specimens resected
T1c: Tumor identified by needle biopsy
(e.g., because of elevated PSA level)
T2: Tumor confined within prostate
T2a: Tumor involves one-half of a lobe
or less
T2b: Tumor involves more than one-
half of a lobe but not both lobes

T2c: Tumor involves both lobes
T3: Tumor extends through the prostatic
capsule
T3a: Unilateral extracapsular ex-
tension
T3b: Bilateral extracapsular extension
T3c: Tumor invades seminal vesicle(s)
T4: Tumor is fixed or invades adjacent
structures other than the seminal
vesicles
T4a: Tumor invades bladder neck, ex-
ternal sphincter, or rectum
T4b: Tumor invades levator muscles,
is fixed to the pelvic wall, or both

Regional Lymph Nodes (N)
N0: No regional lymph node metastasis
N1: Metastasis in a single lymph node
2 cm or smaller in greatest dimension
N2: Metastasis in a single lymph node
larger than 2 cm but not larger than
5 cm in greatest dimension, or multiple lymph node metastases with none
larger than 5 cm in greatest dimension
N3: Metastasis in a lymph node larger
than 5 cm in greatest dimension

Distant Metastasis (M)
M0: No distant metastasis
M1: Distant metastasis
M1a: Nonregional lymph node(s)
M1b: Bone(s)
M1c: Other site(s)

Group Stage
Stage 0: T1a, N0, M0
Stage I: T1a, N0, M0
T1b, N0, M0
T1c, N0, M0,
T1, N0, M0
Stage II: T2, N0, M0
Stage III: T3, N0, M0
Stage IV: T4, N0, any M
Any T, N1, M0
Any T, N2, M0
Any T, N3, M0
Any T, any N, M1

Prostate Cancer American Urologic Staging System

A1: No tumor palpable; focal involvement; well differentiated

A2: No tumor palpable; diffuse involvement; poorly differentiated

B1: Tumor smaller than 2 cm and involving 1 lobe

B2: Tumor larger than 2 cm or diffuse involvement

C: Tumor extension beyond the prostate capsule without evidence of metastases

D1: Tumor of any size involving pelvic lymph nodes below the aortic bifurcation

D2: Tumor of any size involving lymph nodes above the aortic bifurcation, distant metastases to other sites, or both

Nonsmall-cell Lung Cancer—TNM Classification

Primary tumor (T)

T1: Tumor 3.0 cm or smaller in greatest diameter surrounded by lung or visceral pleura and without evidence of invasion more proximal than the lobar bronchus (i.e., not in the main bronchus)

T2: Tumor with any of the following features of size or extent:

Larger than 3.0 cm in greatest dimension

Involving the main bronchus, 2.0 cm or more distal to the carina

Invading the visceral pleura

Associated with atelectasis or obstructive pneumonitis that extends to the hilar region but does not involve the entire lung

T3: Tumor of any size with direct extension to the chest wall (including superior sulcus tumors), diaphragm, mediastinal pleura, parietal pericardium; tumor in the main bronchus less than

2.0 cm distal to the carina but without involvement of the carina; associated atelectasis or obstructive pneumonitis of the entire lung

T4: Tumor of any size that invades any of the following: mediastinum, heart, great vessels, trachea, esophagus, vertebral body, carina; or tumor with a malignant pleural effusion. (In the few patients for whom multiple cytopathologic examinations of pleural fluid are negative for tumor (i.e., fluid is nonbloody and not an exudate) and clinical judgment dictates that the effusion is not related to the tumor, the effusion should be excluded as a staging element and the patient staged as T1, T2, or T3.)

Nodal Involvement (N)

NX: Regional lymph nodes cannot be assessed

N0: No regional lymph node metastasis

N1: Metastasis in ipsilateral peribronchial and/or ipsilateral hilar lymph nodes, including direct extension

N2: Metastasis in ipsilateral mediastinal and/or subcarinal lymph node(s)

N3: Metastasis in contralateral mediastinal, contralateral hilar, ipsilateral or contralateral scalene, or supraclavicular lymph node(s)

Distant Metastasis (M)

M0: No distant metastasis

Group Stage

Stage I: T1, N0, M0

T2, N0, M0

Stage II: T1, N1, M0

T2, N1, M0

Stage IIIA: T1, N2, M0

T2, N2, M0

T3, N0, M0

T3, N1, M0

T3, N2, M0

Stage IIIb: Any T, N3, M0

T4, any N, M0

Stage IV: Any T, any N, M1

REFERENCES

1. Weiss SM, Skibber JM, Rosato FE. Bowel obstruction in cancer patients: performance status as a predictor of survival. J Surg Oncol 1984;25: 15–17.
2. Barnes SG, Sattler FR, Ballard JO. Perirectal infections in acute leukemia. Ann Intern Med 1984;101:515–518.
3. Ginsburg SJ, Comis RL. The pulmonary toxicity of antineoplastic agents. Semin Oncol 1982;9: 34–51.
4. Von Hoff DD, Layard MW, Basa P. Risk factors for doxorubicin-induced congestive heart failure. Ann Intern Med 1979;91:710–717.
5. Gottdiener JS, Mathisen DJ, Borer JS, et al. Doxorubicin cardiotoxicity: assessment of late left ventricular dysfunction by radionuclide cineangiography. Ann Intern Med 1981;94: 430–435.
6. Benoff LJ, Schweitzer P. Radiation therapy-induced cardiac injury. Am Heart J 1995;129: 1193–1196.
7. Dentino M, Luft FC, Yum MN, et al. Long term effect of cis-diamminedichloride platinum (CDDP) on renal function and structure in man. Cancer 1978;41:1274–1281.
8. Lyman NW, Hemalatha C, Viscuso RL, et al. Cisplatin-induced hypocalcemia and hypomagnesemia. Arch Intern Med 1980;140:1513–1514.
9. Marks G, Mohiudden M. The surgical management of radiation-injured intestine. Surg Clin North Am 1983;63:81–96.
10. Lee YN. Bone scanning in patients with early breast carcinoma: should it be a routine staging procedure? Cancer 1981;47:486–495.
11. Ciatto S, Pacini P, Azzini V. Preoperative staging of primary breast cancer. A multicentric study. Cancer 1988;61:1038–1040.
12. Fisher B, Anderson S, Redmond CK, et al. Reanalysis and results after 12 years of follow-up in a randomized clinical trial comparing total mastectomy with lumpectomy with or without irradiation in the treatment of breast cancer. N Engl J Med 1995;333:1456–1461.
13. Winchester DP, Cox JD. Standards for breast-conservation treatment. CA 1992;42:134–162.
14. Fisher B, Constantino J, Redmond C, et al. Lumpectomy compared with lumpectomy and radiation therapy for the treatment of intraductal breast cancer. N Engl J Med 1993;328:1581–1586.
15. Rouesse J, Friedman S, Sarrazin D, et al. Primary chemotherapy in the treatment of inflammatory breast carcinoma: a study of 230 cases from the Institut Gustave-Roussy. J Clin Oncol 1986;4:1765–1771.
16. Hortobagyi GN, Blumenschein GR, Sapnos W, et al. Multimodality treatment of locoregionally advanced breast cancer. Cancer 1983;51: 763–768.
17. McGuire WL, Clark GM. Prognostic factors and treatment decisions in axillary-node-negative breast cancer. N Engl J Med 1992;326:1756–1761.
18. Parl FF, Schmidt BP, Dupont WD, et al. Prognostic significance of estrogen receptor status in breast cancer in relation to tumor stage, axillary node metastasis, and histopathologic grading. Cancer 1984;54:2237–2242.
19. Early Breast Cancer Trialists' Collaborative Group. Systemic treatment of early breast cancer by hormonal, cytotoxic, or immune therapy. Lancet 1992;339:1–15.
20. Rosen PP, Groshen S, Kinne DW, Norton L. Factors influencing prognosis in node-negative breast carcinoma: analysis of 767 T1N0M0/T2N0M0 patients with long-term follow-up. J Clin Oncol 1993;11:2090–2100.
21. Fisher B, Dignam J, Mamounas, EP, et al. Sequential methotrexate and fluorouracil for the treatment of node-negative breast cancer patients with estrogen receptor-negative tumors: eight-year results from National Surgical Adjuvant Breast and Bowel Project (NSABP) B-13 and first report of findings from NSABP B-19 comparing methotrexate and fluorouracil with conventional cyclophosphamide, methotrexate, and fluorouracil. J Clin Oncol 1996;14:1982–1992.
22. Mansour EG, Gray R, Shatila ATL, et al. Efficacy of adjuvant chemotherapy in high-risk node-negative breast cancer. An intergroup study. N Engl J Med 1989;320:485–490.
23. Fisher B, Constantino J, Redmond C, et al. A randomized clinical trial evaluating tamoxifen in the treatment of patients with node-negative breast cancer who have estrogen-receptor-positive tumors. N Engl J Med 1989;320: 479–484.
24. Goldhirsch A, Wood WC, Senn HJ, et al. Meeting highlights: international consensus panel on the treatment of primary breast cancer. J Natl Cancer Inst 1995;87:1441–1445.
25. Kerner BA, Oliver GC, Eisenstat TE, et al. Is preoperative computerized tomography useful in assessing patients with colorectal carcinoma? Dis Colon Rectum 1993;36:1050–1053.
26. Lahr CJ, Soong SJ, Cloud G, et al. A multifactorial analysis of prognostic factors in patients with liver metastases from colorectal carcinoma. J Clin Oncol 1983;1:720–726.
27. Moertel CG, Fleming TR, MacDonald JS, et al. Fluoruracil plus levamisole as effective adjuvant therapy after resection of stage III colon carcinoma: a final report. Ann Intern Med 1995;122: 321–326.
28. Gastrointestinal Tumor Study Group. Prolongation of the disease-free interval in surgically treated rectal carcinoma. N Engl J Med 1985; 312:1465–1472.
29. Krook JE, Moertel CG, Gunderson LL, et al.

Effective surgical adjuvant therapy for high-risk rectal carcinoma. N Engl J Med 1991;324: 709–715.

30. Gastrointestinal Study Group. Radiation therapy and fluorouracil with or without semustine for the treatment of patients with surgical adjuvant adenocarcinoma of the rectum. J Clin Oncol 1992;10:549–557.

31. O'Connell MJ, Martenson JA, Wieand HS, et al. Improving adjuvant therapy for rectal cancer by combining protracted-infusion fluorouracil with radiation therapy after curative surgery. N Engl J Med 1994;331:502–507.

32. Meade PG, Blatchford GJ, Thorson AG, et al. Preoperative chemoradiation downstages locally advanced ultrasound-staged rectal cancer. Am J Surg 1995;170:609–613.

33. Minsky BD, Cohen AM, Kemeny N, et al. Enhancement of radiation-induced downstaging of rectal cancer by fluorouracil and high-dose leucovorin chemotherapy. J Clin Oncol 1992;10: 79–84.

34. Minsky BD, Cohen AM, Enker WE, et al. Sphincter preservation with preoperative radiation therapy and coloanal anastomosis. Int J Radiat Oncol Biol Phys 1995;31:553–559.

35. Armstrong JD, Bragg DG. Thoracic neoplasm: imaging requirements for diagnosis and staging. Int J Radiat Oncol Biol Phys 1984;10: 109–135.

36. Lilenbaum RC, Green MR. Multimodality therapy for non-small cell lung cancer. Oncology 1994;8(5):25–31.

37. Martini N, Kris MG, Flehinger BJ, et al. Preoperative chemotherapy for stage IIIA (N2) lung cancer: the Sloan-Kettering experience with 136 patients. Ann Thorac Surg 1993;55:1365–1374.

38. Rusch VW, Albain KS, Crowley JJ, et al. Surgical resection of stage IIIA and IIIB non-small-cell lung cancer after concurrent induction chemoraditherapy. A Southwest Oncology Group Trial. J Thorac Cardiovasc Surg 1993;105:97–106.

39. Schaake-Koning C, Van Den Bogaert W, Dalesio O. Effects of concomitant cisplatin and radiotherapy on inoperable non-small-cell lung cancer. N Engl J Med 1992;326:524–530.

40. Roth JA, Fossella F, Komaki R, et al. A randomized trial comparing perioperative chemotherapy and surgery with surgery alone in resectable stage IIIA non-small-cell lung cancer. J Natl Cancer Inst 1994;86:673–680.

41. Dillman RO, Seagren SL, Propert KJ, et al. A randomized trial of induction chemotherapy plus high-dose radiation versus radiation alone in stage III non-small-cell lung cancer. N Engl J Med 1990;323:940–945.

42. Rosell R, Gomez-Codina J, Camps C, et al. A randomized trial comparing preoperative chemotherapy plus surgery with surgery alone in patients with non-small-cell lung cancer. N Engl J Med 1994;330:153–158.

43. Bolla M, Gonzalez D, Warde P, et al. Immediate hormonal therapy improves locoregional control and survival in patients with locally advanced prostate cancer: results of a randomized phase III clinical trial of the EORTC Radiotherapy and Genito-urinary Tract Cancer Cooperative Groups. Proc ASCO 1996;15:238.

44. Oesterling JE, Martin SK, Bergstrahl EJ, et al. The use of prostate-specific antigen in staging patients with newly diagnosed prostate cancer. JAMA 1993;269:57–60.

45. Lerner SE, Blute ML, Lieber MM, et al. Morbidity of contemporary radical retropubic prostatectomy for localized prostate cancer. Oncology 1995;9(5):379–386.

46. Catalona WJ, Basler JW. Return of erections and urinary continence following nerve sparing radical retropubic prostatectomy. J Urol 1993; 150:905–907.

47. Herskovic A, Martz K, Al-Sarraf M, et al. Combined chemotherapy and radiotherapy compared with radiotherapy alone in patients with cancer of the esophagus. N Engl J Med 1992; 326:1593–1598.

48. Walsh TN, Noonan N, Hollywood D, et al. A comparison of multimodality therapy and surgery for esophageal adenocarcinoma. N Engl J Med 1996;335:462–467.

49. Khandelwal M. Palliative therapy for carcinoma of the esophagus. Comprehensive Ther 1995;21: 177–183.

50. Tester W, Caplan R, Heaney J, et al. Neoadjuvant combined modality program with selective organ preservation for invasive bladder cancer: results of Radiation Therapy Oncology Group phase II trial 8802. J Clin Oncol 1996;14: 119–126.

51. Schultz PK, Herr HW, Zhang ZF, et al. Neoadjuvant chemotherapy for invasive bladder cancer: prognostic factors for survival of patients treated with M-VAC with 5-year follow-up. J Clin Oncol 1994;12:1394–1401.

52. Kaufman DS, Shipley WU, Griffin PP, et al. Selective bladder preservation by combination treatment of invasive bladder cancer. N Engl J Med 1993;329:1377–1382.

53. Cameron JL. The current management of carcinoma of the head of the pancreas. Annu Rev Med 1995;46:361–370.

54. Gastrointestinal Tumor Study Group. Further evidence of effective adjuvant combined radiation and chemotherapy following curative resection of pancreatic cancer. Cancer 1987;59:2006–2010.

55. Shah JP, Lydiatt W. Treatment of cancer of the head and neck. CA 1995;45:352–368.

56. El-Sayed S, Nelson N. Adjuvant and adjunctive chemotherapy in the management of squamous cell carcinoma of the head and neck region: a meta-analysis of prospective and randomized trials. J Clin Oncol 1996;14:838–847.

57. Leichman L, Nigro N, Vaitkevicius VK, et al. Cancer of the anal canal: model for preoperative adjuvant combined modality therapy. Am J Med 1985;78:211–215.

58. Clarke-Pearson DL, Bandy LC, Dudzinski M, et al. Computed tomography in evaluation of patients with ovarian carcinoma in complete clinical remission. JAMA 1986;255:627–630.

59. NIH Consensus Development Panel on Ovarian Cancer. Ovarian cancer: screening, treatment, and follow-up. JAMA 1995;273:491–497.

60. Minton JP, Hoehn JL, Gerber DM, et al. Results of a 400-patient carcinoembryonic antigen second-look colorectal cancer study. Cancer 1985;55:1284–1290.

61. Moertel CG, Fleming TR, MacDonald JS, et al. The value of serum carcinoembryonic antigen in predicting recurrent disease following curative resection of colorectal cancer. JAMA 1993;270:943–947.

62. McCall JL, Black RB, Rich CA, et al. The value of serum carcinoembryonic antigen in predicting recurrent disease following curative resection of colorectal cancer. Dis Colon Rectum 1994;37:875–888.

63. Putnam JB, Roth JA, Wesley MN, et al. Analysis of prognostic factors in patients undergoing resection of pulmonary metastases from soft tissue sarcomas. J Thorac Cardiovasc Surg 1984;87:260–268.

64. Dresler CM, Goldberg M. Surgical management of lung metastases: selection factors and results. Oncology 1996;10:649–655.

65. Patchell RA, Tibbs PA, Walsh JW, et al. A randomized trial of surgery in the treatment of single metastases to the brain. N Engl J Med 1990;322:494–500.

66. Alexander E III, Moriarty TM, Davis RB, et al. Stereotactic radiosurgery for the definitive, noninvasive treatment of brain metastases. J Natl Cancer Inst 1995;87:34–40.

67. Ahmann FR. A reassessment of the clinical implications of the superior vena caval syndrome. J Clin Oncol 1984;2:961–969.

68. Hausheer FH, Yarbro JW. Diagnosis and treatment of malignant pleural effusion. Semin Oncol 1985;12:54–75.

69. Walker-Renard PB, Vaughan LM, Sahn SA. Chemical pleurodesis for malignant pleural effusions. Ann Intern Med 1994;120:56–64.

70. Ruckdescel J, Moores D, Lee L, et al. Management of malignant pleural effusion: a randomized comparison of tetracycline and bleomycin. Proc ASCO 1990;9:323.

71. Posner MR, Cohen GI, Skavin AT. Pericardial disease in patients with cancer. The differentiation of malignant from idiopathic and radiation-induced pericarditis. Am J Med 1981;71:407–414.

72. Davis S, Rambotti P, Grignani F. Intrapericardial tetracycline sclerosis in the treatment of malignant pericardial effusion: an analysis of thirty-three cases. J Clin Oncol 1984;2:631–636.

73. Lacy JH, Wieman TJ. Management of malignant ascites. Surg Gynecol Oncol 1984;159:397–412.

74. Cheung DK, Raaf JH. Selection of patients with malignant ascites for a peritoneovenous shunt. Cancer 1982;50:1204–1209.

75. Shapirp MJ. Management of malignant biliary obstruction: nonoperative and palliative techniques. Oncology 1995;9:493–499.

76. Harrington KD. The role of surgery in the management of pathologic fractures. Orthop Clin North Am 1977;8:841–859.

77. Townsend PW, Rosenthal HG, Smalley SR, et al. Impact of postoperative radiation therapy and other perioperative factors on outcome after orthopedic stabilization of impending or pathologic fractures due to metastatic disease. J Clin Oncol 1994;12:2345–2350.

78. Rodichok LD, Harper GR, Ruckdeschel JC, et al. Early diagnosis of spinal epidural metastases. Am J Med 1981;70:1181–1187.

79. Maranzano E, Latini P. Effectiveness of radiation therapy without surgery in metastatic spinal cord compression: final results from a prospective trial. Int J Radiat Oncol Biol Phys 1995;32:959–967.

80. Warrell RP. Etiology and current management of cancer-related hypercalcemia. Oncology 1992;6(10):37–43.

81. Theriault RL. Hypercalcemia of malignancy: pathophysiology and implications for treatment. Oncology 1993;7:47–50.

82. Jacoux A, Carr DB, Payne R, et al. Management of cancer pain. Clinical Practice Guideline No. 9: AHCPR Publication No. 94-0592. Rockville, MD: Agency for Health Care Policy and Research, U.S. Department of Health and Human Services, Public Health Service, 1994.

83. Rummanns TA. Nonopiod agents for treatment of acute and subacute pain. Mayo Clin Proc 1994;69:481–490.

17
Infectious Disease

John Stuckey and Richard J. Gross

Both historically and currently, infections have been frequent and major complications of surgical procedures. Postoperatively, infections occur both locally, at the operative as well as distant sites (1–8), and systemically (e.g., bacteremia).

Nosocomial infections occur in approximately 7% of surgical patients, and nosocomial bacteremia occurs in approximately 0.9% of such patients. The reported incidence of localized infections, however, varies widely. Approximately 80% of postsurgical infections involve the superficial wound (24% of such infections), deep wound (i.e., organ/space) (13%), urinary tract (27%), and respiratory tract (15%). (The new terminology of wound infections as surgical site infections is discussed later.) Less frequent are primary bloodstream infections (7%) and those at other sites (15%) (8). Urinary tract infection (UTI) is the most common cause of fever and bacteremia, mainly as a result of catheterization, although such infection has been less frequent in recent studies (27–40%). Whereas respiratory infections are the third most common infection, they are the leading cause of death resulting from nosocomial infection in postoperative patients (8, 9). Wound infection rates have ranged widely, from 3 to 11% in different hospitals and from 0 to 17% for different operations (8, 10–13) (Table 17.1).

The most common organisms involved have been *Staphylococcus aureus* and Gram-negative organisms, and over the past decade, Gram-negative organisms other than *Escherichia coli* have increased in frequency, especially *Pseudomonas*, *Klebsiella*, and *Serratia* sp. An increasing problem has been infection with organisms that are highly resistant to antibiotics, especially methicillin-resistant *Staphylococcus aureus* and vancomycin-resistant *Enterococcus* sp. An increase in fungal infections, especially with *Candida albicans*, also has occurred.

The most important factors contributing to infection are the type of surgery, instrumentation used (especially Foley catheters, endotracheal tubes, and intravenous lines), duration of the procedure, and any underlying medical diseases (discussed later). Other important predisposing factors are previous use of antibiotics and of steroids and immunosuppressives.

This chapter first considers the prevention of surgical infection by use of prophylactic antibiotics. It must not be forgotten, however, that proper surgical technique, postoperative care, and appropriate use of invasive catheters are of primary importance in the prevention of postoperative infection. Treatment of the occasional patient with an infection that is unrelated to the reason for surgery and in whom surgery cannot be postponed also is discussed, as is the diagnosis and management of major infections in the postoperative period.

Table 17.1.   Rate of Wound Infections in Selected Procedures

	Infection Rate (%)	
	Multicenter Study (10)	Cruse (11, 12, 22)
All operations	7.5[a]	5.1
Nonbody cavity		
Mastectomy (modified radical)		4.2
Fractured hip		4.2
Meniscectomy		0.5
Abdominal		
"Negative" laparotomy	1.9	0.5
Partial gastrectomy	10.1	14.4
Partial colectomy	10.0[b]	17.6
Cholecystectomy	6.9	2.0
Inguinal hernia	1.9	0.5
Appendectomy	11.4	6.4
Pelvic		
Abdominal hysterectomy	6.1	4.2
Thoracic		
Pulmonary resection (lobectomy)	6.9	5.5
Vascular		
Femoral-popliteal bypass		8

[a]Range, 3–11% in different hospitals.
[b]Range, 5–20% in different hospitals.

PROPHYLACTIC ANTIBIOTICS

Antibiotics are widely used to prevent postoperative infections. Such infections contribute significantly to the postoperative mortality rate, patient discomfort, late or permanent complications (e.g., enlarged scars or adhesions), prolonged hospitalization (an average of 7–9 days for wound infections), and cost.

The risk of postoperative infection must be balanced against the staggering use of antibiotics for prophylaxis of surgical infection. Prophylactic antibiotics are used in approximately 20% of patients undergoing surgery, and they account for 30% of all antimicrobial drugs used in the hospital setting. In the past, major criticisms of prophylactic antibiotics have included their widespread use for procedures with no apparent benefit and the administration of irrational drug regimens. These criticisms have been largely replaced by issues such as the duration of prophylaxis, the use of cheaper versus more expensive regimens, and use during procedures in which the benefit is small although statistically significant. Internists are increasingly involved in the debate over surgical antibiotic prophylaxis because of questions from antibiotic utilization committees and the need to know the limitations of prophylaxis when providing postoperative consultation.

The definition of *prophylactic antibiotics* is the use of antibiotics *prior* to the establishment of organisms at a given site to prevent clinical infection. Recent contamination is included within the definition of prophylaxis by many authors. Some contaminated and most "dirty" procedures fall in this category (e.g., perforated viscus, abdominal trauma).

There are important theoretic and empirical differences when antibiotics are administered after, rather than prior to, contamination, however, including risk of infection, timing, and duration of "prophylaxis." The effectiveness of antibiotics decreases in a linear fashion with the amount of time since the introduction of bacteria. For example, antibiotics were ineffective when administered 3 hours after contamination in an animal model (14, 15) (Fig. 17.1). Antibiotic treatment may be required for a longer period when gross spillage from a viscus occurs.

The types of infection prevented by prophylactic antibiotics must be clearly understood. Most prophylactic antibiotics used in the surgical setting are given to prevent a single infectious complication (i.e., wound infection). Prevention of deeper infection (e.g., at the site of intestinal anastomosis) is a less common reason. Antibiotics also are administered to prevent both infection at the site of a foreign body or graft insertion and sepsis. Attempts to prevent "all" infections have failed because of the many types of bacteria and the varying times of their introduction. With few exceptions, antibiotics are not effective at preventing infections that are remote from the operative site and not directly related to surgery (e.g., pneumonia, UTI).

Superficial wound infections have a low mortality rate unless other factors (e.g., malnutrition) are present. Morbidity, including discomfort and scarring, is frequent, however. Thus the prevention of morbidity is quantitatively more important than the prevention of mortality. This issue also must be considered when evaluating antibiotic trials, because sample sizes often are not large enough to demonstrate a difference in mortality rates.

Multiple reasons have been cited both for and against the use of prophylactic antibiotics (Table 17.2). However, no convincing decision can be made strictly on the basis of theoretic arguments. The discussion here focuses on wound infection, for which substantial data have been accumulated. (Other types of infections are discussed later under individual headings).

Pathophysiology of Incisional Wound Infection (Surgical Site Infection)

In 1992, the U.S. Centers for Disease Control and Prevention (CDC), the Surgical Infection Society, and others changed the term *wound infections* to *surgical site infections* (SSIs) (16). The new terminology includes both incisional wound infection, including skin and subcutaneous tissues, and deeper "organ/space" infections. In the 1992 modification, three categories of SSI (Fig. 17.2) were defined: *(a)* superficial incisional SSI, *(b)* deep

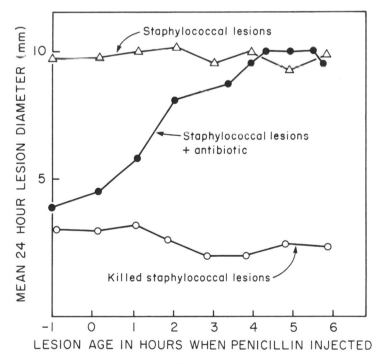

Figure 17.1. Prevention of wound infection by antibiotics in a guinea pig model. The size of the lesion was related to the timing of the antibiotics and infection. The antibiotic (penicillin) was most effective when given before introduction of staphylococci. No difference between treated and untreated animals was seen when antibiotics were given 4 hours or longer after infection. (Reprinted with permission from Burke JF. The effective period of preventive antibiotic action on experimental infections and dermal lesions. Surgery 1961;50:162.)

incisional SSI, and *(c)* organ-space SSI. SSIs represent 37% of all nosocomial infections. Overall rates of SSI are approximately 2.5% but vary depending on several factors. The remainder of this section discusses the pathophysiology of incisional wound infections; that of deeper infections is discussed later.

The development of a wound infection depends on three factors: *(a)* bacterial contamination, *(b)* systemic resistance, and *(c)* local factors (15). A surgical wound may be contaminated by bacteria originating from incompletely prepped skin, breaks in the sterility of the operative technique, surgery performed on infected or contaminated tissue, perforation of viscus, and contamination of the operating room environment. The most common sources of bacteria for wound infection are the patient's own microbial flora; operating room staff are a significantly less common source (and other sources even more uncommon) (17). Bacteremic seeding from distant sites and contaminated prosthetic devices or instruments are also less common sources of bacterial contamination (15).

The quantity of bacteria is a determinant of wound infection, but the type of bacteria also is important. Certain species, such as *Staphylococcus*, are more likely to produce actual infection. Contamination by more than one bacterial species also may influence the development of infection.

The major systemic factor influencing infection rates is nutrition. Other important systemic factors are age of the patient and diseases that decrease the host response to infection (14).

Local defenses at the wound site are important in determining whether infection occurs after contamination. Important local factors are the presence of nonviable tissue, presence of a foreign body or drainage, ability to mount a local inflammatory response, and duration of the surgery. Surgical skill is a real, but poorly defined, factor as well, as shown by the widely varying rates of wound infection between hospitals and surgeons (10–12).

Burke showed the importance of the timing of antibiotic administration in a classic series of experiments (14, 15). When given from 1 hour before to 3 hours after the introduction of bacteria, antibiotics were effective in preventing experimental staphylococcal wound infections.

Table 17.2. Reasons For and Against Use of Prophylactic Antibiotics

For	Against

1. Prevent frequent morbidity and mortality	1. a. Many human trials equivocal or negative
	   b. Increased risk of superinfection and/or resistant organisms
	   c. Toxicity of antibiotics

2. Decrease hospitalization and cost (by preventing complications)	2. High cost of antibiotics; use in large numbers of patients
3. Animal data support efficacy	3. Only good animal model is for wound infection; some experiments negative
4. a. Do no harm b. Avert use of toxic antibiotics for prolonged periods to treat infection	4. Toxicity of antibiotics; use in large numbers of patients
5. Theoretically should work	5. Do not work in practice in many situations
6. Certain patients at high risk of infection (impaired defenses, certain operations)	6. Risk factors and natural history of infections often not well understood (exception: wound infections)

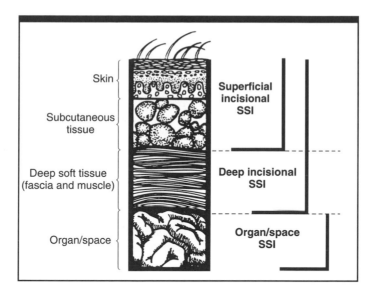

Figure 17.2. Surgical site infection (SSI): anatomy and classification. (Reprinted with permission from Horan TC, Gaynes RP, Martone WJ, Jarvis WR, Emori TG. CDC definitions of nosocomial surgical site infections, 1992: a modification of CDC definitions or surgical wound infections. Infect Control Hosp Epidemiol 1992;13:606–608.)

Animals given antibiotics more than 3 hours after bacterial contamination had similar wound infection rates as the control animals. Infection rates were lowest when antibiotics were given from 1 hour before the introduction of bacteria and rose in a linear fashion until 3 hours after colonization, when infection rates were similar to those of controls (Fig. 17.1).

For many operations, human trials have shown that a single preoperative dose is as effective as continuing antibiotic prophylaxis postoperatively. Data from these experiments have been used to justify the need to start prophylactic antibiotics before the operative procedure and the ineffectiveness of prophylaxis past 0 to 48 hours after the operation.

In clinical (human) studies, contamination of the wound at surgery is the major determinant of wound infection. A standard classification of wounds (**"wound classification"**) is based on the degree of contamination at the time of surgery (Table 17.3). In several studies (10–12), the degree of contamination has closely paralleled the incidence of wound infection (Table 17.4).

Dirty wounds occupy the gray area between prophylaxis and treatment. By definition, bacteria are present in most dirty wounds before surgery but often will present to the physician within the 3-hour period when antibiotics are effective.

Table 17.3.   Classification of Surgical Wounds

Clean: Operation not involving infected areas, traumatic wounds, or entrance into the gastrointestinal, genitourinary, or respiratory tracts. No break in aseptic technique occurred. (If acute inflammation is not present, cholecystectomy, appendectomy, hysterectomy, and urinary tract operations are included in this category.)

Clean-contaminated: The gastrointestinal or respiratory (bronchi or oropharynx) tracts are entered, but no significant spillage or contamination occurs.

Contaminated: Operations involving acute inflammation without pus, major breaks in sterile technique, or fresh traumatic wounds. (Some authors include spillage from a hollow viscus during surgery.)

Dirty: Operations on perforated viscera, abscesses, old (>4 h) traumatic wounds, or where pus is encountered.

Table 17.4. Infection Rates by Wound Classification

	Infection Rate (%)	
	Multicenter Study (10)	Cruse (11, 12, 22)
1. Clean	5.1	1.5
2. Clean-contaminated	10.8	7.7
3. Contaminated	16.3	15.2
4. Dirty[a]	28.6	40.0
Total	7.5	4.7

[a]Dirty wounds occupy the gray area between prophylaxis and treatment. By definition, bacteria are present in most dirty wounds before surgery but often will present to the physician within the 3-hour period when antibiotics are effective. Since antibiotic effectiveness declines even within the 3-hour period after bacterial contamination, we prefer to consider antibiotic therapy of dirty wounds as early treatment.

Since antibiotic effectiveness declines even within that 3-hour period after contamination, we prefer to consider antibiotic therapy of dirty wounds as early treatment rather than as prophylaxis.

Surgical wounds should be classified (Table 17.3) both to decide on the need for prophylaxis in the individual patient and to assess the need for prophylactic antibiotics for a given procedure (18). Other risk factors have been less important than the type of wound, however, in determining the wound infection rate among human studies. Significant determinants include increasing patient age, steroid therapy, obesity, duration of preoperative hospitalization, proper skin preparation, duration of surgery, and number of patients on the ward. Also, certain factors have not been correlated with wound infection, including air colonization (except possibly for clean wounds) and diabetes (10–12, 17).

Two newer classifications have been proposed by the CDC (among others) and are now appearing frequently in the literature. The **SENIC index** (Study on the Efficacy of Nosocomial Infection Control) (19, 20) has shown itself to be a better predictor of wound infection when addi-

tional operative and patient susceptibility factors (Table 17.5) are considered along with the traditional wound classification (Table 17.3). In addition to the wound classification, the SENIC index incorporates the location (abdominal) of surgery, duration of the procedure, and having more than three diagnoses at discharge (i.e., a proxy factor incorporating how "ill" the patient is generally and how susceptible to infection). The index was approximately twice as proficient at predicting wound infection as the traditional wound classification. A few patients undergoing "clean" surgery were at higher risk (because of multiple other risk factors) than patients undergoing contaminated surgery (19, 21).

A newer modification, the **National Nosocomial Infection Surveillance System (NNISS)** index defined an SSI risk index in terms of patient-dependent variables (20, 22). This modified index (1990) is used today to identify patients at risk. The risk index score is calculated from the sum of three variables: (a) the American Society of Anesthesiologists (ASA) risk category, (b) operation class

Table 17.5. Wound Infection Risk (Senic) Index

Factor	Points
1. Abdominal operation	1
2. Operation lasting >2 hours	1
3. Contaminated or dirty infected operation (by traditional wound classification system)	1
4. Having ≥3 diagnoses	1
Total possible points	0–4

Total Points	Wound Infection Risk (%)
0	1
1	4
2	9
3	17
4	27

From Haley RW, Culver DH, Morgan WM, et al. Identifying patients at high risk of surgical wound infection. Am J Epidemiol 1985;121:206–215.

Table 17.6.   National Nosocomial Infection Surveillance System (NNISS) Index

Factor	Points
1. American Society of Anesthesiologists' class 3, 4, or 5	1
2. Operation classified as contaminated or dirty-infected	1
3. Duration of surgery over T hours[a]	1
Total possible points	0–3

Total Points	Wound Infection Risk (%)
0	1.5
1	2.9
2	6.8
3	13.0

From Culver DH, Horan TC, Gaynes RP, et al. Surgical wound infection rates by wound class, operative procedure, and patient risk index. Am J Med 1991;91(Suppl 3B):152S–157S.
[a]T varies with the type of surgery.

(i.e., contaminated or dirty), and *(c)* duration of the operation based on the 75th percentile for that category of procedure (22). Overall rates based on risk category are shown in Table 17.6; rates for selected individual surgical procedures by risk index are shown in Table 17.7. Note that higher infection rates are associated with higher risk indexes. Rates have declined with the widespread use of prophylactic antibiotics.

Prophylactic antibiotics are not indicated for most clean surgeries because of their low rates of infection. By its nature, prophylaxis will only prevent a proportion of infections, so substantial benefit will be difficult to achieve if baseline infection rates are low. For this reason, many experts feel that the benefit of prophylactic antibiotics in this situation is unproven despite the small, statistically significant benefits found in some randomized trials (21).

Principles for Use of Prophylactic Antibiotics

Several factors are frequently cited as common elements of an effective prophylactic antibiotic regimen (Table 17.8). These principles have been developed on the basis of clinical experience and the comparison of successful and unsuccessful prophylactic regimens.

Ideally, prophylaxis is given for infections caused by a single or a few organisms, and it is introduced during a relatively short period of time. The type of infection in question should occur with sufficient frequency or severity that the benefits of prophylaxis outweigh the risks. Wound infections are generally preventable, because they are caused by a few species of bacteria introduced at the time of surgery. Conversely, postoperative UTIs and pneumonia are poor targets for prophylaxis, because they can be caused by a large variety of bacteria at any time during hospitalization.

The antibiotics used should cover most or all of the important organisms, but all possible infecting agents need not—and often cannot—be covered. The antibiotics used should be of the narrowest spectrum possible, the least toxic, and the lowest cost. Whereas multiple-antibiotic regimens are equivalent, "first-line" antibiotics should be avoided to decrease the acquisition of resistance by organisms within the hospital. The antibiotics should be administered for as briefly as possible (usually >1 hour preoperatively and >24 hours postoperatively; one to two doses total often are sufficient), before contamination, and in adequate doses to achieve therapeutic serum-tissue levels throughout the entire operative period. Additional doses may be needed during surgery for prolonged operations or when the half-life of the antibiotic is short.

Despite prophylactic antibiotics, infections will still occur due to local factors and drug-resistant organisms. Infections remote from the site targeted for prophylaxis will not be decreased and may even be increased, especially if prophylaxis is prolonged.

Human Trials

A large number of clinical trials have been conducted in the past 30 years to

Table 17.7. SSI Rates by Operative Procedure and Risk Index Category: Surgical Patient Component, January 1987 to September 1994

	Operative Procedure Category	Duration Cut Point	Risk Index	n	Rate	Risk Index	n	Rate	Risk Index	n	Rate	Risk Index	n	Rate
CARD	Cardiac surgery	5	0.1	5088	2.02	2.3	1191	5.29	—	—	—	—	—	—
CBGB	CABG-chest & leg	5	0	819	1.59	1	32,065	3.15	2.3	7745	5.76	—	—	—
CBGC	CABG-chest only	5	0.1	1046	1.91	2.3	213	5.16	—	—	—	—	—	—
OCVS	Other cardiovascular system	2	0.1, 2.3	4202	0.83		—	—		—	—		—	—
ORES	Other respiratory system	1	0.1, 2.3	929	4.52		—	—		—	—		—	—
THOR	Thoracic surgery	3	0	914	0.44	1	2146	1.82	2.3	660	3.48		—	—
APPY	Appendectomy	1	0	2834	1.27	1	2592	3.36	2.3	920	6.41		—	—
BILI	Liver/pancreas	4	0	262	2.29	1	473	6.13	2.3	200	13.50		—	—
CHOL	Cholecystectomy	2	0	11,491	0.86	1	8060	1.81	2	2167	3.55	3	224	6.25
COLO	Colon resection	3	0	3334	3.99	1	5286	6.47	2	2298	11.27	3	228	17.98
GAST	Gastrectomy	3	0	946	3.59	1	1631	5.89	2.3	603	14.43		—	—
OGIT	Other digestive system	3	0	914	1.97	1	1178	4.24	2.3	351	7.69		—	—
SB	Small bowel surgery	3	0	497	5.03	1	906	8.83	2.3	569	13.18		—	—
XLAP	Laparotomy	2	0	2913	2.06	1	2910	3.51	2.3	1453	9.08		—	—
NEPH	Nephrectomy	3	0.1, 2.3	1004	2.09		—	—		—	—		—	—
OGU	Other genitourinary	2	0	10,288	0.54	1	3608	1.16	2.3	708	5.23		—	—
PRST	Prostatectomy	4	0	984	0.71	1, 2, 3	917	3.16		—	—		—	—
HN	Head and neck	5	0	672	1.49	1	603	4.48	2.3	226	11.95		—	—
OENT	Other ear, nose, and throat	2	0.1	2134	0.47	2	177	3.39	3	14	21.43		—	—
HER	Herniorrhaphy	2	0	3957	1.19	1	2509	1.95	2.3	394	3.81		—	—
MAST	Mastectomy	2	0	2841	1.06	1	2931	1.94	2.3	356	5.34		—	—
CRAN	Craniotomy	5	0.1, 2.3	4350	1.49	1, 2.3	—	—		—	—		—	—

Code	Procedure			N	Rate		N	Rate		N	Rate		N	Rate
ONS	Other nervous system	3	0, 1, 2, 3	1752	1.43	—	—	—	—	—	—	—	—	—
VSHN	Ventricular shunt	2	0, 1, 2, 3	2182	3.90	—	—	—	—	—	—	—	—	—
CSEC	Cesarean section	1	0, 1	33,005	3.41	2, 3	586	7.17	—	—	—	—	—	—
HYST	Abdominal hysterectomy	2	0	10,004	1.51	1	4842	2.50	2, 3	785	5.48	—	—	—
OOB	Other obstetric	1	0	253	0.00	1, 2, 3	66	3.03	—	—	—	—	—	—
VHYS	Vaginal hysterectomy	2	0	3819	0.86	1, 2, 3	1779	2.02	—	—	—	—	—	—
AMP	Limb amputation	1	0, 1, 2, 3	4149	4.48	—	—	—	—	—	—	—	—	—
FUS	Spinal fusion/laminectomy[a]	3	0	19,806	0.91	1	8142	2.24	2, 3	1805	5.54	—	—	—
FUSN	Spinal fusion	4	0	534	0.94	1, 2, 3	423	4.49	—	—	—	—	—	—
LAM	Laminectomy	2	0, 1, 2, 3	1892	1.16	—	—	—	—	—	—	—	—	—
FX	Open reduction of fracture	2	0	5670	0.95	1	7221	1.59	2	1485	2.90	3	135	8.15
OMS	Other musculoskeletal	3	0, 1	13,909	0.73	2, 3	1028	2.43	—	—	—	—	—	—
PROS	Joint prosthesis[b]	3	0	13,666	1.08	1	12,522	1.97	2, 3	1402	4.14	—	—	—
HPRO	Hip prosthesis	2	0	641	0.62	1, 2, 3	1396	1.65	—	—	—	—	—	—
KPRO	Knee prosthesis	2	0, 1	1729	1.04	2, 3	339	2, 65	—	—	—	—	—	—
OPRO	Other prosthesis	2	0, 1, 2, 3	174	1.15	—	—	—	—	—	—	—	—	—
OBL	Other hematologic/lymphatic	3	0	449	0.45	1, 2, 3	420	2.62	—	—	—	—	—	—
OES	Other endocrine system	2	0, 1, 2, 3	1617	0.62	—	—	—	—	—	—	—	—	—
OEYE	Other eye	2	0, 1, 2, 3	1367	0.15	—	—	—	—	—	—	—	—	—
OSKN	Other integumentary system	2	0, 1	4339	1.71	2, 3	731	3.15	—	—	—	—	—	—
SKGR	Skin graft	2	0	779	1.28	1	1158	3.45	2	511	6.65	3	99	12.12
SPLE	Splenectomy	2	0, 1	508	2.56	2, 3	160	6.25	—	—	—	—	—	—
TP	Organ transplant	7	0, 1, 2	1202	6.82	3	192	20.31	—	—	—	—	—	—
VS	Vascular surgery	3	0	2633	1.41	1	12,393	2.03	2	4892	5.50	3	123	12.20

From: Hospital Infections, Program: "National Nosocomial Infections Surveillance (NNIS) Seminannual Report, May 1995." Am J Infect Control 1995;23:377–380.

CABG, Coronary artery bypass graft.

[a]Procedure category was split in June 1994 into FUSN and LAM.

[b]Procedure category was split in June 1994 into HPRO, KPRO, and OPRO.

Table 17.8.   Principles of Successful Prophylactic Antibiotic Regimens

Procedure
1. Infection to be prevented is clearly specified (e.g., wound)
2. Period when bacteria can be introduced is brief
3. One or few organisms cause most infections
4. High enough risk of infection that prophylaxis is beneficial

Antibiotics
5. Antibiotics cover important organisms; narrow spectrum (all organisms need not be covered)
6. Use least toxic drugs
7. Avoid "first line" antibiotics that may be needed for infection, if other agents effective (because of resistance). Use least expensive drugs.
8. Administer before contamination
9. Therapeutic serum-tissue levels through entire period of operation when contamination occurs
10. Administer for as short a duration as possible and only during period when prophylaxis is effective. Avoid administration >1 h preoperatively and prolonged administration (usually >48 hr) postoperatively

determine appropriate indications and use of prophylactic antibiotics. Many older ones, however, had faulty study designs (23), and many recent ones are intended to obtain a U.S. Food and Drug Administration indication for a new antibiotic and contain a sample size that is too small to reach adequate conclusions. In between are the classic, well-controlled studies, mainly from the 1970 to 1980, which form the basis for current recommendations. In reviewing the studies under the individual discussions that follow, the selected major points for adequate study design listed in Table 17.9 should be considered. The most important are representative patient populations, randomization, clear definition of the type of infection to be prevented, and adequate as well as blinded evaluation of the patient.

Because of the many studies comparing new drugs, the fact that many classic studies are now more than a decade old, and space limitations, comprehensive

tables of the clinical trials of prophylactic antibiotics do not appear in this edition. For each type of surgery, a literature review, classic article, or definitive source is cited instead. There is no consensus even among authoritative sources (7, 24–26) on preferred antibiotic choices and indications; the reader should understand this when reading the recommendations. Prophylactic antibiotics for burns, UTIs, and ears, nose, and throat (ENT) procedures are covered elsewhere in this text. Recommended prophylactic antibiotic regimens are summarized in Table 17.10.

Pneumonia

Rationale

Postoperative pneumonia accounts for 15% of postoperative infections, and it is the leading cause of death from nosocomial infection. The mortality rate of noso-

Table 17.9.   Criteria for Adequate Study Design for Clinical Trials of Antibiotic Prophylaxis[a]

1. Prospective, randomized design (includes concurrent controls)
2. Sample stratified by risk or extent of disease before randomization
3. Adequate sample size from a defined, representative population undergoing a single procedure
4. Double-blinded design
5. Antibiotic present before bacteria introduced (prophylaxis vs treatment)
6. Diagnostic criteria for infection objective and specific. Relevant outcomes measured (mortality, number of infections). All possible infections cultured.
7. Antibiotic active against relevant organisms; first dose administered preoperatively; adequate dose and limited duration of administration. Proof target organisms are susceptible.
8. Count antibiotic complications including drug toxicity, superinfection, and change in resistance patterns
9. All patients randomized included in analysis
10. Statistical testing performed

[a]Variables that are not adequate end points are fever, change in colonization, and sterile cultures in absence of clinical infection.

Table 17.10. Recommended Antimicrobial Prophylaxis for Surgery[a, b]

Type of Surgery	Recommended Regimens		Specific Regimens	Postoperative Frequency and Duration[a]	Notes
	First Choice	Alternative			
Gastrointestinal					
Upper gastrointestinal	Cephalosporin	Uncertain	Cefazolin (1 g)	Every 6–8 h for 1 dose to 24 h	Not indicated for uncomplicated peptic ulcer surgery
Colon and rectum	1. Neomycin-erythromycin ± 2. Cephalosporin, high-risk patients only	1. Cephalosporin *or* 2. Metronidazole ± aminoglycoside	Neomycin (1 g) and erythromycin base (1 g) at 1 PM, 2 PM, 11 PM day before surgery Cephalothin (2 g)	None given postoperatively Every 6 h for 1–4 doses	Neomycin and erythromycin preferable for high-risk patients Cefoxitin (2 g)
Cholecystectomy	Cephalosporin	Uncertain	Cefazolin (1 g)	Every 6–8 h for 12–24 h	High-risk patients only
Orthopaedics					
Hip fractures	Cephalosporin	Semisynthetic penicillin	Nafcillin (500 mg–1 g)	Every 6 h for 24 h	
Total hip replacement	Cephalosporin	Semisynthetic penicillin	Cefazolin (1 g)	Every 6 h for 24 h	
Lower extremity amputation for ischemia	Cefoxitin	Uncertain	Cefixitin (2 g)	Every 6 h for 24 h	

Table 17.10. Recommended Antimicrobial Prophylaxis for Surgery *(continued)*

Type of Surgery	Recommended Regimens		Specific Regimens	Postoperative Frequency and Duration[a]	Notes
	First Choice	Alternative			
Otolaryngology	Cephalosporin	Uncertain	Cefazolin (1 g)	Every 6 h for 4 doses	Indicated only for extensive cancer surgery or entry into oropharynx
Pulmonary gynecology					
Vaginal hysterectomy	Cephalosporin	Uncertain	Cephalothin (1–2 g); cefazolin (1 g)	Every 6 h for 12–18 h	? Premenopausal only
Abdominal hysterectomy	Cephalosporin	Uncertain	Cephalothin (1–2 g); cefazolin (1 g)	Every 6 h for 12–18 h	
Urology					
Transurethral prostate resection					Treat preoperative infection by sensitivities; no routine prophylaxis if urine sterile See text
Neurosurgery/vascular surgery	Cephalosporin	Uncertain	Cefazolin (1 g)	Every 6 h for 4 doses	Not indicated for upper extremity procedures

[a]Timing of administration. *Initial dose:* all regimens require one dose preoperatively within 1 hour of surgery; a second dose in the operating room may be necessary for surgery lasting more than 4 hours or the expected duration of action of the antibiotic. *Duration:* most regimens should be stopped within 24 hours postoperatively. Data for most procedures suggest 1–3 total doses (including preoperative dose) are sufficient (see text); colorectal procedures may be an exception.
[b]For most indications, second- and third-generation cephalosporins have not been shown to be superior to first-generation cephalosporins.

comial pneumonia ranges from 30 to 70%. Gram-negative pneumonias carry the highest mortality rate, ranging from 40 to 70%.

High-risk groups include patients who are in coma, in intensive care units (ICUs), and who are on respirators, intubated, using respiratory care equipment, or debilitated. Postoperative pneumonia does not fit the criteria for prophylaxis (Table 17.8) because of the wide variety of possible organisms, the rapid acquisition of new organisms, and the prolonged period in which the patient is at risk.

Clinical Studies

Antibiotics alone do not decrease postoperative production of purulent sputum or the incidence of pneumonia in trials of antibiotic prophylaxis for wound infection. Increased incidences of Gram-negative organisms in pneumonia, drug-resistant organisms causing pneumonia, and increased incidence of pneumonia have been found in various trials.

Recommendations

Antibiotics should not be used for the prophylaxis of pneumonia in surgical patients.

Appendectomy

Rationale

Wound infection is the only common complication of appendectomy that should be considered for antibiotic prophylaxis. Nonperforated appendectomy is classified as clean, contaminated surgery, because the colonized lower bowel is transected. The rate of wound infection after appendectomy is proportionally high, at approximately 10% (Table 17.1). When the appendix is perforated, this rate is much higher and, in addition, peritonitis or abscess may occur. Antibiotics used for perforated appendices should be considered as treatment rather than prophylaxis, because bacteria are present before the antibiotic is administered.

Clinical Studies

Uncontrolled and comparative studies have found conflicting results when using antibiotics for appendectomy (27–29). A randomized trial of ampicillin or tetracycline compared with controls found no effect on the rate of wound infection (15–20%) or the duration of postoperative fever in patients with uncomplicated, acute appendicitis (i.e., normal appendix or acute, unperforated appendix). A higher incidence of intraperitoneal abscess occurred in the patients not receiving antibiotics, but most were in patients with perforated appendices.

Recommendations

Prophylactic antibiotics for uncomplicated, nonperforated appendectomy are recommended by many authorities. The weight of evidence is beginning to favor prophylaxis using a cephalosporin with anaerobic activity (cefotetan or cefoxitin). Antibiotic treatment should be given for the complications of appendicitis, including perforation, peritonitis, and abscess. Antibiotic treatment depends on the sensitivities of any organisms found and is of a longer duration than prophylaxis (24–26, 29).

Cholecystectomy

Rationale

Antibiotics are given to patients undergoing cholecystectomy to prevent wound infection and cholangitis with resulting septicemia. Presumably, cholangitis and septicemia result from instrumentation and manipulation of a previously colonized biliary tract during surgery.

Clinical Studies

The rate of wound infection after cholecystectomy ranges from 1 to 21% (Table 17.1). The risk of wound infection is substantially higher in the presence of infected bile or complications of cholelithiasis. A high-risk group of patients with a wound infection rate of 20 to 27% can be identified by the presence of five factors: (a) age older than 70 years; (b) obstructive jaundice; (c) common duct stones; (d) emergent, acute cholecystitis; and (e) cholangitis (30). Diabetes also may be a risk factor.

Approximately 17% of patients with none of these factors have infected bile. The risk of wound infection with sterile bile or with none of the listed complications ranges from 1 to 2% (11).

The organisms causing wound infection after cholecystectomy are usually the same Gram-negative organisms found in the biliary tree, and a statistically significant reduction in wound infection (from 11–21% to 2–6%) was found in five randomized studies. Two additional studies showed a similar trend favoring antibiotics, but they did not include any separate statistical analysis (30, 31). A single preoperative dose or three doses immediately perioperatively were as effective as a 5-day course of antibiotics.

The incidence of sepsis following cholecystectomy in patients not treated with antibiotics is up to 10%. A decreased rate of sepsis has been shown in three controlled studies of prophylactic antibiotics, but in each study, either no statistical analysis was performed or the sample size was too small to demonstrate any statistical significance. Risk factors for sepsis are similar to those listed above for wound infection.

Many patients with acute cholecystitis have high fever and leukocytosis. Preoperatively, it may be impossible to tell whether cholangitis, sepsis, or biliary infection is present. In this setting, use of antibiotics represents treatment of a suspected infection rather than prophylaxis.

Recommendations

Use of antibiotic is not recommended for patients with uncomplicated cholecystectomy without clinical cholecystitis or other risk factors (i.e., age >70 years, jaundice, common duct stone, cholecystitis, diabetes mellitus). In the presence of these risk factors, prophylaxis is usually administered, but it is not required in all cases. A cephalosporin antibiotic is recommended. Most studies have used this group of antibiotics, and single studies have indicated that both co-trimoxazole and gentamicin are effective. Some authorities recommend a cephalosporin for all biliary surgery.

Most studies have administered one dose preoperatively and continue prophylaxis for 1 to 2 days postoperatively. One to three perioperative doses, however, are just as effective (24–26, 31).

Upper Gastrointestinal Surgery

Rationale

A moderately high rate of wound infection has been reported following gastroduodenal surgery. Other types of infection and sepsis are unusual in the absence of preexisting infection or perforation.

Clinical Studies

The rate of wound infection following surgery on the stomach or duodenum ranges from 10 to 30% (31) (Table 17.1). The risk is much higher for gastric ulcer or cancer (22–23%) than for uncomplicated duodenal ulcer (4–5%), and this difference has been related to the higher incidence and colony count of bacterial colonization in stomachs with low acidity. Some authors have found an increased incidence of wound infection following emergency surgery for actively bleeding ulcers.

Patients with gastroduodenal resections were included in four randomized studies, although only one examined upper gastrointestinal surgery alone. A statistically significant reduction in wound infections (from 20–35% to 0–5%) was found (31). A cephalosporin was given for a duration of three doses to 5 days.

Recommendations

Use of antibiotics is not indicated for patients undergoing surgery for uncomplicated duodenal ulcer. Prophylaxis should be given when surgery is performed for gastric carcinoma, when gastric bypass is performed for obesity, or in the presence of achlorhydria due to other reasons (e.g., atrophic gastritis, prior gastric resection). Inadequate data are available to make a recommendation concerning gastric ulcer or emergency surgery for gastrointestinal bleeding.

The recommended regimen is a single dose of a cephalosporin given 1 hour preoperatively, which is followed postoperatively for a postoperative duration from 2 doses to 1 day (24–26, 31).

Lower Gastrointestinal (Colorectal) Surgery

Rationale

The clearest rationale for use of prophylactic antibiotics is for surgery on the colon and rectum. The most common postoperative infection after colon surgery is wound infection; less common, but more serious, complications are intraperitoneal abscess, anastomotic breakdown, and sepsis. Infectious complications are a significant contributor to the mortality rate after colectomy (31, 32). Although significant colony counts of multiple aerobic Gram-negative organisms may be cultured from the colon, a much larger number of anaerobic organisms are present.

Clinical Studies

The rate of wound infection in patients undergoing elective colectomy without antibiotics ranges from 10 to 60%. Rates of wound infection among hospitals using a variety of prophylactic regimens have ranged from 5 to 20% (Table 17.1). An increased risk of anastomotic breakdown accompanies a local infection of any type, but it is uncertain whether infection of the suture line is the cause or the result of the breakdown. The risk of bacteremia or septicemia after colectomy ranges from 2 to 10%, and a significant proportion of postoperative mortality is related to postoperative infections of the wound, peritoneum, distant organs, and sepsis.

The rate of wound infection has been significantly reduced in randomized studies using neomycin-erythromycin, neomycin–other antibiotic, and cephalosporins (31, 32). Limited evidence suggests that the rates of anastomotic dehiscence and deep intra-abdominal abscess also are reduced by use of prophylactic oral antibiotics.

The careful, randomized Veterans Administration trial (32) demonstrated that a neomycin-erythromycin combination was superior to a cephalosporin, with a 6% versus 30% rate of wound infection, respectively. A statistically significant reduction also was found for all infectious complications combined (39% versus 6%) and for bacteremia-septicemia (7% versus 1%). There was a slight reduction in mortality, from 4 of 67 patients (6%) in the cephalosporin group to 2 of 126 patients (2%) in the neomycin-erythromycin group, but this change was not statistically significant.

Several trials have demonstrated that a cephalosporin will reduce the rate of wound infection compared with that in groups receiving placebo. The degree of reduction differs among various trials, however, in part because of markedly different rates of infection in the control groups studied. A combination of neomycin-erythromycin and a cephalosporin reduced the wound infection rate still further in one study.

Most studies have administered three doses of neomycin-erythromycin within less than 24 hours preoperatively. Cephalosporins have been administered as a single preoperative dose and been continued postoperatively for a total of three doses to 5 days.

Several older trials tested the efficacy of multiple parenteral antibiotics, including an aminoglycoside or combinations of an aminoglycoside with nonabsorbable antibiotics. Most of these studies were inconclusive in demonstrating a therapeutic effect, but an increased rate of staphylococcal enterocolitis was found when parenteral and oral nonabsorbable antibiotics were combined.

Metronidazole decreases the rate of wound infection both when used alone and in combination with aminoglycosides. Metronidazole has not been used widely for prophylaxis in the United States, however, because of fears of carcinogenesis.

Mechanical preparation of the bowel by laxatives and enemas decreases the quantity of feces and the chance of fecal spillage, but not the concentration of bacteria in the colon. Thus mechanical preparation is important in preventing fecal spillage, but it is not equivalent to antibiotic prophylaxis in reducing the bacterial concentration (32).

Antibiotic prophylaxis for local infection does not reduce the rate of distant pulmonary and UTIs. Cephalosporins have been administered from one dose to 5 days, and Stone et al. (33) found similar rates of wound infection for three perioperative doses of cephalosporin compared with 5 days of administration in various types of abdominal surgery. Among patients undergoing colon resection, 5 of 54 patients (9%) in the three-dose group and 5 of 47 patients (11%) in the 5-day group had wound infections. Two of 54 patients (4%) in the three-dose group and 1 of 47 patients (2%) in the 5-day group had intra-abdominal infections. Subsequent studies have shown that approximately 24 hours of postoperative antibiotics is as effective as longer courses. Single-dose prophylaxis give preoperatively is less effective than when the dose is combined with two to four postoperative doses.

Recommendations

Use of antibiotic prophylaxis is clearly indicated for colon surgery because of the high rate of wound infection, peritoneal infection, and sepsis. Multiple trials have shown that antibiotic prophylaxis at least reduces the incidence of wound infection. Neomycin-erythromycin (Table 17.10) is

an effective regimen, and a cephalosporin administered for one dose preoperatively and less than 48 hours postoperatively reduces the rate of wound infection as well. A cephalosporin is probably less effective than neomycin-erythromycin, however, at least in those settings for which a high rate of infection is suspected.

Oral neomycin-erythromycin is the first-choice prophylactic regimen. In high-risk patients, addition of a parenteral cephalosporin for more than one dose but no more than 24 hours seems to provide added benefit. Cephalothin is effective. At least theoretically, a cephalosporin with anaerobic activity should be more effective, but this has not been convincingly demonstrated in clinical trials. Mechanical preparation with laxatives and enemas should be used in all patients. Regimens that should *not* be used are parenteral, nonabsorbable antibiotic combinations (with the possible exception of cephalosporin with neomycin-erythromycin), parenteral aminoglycosides (as first choice), administration of antibiotics only after surgery, and prolonged antibiotic administration beyond 48 hours after surgery.

Abdominal Trauma

Antibiotics are administered for abdominal trauma due to the possibility of gastrointestinal tract perforation. This use of antibiotics represents treatment, because bacterial contamination occurs at the time of trauma, before the institution of antibiotics. Thus antibiotics for abdominal trauma are discussed in detail in the section on peritoneal infections.

Vascular Surgery

Rationale

Infection of synthetic vascular grafts is devastating in terms of mortality and loss of tissue (i.e., amputation) due to the loss of vascular supply. Antibiotic prophylaxis is used to avoid these devastating consequences even though the rate of infection is believed to be low. A secondary consideration is wound infection. The most common organisms are skin and bowel organisms.

Clinical Studies

The incidence of graft infection after vascular surgery is approximately 2%. The rate of wound infection ranges from 5 to 15% (34).

Two of three randomized trials showed that a cephalosporin given as one dose immediately preoperatively and for 24 hours postoperatively reduced the rate of wound, and possibly graft, infection. Vascular surgery on the upper extremity (i.e., brachiocephalic) has a low risk of infection and may not require prophylaxis. Wound infection in ischemic lower-extremity amputations is reduced by use of antibiotics (35).

Recommendations

Use of prophylactic antibiotics is recommended for vascular surgery, with the possible exception of upper extremity procedures, based on the devastating effects of graft infection despite the low rate of occurrence (2%). Administration of a first-generation cephalosporin immediately preoperatively and for 24 hours postoperatively is the recommended regimen. Prophylaxis with cefoxitin for 24 hours is recommended for ischemic lower-extremity amputations (24–26, 34).

Gynecologic Surgery

The following discussion of gynecologic surgery involves both vaginal and abdominal hysterectomy.

Vaginal Hysterectomy

Rationale A high rate of wound infection in the vaginal cuff accompanies vaginal hysterectomy. More serious, but less common, infections are pelvic cellulitis and adnexal abscesses. Prophylactic antibiotics are mainly given to prevent infections of the vaginal cuff.

Clinical Studies Clinical studies have used two criteria for postoperative infections after vaginal hysterectomy because of the difficulty in being certain of infections being present at the end of the vaginal cuff (i.e., wound infection). *Febrile morbidity* has been defined as a temperature greater than 100.4° to 100.6°F on two separate occasions separated by 6 to 24 hours. *Wound infection* has been defined clinically by appearance of the vaginal cuff and culture of pathogenic bacteria from swabs taken of the vaginal apex. The incidence of febrile morbidity has ranged from 28 to 74% and of clinical vaginal cuff infections from 17 to 64%. The risk of both is higher in patients who are premenopausal.

Multiple studies have shown that use of antibiotics reduces the rate of wound infection (36). The most commonly used antibiotics have been the cephalosporins. A single preoperative dose or one dose preoperatively with two doses postoperatively are as effective as a longer duration of therapy.

Use of prophylactic antibiotics have reduced the rate of febrile morbidity (from 32–74% to 0–24%). The rate of clinical wound infection also has been reduced (from 13–64% to 0–20%). Unlike most other surgical procedures, prophylaxis for vaginal hysterectomy also reduces the rate of UTI in most studies (31, 37–43).

Recommendations Antibiotic prophylaxis should be administered to women undergoing vaginal hysterectomy. Cephalosporins have been the most widely evaluated agents, but ampicillin may be adequate as well. Aminoglycosides are not recommended, however, because less toxic antibiotics are effective. Prophylaxis should continue for 12 to 18 hours after surgery (24–26, 36).

Abdominal Hysterectomy

Rationale The rate of wound infection is lower for abdominal hysterectomy compared with that for the vaginal technique. The major use of prophylactic antibiotics in the setting of abdominal hysterectomy has been to prevent wound infection.

Clinical Studies Substantially less information is available on the usefulness of antibiotics after abdominal hysterectomy compared with after vaginal hysterectomy. Similar to vaginal hysterectomy, infectious complications have been defined as febrile morbidity (temperature >100.4°–100.6°F on two occasions) and clinical wound infection. The rate of febrile morbidity after abdominal hysterectomy has ranged from 26 to 41% and that of clinical wound infection from 11 to 22% (Table 17.15) (36). Use of prophylactic antibiotics have reduced the rate of febrile morbidity (from 23–39% to 8–32%) and that of wound infection (from 11–22% to 0–11%).

Authorities recommend antibiotic prophylaxis with cephalosporins for abdominal hysterectomy (24–26, 36) even though the data are less compelling than for vaginal hysterectomy (36).

Recommendations The recommended regimen is one dose of a cephalosporin given preoperatively through 12 to 18 hours postoperatively (24–26, 36).

Transurethral Prostate Resection

Rationale

Traditionally, prostatectomy has been associated with high rates of morbidity and mortality due to sepsis. The high rate of septic complications was seen with open prostatectomy, however, and with transurethral prostatectomy performed using older techniques. Newer techniques of transurethral prostate resection (TURP) have a low, but significant, rate of asymptomatic bacteremia and a lower rate of clinical sepsis compared with the older techniques. The major focus of antibiotic prophylaxis in this setting is postoperative bacteriuria and symptomatic UTI.

Clinical Studies

Infectious morbidity after TURP includes postoperative fever, bacteriuria (positive urine cultures regardless of symptomology), bacteremia (positive blood cultures), and clinical sepsis (positive blood cultures and clinical picture). The rate of bacteriuria after TURP has ranged widely, from 10 to 100% in different studies. A major influence on this rate is the presence or absence of infection in the preoperative urine. When preoperative urine is sterile, the rate of postoperative bacteriuria ranges from 12 to 54%; when preoperative urine is infected, the rate of postoperative bacteriuria ranges from 28 to 100%. If routine postoperative blood cultures are performed in patients with sterile preoperative urine, the rate of bacteremia ranges from 0 to 11% and clinical sepsis occurs in 0 to 6% of patients. An increased incidence of bacteremia would seem to occur in patients with infected preoperative urine, although data are conflicting.

Postoperative bacteriuria is not restricted to those with preoperative infection, however. Infection may be introduced at the time of surgery or during postoperative catheter drainage. Many studies have examined the effectiveness of antibiotics in preventing postoperative bacteriuria and bacteremia, but most studies cannot be evaluated because of the lack of randomization, inadequate control groups, lack of statistical analysis, and inappropriate antibiotic regimens. Those studies that can be evaluated indicate a decreased rate of postoperative bacteriuria with use of antibiotics, but the differences are not convincing. One study found a decreased rate of postoperative bacteriuria only in those patients without preoperative infection. Inadequate data exist to conclude whether antibiotics prevent symptomatic UTI, bacteremia, or clinical sepsis.

Recommendations

A firm recommendation cannot be made because of the lack of data. Patients undergoing TURP should have a preoperative urine culture. If the urine is infected, a therapeutic course of an appropriate antibacterial agent should be given to cure the infection. The chances of sterilizing the urine temporarily are fair in this situation, but the relapse rate will be high. Patients who are infected immediately before the operation should undergo a short course of antibiotics until the catheter is removed (unless catheter drainage is prolonged). Patients with sterile preoperative urine should not receive prophylactic antibiotics, because there is little evidence of any short- or long-term benefit. Following TURP, all patients should be followed closely for sepsis and treated appropriately. Prophylaxis for bacterial endocarditis is indicated in susceptible patients as well (24–26).

Orthopaedics

Areas of concern regarding orthopaedics include fractures, total hip replacement, and clean orthopaedic surgery.

Hip Fracture

Rationale Antibiotics often are used prophylactically in the repair of hip fractures because of the moderate rate of wound infection as well as the risk of infection in an implanted foreign body. Hip fractures represent a heterogenous group. A variety of procedures involve nails, more complex plate-like devices, and total hip replacements.

Clinical Studies The rate of wound infection following repair of hip fracture is approximately 5%. The rate of deep wound and prosthesis infection, however, is not stated separately in most studies. Boyd et al. (44) found that 10 of 13 patients with wound infection had major problems, but the exact incidence of prosthesis infection was uncertain.

The rate of wound infection was reduced (from 5% to 0.8%) in one well-done, randomized study using nafcillin (one dose preoperatively and eight doses postoperatively). A smaller study with oral cloxacillin showed similar results. Total hip replacements may become infected due to sepsis from distant sources, especially the urinary tract.

Recommendations Reviews of antimicrobial prophylaxis for repair of hip fractures have shown conflicting results because of the low rate of infection and the uncertain rate of more serious deep infection. Metallic hardware is placed in all cases, so prophylaxis usually is given. A cephalosporin should be administered for one dose preoperatively and one dose to 24 hours postoperatively. The duration of prophylaxis also will depend on whether a total artificial hip replacement is inserted (discussed later). For patients in whom prolonged surgery exceeds the duration of action for the antibiotic, a second dose may be needed intraoperatively. Distant infection, especially of the urinary tract, should be treated preoperatively because of the risk for hematogenous seeding of prosthetic devices.

Total Hip Replacement

Rationale Infection of a prosthetic joint has serious consequences, including the requirement for removal of the prosthesis and prolonged antibiotic therapy to eradicate the infection.

Clinical Studies Two randomized trials (45, 46) demonstrated decreased rates of wound infection and of late, deep hip infections with antibiotic prophylaxis during total hip replacement. Retrospective studies have shown a decreased rate of infected prostheses when antibiotic prophylaxis is used, but control groups in these studies have not been adequate. A decreased rate of wound infection also was found in one small, randomized study (44).

A total hip prosthesis may be infected by bacteremia from distant infections, especially of the urinary tract and skin. Infection due to seeding from dental and surgical procedures are rare.

Recommendations A cephalosporin (cefazolin) or, as a second choice, a penicillinase-resistant penicillin should be administered preoperatively and for 24 to 48 hours postoperatively. The current distribution of the types of valvular disease among patients with endocarditis probably is different from that of classic studies. Mitral valve prolapse and diseases found in elderly patients are much more common and rheumatic valvular disease less common, but a recent study of this has not been undertaken (24–26). A second dose of the antibiotic should be given intraoperatively if the procedure exceeds 4 hours or the expected duration of action for the antibiotic. Patients with distant infection (especially of the skin and urinary tract) should be treated with antibiotics and have their operations delayed until the infection has been cleared.

Fractures and Clean Orthopaedic Surgery

Rationale Antibiotics are administered after fractures and clean orthopaedic surgery to decrease the chance of wound infection. Antibiotics also are administered to prevent postoperative osteomyelitis, especially after open fractures. Such administration to open fractures should be considered treatment rather than prophylaxis, however, because bacteria are introduced at the time of fracture and before antibiotic administration.

Clinical Studies The rate of wound infection following clean orthopaedic surgery and repair of closed fractures ranges from 1 to 5%. A significant reduction in this rate (from 5% to 3%) was found in one randomized trial using two doses of cephalosporin. This small difference was significant because of the large size of the patient population in the trial. Use of antibiotics reduced the rate of wound, but not deep, infection when metal devices were inserted to repair fractures.

Recommendations Prophylactic antibiotics should not be used in clean orthopaedic surgery or in the repair of closed fractures. The single randomized study showing a benefit is insufficient evidence to recommend such prophylaxis because of the low baseline rate of infection and the small reduction achieved in the infection rate. A

cephalosporin usually is administered when metal devices are inserted.

Otolaryngology

Antibiotic prophylaxis in otolaryngology is discussed in the section on radical neck surgery.

Noncardiac Thoracic Surgery

Rationale

Antibiotics are used to prevent wound infection after thoracic and pulmonary surgery. Some surgeons also use antibiotics to prevent other complications, including pneumonia, empyema, or purulent bronchitis.

Clinical Studies

The rate of wound infection in general hospitals for patients undergoing pulmonary resection is 5 to 6% (Table 17.1). The rate of other types of infection following pulmonary surgery has been 17 to 40% for patients within placebo groups in various trials.

Studies of cephalosporins used for 2 or more days perioperatively have shown conflicting results, in part because of varying underlying infection rates. Most studies have shown at least a trend toward a lower rate of wound infection in those patients receiving prophylactic antibiotics. Consistent lowering of the infection rate, however, has not been shown for more serious infections (e.g., empyema, pneumonia).

Empyema occurs in from 1 to 20% of patients with penetrating chest wounds. The effects of antibiotics in this situation have not been established.

Recommendations

Although the available data are not sufficient to conclusively demonstrate any benefit from prophylactic antibiotics, authorities recommend cefazolin for a total of two or three doses (24–26).

Neurosurgery

Neurosurgical areas of concern include skull fractures and clean neurosurgery.

Skull Fractures

Rationale Prophylactic antibiotics are used after skull fracture to prevent meningitis, especially in the presence of cerebrospinal fluid (CSF) leakage.

Clinical Studies The rate of meningitis after skull fracture has ranged from 0 to 5%. The risk of meningitis is higher if a clinical or subclinical CSF leak is present. No large, randomized trial has separated patients on this basis, and results of available studies conflict on whether antibiotic prophylaxis reduces the rate of meningitis. No study has indicated benefit in patients with skull fractures without CSF leak; the data are inadequate to evaluate the effectiveness of antibiotic prophylaxis in those patients with CSF leak (47).

Recommendations Antibiotics should not be administered to patients with uncomplicated skull fractures without CSF leak. Although antibiotics commonly are used in this setting, data are inadequate to conclude that a benefit exists in patients with CSF leak, and no specific antibiotic regimen can be recommended.

Clean Neurosurgery

Rationale The major consideration for using prophylactic antibiotics in neurosurgery is the prevention of meningitis and infection in prosthetic shunts. Wound infection is a secondary consideration.

Clinical Studies No adequate, randomized study of prophylactic antibiotics in clean neurosurgery (using postoperative meningitis, abscess, or shunt infections as the end result) has been performed. A small study using clindamycin showed a decreased rate of wound infection, but these results were uninterpretable because of an epidemic of infections that occurred during the time of study. Wound infections were confined to patients undergoing surgery with a duration of more than 6 hours. The rate of wound infection was decreased in a meta-analysis (47, 48) of available studies.

Recommendations Use of cephalosporins before craniotomy is recommended. Some authorities also recommend a short course of prophylactic therapy when CSF shunts are inserted (24). No recommendation can be made regarding the type or duration of antibiotics to be used, however, because of the lack of data and the multiple possible infecting organisms.

Subacute Bacterial Endocarditis

Rationale

Antibiotic prophylaxis is recommended for patients at risk of developing bacterial endocarditis because of the devastating consequences of this complication.

Clinical Studies

Despite **uniform agreement that antibiotic prophylaxis is required for patients at risk of bacterial endocarditis**, no retrospective or prospective study has ever demonstrated its effectiveness. The situation is made even more difficult by the lack of data concerning the risk of endocarditis in various patient groups.

The pathogenesis of endocarditis depends on three factors: *(a)* a pre-existing valvular lesion, *(b)* bacteremia, *(c)* and immunologic response. A *bacteremia* is the initiating event in bacterial endocarditis. The most common portals of entry associated with clinical endocarditis are the mouth (i.e., dental work), gastrointestinal tract, and genitourinary tract. An entry site for bacteria, however, can be discovered through a patient history in only 24 to 60% of cases (49). Only in the minority of patients with a clear precipitating event would antibiotic prophylaxis be practical.

Multiple events can cause transient bacteremias (49–51) (Table 17.11). A high rate of bacteremia is associated with the classic precipitating causes of endocarditis. Bacteremias also frequently are seen with procedures not usually associated with endocarditis, such as barium enema and sigmoidoscopy. Transient bacteremia has been reported in 1% of normal persons without mucus membrane trauma (51). The significance of this fact is controversial, however, because the rate approaches the contamination rate of blood cultures and most of the organisms isolated could be considered skin contaminants. Transient bacteremia also has been demonstrated to occur after such routine daily activities as a bowel movement, chewing candy or gum, or teeth cleaning with an irrigation device (51).

Little data are available relating the risk of endocarditis to transient bacteremia (51). One study of 350 children with rheumatic heart disease undergoing tooth extraction showed a 52% rate of streptococcal bacteremia and a 1% rate of endocarditis. The risk of endocarditis may be lower in children than in adults. In addition to the risk of bacteremia, the risk of endocarditis has been thought to depend on the number of organisms present and the duration of the bacteremia (51); however, data to confirm the importance of the duration and intensity of bacteremia are lacking. The nature of the bacteremia also probably depends on the mucosal surface, since bacteremia is seen more frequently in patients with gingival disease.

Only a few Gram-positive organisms commonly cause bacterial endocarditis; these include *Streptococcus viridans*, *Enterococcus* sp., other group D streptococci, and *Staphylococcus* sp. Multiple organisms that do not commonly cause endocarditis also can be recovered during bacteremia, however, including aerobic Gram-negative rods and anaerobes. An important factor may be the immunologic nature of certain Gram-positive cocci, which produce an antibody response that assists adherence to valves or sterile platelet-fibrin vegetations.

Recommendations concerning prophylaxis are made on the basis of the specific organisms from a given site or procedure that pose a major risk of endocarditis. With dental procedures, the most common organism causing endocarditis from dental procedures is *S. viridans*. With gastrointestinal or genitourinary procedures, the most common organism is group D streptococci (which includes the entero-

Table 17.11. Incidence of Bacteremia Following Procedures

High Risk	Intermediate Risk	Low Risk
Prostatectomy (infected urine)	Prostatectomy (sterile urine)	Sigmoidoscopy 2–10%
Transurethral 58%	Transurethral 11%	Colonoscopy 3–6%
Retropubic 82%	Retropubic 13%	Esophageal dilatation, sterile dilator 0%
Esophageal dilatation, unsterile dilator 100%	Barium enema 11%	Fiberoptic bronchoscopy 0%
	Liver biopsy 3–13%	
Tonsillectomy 28–38%	Rigid bronchoscopy 15%	Orotracheal intubation 0%
Dental extraction 18–85%	Nasotracheal intubation 10%	Parturition 0–5%
Periodontal surgery 21–88%	Nasotracheal suctioning, intensive care patients 16%	Intrauterine device insertion 0%
Burn surgery 46%		
Surgery of infected areas 54%		

Reprinted with permission from Flynn NM, Lawrence RM. Antimicrobial prophylaxis. Med Clin North Am 1979;63:1230.

coccus). Subacute endocarditis usually is believed to occur in patients with underlying heart disease; acute endocarditis more frequently occurs on normal valves. In older, classic studies, the most frequent underlying cardiac disease in patients with endocarditis was rheumatic valvular disease, which was present in 40 to 60% of cases. The second most frequent was congenital heart disease, which was present in 7 to 16% of cases. The current distribution of the types of valvular disease among patients with endocarditis probably differs from that in the classic studies. Today, mitral valve prolapse and diseases found in elderly patients are much more common and rheumatic valvular disease less common.

An increasing proportion of patients with endocarditis are elderly (i.e., >60 years) and have degenerative heart disease. Many of these patients have no *clinically* recognizable cardiac disease, although it is difficult to exclude hemodynamically insignificant lesions such as aortic sclerosis. Other degenerative problems in which endocarditis has been reported include bicuspid aortic valves, calcific aortic stenosis, and calcification of the mitral annulus. Endocarditis has been reported in certain lesions, including uncomplicated ostium secundum atrial septal defect and idiopathic hypertrophic subaortic stenosis, but this is rare. Infective endocarditis very rarely occurs in patients with cardiac pacemakers.

Approximately 20 to 40% of all patients with endocarditis have no clinically recognizable cardiac disease. Some of these cases can be explained by inaccurate diagnosis or subclinical heart disease; others can be explained by acute endocarditis with virulent organisms. However, a proportion of cases of subacute endocarditis will have no underlying disease identified.

Finally, the risk of recurrent endocarditis in patients who experience one such attack is 9%. Of those patients who experience a second episode, a third will occur in 25%.

When all available data are summarized, 25 to 60% of patients with endocarditis have a known initiating event and 60 to 80% underlying heart disease. Since only those with both underlying heart disease and an initiating event are practical candidates for antibiotic prophylaxis, **less than one-half of all cases of endocarditis in these patients are potentially preventable by prophylaxis**.

Because of the severe nature of this disease and the ethical considerations resulting from that, no controlled study on the effectiveness of prophylactic antibiotics in preventing endocarditis have been performed. The small number of patients at risk of actually developing endocarditis also make such a trial impractical.

Use of prophylactic antibiotics has been shown to reduce the rate of bacteremia and, possibly, the number of bacteria after certain procedures (49). This reduction is in part an artifact, since bacteria will grow less frequently in blood cultures with an antibiotic present. The rate of bacteremia after use of prophylactic antibiotics rises when penicillinase is added to the blood culture flask.

Prophylactic antibiotics have been tested by evaluating their efficiency in a rabbit model. Older, lower-dose regimens did not prevent endocarditis, whereas higher-dose regimens were effective. The animal model has been criticized, however, both because the concentration of organisms used is much higher than that in human bacteremia and because foreign catheters are used to initiate a valvular nidus.

The only direct evidence in humans for the efficacy of antibiotic prophylaxis comes from reported cases of prophylactic failures (52, 53). Only a few cases of endocarditis have been reported in patients receiving older, lower-dose regimens (49, 52, 53). Many of these patients received doses below what the American Heart Association (AHA) recommends. Failures of prophylaxis also have been reported in patients receiving the newer, higher doses recommended by the AHA (53), but most of these failures were in patients receiving antibiotic regimens other than what the AHA recommends (50, 52). Only limited conclusions can be drawn from these reports of antibiotic failure. This is because of: *(a)* incomplete reporting of cases, *(b)* the fact that only a minority of patients at risk receive prophylaxis, and *(c)* incomplete data in many reports.

Prophylactic antibiotics are not given to many patients who are candidates for prophylaxis. Several studies of dental patients with valvular disease showed that most were unaware of their need for prophylaxis, their dentist was uninformed of their heart disease, and many dentists were not using the recommended antibiotic regimens. That many (or most) patients with underlying heart disease do not receive prophylactic antibiotics indicates a failing of "accepted" care and complicates the interpretation of case reports of antibiotic failure.

Despite gaps in the data, authorities strongly recommend use of prophylactic antibiotics for patients at risk of bacterial endocarditis because of the severe consequences of this disease. Current regimens adopted by AHA expert panels are controversial, however, because of the lack of data. The results of studies using animal models have provided a major impetus for the AHA to switch from lower-dose regimens to the current high-dose regimens.

Recommendations

Most authorities recommend that antibiotic prophylaxis be given to patients who have underlying heart disease on which endocarditis can develop (Table 17.12) and are undergoing procedures (Table 17.13) recognized as carrying a risk of bacteremia related to the development of endocarditis. The **recently revised** prophylactic antibiotic regimens recommended by the AHA Committee on Prevention of Rheumatic Fever and Bacterial Endocarditis are given in Table 17.14. Several

Table 17.12.   Prophylaxis of Bacterial Endocarditis: Underlying Cardiac Disease

---

Endocarditis Prophylaxis Recommended
High-risk category
   Prosthetic cardiac valves, including bioprosthetic and homograft valves
   Previous bacterial endocarditis
   Complex cyanotic congenital heart disease (e.g., single ventricle states, transposition of the great arteries, tetralogy of Fallot)
   Surgically constructed systemic pulmonary shunts or conduits
Moderate-risk category
   Most other congenital cardiac malformations (other than above and below)
   Acquired valvar dysfunction (e.g., rheumatic heart disease)
   Hypertrophic cardiomyopathy
   Mitral valve prolapse with valvar regurgitation and/or thickened leaflets

---

Endocarditis Prophylaxis Not Recommended
Negligible-risk category (no greater risk than the general population)
   Isolated secundum atrial septal defect
   Surgical repair of atrial septal defect, ventricular septal defect, or patent ductus arteriosus (without residua beyond 6 mo)
   Previous coronary artery bypass graft surgery
   Mitral valve prolapse without valvar regurgitation
   Physiologic, functional, or innocent heart murmurs
   Previous Kawasaki disease without valvar dysfunction
   Previous rheumatic fever without valvar dysfunction
   Cardiac pacemakers (intravascular and epicardial) and implanted defibrillators

---

Reprinted with permission from Dajani AS, Taubert KA, Wilson W, et al. Prevention of bacterial endocarditis: recommendations by the American Heart Association. JAMA 1997;277:1794–1801.

qualifications to these recommendations, however, should be noted:

1. The recently released AHA recommendations have multiple major changes from prior recommendations, particularly for dental/respiratory procedures. Changes for dental/respiratory procedures include no

Table 17.13a. Prophylaxis of Bacterial Endocarditis: Procedures—Dental

Endocarditis Prophylaxis Recommended*

Dental extractions

Periodontal procedures including surgery, scaling and root planing, probing, and recall maintenance

Dental implant placement and reimplantation of avulsed teeth

Endodontic (root canal) instrumentation or surgery only beyond the apex

Subgingival placement of antibiotic fibers or strips

Initial placement of orthodontic bands but not brackets

Intraligamentary local anesthetic injections

Prophylactic cleaning of teeth or implants where bleeding is anticipated

Endocarditis Prophylaxis Not Recommended

Restorative dentistry† (operative and prosthodontic) with or without retraction cord‡

Local anesthetic injections (nonintraligamentary)

Intracanal endodontic treatment; post placement and buildup

Placement of rubber dams

Postoperative suture removal

Placement of removable prosthodontic or orthodontic appliances

Taking of oral impressions

Fluoride treatments

Taking of oral radiographs

Orthodontic appliance adjustment

Shedding of primary teeth

Reprinted with permission from Dajani AS, Taubert KA, Wilson W, et al. Prevention of bacterial endocarditis: recommendations by the American Heart Association. JAMA 1997;277:1794–1801.
*Prophylaxis is recommended for patients with high- and moderate-risk cardiac conditions.
†This includes restoration of decayed teeth (filling cavities) and replacement of missing teeth.
‡Clinical judgment may indicate antibiotic use in selected circumstances that may create significant bleeding.

specific recommendation for parenteral regimens for high-risk patients (i.e., prosthetic valves), single dose, and lower doses. These recommendations were published just before publication of this book and are too new to further comment on, but the reader is referred to ref. 50 for their rationale.

2. Patients with prosthetic heart valves may be at a higher risk for

Table 17.13b. Prophylaxis of Bacterial Endocarditis Procedures—GI, GU, Other

Endocarditis Prophylaxis Recommended

Respiratory tract

Tonsillectomy and/or adenoidectomy

Surgical operations that involve respiratory mucosa

Bronchoscopy with a rigid bronchoscope

*Gastrointestinal tract**

Sclerotherapy for esophageal varices

Esophageal stricture dilation

Endoscopic retrograde cholangiography with biliary obstruction

Biliary tract surgery

Surgical operations that involve intestinal mucosa

Genitourinary tract

Prostatic surgery

Cystoscopy

Urethral dilation

Endocarditis Prophylaxis Not Recommended

Respiratory tract

Endotracheal intubation

Bronchoscopy with a flexible bronchoscope, with or without biopsy†

Tympanostomy tube insertion

Gastrointestinal tract

Transesophageal echocardiography†

Endoscopy with or without gastrointestinal biopsy†

Genitourinary tract

Vaginal hysterectomy†

Vaginal delivery†

Cesarean section

In uninfected tissue:

   Urethral catheterization

   Uterine dilatation and curettage

   Therapeutic abortion

   Sterilization procedures

   Insertion or removal of intrauterine devices

Other

Cardiac catheterization, including balloon angioplasty

Implanted cardiac pacemakers, implanted defibrillators, and coronary stents

Incision or biopsy of surgically scrubbed skin

Circumcision

Reprinted with permission from Dajani AS, Taubert KA, Wilson W, et al. Prevention of bacterial endocarditis: recommendations by the American Heart Association. JAMA 1997;277:1794–1801.
*Prophylaxis is recommended for high-risk patients optional for medium-risk patients.
†Prophylaxis is optional for high-risk patients.

Table 17.14a.   Prophylactic Regimens for Dental, Oral, Respiratory Tract, or Esophageal Procedures

Situation	Agent	Regimen
Standard general prophylaxis	Amoxicillin	Adults: 2.0 g orally 1 h before procedure
Unable to take oral medications	Ampicillin	Adults: 2.0 g intramuscularly (IM) or intravenously (IV) within 30 min before procedure
Allergic to penicillin	Clindamycin	Adults: 600 mg orally 1 h before procedure
	or	
	Cephalexin† or cefadroxil†	Adults: 2.0 g orally 1 h before procedure
	or	
	Azithromycin or clarithromycin	Adults: 500 mg orally 1 h before procedure
Allergic to penicillin and unable to take oral medications	Clindamycin	Adults: 600 mg IV within 30 min before procedure
	or	
	Cefazolin†	Adults: 1.0 g IM or IV within 30 min before procedure

Reprinted with permission from Dajani AS, Taubert KA, Wilson W, et al. Prevention of bacterial endocarditis: recommendations by the American Heart Association. JAMA 1997;277:1794–1801.
†Cephalosporins should not be used in individuals with immediate-type hypersensitivity reaction (urticaria, angioedema, or anaphylaxis) to penicillins.

Table 17.14b.   Prophylactic Regimens for Gentiourinary Gastrointestinal (Excluding Esophageal) Procedures

Situation	Agents	Regiment†
High-risk patients	Ampicillin plus Gentamicin	Adults: ampicillin 2.0 g intramuscularly (IM) or intravenously (IV) plus gentamicin 1.5 mg/kg (not to exceed 120 mg) within 30 min of starting the procedure; 6 h later, ampicillin 1 g IM/IV or amoxicillin 1 g orally
High-risk patients allergic to ampicillin/amoxicillin	Vancomycin plus Gentamicin	Adults: vancomycin 1.0 g IV over 1-2 h plus gentamicin 1.5 mg/kg IV/IM (not to exceed 120 mg); complete injection/ infusion within 30 min of starting the procedure
Moderate-risk patients	Amoxicillin or Ampicillin	Adults: amoxicillin 2.0 g orally 1 h before procedure, or ampicillin 2.0 g IM/IV within 30 min of starting the procedure
Moderate-risk patients allergic to ampicillin/amoxicillin	Vancomycin	Adults: vancomycin 1.0 g IV over 1-2 h; complete infusion within 30 min of starting the procedure

Reprinted with permission from Dajani AS, Taubert KA, Wilson W, et al. Prevention of bacterial endocarditis: recommendations by the American Heart Association. JAMA 1997;277:1794–1801.
†No second dose of vancomycin or gentamicin is recommended.

staphylococcal endocarditis when the skin is incised or surgery involves other sites of staphylococcal colonization. Some authorities suggest that these patients receive a parenteral semisynthetic penicillin (e.g., nafcillin) or cephalosporin (e.g., cefazolin) in addition to the other recommendations.

3. Although not included in the AHA

list of recommendations, antibiotic prophylaxis obviously should be given for surgery on infected or contaminated tissue (e.g., abscesses, intra-abdominal emergencies). In these cases, the selected antibiotic will need to be individualized according to the expected bacteriology, but in most instances, antibiotics effective against *S. aureus* should be included.

4. Surgery involving infected areas (e.g., abscesses) should include prophylaxis for suspected or commonly encountered organisms in addition to the listed recommendations.
5. Most authorities do not recommend prophylaxis for procedures carrying a low risk of bacteremia or that are unassociated with clinical endocarditis (e.g., sigmoidoscopy without biopsy). An exception, however, may be patients who also have prosthetic valves.
6. Uncomplicated vaginal delivery had a low rate of bacteremia and only an infrequent occurrence of endocarditis in one large study (54). The risk of endocarditis from dilation, curettage, and manipulation of intrauterine devices is rare, so use of prophylaxis for these procedures is controversial. However, patients with prosthetic valves may receive prophylaxis.
7. Prophylaxis also should be given for several "nonsurgical" procedures, including routine professional cleaning of teeth and Foley catheterization of the urinary tract when infection is present.
8. In patients undergoing prolonged procedures or with a prolonged risk of bacteremia because of delayed healing or infection, antibiotics should be given for a longer period of time than is currently recommended (see ref. 50 for specific recommendations).
9. The indications for and benefits of prophylaxis are not clear in patients with noncardiac vascular devices (e.g., renal dialysis arteriovenous

shunts and fistulae, vascular prostheses, prosthetic joints, CSF shunts). Many authorities recommend prophylaxis for these patients, who incur the risk of infection of the foreign material as well as, in some cases, the risk of endocarditis due to arteriovenous shunts. Although data are lacking, we recommend prophylaxis in patients with both CSF shunts (because of the consequences of infections) and dialysis shunts. Prophylaxis also is provided to recent prosthetic vascular devices less than 6 months old.

10. Prophylactic antibiotics probably are not required for cardiac catheterization, angiography, and angioplasty. Prophylaxis for subacute bacterial endocarditis is not required for most transvenous pacemakers in most situations, but it still may be given. Since the most common infections associated with pacemakers result from staphylococci, coverage for this organism should be considered when antibiotics are used.
11. It should be stressed that prophylaxis against acute rheumatic fever is *inadequate* for bacterial endocarditis because of the substantially lower doses that are used. Patients receiving long-term prophylaxis for rheumatic fever have developed endocarditis with penicillin-resistant organisms, so the use of other antibiotics (e.g., erythromycin, vancomycin, or the addition of an aminoglycoside) in patients receiving long-term penicillin for rheumatic fever prophylaxis should be considered.

Postoperative Respiratory Infections

Epidemiology

Most anesthesia textbooks suggest waiting 2 weeks after an acute upper respiratory infection has cleared before undergoing general anesthesia and elective surgery. This recommendation is based on very old series and case reports of sudden deaths in children. A 1933 series found that postoperative respiratory complications doubled (from 6 to 11%) in the presence of pharyngitis and also rose (6 to 11%) when "oral sepsis" was present. Statistical testing was not done, however, and these findings may not be applicable to modern anesthetic techniques or other types of respiratory infections.

A small number of cases of acute upper airway obstruction (i.e., laryngospasm) and sudden death also have been reported in previously healthy children who underwent elective surgery soon after a respiratory infection. Most of these children were less than 6 months of age. Similar complications have not been reported frequently in adults.

The risk of surgery after pneumonia has not been documented in either a prospective or a retrospective series.

Diagnostic Activities and Approaches

Patients who are to undergo surgery should be asked if they have had symptoms of an acute upper respiratory tract infection within the past 2 weeks. Examination of the ears, nose, and oropharynx may confirm the presence of an infection. The patient's body temperature, white-blood-cell (WBC) count, and differential are useful in ascertaining the activity of respiratory infections.

A chest radiograph should be obtained in patients with recent respiratory symptoms to exclude a mild, resolving pneumonia. Gram stain and culture of sputum should be performed in patients producing purulent sputum. Some patients with respiratory infections who undergo surgery also should have an arterial blood gas to detect unsuspected hypoxemia and to serve as a baseline.

Preoperative Management

Most authorities recommend waiting 2 weeks after an uncomplicated upper respiratory tract infection before undergoing nonemergency surgery. Although empirical documentation is lacking for postpone-

ment of surgery, the medicolegal consequences must be considered should complications occur.

Guidelines for delaying elective surgery in patients with pneumonia are not stated in most anesthesia texts. Surgery should be delayed until all signs and symptoms of pneumonia have cleared, including infiltrates on chest radiographs, sputum production, and abnormal body temperature. Six to eight weeks may be required for chest radiographs to clear.

A few patients will require operation soon after an upper respiratory tract infection or pneumonia, and patients with postoperative pneumonia may require reoperation for intra-abdominal sepsis or for surgical complications. Although documentation is lacking, the risk of postoperative respiratory failure, superinfection, and hypoxia probably is increased. Patients undergoing urgent surgery during a respiratory tract infection should have a baseline preoperative blood gas obtained and, if possible, spirometry performed. These patients need to be closely followed postoperatively for respiratory complications and be observed in an ICU for at least 24 hours after the operation. Therapy for pneumonia should be continued postoperatively with strong emphasis on pulmonary toilet.

Preoperative Urinary Tract Infection

Preoperative UTI is discussed in Chapter 12.

POSTOPERATIVE PROBLEMS

The consulting internist is often called on to evaluate the febrile postoperative patient. The surgeon usually will manage routine infections of the surgical wound, lungs, and urinary tract. Common reasons for a consultation include prolonged fever of undetermined origin, a severely ill or septic patient, interpretation of unusual microbiology results, and use of antibiotics.

The consulting internist requires a background knowledge of both the common and uncommon causes of postoperative fever (Table 17.15) as well as the common reasons for misdiagnosis and failure of the patient to respond to antibiotic therapy (Table 17.16).

The internist's most valuable contributions may involve sorting out causes unrelated to the specific surgical procedure (e.g., drug fever), recognizing a noninfectious cause of fever (e.g., phlebitis, alcoholic hepatitis, gout), or recognizing a

second, complicating infection (e.g., distant seeding from a UTI, infection in a pre-existing vascular graft after prostatic surgery). The internist also may be called on to evaluate of the deteriorating postoperative patient, who usually is already receiving antibiotics, days or weeks after surgery.

The evaluation of a febrile postoperative patient often is an urgent activity. Therefore direct verbal communication between the referring physician and the consulting internist is mandatory so that

Table 17.15. Causes of Postoperative Fever

Diagnostic Possibility	Peak Incidence	Clinical Clue
Most common causes		
Benign postoperative fever	48–72 h	Normal physical examination; temperature, <101° F
Urinary tract infection	48–72 h	Catheter, instrumentation
Wound infection	4–10 d	Purulent drainage
Pulmonary		
Atelectasis	24 h	Rales, decreased breath sounds
Pneumonia	24–48 h	Consolidation, purulent sputum
IV catheter infection	72 h	Unexplained fever, "phlebitis"
Venous thrombosis	7–10 d	+/– leg pain, swelling
Local/regional infection		
Head and neck		
Otitis media	Anytime	Ear pain, nasogastric tube
Sinusitis	Anytime	Nasal discharge, facial pain
Parotitis	48–72 h	Dehydration, parotid swelling
Gastrointestinal		
Intra-abdominal abscess	4 days to weeks	Mass, persistent fever, bacteremia
Pancreatitis	Anytime	Epigastric tenderness, nausea and vomiting
Acute cholecystitis	48 h	Right upper quadrant signs, symptoms
Hepatitis	8–12 wk	Right upper quadrant tenderness, jaundice, AST
Cardiac		
Endocarditis		Peripheral emboli, murmur, anemia
Genitourinary		
Perinephric abscess	5 days after urinary tract infection	"Pyelonephritis" with >5 d fever
Prostatitis	Anytime	Perineal discomfort, boggy prostate
Pudendal/psoas abscess	48 h	Paracervical block, hip pain
Endometritis/salpingitis		
Skeletal		
Vertebral osteomyelitis	Anytime	Low back pain, previous urinary tract infection
Osteitis pubis	Anytime	Pubic tenderness, inner thigh pain
Epidural abscess		Spinal anesthesia, back pain
Skin		
Pressure ulcer	Anytime	Necrotic, devitalized tissue

Table 17.15 *(continued).*   **Causes of Postoperative Fever**

Diagnostic Possibility	Peak Incidence	Clinical Clue
Device related		
Monitoring devices	72 h	Unexplained fever, bacteremia
Prosthetic grafts	Anytime	Bacteremia, gastrointestinal bleeding
Skeletal prostheses	Anytime	Pain, loosening of prosthesis
Vascular access devices	Anytime	Staphylococcus epidermidis bacteremia
Noninfectious causes		
Drug fever	7–10 d	Suspect with any drug
Trauma related	48–72 h	Significant tissue damage
Transfusion reaction	24 h	Abrupt onset posttransfusion
Intramuscular injection	48 h	Fluctuance
Hematoma		Mass
Alcohol/drug withdrawal	2–5 d	History of use
Starch peritonitis		Diffuse abdominal symptoms
		Normal physical examination and
Factitious fever	Anytime	laboratory tests
Endocrine related		
Malignant hyperthermia	Intraoperative	

historical information can be shared and both diagnostic and therapeutic maneuvers coordinated. If reoperation is a possibility, joint planning between the internist and surgeon is required as well.

The internist should be aware of both the local and the national hospital infection rates (1) (Table 17.17), common nosocomial organisms (2), local patterns of susceptibility to antibiotics, and any recent pattern of nosocomial infections or changing patterns of bacterial resistance (3). The hospital epidemiology staff and

Table 17.16.   Common Reasons for Failure to Diagnose Postoperative Fever

1. Incorrect initial diagnosis of prolonged fever
2. Incorrect interpretation of laboratory data
3. Failure to suspect appropriate organisms for clinical situation
4. Drainage of infection not considered or inadequate
5. Remote complication
6. Nonbacterial complication not recognized
7. Superinfection: colonization misinterpreted as infection
8. Preceding disease unrelated to surgery

microbiology laboratory are invaluable resources for additional information, and the internist should be aware of the methods for control of disease transmission and infection in the hospital (4, 5) and the current CDC definitions of nosocomial infections (6).

The Febrile Postoperative Patient

Epidemiology and Pathophysiology

The presence of significant fever usually indicates disease, but the clinical usefulness of this finding in determining the etiology of temperature elevation is very limited. Some understanding of the nature of the febrile response is important when interpreting the significance of fever.

Clinical fever results from biochemical changes in the hypothalamus. Endogenous pyrogens, termed *pyrogenic cytokines*, are polypeptides produced by monocytes, neutrophils, lymphocytes, and other cells in response to stimulation by infectious agents, toxins, injury, and inflammation (55). These pyrogenic cytokines trigger the production of prostaglandin E_2 in the hypothalamic thermoregulatory center. The hypothalamic temperature set-point is reset, thus inducing neuronal transmission from the brain centers to the periphery, which in turn affects heat production and vascular tone, thereby resulting in fever (56). The time of the temperature elevation does not correlate with the peak concentration of circulating cytokines. Aspirin and nonsteroidal anti-inflammatory agents prevent fever by blocking prostaglandin synthesis, but they do not prevent the synthesis and release of pyrogenic cytokines.

The acute-phase protein response to infection also is mediated by pyrogenic cytokines. Acute-phase hepatic proteins, glycoproteins, and globulins are responsible for an elevated sedimentation rate and C-reactive protein.

The biochemical basis for intermittent or remittent fevers remains unknown, but intrinsic circulating neuropeptides such as somatostatin function as natural antipyretics, thus reducing the patient's temperature. It is unknown how much the interplay between naturally occurring peptide antipyretics and sporadic release

of endogenous cytokines affect the fever pattern that is observed during infection (56). The clinical implication is that specific infections cannot be identified by fever patterns.

"Normal" oral temperatures range from 96.6°–99.6°F, with a low occurring in the morning to a high occurring between 4 PM and midnight. In general, elderly patients have lower temperature ranges, such as between a low of 96.6°F to, perhaps, a maximum of 97.6°F late in the day, whereas a 99.6°–100°F range is not unusual for young individuals (with the high occurring in the late afternoon). Diurnal variations range from 0.9°–2.7°F.

Temperature elevation in the postoperative period is very common and, by itself, lacks sensitivity and specificity as an indicator of disease. Early studies by Dykes (57), Livelli et al. (58), Bell et al. (59), and later series by Garibaldi et al. (60) and Giangobbe et al. (61) confirm the existence of a "benign" postoperative fever response. In a study of 871 general surgery patients, 24% developed fever. Of these fevers, 38% were unexplained, 26% resulted from wound infections, 21% from

Table 17.17. Frequency Distribution of Major Sites of Nosocomial Infections by Bedsize and Teaching Affiliation: Hospital-wide Component, January 1993 to April 1995[a]

| Major Site | Nonteaching Hospitals | | Teaching Hospitals | | |
	<200 beds	≥200 beds	<500 beds	≥500 beds	All Hospitals
Urinary tract infection	504 (36.0%)	1560 (33.6%)	3045 (28.2%)	2267 (22.1%)	7376 (27.2%)
Surgical site infection	198 (14.1%)	903 (19.5%)	1934 (17.9%)	2023 (19.7%)	5058 (18.7%)
Pneumonia	261 (18.6%)	779 (16.8%)	1822 (16.9%)	1811 (17.7%)	4673 (17.3%)
Primary bloodstream infection	146 (10.4%)	443 (9.5%)	1647 (15.2%)	2051 (20.0%)	4287 (15.8%)
Other	292 (20.8%)	958 (20.6%)	2356 (21.8%)	2094 (20.4%)	5700 (21.0%)
All infections	1401 (5.2%)	4643 (17.1%)	10,804 (39.9%)	10,246 (37.8%)	27,094 (100%)

Reprinted with permission from Hospital Infections Program, Centers for Disease Control and Prevention. National nosocomial infections surveillance semi-annual report. Am J Infect Control 1995;23:377–385.
[a]Do not use the data in this table for interhospital comparison, because frequencies are not adjusted for risk of infection or intensity of surveillance. The data should be used as a general guide for determining the relative frequency of infection at the major sites.

UTIs, and 13% from respiratory infections. Temperatures up to 102°F are not uncommon, occur up to 2 days postoperatively, and gradually decline over the next several days. Fever that begins or persists after the fourth postoperative day is more likely to represent infection. The exact cause of the temperature elevations is unknown. Roe (62) studied a group of patients in whom an intraoperative drop in temperature was followed by a postoperative rebound to 101°F by 24 hours after surgery and a return to normal by 32 hours. If the intraoperative temperature was controlled and not allowed to decline, no postoperative elevation occurred, thus suggesting to the investigators the presence of an anesthetic "paralysis" of the hypothalamic regulatory mechanism followed by a rebound phenomenon.

Whatever the cause, mild, low-grade fever is expected in the first 24 to 48 hours after surgery, with a gradual decline over 2 to 5 days, but this fever occasionally may persist into the second postoperative week. An arbitrary temperature of 101°F is widely used as an indicator of the need for more in-depth evaluation. Lower temperatures of 99.6°–100°F may have the same significance in elderly and immune-compromised or debilitated patients. Temperatures higher than 102°F within the first 48 hours after surgery are more likely to be caused by atelectasis, invasive wound infection, or leaking viscous (in the case of intra-abdominal surgery), and they should be promptly evaluated.

Musher et al. (63) reviewed the fever patterns of 200 consecutive patients referred to an infectious disease service and concluded that no pattern had diagnostic value. Of these 200 patients, 83% had intermittent or remittent fevers, and of these, 90% had diurnal variations. The lack of diurnal variation was thought to support, at least slightly, a noninfectious cause, since this pattern was seen in approximately 50% of noninfectious febrile entities. Sustained fever was seen in Gram-negative pneumonia and central nervous system (CNS) damage with

enough frequency to suggest one of these diagnoses. Beyond these loose associations, however, the clinician should not look to fever patterns as a clue to the diagnosis. The height of the fever also has variable diagnostic significance.

Diagnostic Approach

Determining the cause of a postoperative fever can be a complex clinical challenge for both the surgeon and internist (62, 64–67) (Table 17.15). **A systematic but individualized approach is suggested.** It is helpful to think in terms of: *(a)* the most common febrile complications of any operation, *(b)* infectious complications of the specific surgical procedure, *(c)* the temporal relation of the fever to the operation, and *(d)* the type and location of the surgery performed (Table 17.18). Beyond this, a systematic, regional approach and a well-planned diagnostic workup appropriate to the condition of the patient are essential (56).

The evaluation and management of individual conditions causing fever are described in subsequent sections. The following is a general approach to the febrile postoperative patient. The **patient history** should be directed toward specific information, such as:

1. *Most Common Causes:* Consider first the most common causes of postoperative fever. A low-grade, self-limited, unexplained fever is common after any major procedure; the cause of such a fever is unknown. Patient temperature usually is less than

Table 17.18. Approach to the Febrile Postoperative Patient

1. Most common febrile complications of surgery (in general)[a]
2. Common infectious complications and sequelae of primary surgical disease
3. Type and location of the surgery
4. The temporal relationship of the fever to the operation
5. Obvious clinical clues

[a]See Table 17.19.

101°F but may reach 102°–103°F for brief periods and then decline gradually over 3 to 4 days. A temperature higher than 102°F on the third or fourth postoperative day should prompt a historical review of the case and a thorough physical examination. Special attention should be directed to the six most common entities: *(a)* pulmonary (e.g., atelectasis, infection, aspiration), *(b)* UTI, *(c)* wound infection, *(d)* thrombophlebitis, *(e)* intravenous access infections, and *(f)* drug allergy (Table 17.19).

2. *Temporal Fever Relationships:* The time of fever onset is relevant but of limited diagnostic value. Early (i.e., within 24 hour after surgery), high fever is likely to result from atelectasis, invasive wound infection, or leaking viscous, whereas fever from the usual wound infection occurs in 4 to 10 days.

3. *Infection Specific to the Procedure:* Look for infections directly related to the procedure, such as toxic shock syndrome following endoscopic sinus surgery (19) or prostatitis after genitourinary surgery.

4. *Type and Location of Surgery:* Look for regional infectious complications of the procedure, such as vertebral disc space infection following spinal or genitourinary surgery.

5. *Clinical Clues:* A focused patient history and physical examination precede laboratory evaluation. Nursing notes should be reviewed for temperature elevations not recorded on the temperature chart. Information also should be obtained regarding pre-existing bacterial or viral infection, drug allergies, any pertinent history of drug use (e.g., alcohol, barbiturates, steroids), prior sensitivities, or presence of indwelling catheters, prosthetic devices, or vascular grafts. Alcohol or other drug withdrawal as well as alcoholic hepatitis may present in the postoperative period. Hepatitis may present postoperatively as a fever of uncer-

Table 17.19.   Most Common Etiologies of Postoperative Fever

Surgical site
Wound
Deep (e.g., abscess, peritonitis)
Specific to the procedure (e.g., infected prosthesis)

Remote
Pulmonary (atelectasis, pneumonia)
Urinary tract infection
Diarrhea (*C. difficile*)
Instrumentation (e.g., intravenous lines[a], central venous lines)

Usually nonbacterial
Drug or anesthetic allergy
Dehydration
Intravenous catheter phlebitis[a]
Thrombophlebitis and pulmonary emboli

Unexplained

[a]Also can be infected (septic phlebitis).

tain origin, and drug-induced hepatitis may present as fever alone.

Anesthesiology and recovery room notes should be reviewed for temperature elevations, drugs or transfusions administered, or notation of aspiration. Clues from these notes and the early postoperative course should point to an endocrine cause, such as thyroid storm or adrenal crises. The medication list should be reviewed and the patient questioned about nonprescription drugs.

The **physical examination** should be systematic and thorough. A depressed level of consciousness may suggest aspiration. The eardrums should be checked for otitis media caused by obstruction from a nasogastric or nasotracheal tube, and the sinuses should be palpated for tenderness and the nose checked for purulent discharge. An ophthalmologic examination may be helpful in selected instances, such as in the presence of candida endophthalmitis or endocarditis. Parotid swelling or submaxillary tenderness should be noted; if present, attempts should be made to express pus from the ducts.

A careful pulmonary examination may reveal atelectasis or consolidation. Atelectasis may be present without causing fever; thus a secondary cause should always be considered. Persistent atelectasis may be a sign of subphrenic or pancreatic abscess or of pulmonary embolism.

New heart murmurs from endocarditis may appear in the postoperative period; if so, a diligent search should be conducted for additional subtle signs of endocarditis. Myocardial infarction may present in elderly patients as fever. Intravenous and arterial cannula sites should be examined for erythema, tenderness, or pus, and all central venous access sites should be examined for exit site, tunnel, or pocket infections. All hyperalimentation lines, central venous access lines, and arterial pressure transducers are potential sources of infection. Abdominal findings of right-upper-quadrant tenderness may suggest postoperative cholecystitis, hepatitis, cholangitis, hepatic abscess, or perihepatic abscess. Although rare, postoperative pancreatitis should not be overlooked. Signs of intra-abdominal abscess may not be present at this point, although a tender mass would be suggestive.

All wounds should be observed for signs of infection, which include purulence, localized swelling, redness, and heat. Recognition of necrotizing soft-tissue infection, which includes bronzing of the skin, induration, crepitance, and cutaneous blistering or necrosis, is particularly important; if major trauma and tissue necrosis have occurred, a temperature of 102°F is not unusual. A rectal examination is mandatory to rule out rectal or prostatic abscess or prostatitis. Suprapubic tenderness or bilateral inner-thigh pain after genitourinary surgery suggests osteitis pubis. The gynecologist will perform postoperative pelvic examinations for cuff abscess, endometritis, pelvic abscess, and septic pelvic thrombophlebitis, but subgluteal or retropsoal abscess after paracervical or pudendal block, especially with hip pain, also should be considered. After spinal anesthesia or back surgery, carefully palpate for tenderness, which would suggest an epidural abscess or vertebral osteomyelitis.

Soft-tissue sites should be examined for intramuscular infection, hematoma, or abscess. The entire skin is observed for pressure ulcers. Tender, swollen joints should be obvious and suggest gout or infection; a septic joint should prompt a search for distant infection. The lower extremities may provide a clue to thrombophlebitis as well. In neurosurgical, orthopaedic, and urologic procedures, the surgeon will be familiar with any causes of fever unique to that procedure.

The initial **laboratory investigation** of suspected infection should include a complete blood count, blood cultures, chest radiography, sputum for Gram stain and culture, urinalysis, urine culture and Gram stain, removal and culture of intravenous catheters, as well as Gram stain and swab culture of any wound drainage (Table 17.20).

The presence of leukocytosis may suggest an infectious cause, especially after the first 24 to 72 hours, but it does not correlate well with infection. Leukocytosis is common in uninfected patients immediately after operation (i.e., <24–48 hours), especially in those who undergo major or intra-abdominal surgery. The absence of leukocytosis or a left shift of the differential, however, does not rule out an infectious cause of postoperative fever.

Clinical judgment guides the initiation of empiric antibiotic therapy. If the patient is clinically ill, has clinical evidence of infection, or a presumptive diagnosis of infection can be made, empiric antibiotics can be initiated based on the site (or sites) of the presumed infection and the most likely organisms involved. If a definite

Table 17.20.   Initial Laboratory Evaluation of Postoperative Fever

1. Complete blood count, differential
2. Chest radiography
3. Febrile blood cultures
4. Urinalysis, culture, Gram stain
5. Intravenous catheter culture
6. Wound swab culture, Gram stain
7. Sputum culture, Gram stain

infection cannot be identified and the patient does not appear to be seriously ill, antibiotics often can be withheld to prevent the masking of abscess, development of drug allergy, and need for further cultures. **Exceptions** include patients with an intravascular prosthesis (e.g., heart valve, vascular graft) or other prostheses, in which bacterial seeding can have devastating consequences, and immunosuppressed or debilitated patients. These patients should be treated empirically as clinical circumstances suggest. Prophylactic antibiotics continued beyond two doses should be stopped.

An **extended workup for fever** should focus on the likely causes as suggested by clinical findings and the type of surgery. Repeated physical examination yields diagnostic clues. Liver function tests and repeat cultures should be obtained, and imaging examinations should be directed at likely causes, especially deep abscess at the operative site.

The diagnosis of occult deep abscesses can be particularly difficult; conversely, extended searches for abscesses often are performed in patients with other readily detectable causes of fever. The most important, common circumstances that should initiate a workup for a deep abscess are: *(a)* a procedure in which abscess is a common complication (e.g., abdominal trauma, colon resection, pelvic surgery, perforated viscus), and *(b)* a prolonged course of disease. If present, localized symptoms and signs are valuable, but these are frequently absent, especially early in the disease course. The development of fever many weeks postoperatively is not specific, and many patients with abscesses will have late postoperative fever for other reasons. The appearance of a fever in a patient who is otherwise well suggests either abscess or a nonbacterial cause (e.g., drug fever). The presence of concomitant, unexplained, multiple-organ failure (e.g., pulmonary, renal, liver, and less commonly, cardiac) as well as fever suggests undrained infection and the need for prompt localization.

Diagnoses that are particularly difficult because of the paucity of signs include suppurative cholangitis, perinephric abscess, retroperitoneal hematoma or abscess, prostatic abscess, pulmonary emboli, and intravenous device infections without obvious suppuration. *Clostridium difficile* colitis may present postoperatively as a fever of uncertain origin. This fever may overshadow minor or atypical (e.g., ileus without diarrhea) gastrointestinal symptoms. A marked leukocytosis may be present as well, and fever with confusion in elderly patients may represent an undetected myocardial infarction.

Failure to determine the cause of prolonged fever usually results from an inadequate patient history, failure to order an important test, or improper evaluation of a previously ordered test (Table 17.16). A complete review should be made of the patient history, hospital course, medication history, and laboratory data, including personal review of radiographs and Gram stains. Four possibilities should be considered:

1. Was an infection common to the operative procedure not considered?
2. Was an infection consistent with the clinical picture not considered?
3. Is this an atypical presentation of a common disease?
4. Is there a noninfectious cause?

Complications that are remote from the operative site (e.g., liver abscess), are nonbacterial (e.g., parapneumonic effusion), or result from inadequate drainage should be considered as well.

In the evaluation of a prolonged postoperative fever, entities unrelated to the surgery or nosocomial infection also must be considered. These include drug allergy, collagen vascular disease, malignancy, drug withdrawal, viral infection, alcoholic hepatitis, and reactivation of tuberculosis. If not already done, all venous access devices should be re-evaluated and unnecessary drugs discontinued.

Factitious fever has been emphasized as a cause of obscure fever. Medical personnel are frequently involved, with additional clues being a well-appearing patient who has a normal physical examination and laboratory studies (including sedimentation rate, C-reactive protein, and WBC count), failure of the fever to follow a diurnal variation, rapid defervescence without diaphoresis, temperature greater than 42°C, and absence of tachycardia. Methods for detection include observed rectal temperatures and measurement of urine temperatures.

At times, abdominal re-exploration must be considered when evaluating a deteriorating patient receiving antibiotics and who has persistent bacteremia; prolonged, unexplained fever; or is at risk for intra-abdominal abscess. The decision to re-explore the patient is surgical and should be made on the basis of all the clinical information.

Intra-abdominal Abscesses

Epidemiology

Intra-abdominal abscesses and intra-abdominal sepsis rank with pneumonia and septicemia as serious causes of morbidity and mortality in the postoperative patient (68). Clearance of bacteria is so efficient that persistent abdominal abscesses will form when hemoglobin, barium, or necrotic tissue persist, thus blocking the lymphatic system, impairing chemotaxis, and providing nutrients for bacterial growth. If bacterial proliferation prevails and inflammation progresses, fibrin formation traps bacteria and seals visceral leaks. Inflammatory capillary permeability may result in an exudate of 300 to 500 mL/h, thus leading to hypovolemia. The sequestered fibrin–bacterial mass and the exudate itself impair phagocytosis and create the environment for abscess formation.

The most common abdominal operations followed by abscess formation are appendectomy, colon resection, pelvic and gynecologic surgery, and surgery for abdominal trauma and perforated viscous (69). Biliary, pancreatic, and genitourinary procedures are less commonly followed by abscess formation.

Abscesses can be intraperitoneal, retroperitoneal, or visceral (Fig. 17.3). The most common postsurgical site is intra-abdominal. The location of the abscess will bear some relation to the site of the primary disease, with the most common, in order of frequency, being right lower quadrant, perihepatic, left lower quadrant, pelvic, and left subphrenic (69, 70). Colonic surgery and trauma are the most frequent causes of subphrenic abscess. Multiple abscesses occur in 20% of abscess patients. Visceral abscesses are uncommon postoperatively but may occur in the liver, pancreas, and kidney.

Bacteriology

The bacteriology of intra-abdominal abscess is polymicrobial. Studies consistently report from three to five, and even up to nine, anaerobes per infection. *Escherichia coli* and *Bacteroides fragilis* are the most frequent isolates, along with *Klebsiella* sp., *Proteus* sp., and *Enterococcus* sp. *Bilophila wadsworthii* (68) is now a frequent isolate as well. Anaerobic organisms predominant in chronic abscesses presenting weeks or months after surgery.

The role of *Enterococcus* sp. is controversial. It is not a vigorous primary pathogen in polymicrobial intra-abdominal infections. It may persist, however, if the initial treatment fails, as occurs in immunocompromised patients, and may become a primary pathogen requiring specific combination therapy (68, 71).

Diagnostic Activities

Improved diagnosis and early intervention have improved considerably the outcome of intra-abdominal abscesses. Previously reported delays in diagnosis of up to 5 weeks are distinctly uncommon in symptomatic patients today. Signs, symptoms, and the diagnostic approach depend on whether the infection has progressed to a discrete fluid collection. In elderly patients, the course of disease may be subtle

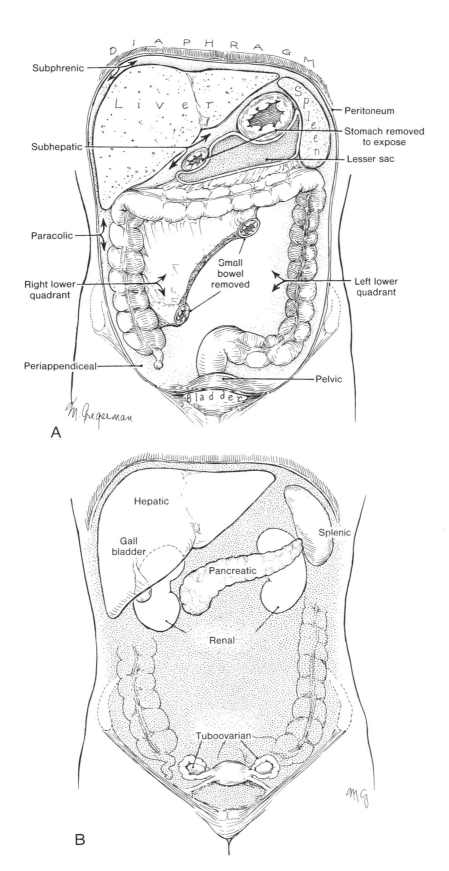

Figure 17.3. For legend see page 38.

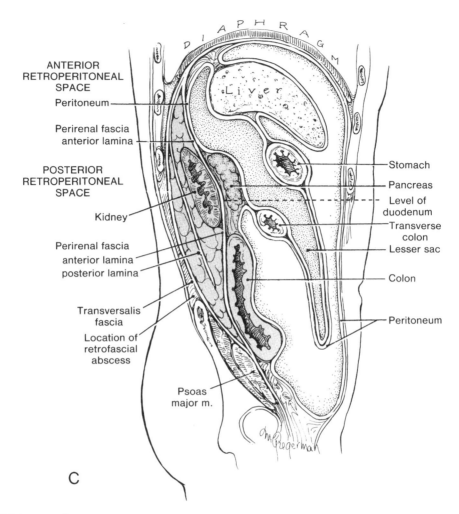

Figure 17.3 *(continued).* The most common locations of abscesses and their anatomic relationships. Abscesses may be **(A)** intraperitoneal (e.g., subphrenic, subhepatic, lesser sac, paracolic, periappendiceal, pelvic), **(B)** visceral (e.g., hepatic, splenic, pancreatic, renal, tuboovarian), or **(C)** retroperitoneal (e.g., anterior/posterior retroperitoneal, perinephric). The retroperitoneal space is bounded by the peritoneum anteriorly and the transversalis fascia posteriorly. The anterior lamina of the perirenal fascia subdivides the anterior and posterior compartments of the retroperitoneal space. (Adapted from Altemeier WA, Alexander JW. Retroperitoneal abscess. Arch Surg 1961;83:512–524; and Altemeier WA, Culbertson WR, Fullen WD, et al. Intraabdominal abscesses. Am J Surg 1973;125:70–78.)

and protracted, with a paucity of findings (72).

The usual clinical scenario involves a patient who undergoes major abdominal surgery, begins to improve or is placed on antibiotics for suspected postoperative infection, and then plateaus or deteriorates into a period of morbidity, with malaise, weight loss, weakness, anorexia, distention, nausea, and vomiting. The other common presentation is fever beginning early in the postoperative course that is unresponsive to antibiotics.

The most relevant circumstance that should initiate a workup for deep abscess is a prolonged course of illness after a procedure in which abscesses are a common complication (e.g., abdominal trauma, colon resection, pelvic surgery, perforated viscus). If present, localized tenderness, fever, and leukocytosis are valuable signs but frequently are absent, especially early in the disease course. Suggestive clues are fever that continues despite use of antibiotics and a persistent, Gram-negative bacteremia.

Multiple-organ failure syndrome is thought to result from a malignant, systemic, inflammatory response syndrome. Different patterns of multiple-organ failure exist depending on the insult (i.e., injury or infection), but otherwise unexplained organ failure (e.g., pulmonary, renal, liver, cardiac) with fever suggest occult infection, often from an intra-abdominal site or abscess (73). The dangers of an unrecognized abscess are sepsis, progressive debilitation, multiple-organ failure, fistula formation, rupture (into the abdomen, a blood vessel, or through the diaphragm, thus producing empyema or pneumonia), and death (68).

Subphrenic abscesses characteristically produce few local signs. They may be suggested, however, by intercostal tenderness, shoulder pain, elevation of a hemidiaphragm, atelectasis, or pleural effusion.

Liver abscesses (74) are related to biliary tract disease in 25 to 40% of cases, but they also have been reported following a wide variety of surgical procedures, with both continuous and hematogenous spread. Single abscesses are more common than multiple abscesses, and they also are more common in older patients. Symptoms tend to be indolent (duration of symptoms, 2–5 weeks), and jaundice, pain, mass, or tenderness may be absent. Malaise, general weakness, anorexia, and weight loss may predominate. Patients often are thought to have fever of unknown origin, pulmonary embolus, cholecystitis, pancreatitis, or some other infection before an enlarged liver or jaundice suggest the diagnosis. On physical examination, only 37% of these patients have fever or right-upper-quadrant tenderness.

Pancreatic abscesses following surgery are rare but have not been eliminated by use of prophylactic antibiotics. Manipulation of the biliary tract, pancreas, or stomach usually precedes this complication, which usually occurs in the setting of postoperative pancreatitis. Fever, leuko-cytosis, abdominal distention, and tenderness are the most frequent findings, but these are nonspecific. Measurement of the serum amylase level is not helpful.

Splenic abscesses only rarely follow intra-abdominal surgery (75). Most cases are related to infective endocarditis, UTI, and nonpenetrating trauma. Symptoms are nonspecific, and only a high degree of suspicion will suggest this diagnosis.

The diagnostic approach to a suspected abscess should begin with plain-film radiography. A chest radiograph may reveal abnormalities suggestive of a subdiaphragmatic process, including pleural effusion, elevated diaphragm, atelectasis, extraluminal air–fluid level, and a subdiaphragmatic gas pattern. For other abscesses, flat, upright, or lateral decubitus abdominal radiographs detect abnormal gas patterns, soft-tissue masses, abnormalities of the psoas shadow, loss of the renal outline, and bony destruction in the spine or twelfth rib.

In patients with localizing pain, fever, and a palpable mass, computed tomography (CT) is the imaging procedure of choice (76). CT has a sensitivity of 78 to 100% depending on the location of the abscess. In contrast, ultrasonography has a sensitivity of more than 90% for abscesses in the right upper quadrant, retroperitoneum, and pelvis, but only of 75 to 82% overall. Ultrasonography also is limited by wounds, dressings, ostomies, and obesity. CT is superior to ultrasonography in all locations, except perhaps the pelvis; sensitivity is lower (60%) in the interloop areas with both modalities. The optimal timing for CT (clinical circumstances permitting) is around the eighth postoperative day, which allows for resolution of tissue swelling and reabsorption of non-suppurative fluid collections (76).

In patients without localizing signs or symptoms, radionuclide scanning is most likely to be helpful (77). Indium-111 oxine, TcHMPAO, and radiolabeled polyclonal IgG have been used, but indium scanning is the most widely available. Indium scanning has a sensitivity of 50 to 75% for chronic infections and of 90 to 100% for acute infections, in which active neutrophilic collections are necessary for detection. Scans are difficult to interpret around the liver and spleen, where neutrophilic activity abounds, but in other regions, these scans can clarify the diagnosis when localization by CT fails.

Treatment

Peritonitis will resolve in most patients who are treated with antimicrobial therapy. When bacteria cannot be contained, a persistent, generalized peritonitis may form, resulting in multiple-organ dysfunction and unresolved sepsis. The bacteria predominating under these circumstances, however, are different from those in early peritonitis and abscess. They include coagulase-negative staphylococci, *Pseudomonas* sp., *Candida* sp., and *Enterococcus* sp. Antimicrobial selection pressure or translocation of bacteria across the bowel wall are postulated mechanisms.

Where bacteria remain, an abscess may form. Once the diagnosis is suspected, every effort should be made to confirm and localize the abscess, which can be treated with use of percutaneous catheter drainage localized by CT or ultrasonography, extraperitoneal surgical drainage, or midline abdominal exploration (78–80). Pelvic abscess may be amenable to transrectal drainage. When surgical intervention is necessary for a single abscess, the extraperitoneal route, if technically possible, is preferred.

Percutaneous catheter drainage is technically possible in 80 to 90% of patients, and is has a success rate of 80 to 90% for well-defined, unilocular abscesses. The success rate is lower for more complex abscesses. The criteria for a successful percutaneous catheter drainage include a well-defined, unilocular cavity; a safe drainage route; an absence of excessive cellular debris; a low fluid viscosity; and immediate surgical access should complications ensue (78).

After aspiration is complete, the catheter is placed for gravity or low-suction drainage until the daily flow is less than 10 mL. After successful drainage, there should be prompt improvement in symptoms, with defervescence of fever in 24 to 48 hours. Repeat scanning determines success and the need for additional catheters or surgical drainage. Complication rates range from 4 to 15%, and complications include bleeding, fistulas, and transgression of the pleural cavity. Pancreatic or complex abscesses increase the complication rate, but comparisons of outcomes with those of historical surgical controls have shown favorable results for PC even though a longer drainage time may be required. Continued catheter drainage at home is possible in selected cases. Fungal abscesses, infected hematomas, and necrotic tissue do not respond well, however, and should be treated surgically. Technical factors such as catheter displacement and poor insertion trajectory may limit success.

Polymicrobial intra-abdominal infection proceeds in a two-stage process, with aerobes predominating in the first 5 days and anaerobes thereafter. The basic requirement when choosing an antibiotic in this situation is activity against both anaerobes and Gram-negative aerobes. The adequacy of penetration by most antimicrobials into the peritoneal cavity has been demonstrated, and all common agents against anaerobes have demonstrated penetration into abscess cavities. The choice of antimicrobials should take into account the severity of illness, risk of toxic side effects (e.g., renal damage with aminoglycosides), previous use of antimicrobials, individual hospital patterns of susceptibility to nosocomial organisms, and degree of immune suppression (24, 71, 81, 82). Use of second-look surgical procedures in the treatment of abdominal infection is beyond the scope of this section.

Bacteremia

Epidemiology

Nosocomial bloodstream infections cause significant morbidity and mortality (83–85). Primary bloodstream infections increased (from 7 to 16% of all nosocomial infections) from the mid-1980s to 1992 (2). This increase largely resulted from Gram-positive bacteria (86). Coagulase-negative staphylococci increased from 9 to 31% of bloodstream isolates, and taken together, coagulase-negative staphylococci and *Staphylococcus aureus* now represent between 38 and 49% of all bacteremias acquired in the hospital (2). During this time, infection with *E. coli* has decreased in frequency (from 23 to 16% of all nosocomial infections), as has infection with *Klebsiella* sp. (from 7 to 5% of all nosocomial infections). Small increases in the rates of infection with *Candida* sp. (from 2 to 5%) and with *S. aureus*, *Enterococcus* sp., *Pseudomonas* sp., and *Enterobacter* sp. (from 1 to 2% each) also have occurred. This marked change in the spectrum of infection has resulted from use of intravascular access devices and appreciation of the pathogenic potential of coagulase-negative staphylococci. Selection pressure from antibiotic prophylaxis also is thought to have contributed to this shift. Characteristically, coagulase-negative staphylococcal infections are nosocomial, usually with *S. epidermitis* (80%), multidrug resistant, indolent (with long periods of latency), and usually involve indwelling foreign devices (87).

Bacteremia occurring on surgical services follows or accompanies postoperative pneumonia, wound infections, UTIs, and most important, is associated with indwelling vascular catheters (2, 87). Other risk factors include manipulative procedures; use of antibiotics, steroids, or antimetabolites; and elderly or severely ill patients.

The most frequent source of Gram-negative bacteremia is the urinary tract. Of those experiencing an infection with a urinary source, 52% have indwelling catheters or have undergone cystoscopy, surgery, or biopsy of the urinary tract. Of those experiencing an infection with a respiratory origin, 70% have endotracheal intubation, respiratory assistance devices, or have undergone tracheostomy, surgery, or biopsy of the respiratory tract.

These statistics emphasize the importance of respiratory and urinary tract instrumentation, but the most recent trend is the large increase in infection with Gram-positive organisms due to intravascular catheters (88). An operative site in the gastrointestinal tract may be the source of bacteremia in postoperative situations, but indwelling catheters, drainage tubes, monitoring devices, diagnostic instruments, inhalation therapy equipment, and hospital food and equipment are more likely sources of colonization and infection. Manipulation of pressure transducers by health care workers also has caused polymicrobial bloodstream infections (89).

Gram-positive bacteremia usually originates from the skin, a wound, or indwelling intravascular lines in surgical patients. Only 2 to 3% of bloodstream bacteremias were anaerobic in a study by Lombardi and Engleberg (90). Between 80 and 90% of these were either from *Clostridium* sp. or *Bacteroides* sp., and most were from a previously suspected gastrointestinal source and were covered by appropriate antibiotics.

Persistent "breakthrough" bacteremia while on antibiotics most frequently is seen in patients using steroids or with diabetes mellitus, moderate renal failure, and leukopenia. Continuing bacteremia suggests the existence of an abscess; other focal, undrained sources of infection (e.g., gallbladder, obstructed urinary tract); other intra-abdominal foci of infection (e.g., biliary or bowel source); endocarditis; or an indwelling vascular device (91).

Increasing resistance to antibiotics over the past 10 to 15 years has resulted in a larger portion of drug-resistant organisms causing serious infection. More than 50% of coagulase-negative staphylococci are now resistant to methicillin, and the resultant increase in the use of vancomycin also has led not only to increasing resistance to vancomycin among coagulase-negative staphylococci but also among *Enterococcus* sp. as well (2). Methicillin-resistant *S. aureus* continue to increase, and penicillin-resistant *Strep-*

tococcus pneumoniae are a major concern. Resistance to third-generation cephalosporins among *Enterobacter* sp., *Proteus* sp., and *Citrobacter* sp., and resistance to imipenem and fluoroquinolone, is rising as well (3). Appropriate selection of antibiotics for resistant organisms is necessary to reduce inadequately treated bacteremia. A recent review by Jones (2) discusses various approaches to these serious infections.

Diagnostic Activities

A frequent problem in postoperative consultation is determining the cause of persistent or recurring bacteremia (91, 92). The most common sources are intravascular foci (e.g., intravenous access devices, prostheses, endocarditis), abdominal abscesses, and gastrointestinal or genitourinary foci. Recent use of surgical instrumentation or manipulation should be considered as a source of transient bacteremia. When the patient has blood cultures that are repeatedly positive for an organism sensitive to the antibiotic being administered, several possibilities should be considered. Intravascular foci should be sought, including tunnel and port infections in venous access devices, prostheses, and bacterial endocarditis. Focal undrained sources of infection also should be considered, including abscesses, undrained infection (e.g., gallbladder or obstructed urinary tract), and intra-abdominal foci (e.g., biliary, bowel). Occult infection in the abdomen should be sought, with special attention to the liver, gallbladder, kidneys, appendix, colon, and intra-abdominal abscesses. Susceptibility testing should be reviewed with the microbiology laboratory and drug resistance monitored as discussed earlier. Both the dose and route of antibiotic administration should be checked as well.

The deteriorating surgical patient who already is on appropriate antibiotics for bacterial sepsis must always be considered to have a surgical lesion requiring drainage or a fungal infection until proven otherwise.

Treatment

Determining the source of bacteremia is particularly important, since elimination of the focus of infection is necessary for cure. Table 17.21 lists the common sources of bacteremia for several organisms. Initial treatment of bacteremia in the surgical patient depends on the most likely site. Current sources on antibacterial coverage (24, 81, 82) should be consulted for antibacterial coverage; those

Table 17.21.   Common Sources of Bacteremia

Staphylococcus aureus	Lung
	Wound
	Intravenous catheter
	Skin
Staphylococcus epidermidis	Prosthetic heart valves
	Ventriculoatrial shunts
	Intravenous catheter
	Urinary procedures
	Valvular heart diseases
	Contaminant
Escherichia coli	Urinary procedures
	Gastrointestinal tract
	Abdominal abscesses
	Peritonitis
Klebsiella sp.	Abdominal wounds
	Gastrointestinal tract
	Intravenous catheter
	Lung
Enterobacter sp.	Contaminated blood products
	Contaminated intravenous fluids
	Intravenous catheter
	Urinary procedures
Serratia sp.	Intravenous catheter
	Urinary procedures
	Pneumonia following respiratory use
Pseudomonas sp.	Respiratory tract
	Urinary tract
	Wound infection
	Intravenous catheter
Proteus sp.	Wound infection
	Urinary tract
Bacteroides sp.	Female genital tract
	Gastrointestinal tract
	Postoperative abdominal abscesses
	Liver abscess
Citrobacter sp.	Urinary tract
Actinetobacter sp.	Intravenous catheter
Erwinia sp.	Intravenous infusion set
Providencia sp.	Urinary tract

with knowledge of individual hospital susceptibility patterns also should be sought.

Fungemia

Epidemiology

The rate of fungemia acquired in the hospital continues to increase with the growing populations of both immunocompromised patients as well as patients requiring prolonged cardiopulmonary support and invasive monitoring, and the use of broad-spectrum antibiotics (93–95). The risk is greatest in critical care units. Fungal species represent 7% of hospital-wide nosocomial pathogens, and they represent 10% of those in ICUs. Candida sp. are the fourth most common bloodstream infection in ICUs, behind *Pseudomonas* sp., *S. aureus*, and coagulase-negative staphylococci. *Candida albicans* has declined in frequency to 50% of candidal isolates, with *C. Tropicalis*, *C. parapsilosis*, and others being identified as well. Bloodstream infections invariably are associated with indwelling vascular catheters. The highest incidence occurs in burn patients with central catheters. Bacteremia precedes or is recognized simultaneously in 88% of patients, and the overall mortality rate for those with established fungemia is high (i.e., 50–80%) (96). The attributable mortality rate of candidemia is 38% (97).

Those typically at risk are severely ill postoperative patients with a serious bacterial infection and who are receiving antibiotics and hyperalimentation, have multiple intravenous lines, and have a Foley catheter. In a study of candidal sepsis among surgical patients (94), the most common preceding procedure was gastrointestinal, involving the small or large bowel. Eighty-five percent were receiving hyperalimentation, 96% had a central catheter, and all received a week of antibiotics. Diabetes, steroid use, or alcohol use did not affect mortality in this study. Approximately 35% of such patients die of their fungemia, 30% of the underlying disease, and 35% recover (97). The best predictors of mortality in this setting are severity of the illness, duration of the candidemia, and prognosis of the underlying illness.

Diagnostic Activities

Clinical clues to the presence of significant fungemia are: (a) any change in the fever pattern, (b) any new, unexplained change in mental status, or (c) any new hypotension. The clinical picture can be indistinguishable from that of Gram-negative septicemia. Many patients have Gram-negative septicemia, are treated, and continue to deteriorate. It is important to recognize that there may be a 2- to 3-week period of latent infection; only after invasion of the bloodstream occurs does the infection become fulminant.

The findings on physical examination are consistent with the presence of sepsis. Especially important features, however, include a cheesy, white exudate that is expressed from the catheter site; erythematous, macronodular skin lesions; and pathognomonic white retinal exudates. A funduscopic examination by an ophthalmologist is strongly recommended if fungemia is suspected. Involvement by other organ systems, especially arthritis, pulmonary disease, osteomyelitis, and myocarditis, may aid in making the diagnosis.

Scrapings from skin lesions should be examined microscopically and cultured. Burn wounds should undergo biopsy for histology and quantitative culture.

Candida sp. may be cultured from wounds, the peritoneum, urine, sputum, or feces. Since colonization of these areas is common, the results of these cultures are not diagnostic of invasive disease. Also, in the presence of a Foley catheter, fungal colony counts cannot distinguish between invasive disease and colonization of the bladder. Renal involvement occurs in 80% of patients with systemic candidiasis, so it is an important but difficult distinction between urinary tract colonization and infection. Serologic tests have not been particularly useful, and research on their usefulness continues. The finding by culture of *Candida* sp. colonizing multiple body sites in a high-risk patient should raise a high suspicion of invasive candidiasis, since a substantial percentage of these patients have invasive infection (98). However, documentation of multiple colonized sites is not sufficient to prove that invasive infection has occurred.

A definitive diagnosis must be made on the basis of a positive tissue biopsy, blood cultures, fundoscopic findings, and skin lesions. Detection times of blood cultures have improved to as soon as 4 days, but a 12% contamination rate remains (99).

Treatment

The difficulty of selecting patients infected with *Candida* sp. for treatment has been reviewed by Edwards and Filler (100). The mortality rate of patients with two or more colonized sites but without fungemia is as high as that for those with fungemia. With an untreated mortality rate of 63% and the difficulty of predicting those with a low probability for invasive disease, several authors have recommended treatment for those at risk. The reader is referred to current references for treatment (100, 101).

Drug Fever

Epidemiology and Pathophysiology

Febrile reactions to drugs, especially antibiotics, complicate evaluation of the postoperative patient. Making the diagnosis of drug fever is difficult in seriously ill patients, in whom withholding possible offending agents may make treatment difficult.

The incidence of drug fever is unknown, but such fever may represent approximately 3 to 5% of adverse drug reactions in hospitalized patients, nearly all of whom receive at least one medication. Approximately 30 to 60% of surgical patients receive antibiotics, of which 10 to 20% receive antibiotics for prophylaxis. Drug fever is a particular problem with

antibiotics, because antibiotics are commonly administered and are a common cause of febrile reactions (102). Implicated agents include penicillins, β-lactam antibiotics, sulfonamides, isoniazid, vancomycin, phenytoin, carbamazepine, procainamide, quinidine, iodides, cimetidine, and barbiturates, though many other drugs have been implicated as well (103).

Hypersensitivity reaction is the best-established mechanism for drug fever, but it does not account for all episodes. Only 18% developed rash and 22% eosinophilia in one large series of patients with drug fever (104). Other postulated mechanisms are: *(a)* direct pyrogenic effect of the injected material (e.g., amphotericin), *(b)* alteration of thermoregulatory mechanisms, *(c)* pharmacologic action, *(d)* side effects (e.g., hemolytic anemia, vasculitis), *(e)* local phlebitis at the site of injection, and *(f)* idiosyncratic responses.

Diagnostic Activities

New fever should prompt a review of the patient's medication record. A thorough patient history of prior allergy to medication, of medication before hospitalization, and of bedside drugs from home should be obtained. All drugs should be suspected, with priority being given to those agents listed earlier. The initial assessment should establish if an infection or other nondrug-related cause is responsible for the fever. Any administration of drugs commonly causing fever, temporal relationship of drug administration to fever, and other signs of drug reaction (e.g., eosinophilia, nephritis) should be established as well.

Isolated drug fever due to antibiotics often begins between the seventh and tenth postoperative days. The fever may begin earlier (median, 5 days) when antineoplastic agents are being used or there has been prior exposure to the agent. Cardiovascular drugs have a median of 10 days to onset of fever (104). Patients with drug fever often appear to be well, without leukocytosis, and without serious toxicity, but high fever and shaking chills are common (53%). Rarely, the patient may appear to be acutely ill, mimicking sepsis with high fever (to 104°F), rigors, hypotension, and hypoxia. Only a few patients (11%) have a relative bradycardia, which is contrary to previous reports. Other organs may be affected (e.g., hepatitis, interstitial nephritis), but this usually occurs later in the course of disease.

No particular fever pattern is characteristic of drug fever. Sustained, intermittent, remittent, and hectic patterns have been described.

Treatment

Most drug fevers will improve within 48 to 72 hours of the offending agent being discontinued. Occasionally, a week or longer is necessary for defervescence, especially if the disease course is complicated by a drug-induced serum sickness or hepatitis.

If drug fever is suspected, the suspected offending drug should be discontinued or substituted. The clinical situation, availability of alternative drugs, and need for medication will determine if all remaining drugs should be stopped, changed together, or if this should be done sequentially. Sequential discontinuation is helpful diagnostically, but it exposes patients to more prolonged risk and lengthens the diagnostic process. Rechallenge will establish the cause, but this should only be done in patients with a major need for the medication.

Rarely, the offending drug cannot be discontinued because it is vital and no alternative exists. The major risk of continuation is end-organ damage, especially exfoliative dermatitis, hepatitis, interstitial nephritis, and vasculitis. Drug fever may be suppressed by salicylates, acetaminophen, steroids, and possibly, antihistamines. Suppression of fever, however, does not eliminate the risk of damage to other organs, and the patient should be closely monitored.

When a drug is identified as causing fever, the patient should be informed. In addition, the drug reaction should be documented in the record so that future administration is avoided.

Pneumonia

Epidemiology

Pneumonia remains a major cause of postoperative morbidity and mortality, representing from 10 to 20% of all nosocomial infections. From 6 to 10 patients per 1000 hospital admissions develop pneumonia in general hospitals, but the rate in ICUs ranges from 8 to 15%. It is the second most common nosocomial infection but has the highest morbidity and mortality rates (105).

Pneumonia in surgical patients varies by category and risk factors. A study of 2969 patients undergoing major abdominal surgery found 45 (1.5%) with postoperative pneumonia (106). Predictors for the progression of atelectasis to pneumonia in this study included blood loss of more than 1200 mL, age older than 65 years, and preoperative use of inhalers. Another study of 107 operations in patients with severe chronic obstructive pulmonary disease (COPD) revealed six deaths and two patients with nonfatal ventilatory failure, thus suggesting that an "acceptable" rate of postoperative pneumonia exists even in patients with significant pulmonary disease (107). Both of these studies highlight the importance of chronic lung disease as a major risk factor in surgical patients. Other studies of postoperative patients relate risk to COPD, length and type of surgical procedure, presence of pathogens in gastric contents at the time of operation, and postoperative colonization with organisms of gastric origin, thus emphasizing the role of gastric microaspiration (37, 38). Other risk factors for pneumonia include patient-related factors such as chronic illness, coma, malnutrition, prolonged perioperative period, and comorbid illness. Infection control factors (i.e., contamination and poor control practices) and intervention-related factors (i.e., surgery, sedatives, tubes and devices, prolonged and inappropriate antibiotic use, prolonged use of H_2-blockers, nasogastric tubes, and enteral feedings) also contribute to morbidity and mortality (38).

Data on the bacteriology of postoperative pneumonia derive mainly from nosocomial pneumonias, in which Gram-negative organisms represent nearly 60% of infections, Gram-positive organisms 20%, and fungi and mixed infections the remainder (105). Studies in trauma and nontertiary care settings report a higher rate of infection with *Haemophilus influenzae* (39, 40). Despite the increase in nosocomial coagulase-positive staphylococcal infections, this organism does not seem to a frequent cause of pneumonia.

Microaspiration of small volumes of oropharyngeal bacteria is the principal mechanism for the acquisition of pneumonia (38), though inhalation from respiratory equipment and hematogenous spread both play a role. Airborne transmission in the hospital is unimportant, however. Normal throat flora of hospitalized patients will convert to Gram-negative colonization, similar to fecal flora, in 27% of patients not receiving antibiotics and in 47% of those receiving antibiotics; in severely ill individuals, this colonization is rapid and approaches 75% in the first few days (38, 105). Combining the high colonization rates of potential pathogens with any of the risk factors described explains the susceptibility of hospitalized patients to pneumonia.

Diagnostic Activities

A standard but useful approach to the diagnosis of hospital-acquired pneumonia has been developed by the American Thoracic Society (38). Patients can be categorized into three groups:

1. Mild to moderate pneumonia without risk factors and with onset at any time during hospitalization, or those with severe pneumonia with onset within 5 days of admission.

2. Mild to moderate pneumonia with risk factors developing any time during hospitalization.
3. Severe pneumonia with late onset (>5 days) or early onset with risk factors.

Patients without risk factors and mild to moderate pneumonia are likely to have one of several "core organisms," which include both the Gram-negative organisms (*Enterobacter* sp., *Escherichia coli*, *Klebsiella* sp., *Proteus* sp., *Serratia* sp., *Haemophilus influenzae*) and the Gram-positive organisms (*Streptococcus pneumoniae* and methicillin-sensitive *Staphylococcus aureus*). In early infection (<5 days), *H. influenzae*, *S. pneumoniae*, and *S. aureus* are isolated more frequently. In patients with mild or moderate pneumonia and specific risk factors such as surgery, altered pathogens include anaerobes because of possible aspiration. In patients with early severe pneumonia or severe pneumonia with onset at any time and with risk factors, drug-resistant Gram-negative organisms, including *Pseudomonas* sp. and *Acinetobacter* sp., as well as methicillin-resistant *S. aureus* are potential pathogens. In ventilator-associated pneumonia, up to 40% of infections are polymicrobial (38).

Criteria for the diagnosis of nosocomial pneumonia (6) include either of the following:

1. Rales or dullness on examination, and either new purulent sputum, positive blood culture, or pathogen from transtracheal aspirate or bronchial washing.
2. New infiltrate, cavitation or effusion, and one of the following: new purulent sputum, positive blood culture, pathogen from transtracheal aspirate or bronchial washing, and histopathologic evidence.

Evaluation should include chest radiography, blood cultures, arterial blood gases, and diagnostic thoracentesis if there is more than 10 mm of effusion on lateral decubitus position. Sputum culture and Gram stain have limited sensitivity and specificity, but they remain an important part of the evaluation as more definitive tests are too invasive for routine use. The main value of a sputum culture is identification of the antibiotic-sensitivity patterns of organisms that are present if drug resistance is suspected. Serologic or urinary antigen studies have only limited value, except perhaps for suspected infection with *Legionella* sp. and for epidemiologic purposes.

For intubated patients, improvements in diagnosis have relied on quantitative cultures from endobronchial aspiration, protected catheter aspiration, protected specimen brush, and bronchiolar alveolar lavage. Studies have shown that endobronchial aspiration compares favorably (84%) with the more invasive techniques (41).

The diagnosis remains challenging, however, as noninfectious infiltrates appear because of atelectasis, pulmonary edema, drug reactions, pulmonary hemorrhage, or acute respiratory distress syndrome (108). Only air bronchograms on chest radiography correlate with the presence of pneumonia. Purulent secretions may represent tracheobronchitis in intubated patients. Blood cultures are positive in only 8 to 20% of cases, and there is another site of infection in up to 50% of patients with severe pneumonia. Cytomegalovirus, influenza, fungi, and tuberculosis must be considered in immunocompromised hosts or clinical circumstances suggesting legionella pneumonia.

Treatment

Interventions to reduce the incidence of pneumonia have been proposed. Placing patients in a semirecumbent position to reduce aspiration and removing subglottic secretions through a special endotracheal tube have had some success. The general approach to treatment, however, is to place the patient in one of the three clinical categories listed earlier. Antibiotics are selected on the basis of the most likely pathogens in each circumstance (24, 68, 81, 82).

Pulmonary Aspiration

The potential aspiration of gastric or oropharyngeal secretions represents a significant risk in the perioperative period. The challenge is to recognize aspiration early and to distinguish it from other postoperative pulmonary complications. Risk factors in the surgical patient include ileus, gastric dilatation, nasogastric feeding tubes, endotracheal tubes, depressed cough and level of consciousness from pain medications, and gastroparesis in patients with diabetes (109).

Epidemiology

The mean interval from operation to aspiration is 1.5 days, though episodes can occur up to 30 days postoperatively. The clinical course of gastric acid aspiration follows one of three patterns:

1. A rapidly progressive, acute course leading to death within 24 hours.
2. Clinical and radiographic improvement over 2 to 16 days after the initial aspiration.
3. Initial improvement followed in 2 or more days by clinical deterioration associated with signs and symptoms of superimposed nosocomial pneumonia (109).

It must be emphasized that infection is not thought to be part of the initial process of gastric aspiration. Infection develops secondarily, probably due to chemical damage or, more insidiously, associated with aspiration of small amounts of colonized oropharyngeal secretions. In intubated patients, secretions that pool around the endotracheal tube can leak into the lung, where the host defenses are compromised. Subclinical aspiration of nasogastric tube feedings, as detected by nonbloody, glucose-positive endotracheal secretions, also contributes to pneumonia (42).

The less fulminant form of pneumonia seldom is witnessed, and it may develop insidiously days to weeks after surgery, with clinical deterioration, weight loss and anemia, putrid sputum, and pulmonary cavitation or abscess. Abrupt onset of a self-limited illness consisting of fever, cyanosis, dyspnea, hypoxemia, and dependent infiltrates suggests aspiration (42). After witnessed aspiration, infection may not develop for 1 to 2 days, though over 50% of cases occurring in 3 to 5 days and some occur as late as 2 or more weeks. The risk of bacterial infection after acid aspiration is 25 to 40% within the first week.

Bacteriology

The bacteriology of in-hospital aspiration is complex, and it largely depends on colonization of the oropharynx. Normal oropharyngeal colonization is replaced by Gram-negative organisms in the hospital, especially in the setting of antibiotic use or intubation. Anaerobic organisms, especially *Bacteroides* sp., play a major role.

Diagnostic Activities

Indicators of infection after aspiration include new or increased fever, leukocytosis, purulent sputum, new or extending pulmonary infiltrate (especially in the posterior segments of the upper lobes or superior segments of the lower lobes) appearing more than 48 hours after aspiration (progression of radiographic findings 36 to 48 hours after witnessed aspiration usually indicates a superimposed infection), increased hypoxia, consistent Gram stain, and unexplained deterioration. Sputum cultures must be interpreted with caution, however, because colonization alone is not indicative of infection. The absence of staphylococci or Gram-negative organisms on culture suggests that these organisms are not involved. A nearly pure growth of one organism means that organism is likely to be causative.

The predictability of the bacteriology of community-acquired aspiration pneumonia means that invasive procedures are indicated only in select cases. In postoperative patients, the bacteriology is less predictable due to colonization by hospital-acquired organisms, and every attempt should be made to identify specific organisms.

Treatment

For witnessed aspiration, supportive care that includes suctioning, oxygen, and volume replacement, preferably in an ICU setting, is desirable until the clinical course becomes clear. Corticosteroids are not helpful. Theoretically, antibiotics should not be given until an infection is documented, but antibiotics are given clinically, however, because of the degree of illness and the precarious situation of most patients who aspirate. Both the decision to administer and the selection of antibiotics are based on the degree of clinical illness, severity of aspiration, Gram-stain results, underlying illness, and general condition of the patient. For most postoperative patients, this means starting antibiotics for all but minor aspirations (110).

The antibiotics used should cover anaerobes and Gram-negative organisms. Other important aspects of care are the recognition of any predisposing causes (e.g, diabetic gastroparesis) and the prevention of repeated episodes of aspiration. Modified video barium swallow tests identify unsuspected aspiration and are the diagnostic procedure of choice.

Atelectasis

Atelectasis is the most common cause of early postoperative fever, and it accounts for up to 90% of postoperative pulmonary complications. Atelectasis occurs in approximately 10 to 20% of patients who undergo abdominal surgery and is more common (20 to 30%) in patients who undergo surgery of the upper abdomen. The contribution of atelectasis to the febrile response is variable, and it may be difficult to interpret clinically in individual patients. Livelli et al. (58) noted segmental or subsegmental atelectasis in 62% of febrile patients and 54% of nonfebrile patients 6 days after cardiac surgery.

Axioms on atelectasis (43) include: *(a)* clinical and radiographic findings of various degrees of atelectasis should be considered cautiously as the cause of early fever; *(b)* fever does not necessarily correlate with the extent of atelectasis and, unless complications occur, should gradually decline as treatment proceeds; *(c)* auscultation may detect atelectasis earlier than radiography, and rales often precede decreased breath sounds; *(d)* atelectasis with fever but normal-appearing radiographs and physical findings can occur; *(e)* infection is not thought to be present in early atelectasis, though unrecognized aspiration could be a common cause of postoperative atelectasis; *(f)* atelectasis could result from other processes (i.e., subdiaphragmatic abscess or pulmonary infarction).

Thus while treatment for atelectasis proceeds, a constant awareness of other febrile conditions must be maintained. Atelectasis in febrile postoperative patients remains common, but it is in part a diagnosis of exclusion. One must avoid ending the search for other causes.

Treatment

See Chapter 7.

Thrombophlebitis and Pulmonary Embolism

Thrombophlebitis and pulmonary embolism are discussed in Chapter 10. Postoperatively, these entities often are in the differential diagnosis of fever. Fever up to 102°F may occur with deep-vein thrombosis; rarely, fever up to 104°F may occur with pulmonary embolism. The frequency of fever in thrombophlebitis is difficult to quantitate. Fever alone may be the sole presenting feature of deep-venous thrombosis, thus prompting duplex compression sonography.

In a review of fever and pulmonary embolism, Murray et al. (111) reported

fever in 64% of angiographically proven cases. Fever was more common with pulmonary infarction. Temperatures up to 40°C are noted early in the course of disease and may persist for more than 1 week. The persistence of (rectal) temperatures of 38.5°C after 4 days or 38°C after 6 days are uncommon and should not be attributed solely to emboli unless evidence for re-embolization exists. Only one patient in the series had hectic fever spikes. The findings of leukocytosis in the range of 10,000 to 20,000 WBCs/mL (and occasionally up to 40,000 WBCs/mL) and empyemalike pleural fluid make these unreliable indicators of infection versus infarction. No patient in this series had shaking chills, though rigors has been reported with pulmonary embolism previously. Thrombophlebitis and pulmonary embolism should be considered in all postoperative febrile patients. The fever itself provides no substantial clues, however, and diagnosis must rely on other parameters.

Urinary Tract Infection

See also Chapter 12.

Epidemiology

Infections of the urinary tract constitute the largest single source of nosocomial infection, and one that is closely related to catheterization. UTIs generally are recognized as the most common nosocomial infection (27%), the most common cause of Gram-negative bacteremia (30 to 40%), and the second or third most common cause of postoperative fever (2). Approximately 15% of hospitalized patients receive indwelling urinary catheters. Currently, the prevalence of infection is approximately 10%, down from the 20 to 25% seen in the 1960s and 1970s (112).

Urethral catheters impair normal defense mechanisms. Their insertion may push organisms into the bladder and serve as a conduit for ascending bacteria, and the catheter surfaces become a niche for adherent bacteria that forms a protective biofilm, thus trapping bacteria in its surface (113). Catheter drainage is imperfect, leading to retained urine, and the catheter may directly damage the urinary epithelium, where normally the protective glycosaminoglycan layer inhibits bacterial adherence. Duration of catheterization is the most important risk factor for bacteriuria. The incidence of bacteriuria is 3 to 10% per day, with most patients being bacteriuric at 30 days (112). Impaired defenses are more important in the pathogenesis of infection than the virulence of the organism.

The risk of infection is related to four factors:

1. Duration of catheterization.
2. Female gender.
3. Catheter care violations.
4. Absence of antibiotics.

Use of sealed-junction catheters reduces the rate of UTIs in catheterized patients as well as the mortality rate in those patients with UTIs who are not receiving antibiotics. Antibiotics administered for 4 to 5 days in catheterized patients have repeatedly reduced the occurrence of UTIs. Lack of hand washing by physicians and nurses causes cross-contamination between catheters and patients (113).

Common morbidity includes asymptomatic bacteriuria, cystitis, and pyelonephritis. From 1 to 4% of patients with UTIs develop bacteremia, with a mortality rate of from 13 to 30% (113). Rarely, complications include perinephric abscess, epididymitis, orchitis, and vertebral osteomyelitis.

In addition to urethral catheterization, surgical instrumentation of the urinary tract and fistulas produced from surgery in adjacent structures also result in UTIs.

Bacteriology

Nearly all studies of nosocomial urinary infections show that E. coli is the most frequent pathogen, ranging from 30 to 50% of isolates. Other frequent pathogens are *Klebsiella-Enterobacter* sp. (13–15%), *Pseudomonas* sp. (10–20%), *Proteus* sp. (3–13%), enterococci (2–10%), and *Candida* sp. (2). Patients with surgical-instrumentation catheters and prior use of antibiotics tend to have a greater incidence of *Pseudomonas* sp., *Serratia* sp., *Providentia* sp., *Citrobacter* sp., *Acinetobacter* sp., and *Candida albicans*. The selective pressure of antibiotic use within a given hospital will contribute to the distribution of bacteria colonizing susceptible patients. Knowledge of the most frequent organisms causing nosocomial UTIs in an individual hospital is important (1).

Diagnostic Activities

In uncatheterized patients, typical symptoms of frequency, urgency, dysuria, and suprapubic discomfort are early clues to the diagnosis, but they also may be caused or obscured by mechanical or chemical irritants in the postoperative period. Fever, flank pain and tenderness, and chills suggest upper respiratory tract infection. In catheterized patients, manifestations may include blood-tinged or turbid urine, bladder spasms with leakage around the meatus, fever, chills, flank pain, and signs of sepsis and shock. In postoperative patients, fever alone may be the sole clinical clue and usually begins at least 48 to 72 hours after surgery or catheterization.

The CDC criteria for urinary infections are listed in Table 17.22. It must be stressed, however, that finding 10^5 organisms/mL in the urine does not guarantee that this is the source of the patient's fever. Because asymptomatic bacteriuria is common, the diagnosis should be based on the clinical situation, culture, and careful follow-up.

Treatment

Therapy for UTI depends on the clinical illness and whether a Foley catheter remains in place. If symptomatic, un-

Table 17.22.   Criteria for Symptomatic Urinary Tract Infection

Must meet criteria 1 or 2
1. One of the following:
   Fever >38° C, urgency, frequency, dysuria, or suprapubic tenderness *and* a culture with >10^5 colonies with no more than 2 species.
2. Any two of the following:
   fever >38° C, urgency, frequency, dysuria, or suprapubic tenderness *and* any of the following:
   a. Positive dipstick test for leukocyte esterase or nitrate
   b. Pyuria >10 WBCs on spun or >3 WBCs in unspun urine
   c. Organisms seen on Gram stain of unspun urine
   d. Two urine cultures on unvoided urine >10^2 with same organism
   e. Urine culture with single organism <10^5 while on antibiotics

Reprinted with permission from Garner JS, Jarvis WR, Emori TG, Horan TC, Hughes JM. CDC definitions for nosocomial infections. Am J Infect Control 1988;16:128–140.

catheterized patients should be treated. Asymptomatic bacteriuria, however, needs to be treated only if it occurs after instrumentation or in pregnant patients.

Patients with indwelling Foley catheters should be treated for symptomatic or febrile urinary infections. Positive cultures in asymptomatic catheterized patients usually should not be treated because of the emergence of drug-resistant organisms. The urine should be routinely cultured either when or shortly after the catheter is removed. At this point, patients can be treated then even if asymptomatic.

The rate of infection can be reduced by proper catheter care (113). The most important measures are to avoid unnecessary catheterization; use a closed, one-way drainage system; ensure proper insertion and daily care; and avoid cross-contamination by hospital personnel.

Special Considerations: Candiduria

A urine culture that is positive for *Candida* sp. occasionally prompts consul-

tation. The spectrum of infections from yeast include asymptomatic candiduria, urethritis, cystitis, primary renal candidiasis, and bacteremic sepsis. Candiduria can, and frequently does, coexist with bacterial infections.

Most urine cultures containing *Candida* sp. represent either contamination or colonization related to use of indwelling catheters, antibiotics, and steroids. The significance of candiduria depends on the presence of infection with tissue invasion, upper urinary tract disease, or systemic illness. The problem of assessing the significance of candiduria relates to the difficulty in proving that tissue invasion or upper tract involvement has occurred; no uniform criteria exist (114).

A urine culture that is positive for *Candida* sp. should not be ignored. If the patient is asymptomatic, the culture should be repeated to minimize contamination and reconfirm the presence of candiduria. Some data suggest that if fewer than 15,000 colonies/mL are present in a midstream urine, renal *Candida* is unlikely. The significance of colony counts is controversial, and colony counts cannot be used in the evaluation of patients with long-term catheters.

In asymptomatic patients, prolonged candiduria may clear with the removal of predisposing factors. Candiduria can be present for 12 months without the manifestation of infection (114).

Tissue invasion usually occurs in patients who are immunocompromised, debilitated, or extremely ill from other causes. The presence of invasive infection with *Candida* sp. is difficult to demonstrate, but positive blood cultures, skin or eye findings, or positive multiple-site cultures will suggest invasive disease. Unreliable indicators of invasion are pyuria, pseudohyphae, and serologic tests.

Treatment of selected at-risk patients with candiduria is controversial but commonly practiced. Amphotericin B bladder washes for 60 to 90 minutes daily for 2 days is most commonly used (115).

In patients who are critically ill, candiduria seems to be an early marker for dissemination. In a group of patients with candidiasis, disseminated infection was not detected and treated for an average of 9 days, with a mortality rate of 53%. A prospective group was treated with systemic fluconazole at the time of candiduria, with a mortality rate of 5%. These statistics have led to the recommendation for systemic treatment of candiduria in those who are critically ill (116).

Perinephric Abscess

Perinephric abscess is an uncommon infection and typically is difficult to diagnose (117). From 70 to 90% of cases follow an upper UTI or urologic surgery with rupture of a parenchymal abscess into the perinephric space. The remainder result from hematogenous spread, usually from the skin. Only in approximately 25% of patients, however, can a history of urinary tract or skin infection be obtained. Renal abscess is more common in the presence of diabetes. Causative bacteria are usually enteric Gram-negative pathogens or *Staphylococcus* sp.; polymicrobial infections are seen in 29% of cases. Urine cultures are positive in 50 to 80% of patients and usually contain the same organism as the abscess. Blood cultures are positive in approximately one-third of cases.

Slightly more than 50% of these patients are febrile, 40% have flank pain or abdominal pain, and most initially are thought to have an upper UTI. Physical examination, maximum temperature, WBC count, and urinary findings do not discriminate between those with pyelonephritis and those with perinephric abscess unless a flank mass is palpated. Abdominal masses may be palpated in approximately 50% of patients; of those with delayed diagnoses, most have no physical findings.

A useful diagnostic clue is that patients with acute pyelonephritis generally are not febrile more than 4 days after the initiation of appropriate antibiotic ther-

apy. Patients with perinephric abscess often are febrile after 5 or more days of antibiotic therapy, and they often remain febrile until surgical drainage has occurred. Abdominal radiographs may show obliterated psoas shadows and loss of renal borders. An intravenous pyelogram may show a perinephric mass, but this may be mistaken for a pseudocyst from the tail of the pancreas. CT scanning is most helpful in making the diagnosis, and CT-guided catheter drainage is usually successful. Sonography provides an alternative imaging modality.

In the postoperative period, most patients who are seen will have been receiving antibiotics for suspected pyelonephritis. If a patient with a UTI has been febrile without other cause after 5 days of appropriate antibiotic therapy, perinephric abscess should be sought.

Treatment is use of antibiotics and drainage, either percutaneous or surgical. Some cases of renal carbuncle, which do not extend into the perinephric space, have been treated successfully with antibiotics alone.

Surgical Site Infections

Epidemiology

See introduction to Chapter 17.

Bacteriology

Representative rates for various organisms causing nosocomial SSI infections are: *S. aureus*, 17%; *Enterococcus* sp., 13%; coagulase-negative staphylococci, 12%; *E. coli*, 10%; *Enterobacter* sp, 8%; *Pseudomonas* sp., 8%; and *Candida* sp., 2% (2). Percentages vary from hospital to hospital, and it must be remembered that from 20 to 60% of SSIs are diagnosed after the patient has been discharged, thus altering hospital statistics. Unusual bacteria, fungi, and anaerobes constitute a small, but probably underreported, percentage of cases. Multiple pathogens are found in a variable percentage of cases.

Diagnostic Activities

The diagnosis of SSI is made clinically according to CDC definitions (16). For example, a diagnosis of superficial incisional SSI is made when the infection occurs within 30 days, is superficial to the fascia, there is purulent drainage or organisms are isolated from aseptically obtained culture, and there is either pain, tenderness, localized swelling redness, or heat. This excludes stitch abscesses and superficial burns.

Much overlap occurs in the appearance of wound infections by different organisms, but some clinical differences between organisms are useful. Staphylococcal infections usually appear in 4 to 6 days with a localized area of induration, cellulitis, and a thick, odorless, creamy yellow pus (118). If there is no drainage, throbbing local pain, redness, and swelling with fever and leukocytosis generally occur. With deep invasion, systemic symptoms appear. Aerobic streptococcal infections usually occur within the first several days postoperatively and with a rapidly progressing cellulitis (86). Early toxic symptoms may be present as well and are indicative of the invasive nature of the infection.

Infections with Gram-negative organisms are more indolent, and their signs are more subtle. The incubation period is generally more than 1 week but can be as long as 1 month, especially if the patient has been on antibiotics. Deep or obscure abscesses are a particular problem with gram-negative wound infections.

Anaerobic streptococcal infections caused by *Peptostreptococcus* sp. may be recognized by a thick, grayish pus that has a fetid odor.

Treatment

Surgical drainage remains the cornerstone of therapy. When needed, antibiotics can be rationally chosen on the basis of the Gram stain, clinical appearance of the wound, and state of the patient. Antibiotics may be started before the wound is drained or debrided but after appropriate specimens for stain and culture are taken. Distant hematogenous complications of wound infection include pneumonitis, meningitis, endocarditis, and major organ abscess (e.g., liver, kidney, spleen).

Special Considerations

Several types of **necrotizing infections of soft tissue** (e.g., skin, subcutaneous tissue, fascia, muscle) may be rarely seen in postoperative patients. Prompt recognition is critical, however, because mortality is high and surgical intervention required (119, 120). Necrotizing infections may complicate even the most minor elective procedures or trauma. The classification and terminology of these diseases vary widely, and individual syndromes are referred to by different names in the literature. All may follow surgery or be seen in patients with trauma.

Clostridial anaerobic cellulitis is an infection of the subcutaneous tissue and usually does not involve the deep fascia and muscle (in contrast to the more well-known clostridial gas gangrene). Onset is gradual. Infected skin is minimally discolored and moderately swollen, and systemic toxicity is absent.

Nonclostridial anaerobic cellulitis is an illness similar to clostridial anaerobic cellulitis, but it is caused by other anaerobic bacteria, often in a mixed infection with multiple Gram-positive and gram-negative anaerobes. Onset may be gradual or abrupt. The appearance of infected skin is similar to that in clostridial cellulitis; differentiation can only be made on the basis of Gram stain. Some systemic toxicity may be present.

Necrotizing fascitis involves the superficial and the deep fascia and is caused by a mixed flora of anaerobes, Gram-positive, and Gram-negative organisms. Onset is abrupt. Infected skin is erythematous and markedly swollen. Systemic toxicity is present and may be marked (121).

Synergistic necrotizing cellulitis also is considered to be a subcategory of necrotizing fascitis, but it involves the skin and muscle as well as the fascia. Infecting bacteria include mixed anaerobes and Gram-negative organisms. Onset is abrupt. Infected skin has scattered areas of necrosis, and swelling is significant. Characteristic "dishwater pus" may be present, and systemic toxicity is marked.

Gas gangrene is a disease that mainly involves muscle. Onset usually is abrupt, and pain is both early and marked. (Moderate pain can be seen with necrotizing fascitis and synergistic necrotizing cellulitis but usually does not occur as early and dramatically). Infected skin is edematous and white early on, which is followed by yellowish-bronze discoloration. Bullae and necrosis may be present, and systemic toxicity is marked and dramatic. Gas gangrene should be contrasted to clostridial anaerobic cellulitis, which is caused by the same species of organism but involves subcutaneous tissues. The lack of systemic toxicity, severe pain, and minimal discoloration of the skin differentiate clostridial cellulitis from gangrene clinically (discussed later).

Infected vascular gangrene is a mixed bacterial infection most commonly due to arteriosclerosis. It involves the devascularized muscle and usually does not spread to more proximal muscle. It is easily distinguished clinically from the other entities discussed.

Despite the differences in clinical presentation listed here, clinical differentiation of these entities often is difficult because of overlapping clinical pictures, the subtle early presentations, and (fortunately) the inexperience of most physicians in dealing with these infections. Needle aspiration of subcutaneous tissue with stat Gram stain is helpful in differentiating clostridial from mixed infections, but failure to obtain pus or a negative Gram stain does *not* exclude infection. Radiography and CT are helpful in establishing the presence of subcutaneous air. The differentiation of muscle involvement often must be made at surgery, however, and is critical because entities involving muscle require more extensive surgery to be lifesaving.

Treatment is administration of appropriate antibiotics and immediate, *adequate* surgical drainage or amputation. The degree of required surgical debridement varies with the different entities depending on involvement of the deep fascia and muscle. Tetanus immunization (i.e., a different clostridium) should not be forgotten.

Fournier's gangrene is considered to be a subcategory of necrotizing fascitis. It is a rare but dramatic syndrome that occurs following surgical procedures involving the perineal area; some authors do not distinguish it from other synergistic necrotizing infections. A mixed aerobic–anaerobic infection with *E. coli*, *Proteus* sp., or *Enterococcus* sp. with *Bacteroides fragilis* causes an obliterative endarteritis and acute dermal gangrene. The syndrome follows herniorrhaphy, hydrocele repair, circumcision, orchiectomy, hemorrhoidectomy, vasectomy, or transrectal prostatic biopsy. Acute onset of genital itching, pain, erythema, swelling, and subcutaneous gas is accompanied by chills, fever, prostration, and toxicity. Involvement may rapidly progress to gangrene and spread to the entire abdominal wall. Aggressive surgical debridement and use of antibiotics directed against **B. fragilis** and enteric Gram-negative rods are essential in preventing high rates of morbidity and mortality. This infection emphasizes the need to examine the skin and soft tissues of the perineal and genital areas in postoperative patients with fever.

Tuberculous, mycotic, and viral infections also occasionally cause wound infections and should be searched for in patients with unresponsive infections. *Candida* sp. are frequent colonizers of wounds, and distinguishing colonization from wound infection with *Candida* sp. is difficult. Demonstration of hyphal forms in biopsy-specimen tissue is the best single criterion of infection.

Toxic Shock Syndrome

Toxic shock syndrome may present a difficult diagnostic problem in the postoperative period because of its lack of localizing, diagnostic symptoms; its rarity; and the similarity of its symptoms with those of other causes of postoperative or postpartum sepsis (122). Graham et al. (123) described only 12 cases (0.003%) in a survey of 390,000 procedures at two hospitals. The syndrome is included in this section, however, because most cases have their origin in a wound "infection," with *Staphylococcus aureus* producing the toxin.

The incidence of toxic shock syndrome after nasal surgery is 16 per 100,000 (67). A high degree of suspicion is needed to make the diagnosis. The rash is diagnostic but occurs late and may be subtle. Other suggestive findings are extremely high temperature (over 104°F) without an obvious source, pharyngeal or conjunctival injection, sore throat, strawberry tongue, severe myalgias (i.e., "respiratory symptoms"), vomiting *and* diarrhea, change in mental status, and multiple-organ dysfunction (e.g., kidney, liver, blood, muscle, CNS). Onset may be insidious with an abrupt worsening or abrupt from the start, with multiple-organ system dysfunction and profound shock. Occurrence of abrupt shock accompanied by multiple-organ system dysfunction, possibly including some of the listed findings that are atypical for surgical sepsis (i.e., respiratory symptoms, watery diarrhea) in the absence of any source of sepsis should raise the possibility of postoperative toxic shock syndrome. The wound may appear to be benign.

Therapy includes mandatory adequate drainage, use of antistaphylococcal antibiotics, and complex supportive care (beyond the scope of this text).

Pelvic Infections

Gynecologists usually treat proven pelvic infections. Consultation with an internist is requested for questions of antibiotic management, persistent fever, and differentiation from other sources of fever.

Puerperal endometritis is the most serious febrile complication of delivery. The diagnosis is made clinically on the basis of the presence of fever, uterine or parametrial tenderness, and abnormal lochia. Unless it is very high, the leukocyte count is less helpful, because postpartum patients may have a moderately elevated WBC count with a left shift as a normal finding. Other common causes of febrile morbidity in the postpartum cesarean patient are urinary tract and wound infections.

In postoperative gynecologic patients, infection can be classified as endometritis (i.e., uterine tenderness), salpingitis (i.e., adnexal tenderness), or peritonitis (i.e., by cul de sac aspiration). During the first 24 hours, infection from group A streptococci, nongroup A streptococci, *Clostridium* sp., or less commonly, Gram-negative rods may produce a rapid toxic picture. A Gram stain for *Clostridium* sp. is important at this stage.

With fever beginning 48 to 72 hours after surgery, the diagnosis of endometritis, vaginal cuff abscess, pelvic cellulitis or abscess, peritonitis, or tubo-ovarian abscess may be made. Pelvic examination identifies the location of the infection and whether drainage is required. Not every mass represents an abscess, however, as matted omentum and bowel may be mistaken for large abscesses.

In patients with continuous fever and appropriate antibiotic coverage for abscess and anaerobes, the internist should be aware of septic pelvic thrombophlebitis as a possibility (124, 125). Septic pelvic thrombophlebitis is a complication of endometritis from any cause and occurs approximately once in every 2000 pregnancies. It is characterized by pain, tachycardia, and antibiotic-resistant fever. A pelvic mass may be present if the ovarian vein is thrombosed, and the diagnosis is suspected by failure to defervesce with 2 to 3 days of antibiotic therapy being initiated. Contrast CT is helpful in making the diagnosis, and the treatment is heparin.

In a review of 77 patients with pelvic infection, there were 14 failures of antibiotic treatment, with 5 of these (36%) resulting from septic pelvic thrombophlebitis and 2 resulting from abscess (126).

Trauma

Trauma is responsible for many admissions to general hospitals, and infections occur in these patients with variable frequency related to the underlying host factors, site of the trauma, extent of the traumatic injury, and degree of contamination. For example, early pneumonia and pulmonary dysfunction following trauma were caused by *Haemophilus* sp. in 37% of patients with pneumonia in one study (40).

Infections following penetrating abdominal trauma are clearly related to the organ that is damaged. Rates of infection are: small bowel, 4%; colon, 15%; pancreas, 15%; and liver, 39%. Abdominal infection after penetrating injury begins with an acute peritonitis due to Gram-negative enteric bacilli and is followed by abscess formation secondary to anaerobic bacteria. Polymicrobial infection is the rule, and abdominal abscesses are the result of aerobic–anaerobic synergism. Other traumatic injuries associated with infectious complications include compound fractures, soft-tissue trauma, skull and facial fractures, and penetrating eye trauma. Multiple-organ failure syndrome (73) is the most important complication, as the mortality rate in these patients approaches 70% (127).

The principles of antimicrobial treatment follow the general rules for "contaminated" and "dirty" surgical cases. Antimicrobial agents in patients with trauma represent treatment (not prophylaxis), since bacteria are introduced before the antimicrobial agents. Use of antibiotics is warranted when the gastrointestinal tract is involved, the wound enters a joint space or involves a tendon, a compound fracture exists, infections with *Clostridium* sp. are likely, or the wound is grossly contaminated. Treatment is continued for 4 to 5 days (127) and is followed by observation except in cases of abdominal trauma with gross contamination, in which case a treatment continues for 7 to 14 days. Continued use of antibiotics may mask late development of an abscess, and such use should not be prolonged without justification.

Fever in the first few days following major trauma is common and does not necessarily indicate infection. Late fever (>3 days) has the same significance as any postoperative fever. Pulmonary embolism should be included in the differential diagnosis of fever in patient with trauma (127).

Diarrhea

Diarrhea resulting from *Clostridium difficile* (i.e., pseudomembranous colitis) is a frequent reason for postoperative consultation, either because of a diagnostic dilemma or questions about therapy. The etiology is a toxin-mediated diarrhea caused by *C. difficile* (128), and predisposing factors are antibiotic therapy and the presence of *C. difficile* in the hospital environment (epidemics have occurred). Most cases on surgical services have followed the use of prophylactic antibiotics, especially with inappropriate, prolonged use (129). Almost all antibiotics have been associated with *C. difficile*.

Presenting symptoms include diarrhea, abdominal pain, discomfort or distention, fever, and leukocytosis. Bacteremia, sepsis, and an acute abdomen also can occur (129). Atypical presentations are fever of uncertain cause and ileus *without* marked diarrhea. The most reliable clinical predictors are diarrhea after 6 days of antibiotics (especially cephalosporins), fecal leukocytosis, a hospital stay of more than 15 days, or readmission to the hospital within 2 weeks (130). Fever, leukocytosis, green diarrheal stool, blood in the stool, and abdominal cramps do not discriminate between infected patients and controls.

Diagnostic Activities

The diagnosis is made by identification of *C. difficile* toxin in the stool by laboratory assay (131). Rapid assays requiring less than 24 hours are now available, and 79% of first specimens are positive, 91% of second specimens, and virtually all of third specimens. Sigmoidoscopy/colonoscopy with biopsy is needed for rapid diagnosis when patients are ill and to rule out other causes. Diagnostic difficulties are posed by the fact that *C. difficile* can colonize the colon (2–10% of patients in some hospitals) and produce positive assays, but not be the cause of the patient's symptoms, and by the nonspecific appearance of the colon, thus requiring biopsy for diagnosis. The diagnosis can be reliably made by using the correlative clinical findings listed earlier, with a maximum of three stool specimens. Colonoscopy with biopsy or an empiric diagnostic trial of therapy sometimes are needed in difficult cases. The differential diagnosis includes other causes of postoperative diarrhea or abdominal symptoms, nonspecific antibiotic-related diarrhea, and nosocomial infectious diarrhea.

Treatment

Treatment includes either metronidazole or vancomycin orally for 10 days; neither drug reaches optimal levels in the colon when given intravenously. Patients unable to take medication by the oral or the nasogastric route postoperatively pose a difficult therapeutic problem; intravenous metronidazole, supplemented by oral drug to the extent that the patient can take it, generally is preferred. Symptomatic improvement is faster with vancomycin (3 versus 4.6 days), which, while more expensive, may shorten the hospital stay. Cholestyramine can be used for symptomatic relief by binding the toxin, but it is not a definitive therapy. The effectiveness of vancomycin and metronidazole may be reduced because of binding to the cholestyramine resin. Alternating doses of antibiotic and cholestyramine may help but does not totally eliminate the problem. The inciting antibiotic should be discontinued.

Recurrence occurs in 7 to 10% of pa-

tients and results from relapse or reinfection. Over 90% of first recurrences can be retreated in the same manner (128). Surgical intervention is required in less than 5% of cases, with a mortality rate of approximately 30% (129).

Vertebral Osteomyelitis and Disc Space Infection

Epidemiology

Postoperative vertebral osteomyelitis is an uncommon infection (accounting for between 2 and 17% of all disc and vertebral infections) following genitourinary instrumentation, UTI, pelvic surgery, back surgery, or a septic process (132). If unrecognized, vertebral osteomyelitis may extend, producing a retroperitoneal abscess. The offending organism reflects the initial site of infection and may be bacterial, fungal, or mycobacterial. Cervical spine infections can occur after tonsillectomy, sinusitis, trauma, dental extractions, or cholecystitis and appendicitis (133).

While *S. aureus* is the most common organism in hematogenously acquired infection, Gram-negative organisms predominate in elderly male patients following genitourinary procedures. Coagulase-negative staphylococci has emerged as a common pathogen when orthopaedic hardware is implanted. Disc space infection from direct inoculation usually follows back surgery.

Diagnostic Activities

Symptoms usually do not appear until after the second postoperative week, and the diagnosis often is delayed or missed (134). Clinical clues include acute or subacute fever, insidious back pain, paravertebral soft-tissue mass, or localized vertebral tenderness. If the onset is insidious, fever may be absent, with anorexia, malaise, and weight loss predominating. Neurologic deficits are rare but, if present, suggest epidural abscess.

The sedimentation rate is elevated above normal, but there may or may not be leukocytosis. When the diagnosis is suspected, cultures of blood, urine, or other infected sites should be obtained. Plain-film radiographs are obtained but may be difficult to interpret postoperatively, and they may take up to 8 weeks to show rarefaction of vertebral bodies, disc space narrowing, vertebral end-plate narrowing, or bony destruction. Magnetic resonance imaging (MRI) is very sensitive (96%) and is the imaging procedure of choice, showing the interruption of end plates, bony destruction, and soft-tissue changes (135). MRI also can distinguish scar tissue from epidural abscess. High-resolution CT also is excellent for defining a specific area known to be infected, but MRI is better for general screening of the spine when the exact location of infection is in doubt. Aggressive attempts should be made to obtain a sample of the organism with CT-guided, needle-aspiration biopsy; if unsuccessful, open biopsy may be required.

Treatment

Use of intravenous antibiotics for 4 weeks is successful in most cases when there is no abscess, the patient feels well, and the sedimentation rate returns to normal (136). Otherwise, a 6- to 8-week course is more appropriate. Surgical intervention is necessary for focal neurologic syndromes or identified paravertebral, psoas, or epidural abscess.

Special Considerations

Osteitis pubis is the painful inflammation of bone, cartilage, periosteum, and ligamentous structures of the anterior pelvic girdle (137). It is a rare complication of prostatectomy, urinary incontinence procedures, pyelonephritis, and abortion. Symptoms begin 2 to 12 weeks after surgery and, without treatment, last for weeks to months. Symptoms are characteristic and consist of suprapubic pain with radiation to the inner thighs that is worsened by abduction of the legs and walking. Findings include intermittent fever in nearly all cases, leukocytosis

in 50%, tenderness over the symphysis pubis, and radiographic evidence of bony destruction and separation of the symphysis.

Most cases result from infection, most commonly *E. coli* or *Pseudomonas* sp., but occasionally, the process is sterile. Diagnosis requires either needle aspiration or biopsy of the bone, since treatment will fail if the specific organism is not identified.

Pressure Ulcers

Epidemiology

Up to 5% of hospitalized patients may develop pressure ulcers, predominantly over the sacrum, ischial tuberosities, greater trochanter, and heels. Orthopaedic and trauma patients are at greatest risk, especially elderly patients with hip fractures. Pressure ulcers may lead to cellulitis, osteomyelitis, joint infections, and sepsis (138).

Bacteriology

A wide variety of both aerobic and anaerobic organisms are cultured from pressure ulcers. While aerobes are more prevalent in the ulcer itself, the resulting bloodstream isolates are more frequently anaerobic, with *B. fragilis* the most common. Group D streptococci frequently are isolated from the wound but rarely cause the bacteremia. Polymicrobial isolates frequently are found in the blood.

Diagnostic Activities

Whether infected or not, all pressure ulcers are colonized with bacteria. Cellulitis may resemble the reactive hyperemia and erythema of normal healing, thus making diagnosis difficult. Significant tissue infection should be obvious, however, with purulent and odiferous exudate and expanding areas of edema, heat, and erythema. A permanent, greenish discharge from the ulcer with green staining of the dressing but no substantial tissue involvement suggests Gram-negative superinfection in necrotic tissue and the need for debridement. Pseudomonas cellulitis and fascitis may result in susceptible patients.

Swab cultures of the wound reflect surface colonization but do not accurately reflect responsible organisms (139). Even so, such cultures are still the most widely used. Quantitative cultures from wound biopsy specimens are possible but not practical. Osteomyelitis may be detected in 26% of nonhealing ulcers. MRI is the procedure of choice for detection, but bone scan in conjunction with indium-111 leukocyte scanning may be helpful. Bone biopsy with quantitative cultures and microscopic examination remains the gold standard.

Sepsis is an infrequent consequence of pressure sores. Bacteremia often will persist without adequate debridement. The size of the ulcer has no bearing on the potential for sepsis, but there usually is marked tissue necrosis. Gram stain of the ulcer has only limited value in documenting the organism causing sepsis.

Treatment

Adequate use of antibiotics, surgical debridement, and further preventive measures are important. Antibiotics should include coverage for Gram-positive organisms, Gram-negative rods, and anaerobes. Local care as well as nutritional support and supplementation are required for healing of the pressure ulcer.

Postoperative Parotitis

Epidemiology

Postoperative parotitis is an acute unilateral or bilateral swelling of the parotid glands that can occur in patients postoperatively. The incidence of parotitis has been estimated to be 1 in 1000 postoperative patients.

Common predisposing conditions are age older than 60 years, debility, dehydration, use of anticholinergics, and alcoholism. The involved parotid gland is infected, usually with S. aureus and Streptococcus sp. and rarely with Gram-negative organisms.

A noninfectious swelling of the parotid gland also may occur in the few hours immediately after operation. Organisms cannot be cultured from the parotid gland, and the etiology is uncertain.

Diagnostic Activities

The usual presentation is unilateral parotid swelling, though bilateral swelling may occur in up to 20% of cases (140). The swelling is painful, but the patient may not complain of pain because of debility or pain medication. Postoperative parotitis usually occurs in patients who are elderly, very debilitated, malnourished, and dehydrated.

Fever is present in some cases. On physical examination, the parotid gland is swollen, firm to hard, and tender. Pus may be expressed from the Stenson's duct but is absent in many patients in whom the duct is totally obstructed.

A Gram stain and culture should be obtained from the drainage from the Stenson's duct. Gentle massage of the parotid gland may produce pus where none is apparent. Plain-film radiographs should be obtained to look for stones in the Stenson's duct and for subcutaneous air.

The major differential diagnosis is benign postoperative parotid swelling (i.e., "anesthesia mumps"). Postoperative, benign, noninfectious swelling usually occurs in the first few hours postoperatively, whereas infectious parotitis occurs 1 to 6 days postoperatively. Pus is not present in benign swelling, and culture of drainage shows only normal flora.

Treatment

Patients with postoperative parotitis should be treated aggressively because of the high mortality rate. An antibiotic that is active against penicillin-resistant staphylococci should be administered and modified according to the result of

Gram stain and culture. *Streptococcus* sp. as well as the anaerobic *Bacteroides* sp., *Peptostreptococcus* sp., and pigmented *Porphyromonas* sp. have been isolated (37).

The patient should be hydrated with intravenous fluids; lozenges should be administered every 2 to 3 hours to promote drainage. If drainage is not seen coming from the Stenson's duct within the first 24 hours, otolaryngological consultation should be obtained as surgical drainage may be needed. Drugs promoting thick secretions should be avoided, especially parasympathomimetic agents.

Benign postoperative parotid swelling can be treated with hydration and lozenges. It does not require surgical drainage or antibiotics.

Indwelling Vascular Catheter Infection

Epidemiology

All peripheral venous and arterial catheters as well as central venous access devices are susceptible to infection. An understanding of the type of catheters used, their infectious complications, and the treatment of suspected infection is helpful when evaluating a febrile surgical patient. The rapid development of new vascular access devices, including novel port-septum designs and catheter-tip location sensors, as well as new infection-resistant biomaterials continues (141).

The types of vascular access devices include acute-care venous catheters, both central and peripheral; transition access devices for short- to intermediate-term use; tunneled catheters; and implanted port systems. Acute-care central and peripheral access devices usually are placed in the arm at the bedside and are intended for short-term use in the hospital. Short- to intermediate-term needs are met with use of a peripherally inserted central catheter line, which is placed at the bedside or procedure room into the subclavian or superior vena cava. A wide variety of tunneled and port devices are implanted surgically for long-term use.

Tunneled catheters are passed subcutaneously to a site 3 to 10 cm from the venous insertion site. Ports are completely implanted under the skin and contain a titanium or plastic reservoir, a silicone access septum, and an attached central venous catheter (141).

Staphylococcal infections usually are introduced from the skin at the insertion site and from hub contamination by medical personnel. Skin organisms migrate along the cannula, and a small fibrin–platelet clot develops. A glycocalyx biofilm layer develops that is conducive to bacterial adherence (142), and *Candida* sp. are thought to seed hematogenously from the gastrointestinal tract and adhere to the fibronectin on the catheter surface. Contaminated infusions are uncommon sources.

Bacteriology

Coagulase-negative staphylococci are the most common organism, followed by *S. aureus*, *E. coli*, *Pseudomonas* sp., *Streptococcus* sp., enterobacteriaceae, and *Candida* sp. Infection in the setting of intravenous infusions are more likely to include *Enterobacter* sp., *Pseudomonas* sp., *Citrobacter* sp., and *Serratia* sp.

Diagnostic Activities

Local, regional, systemic, or combination infections can occur. A local exit-site infection is characterized by erythema, warmth, tenderness, and swelling within 1 to 2 cm of the exit or insertion site, either with or without discharge. As long as the infection remains solely at the exit site, use of antibiotics and local care without catheter removal are possible.

A spreading cellulitis around or along the tunnel tract, usually along its entire course, is called a *tunnel infection*. Tunnel infections involve a more intense reaction, with fever, local pain, swelling, redness, and induration, again with or without purulent discharge at the exit site.

Port-pocket infections have similar symptoms, with pus leaking from needle-access sites after needle withdrawal (141). Systemic line sepsis, or catheter-related septicemia, is potentially the most serious consequence (143).

Fever of uncertain origin commonly is the only symptom; the site may appear normal in the presence of infection. Positive blood cultures with no obvious source, including a normal site, is another frequent presentation. Patients on antibiotics may develop persistent fever, clinical deterioration, or positive blood cultures with no findings at the site. The site of a previously removed catheter may be at fault and frequently is overlooked on physical examination.

Treatment

Suggested catheter management has been outlined by Reed et al. (144). The presence of pus at the exit site is a clear indication for removal. Heat, tenderness, or erythema without pus can be cautiously observed, but there is a low threshold for removal. In cases of suspected sepsis without exit-site signs, a guidewire catheter exchange is performed with semiquantitative cultures using the roll plate technique. If cultures are positive, a new catheter site is chosen. At times, bacteremia can be treated without catheter removal. Blood cultures drawn peripherally with a differential count of 1:10 indicate catheter-related bacteremia. A recent advance in diagnosis has been a fibrin analysis system brush for in situ sampling of the catheter-tip clot (145). Meticulous attention to aseptic technique and removal of all catheters when possible reduces infection. Duration of antibiotic coverage usually is 5 to 7 days, though for deep infections with *S. aureus*, 4 to 6 weeks may be required.

Intravenous Infusion Infections

A brief febrile reaction to blood is common and results from leukoagglutins, platelet agglutinins, or from transfused antigens. The patient temperature usually is less than 102°F, and the patient is not toxic. Flushing and headache may be present, however. Bacterial contamination is rare, but the temporal association of transfusion with the onset of high fever, headache, vomiting, hypotension, and toxicity suggest the diagnosis. Hemolytic or IgA-deficient transfusion reactions are important differential diagnoses. Organisms usually are Gram-negative bacilli, and platelet transfusion and albumin infusions have transmitted infection, mostly in outbreaks of *Salmonella* sp. and *Enterobacter* sp.

Intravenous fluid therapy is associated with infection from the cannula, in-use contamination, and contamination during manufacture. Infusion-related sepsis may present dramatically several hours after an infusion, or it may be masked in a patient who is critically ill by a coexisting disease. These episodes are extremely rare, but they should be kept in mind when no source of infection is apparent or there are clusters of cases.

Procedure- and Device-related Infections

Invasive diagnostic tests, monitoring devices, and therapeutic procedures pose a considerable risk of infection to postoperative patients. Urinary and vascular catheters as well as respiratory devices are discussed elsewhere, but other specialized procedures and devices also can cause infection and bacteremia.

Infection has been caused by contaminated skin grafts, porcine valves, prosthetic devices, and intraocular lenses. Cardiac pacemakers and defibrillators are subject to pocket infections, subcutaneous tract infections, and lead-wire infections involving the vascular structures and epicardium (87). Purulent pocket wound infections that occur within the first 2 weeks mostly result from *S. aureus*. Late infections, often resulting from coagulase-negative staphylococci, may occur after up to 1 year, are insidious, and may migrate along the wire, thus causing endocarditis. A low-grade, coagulase-negative staphylococci periprosthetic infection of silicone breast implants causes a fibrous capsular contracture, thereby requiring removal. Coagulase-negative staphylococci also cause approximately 40 to 80% of penile prosthetic infections, which sometimes can be managed without removal of the prosthesis (87).

Whenever fever or bacteremia is present without explanation, careful consideration must be given to prostheses that were inserted during the surgery in question or any previous surgery. Bacteremia after procedures usually is transient and may go unnoticed. No estimate for the risk of bacteremia has been given because of the wide variation noted in the literature. The actual incidence of established infection after bacteremia is unknown.

Aspiration of a prosthesis or removal with culture of the device may help to prove the source of an infection. Empiric selection of antibiotics depends on the device and the clinical situation, but it usually includes a penicillinase-resistant penicillin and aminoglycoside (87).

Prosthetic Graft Infections

Epidemiology

The internist will encounter patients with prosthetic vascular grafts who are undergoing unrelated surgery. Rates of primary graft infection vary from 0 to 3.5%, with approximately 50% of cases occurring in the first month after the procedure (146). Most occur in aortofemoral or lower extremity grafts; however, carotid and autogenous graft infections do occur. Risk factors for early infection include placement under emergency conditions, a groin location, reoperation for bleeding or thrombosis, and development of a wound infection. Recent notable trends in graft infection include more coagulase-negative staphylococci being identified as pathogens, the delayed appearance of graft infections (sometimes years later), and the failure of prophylactic antibiotics to substantially alter the infection rate. Bacterial contamination at the time of operation remains the most important mechanism, though late infec-

tion does occur secondary to remote infections such as diverticulitis, sepsis, and rarely, procedures involving contaminated areas; other causes are listed in Table 17.23. Early infections (≤30 days) mostly result from *S. aureus* and Gram-negative bacteria, whereas coagulase-negative staphylococci predominate in late infection.

Diagnostic Activities

Early infections with *S. aureus* and Gram-negative organisms present with sepsis, anastomotic bleeding, graft–artery dehiscence, or wound infection. Gram-negative organisms should be suspected when hemorrhage is the presenting sign. Intra-abdominal graft infections present with sepsis, ileus, abdominal tenderness, or pain. Systemic signs frequently are absent in late infection. An inflammatory perigraft mass, sinus tract, pseudoaneurysm, or thrombosis may be suggestive of biofilm graft infection caused by mucin-producing, coagulase-negative staphylococci. Special culture techniques are required to isolate these infections. An aortoprosthetic fistula involves the aorta and a hollow viscus, almost always the fourth part of the duodenum; the most common symptom is gastrointestinal bleeding. A paraprosthetic fistula involves a duodenal erosion with gastrointestinal bleeding, nonspecific (but persistent) abdominal pain, and signs of low-grade infection. An aortoparaprosthetic fistula involves a more extensive virulent infection, and sepsis is the main presenting feature in this situation. Septic emboli,

Table 17.23.   Sources of Prosthetic Graft Contamination

1. Skin flora
2. Direct inoculation at surgery
3. Contaminated instruments or graft
4. Infected lymph nodes
5. Bacteria in diseased arterial walls
6. Postoperative infection (UTI) extended to involve graft

hemorrhage, and remote-organ failure are the more serious consequences of graft infection.

Blood cultures should be obtained but are negative in approximately 50% of patient. All laboratory tests may be normal in late-occurring, coagulase-negative staphylococci infections. Arterial cultures distal to the graft occasionally are positive when venous cultures are negative. CT scanning, duplex ultrasonography, MRI, and arteriography are used diagnostically according to the local preference.

Treatment

Massive bleeding requires immediate surgery without further diagnostic work-up. Most infections require eventual surgical excision to remove the infected prosthesis. Surgery is required for suture-line infection, bleeding, thrombosis, distal embolization, pseudoaneurysm, and fistula (147).

The consulting internist should be aware of the possibility for graft infection when evaluating any patient with a graft who is ill or febrile. An early consultation with a vascular surgeon is recommended.

Prosthetic Valve Endocarditis

Over 100,000 prosthetic valves are implanted each year, with the resultant pool of patients with such valves growing steadily in turn. When these patients are hospitalized for subsequent unrelated surgery, the presence of fever raises the possibility of prosthetic valve endocarditis (148). The overall rate of prosthetic valve endocarditis is 1 to 4%, but much higher rates of 40 to 50% have been seen in *hospitalized* patients with sustained bacteremia (149).

Coagulase-negative staphylococci has emerged as the most common organism infecting prosthetic valves (30–50% of cases). Most cases that occur during the first 12 months probably result from direct inoculation into the wound at the time of surgery and usually involve the sewing ring. Fang et al. (149) studied 115 patients with bacteremia and prosthetic valves and found that 18 (16%) developed subsequent endocarditis that was not present at the onset of bacteremia (mean, 45 days; median, 28 days). All of these cases were nosocomial, with the most common portals of entry being intravascular catheters (6 of 18 patient) and skin and wound infections (5 of 18). No cases of endocarditis were caused by UTIs, whereas 12% of bacteremias without endocarditis were urinary related. A mitral prosthesis and any staphylococcal bacteremia (*S. epidermidis* or *aureus*) were significant risk factors for new endocarditis, and 8 of the 18 cases were caused by *Candida* sp. or Gram-negative organisms.

A new set of criteria has been proposed for the diagnosis of endocarditis that should assist in the proper classification of patients (150). Use of two major criteria (typical blood culture and positive echocardiogram) and six minor criteria (predisposition, fever, vascular phenomena, immunologic phenomena, suggestive echo, and suggestive microbiology) increases the accuracy of diagnoses of prosthetic endocarditis. Coagulase-negative staphylococci presenting within the first year, however, has the following characteristics: valve dysfunction, congestive failure, and fever despite appropriate antibiotics; less than 20% of cases with peripheral findings; and intermittently positive blood cultures despite positive valve ring cultures at surgery. The difficulty of diagnosis stems from false-positive cultures for coagulase-negative staphylococci, patients with only a few blood cultures being positive (i.e., false negatives), and the paucity of peripheral findings. Since infection with this organism involves the valve ring, heart murmurs usually are not detected until late dehiscence occurs.

In surgical patients with intravascular lines and prosthetic valves, a vigorous approach to diagnosis should be made, with strict aseptic drawing of multiple cultures and transesophageal echocardiography in selected cases. Endocarditis may develop later during the hospital stay (median, 28 days after bacteremia), and a high degree of suspicion must be maintained. The duration of antibiotic therapy given in the hospital bears no relation to the development of subsequent endocarditis.

Treatment

Prevention is paramount, because vascular catheters are the source of bacteremia in 33% of all cases of new prosthetic endocarditis. Meticulously sterile placement technique, minimization of catheter use, and prompt removal are important. Antimicrobial and surgical therapy are beyond the scope of this text.

Prosthetic Joint Infections

Large numbers of prosthetic joints continue to be implanted, with an infection rate of from 1 to 2%. In 1989 alone, 1395 procedures were performed on infected total hip prostheses and 1795 on infected knee prostheses (151). The orthopaedist will manage all cases of early infections, but the internist must be aware of late infections and the risks of bacteremia from distant infections or unrelated surgery.

Epidemiology

The rate of infection after total hip and knee arthroplasty averages from 1 to 2%. Many late as well as early hip arthroplasty infections come from the time of the original surgery. Bacteremic infection from distant sites, especially the urinary tract, has been well documented.

Bacteriology

Staphylococcus aureus, coagulase-negative staphylococci, and Gram-negative rods comprise over 80 to 90% of pathogens in infected prostheses. Individually, coagulase-negative staphylococci represent 35% of isolates, *S. aureus* 29%, Gram-negative organisms 15%, and others 7%.

Diagnostic Activities

Prosthetic joint infections can be separated into three groups based on their clinical behavior (152, 153). Group I infections present up to 2 to 3 months after the procedure and usually begin in the first 2 to 5 days with a superficial wound infection or draining hematoma. Local inflammatory signs are present, and areas of marginal wound necrosis should be excised and closed. If early infection is superficial to the fascia lata, decompression and antibiotics may prevent deep extension. If loosening or dislocation of the device occurs, the prosthesis is involved. Group II infections present within 6 months to 2 years and are thought to result from bacterial seeding at the time of surgery. Pain is the primary symptom. Group III infections present after more than 2 years and probably result from hematogenous sources.

The primary late symptoms in all groups are pain in the hip either at rest or with weight bearing, loosening of the prosthesis, and fever. Spontaneous drainage occurs in some. The sedimentation rate is elevated above normal in 84 to 100% of cases, often above 50 (in 80%), but the WBC count is variable. Fever occurs in less than 50% of cases. Plain-film radiographs may show early soft-tissue swelling, periosteal thickening, or focal osteopenia. Ultrasonography can detect effusions around the hip, and indium leukocyte scanning is up to 83% sensitive and 94% specific in detecting infection (154). Direct aspiration, which is only recommended in cases with a strong suspicion of the diagnosis, reveals the causative organism in 66%. The accuracy of preoperative diagnosis with combined sedimentation rate, indium scanning, and aspiration is approximately 80%.

Any patient with a skeletal prosthesis should have the joint carefully examined during evaluation of postoperative fever, because hematogenous seeding from another infected site can occur at any time. The absence of pain or loosening of the prosthesis make infection less likely. Any indication of infection, however, should prompt an orthopaedic consultation.

Treatment of infected prostheses involves complex surgical decision making based on proper patient selection and technical factors (151). A two-stage reimplantation procedure after 5 to 6 weeks of intravenous antibiotics has a success rate of 80 to 90%. Resection arthroplasty, knee arthrodesis, or amputation occasionally are required. Poor surgical candidates have been treated with rifampin and ciprofloxin, with retention of the prosthesis in 60 to 80% (151).

Suppression of infected hips with antibiotics after debridement is successful in approximately 50% of cases. A two-stage reimplantation procedure with a 5–6 month interval between removal and reimplantation has a success rate of 90% (151).

Prevention includes prompt treatment of distant infections, especially those of the genitourinary tract. Detection of asymptomatic bacteriuria and its eradication before implantation is important. Use of prophylactic antibiotics during unrelated surgery is controversial but recommended for gastrointestinal and genitourinary procedures carrying a high risk of bacteremia.

Laparoscopic Surgery

The practice of laparoscopic surgery has advanced rapidly in the past 10 years, with both an increasing number and complexity of procedures and a widening array of conditions becoming amenable to laparoscopic intervention (155). Infectious complications are uncommon because of the exclusion of patients with a greater severity of illness (i.e., COPD) and a reduced potential for wound and pulmonary complications. Foley catheters are removed in the recovery room, and the patient is discharged within 1 to 2 days.

A survey of 77,604 cases of laparoscopic cholecystectomy found there were 33 deaths (156). Only three, however, related to infection: two with pneumonia, and one with necrotizing fasciitis. The conversion to laparotomy rate for complications was 1.2%. The only complication that might be confused with infection was bile duct leak in 0.3%. Cystic duct leaks are most common, with fever, leukocytosis, abdominal pain, nausea, and hyperbilirubinemia.

Other procedures that now can be performed laparoscopically include the Nissen fundoplication antireflux procedure, achalasia procedures, splenectomy, adrenalectomy, colon resection, herniorrhaphy, appendectomy, and lymphadenectomy. The rate of infectious complications in these situations should be low as these procedures are perfected.

REFERENCES

1. Hospital Infections Program, Centers for Disease Control and Prevention. National nosocomial infections surveillance semiannual report. Am J Infect Control 1995;23:377–385.
2. Jones R. Impact of changing pathogens and antimicrobial susceptibility patterns in the treatment of serious infections in hospitalized patients. Am J Med 1996;100(Suppl 6A):3S–12S.
3. Flaherty JP, Weinstein RA. Nosocomial infection caused by antibiotic-resistant organisms in the intensive care unit. Infect Control Hosp Epidemiol 1996;17:236–248.
4. Boyce JB. Treatment and control of colonization in the prevention of nosocomial infections. Infect Control Hosp Epidemiol 1996;17:256–261.
5. Recommendations of the Hospital Infection Control Practices Advisory Committee. Recommendations for preventing the spread of vancomycin resistance. Am J Infect Control 1995;23:87–84.
6. Garner JS, Jarvis WR, Emori TG, Horan TC, Hughes JM. CDC definitions for nosocomial infections. Am J Infect Control 1988;16:128–140.
7. Mandell GL, Bennett JE, Dolin R, eds. Principles and practice of infectious diseases. New York: Churchill Livingstone, 1995:2742–2755.
8. Horan TC, Culver DH, Gaynes RP, et al. Nosocomial infections in surgical patients in the United States, January 1986–June 1992. Infect Control Hosp Epidemiol 1993;14:73–80.
9. Bartlett JG, O'Keefe P, Tally FP, et al. Bacteriology of hospital-acquired pneumonia. Arch Intern Med 1986;146:868–871.
10. National Academy of Sciences–National Research Council. Postoperative wound infections: the influence of ultraviolet irradiation of

the operating room and of various other factors. Ann Surg 1964;160:122–125.

11. Cruse PJE. Surgical wound sepsis. Can Med Assoc J 1970;102:251–258.

12. Cruse PJE. Incidence of wound infection on the surgical services. Surg Clin North Am 1975;55: 1269–1275.

13. Farber BR, Wenzel RP. Postoperative wound infection rates. Am J Surg 1980;140:343–346.

14. Burke JF. Preventive antibiotic management in surgery. Annu Rev Med 1973;24:289–294.

15. Burke JF. The effective period of preventive antibiotic action in experimental incisions and dermal lesions. Surgery 1961;50:161–168.

16. Horan TC, Gaynes RP, Martone WJ, Jarvis WR, Emori TG. CDC definitions of nosocomial surgical site infections, 1992: a modification of CDC definitions of surgical wound infections. Infect Control Hosp Epidemiol 1992;13: 606–608.

17. Ayliffe GAJ. Role of the environment of the operating suite in surgical wound infections. Rev Infect Dis 1991;13(Suppl 10):S800–S804.

18. Society for Hospital Eidemiology of America, et al. Consensus paper on the surveillance of surgical wound infections. Infect Control Hosp Epidemiol 1992;599–605.

19. Haley RW, Culver DH, Morgan WM, et al. Identifying patients at high risk of surgical wound infection. Am J Epidemiol 1985;121: 206–215.

20. Culver DH, Horan TC, Gaynes RP, et al. Surgical wound infection rates by wound class, operative procedure, and patient risk index. Am J Med 1991;91(Suppl 3B):152S–157S.

21. Platt R, Zaleznik DF, Hopkins CC, et al. Perioperative antibiotic prophylaxis for herniorrhaphy and breast surgery. N Engl J Med 1990;322:153–160.

22. Consensus paper on the surveillance of surgical wound infections. Infect Control Hosp Epidemiol 1992;13:599–605.

23. Solomkin JS, Dellinger EP, Christou WV, et al. Design and conduct of antibiotic trials: a report of the scientific studies committee of the surgical infection society. Arch Surg 1987;122: 158–164.

24. Bartlett JG. Pocket book of infectious disease therapy. Baltimore: Williams & Wilkins, 1996.

25. Page CP, Bohnen JMA, Fletcher JR, et al. Antimicrobial prophylaxis for surgical wounds: guidelines for clinical care. Arch Surg 1993;128: 79–88.

26. Antimicrobial prophylaxis in surgery. Med Lett 1995;37:79–82.

27. DiPiro JT, Cheung RPF, Bowden TA, et al. Single dose systemic antibiotic prophylaxis of surgical wound infections. Am J Surg 1986;152: 552–559.

28. Wilson RG, Taylor EW, Dreghaorn C, et al. A comparative study of cefotetan and metronidazole against metronidazole alone to prevent infection after appendectomy. Surg Gynecol Obstet 1987;164:447–451.

29. Gorbach SL. Antimicrobial propylaxis for appendectomy and colorectal surgery. Rev Infect Dis 1991;13(Suppl 10):S815–S820.

30. Chetlin SH, Elliott DW. Preoperative antibiotics in biliary surgery. Arch Surg 1973;107: 319–323.

31. Dellinger EP, Gross PA, Barrett TL, et al. Quality standard for antimicrobial prophylaxis in surgical procedures. Clin Infect Dis 1994;18: 422–427.

32. Condon RE, Bartlett JG, Nichols RL, Schulte WJ, Gorbach SL, Ochi S. Preoperative prophylactic cephalothin fails to control septic complications of colorectal operations: results of controlled clinical trial. Am J Surg 1979;137: 68–74.

33. Stone HH, Haney BB, Kolb LD, et al. Prophylactic and preventive antibiotic therapy: timing, duration and economics. Ann Surg 1979; 189:691–698.

34. Hopkins CC. Antibiotic prophylaxis in clean surgery: peripheral vascular surgery, noncardiovascular thoracic surgery, herniorrhaphy, and mastectomy. Rev Infect Dis 1991;(Suppl 10):S869–S873.

35. Sonne-Holm S, Boeckstyns M, Menck H, et al. Prophylactic antibiotics in amputation of the lower extremity for ischemia. J Bone Joint Surg Am 1985;67:800–803.

36. Hemsell DL. Prophylactic antibiotics in gynecologic and obstetric surgery. Rev Infect Dis 1991;(Suppl 10):S821–S841.

37. Ephgrave KS, Kleiman-Wexler R, Pfaller, M, Booth B, Werkmeister L, Young S. Postoperative pneumonia: a prospective study of risk factors and morbidity. Surgery 1993;114: 815–821.

38. American Thoracic Society. Hospital acquired pneumonia in adults. Diagnosis, assessment of severity, initial antimicrobial therapy, and preventive strategies. A consensus statement. Am J Respir Crit Care Med 1995;153:1711–1725.

39. Schleupper CJ, Cobb DK. A study of the etiologies and treatment of nosocomial pneumonia in a community based teaching hospital. Infect Control Hosp Epidemiol 1992;13: 515–525.

40. Spain DA, Wilson MA, Boaz PW. Haemophilus pneumonia is a common cause of early pulmonary dysfunction following trauma. Arch Surg 1995;130:1238–1231.

41. Marquette CH, Georges H, Wallet F, et al. Diagnostic efficiency of endotracheal aspirates with quantitative bacterial cultures in intubated patients with suspected pneumonia. Comparison with the protected specimen brush. Am Rev Respir Dis 1993:148:138–144.

42. Kingston GW, Phang PT, Leathley MJ. Increased incidence of nosocomial pneumonia in

mechanically ventilated patients with sub-clinical aspiration. Am J Surg 1991;161: 589–592.

43. Schlenker JD, Hubay CA. The pathogenesis of postoperative atelectasis. A clinical study. Arch Surg 1973;107:846–850.

44. Boyd RJ, Burke JF, Colton T. A double-blind clinical trial of prophylactic antibiotics in hip fractures. J Bone Joint Surg Am 1973;55:1251–1258.

45. Doyon F, Evrard J, Mazas F, et al. Long-term results of prophylactic cefazolin versus placebo in total hip replacement. Lancet 1987;i:860–865.

46. Hill C, Mazas F, Flamant R, et al. Prophylactic cefazolin versus placebo in total hip replacement. Lancet 1981;i:795–797.

47. Infection in Neurosurgery Working Party. Antimicrobial prophylaxis in neurosurgery and after head injury. Lancet 1994;344: 1547–1551.

48. Barker FG. Efficacy of prophylactic antibiotics for craniotomy: a meta-analysis. Neurosurgery 1994;35:484–492.

49. Hook EW, Kaye D. Prophylaxis of bacterial endocarditis. J Chronic Dis 1966;15:635–646.

50. Dajani AS, Taubert KA, Wilson W, et al. Prevention of bacterial endocarditis: recommendations by the American Heart Association. JAMA 1997;277:1794–1801.

51. Everett ED, Hirschmann JV. Transient bacteremia, and endocarditis prophylaxis: a review. Medicine 1977;56:61–77.

52. Durack DT, Kaplan EL, Bisno AL. Apparent failures of endocarditis prophylaxis. JAMA 1983;250:2318–2322.

53. Oakley CM, Darrell JH. Antibiotic prophylaxis for bacterial endocarditis. Am J Cardiol 1980;46:1073–1074.

54. Dugrue D, Blake S, Troy P, et al. Antibiotic prophylaxis against infective endocarditis after normal delivery—is it necessary? Br Heart J 1980;44:499–502.

55. Dinarello CA, Cannon JG, Wolff SM. New concepts on the pathogenesis of fever. Rev Infect Dis 1988;10:168–189.

56. Clarke DE, Kimelman J, Raffin TA. The evaluation of fever in the intensive care unit. Chest 1991;100:213–220.

57. Dykes MHM. Unexplained postoperative fever: its value as a sign of halothane sensitization. JAMA 1971;216:641–644.

58. Livelli FD, Johnson RA, McEnany MT, et al. Unexplained in-hospital fever following cardiac surgery. Circulation 1978;57:968–975.

59. Bell DM, Goldmann DA, Hopkins CC, et al. Unreliability of fever and leukocytosis in the diagnosis of infection after cardiac valve surgery. J Thorac Cardiovasc Surg 1978;75:87–90.

60. Garibaldi RA, Brodine S, Matsumiya S, et al. Evidence for the noninfectious etiology of early postoperative fever. Infect Control 1985;6:273–277.

61. Giangobbe MJ, Rappaport WD, Stein B. The significance of fever following cholecystectomy. J Fam Pract 1992;34:437–440.

62. Roe CF. Surgical aspects of fever. Curr Probl Surg 1978;15:1–67.

63. Musher DM, Fainsten V, Young EJ, et al. Fever patterns: their lack of clinical significance. Surgery 1983;94:358–363.

64. Freischlag J, Busutti RW. The value of postoperative fever evaluation. Surgery 1983;94:358–363.

65. Galicier C, Richet H. A prospective study of postoperative fever in a general surgery department. Infect Control 1985;6:487–490.

66. Craig MH, Poole GV, Hauser CJ. Postsurgical gout. Am Surgeon 1995;61:56–59.

67. Younis RT, Lazar RH. Delayed toxic shock syndrome after functional endonasal sinus surgery. Arch Otolaryngol Head Neck Surg 1996;122:83–85.

68. McClean KL, Sheehan GJ, Harding GKM. Intraabdominal infection: a review. Clin Infect Dis 1994;19:100–116.

69. Altemeier WA, Culbertson WR, Fullen WD, et al. Intraabdominal abscesses. Am J Surg 1973;125:70–78.

70. Howard RJ, Simmons RL. Surgical infectious diseases. 3rd ed. Norwalk, CT: Appleton and Lange, 1995.

71. Bohnen JM, Solomkin JS, Dellinger EP, Bjornson HS, Page CP. Guidelines for clinical care: anti-infective agents for intra-abdominal infection. A Surgical Infection Society policy statement. Arch Surg 1992;127:83–89.

72. Cooper GS, Shales DfM, Salata RA. Intra-abdominal infection: differences in presentation and outcome between younger patients and the elderly. Clin Infect Dis 1994;19:146–148.

73. Moore FA, Sauaia A, Moore EE, Haenel JB. Postinjury multiple organ failure: a bimodal phenomenon. J Trauma Injury Infect Crit Care 1996;40:501–512.

74. Seeto RK, Rockey DC. Pyogenic liver abscesses changes in etiology, management, and outcome. Medicine 1996;75:99–113.

75. Ho HS, Wisner DH. Splenic abscess in the intensive care unit. Arch Surg 1993;128:842–846.

76. Montgomery RS, Wilson SE. Intraabdominal abscesses: image guided diagnosis and therapy. Clin Infect Dis 1996;23:28–36.

77. Weldon MJ, Joseph AE, French A, Saverymuttu SH, Maxwell JD. Comparison of 99m technetium hexamethylpropylene-amine oxime labelled leukocyte with 111-indium troplonate labelled granulocyte scanning and ultrasound in the diagnosis of intraabdominal abscess. Gut 1995;37:557–564.

78. Gazelle GS, Mueller PR. Abdominal abscess: imaging and intervention. Radiol Clin North Am 1994;32:913–932.

79. Schecter S, Eisenstat TE, Oliver GC. Computerized tomographic scan guided drainage of intraabdominal abscesses: preoperative and postoperative modalities in colon and rectal surgery. Dis Colon Rectum 1994;37:984–988.

80. Shuler FW, Newman CN, Angood PB, Tucker JG, Lucas GW. Nonoperative management for intraabdominal abscess. Am Surgeon 1996;62:218–222.

81. The choice of antibacterial drugs. Med Lett 1996;38:25–34.

82. Sanford JP, Gilbert DN, Sande MA. Guide to antimicrobial therapy. 26th ed. Dallas: 1996.

83. Pittet D, Tarara D, Wenzel RP. Nosocomial bloodstream infections in critically ill patients. JAMA 1994;271:1598–1601.

84. Gransden WR, Eykyn SJ, Phillips I, Rowe B. Bacteremia due to *Escherichia coli*: a study of 861 episodes. Rev Infect Dis 1990;12:1008–1018.

85. Bone RC. Sepsis and its complications. Crit Care Med 1994;22:S8–11.

86. Lautenschlager S, Herzog C, Zimmerli W. Course and outcome of bacteremia due to *Staphylococcus aureus*: evaluation of different clinical case definitions. Clin Infect Dis 1993;16:567–573.

87. Rupp ME, Archer GL. Coagulase negative staphylococcus associated with medical progress. Clin Infect Dis 1994;19:231–245.

88. Jarvis WJ, Cookson ST, Robles MB. Prevention of nosocomial bloodstream infections: a national and international priority. Infect Control Hosp Epidemiol 1996;17:272–275.

89. Rudnick JR, Bech-Sague CM, Anderson RL, et al. Gram negative bacteremia in open heart surgery patients traced to probable tap water contamination of pressure monitoring equipment. Infect Control Hosp Epidemiol 1996;17:281–285.

90. Lombardi DP, Engleberg NC. Anaerobic bacteremia: incidence, patient characteristics, and clinical significance. Am J Med 1992;92:53–60.

91. Capdevila JA, Almirante B, Pahissa A, Planes AM, Ribera E, Martinez-Vazquez JM. Incidence and risk factors of recurrent episodes of bacteremia in adults. Arch Intern Med 1994;154:411–415.

92. Weinstein MP, Reller LB. Clinical importance of breakthrough bacteremia. Am J Med 1984;76:175–180.

93. Jarvis WR. Epidemiology of nosocomial fungal infections, with emphasis on *Candida* species. Clin Infect Dis 1995;20:1526–1530.

94. Eubanks PJ, de Virglio C, Klein S, Bongard F. Candida sepsis in surgical patients. Am J Surg 1993;166:617–620.

95. Henderson VJ, Hirvela ER. Emerging and reemerging microbial threats. Nosocomial fungal infections. Arch Surg 1996;131:330–337.

96. Tang E, Tang G, Berne TV. Prognostic indicators in fungemia of the surgical patient. Arch Surg 1993;128:759–762.

97. Wenzel RP. Nosocomial candidemia: risk factors and attributable mortality. Clin Infect Dis 1995;20:1531–1534.

98. Slotman GJ, Shapiro E, Moffa SM. Fungal sepsis: multisite colonization versus fungemia. Am Surg 1994;60:107–113.

99. Geha DJ, Roberts GD. Laboratory detection of fungemia. Clin Lab Med 1994;14:83–97.

100. Edwards JE, Filler SG. Current strategies for treating invasive candidiasis: emphasis on infections in non-neutropenic patients. Clin Infect Dis 1992;14(Suppl 1):106–113.

101. Systemic fungal drugs. Med Lett 1996;38:10–12.

102. Weiss ME. Drug allergy. Med Clin North Am 1992;76:857–882.

103. Anderson JA. Allergic reactions to drugs and biologicals. JAMA 1992;268:2844–2857.

104. Mackowiak PA, LeMaistre CF. Drug fever. A critical appraisal of conventional concepts. Ann Intern Med 1987;106:728–733.

105. Craven DE, Steger KA, Barber TW. Preventing nosocomial pneumonia: state of the art and perspectives for the 1990's. Am J Med 1991:91(Suppl 3B):44S–53S.

106. Fujita T, Sakurai K. Multivariate analysis of risk factors for postoperative pneumonia. Am J Surg 1995;169:304–307.

107. Kroenke K, Lawrence VA, Theroux JF, Tuley MR. Operative risk in patients with severe obstructive pulmonary disease. Arch Intern Med 1992;152:967–971.

108. Patton JH Jr, Kudsk KA. Using bronchoalveolar lavage to distinguish nosocomial pneumonia from systemic inflammatory response syndrome: a prospective analysis. J Trauma 1995;39:1134–1139.

109. Finegold SM: Aspiration pneumonia. Rev Infect Dis 1991;13(Suppl 9):737–742.

110. DePaso WJ. Aspiration pneumonia. Clin Chest Med 1991;12:269–284.

111. Murray HW, Ellis GC, Blumenthal DS, Sos TA. Fever and pulmonary thromboembolism. Am J Med 1979;67:232–235.

112. Stamm WE. Catheter associated urinary tract infections: epidemiology, pathogenesis, prevention. Am J Med 1991;91(Suppl 3B):65S–71S.

113. Warren JW. Urethral catheters, condom catheters, and nosocomial urinary tract infections. Infect Control Hosp Epidemiol 1996;17:212–214.

114. Wong-Beringer A, Jacobs RA, Guglielmo BJ. Treatment of funguria. JAMA 1992;267:2780–2785.

115. Sanford JP. The enigma of candiduria: evolution of bladder irrigation with amphotericin B for management—from anecdote to dogma and a lesson from Machiavelli. Clin Infect Dis 1993;16:145–147.

116. Nassoura Z, Ivatury RR, Simon RJ, et al. Candiduria as an early marker of disseminated infection in critically ill surgical patients: the role of fluconazole therapy. J Trauma 1993;35: 290–294.

117. Edelstein H, McCabe RE. Perinephric abscess: modern diagnosis and treatment in 47 cases. Medicine 1988;67:118–131.

118. Sawyer RG, Pruett TL. Wound infections. Surg Clin North Am 1994;74:519–536.

119. Brook I, Frazier EH. Clinical features and aerobic and anaerobic microbiologic characteristics of cellulitis. Arch Surg 1995;130: 786–792.

120. Sutherland ME, Meyer AA. Necrotizing soft tissue infections. Surg Clin North Am 1994;74: 591–605.

121. Mathieu D, Neviere R, Teillon C, Chagnon JL, Lableu N, Wattell F. Cervical necrotizing fascitis: clinical manifestations and management. Clin Infect Dis 1995;21.51–56.

122. Bartlett P, Rengold AL, Graham DR, et al. Toxic shock syndrome associated with surgical wound infections. JAMA 1982;247:1448–1450.

123. Graham DR, O'Brien M, Hayes JM, Raab MG. Postoperative toxic shock syndrome. Clin Infect Dis 1995;20:895–899.

124. Magee KP, Blanco JD, Graham JM. Massive septic pelvic thrombophlebitis. Obstet Gynecol 1993;82(4 Pt 2 Suppl):662–664.

125. Witlin AG, Sibai BM. Postpartum ovarian vein thrombosis after vaginal delivery: a report of 11 cases. Obstet Gynecol 1995;85:775–780.

126. Stovall TG, Thorpe EM, Ling FW. Treatment of post-caesarian section endometritis with ampicillin and sulbactam or clindamycin and gentamicin. J Reprod Med 1993;38:843–848.

127. Fry DE, ed. A symposium: the continued challenge of trauma and infections in surgery. Am J Surg 1993;165:1S–82S.

128. Gerding DN, Johnson S, Peterson LR, Mulligan ME, Silva J Jr. Clostridium difficile associated diarrhea and colitis. Infect Control Hosp Epidemiol 1995;16:459–477.

129. Jobe BA, Grasely A, Deveney KE, Deveney CW, Sheppard BC. Clostridium difficile colitis: an increasing hospital-acquired illness. Am J Surg 1995;169:480–483.

130. Manabe YC, Vinetz JM, Moore RD, Merz C, Charache P, Bartlett JG. Clostridium difficile colitis: an efficient clinical approach to diagnosis. Ann Intern Med 1995;123:835–840.

131. Katz DA, Lynch ME, Littenberg B. Clinical prediction rules to optimize cytotoxin testing for clostridium difficile in hospitalized patients with diarrhea. Am J Med 1996;100: 487–495.

132. Ozuna RM, Delamarter RB. Pyogenic vertebral osteomyelitis and postsurgical disc space infections. Orthop Clin North Am 1996;27:87–94.

133. Ghanayem AJ, Zdeblick TA. Cervical spine infections. Orthop Clin North Am 1996;27: 53–63.

134. Bateman JL, Pevzner MM. Spinal osteomyelitis: a review of 10 years' experience. Orthopedics 1995;18:561–565.

135. Rothman SL. The diagnosis of infections of the spine by modern imaging techniques. Orthop Clin North Am 1996;27:15–31.

136. Sapico FL. Microbiology and antimicrobial therapy of spinal infections. Orthop Clin North Am 1996;27:9–13.

137. Bouza E, Winston DJ, Hewitt WL. Infectious osteitis pubis. Urology 1978;12:663–664.

138. Evans JM, Andrews KL, Chutka DS, Fleming KC, Garness SL. Pressure ulcers: prevention and management. Mayo Clin Proc 1995;70: 789–799.

139. Leigh IH, Bennett G. Pressure ulcers: prevalence, etiology, and treatment modalities: a review. Am J Surg 1994;167(suppl1A): 25S–29S.

140. Brook I. Diagnosis and management of parotitis. Arch Otolaryngol Head Neck Surg 1992; 118:469–471.

141. Whitman ED. Complications associated with the use of central venous access devices. Curr Probl Surg 1996;33:309–378.

142. Raad II, Bodey GP. Infectious complications of indwelling vascular catheters. Clin Infect Dis 1992;15:197–210.

143. Garrison RN, Wilson MA. Intravenous and central catheter infections. Surg Clin North Am 1994;74:557–570.

144. Reed CR, Sessler CN, Glauser FL, Phelan BA. Central venous catheter infections: concepts and controversies. Intensive Care Med 1995; 21:177–183.

145. Heerdon PV, Webb SAR, Fong S, Golledges CL, Roberts BL, Thompson WR. Central venous catheters revisited-infection rates and an assessment of the new fibrin analysing system brush. Anaesth Intensive Care 1996;24: 330–333.

146. Bandyk DF, Esses GE. Prosthetic graft infection. Surg Clin North Am 1994;74:571–590.

147. Lawrence PF. Management of infected aortic grafts. Surg Clin North Am 1995;75: 783–797.

148. Watanakunacorn W, Burkert T. Infective endocarditis at a large community teaching hospital, 1980–1990. A review of 210 episodes. Medicine 1993;72:90–102.

149. Fang G, Keys TF, Gentry LO, et al. Prosthetic valve endocarditis resulting from nosocomial bacteremia: a prospective multicenter study. Ann Intern Med 1993;119:560–567.

150. Durack DT, Lukes AS, Bright DK. New criteria for the diagnosis of infective endocarditis: utilization of specific echocardiographic findings. Duke Endocarditis Service. Am J Med 1994;96:200–209.

151. Wilde AH. Management of infected knee and hip prostheses. Curr Opin Rheumatol 1994;6: 172–176.

152. Salvati EA. Diagnosis and management of the infected hip. Orthopedics 1994;17:811–814.

153. Fitzgerald RH Jr. Diagnosis and management of infected hip prostheses. Orthopedics 1995; 18:833–835.

154. Levine SE, Esterhal JL Jr, Heppenstall R, Calhoun J, Mader JT. Diagnosis and staging osteomyelitis and prosthetic joint infections. Clin Orthop Rel Res 1993;295:77–83.

155. Scott-Conner CH, ed. Laparoscopic surgery. Surg Clin North Am 1996;76(3):436–644.

156. Deziel DJ, Millikin KW, Economou SG. Complications of laparoscopic cholecystectomy: a national survey of 4292 hospitals and an analysis of 77,604 cases. Am J Surg 1993;165: 9–14.

157. Bennet JV, Brachman PS, eds. Hospital infections. 3rd ed. Boston: Little, Brown, 1992.

158. Howard RJ, Simmons RL. Surgical infectious diseases. 3rd ed. Norwalk, CT: Appleton and Lange, 1995.

18

Dermatology

Donald P. Lookingbill and Gregory M. Caputo

Skin disorders are common, and for consultative purposes, they can be categorized as follows:

1. Skin signs of a systemic disease. Examples include rashes associated with febrile illnesses, skin manifestations of acquired immunodeficiency syndrome (AIDS), skin signs of internal malignancy, skin reactions associated with pregnancy, and systemic causes of generalized pruritus.
2. Cutaneous complications of the hospitalization itself and any resultant treatment. This category includes drug rashes and postoperative skin problems.
3. Incidental findings unrelated to either of the first two categories. Skin cancers, including melanoma, are examples.

This chapter also discusses therapy for skin disorders as well as the indications for dermatology consultation.

RASH AND FEVER

Many conditions can cause both rash and fever. Infectious causes, particularly bacterial infections, need to be diagnosed quickly and treated promptly. Noninfectious disorders can also be responsible for rash and fever, and Table 18.1 categorizes many of the infectious and noninfectious causes. The table is organized according to the type of skin lesion; therefore, several definitions are needed. Purpuric rashes result from hemorrhage in the skin, so these lesions do not blanch. Erythematous rashes result from dilated blood vessels, so these rashes do blanch when pressure is applied. Vesicles and bullae are skin lesions that are filled with clear fluid, whereas in pustules, the fluid is opaque.

Infectious Causes of Rash and Fever

Infectious causes of rash and fever include bacteria and rickettsial, spirochetal, mycobacterial, and viral diseases as well as fungal infections.

Bacterial Infections

Cellulitis Cellulitis is the most common of the skin infections with systemic ramifications, but it is not always easy to diagnose. It may sometimes be confused with superficial thrombophlebitis or even with stasis or contact dermatitis. To help in the differentiation, remember that with cellulitis, all four cardinal clinical signs of inflammation—redness, swelling, warmth, and tenderness—are typically present (although tenderness may be absent in neuropathic patients with diabetes). In addition, fever and leukocytosis are often present.

The diagnosis of cellulitis is more secure when an organism is recovered. This is more easily said than done; however, blood cultures are sometimes rewarding. To recover bacteria from the skin, 0.5 to 1.0 mL of nonbacteriostatic saline can be injected into the affected area and the

Table 18.1.   Causes of Rash and Fever

Purpuric Rashes (Do Not Blanch)	
Purpuric macules/papules/bullae (often with necrosis)	Bacterial sepsis
	Neisseria meningococcus
	Staphylococcus aureus
	Streptococci
	Pseudomonas aeruginosa
	Sepsis with disseminated intravascular coagulation
Purpuric macules and papules (without necrosis)	Rickettsial
	Rocky Mountain spotted fever
	Typhus-epidemic
	Candidal sepsis
	Viral
	Enteroviruses
	Hepatitis
	Noninfectious vasculitis:
	Rheumatoid vasculitis
	Systemic lupus erythematosus
	Polyarthritis nodosa
	Wegener's granulomatosis
	Drug-induced vasculitis
	Thrombotic thrombocytopenic purpura
Purpuric ulcerations with eschar (ecthyma gangrenosum)	Pseudomonas sepsis
Erythematous Rashes (Blanchable)	
Generalized erythema	Viral (many types)
	Bacterial
	Typhoid fever
	Typhus-endemic
	Toxic shock syndromes
	Staphylococcal
	Streptococcal
	Noninfectious causes
	Drug reactions
	Systemic lupus erythematosus
	Still's disease
	Erythema multiforme
Localized erythema	Cellulitis
	Streptococcal
	Staphylococcal
	Gram-negative bacteria
	Cryptococcal
Annular erythema	Rheumatic fever (erythema marginatum)
	Lyme disease (erythema migrans)
	Erythema multiforme (target lesions)
Photodistributed erythema	Systemic lupus erythematosus
	Drug reactions
Scaling erythematous papules and plaques	Secondary syphilis
Indurated macules	Candidal sepsis
Indurated papules and nodules	Fungal
	Cryptococcosis
	Histoplasmosis
	Coccidiomycosis
	Mycobacterial
	Lymphoma
Urticaria	Drugs
	Hepatitis

Table 18.1 *(continued).*   Causes of Rash and Fever

Vesicles and Bullae	
Grouped vesicles	Herpes simplex
	Herpes zoster
Generalized vesicles	Varicella
	Enteroviruses
	Rickettsial pox
Generalized blistering	Staphylococcal (scalded skin syndrome)
	Drug-induced erythema multiforme
	Stephens-Johnson syndrome
	Toxic epidermal necrolysis
Pustules	
Hemorrhagic pustules	Gonococcemia
Confluent superficial pustules	Generalized pustular psoriasis

aspirate cultured (1). Usually, this method is not successful, and the microbiology of the cellulitis remains presumptive. In healthy adults, cellulitis is usually caused by Gram-positive cocci, either group A β-streptococci or *Staphylococcus aureus*. With appropriate therapy, fever should resolve in 1 to 2 days and skin inflammation should stop progressing, but it may take several weeks for the erythema to subside completely.

Some strains of streptococci can cause a deep, suppurative cellulitis (e.g., necrotizing fasciitis, pyomyositis). A variety of other bacteria, including *Clostridia perfringens*, can also cause gangrenous or crepitant cellulitis (2). Cellulitis in all of these forms can progress rapidly, resulting in extensive tissue necrosis and, often, death. Magnetic resonance imaging of the cellulitic area can aid in the diagnosis of these serious infections (3), but needle aspiration of purulent fluid is a faster (and less expensive) way to make the diagnosis. Appropriate empiric antibiotics are important, but aggressive, immediate surgical debridement is the most important aspect of managing necrotizing infections.

In immunosuppressed patients, many Gram-negative organisms can cause cellulitis that may be clinically indistinguishable from the Gram-positive variety. Cryptococcal infection can also present with a cellulitis in these same patients

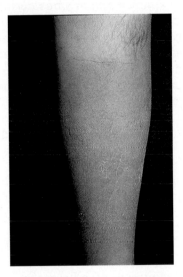

Figure 18.1. Cryptococcal cellulitis. The clinical appearance was identical to that for bacterial cellulitis, but this immunocompromised patient failed to respond to antibiotic therapy. Results of a skin biopsy established the correct diagnosis.

(Fig. 18.1) (4). A skin aspiration or biopsy with appropriate stains and culture is strongly recommended for the microbiologic evaluation of undiagnosed skin lesions in patients experiencing immunosuppression.

Patients with recurrent cellulitis frequently have tinea pedis (i.e., "athlete's foot") where the macerated fissures in the toe webs serve as entry sites for pathogenic bacteria. The legs of coronary artery bypass surgery patients who have had saphenous venectomies are also particularly predisposed to this cellulitis (5).

Bacterial Sepsis Skin lesions associated with bacteremia are caused by a necrotizing vasculitis originating from septic emboli or associated immune complexes. The clinical result is a purpuric macule, papule, or bulla that often becomes necrotic. **Sepsis must always be ruled out when purpuric lesions occur with coexistent fever**. Septic skin lesions occur most commonly with bacteremias resulting from *Neisseria meningitides*, *N. gonorrhoeae*, group A and group D streptococci, *S. aureus*, and *Pseudomonas aeruginosa*.

Purpuric macules and papules frequently occur in patients with meningococcemia and are often important diagnostic findings. As these lesions evolve, they characteristically develop a "gun-metal grey" color in their centers (Fig. 18.2). The lesions usually start on the extremities but can become generalized as the disease progresses. Early diagnosis is important. In an acutely ill, febrile patient, even a few purpuric macules or papules on the extremities should raise the suspicion of meningococcemia. Meningitis is usually, but not always, present.

The triad of fever, polyarthralgia/arthritis, and specific skin lesions characterize the syndrome of gonococcemia. Tenosynovitis may also be present. The skin lesion is a hemorrhagic pustule. There are

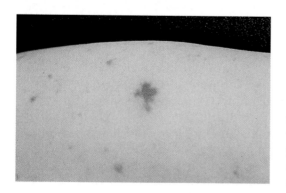

Figure 18.2. Meningococcemia. The center of these purpuric lesions often develop a "gun-metal gray" color.

usually only a handful of such lesions, located in a peripheral distribution (e.g., hands, feet, and distal extremities). Although the skin lesions result from septic emboli to the skin, the organism often cannot be cultured from the pustule. If the patient has been symptomatic for longer than 2 days, blood cultures are also often negative. The organism usually can be recovered from the body orifice that is the primary site of infection.

Staphylococcal septicemia can cause a variety of purpuric skin lesions, ranging from petechiae to purpuric papules to hemorrhagic bullae. Subungual splinter hemorrhages may also be seen, but they are by no means specific for endocarditis and, in fact, are more commonly encountered in a noninfectious setting.

Skin lesions of pseudomonas sepsis can also be expressed in several ways, such as petechiae, hemorrhagic bullae, and less commonly, cellulitis. The lesion specifically associated with pseudomonas sepsis is **ecthyma gangrenosa**, a round, indurated, ulcerative lesion in which a black eschar covers the depressed center. Most frequently, this lesion is found in the axillary or anogenital region. The organism may sometimes be cultured from this lesion, and as with the other bacteremias in which skin lesions appear, blood cultures and early therapy are essential.

Bacterial sepsis can result in **disseminated intravascular coagulation** as well. Cutaneous manifestations include acral cyanosis, livedo reticularis (Fig. 18.3), petechiae, purpuric macules and papules, hemorrhagic bullae, purpura fulminans, dissecting hematomas, and prolonged bleeding from wound sites (6). Clinically, the lesions often appear to be necrotic. Histologically, fibrin thrombi are found in the blood vessels, but in contrast to the findings in vasculitis, only minimal inflammatory infiltrate is present. Results of skin biopsy may suggest the diagnosis; coagulation tests will confirm it. The cutaneous lesions may be the presenting signs for this systemic process, in which sepsis is a frequent cause.

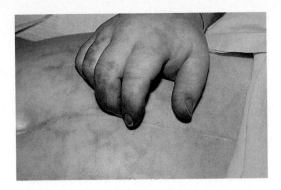

Figure 18.3. Disseminated intravascular coagulation. Note the livedo reticularis on the abdomen and the acral cyanosis and purpura of the fingers.

As discussed, skin lesions from sepsis are usually purpuric in nature. The skin involvement in typhoid fever is an exception, however. Lesions associated with *Salmonella typhi* bacteremia are termed "rose spots" and appear as small, pink macules or papules on the abdomen or lower back. They are few in number and resolve in several days, but they can be important diagnostic clues to this febrile condition.

Toxic Shock Syndrome The toxic shock syndrome was first described in association with certain strains of *S. aureus* that produced a toxin responsible for hypotension and multiorgan involvement (7). More recently, certain strains of streptococci have been shown to produce exotoxins that result in a similar clinical syndrome (8, 9). With either infection, a generalized erythematous eruption can develop, although it is more common in staphylococcal-induced disease, in which the rash is scarlatiniform with flexural accentuation and mucous membrane erythema. In both types, however, delayed desquamation, particularly of the hands and fingers, may occur.

Rickettsial Diseases

A number of rickettsial diseases can cause rash and fever, but in the United States, the most important is Rocky Mountain spotted fever. This disease is characterized by an abrupt onset of fever, headache, and myalgias, followed in several days by development of a rash around the ankles and wrists that subsequently becomes more generalized and involves the palms and soles. As the rash evolves, the macules and papules become purpuric. A biopsy specimen of an early lesion will sometimes show the presence of the responsible microorganisms. Acute and convalescent serologic testing will confirm the diagnosis, but therapy cannot wait for this confirmation. The diagnosis is usually made on a clinical basis, with the rash being very helpful in this regard. Early therapy with tetracycline can be lifesaving.

Spirochetal Diseases

The incidence of syphilis has been increasing. Treponemal septicemia occurs in the secondary form of the disease and results in a systemic disorder with protean manifestations, including fever. The skin rash of secondary syphilis sometimes, but not always, involves the palms and soles, but palmar and plantar involvement is not peculiar to secondary syphilis. For example, the palms and soles can be involved with purpuric lesions in Rocky Mountain spotted fever or with erythematous macules in viral exanthemas and drug eruptions. With secondary syphilis, however, the lesions last for many weeks and usually have a peculiar copper or red-brown color. They often scale as well. The generalized lesions are usually scaling papules and plaques, which sometimes are misdiagnosed as "atypical pityriasis rosea." In any patient with a systemic febrile disease and an accompanying "atypical" rash, a serologic test for syphilis should be done.

Lyme disease is caused by the spirochete *Borrelia burgdorferi*. The characteristic skin lesion associated with the early, localized stage of the disease is termed **erythema migrans**. This lesion originates at the site of the original tick bite and slowly enlarges with time. To qualify as erythema migrans, it must be at least 5 cm in diameter. The lesion is most commonly an erythematous plaque that often develops a pale center as it enlarges (Fig. 18.4). Fever may be present in the early, localized stage of the disease but is more common in the early, disseminated stage, in which secondary annular lesions may occur as well. Neurologic manifestations are common in untreated patients; oligoarthritis occurs in late-stage infection. Antibiotic therapy (e.g., doxycycline) early in the disease can prevent subsequent progression (10).

Mycobacterial Diseases

Although systemic infections with *Mycobacterium tuberculosis* and *M. avium* complex now occur more frequently because of the AIDS epidemic, associated skin lesions are uncommon. Rash with fever, however, is seen with some regularity in patients who are infected with *M. chelonae* (11). This infection occurs most often in immunosuppressed organ-transplant recipients or in patients with autoimmune diseases, especially rheumatoid arthritis. Typically, skin lesions appear as firm papules and nodules, which often drain spontaneously. Abscesses and cellulitis are sometimes found as well. Skin biopsy for appropriate stains and

Figure 18.4. Erythema migrans. The size of this enlarging erythematous lesion meets the criterion of greater than 5 cm. The small, dark area in the center may represent the site of the original tick bite, but this is not always evident.

cultures will reveal the diagnosis, and clarithromycin is useful for therapy (11).

Viral Diseases

A generalized erythematous exanthem is a common skin expression of many viral illnesses. This "morbilliform" eruption is often clinically indistinguishable from a cutaneous drug reaction. Viral exanthems, however, are more frequent in children, usually accompanied by other viral "symptoms," and resolve spontaneously.

Skin lesions in herpetic infections appear as multiple vesicles. In the primary infection (e.g., varicella), vesicles are individual and widespread. In recurrent infections (i.e., recurrent herpes simplex, herpes zoster), vesicles are usually grouped on an erythematous base. Disseminated herpes simplex infection sometimes occurs without skin lesions.

Infections from herpes viruses seldom cause a serious problem in healthy individuals, but in immunosuppressed patients, they can be fatal. If vesicles are present, definitive diagnosis of a herpes infection can be immediately established with the **Tzanck test**. This involves opening a vesicle, scraping the base, smearing the contents on a glass slide, and staining with Wright's, Giemsa, or toluidine blue O stain. Under the microscope, multinucleated giant cells can be seen; this finding is diagnostic for herpes infection but does not specify its type. If available, a fluorescent antibody test for herpes varicella zoster virus can be done on the fluid from a skin vesicle. This test is specific and can provide same-day results. Viral identification can also be made with viral cultures. Herpes simplex virus grows well in 1 to 2 days, but cultures of varicella zoster virus require 7 to 10 days of growth and even then are frequently negative.

Several enteroviruses can cause vesicular skin eruptions as well. For example, Coxsackie A16 virus causes hand-foot-and-mouth disease, which is characterized cutaneously by vesicles in the aforementioned locations. Occasionally, enteroviral and hepatitis virus infections can cause vasculitis appearing as purpuric macules and papules. Hives may also occur in patients with hepatitis.

Fungal Infections

As the number of immunosuppressed individuals has grown, the frequency of systemic fungal infections has increased as well. Systemic candidiasis is most common in patients undergoing treatment for leukemia. The responsible organism is usually either *Candida tropicalis* or *C. albicans*. Associated septic skin lesions occur in a sizable minority (13%) of infected patients (12), and lesions are usually multiple and occur on the trunk and proximal extremities. Generally, they have been described as "maculonodules," a contradiction in terms used to define an indurated papule within an erythematous macule. These lesions are usually less than 1 cm in size and often have a pale center (Fig. 18.5). Unless the patient is thrombocytopenic, however, the lesions are not purpuric. A skin biopsy can be particularly useful; the responsible organism can often be cultured from the specimen as well as seen on pathology sections (especially those stained for fungus).

Disseminated cryptococcosis and histoplasmosis occur in a variety of immunosuppressed patients (including patients with AIDS), and they can involve the skin in several ways. Cryptococcal cellulitis has already been discussed, but *Cryptococcus neoformans* can cause papules that clinically resemble molluscum contagiosum. Firm, erythematous papules and nodules can occur in both histoplasmosis and cryptococcosis. Coccidioidomycosis can produce the same, but less commonly. In a febrile patient with any of these types of lesions, a skin biopsy should be performed and the specimen sent for special stains and for bacterial, mycobacterial, and fungal cultures.

In addition, acute histoplasmosis and coccidiomycosis can cause erythema no-

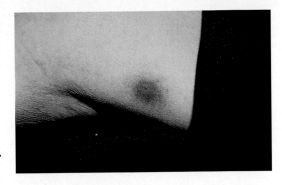

Figure 18.5. Candidal sepsis. This lesion may appear to be macular, but it will feel indurated. In patients with thrombocytopenia, these erythematous lesions may become purpuric.

dosum, which appears as tender, red nodules on the lower legs. These lesions do not contain microorganisms; instead, they represent a reactive, possibly immune complex–mediated phenomenon. Erythema nodosum can also occur as a reaction to drugs, streptococcal infection, sarcoidosis, tuberculosis, colitis caused by *Yersinia* sp., and inflammatory bowel disease.

Noninfectious Causes of Rash and Fever

Drugs

Drugs are the most common cause of skin rashes in hospitalized patients. Drugs can also cause fever, but much less commonly, and not all patients with drug-induced fever have a skin rash. In one survey of 51 episodes of drug-induced fever (13), 39% of patients had an accompanying rash. Such rashes are often, but not always, urticarial in nature. For drug-induced fever, antimicrobials, particularly penicillins, are the most common causes, but methyldopa and quinidine have also been implicated, as have many other agents (1). In most cases, the fever resolves within 48 hours of discontinuing the drug (13, 14).

In addition, drugs can cause severe blistering eruptions, which are grouped under the general category of erythema multiforme. Target lesions of the skin are diagnostic for erythema multiforme, but severe erythema multiforme can also cause marked mucous membrane involvement (i.e., Stephens-Johnson Syndrome) and widespread blistering with skin necrosis (i.e., toxic epidermal necrolysis) (15). Fever commonly accompanies these reactions, which sometimes result in death.

Collagen Vascular Diseases

Autoimmune and rheumatic disease that can result in both fever and rash include systemic lupus erythematosus, rheumatoid arthritis, Still's disease, rheumatic fever, polyarthritis nodosa, and Wegener's granulomatosis. Of these, fever is especially prominent in rheumatic fever and Still's disease. Erythema marginatum is the nonpruritic, annular eruption associated with acute rheumatic fever, but this disease seldom occurs in adults. Still's disease (i.e., juvenile rheumatoid arthritis) is also uncommon in adults. The rash of Still's disease occurs in 90% of patients, and it characteristically appears at the same time as the spiking fevers. The rash consists of small, pink macules or papules on the proximal limbs and trunk or face, and the lesions are often arranged linearly.

Skin manifestations are common in systemic lupus erythematosus, which also is sometimes accompanied by fever. Skin manifestations included in the American Rheumatism Association Diagnostic Criteria include malar rash, discoid rash, photosensitivity, and oral ulcers. In the malar rash of lupus, telangiectasis are often present, but scaling usually is not. These features will help in differentiating lupus from seborrheic dermatitis, which is a red, scaling rash of the face. Seborrheic dermatitis is the most common cause of a "butterfly rash" and often develops in hospitalized patients with a history of dandruff. In the laboratory evaluation of lupus, serologic tests have the most diagnostic value, and they have largely replaced immunofluorescent studies on skin-biopsy specimens.

Cutaneous vasculitis also occurs in some patients with lupus, but it is more common in patients with rheumatoid arthritis, polyarthritis nodosa, and Wegener's granulomatosis. Rheumatoid vasculitis occurs in patients with high titers of rheumatoid factor and causes purpuric lesions in the skin that can ulcerate. Vasculitis in polyarthritis nodosa affects small- to medium-sized arteries, resulting clinically in painful subcutaneous nodules, livedo reticularis, and skin ulcerations. In Wegener's granulomatosis, the inflammation involves small arteries and veins. Cutaneous manifestations include purpuric papules as well as plaques and nodules that are often hemorrhagic and may ulcerate.

Vasculitis

Confusion reigns in the characterization and classification of vasculitis. Strictly speaking, any inflammation of blood vessels could be termed a "vasculitis." More commonly, however, the term is used to describe a necrotizing reaction in blood vessels. When the skin is affected, the clinical appearance is palpable purpura. This is to be distinguished from the macular, nonpalpable, noninflammatory purpura seen in bleeding disorders. One cause for nonpalpable purpura is increased capillary fragility, as seen in the common but benign "senile" purpura or in the less common but more important purpura associated with amyloidosis. In the former, the purpura is confined to the lower arms; in the latter, it is more widespread. With thrombocytopenia, skin lesions are usually small (i.e., petechial).

In vasculitis, the purpuric lesions are elevated because of inflammation both in and around the affected dermal blood vessels. If the process is extensive or large vessels are involved, skin necrosis may occur. Vasculitis is thought to be immune complex–initiated and complement-mediated, and it can occur in a variety of settings. Sepsis and collagen vascular disease have already been discussed;

Table 18.2. Mucocutaneous Manifestations of AIDS

Viral
Herpes simplex, chronic ulcerative[a]
Herpes zoster
Oral hairy leukoplakia
Genital warts
Molluscum contagiosum
Fungal
Candidiasis
Skin papules and nodules from systemic fungal
    infection[a]
Seborrheic dermatitis, severe (*Pityrosporum* sp.)
Bacterial
Staphylococcal abscesses, recurrent and severe
Bacillary angiomatosis
Neoplasms
Kaposi's sarcoma[a]
Lymphoma[a]
Squamous cell carcinoma, oral and rectal
Miscellaneous
Acquired ichthyosis
Pruritic papules/folliculitis
Drug reactions
Psoriasis, explosive and severe

[a]AIDS-defining conditions.

other conditions include cryoglobuline-mia, drug reactions, and occasionally, malignant lymphoma. Some cases of systemic vasculitis are idiopathic.

Whenever purpuric papules appear in the skin, necrotizing vasculitis should be strongly suspected. Confirmation can be obtained with a skin biopsy. When necrotizing vasculitis is diagnosed in the skin, a search should be conducted for the underlying cause and any extracutaneous involvement. Concomitant renal involvement is particularly common. The palpability of vasculitis lesions in the skin may be transient; surprisingly, within a day, a new lesion may have flattened and already begun to fade.

Malignancy

Fever is known to occur in patients with lymphoma, and some of these patients may have skin involvement as well. Patients with cutaneous T-cell lymphoma (i.e., mycosis fungoides) usually do not have fever. In patients with Hodgkin's lymphoma, in which fever is common, skin involvement is rare. Patients with B-cell lymphomas have skin involvement more commonly than those with Hodgkin's disease, but in either setting, skin lesions, if present, appear as nodules that are often firm and violaceous in color. A skin biopsy will confirm the diagnosis.

ACQUIRED IMMUNODEFICIENCY SYNDROME

Skin manifestations are common in AIDS and frequently are the presenting sign (16–18). Because of their immunosuppression, patients with AIDS are susceptible to many mucocutaneous infections (Table 18.2). Cutaneous involvement with systemic fungal infections has already been discussed; in a human immunodeficiency virus (HIV) positive patient, this is an AIDS defining manifestation. **Chronic herpes simplex** is another AIDS-defining illness and appears as an irregular ulcer that has been present for longer than 1 month (Fig. 18.6). **Oral candidiasis** can be the initial manifestation of AIDS, as can **herpes zoster** in young adults who are otherwise apparently healthy. Widespread molluscum contagiosum and warts may occur as well, but these are not specific to AIDS.

Oral "hairy" leukoplakia appears as a white, roughened thickening of the lateral margin of the tongue (Fig. 18.7). It

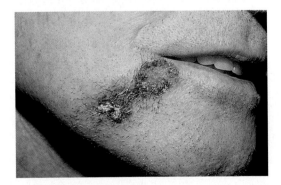

Figure 18.6. Chronic herpes simplex. In immunocompromised patients, persistent erosions should raise the suspicion of chronic herpes simplex.

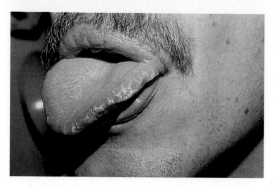

Figure 18.7. Oral hairy leukoplakia. These white, filiform lesions are usually located along the sides of the tongue. (Reprinted with permission from Lookingbill DP, Marks JG. Principles of dermatology. 2nd ed. Philadelphia: WB Saunders, 1993.)

is caused by infection with the Epstein-Barr virus and is commonly found in homosexual patients with AIDS.

Seborrheic dermatitis is another common skin finding in patients with AIDS and frequently appears early in the disease. In one survey, 46% of patients with AIDS had seborrheic dermatitis, compared with 5% of patients without AIDS (16). Seborrheic dermatitis manifests as severe "dandruff" of the scalp accompanied by scaling of the face, particularly in the eyebrows and nasolabial folds. Proliferation of the yeast organism *Pityrosporum ovale* has been implicated in seborrheic dermatitis, and the immunosuppression in patients with AIDS may allow the organism to flourish. This theory is supported by the improvement of the eruption that occurs with ketoconazole therapy.

Other cutaneous manifestations of AIDS include Kaposi's sarcoma as well as other neoplasms and miscellaneous conditions listed in Table 18.2. **Kaposi's sarcoma** was the first cutaneous manifestation to be described in these patients. It is another AIDS-defining manifestation and is most frequently found in homosexual patients infected with HIV. Kaposi's sarcoma probably derives from endothelial cells; therefore, the lesions have a vascular appearance. These red or purple macules, papules, nodules, or plaques (Fig. 18.8) are often benign in appearance and easily misdiagnosed as hemangiomas or bruises. The lesions may be single or multiple, and they can be located anywhere on the skin. In HIV-infected patients, any new red or purple macule, papule, plaque, or nodule should undergo biopsy to rule out Kaposi's sarcoma and to distinguish Kaposi's sarcoma from **bacillary angiomatosis**. Bacillary angiomatosis is caused by organisms of the genus *Bartonella*, which can be detected by lysis-centrifugation culture methods but also can be readily seen in a biopsy specimen. This infection is treated with antibiotics such as doxycycline or erythromycin (19).

SKIN SIGNS OF MALIGNANCY

Malignancy can affect the skin in three ways: *(a)* primary skin cancers, *(b)* metastases to the skin, and *(c)* nonmalignant skin manifestations of internal malignancies.

Primary Skin Cancers

Primary skin cancers are common and often found incidently during a complete

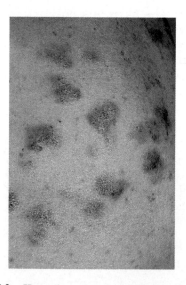

Figure 18.8. Kaposi's sarcoma. The color is purple in Kaposi's sarcoma, as seen in these widespread plaques in a patient with AIDS.

skin examination. This is one of the benefits to examining the entire skin surface in all patients, both hospitalized and ambulatory. In a survey of 1157 new patients in which this was done (20), skin cancers were incidentally detected in 2%. For patients older than 40 years, the frequency of skin cancer was 5%. Most of the skin cancers were basal cell carcinomas, but one patient had melanoma and another Kaposi's sarcoma, which in him was the first sign of HIV infection and AIDS.

Basal cell carcinoma is the most common skin cancer, but it is easily overlooked. The single most important feature is the "pearly" appearance of the papule, plaque, or nodule (Fig. 18.9). This is best appreciated through blanching the affected area by stretching. When this is done, a basal cell carcinoma will appear translucent (i.e., "pearly") compared with the more opaque-appearing, adjacent normal skin.

Squamous cell carcinomas often present as persistent scaling or ulcerated, firm skin nodules or plaques (Fig. 18.10). They most commonly occur on sun-exposed skin or mucous membranes.

Malignant melanoma is the skin tumor most in need of an early diagnosis. For most of these lesions, early diagnosis is possible and consequent surgical cure achievable. The most common type of melanoma is the superficial spreading variety (Fig. 18.11). Seventy percent of all

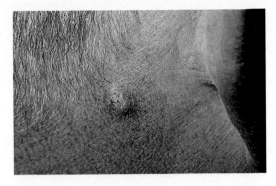

Figure 18.10. Squamous cell carcinoma. This squamous cell carcinoma is, in fact, scaling (i.e., squamous), but these lesions may be ulcerated instead.

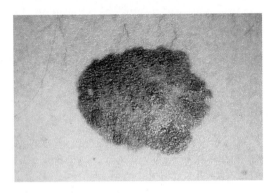

Figure 18.11. Melanoma. Note the asymmetry, irregular border, and varying colors in this superficial spreading melanoma.

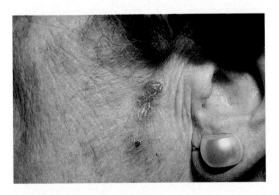

Figure 18.9. Basal cell carcinoma. Note the "pearly" quality of this preauricular nodule.

melanomas fall into this category. Diagnostically, the key word is "irregularity," as expressed in the following "ABCD" features:

A—asymmetry, whereby one-half of the lesion is unlike the other one-half.
B—border irregularity, with a scalloped or notched border.
C—color variation, sometimes including those of the American flag (i.e., red, white, and especially, **blue**).
D—diameter, with melanomas usually being greater than 6 mm.

Nodular melanoma is the next most common type and often appears as a blue/black nodule in the skin. Deep invasion in nodular melanoma often occurs early. A third type of melanoma, lentigo maligna melanoma, usually occurs in the sun-exposed skin of elderly patients. The fourth type of melanoma is the acral lentiginous type, which occurs on the hands and feet and often has a poor prognosis. Superficial spreading melanomas and lentigo maligna melanomas may be present for years before becoming deeply invasive; therefore, **a diagnosis of melanoma should not be excluded because of long-standing duration**.

The reader is encouraged to consult a color atlas on melanoma to become fully familiar with the diagnostic features of this important skin tumor (21). For any lesion carrying a clinical suspicion for malignancy, obtain a dermatology consultation or conduct a biopsy of (or excise) the lesion for a histologic examination. This is particularly critical for suspected melanoma.

Cutaneous Metastases

Metastasis is the most common, and certainly the most unequivocal way, that an internal malignancy is reflected in the skin. Metastatic carcinoma, melanoma, myeloma, as well as lymphoma and leukemia, can infiltrate the skin, and these infiltrates almost always present as firm to hard nodules in the skin, either single or multiple (Fig. 18.12). Less commonly, metastatic cancer in the skin appears as a large area of inflammation, and this can be misdiagnosed clinically as cellulitis. Occasionally, skin metastases are the presenting sign for the internal cancer (22). More commonly, however, skin nodules are noted as a first sign of metastatic disease in a patient with cancer (23).

Skin Signs of Internal Malignancy

Certain skin conditions indicate an underlying internal malignancy. Some of these cutaneous manifestations result from tumor secretory products that interact with the skin. Examples include flushing from vasoactive compounds secreted by carcinoid tumors and addisonian hyperpigmentation from ACTH/MSH polypeptides ectopically produced by certain tumors, especially small-cell carcinomas of the lung.

A variety of idiopathic skin signs have been associated with internal malignancies as well (24, 25). Their occurrence, however, ranges from uncommon to rare. Examples are listed in Table 18.3, and acanthosis nigricans is illustrated in Figure 18.13.

Table 18.3.   Idiopathic Skin Signs of Internal Malignancy

Skin Sign	Tumor Type
Erythematous rashes	
Dermatomyositis	Carcinoma
Erythema gyratum repens	Carcinoma
Necrolytic erythema migrans	Glucagonoma
Scaling rashes	
Acanthosis nigricans, adult onset	Carcinoma (gastric)
Ichthyosis, adult onset	Lymphoma
Acrokeratosis paraneoplastica	Carcinoma (upper respiratory tract)
Skin growths	
Eruptive keratoses (Leser-Trélet)	Carcinoma (gastrointestinal tract)
Multiple sebaceous neoplasms (Torre's syndrome)	Carcinoma (gastrointestinal tract)
Blistering disease	
Paraneoplastic pemphigus	Lymphoma
Acute febrile neutrophilic dermatosis (Sweet's syndrome)	Leukemia

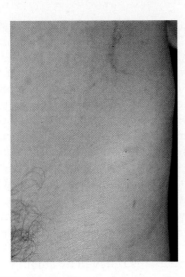

Figure 18.12. Metastatic melanoma. This firm, bluish-colored nodule was the first sign of metastatic disease in this young woman whose primary lesion had been excised 2 years earlier. Results of a skin biopsy established the diagnosis.

SKIN REACTIONS ASSOCIATED WITH PREGNANCY

A variety of skin reactions are associated with pregnancy (26). Table 18.4 lists the most important in descending order of frequency.

Prurigo gravidarum is the most common skin manifestation encountered in pregnancy, with an estimated frequency of up to 2% (26). The pruritus is generalized, caused by cholestasis, and usually develops in the third trimester. Primary lesions are not present. Excoriations may be found, however, and jaundice often develops over time. The process remits within days of delivery but tends to recur in subsequent pregnancies.

As the name implies, pruritic urticarial papules and plaques of pregnancy appears as papules and small plaques resembling hives but that are more persistent (Fig. 18.14). The lesions start on the abdomen and thighs and are extremely pruritic. The rash usually develops during the third trimester, and women in their first pregnancy are most commonly affected. Topical steroids can be helpful, but sys-

temic prednisone is occasionally needed. The condition remits soon after delivery.

Prurigo gestationis of Besnier manifests by small, pruritic, excoriated papules on the proximal limbs and sometimes on the trunk. It most commonly develops in the second trimester, but the cause is unknown. Topical steroids are usually helpful, and the process resolves promptly after delivery.

Herpes gestationis is an uncommon, blistering disorder that may begin anytime during pregnancy and occasionally in

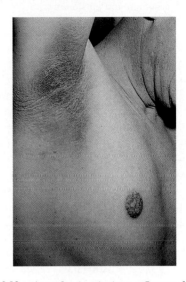

Figure 18.13. Acanthosis nigricans. Internal malignancy should be suspected when acanthosis nigricans develops in mid to late adulthood. Malignancy-associated acanthosis nigricans is often more severe than the "benign" types. Note that in this patient with lung cancer, it even involves the nipples.

Table 18.4. Rash Associated with Pregnancy

Skin Finding[a]	Dermatosis
Pruritus (without primary lesions)	Prurigo gravidarum (Cholestasis of pregnancy)
Erythematous papules	Pruritic urticarial papules and plaques of pregnancy
	Prurigo gestationis
Bullae	Herpes gestationis
Pustule	Impetigo herpetiformis

[a]Findings are listed in decreasing order of frequency.

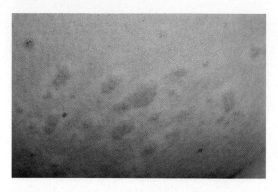

Figure 18.14. Pruritic urticarial papules and plaques of pregnancy, in which the hive-like lesions begin on the lower abdomen and girdle area.

the postpartum period. It is an autoimmune disorder that is virtually identical to bullous pemphigoid. It usually remits after delivery, but the eruptions may recur in subsequent pregnancies. Systemic prednisone in doses of 20 to 40 mg/day is usually required to control the condition.

Impetigo herpetiformis is a rare dermatosis of pregnancy and is a variant of pustular psoriasis. It is a serious condition and may be life-threatening. Fortunately, however, it is extremely rare.

PRURITUS

Itching is the most common dermatologic symptom. Most commonly, the pruritus accompanies a visible skin eruption; therefore, the cause of the pruritus is determined when the rash is diagnosed. Examples include drug eruptions, contact dermatitis, atopic dermatitis, psoriasis, lichen planus, miliaria (i.e., heat rash), folliculitis, candidiasis, and scabies. Of these, scabies is most frequently missed, because the characteristic burrows are not easily found, and may not even be present, so that excoriations may be the only skin findings.

Pruritus may also occur without primary skin lesions. Excoriations may be present, but these will typically spare skin that cannot be reached by the patient (especially the back). Patients with such "rashless" pruritus must be evaluated for

systemic causes (27), which are listed in Table 18.5. In addition to a complete history and physical examination, blood tests will be needed to screen for many of these conditions. Chest radiography is also recommended as part of the screen for Hodgkin's disease, which is the lymphoma most commonly associated with pruritus. The finding of eosinophilia on a complete blood count would suggest a drug or parasitic cause. As previously mentioned, scabies should always be kept in mind, because the diagnostic skin findings are easily missed. Dry skin (i.e., xerosis) in elderly patients can cause itching, and this pruritus is relieved by emollients and low-dose antihistamines. Itching resulting from systemic causes, however, is typically generalized, severe, and unremitting. Psychogenic pruritus should be considered only after all other etiologies are ruled out.

Table 18.5.   Causes of Pruritus without Rash

Hepatic
Biliary obstruction
Renal
Uremia
Endocrine
Hyperthyroidism
Diabetes mellitus[a]
Hypothyroidism[a]
Hematologic
Lymphomas (e.g., Hodgkin's disease)
Polycythemia vera
Leukemia[a]
Anemia[a]
Carcinomas[a]
Lung
Gastrointestinal
Breast
Infestations
Intestinal parasites
Onchocerciasis
Dermatologic
Scabies
Dry skin (xerosis)
Psychogenic
Neurotic excoriations
Delusions of parasitosis

[a]Not well documented.

Therapy for generalized pruritus is directed toward the underlying cause, if one is found. For example, successful treatment of Hodgkin's disease will abolish the pruritus. For symptomatic therapy, ultraviolet light can be beneficial for pruritus associated with renal and hepatic diseases. Antihistamine therapy is usually not helpful.

THE DIABETIC FOOT

Complications of the lower extremities are the most frequent cause of hospitalization in patients with diabetes, and internists are frequently consulted about their treatment. The most frequent problems are:

1. Infection.
2. Neuropathic ulceration.
3. Ischemia.

These complications frequently coexist. The consulting internist must determine the type of problem and participate as a member of a multidisciplinary team (usually including vascular, orthopaedic, reconstructive, or podiatric surgeons) to manage the problem.

Infection

Infectious complications of the diabetic foot are commonly divided into non–limb-threatening and limb-threatening types (28). Non–limb-threatening infection is characterized by shallow ulceration, less than 2 cm of surrounding cellulitis, lack of significant ischemia, and no bone or joint involvement. These infections typically result from *S. aureus* or streptococci organisms. Limb-threatening infections are associated with more extensive cellulitis or lymphangitis, and they may be accompanied by systemic toxicity, full-thickness ulceration, or significant ischemia. These infections are typically polymicrobic and resulting aerobic Gram-positive cocci (e.g., staphylococci, streptococci), anaerobic organisms, and enteric Gram-negative ba-

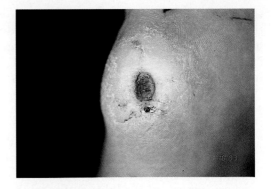

Figure 18.15. Diabetic foot ulcer. An uninflamed neuropathic ulcer under the fifth metatarsal head after debridement that required pressure relief for healing.

cilli (eg., *Escherichia coli*, *Klebsiella* sp., *Proteus* sp.).

The consulting internist must recognize the potential for limb-threatening, and life-threatening, complications and the need for a multidisciplinary approach to management (29). The principles of managing infectious complications are urgent surgical debridement and drainage, appropriate empiric broad-spectrum antibiotics, meticulous local care, and ensuring adequate arterial flow.

Neuropathic Ulceration

Neuropathic ulceration (Fig. 18.15) is a major predictor of subsequent amputation. These lesions may or may not have an associated infection, and they are typically pressure-related, on the plantar surface underneath the metatarsal heads. They must be carefully debrided of devitalized tissue. Plain-film radiographs are recommended to evaluate for soft-tissue foreign bodies and assess bony changes. Those patients without associated cellulitis are treated with local wound care (e.g., saline-damp to dry dressings changed two to three times a day) and by relieving mechanical pressure at the ulcer site. The total-contact cast is a useful modality in relieving pressure (29).

Ischemia

Patients with diabetes characteristically have atheromatous lesions involving the tibial vessels and, contrary to traditional teaching, often have unobstructed pedal vessels. This has resulted in two important bedside principles for evaluating patients with diabetic foot problems:

1. Patients with poor pedal pulses should not be considered to require amputation unless arteriography that carefully evaluates the pedal vessels is performed. Tibial–pedal bypass is an important modality in limb salvage for many such patients.
2. Patients with good pulses should not be considered to have "microvascular disease" in the case of a nonhealing ulcer. Failure to heal most often results from failure to provide adequate pressure relief at the site of the ulcer.

As previously noted, an integrated, multidisciplinary approach is required. Once the lesions have healed, preventive interventions must be instituted; thus, continuity of care after the patient has been released from the hospital is essential.

CUTANEOUS COMPLICATIONS OF HOSPITALIZATIONS

Circumstances associated with hospitalization sometimes result in cutaneous reactions. The following categories will be considered here: *(a)* drug eruptions, *(b)* contact dermatitis, and *(c)* skin infections.

Drug Eruptions

Drug eruptions are easily the most common cutaneous condition for which a consultation is requested. In one large survey (30), cutaneous reactions to drugs occurred in 2.2% of hospitalized patients. This study included only morbilliform eruptions, hives, and generalized itching. Certain drugs (e.g., chemotherapeutic agents) can cause distinctive cutaneous reactions, such as photosensitivity eruptions, radiation recall, hyperpigmenta-

tion, stomatitis, and other mucocutaneous complications (31). For all drugs, the extensive tables in Fitzpatrick's general dermatology text (32) list the different types of eruptions and the drugs most commonly responsible. **Drugs should be considered in the differential diagnosis of any skin rash of uncertain cause.**

The most common cutaneous drug reaction is the morbilliform or so-called "maculopapular" eruption. This is a generalized eruption of erythematous macules and papules that tend to be confluent in large areas (Fig. 18.16). The eruption usually starts proximally and proceeds distally; the legs are usually the last to be involved and, likewise, the last to clear. The erythema is often bright red, which may help to distinguish clinically a drug reaction from a viral exanthem, which it can sometimes mimic. The presence of eosinophilia may also be helpful in this regard. In adults, viral exanthems are much less common than drug reactions as a cause of morbilliform eruptions.

Unfortunately, there is no clinical method or laboratory test to identity which drug is responsible, and because the average hospitalized patient receives nine drugs (30), this poses a problem. To implicate a particular drug, two variables can be considered: the timing of the eruption

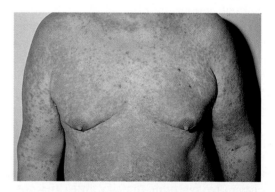

Figure 18.16. Drug eruption. This generalized eruption is comprised of brightly erythematous macules and papules that are confluent in large areas. (Reprinted with permission from Lookingbill DP, Marks JG. Principles of dermatology. 2nd ed. Philadelphia: WB Saunders, 1993.)

in relationship to the initiation of the drug, and the frequency in which specific drugs cause cutaneous reactions. Most drug eruptions occur within several days of initiating the medication. The incidence rates developed in the Boston Collaborative Drug Surveillance Program (30) can serve as guidelines in assessing the statistical likelihood of a given drug causing a rash. Table 18.6 lists some of the most common offending agents based on these data.

Drug reactions occur much more frequently in those infected with HIV than in the general population. For example, in one survey of patients with AIDS (33), eruptions from trimethoprim-sulfamethoxazole occurred in 43%, and skin reactions to aminopenicillins occurred ten times more frequently than in the general population.

It is not always possible to implicate a specific drug in a drug rash. Under these circumstances, reduce the number of drugs being administered to the absolute minimum, and change the most likely drug or drugs to alternative ones if possible.

What are the risks of continuing to administer a drug while a cutaneous reaction is occurring that is caused by that drug? The risks are mainly cutaneous and renal.

The cutaneous risk is possible progression of the inflammatory reaction to an exfoliative erythroderma or toxic epidermal necrolysis. Such progression seldom occurs, however, so a given, essential drug therapy may sometimes be continued in the face of an eruption. In fact, in some cases, a drug rash may resolve despite continuance of the offending agent. This has been documented with ampicillin rashes in immunocompetent patients and also with nonthreatening rashes from trimethoprim-sulfamethoxazole in patients infected with HIV (34). For severe cutaneous reactions, however, it is important to discontinue the implicated drug.

The renal risk is allergic interstitial nephritis, which is a rare complication

Table 18.6. Drug Rash Incidence Rates

Drug	Reaction Rate (Per 100 Recipients)
Amoxicillin	5.1
Trimethoprim-sulfamethoxazole	3.4
Ampicillin	3.3
Ipodate	2.8
Blood, whole human	2.2
Semisynthetic penicillins	2.1
Cephalosporins	2.1
Penicillin G	1.9
Hydralazine	1.9
Sulfisoxazole	1.7
Quinidine	1.3
Cimetidine	1.3
Phenylbutazone	1.2

Reprinted with permission from Bigby M, Jick S, Jick H, Arndt K. Drug-induced cutaneous reactions. A report from the Boston Collaborative Drug Surveillance Program on 15,438 consecutive inpatients, 1975 to 1982. JAMA 1986;256:3358–3363.

most commonly associated with penicillins and cephalosporins. In addition to rash, many of these patients have fever and eosinophilia; the finding of eosinophils in the urine is a valuable diagnostic clue. The condition is usually reversible by discontinuing the offending agent.

Acute anaphylaxis is *not* a hazard when continuing with a drug thought to be responsible for a rash. Anaphylaxis is a consideration when readministering a drug to a patient with a history of cutaneous reaction to that drug, particularly if the eruption was urticarial. In this regard, predictive testing in patients with a history of penicillin allergy can be performed with penicilloyl-polylysine (i.e., major determinant) and minor determinant skin tests. There appears to be good correlation between positive tests and immunoglobulin E–mediated penicillin hypersensitivity (35). Penicillin is the only drug for which these tests are available.

Some patients with penicillin allergy may exhibit cross-reactivity to cephalosporins. The frequency of this has often been placed at 10%, but it may be much lower. In a study of 62 subjects with positive penicillin skin tests (35), only one reacted to a challenging dose of cephalosporin. Nevertheless, if a patient has a history of an *urticarial* or other anaphylactic reaction to penicillin, avoid administration of cephalosporins if possible.

Cross-reactivity can occur with other drugs as well. For example, avoid semisynthetic macrolide antibiotics (e.g., clarithromycin) in patients who are allergic to erythromycin. Patients who are allergic to sulfa drugs may react to thiazides and sulfonylureas (e.g., chlorpropamide).

Drug eruptions clear after discontinuation of the drug, but the time course is important to remember. Eruptions usually take 1 to 2 weeks to clear completely. In fact, the eruption may worsen for several days after the suspected agent has been discontinued. Explaining this to the patient should help to alleviate anxiety when the rash does not clear overnight.

The final aspect of allergic cutaneous drug reactions is what to tell the patient about his or her "allergy." This may be difficult when the reaction was relatively mild or a single drug could not be implicated with certainty. However, patients should be advised, and their charts labeled appropriately, if a cutaneous reaction occurred in which either a specific drug was identified with relative certainty (regardless of the nature of the cutaneous reaction) or a serious (e.g., anaphylactic reaction, erythroderma, extensive blistering reaction) or potentially serious (e.g., urticaria) reaction occurred and one drug was implicated as the most likely cause.

Contact Dermatitis

In allergic contact dermatitis, an offending substance comes into contact with the skin of a sensitized individual and results in a delayed hypersensitivity reaction involving the epidermis, and the underlying dermal blood vessels. Clinically, the epidermal reaction is characterized by vesicles in the acute phase and poorly demarcated areas of confluent, superficial, glistening small papules in the subacute phase. **Itching is invariably present.**

Poison ivy is the prototypic contact allergen. Unless the delivering florist has unusual taste, poison ivy is of course unlikely to be encountered in a hospital setting. Tape, local antiseptics, and other topically applied medications are frequently encountered, however, and these can sometimes induce contact dermatitis in a sensitized individual. The configuration and distribution of the dermatitis often provide clues leading to the diagnosis. For example, square- and rectangular-shaped areas might lead to suspicion of a tape allergy; a large area over the abdomen with streaks extending along the flanks after laparotomy should indicate contact dermatitis to the solution used in preparing the patient for surgery. When localized, contact dermatitis can satisfactorily be treated with cool soaks followed by a topical steroid cream and a systemic antihistamine for the itching. The process usually takes a week or more to resolve.

Miliaria

Miliaria (i.e., "heat rash") occurs on the backs of patients confined to a supine position for extended periods of time. Orthopaedic patients trapped in various devices are frequently affected. The eruption appears as multiple individual erythematous papules or crystal-clear vesicles over the back. Sometimes, an allergy to the bed linen is incorrectly implicated. Such "sheet allergy" is uncommon, although an irritant reaction to detergent remaining in the laundered sheets may sometimes occur. Accordingly, many hospitals provide "hypoallergenic sheets" simply by passing the linens through the rinse cycle an extra time. The lesions in miliaria result from occlusion of the sweat ducts followed by retention of sweat in the skin. Treatment simply involves increased air exposure, and the problem resolves spontaneously.

Skin Infections

Hospitalized patients are at risk for developing superficial as well as deep skin infections. Deep skin infections are most likely to occur as a complication of surgery, and they can evolve to cellulitis and, sometimes, even to a necrotizing fasciitis. As previously discussed, wound debridement, bacterial cultures, and antibiotic therapy are required to treat this serious complication.

The most common hospital-acquired superficial skin infections are of fungal and herpetic cause. Herpes infections have already been discussed; of the superficial fungal infections, candidiasis is the most common. Two factors predispose to *C. albicans* infections: antibiotic therapy, which may suppress the normal bowel flora and allow *Candida* sp. to thrive with resultant oral and perianal infection; and increased heat and moisture in the perineal and perianal areas of patients confined to bed. Clinically, candidiasis appears as a **beefy red eruption** with poorly demarcated borders but with **satellite papules and pustules**. It occurs most commonly in the groin and perianal areas, but in patients confined to bed, lesions may extend up the back as well. The diagnosis can be confirmed by potassium hydroxide preparation of a scraping of superficial pus or scale. Under the microscope, hyphae or pseudohyphae are seen; spores are not diagnostic. Local therapy with a topical agent such as clotrimazole or ketoconazole applied twice daily is usually satisfactory. Widespread or resistant disease can be treated with oral ketoconazole or flucoconazole. Procedures to promote dry skin in susceptible areas are helpful as well.

DERMATOLOGIC THERAPY

Dermatologic therapy is most frequently aimed at infection or inflammation. Skin infections can often be treated topically. Topical imidazoles (e.g., clotrimazole, miconazole, ketoconazole) are effective for both candida and tinea infections, and topical antibiotics are helpful for superficial bacterial infections. Systemic therapy is used for more severe or widespread disease.

Noninfected inflammatory skin conditions are most often treated with a topical steroid, and the bewildering array of available preparations can be divided according to potency (Table 18.7). The selection of an agent depends on both the type of disease and its location. In general, **the weakest effective preparation should be employed**. For example, seborrheic dermatitis can be treated with a mild steroid such as hydrocortisone; psoriasis will respond best to stronger preparations. However, the more potent topical steroids should not be used on "sensitive" skin, such as the face, genitalia, and flexural folds; hydrocortisone is the steroid of choice for these locations. Such sensitive areas of skin are more susceptible to local adverse effects, which include steroid acne (particularly on the face), and skin atrophy, which sometimes results in skin breakdown. Occurrence of these local side effects increases with the potency of the topical steroid.

Topical steroids are available in several vehicles, including creams, ointments, lotions, and solutions. Creams are most commonly employed and easy to use, because they are in a water base and not "greasy." Ointments are in an oil base and, therefore, more occlusive and more effective. They are particularly useful for dry, scaly conditions. Lotions are sometimes employed when large areas of skin are involved, and solutions are used for conditions involving the scalp.

Plastic-wrap occlusion will increase the potency of topical steroids tenfold, but wraps are awkward to use and increase the risk of both local and systemic side effects. Thus, they are not generally recommended. Even without plastic occlusion, adrenal-suppressive doses of corticosteroids can be absorbed from the application of a moderate-strength topical steroid that is applied to inflamed skin if

Table 18.7.   Topical Steroid Preparations

Potency	Brand	Generic	% Steroids
Lowest	Hytone	Hydrocortisone	1.0
			2.5
Low	Tridesilon	Desonide	0.05
Medium	Valisone	Betamethasone valerate	0.1
	Synalar	Fluocinolone acetonide	0.025
	Westcort	Hydrocortisone valerate	0.2
	Aristocort, Kenalog	Triamcinolone acetonide	0.1
High	Cyclocort	Amcinonide	0.1
	Diprosone	Betamethasone dipropionate	0.05
	Topicort	Desoximethasone	0.25
	Lidex	Fluocinonide	0.05
	Halog	Halcinonide	0.1
Super-high	Diprolene	Betamethasone dipropionate	0.05
	Temovate	Clobetasol propionate	0.05
	Ultravate	Halobetasol propionate	0.05

Reprinted with permission from Lookingbill DP, Marks JG. Dermatologic therapy. In: Principles of dermatology. 2nd ed. Philadelphia: WB Saunders, 1993:53–63.

the entire skin surface is involved or from the application of one of the newer, "superpotent" steroids (e.g., Diprolene, Temovate) to more limited areas. For preoperative purposes, patients using long-term, large amounts of topical steroids should be treated in the same way as patients who have been on systemic-suppressive doses.

Systemic steroids are sometimes needed for severe or extensive inflammatory conditions, such as severe contact dermatitis and autoimmune blistering diseases (e.g., pemphigus). Systemic steroids should only be employed when the dermatologic diagnosis is certain, however, and when the benefits outweigh the risks. If in doubt, a dermatology consultation should be obtained.

WHEN TO CONSULT A DERMATOLOGIST

Many of the disorders covered in this chapter can be addressed without consulting a dermatologist. There are some circumstances, however, when a dermatology consultation is desirable. Examples include: (a) for growths that might be malignant; (b) for rashes of uncertain cause, particularly in patients with acute febrile illness; (c) whenever need for a biopsy is in doubt; (d) for rashes that do not respond to therapy; and (e) when systemic steroid therapy is being considered for a dermatologic condition.

Atypical pigmented lesions and persistent, firm nodules in the skin should raise the suspicion of possible malignancy. Biopsy or excision will answer the question, but neither may be needed. For example, the pigmented lesion may be a dark seborrheic keratosis rather than a melanoma, and if a dermatologist can make this diagnosis clinically, the patient can be spared an unnecessary procedure (36). Conversely, performing a "blind" biopsy of a rash will frequently be unrewarding unless the dermatopathologist is provided with a differential diagnosis. Additionally, it takes several days before the results will be available. Therefore, with an undiagnosed rash, particularly in an acutely ill patient, a consultation with a dermatologist should be obtained to determine if the rash represents a clue to the diagnosis of a systemic illness and if a biopsy will be helpful. In general, when the need for a

biopsy is in question, a consultation is recommended to determine if the biopsy is needed and, if it is, how best to perform it and interpret its results.

In terms of dermatologic therapy, a consultation should be considered if a skin eruption is not responding to a prescribed therapy. For example, a crusting erosion will not respond to an antibiotic if it is caused by herpes simplex. Similarly, a dermatologist's opinion should be sought in most cases before prescribing systemic steroids for a skin condition in a hospitalized patient. This is particularly important if any question exists regarding the cause of the rash.

REFERENCES

1. Hook EW, Hooton TM, Horton CA, Coyle MB, Ramsey PG, Turck M. Microbiologic evaluation of cutaneous cellulitis in adults. Arch Intern Med 1986;146:295–297.
2. Feingold DS. Gangrenous and crepitant cellulitis. J Am Acad Dermatol 1982;6:289–299.
3. Saiag P, Le Breton C, Pavlovic M, Fouchard N, Delzant G, Bigot JM. Magnetic resonance imaging in adults presenting with severe acute infectious cellulitis. Arch Dermatol 1994;130:1150–1158.
4. Carlson KC, Mehlmauer M, Evans S, Chandrasoma P. Cryptococcal cellulitis in renal transplant recipients. J Am Acad Dermatol 1987;17:469–472.
5. Baddour LM, Bisno AL. Recurrent cellulitis after coronary bypass surgery. Association with superficial fungal infection in saphenous venectomy limbs. JAMA 1984;251:1049–1052.
6. Robboy SJ, Mihm MC, Colman RW, et al. The skin in disseminated intravascular coagulation. Br J Dermatol 1973;88:221–229.
7. Resnick SD. Medical progress. Toxic shock syndrome: recent developments in pathogenesis. J Pediatr 1990;116:321–328.
8. Stevens DL, Tanner MH, Winship J, et al. Severe group A streptococcal infections associated with a toxic shock-like syndrome and scarlet fever toxin A. N Engl J Med 1989;321:1–7.
9. The Working Group on Severe Streptococcal Infections. Defining the group A streptococcal toxic shock syndrome. JAMA 1993;269:390–391.
10. Malane MS, Grant-Kels JM, Feder HM, Luger SW. Diagnosis of lyme disease based on dermatologic manifestations. Ann Intern Med 1991;114:490–498.
11. Wallace RJ, Brown BA. Skin, soft tissue, and bone infections due to *Mycobacterium chelonae*: importance of prior corticosteroid therapy, frequency of disseminated infections, and resistance to oral antimicrobials other than clarithromycin. J Infect Dis 1992;166:405–412.
12. Grossman ME, Silvers DN, Walther RR. Cutaneous manifestations of disseminated candidiasis. J Am Acad Dermatol 1980;2:111–116.
13. Mackowiak PA, LeMaistre CF. Drug fever: a critical appraisal of conventional concepts. An analysis of 51 episodes in two Dallas hospitals and 97 episodes reported in the English literature. Ann Intern Med 1987;106:728–733.
14. Lipsky BA, Hirschmann JV. Drug fever. JAMA 1981;245:851–854.
15. Roujeau JC, Stern RS. Medical progress. Severe adverse cutaneous reactions to drugs. N Engl J Med 1994;331:1272–1285.
16. Smith KJ, Skelton HG, Yeager J, et al. Cutaneous findings in HIV-1-positive patients: a 42-month prospective study. J Am Acad Dermatol 1994;31:746–754.
17. Dover JS, Johnson RA. Cutaneous manifestations of human immunodeficiency virus infection. Part I. Arch Dermatol 1991;127:1383–1391.
18. Dover JS, Johnson RA. Cutaneous manifestations of human immunodeficiency virus infection. Part II. Arch Dermatol 1991;127:1549–1558.
19. Koehler JE, Quinn FD, Berger TG, LeBoit PE, Tappero JW. Isolation of *Rochalimaea* species from cutaneous and osseous lesions of bacillary angiomatosis. N Engl J Med 1992;327:1625–1631.
20. Lookingbill DP. Yield from a complete skin examination. J Am Acad Dermatol 1988;18:31–37.
21. Sober AJ, Fitzpatrick TB, Mihm MC, et al. Early recognition of cutaneous melanoma. JAMA 1979;242:2795–2799.
22. Lookingbill DP, Spangler N, Sexton FM. Skin involvement as the presenting sign of internal carcinoma. J Am Acad Dermatol 1990;22:19–26.
23. Lookingbill DP, Spangler N, Helm KF. Cutaneous metastases in patients with metastatic carcinoma: a retrospective study of 4020 patients. J Am Acad Dermatol 1993;29:228–236.
24. Poole S, Fenske NA. Cutaneous markers of internal malignancy. I. Malignant involvement of the skin and the genodermatoses. J Am Acad Dermatol 1993;28:1–13.
25. Poole S, Fenske NA. Cutaneous markers of internal malignancy. II. Paraneoplastic dermatoses and environmental carcinogens. J Am Acad Dermatol 1993;28:147–164.
26. Winton GB, Lewis CW. Dermatoses of pregnancy. J Am Acad Dermatol 1982;6:977–998.
27. Kantor GR, Lookingbill DP. Generalized pruritus and systemic disease. J Am Acad Dermatol 1983;9:375–382.

28. Gibbons G. Diabetic foot sepsis. Semin Vasc Surg 1992;5:244–248.

29. Caputo GM, Cavanagh PR, Ulbrecht JS, et al. Assessment and management of foot disease in patients with diabetes. N Engl J Med 1994;331:854–860.

30. Bigby M, Jick S, Jick H, Arndt K. Drug-induced cutaneous reactions. A report from the Boston Collaborative Drug Surveillance Program on 15,438 consecutive inpatients, 1975 to 1982. JAMA 1986;256:3358–3363.

31. Bronner AK, Hood AF. Cutaneous complications of chemotherapeutic agents. J Am Acad Dermatol 1983;9:645–663.

32. Fitzpatrick TB, Eisen AZ, Wolff K, et al., eds. Dermatology in general medicine. 4th ed. New York: McGraw-Hill, 1993.

33. Coopman SA, Johnson RA, Platt R, Stern RS. Cutaneous disease and drug reactions in HIV infection. N Engl J Med 1993;328:1670–1674.

34. Sattler FR, Cowan R, Nielsen DM, et al. Trimethoprim-sulfamethoxazole versus pentamidine for therapy of pneumocystis pneumonia: a prospective, crossover study in patients with AIDS. Ann Intern Med 1988;109:280–287.

35. Saxon A, Beall GN, Rohr AS, Adelman DC. Immediate hypersensitivity reactions to beta-lactam antibiotics. Ann Intern Med 1987;107:204–215.

36. Federman D, Hogan D, Taylor JR, Caralis P, Kirsner RS. A comparison of diagnosis, evaluation, and treatment of patients with dermatologic disorders. J Am Acad Dermatol 1995;32:726–729.

RECOMMENDED READINGS

1. Lookingbill DP, Marks JG. Principles of dermatology. 2nd ed. Philadelphia: WB Saunders, 1993.

2. Moschella SL, Hurley HG. Dermatology. 3rd ed. Philadelphia: WB Saunders, 1992.

19

Orthopaedics and Rheumatology

Richard J. Gross and Brent G. Petty[1]

This chapter focuses on: *(a)* the medical evaluation of patients requiring bone and joint surgery and, *(b)* the care of concomitant joint disease in patients requiring unrelated surgery. Risk factors pertaining to these two groups and ways to minimize morbidity and mortality also are discussed.

HIP FRACTURES

More than 1.6 million hip fractures occur in the United States each year, and surgical repair of a fractured hip is one of the five most common procedures performed in Medicare beneficiaries. Seventy percent of these operations involve patients older than 70 years. Most commonly, the patient is a white woman with osteoporosis, which occurs much less frequently in blacks and in men.

Approximately 6 to 10% of patients operated on for hip fractures die within 30 days (1, 2), and 20% die within 3 months. This high mortality rate results from the combination of preexisting disease and concomitant, acute medical problems superimposed on the fracture.

Certain patient characteristics define a particularly high-risk group (Table 19.1). Each of the following is considered to at least double the risk of mortality: *(a)* age older than 65 years, *(b)* male gender, *(c)* nonambulatory status before fracture,

(d) history of congestive heart failure, *(e)* 24- to 48-hour delay between injury and hospitalization, *(f)* history of angina, *(g)* chronic obstructive pulmonary disease, and *(h)* malnutrition. Investigation at our institution suggests that nine preoperative risk factors predict most deaths (Table 19.2). Postoperative hypotension and upper gastrointestinal bleeding are additional contributors to mortality, but they not predictable by preoperative assessment (3). Deaths are uncommon in the immediate perioperative period, but begin to occur more frequently in the first postoperative week, peaking in the second to fourth postoperative weeks.

The three major causes of mortality are pneumonia, heart failure, and pulmonary emboli (Table 19.3). A review of the medical risk factors and causes of death listed here suggests that prudent preoperative evaluation and management, in addition to intensive postoperative follow-up, may influence postoperative morbidity and mortality. A few interventions seem to have the most impact: *(a)* early detection and treatment of infection (especially of urinary tract infection and pneumonia), *(b)* optimizing volume status (avoiding volume depletion due to bleeding into the fracture or limited intake, and avoiding fluid overload, particularly in patients with a history of congestive heart failure), and *(c)* optimizing cardiac function (reducing symptoms or signs of congestive heart failure, and minimizing episodes of myocardial ischemia).

---

[1]John W. Burnside contributed to this chapter in the first and second editions.

Table 19.1.   Hip Fractures: Risk Factors for Mortality[a]

1. Age >65 years
2. Male
3. Nonambulatory before fracture
4. 24- to 48-hour delay from injury to hospital admission
5. History of congestive heart failure
6. History of angina
7. Malnutrition
8. Chronic obstructive pulmonary disease

[a]Each factor at least doubles the expected mortality rate.

Table 19.2.   Medical Conditions Related to Perioperative Hip Fracture Mortality[a]

1. Electrocardiogram showing myocardial infarction or definite ischemic change
2. Congestive heart failure (decompensated)
3. Noncardiac dyspnea
4. Cerebrovascular accident
5. Renal failure
6. Sepsis
7. Hepatomegaly
8. Alkalosis
9. Not undergoing surgery due to severe medical problems

Reprinted with permission from Gross R, Curtis J, Brooker A. Effect of coexisting medical illness on mortality of hip fracture repair. Clin Res 1986;34: 819A.
[a]Postoperative hypotension and upper gastrointestinal bleeding are additional factors contributing to mortality but are not predictable from preoperative factors.

Preoperative Evaluation

Begin assessment of a patient with an inquiry regarding the accident. Hip fractures generally occur because of a fall, though most patients cannot tell you why they fell. Try to determine why the patient fell. If a history of seizure or syncope emerges, investigate the usual cardiac and neurologic causes. With the exception of patients with obvious arrhythmia or myocardial infarction, a full evaluation usually can be deferred to the postopera-

tive period. Twenty-five percent of patients will report feeling dizzy before the fall.

Certain aspects of the patient history and physical examination deserve special attention. First, assess volume status. Keep in mind that 500 to 1500 mL of blood may be lost into the thigh, and that the thirst mechanism of elderly patients often does not function well. A full test for orthostatic hypotension usually is not possible, and skin turgor is a frequently unreliable indicator in elderly patients. Signs of congestive heart failure that should be assessed include rales, edema, gallops, and distended neck veins. Again, the specificity of this examination is compromised in patients with hip fracture (e.g., by the presence of rales due to atelectasis or aspiration, or the inability to hear rales due to poor inspiration or the inability to sit up). A careful neurologic examination also is important. Postoperative confusion, fat emboli, and cerebral vascular accident are most accurately evaluated if a good baseline has been recorded, and note carefully the presence or absence of peripheral pulses (again for subsequent reference). A careful search for symptoms or subtle signs of infection, especially for pneumonia or urinary tract infection, should be performed as well.

Certain laboratory tests are important to help with these preoperative assessments. The urine specific gravity is a fair test of both intravascular volume and renal-concentrating ability, and chest radiography will help to determine whether congestive heart failure or parenchymal

Table 19.3.   Hip Fractures: Causes of Mortality

Cause	% of Mortality
Pneumonia	40
Congestive heart failure	20
Pulmonary emboli	15
Myocardial infarction	10
Sepsis (any source)	10
Cerebrovascular accident	5

lung disease is present. Electrocardiography, including rhythm strip, can show evidence of myocardial infarction or arrhythmia.

The elderly lung provides good soil for pathogens. When properly performed, the best preoperative test of pulmonary function is the maximum breathing capacity. It not only tests volumes but the entire mechanical capacity of the lungs, and it relates to the patient's ability to generate an effective cough. A value of less than 40 L/min indicates increased risk. Measurement of arterial blood gases is useful in elderly or debilitated patients as well. If the patient has chronic bronchitis or is producing any sputum, Gram stain and culture may guide antibiotic therapy (see Chapter 17). Poor dentition in elderly patients may break with intubation, and full-stomach contents might wind up in the airways.

Most patients will have a Foley catheter inserted for the evaluation of fluid volumes and for comfort. Initial specimens should be cultured, because urinary tract infection is common and a source of significant morbidity in patients with hip fracture. Scrupulous care of the catheter also is important.

Whether and When to Operate

There are no good data on patients randomized to surgical and conservative treatment. In almost all cases, the patient will undergo surgery because of the high mortality rate for nonoperated hip fractures in older series and the prolonged immobility of untreated fractures. A conservative approach is justified in patients who are terminally ill or have a high perioperative risk, especially if the fracture is a nondisplaced, intertrochanteric fracture the surgeon feels has a chance of healing with sufficient function to allow activities of daily living.

There probably is an optimal time for surgery for individual patients, but no ideal time has been reported in the literature. Hip fracture repair is not an emergency procedure, and the mortality rate may be higher in medically unstable patients taken directly from the emergency room to the surgical suite. Sufficient time should be taken to stabilize medical problems as quickly as reasonable, but surgery should not be unduly delayed by slowness in attending to medical problems. Proceeding with surgery from 24 to 48 hours after admission frequently allows sufficient time to correct volume status, congestive heart failure, cardiac ischemia, infection, and other medical problems. Delays of up to 3 to 5 days, when indicated by severe medical problems, probably do not increase mortality significantly, but after 5 to 7 days, prolonged immobility significantly increases the complication rate. For patients with significant, improvable medical problems on admission, the optimal time for surgery is when: (a) the patient appears to have made major improvement, (b) the patient appears to have been medically stable for 12 to 24 hours, and (c) no further, substantial improvement within a reasonably brief period of time seems likely. For patients without medical problems or with problems that cannot be improved in a few days, the timing of surgery is a surgical decision; orthopaedic surgeons usually prefer taking the patient to the operating room as soon as feasible, either on admission or within 12 hours, to allow mobilization as soon as possible and to minimize any complications of immobility.

Operative Care

The choice of anesthesia, of course, is a decision for the anesthesiologist. The conventional wisdom that spinal or epidural anesthesia is safest may not be true. Hypotension probably is more common with such anesthesia, agitation and anxiety may be greater, and pulmonary toilet is difficult. The most common intraoperative complication is hypotension; adequate volume replacement with colloid and crystalloid is the best prophylaxis.

Use of prophylactic antibiotics is effective in reducing the incidence of wound infections. Cefazolin, 1 g preoperatively and every 6 hours for three additional doses, is recommended (4). There is no documented, beneficial effect on mortality, however, or on morbidity other than wound infection (5).

Coumarin (Coumadin), adjusted-dose heparin, and enoxaparin are effective prophylaxis for thromboembolic disease (6–9). Aspirin has been effective in some studies and may reduce the overall mortality rate in this population (2). Fixed, low-dose heparin, however, is ineffective as thromboembolic prophylaxis (see Chapter 9).

Postoperative Care

Table 19.4 lists the rate of postoperative complications in patients with hip fractures. About half of these patients will develop a postoperative fever, and half of these will be pyogenic. The most common infectious causes of fever are pneumonia and urinary tract infection. Pneumonia often has few clinical signs other than fever, and rales may be absent due to poor inspiration, inability of the patient to sit up for the examination, and dehydration. Sputum Gram stain and culture can be helpful. Urinalysis and Gram stain of unspun urine can aid in rapidly establishing the presence of urinary tract infection; if the urine specimen is negative in pa-

Table 19.4. Hip Fracture: Postoperative Complications

Complication	Patients (%)
Fever (all sources)	50
Intra- and immediate postoperative hypotension	20
Infection: lung, bladder, wound	16
Altered mentation	14
Gastrointestinal bleeding	6
Acute renal failure	4
Congestive heart failure (uncompensated)	2
Pulmonary embolism (clinically evident)	2

tients with a fever that seems clinically due to a bacterial infection, an occult pneumonia is likely than other causes of fever. The cause of fever cannot be found in many patients, in whom it presumably results from noninfectious causes such as hematoma, atelectasis, drugs, blood transfusion, and anesthesia.

Pulmonary emboli cause 15 to 30% of deaths in patients with hip fracture, and they are present in 50% or more at autopsy. Prophylaxis, early ambulation, and vigilant follow-up remain the best approach (9) (see Chapter 9).

A relaxation of clinical scrutiny often sets in after the first few postoperative days; in fact, this is the most dangerous time. The conscientious consulting internist will reassess the patient with particular care at this time as well as throughout his or her entire hospital stay.

JOINT REPLACEMENTS

Approximately 90,000 total hip replacements (THR) are performed each year. This major surgical advance regularly yields a high-quality, functional result. It appears that THR is cost-effective as well, comparing favorably with coronary artery bypass graft surgery and renal dialysis in terms of the cost for each quality-adjusted life-year. In some situations, it even appears to be cost-saving, reducing or eliminating the high cost of custodial care and extending quality-adjusted life expectancy by 7 years (10).

The primary indications for THR are pain, diminished range of motion, and altered mechanics producing disability and damage to other joints. Major complications of the procedure are thromboembolic disease, sepsis, dislocation of the prosthesis, and heterotropic ossification (particularly in patients with ankylosing spondylitis). Chances of surgical success can be increased by prudent treatment of concomitant medical problems; still, one-fourth of these patients will have medical complications during hospitalization

Table 19.5. Medical Complications of Total Hip Replacement

Complication	Patients (%)
Urinary retention and/or infection	22
Thrombophlebitis (clinically evident)	13
Pneumonia/atelectasis	10
Pulmonary embolus (clinical evident)	6
Gastrointestinal bleeding	4
Myocardial infarction	1.6
Wound infection	1.3
Death	1.0

(Table 19.5). Unlike the situation with fractured hips, young patients with THR seem to have higher morbidity rate than older patients (65% of patients with complications are younger 60 years, and 35% are older than 60). Perhaps this is proof that advanced years testify to some degree of durability, though many younger patients with THR also have chronic systemic diseases such as rheumatoid arthritis or trauma. The success rate with hip surgery has led to the replacement of knees and, less often, shoulders, elbows, wrist bones, and fingers. As the techniques improve, these will become more frequent. With all of these procedures, however, it serves physicians well to recall they are elective procedures; none are emergent (or even urgent).

Usually, there is no point beyond which a hip cannot be replaced. Therefore, utilization reviews and surgical schedules notwithstanding, there is no excuse for allowing surgery on a patient who is poorly prepared. Furthermore, in an era of increasing pressure to reduce costs by reducing length of stay, concern has arisen over just how far this process can be taken without compromising quality of care. Especially worrisome is the specter of increasingly elderly and less healthy patients being treated with the same approach as that used for younger, more fit patients (11). In patients with rheumatoid arthritis undergoing hip or knee replacement, length of stay is prolonged with a patient age of 55 years or older, female sex, nonwhite ethnicity, poor functional status, positive rheumatoid factor, and an operating room time of longer than 6 hours (12).

The perioperative (i.e., 30-day) mortality rate of THR, unlike that for hip fracture surgery, is low (0.5–2.8%) (1). Mortality increases threefold for each 10-year increase in age over 65 years. The survival rate is 96.3% at 1 year and 93.6% at 2 years after hip replacement. Not surprisingly, pulmonary embolus leads the list of fatal complications (1%) (13). There are few clinical predictors of this complication. Obesity and previous thrombophlebitis correlate with the development of phlebitis, and patients with previous symptomatic venous thromboembolic disease have a significantly increased risk of pulmonary embolus. Age older than 60 years and congestive heart failure also are factors that appear to increase risk. Patients in congestive heart failure should be optimally compensated before surgery to help reduce the risk of emboli.

Long-term functional outcomes and postoperative hospital complications after hip replacement surgery are predicted by the presence and amount of preexisting disease (14). As with some other surgical procedures, the number of THR procedures performed by the surgeon is related to the outcome. Specifically, patients undergoing surgery by surgeons who perform less than 10 THRs per year have higher mortality rates, more infections, more serious complications, and undergo more revision operations. In addition, patient age, comorbidity, and male gender are significantly related to the probability of dying within 3 weeks after total hip arthroplasty (15).

Various prophylactic anticoagulation programs are available for patients undergoing orthopaedic surgery. Low-molecular-weight dextran interferes with platelet function and fibrin bridging. In our experience, dextran causes the highest rate of postoperative bleeding (16%), full-dose heparin or warfarin combined with aspirin or dextran cause excessive bleeding (15–25%), and warfarin alone provides the best protection and fewest bleeding episodes. Others also have concluded that warfarin is safe and effective for the prevention of pulmonary embolism after total hip arthoplasty (13). Low-molecular-weight heparin (enoxaparin) has been shown to prevent thromboembolic disease as well. A randomized, controlled study of enoxaparin showed significant reduction of proximal vein thrombosis compared with placebo controls; in addition, there was no increase in bleeding complications (16).

Total knee replacements also are complicated by thrombosis. Because the procedure includes application of a tourniquet, thrombosis below the knee is frequent (57% of those receiving heparin prophylaxis, and 72% of those treated with aspirin alone) (17). Several studies have produced the conclusion that while prophylaxis is indicated, full anticoagulation postoperatively should be used only in those with clots extending into the thigh.

Superficial wound infection occurs in 1.3% of patients. Local measures and appropriate antibiotics are effective within 7 days. Prophylaxis with perioperative antibiotics reduces the risk of deep wound infection, and the effects of ultraclean air are additive (5).

Deep-wound sepsis occurs in 1% of patients with THR; interestingly, half of these appear between 3 months and 2 years of surgery. Of 87 patients of prosthetic joint infection reported since 1975, 52 had established infections elsewhere, generally in the urinary and respiratory tract. Most of the pathogens were *Staphylococcus* sp., few of which were sensitive to penicillin. Antibiotic prophylaxis at the time of surgery substantially reduces late infections up to 5 years later. The combination of prevention of infection at the time of surgery and the predominant organism being *Staphylococcus* sp. suggests that most late infections either relate to hematogenous seeding that is unrelated to the surgical procedure or are introduced at the time of surgery, lay dormant, and then reactivate years later. Both mechanisms probably contribute to late infection. The usual prophylactic program recommended for patients with valvular heart disease may be inadequate to cover the usual organisms causing late artificial-joint infection.

Postoperative infections occur in 12% of patients, with the most common site being the urinary tract. Prolonged postoperative bladder infection may provide a source of sepsis for the hip. No patient should go to the operating room with an untreated urinary tract infection. Bladder catheterization causes most postoperative genitourinary tract infections, and urinary tract infections can be prevented by sealed catheter–drainage systems, meticulous catheter care, and using the shortest duration of catheterization possible. Preoperative prostatism presages postoperative obstruction. Many patients enter the hospital to have a hip replacement and leave having not only a prosthetic hip but also a transurethral prostatectomy. Substantial evidence of outlet obstruction might prompt elective prostatectomy in advance of joint replacement.

Myocardial infarction or congestive heart failure will occur in 2% of patients. A previous myocardial infarction within 3 to 6 months is sufficient cause to postpone surgery, because the risk of a perioperative myocardial infarction is 6%. Average intraoperative blood loss is 1500 mL, which needs to be adequately replaced. The intake and output sheet assumes great importance in patients with cardiac or renal disease.

Similar to damaged or prosthetic heart valves, prosthetic joints can be a site for adherence of blood-borne bacteria. Nevertheless, whether patients with indwelling prosthetic joints require antibiotic prophylaxis when undergoing dental, gastrointestinal, or genitourinary procedures remains controversial. Many experts do not believe that such prophylaxis is necessary (18). If prophylaxis is elected, however, the generally suggested program differs somewhat from heart valve prophylaxis (Table 19.6). Patients admitted to the hospital for procedures involving infected sites (e.g., drainage of abscesses, including skin boils) should receive prophylaxis to avoid late joint infection.

FAT EMBOLIZATION

Fractures of long bones, burns, and rapid decompression sickness predispose patients to fat embolism. Perhaps 5% of deaths from multiple trauma are caused by fat embolism. When recognized clinically, this syndrome carries a 15% mortality rate.

The usual clinical picture consists of rapidly progressive respiratory embar-

rassment, truncal and retinal petechiae, fat globules in the blood and urine, a rising serum lipase level, and electrocardiographic changes of acute right-heart strain. Thrombocytopenia, anemia, and pyrexia soon follow, and central nervous system changes ranging from confusion to stupor are common. The most consistent clinical findings include tachycardia, tachypnea, pyrexia, central nervous system changes, and significant hypoxemia ($P_{O_2} < 50$ mm Hg).

The mainstay of therapy is respiratory support to ensure adequate oxygenation. Corticosteroids are used to reduce cerebral edema, to preserve platelets, and to blunt the effect of vasoactive substances on the lungs. Alcohol, heparin, and dextran are ineffective and may even be contraindicated.

RHEUMATOLOGIC CONSIDERATIONS IN SURGICAL PATIENTS

Drugs

Almost all patients with rheumatic diseases will be taking at least one drug when admitted to a hospital. The drugs used to treat rheumatologic illness range from relatively safe nonsteroidal anti-inflammatory drugs (NSAIDs) to cytotoxic and immunosuppressive compounds (e.g., methotrexate, cyclophosphamide, cyclosporine). The therapeutic armamentarium allows a more aggressive medical approach to rheumatologic diseases, a posture that now is being taken increasingly frequently, especially in patients with serious illness. The particular drug toxicities to assess in patients presenting for surgery are listed Table 19.7 (19). Perioperative treatment of patients taking corticosteroids is covered in Chapter 13.

Nonsteroidal anti-inflammatory drugs share certain characteristics worth remembering when dealing with surgical patients. Almost all have an effect on prostaglandins and may alter renal function with resultant accumulation of fluid; congestive heart failure may be the un-

Table 19.6. Antibiotic Prophylaxis for Patients with Prosthetic Joints[a]

I. Oropharyngeal procedures: same as endocarditis prophylaxis (see Chapter 17).[b]

II. Genitourinary or gastrointestinal procedures: same as endocarditis prophylaxis (see Chapter 17).[b]

III. Procedures in which infection with *Staphylococcus aureus* is a risk:[c]
   A. Cefazolin, 1 g intravenously 1 hour preoperatively and repeated in 8 hours.
   B. Vancomycin, 1 g intravenously 1 hour preoperatively
      or
      Clindamycin, 300 mg intravenously 30 minutes preoperatively and 150 mg intravenously 6 hours after initial dose.

IV. Procedures on infected tissue: variable depending on anticipated pathogens and sensitivities in local area.

---

[a]Use of antibiotic prophylaxis in patients with indwelling prosthetic joints is controversial. Prophylaxis sometimes is recommended more for recently inserted joints. Most authorities agree that antibiotics should be given for surgery on infected areas (e.g., abscesses).
[b]Some authorities recommend additional doses.
[c]*Staphylococcus* sp. probably represent the largest risk to prosthetic joints. Alternative regimens ("B") are recommended in patients allergic to cephalosporin. Vancomycin is recommended when methicillin-resistant *S. aureus* is a risk.

Table 19.7. Toxicities of Some Drugs Used to Treat Rheumatologic Diseases

Drug	Potential Toxicities	Laboratory Evaluation
Salicylates	Gastrointestinal ulcerations and bleeding Renal insufficiency	CBC Fecal occult blood testing Creatinine, BUN
Methrotrexate	Myelosuppression Hepatic dysfunction Pulmonary infiltrates or fibrosis	CBC LFTs Chest radiography
Azathioprine	Myelosuppression Hepatotoxicity	CBC LFTs
Corticosteroids	Hypertension Hyperglycemia Hypothalamic-pituitary-adrenal axis suppression	Serum glucose
Cyclophosphamide	Myelosuppression Hemorrhagic	CBC Urinalysis
Cyclosporine	Renal insufficiency Anemia Hypertension	CBC Creatinine, BUN

BUN, blood urea nitrogen; *CBC*, complete blood count; *LFTs*, liver function tests.

happy consequence. These drugs also impair platelet function and can cause gastrointestinal ulceration and bleeding. Up to 17% of patients taking at least eight aspirin a day for 3 months or more will have gastric ulcers, and 40% will have gastric erosions. Fully one-third of these ulcers will be asymptomatic; thus the risk of upper gastrointestinal bleeding with additional stress from a surgical procedure becomes a real concern. The role of prophylaxis in such patients (i.e., those not diagnosed as having a lesion but who are at risk for it) and the indicated prophylactic regimen have not been established (see Chapter 12).

Most NSAIDs are unavailable in parenteral form, and their use therefore is precluded in patients who can have nothing by mouth. Ketorolac is available in an intramuscular form but lacks anti-inflammatory activity, is recommended for brief use only, has a significant risk of gastrointestinal bleeding, and has received U.S. Food and Drug Administration approval only for pain indications; therefore it is not indicated as a substitute for long-term use of NSAIDs while the patient

cannot take oral medication. Parenteral analgesics may be used to control pain but will not provide an anti-inflammatory effect.

Methotrexate is being used more frequently in patients with rheumatoid arthritis, especially those with severe disease. While serious adverse events from such aggressive treatment are possible, the overall experience with methotrexate has shown it to be acceptably safe, even after many years of treatment (20). Drugs such as cyclosporine are used in patients with systemic lupus erythematosus who have responded inadequately to steroids and standard cytotoxic drugs (21).

Issues of Underlying Rheumatic Disease

There is no unanimity of opinion regarding the effect of prolonged bed rest on patients with rheumatic diseases. Although the potential for stress-induced flare in any particular joint may decrease, the known effects of calcium loss from bone, flexion contractures, and muscle wasting clearly are detrimental. If more than brief postoperative bed rest is anticipated, early involvement of the physical therapy department should be part of the preoperative planning. Range-of-motion exercise devices and splints are available to maintain muscle tone and either delay or prevent contractures.

Acute postoperative flares of arthritis may have an infectious cause; it is unwise to assume they always result from the underlying arthritis. This especially pertains to contaminated surgery, in which an abnormal or artificial joint provides the same attractiveness to circulating bacteria as a diseased or artificial heart valve. Compounding the diagnostic dilemma of infection in a joint (or elsewhere) is the immunosuppression that frequently exists in patients with long-standing rheumatic diseases treated using corticosteroids, cytotoxic agents, or both.

One fatal complication of rheumatoid arthritis is atlanto-occipital subluxation. Procedures requiring hyperextension of the neck, including endotracheal intubation or certain surgical procedures such as rigid bronchoscopy, may be hazardous because of instability of the atlantoaxial joint. Preoperative neck radiographs (lateral views in flexion and extension) should be part of the preoperative evaluation in patients with rheumatoid arthritis. Similarly, endotracheal intubation may prove to be difficult in patients with ankylosing spondylitis in whom the cervical spine has become fused. Respiratory insufficiency may occur due to rheumatoid lung disease or restricted mobility of the rib cage. In addition, several other anatomic and physiologic changes of rheumatoid arthritis, as summarized in Table 19.8, can complicate perioperative and anesthetic treatment. The anesthesiologist is well served when he or she is alerted to these potential problems.

Crystal-induced Arthritis

Surgery has long been recognized as a precipitating factor for acute gout. Likewise, the acute inflammation of pseudogout (i.e., chondrocalcinosis) may appear in the postoperative period. These problems often occur 5 to 7 days after surgery.

The definitive diagnostic procedure is examination of the synovial fluid, with attention given to the presence of birefringent crystals characteristic of the disease: *(a)* weakly positive, blunt rods and rhomboids of calcium pyrophosphate; or *(b)* strongly negative, birefringent needles of sodium urate crystals. The synovial analysis also is important to exclude septic arthritis.

If the patient is unable to take oral medications for acute crystal-induced gout, the treatment of choice probably is parenteral steroids. Intravenous colchicine has been used in the past to provide prompt (i.e., 24 hours) relief from gout and may have a mild effect on pseudogout, but its use carries more risk than a short course of parenteral steroids. The oral treatment of choice for either disorder in the acute phase is indomethacin.

The most important approach to preventing perioperative gout attacks is prophylaxis. For most patients with this disease, there is an appropriate history. Medications stopped in advance of surgery often are forgotten postoperatively, and the attack then occurs.

Felty's Syndrome

Patients with rheumatoid arthritis may display this syndrome of splenomegaly and granulocytopenia. As a group, they are susceptible to infection, but the correlation between the level of white-cell depression and that risk is poor. The best guide in evaluating individual patients is the history. A low white-blood-cell count with no history of recurrent infection should not be interpreted as call for extra measures (e.g., splenectomy, prophylactic antibiotics) through pregnancy or surgery. Those with frequent infections require very careful culture techniques and prophylactic antibiotics and may respond to splenectomy, though the leukopenia may recur. The predictability of success with splenectomy for any one individual, how-

Table 19.8.   Anaesthetic Hazards in Patients with Rheumatoid Arthritis

Respiratory	
Airway	Ventilation
Hypoplastic mandible	Rheumatoid nodules in lung
Temporomandibular ankylosis	Chronic diffuse interstitial fibrosis
Restriction cervical spine motion	Caplan's syndrome
Atlantoaxial subluxation	Costovertebral joints
Cricoarytenoid arthritis	Thoracic vertebrae flexion deformity
Laryngeal tissue damage	Tuberculous lung

Cardiovascular
Pericardial, myocardial, coronary arteries
Aortic insufficiency
Arhythmias
Disseminating necrotizing arteries

Haemopoietic, Hepatic, and Renal
Anemia
Leukopenia
Bleeding tendency (decreased platelets)
Renal amyloidosis

Posture
Skin fragility
Postoperative chest complications
Multiple joint disease
Recent surgical site healing

Adapted with permission from Jenkins LC, McGraw RW. Anaesthetic management of the patient with rheumatoid arthritis. Can Anaesth Soc J 1969;16:407–415.

ever, is not great enough to justify the additional surgical risk of performing a splenectomy at the time of other indicated surgery, even if the latter is associated with a high incidence of infection.

Shoulder-hand Syndrome

Shoulder-hand syndrome is the most common reflex neurovascular dystrophy. Twenty percent of these cases occur after myocardial infarction, and 20% are com-

plications of cervical spine disease. The onset may be insidious or acute, and it is characterized by marked vasomotor instability with variable pallor, erythema, livedo reticularis, and swelling. The pain is diffuse, poorly localized, and is shortly followed by rapid, significant osteoporosis of the upper-extremity bones. The best treatment is vigorous physical therapy, analgesics for pain, and occasionally, neural blockade. Corticosteroids or indomethacin also frequently are of great help.

REFERENCES

1. Whittle J, Steinberg EP, Anderson GF, et al. Mortality after elective total hip arthroplasty in elderly Americans. Clin Orthop 1993;295:119–126.
2. Nettleman MD, Alsip J, Schrader M, Schulte M. Predictors of mortality after acute hip fracture. J Gen Intern Med 1996;11:765–767.
3. Gross R, Curtis J, Brooker A. Effect of coexisting medical illness on mortality of hip fracture repair. Clin Res 1986;34:819A.
4. Kernodle DS, Kaiser AB. Postoperative infections and antimicrobial prophylaxis. In: Mandell GL, Bennett JE, Dolin R, eds. Principles and practice of infectious diseases. 4th ed. New York: Churchhill Livingstone, 1995:2742–2756.
5. Norden CW. Prevention of bone and joint infections. Am J Med 1985;78(Suppl B):229–234.
6. Bergovist D, Benoni G, Bjorgell O, et al. Low-molecular-weight heparin (enoxaparin) as prophylaxis against venous thromboembolism after total hip replacement. N Engl J Med 1996;335:696–700.
7. Jorgensen LW, Wille Jorgensen P, Hauch O. Prophylaxis of postoperative thromboembolism with low molecular weight heparins Br J Surg 1993;80:689–704.
8. Mohr DN, Silverstein MD, Murtaugh PA, Harrison JM. Prophylactic agents for venous thrombosis in elective hip surgery: meta-analysis of studies using venographic assessment. Arch Intern Med 1993;153:2221–2228.
9. Wells PS, Lensing AW, Davidson Prins MH, et al. Accuracy of ultrasound for the diagnosis of deep venous thrombosis in asymptomatic patients after orthopedic surgery. Ann Intern Med 1995;122:47–53.
10. Chang RW, Pellissier JM, Hagen GB. A cost-effectiveness analysis of total hip arthroplasty for osteoarthritis of the hip. JAMA 1996;275:858–865.
11. Johanson NA. The hospital course in total hip and knee arthroplasty: which length of stay is right? J Rheumatol 1997;24:1–2.
12. Escalante A, Beardmore TD. Predicting length of stay after hip or knee replacement for rheumatoid arthritis. J Rheumatol 1997;24:146–152.
13. Lieberman JR, Wollaeger J, Dorey F, et al. The efficacy of prophylaxis with low-dose warfarin for prevention of pulmonary embolism following total hip replacement. J Bone Joint Surg Am 1997;79:319–325.
14. Greenfield S, Apolone G, McNeil BJ, Cleary PD. The importance of co-existent disease in the occurrence of postoperative complications and one-year recovery for patients undergoing total hip replacement. Med Care 1993;31:141–154.
15. Kreder HJ, Deyo RA, Koepsell T, et al. Relationship between the volume of total hip replacements performed by providers and the rates of postoperative complications in the state of Washington. J Bone Joint Surg Am 1997;79:485–494.
16. Turpie AGG, Levine MN, Hirsh J, et al. A randomized controlled trial of a low-molecular-weight heparin (enoxaparin) to prevent deep-vein thrombosis in patients undergoing elective hip surgery. N Engl J Med 1986;315:925–929.
17. Stulberg BN, Insall JN, Williams GW, et al. Deep-vein thrombosis following total knee replacement. J Bone Joint Surg Am 1984;66:194–201.
18. Wahl MJ. Myths of denal-induced prosthetic joint infections. Clin Infect Dis 1995;20:1420–1425.
19. American College of Rheumatology Ad Hoc Committee on Clinical Guidelines. Guidelines for monitoring drug therapy in rheumatoid arthritis. Arthritis Rheum 1996;39:723–731.
20. Kremmer JM. Safety, efficacy, and mortality in a long-term cohort of patients with rheumatoid arthritis taking methotrexate: follow-up after a mean of 13.3 years. Arthritis Rheum 1997;40:984–985.
21. Caccavo D, Lagana B, Mitterhofer AP, et al. Long-term treatment of systemic lupus erythematosus with cyclosporin A. Arthritis Rheum 1997;40:27–35.

20

Perioperative Management of Neurologic Conditions and Complications

Mohamad Ghias Arar, Yousef Dairi, and Lourdes C. Corman

Surgical risk in patients with neurologic conditions, as in patients with other conditions, depends on the patient's age and overall health, cardiovascular reserve, quality of the operative and perioperative care, and the type, extent, and urgency of the planned surgery. The neurologic condition may raise some specific concerns as well, as, for example, in patients with Parkinson's disease. The most important questions to answer, as in any other patient, are:

1. **How stable is the patient's clinical condition?**
2. **Can the clinical condition be further stabilized or improved before the scheduled surgery?**
3. **Are any changes in the patient's surgical or anesthetic care required?**
4. **Which postoperative complications can occur, and which can be prevented?**
5. **In a patient with recent stroke, how long should the surgery be delayed?**

PATIENTS WITH PREEXISTING NEUROLOGIC CONDITIONS

Cerebrovascular Disease

Cerebrovascular disease (CVD), coronary atherosclerosis, and cancer are the top three killers in the Western world. The prevalence of CVD increases exponentially with each decade of life after age 50. For this reason, asymptomatic CVD should be suspected in all patients older then 50 years, particularly if hypertension, smoking, or diabetes is present as well (1, 2). These patients must also be carefully evaluated and treated for **cardiovascular disease**, because these two conditions *always* coexist. By definition, patients with known CVD are considered to be at risk for stroke even without any surgical intervention. When undergoing surgery, however, their postoperative risk depends on the extent of the coronary and cerebral atherosclerosis.

Postoperative Strokes

Postoperative strokes occur in two distinct time periods: early (i.e., within 5 days of surgery) or late (i.e., 5 days to 2 years after surgery). Early or perioperative strokes usually occur within the first 2 to 5 days after surgery rather than during the procedure itself (3). Procedures that carry the highest risk of stroke are carotid endarterectomy (CE) and cardiac surgery. Currently, the risk of stroke following CE is less than 2.5% in good centers with a high volume of surgical cases (4). In elderly patients, the risk of stroke following cardiac surgery is less than 2.9% (3).

Cervical Bruit and Risk of Postoperative Stroke

Cervical bruit was first described by C.M. Fisher in the early 1950s as indicating increased arterial flow contralateral to an occluded carotid artery. Since then, it has been correctly viewed as a marker for increased risk of future stroke (5). In adults, the prevalence of cervical bruits is close to 5%, and this rate increases with age and in those with hypertension (6). Prevalence also increases when the underlying carotid artery is stenosed or occluded, but reported frequencies of underlying vessel abnormalities vary greatly. In fact, a cervical bruit by itself is *not* a reliable indicator of occlusive disease in the ipsilateral or contralateral carotid arteries (7). Among 241 nursing home residents over 75 years of age, the presence or absence of a cervical bruit did not change the 3-year cumulative risk of stroke of 10 and 9%, respectively (8).

Community dwelling individuals over age 45, without prior stroke, and with asymptomatic cervical bruits followed prospectively had an incidence of stroke of 31.9%, compared with 3.4% among those without a bruit (6). However, stroke was ipsilateral to the bruit in only one-third of cases, and the presence of a bruit was as good (or better) a marker for cardiac morbidity. This role of cervical bruits as a marker of ischemic cardiac disease has been confirmed in other studies (5, 9). In the Framingham cohort, a carotid bruit indicated increased risk for stroke, myocardial infarction, and death rather than ipsilateral arterial stenosis leading to cerebral infarction (5).

Another study followed 500 asymptomatic patients with cervical bruits using clinical and Doppler ultrasonographic assessments. At 1 year, the incidence of cardiac ischemic events and death were 7 and 4%, respectively, and that of transient ischemic attack (TIA) plus stroke 6%. The overall 1-year incidence of stroke was 1.7%, and these usually occurred after warning TIAs. The degree of carotid artery stenosis at initial presentation and the rate of progression of carotid arterial stenosis were powerful predictors of neurologic sequelae; however, less than one-half of those in whom stenosis progressed to complete occlusion became symptomatic (9). Again, cardiac ischemic events, cardiac death, and sudden death were more common than TIA or stroke in this population. From these data, the risk of disabling stroke occurring without warning TIAs has been estimated at less than 2% (5, 6, 9). Given this knowledge, there is no rationale to recommend CE in asymptomatic patients with cervical bruits before other scheduled surgery. Unfortunately, however, carotid bruits were not helpful in identifying patients with more than 70% stenosis for whom CE has been shown to be protective regarding prior stroke in other studies (10).

Patients with Previous Stroke or TIA

Risk of postoperative stroke in patients with prior stroke or TIA may be higher than in those without. However, this has not been confirmed, consistently.

Establishing the cause of the prior stroke or TIA helps in identifying appropriate prophylactic treatment. In the postoperative setting, new onset of atrial fibrillation is associated with an increased risk of stroke (11). In nonsurgical patients, multiple processes may result in stroke, but the most common is thromboembolic infarction secondary to atherosclerosis and hypertension. Classifying the stroke as either thrombotic, embolic, or lacunar helps to define the prognosis and treatment. For example, a lacunar infarction usually involves small areas in the deep substance of the brain, occurs in patients with hypertension, can be prevented by long-term control of blood pressure, and as a rule, is associated with good recovery. In the acute setting of stroke, however, overtreatment of hypertension may be deleterious. Embolism from a cardiac source in association with abnormal heart rhythms or valvular disease requires evaluation to determine the need for antiarrhythmic medication, anticoagulation, or valvular replacement, and the prognosis in this situation is more serious. Stroke secondary to intracerebral bleeding accounts for approximately one-fifth of all strokes and are usually catastrophic. On the other hand, embolism from atheromatous plaque in the cervical carotid or a transient neurologic deficit occurring in association with stenosis or occlusion of the ipsilateral artery has a varied prognosis.

In patients with a known prior stroke, there are no definitive data to establish how long to wait after the stroke before proceeding with nonneurologic surgery. It is reasonable to expect that delaying nonemergency surgery should result in a more clinically stable patient (which, by definition, would include only those well enough to stabilize after and survive the acute stroke). An acceptable waiting period is 6 to 12 weeks, because the clinical condition has often been established by then. However, this can (and should) be modified as necessary for each patient depending on the type of surgery being contemplated and how urgently it is needed.

Therapy for postoperative stroke appears to have little effect on final outcome, and it consists mainly of treating any associated conditions (e.g., arrhythmias). Administering low-molecular-weight heparin within 48 hours of symptom onset improves outcome at 6 months (12). For acute perioperative stroke, other

therapeutic modalities may yet emerge, including calcium channel blockers and hemodilution, but in general, meticulous anesthetic, surgical, and medical management both intraoperatively and perioperatively are the best treatment. For patients outside the operative setting and without contraindications to thrombolytics, tissue plasminogen activator (tPA) increases the likelihood of minimal or no disability at 3 months by 30%. This effect was seen if tPA was given within 3 hours of symptom onset, however, and at the expense of increasing the risk of symptomatic intracranial bleeding to 6.4% (from 0.6% for the placebo group) (13). Table 20.1 summarizes our recommendations for the perioperative care of patients with CVD.

Patients on antiplatelet therapy with aspirin, dipyridamole, or both, or on warfarin for TIAs, may require discontinuation of treatment 1 week before scheduled elective surgery that is associated with a high risk of bleeding in a critical anatomic site. Otherwise, antiplatelet therapy is best continued until 2 to 3 days before surgery. Warfarin may be discontinued 24 to 48 hours before surgery, and its anticoagulation effect can be reversed by oral or parenteral vitamin K.

In **symptomatic patients or those with a cervical bruit** you wish to evaluate further, duplex ultrasonography has been recommended, with confirmation of moderate- or high-grade stenosis by arteriography. Ultrasonography has a sensitivity and specificity of only 67% and close

---

Table 20.1. Perioperative Care of Patients with Cerebrovascular Disease

1. In a patient with recent stroke or TIA, establish the most likely etiology, treat appropriately, and delay elective surgery until the neurologic status has stabilized and maximum recovery of function occurred (a minimum of 6–12 weeks).
2. For patients with stroke-in-evolution, postpone nonemergency surgery until stable.
3. Patients with an asymptomatic cervical bruit should be assessed for generalized atherosclerosis. No evidence supports the use of simultaneous or staged carotid endarterectomy and coronary artery bypass graft in asymptomatic patients.
4. Patients who are bedridden or likely to be confined to bed postoperatively should receive appropriate prophylactic anticoagulation or intermittent external pneumatic calf compression to prevent deep-venous thrombosis.

to 80%, respectively, and correlation with arteriography remains imprecise (14). Two studies from the last 5 years, the North American Symptomatic Carotid Endarterectomy Trial (NASCET) (15) and the European Carotid Surgery Trial (ESCT) (16), have established **the efficacy of CE in symptomatic patients with significant carotid stenosis of greater than 70%**, with absolute differences in the ipsilateral stroke rate of 17 and 14% at 2 and 3 years after the procedure, respectively (17). The degree of **benefit** in both trials **was inversely related to the diameter of stenosis;** the greater the blockage, the better the results with CE. The results of CE in **patients without symptoms of TIA or stroke** are more controversial, but recent studies tend to favor CE in greater than 70% stenoses in institutions with low morbidity rates for CE.

There is no evidence that prophylactic CE is indicated in patients undergoing coronary artery bypass surgery (18). Studies of cerebral blood flow have shown that neither the percentage stenosis nor the size of the residual lumen is a reliable indicator of the hemodynamic status of cerebral circulation (19). In our opinion, **combined cardiac and carotid surgery only succeeds in adding the short-term risk of stroke and death from CE to the risk of death and stroke associated with coronary bypass.** Most patients with strokes have warning TIAs, so close follow-up after vascular or coronary surgery appears to be the best approach.

SEIZURE DISORDERS

Up to 0.5% of the general population have been estimated to suffer from some form of epilepsy or seizure disorder at some time in their lives. With these patients, the most important questions to answer are:

1. How recent are the seizures?

2. What is causing the seizures?
3. Are the seizures well controlled?

A seizure disorder does not require any special anesthetic management, but good seizure control is important to decrease perioperative morbidity from breakthrough seizures. The extent and force of involuntary muscle contraction during seizures can disturb the surgical wound. In addition, cerebral anoxia and aspiration during the seizure can markedly impair recovery from surgery (20).

In only 25% of patients do recurrent seizures have an identifiable cause. Drugs, neoplasms, vascular injury, metabolic derangements, and trauma are the most common. Drugs can cause seizures either as a toxic effect from large doses (i.e., meperidine, lidocaine, penicillin, propoxyphene, and so on) or secondary to acute withdrawal after previous excessive use (i.e., alcohol, diazepam, chlordiazepoxide, barbiturates, and so on) (21). As a rule, focal seizures result from structural lesions, but in nonketotic hyperglycemia, 75% of motor seizures are focal in nature. Most patients with recurrent seizures have idiopathic epilepsy; once diagnosed, treatment is guided by the type of epileptic syndrome the patient manifests.

In alcoholics, "rum fits" usually occur within 48 hours of stopping their alcohol intake and consist of one or two generalized tonic-clonic seizures without lateralizing signs. Rum fits do not recur except in the setting of withdrawal, and they do not require anticonvulsant medication. **Continuing seizure activity** suggests a structural lesion of the central nervous system and should be evaluated further. Patients at risk for rum fits are also at high risk for injury, and a subdural hematoma should be excluded. They may be abusing other drugs that can produce seizures as well. A drug screen is worth obtaining when seizures persist or are difficult to control. This is the same patient population that may also develop delirium tremens, and tranquilizers (i.e., chlordiazepoxide, benzodiazepines), β-blockers, and clonidine have been advocated for management. **Comorbidity is common in patients who abuse alcohol.** Alcohol-induced hepatic disease of varying degree often coexists, and these patients are usually long-term, heavy smokers and may have previously unrecognized chronic obstructive pulmonary disease. Impairment of lung or hepatic function may require modifications in intraoperative and postoperative care. Nutritional status is often borderline as well, and we recommend parenteral thiamine, 100 mg/day for 1 week, plus supplementation with other B vitamins at the time of hospital admission.

Patients with well-controlled seizures should remain on their anticonvulsant regimen through the morning of surgery and resume their medications immediately following. Table 20.2 reviews the doses and routes of administration for

these drugs (22–24). If the patient's epilepsy is poorly controlled, therapy should be started or optimized before surgery, and the procedure should be delayed if possible. Other antiepileptic drugs currently available in Europe, Canada, Japan, or that are being tested in United States, might soon be available.

Women of childbearing age with idiopathic seizures requiring anticonvulsant treatment may also be referred for consultation. Careful control of the serum level is usually needed because of changes in the protein-binding and metabolism of these drugs during pregnancy. The relative risk of fetal malformation in this population is two to three times that in the general population, but the risk of recurrent seizures poses greater risk to the mother and unborn child than the possible increased risk of teratogenicity. Mothers with epilepsy have no greater risk of

Table 20.2. Anticonvulsant Drugs

Drug	Usual Daily Dose	Route of Administration	Serum Half-life (h)	Therapeutic Blood Levels (mg/L)
Fhosphenytoin (Cerebyx)[a]	15–20 Phenytoin/kg equivalent (22.5–30.0 mg/kg)	IV, IM	26	—
Phenobarbital	120–250 mg qd (3–5 mg/kg)	Oral, IV	96 + 12	15–35
Primidone (Mysoline)	250 tid (to 1500 mg qd)	Oral	12 + 6	6–12
Carbamazepine (Tegretol)	200 mg bid or tid (to 1200 mg qd)	Oral	15 + 2	6–12
Ethosuximide (Zarontin)	750 mg qd (to 2000 mg qd)	Oral	60 + 6	40–100
Sodium valproate (Depakene)	500 mg bid (to 1000 mg tid)	Oral	6 + 20	50–100
Diazepam (Valium)[b]	10 mg, may repeat every 20 min for two doses	IV[c]	24–48	—

IM, intramuscular; *IV*, intravenous.

[a]IV phenytoin might be replaced by Fosphenytoin, which has much more advantage on phenytoin, resulting in significantly less venous irritation and phlebitis at the site of IV injection and could be given IM in case IV access is difficult to obtain. Careful studies of IV Fosphenytoin infusion up to 150 mg/min in healthy volunteers revealed no evidence of clinically significant hypotension or electrocardiographic changes, and it does not cause respiratory or central nervous system depression. One-hundred patients have recovered with an IV loading dose of 13.3 to 20.0 mg/kg at a rate of 180 mg/min without significant cardiovascular or adverse side effects.

[b]Used only in status epilepticus.

[c]Must be given slowly (1–2 mg/min).

Table 20.3. **Perioperative Care of Patients with Seizures**

1. If seizures are controlled, continue the same medications through the morning of the surgery and resume postoperatively. If drugs must be given parenterally, intravenous phosphenytoin, phenobarbital, diazepam, or a combination may be used.
2. If seizures are poorly controlled, postpone elective procedures until better control is achieved.
3. Identify drug and alcohol users at the time of admission to prepare for withdrawal seizures.

toxemic seizures than normal women. A megaloblastic anemia responsive to folic acid may develop after long-term treatment with hydantoin. Newborn children of women on anticonvulsants are at risk for bleeding secondary to a deficiency of vitamin K–dependent clotting factors induced by some of these drugs, especially hydantoin, phenobarbital, and primidone.

Table 20.3 summarizes our recommendations for the perioperative care of patients with seizure.

DEMENTIA

Dementia is a syndrome characterized by chronic, progressive failure of intellectual function that is severe enough to interfere with normal social and work activities. It may occur at any age and result from more than 60 different disorders. The dementia syndrome can be classified into two major categories depending on the neuroanatomic areas affected. Cortical dementia is the most common and is typified by Alzheimer's disease. In this syndrome, aphasia, amnesia, apraxia, cognitive impairment, and abnormalities in visual-spatial relationships occur early, but abnormalities of gait and movement do not occur until quite late in the illness. In contrast, subcortical dementia manifests dysarthria, hypophonic speech, abnormal posture, tremor, and gait disturbance. Subcortical dementia is associated with Parkinson's disease, progressive supranuclear palsy, Huntington's disease, normal pressure hydrocephalus, and so on. Multi-infarct dementia presents with features of both cortical and subcortical disease.

Mild dementia may go unrecognized until the patient is stressed, as occurs with hospitalization and surgery. Elderly patients may develop changes in mental status during the postoperative period as the first manifestation of dementia. Changes mimicking dementia may also be caused by drugs. Commonly used drugs that can interfere with cognition include anticholinergic, antihypertensive, psychotropic, sedating, and hypnotic agents (25). Even drugs such as digoxin have a central neural effect, even in therapeutic doses. Multi-infarct dementia is potentially treatable when diagnosed early, as is dementia resulting from many of the less common causes, such as vitamin B_{12} deficiency and endocrinopathies. In addition, depression and other affective disorders can mimic idiopathic dementia yet respond to medications. Unfortunately, however, it appears that the prevalence of potentially reversible causes of dementia has been overestimated in the past (26, 27).

The most common cause of dementia is Alzheimer's disease, the prevalence of which increases with age and has been estimated at 15% in those over 65 years (10% with mild dementia, 4–5% with severe symptoms). Either alone or in combination with other illnesses, Alzheimer's disease accounts for approximately 70% of dementia cases, with an average survival time of 8 to 10 years (25, 28). In patients who appear otherwise normal, Alzheimer's disease is suspected in the presence of amnesia, inability to compose and write a sentence, or in the presence of frontal-release signs (e.g., the snout and grasp reflexes). Mild disorientation is not specific enough to diagnose dementia. A variety of neuropsychologic tests are available for more formal testing, and sequential bedside testing of intellectual function with a mini-mental status examination is useful to follow any suspected decline during the perioperative period. **A multitude of pharmacologic agents** are under consideration for the treatment of dementia (28). Alzheimer's disease has been consistently associated with diminished levels of acetylcholine and somatostatin in the cortical areas of the brain. Results of trials using large doses of acetylcholine precursors in the form of lecithin in conjunction with centrally acting acetylcholinesterase inhibitors (e.g., tetrahydroaminoacridine) appear encouraging (29), but further testing is needed.

Operative risks in patients with dementia are the same as in patients without dementia. However, the underlying cause of the dementia may introduce a risk that is specific to that condition. For example, a patient with dementia from unrecognized hypothyroidism may develop myxedema coma in the postoperative period. On the other hand, treatment of the dementia may carry a high risk of morbidity, as occurs with shunting procedures for normal-pressure hydrocephalus. Mortality and morbidity in this setting are reported as between 10 and 40%. Inability of the patient to cooperate may impair recovery as well. In general, perioperative care of patients with dementia is straightforward, and Table 20.4 summarizes our recommendations.

When there is a family history of Alzheimer's disease, and especially of early onset, tests for specific mutations on chromosomes 1, 14, and 21 may be useful at some point in the future. Patients with Alzheimer's disease have a higher frequency of apolipoprotein E^4 alleles, thus suggesting that genotyping could assist in making the diagnosis (25).

MYASTHENIA GRAVIS

Myasthenia gravis is a disorder of the neuromuscular junction that is characterized by the sudden or insidious onset of muscle weakness associated with exertion. The bulbar and ocular muscles are preferentially affected, but any muscle group can be involved (30). The diagnosis is confirmed by electromyographic demonstration of decreased muscle action potentials, by the resolution of muscle weakness within 30 to 60 seconds following parenteral administration of edrophonium (Tensilon), and by increased levels of antibodies to the acetylcholine receptor. Prevalence is low, at 33 per 1 million population. It can occur at any age but appears most commonly in young females and older males. Among younger females, lymphocyte typing has revealed an overrepresentation of HLA-B8. Patients with myasthenia gravis often have findings suggestive of autoimmunity. **Antibodies to the acetylcholine receptor** of skeletal muscle are present in 80 to 90% of patients with generalized myasthenia (30), antinuclear antibodies in 20%, and

Table 20.4. Perioperative Care of Patients with Dementia

1. Elderly patients require smaller doses of most medications, and all medications may worsen an already compromised intellect.
2. Acute anxiety, restlessness, agitation, or combative behavior in the postoperative period should *always* be considered secondary to a correctable cause rather than to the underlying demented state.
3. If the altered behavior has no correctable causes, therapy with psychotropic agents may be indicated. This is more likely to occur in patients who required these drugs preoperatively, for whom the same drug in an equivalent oral or parenteral dose should be given.

antibodies to common antigens present in skeletal muscle, gastric mucosa, and thymus in 30%. Thymoma occurs in 10 to 15% and thymic hyperplasia in more than 50%. Hyperthyroidism occurs in 5%. Systemic lupus erythematosus and other rheumatic diseases with a suspected autoimmune etiology have also been reported to occur in these patients more commonly than expected.

Drug therapy involves steroids, cytotoxic drugs, and those that inhibit acetylcholinesterases. Thymectomy is recommended mostly in young adults when the response to anticholinesterases is unsatisfactory. **Myasthenic "crisis,"** which manifests with sudden onset of difficulty in breathing severe enough to require mechanical ventilatory support, occurs in up to 25% of these patients. Overtreatment with cholinesterase inhibitors can cause weakness; therefore, careful titration of the dose is important. Steroid therapy is generally initiated with low doses and under careful medical supervision to minimize the worsening of symptoms often seen during the first days of treatment. Patients resistant to steroids or with high morbidity from this hormone have been managed successfully with azathioprine or cyclophosphamide (31). Plasmapheresis appears to be superior to intravenous γ-globulin for the treatment of myasthenic crisis in some patients (32). There are also reports of continuous pyridostigmine infusion being successful in the management of myasthenic crisis (33). In most patients, plasma exchange produces rapid and consistent improvement that is accompanied by transitory reduction in serum levels of acetylcholine-receptor antibody. When the exchanges are discontinued, however, antibody levels rise to pretreatment levels or higher, and this may be accompanied by clinical worsening. Therefore, immune suppression is instituted concurrently with plasma exchange. Before thymectomy, plasma exchange produces rapid improvement and reduces perioperative morbidity (31). A milder form of the disease, limited to the ocular muscles, is easier to treat and has a better prognosis.

Anesthesia and surgery should be performed by a team experienced in the care of patients with myasthenia gravis. The major risks are pulmonary complications, including apnea, prolonged need for mechanical ventilatory support, and excessive secretions. Preoperative sedation, induction with thiopental, tracheal intubation, succinylcholine in conventional doses, and nitrous oxide or halothane anesthesia have been given without any adverse effects. Management is aimed at reducing the risk of inadequate ventilation and avoiding drugs or conditions that may worsen the neuromuscular abnormalities. Several clinical features have been suggested as predictive of postoperative complications: long-standing disease, coexistent pulmonary disease, high maintenance dose of acetylcholinesterase inhibitors, and low preoperative vital capacity. Table 20.5 summarizes our recommendations for the perioperative care of these patients.

THE EXTRAPYRAMIDAL DISORDERS

The extrapyramidal disorders are characterized by a combination of abnormal involuntary movements, altered muscle tone, and impaired postural reflexes. They include the parkinsonian syndromes, dystonias, choreas, hemiballismus, and athetosis. The parkinsonian syndromes are by far the most common of the extrapyramidal disorders, with a prevalence in the United States of 1% in those older than 60 years and a yearly incidence of 50,000 new cases. The total U.S. prevalence is estimated at over 1 million people. Most cases are idiopathic, but there are several primary causes, including carbon monoxide or heavy metal (especially manganese) poisoning, late consequence of the 1918 encephalitis lethargica epidemic (possibly resulting from influenza A virus), trauma, hypoparathyroidism and associated calcifications of

Table 20.5. Perioperative Care of Patients with Myasthenia Gravis

1. Check thyroid function.
2. Preoperatively measure the vital capacity. Postoperatively, follow the patient with bedside spirometry to monitor peak flow rates.
3. Continue cholinesterase inhibitors through the day before surgery, and discontinue on the day of surgery to avoid muscarinic side effects (e.g., increased secretions, facilitated cardio-inhibitory reflexes, and so on).
4. If the patient is currently (or has recently been) on steroids, provide perioperative parenteral corticosteroids.
5. Be prepared to continue mechanical ventilation postoperatively for as long as necessary.
6. Withhold cholinergic therapy until patient's condition stabilizes, then begin at one-half the preoperative dose before extubation. If the drug is given parenterally, give one-tenth the oral dose intramuscularly or one-thirtieth the oral dose intravenously.
7. Avoid drugs with a known potential for aggravating neuromuscular blockade.
8. If the patient is on cholinergic medication, avoid stimuli that would further exacerbate cardioinhibitory vagal reflexes (i.e., enemas and Valsalva maneuver).

the basal ganglia, and cerebral arteriosclerosis. In addition, a parkinsonian syndrome and tardive (or late-onset) dyskinesias can occur in patients on neuroleptic drugs. In younger adults with slow onset of parkinsonian symptoms, Wilson's disease must be excluded.

Major advances in our understanding of Parkinson's disease have developed from the observation (34) that severe, acute symptoms resulted from the ingestion of contaminated synthetic heroin. The contaminating toxin, MPTP (1-methyl-4-phenyl-1,2,5,6-tetrahydropyridine), exerts its damage through selective killing of the substantia nigra cells by its oxidation product, MPP^{++}. In an experimental primate model, damage can be prevented by administration of selegiline (Deprenyl), a selective inhibitor of monoamine oxidase B. Another breakthrough came with discovery of the pathogenesis of a similar syndrome in Guam, where chronic exposure to small amounts of a nonphysiologic amino acid present in a local food staple produced a parkinsonian syndrome. Higher doses of the same product over shorter periods produced a syndrome similar to amyotrophic lateral sclerosis (35).

Several classes of drugs are available to treat the Parkinson's disease

(36), and Table 20.6 summarizes the recommended dosages. The major toxic side effects for these drugs are dry mouth, blurring of vision secondary to cycloplegia, urinary and fecal retention, worsening of glaucoma, confusion, and hallucinations. Because of marked variation in individual responsiveness, the dose ranges are wide. Since the advent of levodopa, most patients sooner or later have this drug added as the mainstay of therapy (37). Before the advent of this drug, disability occurred in 90% of patients affected with Parkinson's disease for longer than 15 years, and mortality was three times higher than in a matched control population. The major causes of death were aspiration pneumonia and respiratory insufficiency secondary to an inability to swallow secretions and rigidity of the chest wall musculature; generalized rigidity and associated immobility continue to be a common prelude to death.

Treatment with levodopa, although ineffective in preventing progression of the disease, has improved the quality of life and prolonged survival by 3 or more years in the 80% who respond to the drug. The dramatic response of muscle rigidity to this drug and the decrease in cardiovascular and gastrointestinal side effects when combined with the peripheral dopa

Table 20.6.   Perioperative Care of Patients with Parkinson's Disease

1. Pharyngeal dysfunction leads to decreased spontaneous swallowing and increases the risk of aspiration. Frequent and extended suctioning is needed.
2. Pulmonary function tests often reveal restrictive deficits secondary to chest wall muscular rigidity. Oxygen saturation should be monitored.
3. Preoperative and perioperative nasogastric suction may help to reduce nausea and vomiting. Antiemetics are contraindicated.
4. Postoperative dysphagia or unconsciousness may prohibit oral therapy. Levodopa/carbidopa solution can be fed through a silastic tube with a weighted mercury tip and given directly into the duodenum. The solution may be prepared by pulverizing and dissolving 10 tablets of regular carbidopa/levodopa (10/100) or four tabs (25/250) in 1000 mL of tap water with 1 g of ascorbic acid to yield a 1 mg/mL solution of levodopa. (Ascorbic acid acidifies the solution and prevents oxidation.) The infusion rate can start at 25 mL/h and be adjusted according to clinical response. The solution should be protected from light (e.g., a dark bottle) and kept refrigerated.
5. Sudden withdrawal of anti-Parkinson therapy can lead to a dopamine withdrawal syndrome resembling the neuroleptic malignant syndrome. Therapy involves aggressive cooling measures, hydration, and medications. Bromocriptine, up to 100 mg/day, has been recommended. Alternatives include diazepam 3–5 mg intravenous; or dantrolene, 1 mg/kg intravenous push to a maximum of 10 mg/kg.
6. End-of-dose dystonia can occur in the postoperative period. It is treated with Benadryl IV.

decarboxylase inhibitor carbidopa (as in Sinemet) produced an enthusiastic era in the treatment of Parkinson's disease. Unfortunately, side effects of central origin, including mental aberrations, tardive dyskinesias, and hypotension, were not eliminated by the addition of carbidopa. As treatment progresses, a greater number of patients develop these side effects; for example, after 2 years, abnormal movements are noted in 70%. The "on-off" phenomenon, a very disabling side effect, occurs after long-term therapy with levodopa, with or without carbidopa, in 50%. Although of some benefit, limiting the patient's protein intake to suppertime, varying the time of dosing, and slowly reducing the daily dose to the minimum effective level, have not eliminated the occurrence or severity of these attacks. Lithium salts and estrogens have also been tried without effect. "Drug holidays," which were popular for a time, appear to worsen the condition of patients with severe disease. Gradual dose reduction and combination therapy with other dopaminergic agents (e.g., pergolide and bromocriptine) appear to be more useful (36). When administered subcutaneously,

the antiemetic domperidone can be an effective "rescue" therapy in patients who are intermittently "trapped" in unpredictable "off" periods. Optimal therapeutic benefit from levodopa occurs in the first 3 years of therapy and then declines, often to pretreatment levels, over the next 3 to 4 years. Initial response to levodopa is independent of the duration or severity of the disease and of the age of the patient.

Drug therapy for Parkinson's disease is aimed at neuroprotection and control of symptoms. The decision to begin symptomatic therapy depends on how disabling or troublesome the symptoms are to the patient. In early disease, when functional impairment is not present, selegiline at doses of 10 mg/day slows the progression of symptoms and the need for administration of carbidopa/levodopa by 50%. When functional impairment finally occurs, symptomatic therapy is initiated. In patients 60 years or younger, with mild akinesia and rigidity, and in whom tremor is not a major problem, 100 to 300 mg/day of amantadine administered in divided doses twice daily can be used; larger doses provide no additional benefit and increase the likelihood of adverse effects. If tremor is predominant, anticholinergics, such as trihexyphenidyl initiated at 0.5 to 1.0 mg twice daily and increased gradually to 2 to 3 mg three times a day, are helpful. Benzotropin is given concurrently as 0.5 to 1.0 mg twice daily because of the high incidence of peripheral and central nervous system side effects associated with these drugs. Their use in patients without tremor and those 60 years or older with dementia is not recommended. In patients older than 60 years, dopamine agonists are reserved for those with declining response to levodopa, motor fluctuations, dyskinesias, or other adverse effects from levodopa. Patients treated with bromocriptine and levodopa show an equivalent therapeutic benefit as well as less motor fluctuations and dyskinesias than patients treated with levodopa alone. The dose for bromocriptine starts at 1.25 mg daily and is titrated slowly to 10 to 25 mg daily. Pergolide is more potent and has a longer duration of action; the initial dose of pergolide is 0.05 mg daily and is titrated slowly to 2 to 3 mg daily in divided doses (36). Pallidotomy has reportedly produced major improvements in akinesia and dyskinesia, but it is still being studied. Transplantation of autogenous adrenal medulla to the neostriatum is also being studied.

Postoperative complications are common in untreated patients with Parkinson's disease because of widespread muscle rigidity. Involvement of the chest muscles (i.e., "wooden chest") may lead to secondary ventilatory insufficiency. Rigidity of the muscles of deglutition prevents normal swallowing of food and saliva, and this often leads to aspiration. Rigidity of other muscle groups prevents frequent changes of position and normal gastrointestinal and urinary emptying. In addition, patients have a markedly increased risk of confusion and hallucinations in the postoperative period (37). Table 20.6 summarizes our recommendations for the perioperative care of these patients.

MYOTONIC DYSTROPHY

Myotonic dystrophy and some of the limb-girdle dystrophies are the only dystrophies that present during adulthood. Myotonic dystrophy is an autosomal dominant, multisystem disease with a highly variable clinical expression. Patients with myotonic dystrophy are at high risk for complications in the perioperative period (38, 39). Myotonia is a characteristic finding, and it may be the only clue to presence of the disease in undiagnosed patients. Muscle weakness and atrophy, cardiac and endocrine abnormalities, cataracts, testicular atrophy, mental deterioration, and frontal baldness, whether singly or in combination, may complete the clinical picture. Abnormal membrane function leading to repetitive depolarization is responsible for the characteristic myotonia and weakness. The condition is worsened by cold ambient temperatures, and it improves with continued muscular activity. A beneficial effect from class I antiarrhythmic agents, such as procainamide, phenytoin, and quinidine, as well as from calcium channel blockers has been reported.

Perioperative complications tend to occur in the intraoperative and immediate postoperative periods because of adverse reactions to drugs. Delayed complications occur in proportion to the severity of the disease. Depolarizing neuromuscular blockers such as succinylcholine and decamethonium should be avoided, whereas nondepolarizing drugs such as curare appear to be tolerated. As with other preexisting neurologic illnesses, making the diagnosis before surgery is the best way to avoid complications.

POSTOPERATIVE NEUROLOGIC COMPLICATIONS

Multiple factors contribute to postoperative neurologic morbidity. General, spinal, and local anesthesia can result in transient or permanent neurologic deficits (40, 41). Drugs used in the perioperative

Table 20.7. Postoperative Neurologic Complications

1. Ischemic injury to the brain.
2. Altered mental status, delirium, and coma.
3. Seizures of new onset.
4. Cauda equina syndrome.
5. Peripheral nerve palsies.

period may also contribute to alterations in nervous system function. Table 20.7 lists some of the more common and devastating postoperative neurologic complications.

Localized ischemia of the central nervous system leading to strokes in the perioperative period was discussed earlier. In summary, early postoperative strokes occur within the first days after surgery. Most postoperative strokes are embolic, although hypercoagulability associated with surgical manipulation of certain tissues may play a role as well. Prevention is the best treatment, and this is best done by treating arrhythmias and preventing contamination of the blood with air, clots, or foreign substances during cardiopulmonary bypass. Postoperative prophylactic anticoagulation for deep-venous thrombosis with low-dose heparin may also be beneficial in preventing postoperative stroke in this period.

Altered mental status, delirium, and coma in the postoperative period **should be considered as resulting from a complication** of drug therapy, a metabolic abnormality, or sepsis. Persistent treatment with neuroleptics is not advised, however, except as a temporary measure while further diagnostic studies are conducted. In elderly patients, over-medication with "usual" doses of analgesics can lead to apnea. In obese patients, delayed recovery from anesthesia because of continued slow release of fat-soluble inhalational agents accumulated in fatty depots is common. Underlying mild or unrecognized liver or kidney impairment

can precipitate altered mental status, and in patients with recent trauma, fat embolism should be considered, especially if the trauma is associated with fractures of the long bones. Altered mental status secondary to global ischemia occurs most commonly in patients undergoing valvular or other cardiac surgery, and it is related to the length of time that the patient is kept on bypass.

Seizures of new onset in the postoperative period may occur secondary to alcohol, from drug withdrawal in unrecognized abusers, or from fluid or electrolyte abnormalities. When these seizures are associated with acute hyponatremia from excessive administration of hypotonic fluids, mortality and severe morbidity approach 100% in women (42, 43). In these patients, grand mal seizures develop 2 to 3 days postoperatively in association with serum sodium values of less than 110 mmol/L and other laboratory evidence for inappropriate secretion of antidiuretic hormone. Rapid correction of the serum sodium restores normal brain function for only a few hours or days, but with recurrence of seizures, coma, and death from irreversible central or extrapontine myelinolysis. The syndrome has been variously ascribed to an overly long period of hyponatremia, overly fast correction of hyponatremia, or attainment of an overly high level of sodium (44). Prompt identification of hyponatremia and cautious treatment with normal saline are recommended. Since this syndrome is mostly iatrogenic, prevention should be the cornerstone of treatment in this devastating complication.

Cauda equina syndrome secondary to ischemic injury of the spinal cord presents with bowel and bladder difficulties, sensory abnormalities, and autonomic dysfunction. Although it is uncommon, the syndrome occurs in association with aortic/cardiac surgery in elderly patients or from local trauma caused by spinal or epidural anesthesia. A history of poliomyelitis, disc disease, or other diseases of the central nervous system correlates with a higher risk of complications from spinal anesthesia (40).

Peripheral nerve palsies can result from prolonged pressure on or stretching of a peripheral nerve and associated ischemia. When the ischemic episode is short-lived, paresthesias result. During sleep, these sensations allow us to shift position to avoid pressure damage to the nerve. Under anesthesia, however, prolonged pressure on a peripheral nerve can occur and result in axonal degeneration (i.e., axonotmesis) or death of the axon and Schwann cells that envelop it (i.e., neurotmesis). Whereas axonal degeneration is slowly reversible, neurotmesis can be irreversible (45). Patients with underlying neuropathy, particularly diabetes, are at higher risk for this complication.

The optic nerve can be permanently injured when undue pressure is applied around the orbit, leading to increased intraocular pressure and ischemia, as can occur when the patient is positioned facedown (e.g., for craniotomy). If the ischemic episode lasts longer than 4 minutes, blindness results. Reversible damage to the superficial branches of the trigeminal nerve can occur from a tight-fitting face mask (e.g., for anesthesia). Retainers to hold the mask in place can compress the facial nerve at the lower edge of the mandibular rami and produce palsy. The sciatic nerve is most often injured by intramuscular injections in the buttocks outside of the recommended upper, outer quadrants. Malposition of the legs or arms can result in foot drop and sensory deficits or in ulnar and radial nerve palsies (45).

Damage to the brachial plexus is the single most common serious injury in the postoperative period; it occurs following open heart surgery and was reported in 5% of patients studied prospectively at the Cleveland Clinic (46). Several different mechanisms may cause the injury. Direct compression, excessive depression of the shoulder girdle in the Trendelenburg position, hyperabduction of the arm, cannulation of the internal jugular vein, and penetration of the plexus by a first rib

fractured during sternotomy have all been implicated.

Injury of cranial or peripheral nerves is best treated by prevention. This is achieved by paying meticulous attention to the positioning of all body parts throughout the procedure to avoid direct pressure on any nerve.

REFERENCES

1. Bonita R. Epidemiology of stroke. Lancet 1992; 339:342–347.
2. Bronner LL, Kanter DS, Manson JE. Primary prevention of stroke. N Engl J Med 1995;333: 1392–1400.
3. Reed GL III, Singer DE, Picard EH, et al. Stroke following coronary-artery bypass surgery. N Engl J Med 1988;319:1246–1250.
4. Brott T, Toole JF. Medical compared with surgical treatment of asymptomatic carotid artery stenosis. Ann Intern Med 1995;123:720–722.
5. Wolf PA, Kannel WB, Sorlie P, et al. Asymptomatic carotid bruit and risk of stroke: the Framingham study. JAMA 1981;245:1442–1445.
6. Heyman A, Wilkinson WE, Heyden S, et al. Risk of stroke in asymptomatic persons with cervical arterial bruits: a population study in Evans County, Georgia. N Engl J Med 1980;302: 838–841.
7. Corman LC. The preoperative patient with an asymptomatic bruit. Med Clin North Am 1979; 63:1335–1340.
8. Van Ruiswyk J, Noble H, Sigmann P. The natural history of carotid bruits in elderly persons. Ann Intern Med 1990;112:340–343.
9. Chambers BR, Norris JW. Outcome in patients with asymptomatic neck bruits. N Engl J Med 1986;315:860–865.
10. Sauve JS, Thorpe KE, Sackett DL, et al. Can bruits distinguish high-grade from moderate symptomatic carotid stenosis? Ann Intern Med 1994;120:633–637.
11. Taylor GJ, Malik SA, Colliver JA, et al. Usefulness of atrial fibrillation as a predictor of stroke after isolated coronary artery bypass grafting. Am J Cardiol 1987;60:905–907.
12. Kay R, Wong KS, Yo YL, et al. Low-molecular-weight heparin for the treatment of acute ischemic stroke. N Engl J Med 1995;24:1588–1593.
13. The National Institute on Neurological Disorders and Stroke rt-PA Sroke Study Group. Tissue plasminogen activator for acute ischemic stroke. N Engl J Med 1995;24:1581–1587.
14. Barnett HJM, Haines SJ. Carotid endarterectomy for asymptomatic carotid stenosis. N Engl J Med 1993;328:276–279.

15. Executive Committee for the Asymptomatic Carotid Atherosclerosis Study. Endarterectomy for asymptomatic carotid artery stenosis. JAMA 1995;273:1421–1428.

16. European Carotid Surgery Trialists' Collaborative Group. Endarterectomy for moderate symptomatic carotid stenosis: interim results from the MRC European Carotid Surgery Trial. Lancet 1996;347:1591–1593.

17. Barnett HJM, Eliasziw M, Meldrum HE. Drugs and surgery in the prevention of ischemic stroke. N Engl J Med 1995;332:238–248.

18. Ad Hoc Committee, American Heart Association. Guidelines for carotid endarterectomy—a multidisciplinary consensus statement. Circulation 1995;91:566–579.

19. Powers WJ, Press GA, Grubb RL Jr, et al. The effect of hemodynamically significant carotid artery disease on the hemodynamic status of the cerebral circulation. Ann Intern Med 1987;106:27–35.

20. Roizen MF. Anesthetic implications of concurrent disease. In: Miller RD, ed. Anesthesia. 2nd ed. New York: Churchill Livingstone, 1986:1:255–357.

21. Messing RO, Simon RP. Seizures as a manifestation of systemic disease. Neurol Clin 1986;4:563–584.

22. Dichter MA, Brodie MJ. New antiepileptic drugs. N Engl J Med 1996;334:1583–1590.

23. Brodie MJ, Dichter MA. Antiepileptic drugs. N Engl J Med 1996;334:168–175.

24. Anonymous. Drugs for epilepsy. Med Lett Ther 1995;37:37–40.

25. Geldmacher DS, Whitehouse PJ. Evaluation of dementia. N Engl J Med 1996;335:330–336.

26. Barry PP, Moskowitz MA. The diagnosis of reversible dementia in the elderly: a critical review. Arch Intern Med 1988;148:1914–1918.

27. Clarfield AM. The reversible dementias: do they reverse? Ann Intern Med 1988;109:476–486.

28. Writing Committee, Lancet Conference. The challenge of the dementias. Lancet 1996;347:1303–1307.

29. Davis KL, Powchik P. Tacrine. Lancet 1995;345:625–630.

30. Phillips LH II. The epidemiology of myasthenia gravis. Neurol Clin North Am 1994;12:263–271.

31. Sanders DB, Scoppetta C. Management of myasthenia gravis. Neurol Clin North Am 1994;12:343–368.

32. Stricker RB, Kwiatkowska BJ, Habis JA, Kiprov DD. Myasthenic crisis—response to plasmapheresis following failure of intravenous γ-globulin. Arch Neurol 1993;50:837–840.

33. Saltis LM, Martin BR, Traeger SM, Bonfiglio MF. Continuous infusion of pyridostigmine in the management of myasthenic crisis. Crit Care Med 1993;21:821–822.

34. Lewin R. Trail of ironies to Parkinson's disease. Science 1984;224:1083–1085.

35. Anonymous. A poison tree. Lancet 1987;ii:948–948.

36. Koller WC, Silner DE, Lieberman A. An algorithm for management of Parkinson's disease. Neurology 1994;44(Suppl 10):S5–S51.

37. Golden WE, Lavender RL, Metier WS, et al. Acute postoperative confusion and hallucinations in Parkinson disease. Ann Intern Med 1989;111:218–222.

38. Aldridge LM. Anaesthetic problems in myotonic dystrophy. Br J Anaesth 1985;57:119–130.

39. Anonymous. Treatment of myotonia. Lancet 1987;i:1242–1244.

40. Vandam L. Neurological sequelae of spinal and epidural anesthesia. Int Anesthesiol Clin 1986;24:231–255.

41. Seibert CP. Recognition, management and prevention of neuropsychological dysfunction after operation. Int Anesthesiol Clin 1986;24:39–58.

42. Arieff AI. Hyponatremia, convulsions, respiratory arrest, and permanent brain damage after elective surgery in healthy women. N Engl J Med 1986;314:1529–1535.

43. Stem RH, Riggs JE, Schochet SS Jr. Osmotic demyelination syndrome following correction of hyponatremia. N Engl J Med 1986;314:1535–1542.

44. Narins RG. Therapy of hyponatremia. Does haste make waste? N Engl J Med 1986;314:1573–1575.

45. Dornette WHL. Compression neuropathies: medical aspects and legal implications. Int Anaesthesiol Clin 1986;24:201–229.

46. Hanson MR, Brever AC, Furlan AJ, et al. Mechanism and frequency of brachial plexus injury in open-heart surgery: a prospective analysis. Ann Thorac Surg 1983;36:675–679.

21

Medical Illness in the Psychiatric Patient

Noel Ballentine and Paul Kettl

In a case presenting any mental abnormality the first essential is a thorough physical examination in order to discover the causal factors and if possible eliminate them. Too often it is assumed that the physical condition of a mental patient is good; thus the examination is far too brief and cursory.

—R.J. Phillips, 1937

Psychiatric patients frequently are treated without careful attention being given to their medical problems. When studied with a structured patient history and physical examination, however, it was discovered that in 224 consecutive psychiatric admissions, 9% had a medical condition presenting with psychiatric symptoms and 44% had concomitant medical illness requiring treatment (1). The physical examination appeared to be the most sensitive determinant. Depending on the psychiatric diagnosis (e.g., psychosis), the medical history may be virtually impossible to obtain (or unreliable). To obtain a comprehensive medical history and perform a thorough physical examination in an anxious, demented, or manic-depressive patient may require some ingenuity, and specific aspects of the psychiatric disease that is present may need to be taken into account. Frequently, symptoms are observed by attending personnel rather than reported by the patient. Many specifics relating to the evaluation of physical disease in patients who are mentally ill are well described in the classic treatise by Kampmeier (2).

Many psychiatrists do not perform a complete physical examination, either because of a conviction that it is not helpful, a feeling of incompetence, a belief it has been performed adequately elsewhere, or a concern for violating a mentally ill patients' sensitivities. This latter issue deserves consideration, particularly in patients who are psychotic, and coordination between psychiatrists and the consulting internist is important. However, investigation for medical problems is worthwhile. Two studies of chronically ill psychiatric patients showed that most (69%) had medical diagnoses that were not detected by the referring physician (or they had no primary care physician) (3, 4). One study in a psychiatric hospital showed that approximately 50% of patients' physical problems were not addressed, but that when they were, resolution or improvement of the problem occurred in 94% of cases (5).

Various studies show the importance of several factors in predicting medical illness among patients with psychiatric symptoms. Increasing age, a history of neurologic disease, and an abnormal neurologic examination are among the most important (1). Other studies show that endocrine and cardiac diseases frequently account for psychiatric symptoms. Diabetes, asthma, hypertension, and dermatologic as well as orthopaedic conditions frequently are concomitant diseases in patients with psychiatric illness.

Evaluation beyond a complete medical history, review of systems, and physical examination remains somewhat controversial. Screening laboratory studies are routinely obtained in the belief that unsuspected medical illness will be detected (6, 7). Some studies show no benefit to this practice, however, in that screening with blood chemistries, blood counts, and thyroid function tests have added no diagnostic information to the history and physical examination (8). Evaluation of a problem that is discovered (e.g., dementia) or of a symptom (e.g., ataxia possibly suggesting Wilson's disease) probably has merit. Hollister (8a) studied electrocardiograms (ECGs) in 1006 consecutive psychiatric admissions; as in the general population, few abnormalities were found in patients younger than 50 years of age with no history or physical findings suggestive of cardiovascular disease. The conclusion was that ECG is useful in

Table 21.1.   Format for the Evaluation of Psychiatric Patients

History Points to Stress in Addition to General Medical History	If History Is Suggestive
1. Drug history	Evaluate for toxicity
Prescribed?	
Over-the-counter, topical?	
Home remedies, alternative (complementary) medicine, herbal teas, caffeine?	
Vitamins, tonics?	
Tranquilizers, nerve pills?	
Illicit drugs?	
2. Potential toxin exposure	Evaluate for toxicity
Occupational: mining, metals, plastics, other industry, paints, mercury, insecticides	
Hobbies: lead (ceramics), metals, hydrocarbons	
Home: cleaning fluids, space heaters (carbon monoxide)	
3. Family history	
Neurologic disease?	
Wilson's disease? (liver disease)	
Porphyria?	
Huntington's chorea?	
4. Dietary history	
Alcoholism	Administer thiamine
	Consider deficiency diseases
Bizarre diet, vegetarianism, bulimia, anorexia, chronic vomiting	Consider deficiency diseases
5. Psychiatric history	
Abrupt onset?	Evaluate for delirium
Visual hallucinations only?	Suspect organic cause
6. History of trauma, falls, unexplained injuries	Consider subdural hematoma
7. Somatization, chronic pain syndromes	Consider abuse (domestic violence)
8. Psychiatric symptoms accompanied by multiple somatic symptoms in older patient?	Probable organic disease, consider depression, evaluate thyroid
9. History of changes in consciousness, memory losses, fugue states, repetitive episodes?	Evaluate for psychomotor epilepsy

Table 21.1. (continued)   **Format for the Evaluation of Psychiatric Patients**

Physical Examination: Emphasize in Addition to General Examination	If Findings Are Positive
1. Mental status	
Altered state of consciousness obtundation?	Evaluate for delirium and serious medical illnesses
Cognitive function decreased?	Suspect delirium or dementia, consider formal psychometric testing
2. Neurologic examination	
Tremor, asterixis	Suspect delirium
Myoclonus about face and neck	Almost pathognomonic for delirium
Specific neurologic findings, focal deficits?	Evaluate appropriately for neurologic disease
Peripheral neuropathy?	Consider vitamin deficiency, diabetes, lead poisoning, alcoholism
3. Standard screening tests	
Complete blood count with differential	
Sedimentation rate	
Urinalysis	
Blood chemistries, including: electrolytes, calcium, renal function, liver function, glucose	
Thyroid function tests, especially TSH screen	
Serologic test for syphilis	
When appropriate: HIV antibody	
4. Further evaluation	
Acute psychosis:	
Send urinary and blood drug screens	
In older patient: ECG, chest radiography, CNS imaging (CT/magnetic resonance imaging)	
EEG	
In appropriate clinical situation: screen for porphyria, Wilson's disease	
Delirium	
Anticholinergic signs: flushing, fever, tachycardia, dilated pupils?	
If alcoholism, malnutrition, chronic vomiting: administer thiamine	
Chest radiography, ECG, blood gases and carboxyhemoglobin level, urine and blood drug screen, EEG	
If EEG shows diffuse slowing, treat supportively for delirium and investigate further for underlying disease	
Lumbar puncture	

older patients, in those with possible cardiovascular disease, and in those needing drugs that can affect cardiac function or conduction times.

Table 21.1 presents a format for the evaluation of psychiatric patients.

MANAGEMENT OF CONCOMITANT MEDICAL ILLNESS

Existing psychiatric problems can be exacerbated by medical illness; for example, thyroid disease, asthma, drug therapy, or infection may affect psychiatric symptomatology. On the other hand, psychiatric symptoms also may obfuscate or alter the underlying medical condition. Further, psychiatric disease may cause self-neglect, poor compliance, or deceit by the patient that interferes with therapy for the medical condition. To be effective, therapy must address these factors that complicate optimal care. Some common and important clinical situations that require an integrated approach are discussed here.

Patients with Hypertension

Because of the high prevalence of hypertension in the general population, psychiatric patients with concomitant hypertension are commonly encountered. Three major points must be considered in psychiatric patients: *(a)* evaluation, *(b)* side effects, and *(c)* drug interactions.

Most patients with hypertension do not require evaluation for secondary causes of hypertension. If measured in consideration of pheochromocytoma, levels of serum catecholamines are elevated in highly anxious or manic patients. Neuroleptic agents and tricyclic antidepressants elevate catecholamines as well, and unsuspected pheochromocytoma may become symptomatic with use of tricyclic antidepressants (9). When evaluating patients for hypercortisolism, it must be recognized that depression can result in elevated random and fasting cortisol levels as well as in a blunted response to dexamethasone suppression. A number of approaches also have attempted to differentiate pseudo-Cushing's states such as depression, alcoholism, and obesity. Clinical suspicion remains important, however, and can be supported by results of the 48-hour, low-dose dexamethasone suppression test and urinary free cortisol measurements (10). Another test, corticotropin-releasing hormone stimulation following low-dose dexamethasone administration (the so-called *dexamethasone-CRH test*), may be more specific (11). Successful therapy for depression will correct the elevated cortisol level.

β-Blockers, reserpine, and α-methyldopa can cause depression that is reversible on discontinuation of the drug. Carney et al. (12), however, studied depression in cardiac patients undergoing elective cardiac catheterization and found no difference between depression scores in patients on β-blockers and those in patients receiving other medications. β-Blockers as well as α-blockers can cause fatigue and lassitude, which may contribute to symptoms of depression, and β-blockers, particularly those such as propranolol, which is more lipid (i.e., brain) soluble, also may result in insomnia, vivid dreams, or hallucinations as well as memory loss or confusion. The central nervous system (CNS) effects of β-blockers occasionally can benefit patients by suppressing symptoms of anxiety, thus showing clinical efficacy in panic disorders and stage fright (13, 14). Many antihypertensive agents cause impotence as well, which may contribute to depression. Studies on the quality of life in patients taking antihypertensives have shown adverse effects from many drugs, a frequent cause of noncompliance. The results of one study suggested that angiotensin-converting enzyme (ACE) inhibitors result in significantly improved measures of quality of life, work performance, and sexual function (15). Orthostatic hypotension is a frequent problem during use of antidepressants having significant anticholinergic effects, and this can be exacerbated by treatment with antihypertensives. Table 21.2 summarizes drug therapy in psychiatric patients with hypertension.

Hypertension itself also can lead to neuropsychiatric changes, which may be wrongly attributed to antihypertensive medication (16). There may be an association between depression and hypertension that is unrelated to adverse drug effects. A study of 452 outpatients found that major depression was three times more common in those with hypertension than in those without (17); age, sex, other chronic medical illness, and current use of antihypertensive medication did not account for the difference.

Table 21.2. Drug Interactions in the Psychiatric Patient with Hypertension

Antihypertensive Drug	Tricyclic Antidepressants	Lithium	Antipsychotic Agents	Psychiatric Effects
ACE inhibitors	None	None	None	Improved quality of life
α-Methyldopa	Diminished tricyclic efficacy possible. Usually not clinically significant	Enhanced lithium CNS toxicity (rare)	Delirium reported with combined therapy (rare)	Depression Delirium
β-Blockers	May decrease efficacy of tricyclics. Clinical relevance not clear	None	Metabolic interaction with phenothiazines results in increased blood levels of both	Energy loss, fatigue may enhance depression Hallucinations, delirium (rare)
Calcium channel blockers	Possible orthostatic hypertension	Neurotoxicity	Possible orthostatic hypotension	Low incidence depressive effects
Clonidine	Antihypertensive effects partially antagonized. May interfere with tricyclic therapy. Enhanced rebound hypertension	None	Hypotension (occasional). Delirium reported with combined therapy (rare)	Delirium Depression
Diuretics	Increased orthostatic hypotension	Altered renal excretion	Increased orthostatic hypotension	Symptomatic Hypokalemia
Guanethidine	Antihypertensive effects blocked	None	Antihypertensive effect blocked	Depression
Vasodilators	Increased orthostatic hypotension	None	Increased orthostatic hypotension	None

Lithium therapy is affected by use of diuretic drugs. Renal excretion is decreased and may result in toxicity. Lithium levels must be measured frequently when simultaneous therapy is necessary, and particularly during the initiation of diuretics. In addition, use of ACE inhibitors can significantly elevate lithium levels (18).

Several case reports have suggested beneficial CNS effects of calcium channel blockers, specifically in the treatment of acute mania and tardive dyskinesia. There also is evidence that calcium channel blockers can worsen hostility in patients who are schizophrenic (19).

In addition, psychotic reactions can occur in patients (especially elderly patients) taking antihypertensive drugs.

Psychiatric Illness and Cardiovascular Disease

Until recently, there has been little evidence that underlying or concurrent psychiatric disease is a risk factor for coronary artery disease. However, data from the Systolic Hypertension in the Elderly Program (SHEP) show that worsening of a depression score over time, as opposed to the baseline depression score, predicted an 18 to 26% increased risk of subsequent stroke, myocardial infarction, or death from any cause (19a). Phobic anxiety has been associated with cardiovascular disease, particularly sudden death. Beyond this, however, studies show little association despite clear evidence that risk factors for coronary disease risk factors (particularly smoking but also probably hypertension, hyperlipidemia, and physical inactivity) are significantly more common in some mental disorders. There is little prospective information.

Clearly, cardiac disease can result in depression, which often goes unrecognized and untreated. Carney et al. (12) studied patients with angiographically proved coronary artery disease and found the lifetime prevalence of major depression in these patients to be 26%. The presence of depression predicted the occurrence of major cardiac events better than traditional risk factors independent of severity of underlying coronary artery disease or functional capacity of the heart.

The cardiac effects of psychoactive drugs are fully addressed in the psychopharmacology section of this chapter.

CONSULTATION TO SURGICAL SERVICES: PSYCHIATRIC ISSUES

Multiple psychiatric issues face the consulting internist who is involved in caring for surgical patients. Most patients facing surgery experience issues of anxiety, stress, fear, and loss of control. One role of the consultant, who may be the patient's primary care physician as well, is to assess the patient's coping mechanisms and determine if the stress of preoperative evaluation, surgery, and postoperative recovery will so deplete his or her physiologic and psychologic reserves as to make them decompensate mentally after surgery. The significance of the surgery to the patient may vary tremendously depending on his or her prior experience, the specific surgery and the reason for it, the support systems available, and the patient's perception of what will happen. The ability of the consultant—and of the responsible surgeon—to understand and address these issues will go further toward making the outcome satisfactory than any test that is available.

Postoperative confusional states are common, and a prevalence of approximately 20% is a reasonable estimate. The prevalence after cardiac surgery may be significantly higher, and perhaps even doubled. Clearly, many mental derangements that occur after surgery go unrecognized by caregivers (20). Of 150 surgical patients seen in psychiatric consultation during a 2-year period at the Johns Hopkins Hospital, cognitive impairment (usually delirium) was diagnosed in approximately one-quarter of patients, and affective disorders, some of which were associated with delirium, affected over one-third of patients. Adjustment disorders affected approximately one-quarter of patients who required consultation and depression approximately one-tenth (20a).

PREOPERATIVE EVALUATION AND PREPARATION FOR SURGERY

Risk Factors for Psychiatric Complications

The extent of psychiatric appraisal before surgery depends on the underlying and associated conditions and the known coping mechanisms of the patient. A prior history of psychiatric complications, with or without surgical associations, is most important. However, patients with no prior history of psychiatric problems may be at risk for complications in the postoperative period. Attention to any risk factors associated with psychiatric complications in the surgical situation will improve outcome and help to prepare patients for psychic stress and to deal with stress in the recovery period (21, 22).

Etiologic factors associated with neuropsychiatric complications after surgery have been evaluated, but different age and socioeconomic groups, the surgical procedure or disease involved, underlying medical or comorbid psychiatric conditions make generalizing the information gleaned from the various studies difficult. This puts the burden on the consulting internist to investigate the constellation of potential risk factors that may be present in the patient with a specific clinical situation. When evaluating the risk for neuropsychiatric complications, it must be appreciated that both low- and high-risk patients coupled with low- and high-risk surgical situations exist in a context of low- and high-stress clinical situations. For example, an emotionally stable patient seeking an elective hernia repair might represent one end of the spectrum and a highly anxious young mother of four who is facing a disfiguring breast surgery the other.

Anxiety

Most patients face surgery with an appropriate, moderate, "healthy" level of anxiety that works to mobilize their coping resources. Fear of pain, death, loss, suffering, or disfigurement often are sources of anxiety. Some patients may worry about the loss of control that occurs with anesthesia or dependency during the postoperative recovery. Since anxiety is inextricably linked with pain, acknowledging and reducing anxiety will in turn diminish pain. Conversely, effective treatment of pain will serve to diminish anxiety (22).

Some patients have premorbid anxiety disorders or panic states and are at higher risk for anxiety complications postoperatively. Occasionally, patients will develop incapacitating anxiety preoperatively. Many hyperanxious patients will respond well to careful reassurance and the provision of information; sometimes surgery will need to be delayed to accomplish this. When necessary, pharmacologic therapy with benzodiazepines in adequate and regular doses to treat anxiety, but not to overly sedate, is effective.

Patients who do not respond adequately to these measures can be at a particularly high risk and may need further evaluation. Occasionally, psychotic patients may present with anxiety, and patients with mild dementia may present similarly. **Patients with agitated depression may simply appear to be anxious, and therapy with anxiolytics may worsen their depression.**

When patients have no apparent anxiety, the physician should be alert that there may be a problem. The most common reason for such an appearance is massive denial. This needs to be addressed preoperatively with counseling, since the denial defense mechanisms generally will break down postoperatively—with severe consequences. Patients may develop a number of behavioral problems, including anger, panic, or depression.

Other patients with no apparent anxiety have hidden agendas leading them to surgery. Some have psychotic delusional needs that they believe will be fulfilled by the procedure (22, 23). The Munchausen syndrome is the most exaggerated version, but less extreme, dependent patients seek surgery to assume "the sick role" (22). The physician should be alert for patients who have had multiple surgeries, especially if the indications for these procedures seem vague. Patients with chronic pain syndromes or somatization disorder are at high risk for inappropriate surgery with unsatisfying outcomes. Patients who state dissatisfaction with previous physicians may simply have had a difficult experience, but some have litigious natures or unreasonable expectations that may create problems postoperatively.

Depression

Major depression increases the risk of postoperative morbidity and mortality. Many patients with chronic disease have depressed mood, but in patients with vegetative signs of depression, such as poor sleep, crying, poor appetite, poor motivation, and fatigue, clinical depression must be considered and treated effectively. This may require a delay in surgery, therapy with antidepressant medication, or electroconvulsive therapy (ECT). Suicide is a frequent complication in patients with physical illness associated with depression, and a psychiatric assessment of risk and appropriate suicide precautions should be undertaken.

Other Psychiatric Risks for Surgery

Prior psychiatric complications, including delirium, psychotic reactions, severe anxiety, and depression, following previous surgery represents an important risk. Dementia is a major risk factor for postoperative complications, particularly delirium, and patients who are only mildly demented may escape detection without a careful assessment. Suspicion of possible dementia is necessary in elderly patients who are vague or confused. Evaluation by psychologic testing such as the Mini-Mental Status Examination by Folstein et al. (24) will determine if the patient has dementia, and careful attention to possible postoperative delirium is necessary.

Elderly patients are at higher risk for delirium and acute confusional states, and these patients are associated with a higher mortality rate and loss of ability to live independently after hospitalization.

Habituating substances deserve special attention. Withdrawal of alcohol, benzodiazepines, or narcotics places postoperative patients at increased risk. Symptoms of withdrawal may be mistaken for anxiety or delirium, and the specific nature of the problem may not recognized. In general, when drug dependency is recognized preoperatively, it can be dealt with appropriately. In elective situations, withdrawal and detoxification can precede surgery. In emergent situations, maintenance with benzodiazepines or opiates perioperatively will suffice until formal withdrawal can be addressed.

The greatest risk surrounding habituating substances is when the patient's dependency is not recognized. Patients can be deceptive regarding use of illicit substances or alcohol abuse; however, patients not infrequently lack understanding of the habituating nature of some substances, particularly benzodiazepines used for insomnia or chronic anxiety but also drugs used for pain conditions, opiates, or barbiturates. Many patients who would consider themselves to be "social drinkers" consume enough alcohol to undergo withdrawal, and it is necessary to be specific in questions regarding the frequency and quantity of alcohol consumed. Because patients with alcohol overuse will almost always underreport how much they actually drink, careful attention for the signs of withdrawal during the postoperative period is still necessary. Careful, nonjudgmental questioning with an appropriate level of suspicion usually will lead to appropriate responses from patients, especially when they understand the reasons behind the evaluation.

Patients who are addicted to narcotics present special concerns. These patients may be habituated, might not respond to the usual doses of narcotics, and may

legitimately require higher doses for adequate control of pain. However, inordi-
nate demands for pain medication, including higher doses or frequency of
administration, specific preparations or
routes of administration, or prolonged
administration, should raise the suspicion
of drug addiction or drug-seeking behavior. Addicted patients occasionally will
approach surgery for drug-seeking purposes, either undergoing a procedure or
seeking an evaluation because of a pur-
portedly painful condition.

Preoperative Assessment of Patients with Known Psychiatric Illness

Most patients with psychiatric disorders, including those that are severe and
chronic, are not at higher risk for surgery
than patients without mental disorders.
The risks of mortality and morbidity increase when psychiatric patients are unstable (i.e., with unpredictable, uncooperative behavior).

The major concerns regarding preoperative assessment of psychiatric patients
include risk evaluation for postoperative
behavior problems and treatment of patients with acute psychosis, mania, or
depression who require surgery and drug
therapy. The issue of informed consent
also must be addressed.

Patients with schizophrenia who are
effectively treated and cooperative are not
"higher-risk" patients for surgery. In fact,
psychotic symptoms appear to improve in
the time surrounding surgery, probably
because of the increased focus on physical
illness (23). When not symptomatic, patients with mania, bipolar disorders, or
depression are not at higher-than-average
risk.

However, the actively psychotic, depressed, or agitated patient presents a
major risk postoperatively. Self-harm, suicide, or elopement may occur if patients
are not effectively treated, preferably
before surgery. Continuous, one-to-one
nursing is required. Psychotic or actively
hallucinating patients may not report

symptoms, including severe pain, the need
to void, or other physical sensations.
Whereas insomnia and sleep deprivation
have not been associated with adverse
outcomes, the potential for increased agitation and delirium exists. Patients with
severe depression, and especially those
with a diminished will to live, are at
higher risk for adverse outcomes. These
patients may view surgery as a potential
suicide attempt, and they must be treated
appropriately and observed closely (22).

Psychiatric patients who are chronically ill, and especially those who are
institutionalized, present unique diagnostic and treatment problems (2). Most of
these patients have chronic schizophrenia, dementia, or mental retardation. Obtaining a patient history may be impossible, because these patients often are
noncommunicative, paranoid, hallucinating, inattentive, or demented. The historical perspective generally is provided by
staff who know the patient's behavior and
observe a change that is interpreted as a
new symptom. Patients may be unable to
appreciate or report symptoms (including
pain), but distress, increased agitation, or
fretfulness suggests that something is
wrong. Physical examination may be extremely difficult and may yield little or no
relevant information. Patients often are
uncooperative and extremely resistant to
attempts at examination, and they may
grow agitated and combative. Physical
injury to the examiner and patient may
occur. Attempts to perform diagnostic testing may be met with similar problems,
and only those tests that are critically
necessary should be considered. Usually,
diagnostic tests can be completed with
special precautions, which may involve
sedation, extra attendants, and additional
planning.

The ability to give informed consent is
maintained in most patients with psychiatric disease. The elements of informed
consent in these patients are no different
from those in any other. Whereas the
responsibility of obtaining consent is
placed on the operating surgeon, the con-

sulting internist often is in the best position (perhaps in coordination with the primary care physician) to help the patient develop a full understanding of the risks, benefits, and nature of the procedure so that he or she can make a proper decision. Rockwell and Pepitone-Rockwell (22) have written eloquently on aspects of consent and the psychiatric value of proper informed consent in improving outcome during the postoperative period. Psychiatric patients may need more consideration and time to achieve an informed consent because of their emotional or cognitive difficulties. Actively psychotic, depressed, confused, or demented patients may be unable to understand the nature of their physical disease, the importance of therapy, or the risks, benefits, and potential outcomes of treatment. When this is the case, they cannot give consent. In all but emergency surgery, consent will need to be obtained from a proxy or treatment delayed until the underlying psychiatric condition is stabilized and the patient is able to provide consent.

Psychotherapeutic drugs must be addressed preoperatively. Three issues are involved: *(a)* potential drug interactions with anesthetic and other perioperative drugs, *(b)* drug withdrawal side effects, and *(c)* adverse psychiatric effects of drug withdrawal.

Monoamine oxidase (MAO) inhibitors present the most dangerous interactions with anesthetic agents. Traditionally, these agents have been viewed as second-line drugs, but they sometimes are required in the treatment of psychiatric patients. Life-threatening hypertensive responses to pressor agents may result. These drugs need to be discontinued at least 2 weeks before surgery. Abrupt withdrawal is not associated with symptoms. When faced with emergency surgery, great care in providing anesthetic agents and other drugs is necessary. Many drugs will have a prolonged and potentiated effect. Fatal hyperpyrexic reactions have occurred with narcotic agents, and meperidine appears to be the most dangerous. Pressors should be avoided, and when necessary, extreme caution in dosing is required to prevent exaggerated effects (23). Anesthesiologists will be responsible for most such decisions in the perioperative period and are well aware of the difficulties with MAO inhibitors.

Tricyclic antidepressants have anticholinergic, cardiodepressant, and α-adrenergic blocking activity that can affect the action of anesthetic agents. Several days before surgery, they can be discontinued abruptly with few symptoms. Withdrawal symptoms include dizziness, headache, and gastrointestinal complaints of diarrhea, abdominal pain, and nausea. Generally, these drugs can be restarted several days postoperatively with no danger of precipitating depression. Patients who experience postoperative urinary retention or ileus or who have cardiac complications should not be restarted on these drugs until those conditions have resolved.

The new serotonin reuptake inhibitors may be less complicated. Anecdotal experience (personal communication, Kane High, MD, Dept. of Anesthesiology, Hershey Medical Center) suggests that anesthesiologists frequently administer anesthetic agents without preoperative discontinuation of selective serotonin reuptake inhibitors (SRRIs), and that SSRIs are free of the cardiac side effects of tricyclic agents. Brief periods of withdrawal from SSRIs do not appear to affect depressive symptoms adversely.

The actions of phenothiazines and butyrophenones are well known to anesthesiologists due to their frequent use as preoperative sedative agents. These drugs generally are stopped briefly during the postoperative period with no adverse effects. If they are withheld postoperatively, especially in patients who have required long-term administration, tardive dyskinesia can be precipitated, with resolution on reinstitution of the drug (23). Patients who require short-term antipsychotics postoperatively usually require parenteral administration. Anticholinergic withdrawal in patients requiring treatment for antipsychotic-induced parkinsonism can lead to symptoms of rigidity. Abrupt withdrawal of clozapine can induce symptoms of diaphoresis, flushing, diarrhea, and hyperactivity; therefore gradual reduction is preferable. There have been several reports of abrupt relapse after the withdrawal of clozapine, but other physicians who have withdrawn clozapine because of agranulocytosis have not observed this (25).

Therapeutic lithium levels potentiate the effects of anesthetic agents (23), thus requiring adjustment of the anesthetic dose. Lithium can be abruptly discontinued several days before elective surgery with no ill effects, and it should be withheld postoperatively until the patient's fluid and electrolyte status has stabilized. Manic-depressive patients can relapse if lithium is stopped for as little as several weeks.

POSTOPERATIVE DELIRIUM

Postoperative delirium is a common and dangerous condition that is associated with increased hospital mortality and morbidity. Delirium is a syndrome of altered consciousness with cognitive impairment associated with disorders of attention, thought perception, and sleep–wake cycle. It is important to contrast this condition with that of dementia, in which consciousness is retained in the face of cognitive impairment. With delirium, disorientation and psychomotor activity are impaired, as is memory. The onset is abrupt, usually in the first few days after surgery, and it usually does not last more than several days to a week (and rarely longer than a month). While the specific cause is unknown, there are multiple risk factors and precipitating factors (Table 21.3). Multifactorial conditions also are involved in many patients with delirium. The importance of making the diagnosis and treating the underlying causes is that delirium may represent the most obvious manifestation of serious underlying disease or a complication of surgery such as infection, perioperative infarct, or heart failure.

In a prospective survey of delirium among 1341 surgical patients, Owens and Hutelmyer (26) found that 9% developed postoperative delirium. Advanced age, alcohol use, poor cognitive status, poor general health, and electrolyte disturbances were risk factors. Delirium is a poor prognostic sign, with higher rates of major complications, longer lengths of hospital stay, and higher rates of discharge to a nursing home.

Terminology is not uniform among researchers. Whereas *delirium* is the term used in the *Diagnostic and Statistical Manual of Mental Disorders, Third Edition*, many other terms, such as *acute confusional state*, *postoperative psychosis*, *intensive care unit psychosis*, *metabolic encephalopathy*, and *cardiac psychosis*, have been applied. Some studies have concentrated on floridly symptomatic patients, and some have trained patients preoperatively to report any unusual sensory or cognitive experiences, however brief or mild, during the postoperative period (27). The percentage of postoperative patients with delirium relates to many factors in the population being studied, including age, medications, previous conditions, and the surgical procedure.

Golinger (20a) studied 150 consecutive psychiatric consultations on the surgery service at the Johns Hopkins Hospital over a 2-year period. Delirium was found in 20.7% of these patients. When the reason for consultation was listed as mood disturbance (39% of consultations), delirium was diagnosed in 26.3% of patients. Dyer (27a) reviewed this subject as well and found that of the 26 relevant and valid studies, the incidence of postoperative delirium in all age groups was 36.8%, with a reported range of from 0 to 73.5%. The incidence is highest in elderly patients and appears to be between 25 and 50%.

Postoperative confusion often is underdiagnosed. Golinger noted that delirium

Table 21.3. Organic Causes of Delirium

I. Intoxication
   A. Alcohol: ethyl and methyl
   B. Drugs: anticholinergic agents, sedative–hypnotics, digitalis derivatives, opiates, corticosteroids, salicylates, antibiotics, anticonvulsants, antiarrhythmic and antihypertensive drugs, antineoplastic agents, cimetidine, lithium, antiparkinson agents, disulfiram, indomethacin
   C. Inhalants: gasoline, glue, ether, nitrous oxide, nitrites
   D. Poisons:
      1. Industrial: carbon disulphide, organic solvents, methylchloride and bromide, heavy metals, organophosphorus insecticides, carbon monoxide
      2. Plants and mushrooms
      3. Toxins (e.g., snakebite)
II. Withdrawal syndromes
   A. Alcohol (delirium tremens)
   B. Sedatives/hypnotics: barbiturates, chloral hydrate, chlordiazepoxide, diazepam, ethchhlorvynol, glutethimide, meprobamate, methyprylon, paraldehyde
   C. Amphetamines
III. Metabolic disorders
   A. Hypoxia
   B. Hypoglycemia
   C. Hepatic, renal, pancreatic, pulmonary insufficiency (encephalopathy)
   D. Errors of metabolism: porphyria, carcinoid syndrome, hepatolenticular degeneration (Wilson's disease)
IV. Nutritional disorders
   A. Vitamin deficiency: nicotinic acid, thiamine, cyanocobalamine (vitamin B_{12}), folate, pyridoxine
   B. Hypervitaminosis: intoxication by vitamins A and D
   C. Disorders of fluid and electrolyte metabolism: dehydration, water intoxication, alkalosis, acidosis, hypernatremia, hyponatremia, hyperkalemia, hypokalemia, hypercalcemia, hypocalcemia, hypermagnesemia, hypomagnesemia
V. Hormonal disorders: hyperinsulinism, hyperthyroidism, hypothyroidism, hypopituitarism, Addison's disease, Cushing's syndrome, hypoparathyroidism, hyperparathyroidism
VI. Infections
   A. Systemic: pneumonia, typhoid, typhus, acute rheumatic fever, malaria, influenza, mumps, diphtheria, brucellosis, infectious mononucleosis, infectious hepatitis, malaria, subacute bacterial endocarditis, bacteremia, septicemia, Rocky Mountain spotted fever, legionnaires' disease
   B. Intracranial (acute, subacute, and chronic): viral encephalitis, aseptic meningitis, rabies, herpes; bacterial meningitis–meningococcal pneumococcal, *Haemophilus influenzae,* granulomatosus angiitis
VII. Neoplasms
   A. Metastasis
   B. Remote effects (toxins?)

---

may not be appreciated by the surgeon, because one-word associated symptoms of the major presenting illness are given undue emphasis. Studies that use a self-report of confusion have had a significantly higher incidence (58%) of delirium. Gustafson et al. showed underdiagnosis and poor documentation of delirium by both nurses and physicians (20), then proved a reduction in the incidence of delirium from 61.3 to 47.6% when a comprehensive evaluation and prevention program was instituted (28). Another study of general medicine patients showed that 32% of cases went undiagnosed (29). Some patients with delirium are not agitated, loud, and rambunctious (i.e., the so-called *quiet presentations*); these patients are more frequently underdiagnosed by physicians yet also have a poor prognosis.

Outcome studies showed that patients with delirium demonstrate increased mortality, loss of independence, nursing home placement, and mental decline compared with those without delerium. Delirium is an important entity to identify correctly for a variety of reasons besides simply relieving a patient from a troubling and confusing illness. Delirium sometimes is the first presenting symptom of an electrolyte disturbance, medical illness, or trouble with legal or illicit drugs. Pompei et al. (28a) found that delirious patients had an increased risk of hospital death, and Rockwood (28b) found that among his series of delirious patients, only 52% experienced complete symptom recovery. Inouye et al. (29) reported case fatality rates of between 25 and 33%. Various studies document a range of increased hospital mortality, from 2 to 20 times that of controls. Patients who experience delirium and are followed after hospital discharge show excess mortality and functional decline when followed for several years. It is unclear, however, whether delirium directly causes functional decline or is simply a marker for underlying causal conditions. It is equally unclear whether intervention will diminish the risk of mortality and morbidity. One study showed a length of hospitalization four times longer in patients with postoperative confusion and femoral neck fractures (30). Orthopaedic patients with postoperative confusion had a lessened potential for postoperative rehabilitation. In a study of 1285 patients with delirium on medical and surgical services, Levkoff (30a) found an increased mortality rate (13% versus 5% in controls), length of stay (23.7 days versus 13.6 days in controls), and total charges ($17,377 versus $11,946 in controls).

Risk factors for postoperative delirium are identified in a major review by Dyer et al. (27a). Age has emerged as a factor in many studies. Studying both medical and surgical patients, Schor et al. found that age older than 80 years was associated with delirium (30b). Mental status before surgery also plays a role, as does institutionalization before hospital admission. Multiple studies have identi-

fied the risk of dementia for postoperative delirium, and in fact, delirium can be a sign of early dementia. Depression that occurs preoperatively increases risk as well.

A number of laboratory abnormalities are predictive of postoperative confusion. These include albuminuria, alkalosis, anemia, azotemia, electrolyte abnormalities, and leukocytosis. Hypoxemia also is a risk factor. Levkoff (30a) showed that four factors were associated with 80% of postoperative delirious states in one large series; these were development of a urinary tract infection at any time during the hospital stay, or low serum albumin, leukocytosis, and/or proteinuria on admission. This retrospective analysis then was validated prospectively and was found to be predictive. In addition, Schor (30b) found that any symptomatic infection or temperature greater than 37.2° C also identified patients at risk.

Other conditions are associated with increased risk of confusion. Fracture on admission and uncontrolled pain increase the risk of delirium, and there may be an increased risk for intracardiac versus extracardiac procedures (31). The method of anesthesia (i.e., general versus epidural) is not associated with postoperative cognitive changes in prospective, randomized trials (30). A prospective study evaluated adverse cerebral outcomes after cardiac surgery and found that overall, 6.1% of patients had serious cerebral outcomes, ranging from stroke and death to seizures and deterioration of intellectual function (32).

Drug-related risk factors are among the most important and potentially controllable. One study found that the absolute number of drugs being administered simultaneously related to postoperative confusion, with five or more being significant (33). Some data implicate anticholinergic agents specifically, but a recent study by Marcantonio et al. (26) showed that no confusion occurring postoperatively related to use of anticholinergics. Tune et al. (34) showed a dose-related association with drugs binding to the muscarinic acetylcholine receptor (i.e., anticholinergic drugs).

Schor found no statistically significant relationship between use of narcotics and delirium, but Marcantonio et al. (26) found that meperidine caused delirium. In this same study, patient-controlled intravenous administration of narcotic for pain control was not associated with delirium, but epidural analgesia was. In addition, Schor found a decreased incidence of benzodiazepine-related delirium, whereas Marcantonio et al. found a dose-related increase, particularly with the long-acting agents, which doubled the risk over short-acting agents. Zolpidem, which is a non-benzodiazepine hypnotic agent, is selectively bound to the type 1 benzodiazepine receptor subtype. Unlike other benzodiazepines, it does not suppress deep sleep and REM sleep. Some studies have shown efficacy as a hypnotic with little development of tolerance (34a). No clear data are available for hospitalized patients and delirium using this relatively new agent.

Table 21.4 summarizes the evaluation of patients with postoperative delirium. A history will not be available directly from the patient, but it can be put together from the preoperative history, relatives, friends, or the previous record. Risk factors, particularly mental status and drugs, are especially important. The physical examination needs to specifically address the neurologic state, evaluation for infection, and cardiorespiratory status. Laboratory testing for metabolic abnormalities is important, and the CNS may require imaging studies performed on the basis of the history or physical examination. Delirium presents with an electroencephalogram (EEG) that is characterized by diffuse, symmetrical slowing; therefore when the diagnosis is in doubt, an EEG may be useful. EEG changes in delirium are nearly ubiquitous, are more sensitive than changes in the physical examination, and may precede apparent changes in cognitive function. When delirium results

Table 21.4.   Evaluation of the Patient with Postoperative Delirium

1. Mental status and neurologic examination
   Distinguish delirium from psychiatric or neurologic complications
2. General physical examination
   Fever
   Papilledema
   Meningismus
   Cardiopulmonary dysfunction
   Stigmata of liver disease
3. Review preoperative course
   Did nurses note disorientation or "sundowning"?
   Possibility of head trauma
   Prolonged malnutrition, hyperlimentation
   Fever preoperatively
4. Review current medications
   Intraoperative hypoxemia or hypotension
   Hypothermia
   Drugs
   Complications
5. Review current medications
6. Historical factors (obtain from friends, relatives)
   Pre-existing dementia: forgetfulness, wandering, confusion, emotional lability
   Alcoholism
   Other substance abuse
   Prescription drugs
7. Laboratory studies
   Electolytes
   Glucose
   Blood urea nitrogen
   CBC and differential
   If clinically indicated: drug screens
   Calcium
   Magnesium
   Phosphate
   Blood gases
   Urinalysis
   All should be done, and if clinically indicated; drug screens should be done.
8. Chest radiography, ECG, imaging studies
   Obtain EEG if required for confirmation of delirium
9. Lumbar puncture if infection suspected

from alcohol or sedative drug withdrawal, the EEG shows fast, low-amplitude activity. Occasionally, seizures can present as delirium. EEG can identify status epilepticus or partial complex seizures; patients with psychosis or affective disorders usually have a normal EEG. If no contraindication exists, obtaining cerebrospinal fluid by lumbar puncture should be considered for patients in whom delirium remains unexplained.

Once the diagnosis of delirium is made, the underlying cause must be specifically sought and treated. Since delirium so often suggests the occurrence of a serious, acute physical illness or preoperative complication, failure to treat the specific cause can lead to disastrous results, particularly in elderly patients. Causes can include infection, including sepsis, thromboembolic disease, myocardial infarction or congestive heart failure, hypoglycemia, hypoxia, and drug intoxication.

Several general treatment considerations are important when delirium is first recognized. All drugs, and particularly those with anticholinergic activity, must be carefully reviewed for appropriateness and, if necessary, discontinued or reduced if possible. Fluid and electrolytes must be balanced, severe anemia corrected, and nutritional status and vitamins addressed as supportive treatment. Nursing care is important as well, not only in the initial recognition of the disorder but in reorienting and reassuring the patient. Sensory deprivation contributes to delirium, and good lighting, including exposure to outside sunlight, may help. Close observation, attendance by friends or relatives, availability of a clock or a calendar and orienting messages, quiet at night, and familiar objects also will reduce anxiety and disorientation.

Drug therapy frequently is necessary in patients who are severely agitated, especially when there is risk of pulling out intravenous lines or catheters, climbing out of bed or elopement, or tearing apart dressings and sutures. Haloperidol, whether orally or intramuscularly, in doses of from 1 to 5 mg repeated hourly until calming occurs usually is the therapy of choice for acute delirium, because it is the safest and least interactive with other drugs and medical conditions. In elderly patients or those with mild delirium, lower doses (e.g., 0.5 mg every hour until symptoms subside) often suffice (35). Some physicians prefer phenothiazines (e.g., chlorpromazine), which are more sedating though associated with more cholinergic activity and cardiovascular effects. Often, the latter agents are better used in younger, stronger, and more physically fit patients who are severely agitated postoperatively. Intravenous sedation is effective and safe in agitated patients who are critically ill (36, 37).

For alcohol and sedative–hypnotic withdrawal, benzodiazepines are the drugs of choice. These can be titrated orally at 30-minute intervals until agitation is relieved. Intramuscular diazepam is erratically absorbed; lorazepam, 1 to 4 mg, is better in this regard. Attention to excessive sedation and airway obstruction is important, and titration of the dosage is beneficial (recognizing that some patients with delirium tremens may require high doses initially). Because of renal clearance, oxazepam and lorazepam are preferred agents with coexisting hepatic disease or hepatic encephalopathy. In patients with alcoholism, thiamine also must be administered to prevent the Wernicke-Korsakoff syndrome. Antipsychotic agents lower seizure thresholds and therefore are relatively contraindicated in withdrawal states.

Physostigmine has been shown to reverse some cases of delirium caused by anticholinergic toxicity. Physostigmine salicylate, 1 to 2 mg given slowly intravenously or intramuscularly and repeated after 15 minutes with careful monitoring, may be considered in severe anticholinergic intoxication. It must be given cautiously, however, because of its potential to induce seizures or cardiac arrhythmia. Contraindications include cardiac disease, asthma, diabetes, peptic ulcer, and bowel or bladder obstruction.

Perioperative treatment of delirium optimally will include prevention. Eliminating noncritical medication, general supportive measures, good nursing care, and postoperative monitoring are important.

Early recognition of delirium will lead to prompt intervention and decreased potential for harm.

MEDICAL EVALUATION FOR ELECTROCONVULSIVE THERAPY

Electroconvulsive therapy is perhaps the least understood medical treatment in use today. Before the onset of effective psychiatric medications, it was often overused. Over the decades since then, however, its popularity has varied (38). Even today, use of ECT varies from place to place across the United States (39).

Electroconvulsive therapy represents an effective treatment for major depression and bipolar disorder. Success rates are at least as good as those with medication and often are superior. Many studies show that ECT is effective in patients for whom medications or other treatments are not effective (40). This treatment seems to be especially useful in elderly patients, who sometimes have difficulty tolerating the side effects of antidepressant medication. Elderly patients who receive ECT demonstrate greater clinical improvement than patients on medication and, in fact, are more likely to be alive at follow-up compared with patients on pharmacotherapy (41). Despite these remarkable results, however, it sometimes is difficult to obtain patient consent for ECT. Videotapes showing the treatment and giving information about it can be helpful, as can testimonials from other patients who have received the treatment.

Patients with major depression and psychotic features seem to benefit most from ECT (40), perhaps because pharmacologic measures are relatively ineffective. Bipolar disorder and, occasionally, schizophrenia that is resistant to medication also have been treated with ECT. Patients with schizophrenia and prominent mood symptoms may be the subgroup of those suffering from schizophrenia most likely to benefit (42). In addition, maintenance ECT, given periodically on an outpatient basis, can help to maintain remission from further episodes of illness (44).

In ECT, the patient fasts after midnight of the night before the treatment. Electrodes are placed either on each temple for bilateral treatment, which usually leads to quicker response (45) and is better generalized throughout the brain (46) than is unilateral treatment. However, there are concerns that bilateral ECT may be associated with higher rates of reversible memory impairment as an unwanted side effect. ECG leads are applied, as are a pulse oximeter and a blood pressure cuff. EEG monitoring is used to verify the occurrence of a seizure and to determine its length. Ultrabrief, light general anesthesia (usually with methohexital) is then given to the patient (47), and the patient then receives succinylcholine to relax his or her skeletal muscles.

If the patient is unable to have a seizure of sufficient length, the electrical energy delivered by the ECT stimulus machine is increased. If a seizure of sufficient length still is not obtained, caffeine can be given intravenously to lower the seizure threshold (48–50). The patient is monitored during the recovery period for changes in oxygenation, blood pressure, and cardiac rhythm.

Medical Evaluation before ECT

The consulting internist often is asked to evaluate a patient to help determine the risk of proceeding with ECT. Death occurs in approximately 1 to 4 per 100,000 treatments (40, 42, 51), which is comparable to the death rate for anesthesia in minor surgery.

There are no absolute contraindications for ECT (47). A wide array of conditions present relative contraindications, however, and certain conditions also require further evaluation before anesthesia.

A space-occupying lesion or other condition that could increase intracranial pressure are relative contraindications for ECT (47). Likewise, a recent stroke (i.e., within the last 6 months) also places the patient at substantially higher risk during

ECT (47). During the seizure, the systolic blood pressure usually rises, often by 40 to 50 mm HG, which could cause another stroke.

An unstable vascular aneurysm or malformation also places the patient at increased risk during ECT. A retinal detachment as well as a pheochromocytoma are conditions that place the patient at higher risk for the treatment as well because of the associated risk of a sudden rise in blood pressure with the treatment itself (47).

Most often, however, the consultant will be called on to assess the cardiac risk of ECT. Especially in elderly patients, an assessment of cardiac risk should be done before ECT is performed. At minimum, this should include a physical examination and ECG as well as electrolyte levels and complete blood count.

A myocardial infarction within the previous 6 months is a relative contraindication for the treatment (47). Abrupt increases in heart rate, blood pressure, and cardiac contractility also occur during ECT and are more pronounced in elderly patients (52). In addition, asystole for several seconds following the electrical stimulus can occur (53, 54), but this usually resolves spontaneously without the need for treatment.

A cardiac pacemaker is not a contraindication for ECT; however, the cardiac function of patients with pacemakers must be carefully evaluated before ECT. Pacemaker functioning should be documented by ECG, and the structural integrity of the pacemaker wire should be verified by chest radiography (23). If the patient has a demand pacemaker, an external magnet may be required to convert the device to fixed mode.

Of the patients with pre-existing cardiac disease in one study, 55% had at least one cardiac complication following ECT (55). Most were transient, such as transitory arrhythmias or ST-T wave changes on the ECG. In addition, 20% of the patients in this study had persistent ECG changes associated with chest pain.

There were no deaths associated with ECT in this study.

Even in those patients with cardiac disease, ECT remains remarkably safe. A study of 26 "high risk" patients for ECT found they did not suffer more major complications from the procedure than did those without cardiac disease (55). A similar study of 40 patients with cardiovascular disease found a higher rate of cardiac complications than that among matched patients without cardiac disease, but most of these complications were transitory (56). Interestingly, 21 of the 40 patients with cardiovascular disease in this study had undergone trials of tricyclic antidepressants before ECT; of these, 11 had to discontinue treatment with the drug. Thirty-eight of the 40 patients with cardiac disease were able to finish their course of ECT despite their medical illness.

Headaches may occur after the ECT treatment (57). Use of acetaminophen or nonsteroidal anti-inflammatory agents usually are effective.

Delirium also may occur after ECT, and different studies have shown that occurrence rates for delirium and memory disturbances with ECT vary from 11 to 39% (58–60). Rates of delirium persisting after ECT are not higher in patients who have suffered a cerebrovascular accident in the past, ranging from 15 to 28.5% (61, 62). Patients with Parkinson's disease as well as those with pre-existing cognitive impairment may be at higher risk for delirium (63). Cognitive problems with ECT are greater if the treatment is given three times a week (as typically performed in the United States) than if given twice a week (as often performed in the United Kingdom) (64). The rate of response, however, is faster if the treatment is given three times per week. Although the patient may experience spotty memory loss for events surrounding the treatment, cognitive changes, including memory loss, are fully reversible. Also, there is no evidence that ECT causes any structural damage to the brain (65).

MEDICAL ILLNESS PRESENTING WITH PSYCHIATRIC SYMPTOMS

Medical illness often presents with clouded sensorium, thought disorder, anxiety, and depressive symptoms. A thorough medical evaluation to elucidate medical conditions that explain the symptoms, or part of the presentation, is necessary before making a primary psychiatric diagnosis and embarking on treatment.

Table 21.5 presents several examples of medical illnesses that cause psychiatric symptoms. Much of the information summarized in this section is available from general medical texts (66, 67). The following examples of medical disease presenting with psychiatric symptoms have been chosen because of their relative frequency, the importance of treatment that is different from psychiatric therapy, general interest, or important conceptual information.

Endocrinopathies

Thyroid dysfunction is common and can mimic a number of psychiatric dis-

Table 21.5. Some Medical Illnesses Presenting with Psychiatric Symptoms

1. Endocrine
   Hyperthyroidism
   Hypothyroidism
   Pheochromocytoma
   Hyperparathyroidism
   Addison's disease
   Cushing's syndrome
2. CNS
   Dementia, Alzheimer's disease
   Space-occupying lesions
   MS, parkinsonism, Huntington's disease
   Seizures
3. HIV-related
4. Metabolic
   Wilson's disease
   Porphyria
5. Toxic
6. Deficiency states
7. Cardiac/pulmonary/renal/rheumatologic/infectious

orders. Hyperthyroid conditions may present with neurotic symptoms, agitation, insomnia, or anxiety as well as somatic complaints, with weight loss, chronic diarrhea, or palpitations. Cognitive and psychologic symptoms such as impaired concentration and memory as well as paranoia, hallucinations, and delusions can occur. Hypothyroid conditions can present with symptoms of depression or dementia, and evaluation of the thyroid status is undertaken in any patient with psychiatric or somatic complaints. Laboratory measurements of triiodothyronine (T_3), thyroxine (T_4), and thyroid-stimulating hormone (TSH) are normal in patients with depression (68).

The highly sensitive TSH test is the best method to evaluate patients initially. The T_4 level is elevated in 90% of patients with hyperthyroidism, but many patients with an elevated T_4 level are not hyperthyroid (they will have a normal TSH). The occasional patient with either hyperthyroidism and a normal T_4 or T_3 thyrotoxicosis will have a depressed TSH level. A low TSH level should be evaluated further with a free T_4 measurement.

An elevated or depressed T_4 level frequently results from drugs or illness by alteration in T_4 binding. The TSH test can be used in almost all clinical situations to confirm hyper- or hypothyroidism (69–71).

Elderly patients with hyperthyroidism may have neuropsychiatric manifestations, but these may be overlooked because of the prominence of the cardiac presentation (72). It is not unusual for the consultant to be asked to evaluate the patient because of his or her heart problem.

Long-term lithium therapy can induce hypothyroidism. One study of 19 manic-depressive (i.e., bipolar disorder) patients, 15 of whom were women, receiving therapeutic dosages of lithium carbonate for 10 to 20 years included 8 patients (42%) who required therapy for hypothyroidism (73).

Factitious hyperthyroidism is an important, though uncommon, psychiatric condition presenting with medical symptoms. Classically described in patients with some medical background, it must be recognized that some practitioners of diet therapy occasionally prescribe thyroid preparations as appetite suppressants and stimulants, as do psychiatrists attempting to treat recalcitrant depression. Small, daily supplementation with T_3 potentiates the action of tricyclic antidepressants (68). The autoimmune signs of Grave's disease, such as ophthalmopathy, lid lag, and stare, are absent. Tachycardia or headaches are prominent presenting complaints. Patients characteristically are reluctant to disclose T_4 abuse, so the diagnosis is made by clinical suspicion in a patient with prominent neurotic symptoms. Laboratory testing will show elevated T_3 and T_4 and suppressed TSH levels.

Hypothyroidism may be mild or severe and diagnosed by an elevated TSH level. In ambulatory patients who are 65 years and older, the incidence of hypothyroidism is between 3 and 10% (74, 75). Severe hypothyroidism results in apathy, retarded speech and reactions, dry and coarse skin, hoarse voice, cold intolerance, and constipation. Depression and dementia are common psychiatric manifestations. Symptoms often develop gradually, and this may interfere with their recognition by medical personnel and caregivers, including the patient's family.

Subclinical hypothyroidism is a common consultation question. Because of the relatively high incidence of the condition, patients will be discovered with mild to moderate elevations in the TSH level and a normal T_4 measurement. The value at which the TSH elevation is high enough to result in symptoms is arguable. Some consider values between 5 and 10 µm/mL to be treatable. One rationale for initiating replacement therapy is that eventual symptomatic hypothyroidism is inevitable and replacement helps to assure follow-up evaluation and treatment.

Parathyroid disorders may cause psychiatric symptoms when hypercalcemia is severe. Symptoms range from mild personality changes to severe psychiatric disorders, including coma and obtundation. With mild elevations in the calcium level, vague complaints such as anxiety, fatigue, depression, and inability to concentrate may suggest psychoneurosis. At higher levels, patients may show confusion, agitation, paranoia, hallucinations, and delusions before progressing further to stupor and coma. Neuromuscular involvement with hyperparathyroidism may result in weakness, fatigue, and muscle atrophy.

Because of the relative frequency of both mild hypercalcemia and depression in the general population, patients often will have both conditions. Depressive symptoms should not necessarily be considered an indication for operative intervention.

Other Endocrine Disorders

Endogenous **hypercortisolism**, including Cushing's disease, can result in depression, psychosis, weakness, agitation, paranoia, or mania. Hypofunction of the pituitary or adrenal glands may present with nonspecific mental symptoms, including weakness, anorexia, nausea and vomiting, apathy, memory loss, depression, disorientation, and psychosis.

Patients with depression may have excessive secretion of adrenocorticoids. Overnight dexamethasone testing does not suppress the plasma cortisol level in these patients, but it does suppress the plasma cortisol level in patients with schizophrenia or acute psychosis. The 24-hour urinary cortisol level should be normal in patients with depression who are not cushingoid (68).

Hypoglycemia produces central nervous symptoms when it is profound (i.e., <30 mg/dL). Classic adrenergic symptoms of hypoglycemia, such as diaphoresis, tremor, palpitations, flushing, hunger, headache, and weakness, are related to the rapidity of the fall in serum glucose, not to the degree of hypoglycemia. Symptoms of classic hypoglycemia may not arise if the drop is gradual. CNS symptoms of mild confusion and delirium may occur in mild hypoglycemia, but with more profound drops, seizures may result. Coma develops at serum glucose levels of 10 mg/mL and may be irreversible if not treated. Multiple other symptoms also can be seen, including hemiparesis, monoparesis, paresthesia, ataxia, dysarthria, profound confusion, and emotional liability. Patients occasionally will appear to be intoxicated.

Hypoglycemia with hyperosmotic states may present as confusion, dysarthria, or fatigue. Generally, making the diagnosis is not difficult.

Pheochromocytoma presents with clinical manifestations relating to the elevated levels of epinephrine and norepinephrine. Paroxysms of headache, anxiety, diaphoresis, tachycardia, epigastric pain, pallor, and syncope may occur. Hypertension can be sustained or episodic. Patients frequently are misdiagnosed as having anxiety or panic disorders, and pheochromocytoma must be considered in any patient with hypertension and paroxysmal symptoms.

Neurologic Illness

Parkinson's disease often presents with a number of psychiatric manifestations, and therapeutic agents cause adverse reactions that often suggest psychiatric disease. The clinical presentation of parkinsonism with bradykinesia, muscle rigidity, and tremor are gradually progressive; when established, these usually suggest the correct diagnosis. Occasionally, patients with bradykinesia may appear to have psychiatric disease, as suggested by hesitation in speech or movement. Mild dementia and depression are not infrequent. Depression may occur in as many as 50% of these patients and should be treated in the usual fashion. The prognosis of the underlying parkinsonism is not affected, but the patient's quality of life would be expected to improve (as occurs with other depressive states). Alzheimer's disease may coexist with parkinsonism.

Drugs, including phenothiazines, butyrophenones (e.g., haloperidol), and reserpine, may bring on a syndrome of parkinsonism. Discontinuation or decreased dosage may decrease the symptoms; however, tardive dyskinesia may persist. Neuroleptic agents will worsen existing parkinsonism and are contraindicated. A meperidine analogue, MPTP (1-methyl-4-phenyl-1,2,3,6,-tetrahydropyridine), taken in accidental administration by intravenous drug abusers, causes an irreversible Parkinsonian-like state due to selective destruction of substantial nigra dopaminergic neurons (76, 77).

Psychiatric symptoms related to levodopa occur in approximately 30% of treated patients and include confusion, depression, agitation, hallucinations, and insomnia. Other agents such as pergolide and selegiline also may have neurologic symptoms, though perhaps less frequently.

Huntington's disease clinically consists of progressive dementia associated with choreoathetosis. Generally, the disease is not difficult to recognize, especially with a positive family history. However, the clinical aspects of this disease may not progress at similar rates, and when dementia and depression predominate, there may be difficulty making the diagnosis.

Dystonias may suggest psychiatric disease, because the movement disorder may appear bizarre. Interestingly, when 100 musicians with hand difficulties were studied by Hochberg et al. (78), tendinitis or nerve entrapment accounted for all complaints, with the possible exception of two musicians who were diagnosed as manic-depressive. Drug-induced dystonia may consist of three distinct syndromes. First, acute dystonia may follow a short course of an antipsychotic drug, or even a single dose. This is most common in adolescents. Therapy consists of intravenous diphenhydramine, 25 to 50 mg, and discontinuation of the neuroleptic agent. Second, parkinsonism occurs in 10% of patients receiving long-term antipsychotic therapy. Anticholinergic therapy is beneficial. The neuroleptic agent should be discontinued, or if this is not possible, reduction in dosage must be considered. Third, tardive dyskinesia occurs in approximately 20% of patients receiving long-term therapy, and its treatment is problematic (3). Withdrawal of antipsychotic drugs may result in improvement over weeks or months; however, extrapyramidal side effects may be irreversible and even may worsen on withdrawal. If movements worsen or persist, or if the underlying psychiatric problem becomes unmanageable, one must reinstitute the smallest effective dose of antipsychotic medication.

Gilles de la Tourette's syndrome is a condition of unknown cause that presents with multiple facial tics and involuntary vocalizations. It begins in childhood and may be progressive. Behavioral symptoms may include compulsive touching of others and coprolalia (i.e., explosive utterance of obscenities). It may remit, but severe disability can occur. Therapy with haloperidol or clonidine is partially effective (79).

Multiple sclerosis, especially early in its course, frequently is mistaken for psychiatric disease. It can have a myriad of presentations depending on the location of demyelinization within the CNS. Criteria to establish the diagnosis require at least two clinical episodes of neurologic deficit. It is not unusual to have one or more clinical episodes so subtle that they go unrecognized. Laboratory tests (i.e., computed tomography [CT], magnetic resonance imaging) can be misleading. Symptoms may wax and wane in severity; therefore if symptoms are bizarre or when complaints are vague and neurologic findings minimal, multiple sclerosis may be mistaken for a conversion reaction (e.g., hysteria). On the other hand, it is important to remember that the diagnosis carries significant implications, and the clinical criteria for diagnosis need to be respected.

In patients with known multiple scle-rosis, several psychiatric manifestations may occur. The psychiatric response to chronic disease is potentially a component, but manifestations mostly result from direct CNS pathology. Depression is the most common emotional disorder and may be bipolar. Intellectual decline or dementia may occur, and patients may develop a superimposed hysterical component that complicates the clinical presentation. Further, patients may develop an inappropriate euphoria; when this coexists with depression, it is important to ask the patient specifically about his or her mood and the cardinal features of depression.

Central Nervous System Diseases

Dementia affects approximately 15% of those older than 65 years. The most common treatable causes, including hydrocephalus, hypothyroidism, and brain tumor, tended to occur in patients younger than 65 years old. In another series of 500 patients with dementia who were evaluated with use of CT, potentially treatable causes were found in 10% (80). The long-term outcome of these treatable cases, however, has not been well studied.

At onset, the symptoms of Alzheimer's disease may suggest depression. Intellectual decline gradually becomes apparent, and difficulty in decision making and poor judgment are characteristic. The onset of symptoms may be so gradual that even close contacts of the patient, such as immediate family members, may be less sensitive to its progression than occasional contacts. Advanced disease may be characterized by aphasia, myoclonic jerks, psychosis, and occasionally, seizures.

Evaluation of dementia should include a careful patient history and physical examination, nutritional evaluation, serology for syphilis, thyroid function studies, and general blood chemistries to screen for diabetes mellitus, renal disease, hyperparathyroidism, and electrolyte disturbances. Results of a complete blood count may suggest an underlying infectious disease or abnormal red blood cell indices, such as megaloblastic changes, or a nutritional disorder. CT may disclose or confirm causes in a significant proportion of patients, and it should be considered in patients when CNS infection, neoplasm, or multi-infarcts are possible. Testing for infection with human immunodeficiency virus (HIV) is important if the history suggests the patient is at risk. Examination also should include a careful mental status examination. Depression may cause pseudodementia. More commonly, however, mild to moderate dementia is accompanied by depression, which when treated can result in improved quality of life. Patients with pseudodementia tend to be more cognizant and therefore disturbed by their symptoms; for example, they may complain more actively about memory loss (81) On Folstein (Mini-Mental Status) testing, patients with dementia tend to score lower than 24 (out of a possible 30), and usually much lower, whereas patients with depression will score higher than 24 (24).

Pick's disease is a rare form of dementia that is similar clinically to Alzheimer's dementia. The progression may be more rapid, however, and focal signs such as aphasia and hemiparesis are more prominent. On CT scans, frontal or temporal atrophy usually is apparent.

Multi-infarct dementia results from multiple small cerebral infarctions due to diffuse, small-artery atherosclerotic disease. The onset may appear to be stepwise, with progression occurring in recognizable episodes of decline with periods of stable function between. Localizing neurologic signs are more prominent than with Alzheimer's disease. Other signs of vascular disease, diabetes mellitus, hypertension, and a history of smoking may be associated. Early recognition and attention to risk factors may be beneficial.

Hydrocephalus (i.e., normal pressure hydrocephalus), is an important cause of dementia, because progression or reversal of dementia is possible with ventricular

shunting procedures. The cause is unknown, but patients generally have a defect in CSF resorption that results in gradual ventricular dilatation. Occasionally, this may follow traumatic head injury, subarachnoid hemorrhage, or meningitis. Symptoms include progressive dementia and gait disturbance. Urinary incontinence frequently accompanies the disorder but is present in less than 50% of patients. Approximately 50% of patients show improvement following shunting procedures. Those with mild symptoms, who are treated earlier, seem to do better, as do those who respond to CSF removal (82). Shunting is not without risk, however, and shunt malfunction is common (83).

Neuropsychiatric Manifestations of HIV Infection 1

The neuropsychiatric manifestations of HIV infection have been extensively reviewed by Atkinson et al. (84). Some persons at high risk for HIV infection, specifically homosexual men and intravenous drug users, may be at higher-than-average risk for psychopathology (33, 85). Infected patients may have psychiatric illness and adjustment reactions found in the general population and with other medical illness. Psychiatric symptoms may be part of the expression of HIV-related complications (e.g., CNS infection) or result from therapy (e.g., drug side effects). A large prospective study showed an identical prevalence of neuropsychologic abnormalities in healthy homosexual and bisexual seropositive men versus seronegative homosexual men (86, 87). Finally, specific HIV-related neuropsychiatric conditions, such as delirium and dementia, also exist.

Issues of anxiety, fear, anger, and denial present early on, and they often accompany the behavioral response to seroconversion. In the later stages of HIV disease, issues of pain, dementia, and terminal care predominate.

Anxiety episodes appear to be more common in patients with HIV but do not occur more frequently than in seronegative homosexual men. Therapy for anxiety, as in non-HIV illness, is appropriate when symptoms interfere with function (e.g., work, social interactions) or when anxiety is distressing. If pharmacologic therapy is necessary, benzodiazepines generally are used, but the specific drug chosen will depend on any underlying, concomitant medical problems and the specific anxiety situation to be treated. Alternatives to benzodiazepines include hydroxyzine and buspirone. The advantage of these alternatives is that they are nonaddictive.

Rates of **depression** are elevated to levels equal to those in individuals with non-HIV chronic medical illness (approximately doubled, to 5–8%). Rates are higher (up to 40%) for hospitalized HIV-positive patients, but this also appears to be equal to those in non-HIV-positive hospitalized patients. Making the diagnosis may be difficult, because so many symptoms that are useful in the diagnosis of depression also are common in symptomatic HIV-positive patients.

Selection of an appropriate drug in patients with HIV infection may need to take into consideration that patients with AIDS may be at greater risk for the anticholinergic side effects of tricyclics. For this reason, newer SSRIs may be more attractive, but they are no more effective. Occasional weight loss, anxiety, and insomnia may be a problem with the new agents and not with the tricyclics. Bupropion can lower the seizure threshold more than other anti-depressants. When ECT is considered, no specific contraindications apply to patients with HIV infection (88).

Mania rarely has been associated with HIV infection. Case reports of mania secondary to complications of HIV infection exist, involving the use of cryptococcal meningitis therapy, corticosteroids, or antiretroviral therapy (see Appendix) (89, 90). Mania can be treated with low-dose neuroleptic agents, lithium in standard doses, or clonazepam.

HIV infection, especially when advanced, may cause **psychosis** in as many as 5% of patients. A significant proportion of these patients show rapid deterioration of mental and medical status (91). Other causes of psychosis include use of prescription or illicit drugs.

Neuroleptic agents, such as chlorpromazine or haloperidol, are useful in treatment of psychosis. Dosages should be reduced in patients with AIDS, because extrapyramidal effects are common (30–50%). Many patients with AIDS will not tolerate anticholinergic side effects such as xerostomia and constipation. In addition, patients with AIDS, especially those with the cognitive disorders, appear to be at greater risk for malignant neuroleptic syndrome (92).

The lifetime risk of **alcohol abuse** is two to three times higher (approaching 40%) in both seronegative and seropositive homosexual men compared with that in heterosexual men, whereas current use appears to be equal in each group (93). Further, infection with HIV does not appear to increase the risk of alcohol abuse. The importance of identifying and treating alcohol and drug abuse has been emphasized because of the concern that impaired judgment may predispose a person to behavior that will increase the risk of acquiring or transmitting HIV, noncompliance with therapy for HIV, or complications (e.g., tuberculosis chemotherapy).

HIV-associated dementia (HAD) may result in cognitive impairment (94, 95). Motor function may be impaired, thus resulting in ataxia and incoordination. Affect may be altered as well and result in inappropriate behavior, including violence, labile mood and irritability, and apathy.

The incidence and prevalence of HAD is not clear. At one time, it was believed that up to two-thirds of symptomatic patients with HIV infection would develop this complication; however, several studies now show that the incidence is less, between 7 and 14%, even in advanced cases of HIV infection. It is believed that earlier treatment with zidovudine (AZT) may account for this declining incidence (86, 87, 96, 97).

Mild neurocognitive disorder refers to the more common impairment (approximately 50% of symptomatic patients with HIV infection) (98). Making the diagnosis requires involvement in cognition, as in HAD, but the defects are only so severe as to produce mild interference with social or occupational abilities. It is unclear if mild neurocognitive disorder progresses to HAD.

Psychostimulants, such as methylphenidate and dextroamphetamine, have been advocated for therapy, but no controlled studies on their use are available. The significant potential for abuse of these drugs must be taken into account. Treatment with N-methyl-D-aspartate (NMDA) antagonists and netroglycepine also may prove to be beneficial (95).

The wide range of associated complications and therapies associated with a chronic disease as complicated as AIDS places these patients at high risk for **delirium**. The evaluation should proceed along the same lines as that for any patient, with special attention being given to the myriad of potential etiologic factors such as infection, CNS complications such as tumors, metabolic derangements, and medications.

Inadequate diagnosis and management of **pain** is a common problem with treatment for HIV infection. Persistent barriers to pain control, as in cancer pain management (95a), may be higher in patients with HIV. These patients often hesitate to ask for relief under the perception that the request will be misinterpreted by caregivers, that they will become addicted or that the pain is inevitable or untreatable, or that their pain is deserved. Physicians also often underestimate the pain or are overly concerned with addiction or habituation.

Metabolic Diseases

Wilson's disease is a rare, autosomal recessive trait that results in excessive deposition of copper in tissues, including the brain, liver, kidney, and cornea. Neurologic symptoms may appear identical to those of schizophrenia, manic-depressive psychoses, neuroses, dystonias, or other bizarre manifestations. The importance of recognizing the diagnosis lies in the fact that Wilson's disease is associated with a severe outcome when untreated. Low ceruloplasmin levels are found in 95% of patients.

The **porphyrias** are a group of disorders of heme biosynthesis that may be either inherited or acquired. Neurologic manifestations during acute attacks include behavioral changes ranging from severe anxiety to delirium or frank psychosis. Between acute episodes, patients may have depression, anxiety, or vague somatic complaints. The pathophysiology leading to neurologic symptoms is unknown. Laboratory diagnosis relies on the measurement of increased aminolevulinic acid or porphobilinogen excretion in urine. During acute attacks, when neuropsychiatric symptoms are apparent, levels usually are elevated, but the magnitude of the elevation does not correlate with the severity of the symptoms.

Nutritional Diseases

Wernicke's encephalopathy results from thiamine (i.e., vitamin B_{12}) deficiency. Classically seen in alcoholics, other people suffering from severe malnutrition, such as patients with AIDS, cancer, starvation, or on fad diets (including poorly educated vegetarians), also are at risk. The classic triad consists of ataxia, ophthalmoplegia, and obtundation. Mental changes are observed in 90% of patients and include a global confusional–apathetic state with listlessness, disorientation, and indifference. Symptoms may accompany alcohol withdrawal. Underdiagnosis is common, and a high degree of suspicion is required. This is because immediate therapy will restore function and prevent permanent sequelae (99). Therapy with thiamine, 50 to 100 mg intravenously daily for 5 days, will promptly (in hours to days) correct the ocular abnormalities and replenish the thiamine stores. Particular attention must be given to intravenous glucose, which when provided in the face of thiamine deficiency will either precipitate or worsen Wernicke's disease.

Recovery from Wernicke's encephalopathy may reveal underlying **Korsakoff's psychosis** characterized by defective learning and memory, in which case the condition is referred to as **Wernicke-Korsakoff syndrome**. Complete recovery from Korsakoff's psychosis usually occurs in less than 20% of patients. The remainder may have some recovery, but the residual defect in memory and judgment frequently requires long-term institutional care.

Niacin deficiency results in pellagra. However, it also can result in an encephalopathy with prominent mental symptoms, including anxiety, depression, fatigue, and apathy, which may progress to confusion, disorientation, hallucinations, and psychosis.

Vitamin excess occasionally causes symptoms that can be confused with psychiatric disease. Vitamin A toxicity may result in dizziness, fatigue, anorexia, and abdominal as well as musculoskeletal pain. In excess, vitamin E can cause similar nonspecific complaints.

Occasionally, psychiatric symptoms are caused by toxicity from **trace metals**. Aluminum toxicity has been reported in patients undergoing renal dialysis who present with an encephalopathy and symptoms of malaise, memory loss, dementia, asterixis, twitching, and seizures. Zinc can cause lethargy, and miners inhaling manganese over long periods of time can present with asthenia, anorexia, apathy, and psychosis.

Carbon monoxide toxicity may result in headache, confusion, or malaise. When chronic, it may be diagnosed erroneously neuropsychiatric disease. Diagnosis and treatment are straightforward if carbon monoxide toxicity is suspected.

ALCOHOL ABUSE

Few problems are so common, and so often ignored, as alcohol abuse. Since one in five hospitalized patients suffers from alcohol abuse (100), the consulting internist frequently will see alcohol-related health difficulties: 43% of head trauma cases admitted to a university rehabilitation program and 38% of new spinal cord injuries suffer from alcoholism (101, 102). The overall prevalence of women drinking during pregnancy has been declining (32% of pregnant women in 1985 versus 20% in 1988), but there has been no decline in alcohol consumption among young mothers under the age of 25 during pregnancy or in the less well educated (103).

In one study, however, only 45% of patients suffering from alcoholism were asked about their drinking by their doctor (104). Of those who were asked, only 25% were told to reduce their alcohol intake or were warned about the hazards of drinking, and only 3% were referred to an alcohol treatment program. An alcohol assessment should be part of the evaluation for every new patient seen by the consultant.

Problem drinking may occur with as little as 14 drinks per week (105). The "CAGE" questionnaire, which was developed by John Ewing (106), is quite helpful. In it, the interviewer asks only four questions:

1. Have you ever felt you should cut down on your drinking?
2. Have people annoyed you by criticizing you about your drinking?
3. Have you ever felt guilty about your drinking?
4. Have you ever taken a drink first thing in the morning as an eye opener?

If the patient answers yes to any two of these questions, he or she probably has a drinking problem and should be referred for additional evaluation or treatment.

More complete questionnaires also are available. These include the Michigan Alcoholism Screening Test (MAST) (107) and The Alcohol Use Disorders Identification Test (AUDIT) (108).

The consultant often is the first caregiver to recognize alcoholism in the patient. These patients may have been admitted for elective surgery or for surgery after trauma, and 3 to 5 days after admission, after the surgical procedure and postoperative period seemed to be going well, they will develop a delirium. Any new delirium in this period must include alcohol withdrawal in the differential diagnosis.

Hallucinations can occur secondary to alcohol at almost any time, but they typically occur during the first 24 hours after cessation of drinking. In one series of psychiatric examinations following arrest for alcohol-related misdemeanors (e.g., driving while intoxicated), the most common major psychiatric disturbance was alcohol hallucinosis, which affected 9% of those referred for treatment at some time in their past (109).

The clinical course to follow in beginning treatment with any patient afflicted by an alcohol problem is described by the mnemonic device "TAR and feather." *TAR* comes from the triad of steps to *TELL* the patient you are concerned about his or her alcohol abuse, advise *ABSTINENCE*, and *REFER* for further alcohol counseling.

First, tell the patient you are concerned that his or her drinking has led to problems (often the one that landed him or her in the hospital or your clinic). Next, advise abstinence to the patient; however, the patient often will fight this advice. In one study of 1289 alcoholics who were evaluated at a 5- to 7-year follow-up, only 1.6% had stable, moderate drinking and only 4.6% were abstinent with occasional drinking (110). Therefore only approximately 6% of alcoholics can

drink moderately, so total abstinence from alcohol remains the goal for treatment. Finally, refer the patient for further care to AA (Alcoholics Anonymous) as well as to an appropriate treatment program, whether inpatient, day treatment, or outpatient.

Feather refers to medication to soften alcohol withdrawal and help prevent relapse. As for the proper "feather," benzodiazepines remain the cornerstone of therapy. The alcoholic patient should hardly ever be maintained on long-term benzodiazepine therapy, but brief use (1–2 weeks) is helpful in the treatment of alcohol withdrawal. These medications will help to decrease the risk of seizure, CNS symptoms of delirium, and muscle tremor, anxiety, or other psychologic disturbances. Elderly individuals or those with impaired hepatic function should be given shorter-acting benzodiazepines with less dependence on hepatic metabolism (e.g., lorazepam, oxazepam) (111).

After detoxification, each patient should be evaluated for use of naltrexone. In one series, naltrexone, 50 mg/day, cut relapse rates in half among alcoholic patients who received the it (112). In another study, naltrexone also substantially reduced relapse rates, but this improvement was seen only when the patient received supportive psychotherapy as well (113). Thus naltrexone may not reduce relapse, but it probably does the best job when used as part of a multimodal treatment program.

EATING DISORDERS AND THEIR MEDICAL COMPLICATIONS

Treatment of patients with eating disorders can be one of the most challenging situations for the consulting internist. When dealing with a young woman who has caused her own medical problems by refusing to eat or by purging food, the consultant is faced with a series of problems that often are chronic, resistant to treatment, and potentially fatal. In anorexia nervosa, mortality rates can range up to 22%. While suicide claimed 258 of these deaths, at least one-half were from the direct effects of anorexia nervosa (113a). Death rates for bulimia are not as clear, because it appears to be a rampant disorder among college-age women, with the prevalence estimated to be between 4.58 and 18% of this group (114). Bulimia can certainly be fatal, and it also can present a wide array of medical complications in young women being seen for other chief complaints and who otherwise look "normal."

Anorexia nervosa is an illness that typically strikes young women in their teens. Patients refuse to maintain their body weight above a minimally normal level, yet they have a fear of becoming overweight and go to great lengths to avoid even the slightest weight gain or appearance of any body fat. They may choose to keep their weight low by restricting their food intake; vomiting; using laxatives, diurctics, or enemas; or by some combination of these.

Bulimia also presents with a preoccupation about weight and eating, but here, the patient's weight is normal or a bit above normal. The abnormal eating behavior is characterized by "binges" of eating large, and sometimes massive, amounts of food at one setting, which then is followed by a "purge." Medical problems develop from the constant stress of these large fluid changes and losses, related electrolyte disturbances, and nutritional deficiencies. Ninety percent of bulimic patients are female.

Medical complications from these conditions are legion, severe, and sometimes fatal. Laboratory abnormalities often occur, but no single test is diagnostic. Hematologically, leukopenia and mild anemia are common (115). Fluid shifts can cause dehydration, yielding a high blood urea nitrogen, hypokalemia, and hypochloremia. Vomiting often produces a metabolic alkalosis as well (116). Low serum levels of phosphate, magnesium, and zinc can accompany these abnormal eating behaviors. Laxative abuse can

cause a metabolic acidosis, and the secretion of luteinizing hormone returns to prepubertal levels. Females also experience lower estrogen levels, and males develop lower testosterone levels (115). On the ECG, sinus bradycardia can occur, and arrhythmias are possible, especially if potassium levels are critically low. CT scans of the brain show more cerebral atrophy than found in normal controls, presumably secondary to starvation.

The serum amylase level frequently is elevated in patients with bulimia, but the ability of this one test to discriminate between these patients and normal controls is limited (117, 118). In one study, a statistically significant, positive relationship between binge frequency and serum amylase level was found in only 25% of patients (118).

The physical examination may produce important clues to the presence and severity of eating disorders. In anorexia nervosa, starvation can lead to a low heart rate, low blood pressure, and at times, a yellowing discoloration of the skin. Some patients also develop soft, fine hair covering their skin, reminiscent of the small hairs covering a newborn (i.e., lanugo). Peripheral edema may be present secondary to low serum protein levels; congestive heart failure may occur as well. Osteoporosis from calcium resorption may occur as well. Delayed pubertal development and amenorrhea are fairly common, and constipation as well as poor gastrointestinal motility also are seen.

The physical examination of patients with suspected bulimia should begin with the mouth. There, the constant washing of gastric acid past the teeth will lead to dental erosion and dental caries. Parotid and submaxillary salivary glands can be enlarged or swollen. Examination of the hands may reveal scarring or callous formation at the knuckles of the dominant hand, which are caused by scraping the hand by the teeth to induce vomiting. Potentially fatal esophageal tears, unfortunately, cannot be detected on the physical examination.

The endocrine disturbances in anorexia are legion. Starvation and weight loss lead to amenorrhea. The sex hormones and responses of luteinizing hormone and follicle-stimulating hormone resemble those of prepubertal individuals (114). Because these patients can have persistent or recurrent wide swings in weight and eating behavior, their endocrine systems sustain repeated trauma from this abnormal behavior; therefore some patients may continue to have disturbances in their endocrine regulation even after they have achieved and maintained a normal weight. One study documented that one-third of women had persistent amenorrhea despite a normal weight (114). The starved state also leads to low levels of thyroid hormones. T_3 often is low, but T_4 often is normal (116). This decrease in T_3 may be adaptive in the induced, starved state of an eating disorder, helping to reduce the metabolic rate, conserving energy, and reducing muscle catabolism (114). This relative hypothyroidism, however, is associated with cold intolerance, dry skin and hair, and sometimes, slow reflexes. Approximately 50% of patients with anorexia nervosa have elevated levels of growth hormone, but these levels usually return to normal during refeeding. Vasopressin also can be reduced in a minority of patients, leading to some polyuria.

Anorexia nervosa may develop fatal cardiac complications. The muscle mass of the left ventricle thins, and the chamber size of the left ventricle can be reduced as well (114). The combination of these factors can lead to congestive heart failure, which especially can be a problem during the refeeding of treatment in which larger fluid and protein loads can be thrust on the still weak left ventricle. Weight gain in treatment therefore should therefore be limited to 2 pounds per day. If the patient with anorexia nervosa engages in various purging strategies, electrolyte disturbances can emerge, and hypokalemia frequently occurs, which can lead to cardiac arrhythmias that may be fatal.

Starvation often is associated with dehydration. A reduced glomerular filtration rate can occur, which may predispose patients to the development of renal stones (114). Abuse of diuretic agents can further complicate renal health, along with causing electrolyte disturbances.

Starvation also takes its toll on the gastrointestinal system. Decreased gastric motility and emptying often occur, and they frequently are associated with constipation. This leads to a sensation for the patient of stomach fullness or distention, which leads them to believe that they are "stuffed" or "fat," which in turn leads them to restrict their food intake still further. Patients also may treat this "fullness" with cathartics, frequently leading to cathartic abuse. The diarrhea that follows can contribute to the patient's dehydration, complicated acid/base balance, and electrolyte disturbances (114). In addition, starvation can lead to fatty infiltration of the liver, which can be associated with elevated liver function tests.

Patients with bulimia can die suddenly from a wide array of complications. Large binges can occur in amazingly small periods of time, leading to sudden stomach distention or rupture. Repeated binging can be associated with Mallory-Weiss tears or gastric bleeding. which can lead to an acute gastrointestinal bleeding and death. Vomiting also can be associated with aspiration, which can lead to pneumonia or asphyxia. If patients use ipecac to induce vomiting, they can run into cardiac trouble as ipecac has been associated with potentially fatal myocardial dysfunction (114). Vast fluid changes and electrolyte disturbances can lead to seizures in some patients as well (119).

The more common physical complications of bulimia come from the chronic binge–purge phenomenon. The sometimes massive fluid shifts in these episodes often are associated with a loss of potassium, which then requires supplementation. This situation can be worsened if the patient with bulimia also is using diuretics to lose weight or is abusing laxatives in the mistaken notion that they may help in weight loss. Weight changes lead to menstrual irregularities in 40% of patients with bulimia (114). Constant purging also can lead to decreased gastric emptying, which can take time to resolve even after the patient has resumed normal eating. As mentioned, dental disease is common in these patients and is another chronic medical complication of bulimia.

All of these medical complications of eating disorders are serious enough by themselves, but they frequently are complicated further by substance abuse, often coexisting with the eating disorder (120). Cocaine or amphetamines may be used to lose weight, and this can be especially dangerous in combination with an eating disorder. The cardiac and electrolyte disturbances already present can be dangerously exacerbated by these stimulants as well.

The challenge to the consulting internist as part of the treatment team caring for a patient with an eating disorder is more than understanding the wide array of medical complications. The internist is confronted by a patient who is responsible for her own medical condition—and who is also fighting to further worsen her own health by continuing to lose weight, purging, and binging. Feelings of frustration and anger toward a patient, who sometimes is close to self-induced death, must be understood. It is important to realize that the patient's unreasonableness and inability to understand the nature of the illness is, in fact, the essence of the disorder.

PSYCHIATRIC PROBLEMS IN ELDERLY PATIENTS

Elderly patients may be at particular risk for certain conditions such as anxiety and depression because of a reaction to chronic disease, loss and grief, or functional decline. Psychopharmacology in geriatric patients has important differences in absorption, distribution, metabolism, excretion, and receptor sensitivity as compared with younger patients (121). Concomitant chronic health problems and polypharmacy, including over-the-counter drugs, complicate the problem. **The key concepts in prescribing psychoactive agents for elderly patients is to start at low doses, to increase the dose slowly and gradually until the therapeutic end point (which may not result in total elimination of symptoms) is achieved, to watch carefully for side effects, and to discontinue or change the medication if a therapeutic effect is not achieved.** Dosage reduction or drug elimination after several months of therapy should always be a consideration.

Depressive symptoms in elderly patients may be wrongly attributed by patients, their families, and caregivers as part of the normal aging process. Depression may accompany dementia, or dementia may appear to be the most prominent symptom of depression (the so-called *pseudodementia of depression*). Drug side effects are a common, reversible cause. In elderly patients with depression, suicide is common. White widowers who live alone, suffer from chronic medical disease, and are recently widowed or who abuse sedatives or alcohol are particularly at risk (121).

Because the classes of relevant drugs are equally effective, the major pharmacologic consideration involves the side effect profile. Tricyclic antidepressants may be more problematic in elderly patients because of orthostatic hypotension and anticholinergic properties. Newer agents, such as the SSRIs, have fewer side effects. Anxiety (the so-called *serotonin syndrome*) may be a problem, but it usually can be avoided by use of lower starting doses. The older heterocyclic antidepressants nortriptyline and desipramine may be useful, and despite having little anticholinergic effect (though orthostatic hypotension can be a problem), trazodone is useful in that it is sedating and can be useful when agitation or insomnia are prominent features of depression. When one or two agents have proved to be ineffective after an adequate therapeutic trial, other options include dual therapy, augmentation with thyroid hormone or lithium, use of MAO, methylphenidate, or ECT (122).

Table 21.6 summarizes the clinical features of delirium, dementia, and acute functional psychosis. Anxiety and insomnia are common in elderly patients, and benzodiazepine therapy often is hazardous. Increased incidence of falls, cognitive decline, depression, oversedation, dementia, delirium, rebound insomnia, and withdrawal must be considered. Therapy should be of short duration and use smaller doses than for younger patients. CNS effects are exaggerated, and the half-lives of many preparations essen-

tially are doubled (123). Lorazepam, oxazepam, and alprazolam have shorter half-lives and seem to be the preferred agents. Nonpharmacologic therapies, including sleep hygiene, counseling, exercise, and avoidance of stimulants and alcohol, are important adjuncts. Other agents include zolpidem, buspirone, low-dose sedative antidepressants, β-blockers, and carbamazepine, which has been shown to be useful in agitated nursing home patients with dementia.

Psychosis in elderly patients most commonly results from dementia. Therapy with neuroleptic agents often is necessary. The major difficulties include tardive dyskinesia, anticholinergic effects, and orthostatic hypotension. Therapy should be of short duration when possible, and dosage

Table 21.6. Clinical Features of Delirium, Dementia, and Acute Functional Psychosis

Characteristic	Delirium	Dementia	Acute Functional Psychosis
Onset	Sudden	Insidious	Sudden
Course over 24 hours	Fluctuating, with nocturnal exacerbation	Stable	Stable
Consciousness	Reduced	Clear	Clear
Attention	Globally disordered	Normal, except in severe cases	May be disordered
Cognition	Globally disordered	Globally impaired	May be selectively impaired
Hallucinations	Usually visual or visual and auditory	Often absent	Predominantly auditory
Delusions	Fleeting, poorly systematized	Often absent	Sustained, systematized
Orientation	Usually impaired, at least for a time	Often impaired	May be impaired
Psychomotor activity	Increased, reduced, or shifting unpredictably	Often normal	Varies from psychomotor retardation to severe hyperactivity, depending on the type of psychosis
Speech	Often incoherent, slow or rapid	Patient has difficulty finding words, perseveration	Normal, slow or rapid
Involuntary movements	Often asterixis or coarse tremor	Often absent	Usually absent
Physical illness or drug toxicity	One or both are present	Often absent, especially in senile dementia of the Alzheimer's type	Usually absent

reduction or drug elimination is a key consideration. Lower-potency agents such as chlorpromazine or thioridazine have less potential for tardive dyskinesia and extrapyramidal symptoms, but they are more sedating and have more autonomic side effects than more-potent agents such as haloperidol or risperidone.

Geriatric patients, and especially those with dementia, are at particular risk for elder abuse. Violent behavior and violent feelings toward the patient among family caregivers are relatively common. A high degree of suspicion and a proactive, nonjudgmental approach likely will allow appropriate intervention to be made. One study (125) examined caregivers (including adult children) caring for parents (55%), spouses caring for spouses (37%), and other relatives providing care (8%). Based on self-reporting, physical abuse of patients was discovered in 12% and abuse of caregivers in 33%. Caregivers who reported abusive behavior directed at them by patients also reported a higher rate of elder abuse (124, 125). In general, abusive caregivers were involved in the care of patients who had mild dementia, who were older, and who reported more deteriorating health (126). Strategies for help include providing respite care for the patient, reducing stress and fatigue for the caregiver, and counseling and therapy for specific behaviors, particularly aggressive behavior by the patient.

ANTIPSYCHOTIC DRUGS

As a general rule, more-potent antipsychotic drugs have a greater potential to cause acute dystonic reactions, parkinsonian side effects, and akathisia. Less-potent drugs have a greater propensity to cause sedation, cardiac side effects, and anticholinergic side effects. Because sedation is such a problem in the long-term use of these agents, higher-potency (and less-sedating) drugs such as haloperidol and thiothixene are most commonly used.

Acute dystonic reactions are muscle contractions of virtually any voluntary muscle, which usually occur in the first few days of treatment with antipsychotic drugs. Young men are especially vulnerable to these effects. Musculature of the neck, face, back, and tongue most often are affected; rarely, laryngeal dystonia may occur, causing compromise of the airway (127). Because these symptoms often occur in those who are beginning treatment and in those who are already suffering from a frightening psychotic illness, prompt treatment of these distressing symptoms is essential. Use of diphenhydramine, 50 mg intramuscularly or intravenously, often is quite effective, and it can be repeated every hour as needed to control the symptoms. Anticholinergic medication such as benztropine, 1 to 2 mg, or trihexyphenidyl, 2 to 4 mg, also can be given intramuscularly to help alleviate symptoms. Once these symptoms occur, patients are given standing doses of anticholinergic medications to prevent recurrences.

Parkinsonian side effects are common with these drugs, affecting approximately two-thirds of patients who first take the medication. These symptoms are caused by the dopamine blockade of the drugs, and they can mimic virtually any symptom of Parkinson's disease. Tremor, rigidity, cogwheel rigidity, masked facies, flat affect, micrographia, drooling, festinating gait, and even mental slowness are common. It sometimes is difficult to determine which symptoms are side effects of medication and which are from the original illness; symptoms such as flat affect, mental slowness, and masked facies can come from either source. Fortunately, treatment for these symptoms is quite effective. Typically, anticholinergic agents such as benztropine, biperiden, and trihexyphenidyl are used at gradually progressive doses until the symptoms are controlled. Typical antiparkinsonian agents such as carbidopa or even amantadine usually are avoided, however, because dopaminergic agents may worsen psychotic symptoms.

Akathisia is an intense, uncomfortable sensation of feeling the need to move. Patients appear to be restless and often pace during the course of your interview. It may be impossible to determine whether a patient is suffering anxiety from their psychiatric disorder or akathisia from their medication; however, if the patient identifies ambulation as helping with the symptoms, it is more likely akathisia. Use of medication for this side effect is less successful than for the other side effects previously mentioned. Anticholinergic medications such as benztropine or trihexyphenidyl usually are attempted first. Propranolol generally is the drug of second choice. Benzodiazepines at bed time can be of some use for this troublesome side effect. Fortunately, the half-life of these agents is long enough to allow once-a-day dosing.

Cardiac side effects mainly occur with low-potency antipsychotic medications. Especially in the setting of an overdose, these side effects can be dangerous and even lethal. Tachycardia and hypertension (especially postural hypertension) are the usual side effects. In addition, cardiac conduction can be slowed in a quinidine-like fashion, and cardiac conduction may be prolonged (128).

Anticholinergic side effects such as dry mouth, blurry vision, and urinary retention are common, especially with low-potency drugs. Severe tachycardia or urinary retention in older men with prosthetic hypertrophy, however, can represent dangerous or emergency-level side effects and are more common with lower-potency drugs.

One of the more unfortunate side effects of typically used antipsychotic agents, tardive dyskinesia is the involuntary muscle movement of any muscle group. Usually, however, it involves the oral–buccal musculature. Muscles of the trunk can be involved as well, thus producing choreiform movements. The cause of this side effect likely is related to persistent dopamine blockade that results in dopamine-receptor supersensitivity to any remaining dopamine in the synapse. This causes excitation or extra movements from any dopamine that is transmitted (129).

Tardive dyskinesia occurs in 4% of patients per year of treatment. Elderly patients are at greater risk (130), and using lower doses of antipsychotic medication probably is protective (131, 132). To screen for tardive dyskinesia, the Abnormal Involuntary Movement Scale (AIMS) is helpful both in making the diagnosis and in documenting the severity of the disorder (133). No good treatment for tardive dyskinesia is available. Once recognized, however, the risks of continuing with the medication versus the risks of the tardive dyskinesia must be assessed and discussed with the patient. Addition of benzodiazepines and withdrawal of accompanying anticholinergic medications can be helpful. It should be noted that not all dyskinesias caused by the antipsychotic medications are "tardive" dyskinesia, and that immediately on discontinuation of antipsychotic agents, some patients experience dyskinetic movements, which typically resolve over several weeks.

Neuroleptic malignant syndrome is a potentially lethal complication of treatment with antipsychotic drugs that is characterized by fever, muscular rigidity, delirium, and autonomic dysfunction (134). Neuroleptic malignant syndrome must be included in the differential diagnosis of any patient receiving antipsychotic medications who has extrapyramidal symptoms and fever. Fortunately, this is a relatively uncommon situation, however, with rates estimated at from 0.2 to 1% (135–137). Muscular stiffness and stress can be quite severe, causing large elevations in the creatine phosphokinase level and significant myoglobinuria (138). Autonomic instability and even heat stroke can occur (139). Treatment with dantrolene (for drug fever), bromocriptine (for the dopamine blockade from antipsychotic drugs), or both has been helpful (140, 141). For dantrolene, 1 to 3 mg/kg per day given orally or intravenously in four divided doses generally has been used. Bromocriptine is begun at 2.5 mg orally three times a day and is increased to 5 to 10 mg orally three times a day as tolerated by the patient (127). These doses are continued for 1 week following resolution of the symptoms. Supportive measures, including fluids, attention to the patient's airway and need for oxygen, and ice packs or cooling blankets to bring down the patient's temperature, are essential. The patient's cardiovascular and renal status must be carefully monitored and supported, and subsequent treatment with antipsychotic medications should be avoided. If retreatment is chosen, the patient should be followed carefully for any reemergence of neuroleptic malignant syndrome (142–144). If patients cannot be sustained without antipsychotic treatment, the drug treatment with thioridazine (i.e., a low-potency antipsychotic), risperidone, or clozapine should be considered.

Antipsychotic medications also inhibit prolactin-inhibiting factor in the brain, which leads to a peripheral increase in prolactin. Lactation in women and gynecomastia in men can develop, and sexual side effects of virtually any kind can occur as well. Men suffer from erectile dysfunction and anorgasmia. Women may develop problems with arousal and vaginal lubrication as well as anorgasmia.

Central changes in temperature regulation also can occur, thus making heat stroke more likely. Therefore, especially in the summer months, patients need to be cautioned about proper sun protection. Changes in retinal pigmentation can occur as well, especially with doses of thioridazine greater than 800 mg/day.

Antipsychotic medications can be dangerous when overdose occurs, and because they are given to patients who are more likely to commit suicide, this is a strong concern. The major danger results from cardiac effects. Low-potency drugs in particular can cause hypertension as well as widening of the QRS complex, even lead-ing to full heart block. Hypotension is best treated with volume expansion. β-Adrenergic agonists should be avoided (23). Hypotension that does not respond to fluids can be treated with vasopressors such as norepinephrine (Levophed) or phenylephrine (Neo-synephrine) (127).

Antipsychotic agents lower the seizure threshold, and in an overdose, they may produce marked CNS excitation. Treatment of CNS excitation in the setting of an overdose can be accomplished through use of benzodiazepines.

Newer Agents

Approximately one-third of previously unresponsive patients will improve in the first 6 weeks of treatment with clozapine (145). In addition, clozapine often is better tolerated than traditional antipsychotic medications. It has a low rate of extrapyramidal symptoms or tardive dyskinesia, probably because it seems to target dopamine systems in the cortical and limbic regions rather than the nigrostriatal or tuberoinfundibular regions of the brain (146). Use of this drug is associated with a 1% risk of agranulocytosis, however, and mandatory weekly checks of white blood cell counts are required (147). There is a dose-related, increased risk of seizure, ranging from 0.6% in patients receiving less than 300 mg/day to 14% in patients receiving greater than 600 mg/day (146).

Because of the cost and monitoring problems associated with its use, clozapine usually is reserved for those patients who are severely ill from schizophrenia and who have not responded to other medications (148). It sometimes is used to treat psychotic symptoms in bipolar disorder or resistant agitation in dementia. Its lack of extrapyramidal side effects made it a drug to consider in elderly patients or those suffering from psychotic symptoms or Parkinson's disease (149, 150).

Risperidone is another useful antipsychotic medication. At least in low doses, the drug is more free of the traditional side effects associated with antipsychotic medications. Starting doses begin at 1 mg orally twice a day and then increase gradually to 3 mg orally twice a day as needed. At doses greater than that amount, the drug can carry significant muscular side effects (similar to those with haloperidol), and maximal antipsychotic efficacy in most patients is within that 1 to 3 mg dosage range. Hypotension as well as insomnia, agitation, anxiety, headache, and extrapyramidal reactions can occur, but risperidone generally is better tolerated than traditional drugs.

Blanzapine, sertindole, seroquel, and ziprosirosidone are other potentially effective agents with lower rates of side effects.

Medications for Bipolar Disorder

Lithium carbonate remains the cornerstone of treatment for bipolar disorder. It is helpful in relieving the symptoms of an acute episode and in maintaining a stable mood. Because it is a "maintenance drug," those suffering from this disorder often continue taking the drug for years.

Lithium has a narrow therapeutic window, so frequent measurements of blood levels should be done (at least every 2 months). For an acute episode of mania, the patient's blood level should be 1.0 to 1.5 mEq/L, but for maintenance therapy, a blood level of 0.45 to 0.8 mEq/L often is sufficient (151, 152). Blood levels are drawn 12 hours after the last dose.

Gastrointestinal symptoms are the most commonly encountered side effects and include nausea, vomiting, diarrhea, cramps, and anorexia (128). Usually, these symptoms will diminish over time; use of postprandial dosing may help.

Lithium therapy also can lead to a decline in the glomerular filtration rate (153). Measuring the 24-hour urinary creatinine clearance is a good way to monitor renal functioning. Even if the patient's renal concentrating ability is decreased, it is not necessary to stop lithium therapy, because no death from lithium-induced renal insufficiency has ever been reported (154).

Hypothyroidism can be a side effect of lithium as well, occurring in one survey among 7.8% of patients on lithium (155). In general, if hypothyroidism appears de novo with lithium therapy, it is better to add thyroid supplementation than to remove lithium treatment when the patient clearly is benefiting.

Weight gain, which sometimes is significant, can occur with lithium therapy. If this is a problem, the patient should be checked for lithium-induced hypothyroidism.

Cardiac side effects of lithium usually are benign. They include ECG changes such as T-wave flattening and QRS widening (128).

When lithium is being administered, nonsteroidal antiinflammatory agents or angiotensin-converting inhibitors should be used with caution, because both can increase lithium levels to a potentially toxic range (151, 152). Thiazide diuretics can raise lithium levels as well (154). Lithium may also prolong the neuromuscular blockade of both depolarizing and nondepolarizing anesthetic agents; therefore lithium should be stopped, if possible, 2 to 3 days before anesthesia (128).

Lithium use has been associated with cardiac malformations in the fetus. In addition, widely varying lithium levels in both the mother and the fetus can be found at birth because of the wide fluid shifts that occur surrounding delivery. However, removal of lithium therapy in a woman with recurrent affective disorder may place both mother and baby at risk for a recurrence of the mood disorder and any associated behavioral consequences.

If lithium use is maintained during pregnancy, it is wise to stop it 2 weeks before the anticipated delivery date to avoid wide shifts of drug levels in the blood. Carbamazepine or valproate sometimes are used instead of lithium in patients with bipolar disorder; however, when used during pregnancy, both drugs are associated with higher rates of spina bifida in infants. If a woman has been stable on lithium for years and suffered severe episodes of illness before such therapy, both she and her physician sometimes simply agree to continue therapy during pregnancy while carefully monitoring the fetus.

Lithium intoxication can be a medical emergency. Hemodialysis can be used to quickly clear lithium from the body if blood levels are greater than 2.5 mEq/liter or if the patient is severely ill. After hemodialysis is stopped, there may be a rebound increase in lithium level from the drug pouring out of the intracellular space into the extracellular space. Lithium levels should be monitored in the hours following hemodialysis, and if the levels rise, hemodialysis may be needed again (156). Intravenous fluids are necessary if lithium toxicity has induced vomiting, thus leading to volume depletion (151, 152, 154).

If lithium intoxication results from an acute overdose, vomiting should be induced to remove lithium from the stomach. Even after lithium levels are low or reach zero, which can occur quickly with hemodialysis, the patient may continue to suffer from a resolving delirium that could take weeks to fully clear.

Lithium also sometimes is used as an augmentation strategy in patients with unipolar depression if the original antidepressant drug is not effective (157–159).

The second-line drug for treatment of bipolar disorder is carbamazepine. Since 1980, it has been used either alone or in combination with lithium when lithium alone has been ineffective. Approximately two-thirds of patients with treatment-resistant bipolar disorder show a favorable response to carbamazepine (160–162). Clinicians generally aim for a blood level of between 4 and 12 vg/mL. Carbamazepine generally is well tolerated, but it can lead to drowsiness and ataxia, especially in elderly patients

(128). Blurred vision, nausea, and vomiting also can occur. White blood cell counts may transiently decrease, especially at the beginning of therapy, but agranulocytosis and aplastic anemia are rare, only occurring in approximately 1 per 125,000 patients.

Several drug interactions with carbamazepine should be noted. Erythromycin, verapamil, diltiazem, and propoxyphene can raise carbamazepine levels. Carbamazepine can decrease the levels of haloperidol and birth control pills. Perhaps the most common drug interaction of carbamazepine, however, is with itself: carbamazepine can autoinduce its own enzymes and cause blood levels of the drug to drop after several weeks of treatment.

Medication for Major Depression

There is a 4% prevalence rate of major depression in the United States. All of the newer drugs work equally well, and all work as well as the older tricyclic antidepressants. The major advantage of the newer agents is a more favorable side effect profile, especially in those patients with severe or chronic medical illnesses.

Currently, SSRIs available for use in the United States include: (a) fluoxetine (Prozac), (b) sertraline (Zoloft), (c) paroxetine (Paxil), and (d) fluvoxamine (Luvox). Fluvoxamine has been approved for use only in patients with obsessive–compulsive disorder. These four drugs are quite similar, however, and vary mainly in their half-lives. Fluoxetine has the longest half-life (2–3 days) and fluvoxamine the shortest (approximately 12 hours).

The SSRIs effectively treat approximately 70% of patients with major depression. They usually are well tolerated, but gastrointestinal upset, nausea, anorexia, or weight gain affects perhaps 20% of patients. Nervousness or agitation affects somewhat fewer patients. A few will find sleeplessness to be a persistent problem, whereas others will complain of sedation. Sexual side effects of all kinds commonly occur with both sexes, and while the exact prevalence is unknown, problems in sexual functioning may be the most common side effect of these drugs. Because they have little effect on the heart, they have become the drugs of choice in those patients with cardiac disease (163). For the same reason, these agents also are remarkably safe during an overdose (164). Elderly patients typically tolerate the SSRIs well and therefore can take the medication long enough to receive the benefit of drug treatment (165, 166).

Use of MAO inhibitors with fluoxetine can be fatal (167); thus, because of the long half-life of fluoxetine, one should wait 6 weeks after stopping fluoxetine (or 2 weeks after stopping other SSRIs) before beginning an MAO inhibitor. Fluoxetine should not be used with terfenadine (Seldane), astemizole (Hismanal), or cisapride (Propulsid). Using fluoxetine in combination with these drugs can lead to increased an plasma concentration of these substances, which in turn can lead to QT prolongation and possible torsades de pointes–type ventricular tachycardia. It probably is wise to avoid use of these other drugs with the other SSRIs as well.

Sertraline (Zoloft) is another novel, specific SSRI. The main difference between this drug and fluoxetine is in its shorter half-life (26 hours) (168).

Shortly after bupropion (Wellbutrin) was introduced in 1986, it was quickly withdrawn from the market, because a relatively large percentage of patients with bulimia suffered seizures during a trial with the drug (169). Bupropion then was extensively studied for seizure risk. If the dosage is kept below the recommended maximum 450 mg/day, the risk of seizure varies from 0.35 to 0.44% (170), compared with a risk for fluoxetine or tricyclic antidepressants of approximately 0.28%. Its efficacy is similar to that of fluoxetine or doxepin (i.e., a tricyclic antidepressant), and its side effects are similar to those of fluoxetine in many respects (171, 172). Bupropion has few cardiac side effects and is safe to use in patients with congestive heart failure (173, 174), and it produces remarkably few sexual side effects (175). Bupropion thus may be the drug of choice for patients who have experienced sexual side effects on other antidepressants.

Venlafaxine (Effexor) is another novel antidepressant agent that inhibits the reuptake of serotonin and norepinephrine, and it has some effect blocking the reuptake of dopamine as well (176). It offers a very favorable cardiac side effect profile as well (177, 178). When used in a dosage greater than 200 mg/day, however, hypertension becomes a problem in more than 5% of patients.

Nefazodone (Serzone) is another novel antidepressant compound that is similar chemically to trazodone. Nefazodone is another well-tolerated and effective drug in the treatment of depression, but it produces less sedation than trazodone (179, 180). Nefazodone also may produce less sexual side effects than other antidepressant agents, but clinical experience with the compound is not sufficient to document this clearly.

Trazodone (Desyrel) is an effective antidepressant agent. It most often is used as a sleeping aid, however, usually in combination with one of the newer antidepressant drugs.

In some clinical situations, the tricyclic antidepressants continue to have advantages. Because these agents have been used clinically for decades, generic brands are available that cost much less than brand-name antidepressants. Also, the tricyclic antidepressants are quite sedating, which usually is a problem but sometimes can be a benefit in patients with chronic sleep problems. In addition, clear therapeutic ranges have been established for the blood levels of these compounds (181), and they are helpful in the setting of chronic neurogenic pain as well.

The tricyclic antidepressants include amitriptyline, nortriptyline, protriptyline, imipramine, desipramine, chlorimipramine, and doxepin. Because of their many side effects, they typically are started at low doses and increased incrementally every 3 to 4 days until the level of 150 to 300 mg/day of amitriptyline or imipramine is reached. Typical side effects, which have made these agents less popular today, are sedation and a wide array of anticholinergic side effects, including dry mouth, blurry vision, constipation, and urinary retention.

Weight gain and sexual side effects also occur with these agents (182). The main concern, however, with tricyclic antidepressants is that they produce a number of significant cardiac effects. These drugs prolong cardiac conduction, as manifested by increased PR, QRS, or QT intervals (183), and they can cause significant orthostatic hypotension (184). Nortriptyline seems to be the tricyclic antidepressant that produces the least orthostasis (185). Unexplained death has been reported as well.

Treatment of overdose involves gastric lavage and use of activated charcoal to prevent absorption of these agents. The cardiac effects of these drugs mandate close cardiovascular monitoring, and the hypotensive effects of these agents often require fluids to be given to raise the patient's blood pressure. Increased QRS duration alerts the clinician to a toxic effect on cardiac conduction and should be monitored. Supraventricular tachycardia may respond to use of propranolol, but use of digoxin should be avoided as it may precipitate heart block (127). Likewise, use of quinidine, procainamide, and disopyramide should also be avoided, because these agents may further prolong the QRS interval.

The MAO inhibitors remain effective drugs. However, because of the need to maintain a tyramine-free diet with their use as well as concern about drug interactions, they are not typically first-line agents in the treatment of depression. Only 25% of psychiatrists regularly prescribe these drugs (186). To use them, the patient must agree to avoid food with a high tyramine content (e.g., cheeses, liver, smoked or pickled fish, red wine, beer, excessive amounts of caffeine). Still, the "cheese reaction," which can lead to a hypertensive crisis, is relatively uncommon (187). More worrisome are drug interactions, which can lead to unpredictable rises in blood pressure. Combining MAO inhibitors with sympathomimetic agents (e.g., amphetamines) or with narcotic analgesic agents (e.g., meperidine) can cause a hypertensive crisis. MAO inhibitors combined with guanethidine can cause severe hypotension, and because MAO inhibitors commonly cause orthostatic hypotension, combining them with antihypertensive agents can be risky as well. Combined use of tricyclic antidepressants and MAO inhibitors are used occasionally and cautiously in patients who are treatment resistant, but MAO inhibitors should never be combined with SSRIs or other, newer agents (188).

Light therapy is being increasingly used to treat seasonal affective disorder, in which depressive symptoms are experienced at the same time each year (usually during the fall and winter months) and the patient is well at the same time each year. The incidence of seasonal affective disorder rises with increasing geographic latitude, and the disorder generally is not as disabling as typical major depression. Seasonal affective disorder can cause significant symptoms, however. Treatment of this disorder generally involves the patient being exposed to a bright light (10,000 lux, or approximately 20 times as bright as ordinary room light) for 2 hours from 6 to 8 AM. If morning light exposure is not effective, using light in the evening can be considered (189). Alternatively, a "dawn simulator," which gives gradually increasing light leading to awakening, also is an effective treatment for winter depression (190). Light therapy usually is well tolerated, producing only occasional headaches or eyestrain (191). Its effectiveness probably is not due to simple light exposure but rather to the light retraining the intrinsic brain rhythms, which may be thrown out of rhythm by the shorter winter days. Thus, in effect, lengthening days by extending the exposure of the brain to bright light may reset these rhythms and the brain, thus resolving depressive symptoms.

TREATMENT OF ANXIETY DISORDERS

Pharmacologic treatment of certain anxiety disorders, such as obsessive–compulsive or panic disorder, often involves the use of antidepressant agents. Chlorimpramine or fluoxetine often are used in the treatment of obsessive–compulsive disorder. Many antidepressant drugs are useful in the treatment of panic disorder, and the MSO inhibitors are the most effective drugs for this condition. Because of their many troublesome side effects, however, MAO inhibitors usually are not first-choice drugs for this condition. SSRIs typically are used first in panic disorders, and tricyclic antidepressants often are used as well.

The most common drugs used in the treatment of generalized anxiety disorder remain the benzodiazepines. Buspirone, however, which is a nonbenzodiazepine compound, also is available to treat anxiety (192). A controlled comparison of buspirone with diazepam showed that buspirone has anxiolytic properties similar to those of diazepam (193). Diazepam seemed to be more effective in treatment of the somatic symptoms of anxiety, however, and buspirone was more effective in treatment of the cognitive and interpersonal problems associated with anxiety. In addition, buspirone clearly is not a readily abusable drug (194). However, because the agent takes several weeks to become fully effective, buspirone is not effective as am "as needed" medication, and it does not give an immediate calming sense. Thus many patients prefer the wide array of benzodiazepines as treatment for anxiety symptoms, and these agents are the mainstay pharmacologic treatment for acute anxiety or generalized anxiety disorder.

An agent also is now available to reverse the effects of benzodiazepines in the event of overdose or oversedation. Flumazenil typically is given intravenously at an initial dose of 0.2 mg. The onset of action is rapid and dramatic, with reversal of sedation often occurring within 1 to 2 minutes. Because the duration of action often is less than 1 hour, however, it is significantly shorter than the half-life of the benzodiazepine being blocked. Thus successive doses often are needed until the patient has recovered from the benzodiazepine overdose or oversedation.

Appendix
Some Drugs that Cause Psychiatric Symptoms

Drug	Reactions	Comments
Acyclovir	Hallucinations, fearfulness, confusion, insomnia, hyperacusis, paranoia, depression	At high doses, particularly in patients with chronic renal failure
Amantadine (Symmetrel)[a]	Visual hallucinations, paranoid delusions, nightmares, mania, exacerbation of schizophrenia	Several reports: more frequent in elderly
Amphetamine-like drugs	Bizarre behavior, hallucinations, paranoia, agitation, anxiety, manic symptoms	Usually with overdose or abuse; can occur with **inhaler abuse**
Amphotericin B (Fungizone)	Delirium	With intravenous and intrathecal use
Anabolic steroids	Aggression, mania, depression, psychosis	Several reports
Anticonvulsants	Agitation, confusion, delirium depression, psychosis, aggression, mania, toxic encephalopathy	Usually with high doses or high plasma concentrations
Antidepressants, tricyclic	Mania or hypomania, hallucinations, paranoia	Mania or hypomania in approximately 10% of patients; also after withdrawal
Antihistamines	Anxiety, hallucinations, delirium	Especially with overdosage
Atropine and anticholinergics	Confusion, memory loss, disorientation, depersonalization, delirium, auditory and visual hallucination, fear, paranoia, agitation, bizarre behavior	More frequent in elderly and children with high doses; has occurred with transdermal scopolamine
Barbiturates	Excitement, hyperactivity, visual hallucinations, depression, delirium tremens–like syndrome	Especially in children and elderly patients or on withdrawal
Belladonna alkaloids	See "Atropine and anticholinergics"	
Benzodiazepines	Rage, hostility, paranoia, hallucinations, depression, insomnia, nightmares, anterograde amnesia	During treatment or on withdrawal; may be more common in elderly patients
β-Adrenergic blockers	Depression, confusion, nightmares, hallucinations, paranoia, delusions, mania, hyperactivity	With usual doses, including ophthalmic use
Captopril	Severe anxiety, hallucinations, insomnia, mania	Especially in depressed patients
Cimetidine (Tagamet)	See "Histamine H_2-receptor antagonists"	

605

Drug	Reactions	Comments
Cocaine	Anxiety, agitation, psychosis	Can occur with topical use
Codeine	See "Narcotics"	
Contraceptives, oral	Depression	In 15% in one study[1]
Corticosteroids (prednisone, cortisone, ACTH, others)	Mania, depression, confusion, paranoia, hallucinations, catatonia	Especially with high doses; can occur on withdrawal or with inhalation
Cyclobenzaprine	Mania, hyperactivity, psychosis	In several reports[2]
Dapson	Insomnia, agitation, hallucinations, mania	Several reports; may occur even with low doses
Deet (Off)[a]	Toxic encephalopathy, mania, hallucinations	With excessive or prolonged use, particularly in infants and children
Digitalis glycosides	Nightmares, euphoria, confusion, amnesia, aggression, psychosis, depression	Especially high doses or high plasma levels and in elderly patients
Disopyramide (Norpace)[a]	Agitation, panic, depression, psychosis	Within 24–48 hours after starting
Ephedrine	Hallucinations, paranoia	Excessive dosage
Histamine H_2-receptor antagonists	Hallucinations, paranoia, bizarre behavior, delirium, disorientation, depression, mania	Usually with high dosage; more often in elderly patients; renal dysfunction
Interferon alfa (Roferon-A; Intron A)[a]	Delirium, paranoia, depression, suicidal thoughts, anxiety	In 10 of 58 patients with viral hepatitis[3]
Isoniazid (INH)[a]	Depression, agitation, hallucinations, paranoia	Several reports
Isotretinoin (Accutane)	Depression	In several reports[4]
Levodopa (Dopar)[a]	Delirium, depression, agitation, hypomania, nightmares, night terrors, hallucinations, paranoia	More frequent in elderly patients or with prolonged use
Methyldopa (Aldomet)[a]	Depression, amnesia, nightmares, psychosis	Several reports
Methylphenidate (Ritalin)[a]	Hallucinations, paranoia	Several reports in children
Methysergide (Sansert)	Depersonalization, hallucinations, agitation	Several reports
Metoclopramide (Reglan)[a]	Mania, severe depression, crying, delirium	Several reports
Narcotics	Nightmares, anxiety, agitation, euphoria, dysphoria, depression, paranoia, hallucinations	Usually with high doses
Nonsteroidal anti-inflammatory drugs	Paranoia, depression, inability to concentrate, anxiety, confusion, hallucinations, hostility	Not reported with all drugs in this class
Phenelzine (Nardil)	Paranoia, delusions, fear, mania, rage	Mania or hypomania in approximately 10% of depressed patients
Phenylephrine (Neo-Synephrine)[a]	Depression, hallucinations, paranoia	Overuse of nasal spray
Prazosin (Minipress)[a]	Hallucinations, depression, paranoia	In four patients; two had renal failure[5]
Procaine derivatives	Terror, confusion, psychosis, agitation, bizarre behavior, depression, panic	Many reports, especially with penicillin G procaine
Quinidine	Confusion, agitation, psychosis	Usually dose related
Reserpine (Serpasil)[a]	Depression, nightmares	Common with >0.5 mg/day

Drug	Reactions	Comments
Salicylates	Agitation, confusion, hallucinations, paranoia	Chronic intoxication
Theophylline	Withdrawal, mutism, hyperactivity, anxiety, mania	Usually with high serum concentrations
Thyroid hormones	Mania, depression, hallucinations, paranoia	Initial doses in susceptible patients
Tranylcypromine (Parnate)	Mania or hypomania	In approximately 10% of depressed patients

Modified with permission from Med Lett 1993;35:65–70.
[a]Also available with other brand names or generically.
[1]J Leeton, Aust NZ. J Obstet Gynaecol 1993;13:115–118.
[2]AR Beeber, JM Manring, Jr. J Clin Psychiatry 1983;44:151–152; HH Harsch, Psychosomatics 1984;25:791–793. PA Engel, D Chapron, J. Clin Psychiatry 1993;54:39.
[3]PF Renault et al. Arch Intern Med 1987;147:1577–1580. JL Levenson, HJ Fallon. Am J Gastroenterol 1993;88:760–761.
[4]PG Hazen et al. J Am Acad Dermatol 1983;9:278–281. PL Scheinman et al. J Am Acad Dermatol 1990;22:1112–1117.
[5]DKF Chin et al. Br Med J 1986;293–297. JF Patterson. J Clin Psychopharmacol 1988;8:228–233.

REFERENCES

1. Chandler JD, Gerndt JE. The role of the medical evaluation in psychiatric inpatients. Psychosomatics 1988;29:410–416.
2. Kampmeier RH. Diagnosis and treatment of physical disease in the mentally ill. Ann Intern Med 1977;86:637–645.
3. Barnes RF, Mason JC, Greer C, et al. Medical illness in chronic psychiatric outpatients. Gen Hosp Psychiatry 1983;5:181–195.
4. McCarrick K, Manderscheid HW, Bertolucci E, et al. Chronic medical problems of the chronic mentally ill. Hosp Community Psychiatry 1986;37:289–291.
5. McMahon LM, Longabaugh R, Desrosiers M, Kriebel GW Jr. Management of physical problems in a psychiatric hospital: a study of problem-oriented patient care. Quality Rev Board 1981;7(8):13–19.
6. Hall RCW, Popkin MK, Devaul RA, et al. Physical illness presenting as psychiatric disease. Arch Gen Psychiatry 1978;35:1315–1320.
7. Koranyi EK. Morbidity and rate of undiagnosed physical illnesses in a psychiatric clinic population. Arch Gen Psychiatry 1979;38:414–419.
8. Dolan JG, Muchlin Al. Routine laboratory testing for medical disorders in psychiatric inpatients. Arch Intern Med 1985;145:2085–2088.
8a. Holister LE. Electrocardiographic screening in psychiatric patients. J Clin Psychiatry 1995;56(1):26–29.
9. Achong MR, Keane PM. Pheochromocytoma unmasked by desipramine therapy. Ann Intern Med 1981;94:358–359.
10. Trainer PJ, Grossman A. The diagnosis and differential diagnosis of Cushing's syndrome. Clin Endocrinol 1991;34:317–330.
11. Yanovski JA, Cutler GB, Chrousos GP, Nieman LK. Corticotropin-releasing hormone stimulation following low-dose dexamethasone administration: a new test to distinguish Cushing's syndrome from pseudo-Cushing's states. JAMA 1993;269:2232–2238.
12. Carney RM, Rich MW, teVelde A, Saini J, Clark K. Prevalence of major depressive disorder in patients receiving beta-blocker therapy versus other medications. Am J Med 1987;83:223–226.
13. Peet M. The treatment of anxiety with beta-blocking drugs. 1988;64(Suppl 2):45–49.
14. Brantigan CO, Brantigan TA, Joseph N. Effect of beta blockade and beta stimulation on stage fright. Am J Med 1982;72:88–94.
15. Crogg SH, Levin S, Tevta MA, et al. The effects of antihypertensive therapy on the quality of life. N Engl J Med 1986;314:1657–1664.
16. Kvasnicka J, Flack JM, Grimm RH. Treatment of hypertension in the presence of coexisting medical conditions. Drugs Aging 1994;4:304–312.
17. Rabkin JG, Charles E, Kass F. Hypertension and DSM-III depression in psychiatric outpatients. Am J Psychiatry 1983;140:1072–1074.
18. Teitelbaum M. A significant increase in lithium levels after concomitant ACE inhibitor administration. Psychosomatics 1993;34:450–453.

19. Kushnir SL, Ratner JT. Calcium channel blockers for tardive dyskinesia in geriatric psychiatric patients. Am J Psychiatry 1989;146:1218–1219.

19a. Wassertheil-Smoller S, et al. Change in depression as a precursor of cardiovascular events. Arch Intern Med 1996;156:553–561.

20. Gustafson Y, Brannstrom B, Norberg A, Bucht G, Winblad B. Underdiagnosis and poor documentation of acute confusional states in elderly hip fracture patients. J Am Geriatr Soc 1991; 39:760–765.

20a. Golinger RC. Delirium in surgical patients seen at psychiatric consultation. Surg Gynecol Obstet 1986;163:104–106.

21. Butler DJ, Turkal NW, Seidl JJ. Amputation: preoperative psychological preparation. J Am Board Fam Pract 1992;5:69–73.

22. Rockwell DA, Pepitone Rockwell F. The emotional impact of surgery and the value of informed consent. Med Clin North Am 1979;63: 1341–1351.

23. Havdala HS, et al. Potential hazards and applications of lithium in anesthesia. Anesthesiology 1979;50:534–537.

24. Folstein MF, Folstein SE, McHugh PR. "Mini-Mental State": a practical method for grading the cognitive state of patients for the clinician. J Psychiatry Res 1975;12:189–198.

25. Lieberman, JA, Kane JM, Johns CA. Clozapine: guidelines for clinical management. J Clin Psychiatry 1989;50:329–338.

26. Marcantonio ER, Golman L, Mangione CM, et al. A clinical prediction rule for delirium after elective noncardiac surgery. JAMA 1994;271: 131–139.

27. Owens JF, Hutelmyer CM. The effect of preoperative intervention on delirium in cardiac surgical patients. Nurs Res 1982;31:60–62.

27a. Dyer CB, Ashton CM, Teasdale TA. Postoperative delirium—a review of 80 primary data-collection studies. Arch Intern Med 1995; 155:461–465.

28. Gustafson Y, Brannstrom B, Berggren D, et al. A geriatric-anesthesiologic program to reduce acute confusional states in elderly patients treated for femoral neck fractures. J Am Geriatr Soc 1991;39:655–662.

28a. Pompei P et al. Delirium in hospitalized older patients: outcomes and predictors. J Am Geriatr Soc 1994;42(8):809–815.

28b. Rockwood K. The occurence and duration of symptoms in elderly patients with delirium. J Gerontol 1993;48(4):M162–M166.

29. Inouye SK, van Dyck, Alessi CA, Balkin A, Siegal AP, Horowitz RI. Clarifying confusion: the Confusion Assessment Method: a new method for detection of delirium. Ann Intern Med 1990;113:941–948.

30. Berggren D, Gustafson Y, Eriksson B, et al. Post-operative confusion after anesthesia in elderly patients with femoral neck fractures. Anesth Analg 1987;66:497–504.

30a. Levkoff SE, et al. Identification of factors associated with the diagnosis of delirium in elderly hospitalized patients. J Am Geriatr Soc 1988;36:1099–1104.

30b. Schor JD, et al. Risk factors for delirium in hospitalized elderly. JAMA 1992;267(6): 827–831.

31. Slogoff S, Girgis KZ, Keats AS. Etiologic factors in neuropsychiatric complications associated with cardiopulmonary bypass. Anesth Analg 1982;61:903–911.

32. Roach GW, Kanchuger M, Mangano CM, et al. Adverse cerebral outcomes after coronary bypass surgery. N Engl J Med 1996;335:1857–1863.

33. Williams RB Jr, Sherter C. Cardiac complications of tricyclic antidepressant therapy. Ann Intern Med 1971;74:395–398.

34. Tune LE, Holland A, Folstein MF, et al. Association of postoperative delirium with raised serum levels of anticholinergic drugs. Lancet 1981;ii:651–653.

34a. Scharf M, et al. ??? J Clin Psychiatr 1994; 55:192.

35. Steinhart MJ. The use of haloperidol in geriatric patients with organic mental disorder. Curr Therapeutic Res 1983;33:132–142.

36. Seneff M, Mathews R. Use of haloperidol infusions to control delirium in critically ill adults. Ann Pharmacother 1995;29:690–693.

37. Shapiro B, Warren J, Egol A, et al. Practice parameters for intravenous analgesia and sedation for adult patients in the intensive care unit: an executive summary. Crit Care Med 1975;23:1596–1600.

38. Thompson JW, Blaine JD. Use of ECT in the United States in 1975 and 1980. Am J Psychiatry 1987;144:557–562.

39. Hermann RC, Dorwart RA, Hoover CW, Brody J. Variation in ECT use in the United States. Am J Psychiatry 1995;152:869–875.

40. Consensus conference: electroconvulsive therapy. JAMA 1985;254:2104–2108.

41. Philbert RA, Richards L, Lynch CF, Winokur G. Effect of ECT on mortality and clinical outcome in geriatric unipolar depression. J Clin Psychiatry 1995;56:390–394.

42. Coffey CE, Weiner RD. Electroconvulsive therapy: an update. Hosp Comm Psychiatry 1990; 41:515–521.

43. deleted

44. Monroe RR. Maintenance electroconvulsive therapy. Psych Clin North Am 1991;14: 947–960.

45. Gregory S, Shaweross CR, Gill D. The Nottingham ECT study. A double-blind comparison of bilateral, unilateral and simulated ECT in depressive illness. Br J Psychiatry 1985;146: 520–524.

46. Swartz CM, Larson G. Generalization of the effects of unilateral and bilateral ECT. Am J Psychiatry 1986;143:1040–1041.

47. American Psychiatric Association. Task force on electroconvulsive therapy. Washington, DC: American Psychiatric Press, 1990.

48. Shapira B, Lerer B, Gilboa D, Drexler H, Kugelmass S, Calev A. Facilitation of ECT by caffeine pretreatment. Am J Psychiatry 1987;144:1199–1202.

49. Lurie SN, Coffey CE. Caffeine-modified electroconvulsive therapy in depressed patients with medical illness. J Clin Psychiatry 1990;51:154–157.

50. Hinkle PE, Coffey CE, Weiner RD, Cress M, Christison C. Use of caffeine to lengthen seizures in ECT. Am J Psychiatry 1987;144:1143–1148.

51. O'Connell RA. A review of the use of electroconvulsive therapy. Hosp Comm Psychiatry 1982;33:469–473.

52. Welch CA, Drop LJ. Cardiovascular effects of ECT. Convulsive Ther 1989;5:35–43.

53. Kaufman KR. Asystole with electroconvulsive therapy. J Int Med 1994;235:275–277.

54. Rasmussen KG, Zorumski CF, Jarvis MR. Asystole in ECT (letter). J Clin Psychiatry 1994;55:313–314.

55. Rice EH, Sombrotto LB, Markowitz JC, Leon AC. Cardiovascular morbidity in high-risk patients during ECT. Am J Psychiatry 1994;151:1637–1641.

56. Zielinski RJ, Roose SP, Devanand DP, Woodring S, Sackeim HA. Cardiovascular complications of ECT in depressed patients with cardiac disease. Am J Psychiatry 1993;150:904–909.

57. Weiner SJ, Ward TN, Ravaris CL. Headache and electroconvulsive therapy. Headache 1994;34:155–159.

58. Figiel GS, Coffey CE, Djang WT, Hoffman G, Doraiswamy PM. Brain magnetic resonance imaging findings in ECT-induced delirium. J Neuropsychiatry 1990;2:53–58.

59. Mulsant BH, Rosen J, Thornton JE, Zubenko GS. A prospective naturalistic study of electroconvulsive therapy in late-life depression. J Geriatr Psychiatry Neurol 1991;4:3–13.

60. Sanchez A, Kettl PA. Incidence of post-ECT delirium in geriatric patients (Abstract). In: Program and abstracts on new research. Washington, DC: American Psychiatric Press, 1994.

61. Currier MB, Murray GB, Welch CC. Electroconvulsive therapy for post-stroke depressed geriatric patients. J Neuropsychiatry Clin Neurosci 1992;4:140–144.

62. Martin M, Figiel G, Mattingly G, Zorumski CF, Jarvis MR. ECT-induced interictal delirium in patients with a history of a CVA. J Geriatr Psychiatry Neurol 1992;5:149–155.

63. Figiel GS, Hassen MA, Zorumski C, et al. ECT-induced delirium in depressed patients with Parkinson's disease. J Neuropsychiatry Clin Neurosci 1991;3:405–411.

64. Lerer B, Shapira B, Calev A, et al. Antidepressant and cognitive effects of twice- versus three-times-weekly ECT. Am J Psychiatry 1995;152:564–570.

65. Devanand DP, Dwork AJ, Hutchinson ER, Bolwig TG. Does ECT alter brain structure? Am J Psychiatry 1994;151:957–970.

66. Isselbacher KJ, Braunwald E, Wilson JD, et al. Harrison's principals of internal medicine. 13th ed. New York: McGraw-Hill, 1994.

67. Dale DC, Federman DD. Scientific American Medicine. New York: Scientific American Inc., 1978–1997.

68. Gruen PH. Endocrine changes in psychiatric diseases. Med Clin North Am 1978;62:285–296.

69. Ross DS, Daniels GH, Gouveia D. The use and limitations of a chemiluminescent thyrotropin assay as a single thyroid function test in an out-patient endocrine clinic. J Clin Endocrinol Metab 1990;71:764–769.

70. Spencer CA, LoPresti JS, Patel A, et al. Applications of a new chemiluminomctric thyrotropin assay to subnormal measurement. J Clin Endocrinol Metab 1990;70:453–460.

71. Surks MI, Chopra IJ, Mariash CN, et al. American Thyroid Association guidelines for use of laboratory tests in thyroid disorders. JAMA 1990;263:1529–1532.

72. Woeber KA. Thyrotoxicosis and the heart. N Engl J Med 1992;327:94–98.

73. Stancer HC, Forbath N. Hyperparathyroidism, hypothyroidism and impaired renal function after 10 to 20 years of lithium treatment. Arch Intern Med 1989;149:1042–1045.

74. Bagchi N, Brown TR, Parish RF. Thyroid dysfunction in adults over 55 years: a study in an urban US community. Arch Intern Med 1990;150:785–787.

75. Sawin CT, Castelli WP, Hershman JM, et al. The aging thyroid: thyroid deficiency in the Framingham study. Arch Intern Med 1985;145(8):1386–1388.

76. Langston JW, Ballard P. Parkinsonism induced by 1-methyl 4-phenyl-1,2,3,6-tetrahydropyridine (MPTP): implications for treatment and pathogenesis of Parkinson's disease. Can J Neurol Sci 1984;11:160–165.

77. Langston JW, Ballard P, Tetrud JW, et al. Chronic parkinsonism in humans due to a product of meperidine-analog, synthesis. Science 1983;219:979–980.

78. Hochberg FH, Leffert RD, Heller MD, Merriman L. Hand difficulties among musicians. JAMA 1983;249:1869–1872.

79. Leckman JF, Cohen DJ. Recent advances in Gilles de la Tourette syndrome: implications for clinical practice and future research (review). Psychiatric Developments 1983;1(3):301–306.

80. Bradshaw Jr, Thomson JLG, Campbell MJ. Computed tomography in the investigation of dementia. BMJ 1983;286:277–286.

81. Arie T. Pseudodementia. BMJ 1983;286:1301–1302.

82. Wikkelso C, Anderson H, Blomstrand C, Lindqvist G. The clinical effect of lumbar puncture in normal pressure hydrocephalus. J Neurol Neurosurg Psychiatry 1982;45:64–69.

83. Hughes CP, Siegel BA, Coxe WS, et al. Adult idiopathic communication hydrocephalus with and without shunting. J Neurol Neurosurg Psychiatry 1978;41:961–971.

84. Atkinson JH, Grant I, Kennedy CJ, et al. Prevalence of psychiatric disorders among men infected with human immunodeficiency virus. Arch Gen Psychiatry 1988;45:859–864.

85. Williams JB, Rabkin JG, Remien RH, et al. Multidisciplinary baseline assessment of homosexual men with and without human immunodeficiency virus infection. II. Standardized clinical assessment of current and lifetime psychopathology. Arch Gen Psychiatry 1991;48:124–130.

86. McArthur JC, Cohen BA, Selnes OA, et al. Low prevalence of neurological and neuropsychological abnormalities in otherwise healthy HIV-1 infected individuals: results from the Multicenter AIDS Cohort Study. Ann Neurol 1989;26:601–611.

87. McArthur JC, Hoover DR, Bacellar H, et al. Risk factors for development of HIV dementia in homosexual men: report from the Multicenter AIDS Cohort Study. Presented at the 8th International Conference on AIDS, Amsterdam, The Netherlands, July 1992:19–24.

88. Schaerf FW, Miller RR, Lipsey JR, et al. ECT for major depression in four patients infected with human immunodeficiency virus. Am J Psychiatry 1989;146:782–784.

89. Johannessen DJ, Wilson LG. Mania with cryptococcal meningitis in two AIDS patients. J Clin Psychiatry 1988;49:200–201.

90. O'Dowd MA, McKegney FP. Manic syndrome associated with Zidovudine. JAMA 1988;260:3587.

91. Harris J, Jeste DV, Gleghorn A, et al. New-onset psychosis in HIV- infected patients. J Clin Psychiatry 1991;52:369–376.

92. Breitbart W, Marotta RF, Call P. AIDS and neuroleptic malignant syndrome. Lancet 1988; ii:1488–1489.

93. Perry S, Jacobsberg LR, Fishman B, et al. Psychiatric diagnosis before serological testing for the human immunodeficiency virus. Am J Psychiatry 1990;147:89–93.

94. Lunn S, Skydsbjerg M, Schulsinger H, et al. A preliminary report on the neuropsychologic sequelae of human immunodeficiency virus. Arch Gen Psychiatry 1991;48:139–142.

95. Lipton SA, Gendelman HE. Seminars in medicine of the Beth Israel Hospital, Boston. Dementia associated with the acquired immunodeficiency syndrome. N Engl J Med 1995;332:934–940.

95a. Von Roenn JH, et al. Physician attitudes and practice in cancer pain management. Ann Intern Med 1993;119:121–126.

96. Navia BA, Jordan BD, Price RW. The AIDS dementia complex: I. Clinical features. Ann Neurol 1986;19:517–524.

97. Navia BA, Prich RW. The acquired immunodeficiency dementia complex as the presenting or sole manifestation of human immunodeficiency virus infection. Arch Neurol 1987;44:65–69.

98. Grant I, Heaton RK, Velin R, et al. Rates of cognitive impairment and prediction of neuropsychological decline in HIV + persons: a 2-year follow-up. Presented at the Ninth International Conference on AIDS, Berlin, June 7–11, 1993.

99. Harper CG, Giles M, Finlay-Jones R. Clinical signs in the Wernicke-Korsakoff complex: a retrospective analysis of 131 cases diagnosed at necropsy. J Neurol Neurosurg Psychiatry 1986; 49:341–345.

100. Moore RD, Bone LR, Geller G, et al. Prevalence, detection and treatment of alcoholism in hospitalized patients. JAMA 1989;261:403–407.

101. Kettl PA. Basic rules for managing dementia. Patient Care 1993;27:79–92.

102. Kettl PA, Bixler EO. Prevalence of alcoholism in spinal cord injury (abstract). In: Proceedings of the American Spinal Injury Association, 15th Annual Meeting, Las Vegas, Nevada, 1989:30.

103. Serdula M, Williamson DF, Kendrcik JS, Andu RF, Byers T. Trends in alcohol consumption by pregnant women: 1985 through 1988. JAMA 1991;265:876–879.

104. Hingson R, Mangione T, Meyers A, et al. Seeking help for drinking problems: a study in the Boston metropolitan area. J Stud Alcohol 1982;43:273–288.

105. Buschsbaum DG, Welsh J, Buchanan RG, et al. Screening for drinking problems by patient self report: even "safe" levels may indicate a problem. Arch Intern Med 1995;155:104–108.

106. Ewing JA. Detecting alcoholism: the CAGE questionnaire. JAMA 1984;252:1905–1907.

107. Selzer ML. The Michigan alcoholism screening test: the quest for a new diagnostic instrument. Am J Psychiatry 1971;127:89–94.

108. Babor TF, Ramon de la Fuente J, Saunders J, et al. AUDIT: the alcohol use disorders identification test: guidelines for use in primary health care. Document no. WHO/MNH/DAT 89.4. Geneva: World Health Orqanization, 1992.

109. Kettl PA, Bixler EO, Lyerly J. Prevalence of depression in DWI problem drinkers. In: Perrine MWB, ed. Alcohol, drugs, and traffic

safety. Chicago: National Safety Council, 1990: 667–672.

110. Helzer JE, Robins LN, Taylor JR, et al. The extent of long term moderate drinking among alcoholics discharged from medical and psychiatric treatment facilities. N Engl J Med 1985; 312:1678–1682.

111. Kettl PA, Schroeder-Mullen H. Detecting problem drinkers in your practice. Patient Care 1995;29:27–41.

112. Volpicelli JR, Alterman AI, Hayashida M, et al. Naltrexone in the treatment of alcoholism dependence. Arch Gen Psychiatry 1992;49: 876–880.

113. O'Malley SS, Jaffe AJ, Chang G, et al. Naltrexone and coping skills therapy for alcohol dependence: a controlled study. Arch Gen Psychiatry 1992;49:881–887.

113a. Herzog DB, Keller MB, Lavari PW. Outcome in anorexia nervosa and bulimia nervosa—a review of the literature. J Nerv Mental Dis 1988;176:131–143.

114. Herzog DB, Copeland PM. Eating disorders. N Engl J Med 1985;313:295–303.

115. American Psychiatric Association. Diagnostic and statistical manual of mental disorders. 4th ed. Washington, DC: American Psychiatric Association, 1994.

116. Andreasen NC, Black DW. Introductory textbook of psychiatry. Washington, DC: American Psychiatric Press, 1991.

117. Gwirtsman HE, Kaye WH, George DT, Carosella NW, Greene RC, Jimerson DC. Hyperamylasemia and its relationship to binge-purge episodes: development of a clinically relevant laboratory test. J Clin Psychiatry 1989;50:196–204.

118. Walsh BT, Wong LM, Pesce MA, Hadigan CM, Bodourian SH. Hyperamylasemia in bulimia nervosa. J Clin Psychiatry 1990;51:373–377.

119. Yager J. Eating Disoders. In: Stoudemire A, ed. Clinical psychiatry for medical students. Philadelphia: JB Lippincott, 1990.

120. Hudson JI, Pope HG, Yurgelun-Todd D, Jonas JM, Frankenburg FR. A controlled study of lifetime prevalence of affective and other psychiatric disorders in bulimia outpatients. Am J Psychiatry 1987;144:1283–1287.

121. Thompson II TL, Moran MG, Nies AS. Psychotropic drug use in the elderly (second of two parts). N Engl J Med 1983;308:194–199.

122. Thompson II TL, Moran MG, Nies AS. Psychotropic drug use in the elderly (first of two parts). N Engl J Med 1983;308:134–138;194–199.

123. Greenblatt DJ, Allen MD, Shader RI. Toxicity of high-dose flurazepam in the elderly. Clin Pharmacol Therapeutics 1976;21:355–361.

124. Pillemer K, Suitor JJ. Violence and violent feelings: what causes them among family caregivers? J Gerontol 1992;47:S165–172.

125. Coyne AC, Reichman WE, Berbig LJ. The relationship between dementia and elder abuse. Am J Psychiatry 1993;150:643–646.

126. Grafstrom M, Nordberg A, Winblad B. Abuse is in the eye of the beholder. Report by family members about abuse of demented persons in home care. A total population-based study. Scand J Social Med 1993;21:247–255.

127. Arana GW, Hyman SE. Handbook of psychiatric drug therapy. Boston: Little, Brown, 1991.

128. Miller FE, Boshes RA. Side effects of psychotropic drugs. In: Flaherty JA, Channon RA, Davis JM, eds. Psychiatry diagnosis and therapy. Norwalk, CT: Appleton and Lange, 1988.

129. Lieberman J. Dopamine pathophysiology in tardive dyskinesia. Psych Ann 1989;19: 289–296.

130. Rabins PA, Tune LE, McHugh PR. Tardive dyskinesia. Johns Hopkins Med J 1981;148: 206–211.

131. Ko GN, Zhang LD, Yan WW, et al. The Shanghai 800: prevalence of tardive dyskinesia in a Chinese psychiatric hospital. Am J Psychiatry 1989;3:387–389.

132. Yassa R, Nair NPV, Iskandar H, Schwartz G. Factors in the development of severe forms of tardive dyskinesia. Am J Psychiatry 1990;147: 1156–1163.

133. Munetz MR, Schulz SC. Screening for tardive dyskinesia. J Clin Psychiatry 1986;47: 75–77.

134. Lazurus A. Neuroleptic malignant syndrome: detection and management. Psych Ann 1985; 15:706–712.

135. Keck PE, Sebastianelli J, Pope HG, McElroy SL. Frequency and presentation of neuroleptic malignant syndrome in a state psychiatric hospital. J Clin Psychiatry 1989;50: 352–355.

136. Janicak PG, Bresnahan DB, Comaty JE. The neuroleptic malignant syndrome: a clinical update. Psych Ann 1987;17:551–555.

137. Denk MZ, Chen GQ, Phillips MR. Neuroleptic malignant syndrome in 12 of 9,792 Chinese inpatients exposed to neuroleptics: a prospective study. Am J Psychiatry 1990;147:1149–1155.

138. Mueller PS. Neuroleptic malignant syndrome. Psychosomatics 1985;26:654–662.

139. Abbott RJ, Loizou LA. Neuroleptic malignant syndrome. Br J Psychiatry 1986;148:47–51.

140. Granato JE, Stern BJ, Ringel A, et al. Neuroleptic malignant syndrome: successful treatment with dantrolene and bromocriptine. Ann Neurol 1983;14:89–90.

141. Rosebush P, Stewart T. A prospective analysis of 24 episodes of neuroleptic malignant syndrome. Am J Psychiatry 1989;146:717–725.

142. Levenson JL, Fisher JG. Long-term outcome after neuroleptic malignant syndrome. J Clin Psychiatry 1988;49:154–156.

143. Gelenberg AJ, Bellinghausen B, Wojcik JD, Falk WE, Farhadi AM. Patients with neuroleptic malignant syndrome histories: what happens when they are rehospitalized? J Clin Psychiatry 1989;50:178–180.

144. Pope HG, Aizley HG, Keck PE, McElroy SL. Neuroleptic malignant syndrome: long term follow up of 20 cases. J Clin Psychiatry 1991; 52:208–212.

145. Kane J, Honigfeld G, Singer J, et al. Clozapine for the treatment-resistant schizophrenic. Arch Gen Psychiatry 1988;45:789–796.

146. Cadoret RJ, Cain CA, Grove WM. Development of alcoholism in adoptees raised apart from alcoholic biological relatives. Arch Gen Psychiatry 1980;37:561–563.

147. Wagner RL. Mandatory WBC monitoring in severe, refractory schizophrenia. J Clin Psychiatry Monograph 1990;8:30–36.

148. Marder SR, Van Putten T. Who should receive clozapine? Arch Gen Psychiatry 1988;45: 865–867.

149. Oberholzer AF, Hendriksen C, Monsch AU, Heierli B, Stahelin HB. Safety and effectiveness of low-dose clozapine in psychogeriatric patients: a preliminary study. Int Psychogeriatrics 1992;4:187–195.

150. Friedman JH, Lannon MC. Clozapine-responsive tremor in Parkinson's disease. Movement Disorders 1990;5:225–229.

151. Jefferson JW. Lithium: a therapeutic magic wand. J Clin Psychiatry 1990;50:81–86.

152. Jefferson JW. Lithium: the present and the future. J Clin Psychiatry 1990;51(Suppl):4–8.

153. DePaulo JR, Correa EL, Sapir DG. Renal glomuerular function and long-term lithium therapy. Am J Psychiatry 1981;138:324–327.

154. Schou M. Lithium treatment. Br J Psychiatry 1986;149:541–547.

155. Yassa R, Saunders A, Nastase C, Camille Y. Lithium induced thyroid disorders: a prevalence study. J Clin Psychiatry 1988;49:14–16.

156. Karki SD, Holden JMC. Treatment of lithium intoxication. Psych Ann 1988;18:708–712.

157. DeMontigny C, Grunberg F, Mayer A, Deschenes JP. Lithium induces rapid relief of depression in tricyclic antidepressant drug non-responders. Br J Psychiatry 1981;138: 252–256.

158. Garbutt JC, Mayo JP, Gillette GM, Little KY, Mason GA. Lithium potentiation of tricyclic antidepressants following lack of T3 potentiation. Am J Psychiatry 1986;143:1038–1039.

159. Kettl PA. Lithium augmentation in geriatric major depression (abstract). In: Program and abstracts on new research. Washington, DC: American Psychiatric Press, 1994:187.

160. Ballenger JC, Post RM. Carbamazepine in manic-depressive illness: a new treatment. Am J Psychiatry 1980;137:782–790.

161. Elphick M. An open clinical trial of carbamazepine in treatment-resistant bipolar and schizo-affective psychotics. Br J Psychiatry 1985;147:198–200.

162. Placidi GF, Lenzi A, Lazzerini F, Cassano GB, Akiskal HS. The comparative efficacy and safety of carbamazepine versus lithium: a randomized, double-blind 3-year trial in 83 patients. J Clin Psychiatry 1986;47:490–494.

163. Fisch C. Effect of fluoxetine on the electrocardiogram. J Clin Psychiatry 1985;46:42–44.

164. Borys DJ, Setzer SC, Ling LJ, Reisdorf JJ, Day LC, Krenzelok EP. Acute fluoxetine overdose: a report of 234 cases. Am J Emerg Med 1992;10: 115–120.

165. Feighner JP, Boyer WF, Meredith CH, Hendrickson G. An overview of fluoxetine in geratric depression. Br J Psychiatry 1988;153: 105–108.

166. Altamura AC, DeNovellis F. Guercetti GT, Invernizzi G, Percudani M, Montgomery SA. Fluoxetine compared with amitriptyline in elderly depression: a controlled clinical trial. Int J Clin Pharm Res 1989;9:391–396.

167. Feighner JP, Boyer WF, Tyler DL, Neborsky RJ. Adverse consequences of fluoxetine-MAOI combination therapy. J Clin Psychiatry 1990; 51:222–225.

168. Berman I, Sapers BL, Salzman C. Sertraline: a new serotonergic antidepressant. Hosp Comm Psych 1992;43:671–672.

169. Weisler RH. A profile of buproprion: a nonserotonergic alternative. J Clin Psychiatry Monograph 1991;9:29–35.

170. Davidson J. Seizures and buproprion: a review. J Clin Psychiatry 1989;50:256–261.

171. Feighner JP, Gardner EA, Johnston JA, et al. Double-blind comparison of buproprion and fluoxetine in depressed outpatients. J Clin Psychiatry 1991;52:329–335.

172. Feighner J, Hendrickson G, Miller L, Stern W. Double-blind comparison of doxepin versus buproprion in outpatients with a major depressive disorder. J Clin Psychopharmacol 1986;6: 27–32.

173. Roose SP, Dalack GW, Glassman AH, Woodring S, Walsh T, Giardina EGV. Cardiovascular effects of buproprion in depressed patients with heart disease. Am J Psychiatry 1991;148: 512–516.

174. Cardiovascular effects of imipramine and buproprion in depressed patients with congestive heart failure. J Clin Psychopharmacol 1987;7: 247–251.

175. Walker PW, Cole JO, Gardner EA, et al. Improvement in fluoxetine-associated sexual dysfunction in patients switched to buproprion. J Clin Psychiatry 1993;54:459–465.

176. Mendels J, Johnston R, Mattes J, Riesenberg R. Efficacy and safety of bid doses of venlafaxine in a dose-response study. Psychopharmacol Bull 1993;29:169–174.

177. Shrivastava RK, Cohn C, Crowder J, et al. Long-term safety and clinical acceptability of venlafaxine and imipramine in outpatients with major depression. J Clin Psychopharmacol 1994;14:322–329.

178. Clerc GE, Ruirny P, Verdeau-Pailes J. A double-blind comparison of venlafaxine and fluoxetine in patients hospitalized for major depression and melancholia. Int Clin Psychopharmacol 1994;9:139–143.

179. Fontaine R, Ontiveros A, Elie R, et al. A double-blind comparison of nefazodone, imipramine, and placebo in major depression. J Clin Psychiatry 1994;55:234–241.

180. Rickels K, Schweizer E, Clary C, Fox I, Weise C. Nefazodone and imipramine in major depression: a placebo-controlled trial. Br J Psychiatry 1994;164:802–805.

181. Preskorn SH. Tricyclic antidepressants: the whys and hows of therapeutic drug monitoring. J Clin Psychiatry 1989;50(Suppl):34–42.

182. Kowalski A, Stanley RO, Dennerstein L, Borrows G, Maguire KP. The sexual side effects of antidepressant medication: a double-blind comparison of two antidepressants in a nonpsychiatric population. Br J Psychiatry 1985;147:413–418.

183. Glassman AH, Roose SP. Cardiovascular effects of tricyclic antidepressants. Psych Ann 1987;17:340–342.

184. Roose SP, Glassman AH. Cardiovascular effects of tricyclic antidepressants in depressed patients with and without heart disease. J Clin Psychiatry Monograph 1989;7:1–18.

185. Roose SP, Glassman AH, Giardina EGV, et al. Nortriptyline in depressed patients with left ventricular impairment. JAMA 1986;256:3253–3257.

186. Clary C, Mandos LA, Schweizer E. Results of a brief survey on the prescribing practices for monoamine oxidase inhibitor antidepressants. J Clin Psychiatry 1990;51:226–231.

187. Pare CMB. The present status of monoamine oxidase inhibitors. Br J Psychiatry 1985;146:576–584.

188. Feighner JP, Herbstein J, Damlouji N. Combined MAOI, TCA, and direct stimulant therapy of treatment-resistant depression. J Clin Psychiatry 1985;46:206–209.

189. Rosenthal NE. Diagnosis and treatment of seasonal affective disorder. JAMA 1993;270:2717–2720.

190. Avery DH, Bolte MA, Dager SR, et al. Dawn simulation treatment of winter depression: a controlled study. Am J Psychiatry 1993;150:113–117.

191. Levitt AJ, Joffe RT, Moul DE, et al. Side effects of light therapy in seasonal affective disorder. Am J Psychiatry 1993;150:650–652.

192. Eison AS, Temple DL. Buspirone: review of its pharmacology and current perspectives on its mechanism of action. Am J Medicine 1986;80(Suppl 3B):1–9.

193. Rickels K, Weisman K, Norstad N, et al. Buspirone and diazepam in anxiety: a controlled study. J Clin Psychiatry 1982;43:81–86.

194. Cole JO, Orzack MH, Beake B, Bird M, Bar-Tal Y. Assessment of the abuse liability of buspirone in recreational sedative users. J Clin Psychiatry 1982;43:69–74.

22
Special Topics

Richard J. Gross[1]

The preceding chapters have examined the effect of a single medical problem on a patient's overall risk from anesthesia and surgical procedures. This chapter uses the opposite approach, discussing how the risks to a patient from selected operations are affected by common medical problems.

The procedures were selected based on the prevalence of significant medical problems unrelated to the primary surgical disease and the availability of literature relating medical risk to the specific surgery. Preoperative problems that are not discussed in standard textbooks are emphasized. In addition, several special problems that do not fit elsewhere in this book are included, such as surgery in elderly patients (i.e., >65 years) and consultation on patients with burns.

SURGICAL PROBLEMS IN ELDERLY PATIENTS

The evaluation of elderly patients for surgery has become increasingly important as those older than 65 years account for more and more major, complex surgical cases and the factors accounting for the increased surgical risks in this group are better defined (1). Improvements in both surgical and anesthesiologic techniques have greatly reduced the risk of

surgery in these patients, even in those who are very old (i.e., >80 years) (2), though some authorities have questioned whether a decrease in risk actually has occurred (3–5).

The mortality rate is increased for elderly patients in certain operations. In most cases, however, age itself is a relative—and not a prohibitive—risk factor. The effect of age on operative risk varies widely between different procedures, ranging from a very small increase in risk during a cataract extraction to a major increase during partial gastrectomy (Table 22.1).

Many physicians are not aware how the effect of age on operative risk has changed over the past 30 years, or of the different factors contributing to this increased risk. Most of this section outlines the effect of age on the risk of different operative procedures, the proportion of increased risk due to age itself versus that from concomitant disease, the interaction of age with other risk factors, and the degree to which this increased risk can be reduced (see also Chapter 3). A consistent theme throughout this section is that **a patient should neither be rushed into nor denied surgery solely because of his or her age.**

The risk from many operations is increased for patients in the older age groups. This increased risk results both from age itself and from other accompa-

---

[1]William S. Kammerer contributed to this chapter in the first and second editions.

Table 22.1.　Representative Mortality for Selected Common Surgical Procedures in the Elderly[a,b]

Operation	Mortality (%)[b]	
	All Adult Patients (age 20-up)	Elderly (age 65+)
All procedures	2 (.9% excluding age 65+)	5–10%
Non-body cavity		
Amputation	2–4	3–17
Cataracts	0.01–0.05	0.01–0.2
Hernia		
Elective	0.01	0.3
Emergency	0.1	1–3
All	0.05	1
Mastectomy (modified radical)	0.1	0.6
Radical neck dissection	0.1–1	11
Transurethral resection prostate	<0.09	<0.33
Total hip replacement		5
Abdominal		
Appendectomy		
Without perforation	0.01	0.6
Perforated	0.1	6
Cholecystectomy (elective)	0.3–7	3–7
Colon resection (cancer)	5	10
Gastric		
Vagotomy-pyloroplasty	0.6	3–18
Partial gastrectomy	1–3	3–18
Thoracic and Cardiac		
Pneumonectomy	3–6	10–20
Aortic valve	5–10	15–20
Mitral valve	10	15–20
Coronary artery bypass graft	7	3–5
Vascular		
Aortic aneurysm (elective)	5	5–10%
Major bypass for peripheral vascular disease	5	15

[a]Derived in part from Refs. 3, 4, 18, 21, 26, 29, 33, 130, 174–182.

[b]The mortality figures cited above are from representative series in the literature. The relative differences can be taken as accurate. The absolute mortality should NOT be considered definitive because of wide variation in series in the literature, recent improvements in mortality that have not appeared in the literature, and differences in patient population, severity of disease, and expertise between different centers.

nying diseases found in older patients. Some empiric data now suggest that the severity of associated illnesses may contribute more than age to the increased perioperative risk in elderly patients (6).

Age

The age above which the risk of surgery is markedly increased has been moved back from 50 to 60 years in the 1940s to the current 65 to 80 years. Major surgery also now is performed with acceptable risk in healthy patients older than 80 years (7–15). It is not likely, however, that the age contraindicating major surgery can be moved back much further because of the small proportion of patients older than 90 years. A more likely occurrence will be the use of age as a relative rather than an absolute risk factor.

The risk of surgery is still increased in elderly patients compared with that in other age groups. The overall risk for all operations in adults younger than 65 years is 0.9%, compared with 5 to 10% for patients older than 65 years (Table 22.1).

Table 22.2.   Surgical Mortality in the Very Old

Study	Control Group (<age)	Age >80	>90
Denney (1972)			29%
Djokovic (1979)			6.2%
Adkins (1984)			13.4%
Michael (1984)			7.5%
Pollock (1987)	5%	20%	
Hosking (1989)			8.4%
Median	—	—	8.4%

Table 22.1 should be interpreted as showing only relative differences, however, because there is wide variation in mortality rates depending on the year of the study and the center at which it was performed.

In very old patients (i.e., >80 years), surgical risk is elevated (approximately 10%) (Table 22.2) compared with that in patients younger than 65 years (0.9%) and between 65 and 80 years (approximately 5%), but the risk is not prohibitive. Reports on small numbers of patients 100 years or older (11, 15) show acceptable risks, but most of these procedures have been minor.

The risk of anesthesia increases with age, with the largest difference occurring between those younger than and those older than the 60- to 65-year age group (Table 22.3, Fig. 22.1). Current series indicate overall mortality due to anesthesia and surgery is 1 to 2% in those younger than 60 years and increases to between 5 and 15% in those older than 65 years. Within the group defined as "elderly" above age 65, there seems to be similar mortality between ages 65 and 80 (Table 22.3). The risk then increases from approximately 5 to 10% to from 10 to 20% in those aged 80 years and older. However, more recent data suggest that surgery can be done in those aged 80 to 90 with a 5 to 10% mortality rate (8, 10–13). Thus current evidence suggests an increment in risk above age 60 to 65, but risk does not necessarily increase in a linear fashion thereafter.

The increased surgical risk in elderly patients is related to the type of surgery being performed. With the exception of radical neck dissection, the risk from surgery not involving body cavities is not increased, or is only slightly increased, in patients older than 65 (Table 22.1).

Major abdominal and thoracic surgery carry significantly increased risk in elderly patients. An important factor in this

Table 22.3.   Anesthesia—Surgical Mortality in the Elderly

Study	Age ≤65	65–70	70–80	80–90	90+
Djokovic, 1979				5%	9%
Marx, 1973	1–3%	4.3%	6.6%	7.8%	
Burnett, 1972				7–13%	
Kohn, 1973 (all ages)[a]	≈5%[b]	5%		12%	
Marshall, 1964				20%	13.5%
Lassen, 1962	2.5%	10.9%	14%	25%	
Coghill, 1967					
Elective surgery	8%		18%		
Emergency surgery	10%		23%		

[a]Age 70–75, 5%; age 75–90+, 12%.
[b]Age 60–70.

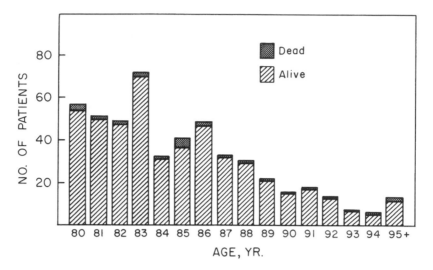

Figure 22.1. Perioperative mortality by age for patients older than 80 years (the "very elderly"). There is no increase in the mortality rate with increasing age over 80. Note the "surprisingly" low mortality for such an elderly group of patients. (Reprinted with permission from Djokovic JL, Hedley-Whyte J. Prediction of outcome of surgery and anesthesia in patients over 80. JAMA 1979;242:2301–2306. Copyright 1979, American Medical Association.)

increased risk is the higher incidence of emergency procedures and the markedly increased risk from emergency procedures in elderly patients.

A number of other factors beside age contribute to the increased operative risk in elderly patients as well (Table 22.4). An understanding of these factors is crucial, because they determine the very wide variation in operative risk between patients of the same age. The most important factors are sex, type of anesthesia and surgery, overall medical condition, certain specific diseases (e.g., heart or lung disease), and the patient's general physical and psychologic status.

Sex

Perioperative mortality was 6.6% for females and 5.6% for males in a study of patients older than 80 years. There are suggestive data, however, that risk may be lower for females under certain circumstances. Females may have a lower anesthetic mortality rate (16), and pulmonary disease may represent a lower risk in females (17). Females undergoing cholecystectomy also may have a lower mortal-

ity rate than that in males (18). Adequate controls have not been examined to determine whether these associations are real or result from confounding variables.

Table 22.4.   Known Factors Increasing Operative Risk in the Elderly (in addition to age)

A. **Patient**
   1. ? Sex
   2. General health (ASA status; healthy vs. chronic disease)
   3. General condition
      Nutrition (malnutrition)
      Activity (debility, inanition)
      Psychological status (attitue toward surgery, will to live, social situation)
B. **Specific organ disease**
   1. Cardiac (coronary artery disease, congestive heart failure)
   2. Infection or sepsis (especially pneumonia)
   3. Renal disease
   4. Less important or common: COPD, liver disease, congestive failure, dementia
C. **Type of surgery**
   1. Body cavity vs. non-body cavity
   2. Elective vs. emergency
   3. Type of anesthesia
   4. Finding of surgically uncorrectable disease or malignancy

Types of Anesthesia

Spinal anesthesia does not necessarily offer a lower risk than general anesthesia (7, 19). Local anesthesia or regional block carries a very low risk. The anesthesia literature indicates a higher mortality rate in procedures done under local compared with other types of anesthesia, but this results from selection of the worst cases for local procedures. Generally, there has been a very small increment in operative mortality with age for elective procedures under local anesthesia (e.g., cataract extraction).

Surgical Procedure

Major determinants of surgical risk in elderly patients are the urgency of the procedure and the need to enter the peritoneal or pleural cavities. Emergency or urgent surgery consistently has a much higher (i.e., three times) mortality rate than the same surgery performed electively (4, 5). The increment in risk for emergency surgery is proportionately much higher for elderly than young patients. The higher risk for emergency surgery has been supported by mortality rates in general surgical series (Table 22.1, Fig. 22.2) and series for specific operations (Tables 22.5 and 22.6).

Abdominal or thoracic surgery has a much greater increment in risk (as well as an absolutely high risk) than surgery not involving body cavities (Table 22.1) (20). There is only a slightly increased risk to non–body cavity surgery, especially if it is performed under local or regional anesthesia (e.g., cataract extraction, elective hernia repair). Notable exceptions are neurosurgery and radical neck dissection (1, 21). Repair of hip fracture carries a significant risk in elderly patients, though much of this increased risk may result from concomitant medical problems rather than from age (22) (see also Chapter 18). Pneumonectomy also is performed with increased risk in elderly patients, though the effect of age on less-extensive resection is not as well documented. The

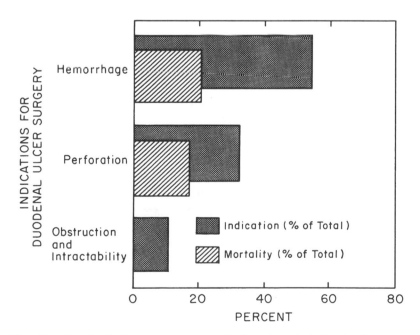

Figure 22.2. Mortality of duodenal ulcer surgery among elderly patients by indication for surgery. Emergency indications for surgery carry a higher mortality. (Reprinted with permission from Ferris P. Surgical management of the elderly. Hosp Prac 1976;11:68 [chart by A. Miller].)

Table 22.5.   Elective versus Emergency Surgery in the Elderly

	Elective Operations	Emergency Operations	Age Group
Cole			
Three series prior to 1960	6.5%	18.5%	>60
Two series— 1957, 1965	5.0	24%	>70
Marshall, 1964	10%	20%	>80

risk of major vascular surgery in elderly patients has fallen greatly and now approaches that of younger patients if proper patient selection and appropriate procedures are used.

Thus, elective surgery not involving body cavities can be performed at a relatively low risk in elderly patients. A major decrement in risk also can be obtained by performing body cavity surgery electively rather than urgently.

The finding of surgically uncorrectable disease at the time of surgery (e.g., extensive mesenteric infarction, disseminated cancer) greatly increases the surgical risk and accounts for a significant proportion of the perioperative mortality in elderly patients (1, 23). Surgery for malignancy in elderly patients carries a higher risk than surgery for other conditions. These factors usually cannot be modified, but they do affect surgical risk.

General Health

Overall scales of illness severity, which are independent of specific organ system disease, are important measures of operative risk. These scales have graded the severity of an illness in a spectrum ranging from healthy to terminally ill. The best-known general measure is the American Society of Anesthesiologists (ASA) scale, in which operative mortality increases as the ASA status declines from healthy (i.e., class I) to moribund (i.e., class V). There is some evidence support-

ing ASA status as a risk factor independent of age (Fig. 22.3) (1, 18). A healthy elderly patient is at less risk than a patient rated moderately to severely ill overall (without making specific reference to the organ system involved).

General Condition

Whereas "general health" refers to the patient's overall severity of illness, the patient's "general condition" refers to his or her overall physical and psychologic status as assessed by factors such as nutrition, debility, and daily activities. The physician's overall general opinion of patient status is still important. Some authors have contrasted the terms *physiologic age* with *chronologic age* to describe the differences in physical conditioning and activity of older patients at the same age. It is important that the physician's overall assessment be factual, objective, and accurate; too often, physicians make a quick, poorly thought-out statement about the patient's general condition on which life and death decisions are made. From my experience and review of the literature, most physicians base their assessment of a patient's general condition on three factors: (a) nutrition, (b) activity, and (c) psychologic status. The more commonly used negative terms are: (a) malnutrition, (b) debility (or inanition), and (c) will to live.

Table 22.6.   Mortality for Elective versus Emergency Surgery in the Elderly—Selected Procedures

	Mortality	
	All Patients	Elderly (age 65+)
Appendectomy		
Elective	0.01%	0.2–0.8%
Emergency	0.03%	4–20%
Cholecystectomy		
Elective	0.2%	3%
Emergency	2%	5–10%

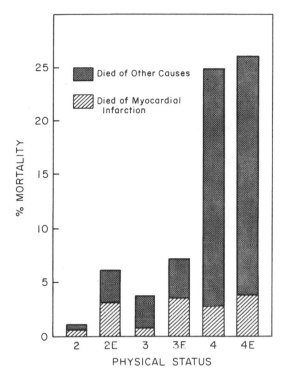

Figure 22.3. Perioperative mortality in elderly patients older than 80 years according to ASA class. The ASA class is a reasonable predictor of risk for perioperative death. Note the very high mortality rate for class IV patients and the increment in mortality for emergency surgery in class II and III patients. (Reprinted with permission from Djokovic JL, Hedley-Whyte J. Prediction of outcome of surgery and anesthesiology in patients over 80. JAMA 1979;242:2301–2306. Copyright 1979, American Medical Association.)

The objective measures of **nutritional status** previously given (Chapter 6) are applicable to older patients. Many of these measures were validated on elderly, hospitalized populations. It is important that multiple objective measures be used, however, and then combined with the physician's own assessment, because no single measure now available is accurate.

Activity level (24, 25) is best described by contrasting the example of a 70-year-old patient who is active in family life, gardening, and tennis, with the bedridden, nursing home patient of the same age with dementia. Assessment of activity should include the patient's daily activi-

ties, whether the patient lives or can live alone, his or her level of independence for activities of daily living, and muscle mass. The term *debility* is used to describe a patient with loss of muscle mass and ability to perform activities. The term *inanition* refers to the loss of interest in doing daily activity and ability to do them.

Several factors contribute to a patient's **psychologic status** before surgery. The patient's attitude toward surgery and his or her feelings about its outcome are important. No study has proved that the patient's predictions of surgical outcome correlate with the actual results, but most clinicians dealing with elderly patients have found such a correlation. The patient's overall will to live is important, as are both his or her previous living (i.e., social) situation and the situation to which he or she will return postoperatively, "quality of life."

SPECIFIC ORGAN SYSTEM DISEASE

Dysfunction of several organ systems is responsible for much of the perioperative mortality in elderly patients. Unrelated organ system disease contributes substantially to the increased surgical risk of these patients as well (5, 23, 25–28).

Pre-existing **cardiac disease,** especially coronary artery disease or congestive heart failure, increases operative risk (8, 29, 30–32). Age older than 70 years is a risk factor independent of pre-existing heart disease for postoperative cardiac complications (32). Weaker associations have been made between preoperative **pulmonary disease,** age older than 70 years, and postoperative morbidity (16, 18, 29, 33). Pre-existing **infection** increases operative risk as well as the risk of postoperative infection at sites remote from the preoperative infection; infection carries a high risk in elderly patients.

Table 22.7 provides **"causes"** of postoperative mortality in elderly patients. Cardiac disease is the most frequent cause of mortality; infection and sepsis are the

Table 22.7. "Causes" of Mortality Postoperatively in Elderly Patients[a]

Cause	Djokovic (1979)	Cole (1950–1952)[b]	Randall (1968)	Kohn (1973)	Miller (1977)	Palmberg (1979)
Heart disease (all)	32%	24%	12%	12%	17%	13%
Myocardial infarction	29%				17%	2%
Congestive heart failure	3%					
Pulmonary emboli	3%	11.6%	5.5%	12%	6%	33%
Chronic obstructive lung disease	3%	—[c]	—[c]			
Infection (total)	26%	33%	56%	16%		
Pneumonia (± sepsis, atelectases)	26%	18%	28%	16%	56%	26%
Sepsis (includes peritonitis)		15%	28%		22%	
Gastrointestinal						
Liver disease				4%		
Bleeding					6%	6%
Renal failure	3%	7.5%	0%	8%		
Miscellaneous (total)	34%	23%	18%	38%		10%
Carcinoma	6%	12%	18%	16%		
Subarachnoid hemorrhage	6%					
Mesenteric infarction	19%					
Ruptured aortic aneurysm	3%					

[a]Compiled from series in the bibliography.
[b]Average of three series.
[c]Pulmonary deaths included in pneumonia mortality.

second most common causes. Renal failure is a significant contributing factor to mortality in elderly patients, but inadequate data are available on whether preoperative renal disease or intraoperative acute renal failure is the more important determinant of postoperative morbidity.

Among the types of postoperative **morbidity** that are increased in elderly patients, delirium or confusion has been among the least understood. Two recent prospective studies (34, 35) identified risk factors for delirium in addition to age (see Table 22.8). Disappointingly, most of these risk factors were not modifiable. In a small series of 50 patients older than 70 years with delirium, only approximately one-third had a single, identifiable cause of delirium, and no information was given on whether correction of this "cause" also corrected the delirium. This mirrors clinical experience, in which most elderly patients with postoperative delirium have multiple possible "causes" not clearly related to the delirium, which does not

necessarily clear promptly with correction of the "cause" (see also Chapter 20).

Diagnostic Activities and Approaches

A comprehensive preoperative evaluation (see Chapter 23) is necessary because

Table 22.8. Risk Factors for Delirium Postoperatively*

1. Age >70 years**
2. Alcohol abuse**
3. Poor cognitive status or dementia****
4. Poor functional status**
5. Markedly abnormal preoperative sodium, potassium, or glucose****
6. Noncardiac thoracic surgery**
7. Aortic aneurysm surgery**
8. Illness severity***
9. Fever or hypothermia***
10. Psychoactive drug use***
11. Azotemia***

*From refs. 34, 35.
**Risk factor found in ref. 34 only.
***Risk factor found in ref. 35 only.
****Risk factor found in both studies; ref. 34 and 35.

of the wide variety of concomitant medical conditions and the need for general health information in elderly patients. The information from this initial evaluation should be reviewed for established, preoperative risk factors when the database is complete. In my experience, risks are commonly misjudged in elderly patients unless clinicians review the patient record with specific risk factors in mind (see Chapter 3).

The record should be examined for two sets of risk factors (Table 22.4). First are diseases of *organ systems* that place the elderly at particularly high risk, such as cardiac disease (especially coronary artery disease), infection or sepsis (especially pneumonia), chronic obstructive lung disease, or chronic renal failure. Second are *general risk factors* characteristic of the patient and the type of surgery (Table 22.4).

Finally, an assessment of benefit to the patient in terms of quality of life and, if applicable, longevity is even more crucial in the elderly than in other age groups (see Chapter 3). Assessment of cardiac status is discussed on p. 107.

Patients older than 60 to 65 years who are undergoing major surgery should have spirometry routinely considered because of the increased frequency and severity of pulmonary complications in this age group. In addition, the results of spirometry correlate with the overall mortality.

Routine tests of renal function using the serum creatinine level and blood urea nitrogen are needed because of the frequent mild to moderate renal dysfunction that occurs with aging. Glomerular filtration rate falls with increasing age, and the serum creatinine level may be falsely low due to reduced muscle mass. The urea nitrogen may be falsely low due to poor intake or falsely high due to volume depletion. A normal serum creatinine level of 1.0 mg/dL in an 80-year-old patient may be found even as renal function is being lost (i.e., 50% of renal function is lost before the creatinine level rises). Serum blood urea nitrogen and creatinine level may be a misleading estimate of renal function in aged patients. A measurement of the creatinine clearance can resolve questions if renal function is an important issue.

Infection or sepsis may be clinically subtle in sick elderly patients. Infection often is difficult to detect because the physical signs are masked (e.g., the absence of rales due to dehydration, poor inspiration, or inability to sit up). In elderly patients, a careful and often-repeated search for infection should be made in the presence of even nonspecific signs of infection (e.g., unexplained low-grade fever, unexplained leukocytosis, or "downhill" course).

A baseline formal mental status examination should be done as part of the neurologic examination of elderly surgical patients. The "Mini-Mental Status" scale is a semiquantitative questionnaire that can be administered repetitively and by a nonphysician in a short period of time. It has been well validated, but it has limited sensitivity. The physician's general impression of the patient based on conversation or history taking is an inaccurate way to assess mental status.

Preliminary studies have indicated that surgical risk in elderly patients may be measured more precisely by invasive assessments of cardiac and pulmonary function (36, 37). Very high mortality was confined to patients with poor ventricular function and large differences in A-V oxygen. These assessments are not widely done, but they are frequently quoted. I do not recommend routine catheterization to define surgical risk, however, because of a lack of data on the validity of these measurements and the risk of right heart catheterization. Even so, determination of cardiac output and A-V oxygen differences as measured through right heart catheterization may be worthwhile *additional* data to obtain in patients for whom the decision regarding major surgery is borderline. Until further information is available on the validity of these measurements, they should not be the *sole* reason behind a decision for or against surgery.

Treatment Principles

Preoperative Treatment

The decision to operate on an elderly patient remains a difficult clinical problem (38). There is an increased surgical risk to the patient, but also less tolerance by the patient of the effects of surgically uncorrected disease and emergency surgery.

In judging the effect of surgery on longevity, most clinicians do not recognize that the average 70- to 80-year-old patient has a *mean* life expectancy of 8 years (39) (see also Chapter 24). Too often, elderly patients are refused surgery because "they only have 1 or 2 years to live." The other major consideration in elderly patients is that the end point often is not a major increase in longevity, as it is in younger patients, but rather an improvement in the quality of life or his or her degree of functioning in daily activities.

The balance of benefit versus risk of surgery in elderly patients usually can be determined with use of the general guidelines previously given. In using this schema, the benefits considered must include *accurate* assessment of longevity and quality of life, including the *patient's* feelings about his or her future and the surgery. This assessment must focus on those general factors and any specific organ diseases (Table 22.4) that most affect mortality in this age group, any specific medical risk factors applicable to all patient groups (23), and age.

The age at which surgical risk increases has changed over the past 30 years. The degree of risk has changed as well, from a prohibitive 25+% to from 5 to 10%. The 5 to 10% range, however, still indicates a significantly higher risk than the 0.9% for young patients. Another perspective can be obtained by realizing that while a 5 to 10% risk is regarded as large by today's standards, it was a quite acceptable only 20 to 30 years ago. As discussed earlier, the data show that this major increase of risk may not occur until 65 or 70 years of age rather than 55 or 65 years.

Deciding whether to perform surgery on the basis of the factors listed earlier (Table 22.4) seems complex because the risk factors listed are not familiar to most physicians outside the geriatric specialty. Once the list is mastered, however, the decision is no more complex than other medical decisions. These risk factors provide a more precise estimate of surgical risk, but they should complement, not supplant, the clinician's overall judgment.

Nutritional supplementation by oral, nasogastric, or intravenous hyperalimentation should improve surgical risk due to malnutrition in elderly patients. When using these modalities, the risks of nutritional interventions, particularly aspiration pneumonia and sepsis, should be recognized.

Preoperative management of specific organ system problems in elderly patients is covered in the preceding chapters on each system (e.g., cardiovascular disease).

Postoperative Treatment

Several considerations are important in the postoperative treatment of elderly patients. Such patients are more often confused (i.e., suffering delirium) postoperatively, with possible underlying "causes" including fever, anemia, fluid and electrolyte disturbances, hypoxia, hypotension, and residual effect of anesthetics or analgesics. As described earlier, however, most patients do not have a single cause, and correction of underlying "causes" frequently does not result in rapid clearing of the delirium, thus suggesting either no relationship, multiple causes, or a prolonged delay in recovery from delirium once the cause has been corrected. It is not known which of these factors is operative in most patients.

The stress of surgery and unfamiliar surroundings are frequent precipitating causes as well, and unless they are specifically sought, postoperative changes in mental status often are missed until they are severe. Simple measures to prevent confusion include returning the patient to the same room he or she occupied preoperatively, allowing the presence of familiar objects and relatives, and avoiding the use of unnecessary instrumentation. If possible, using smaller doses of narcotic analgesics and hypnotics (or avoiding them altogether) is among the most helpful interventions. Avoidance of narcotics with anticholinergic activity (e.g., meperidine) has been suggested by one author (34) and, in my own experience, has been helpful, but this has not yet been tested in clinical trials. Epidural pain management also may reduce postoperative confusion, but again, documentation is lacking. It is not known whether constant subcutaneous infusion of low-dose narcotics by one of several available devices reduces postoperative delirium, but the avoidance of peak levels suggests that it might help.

After prolonged bed rest, mobilization is more difficult for elderly than for younger patients. Elderly patients should be gotten out of bed and ambulated as quickly as possible. Judgment should be used, however, in not ambulating patients with inadequate pain relief or who are too weak for such activity. Before ambulation, blood pressure should be taken while lying, sitting, and standing in elderly patients who have been at bed rest for more than 2 or 3 days because of the frequent occurrence of orthostatic hypotension. In the absence of volume depletion, patients suffering from mild orthostatic hypotension and who have either no or minimal symptoms may be helped out of bed more slowly and with use of elastic leg stockings. Severe orthostatic hypotension with marked symptoms may require use of tilt tables and physical therapy.

More meticulous attention than usual should be paid to maintaining fluid and electrolyte balance and oxygenation. Major complications may result from small errors in the treatment of elderly patients that would not affect younger patients.

Postoperative infections often present subtly in elderly patients, who also tolerate poorly untreated infections and undrained abscesses. The lack of tolerance is for both the acute development of septic shock and for development of a chronic, downhill course. Even with vigorous therapy and nutritional support, elderly patients may not recover from subacute infection if discovered late in its course. Subtle signs that should lead to a careful search for infection include low-grade fever, leukocytosis, or unexplained downhill course. One should not expect to find all the unusual signs of infection in any given elderly patient.

Special Considerations

Several operations are frequently performed in elderly patients and have special considerations besides those discussed already.

Cataracts

See page 641.

Hernia (Elective)

Elective hernia repair carries a slightly increased risk in elderly patients. Uncomplicated hernia repair usually can be done under local anesthesia with sedation. While the operative risk with local anesthesia is small in patients without unstable coronary artery disease, the benefit of performing elective surgery on asymptomatic hernias in elderly patients still is controversial (18, 40).

Transurethral Prostate Resection

See page 641.

Partial Colectomy

Colon resection for cancer carries an increased operative risk in elderly patients because of the major intraabdominal nature of the procedure and the risk of infection (28, 41, 42). Risk also is increased by the greater frequency of emergency operations and complicated presentations (e.g., obstruction, perforation) as compared to other procedures. The operation usually is undertaken in all but very poor risk patients because of the ultimately fatal nature of the disease and the lack of available alternative procedures. Possible alternatives for low-lying rectal carcinoma are fulguration and laser therapy, but these often require multiple applications of general anesthesia and are not curative.

Ulcer Operations

The mortality rate for ulcer operations is markedly increased in elderly patients. This increased risk results in part from more elderly patients being operated on for complications and having emergency surgery (Fig. 22.2) (43). Other contributing factors are the major intra-abdominal nature of the procedure and the closeness of the operative site to the diaphragm (with resulting pulmonary compromise). Medical treatment should be used for peptic ulcer disease in elderly patients unless complications supervene. In elderly patients who require surgery, most surgeons perform the simplest definitive procedure for the complication rather than an extensive, "curative" surgery. Cardiac and pulmonary complications are the most common.

Appendicitis

Appendicitis retains its classic reputation as an operation with a greatly increased mortality rate in elderly patients, whether it is uncomplicated or for perforation (Table 22.1). Although British studies indicate that medical therapy may be an viable alternative in *some* patients, operation remains the treatment in the United States for all patients. Early diagnosis and operation are essential, however, because the risk is much higher if perforation occurs (0.6% versus 6–10%, respectively).

Aortic Aneurysm

See page 641.

Gynecologic Surgery

Gynecologic procedures have been performed with a low mortality rate in elderly women (3, 44). Many of the procedures reported in the literature, however, have been through a vaginal rather than abdominal approach.

Thoracotomy

In the past, age older than 70 years has been considered a relative contraindication to lung resection. More recent studies, however, have reported an acceptable operative mortality rate, such as 4% among patients older than 70 years with lung resection, though approximately 50% of those patients had conservative amounts of lung resected (e.g., segmental or wedge resection) rather than undergoing pneumonectomy (45). In addition, 20% of patients had major complications. This compares with a 17% operative mortality rate in prior studies (45). Risk factors for perioperative morbidity were congestive heart failure, previous pulmonary resection, and the extent of lung resected. Lung resection can be performed in selected patients older than 70 years with an acceptable mortality rate if proper patient selection, certain lung-sparing operative techniques, and good supportive medical care are used.

Abdominal Aortic Aneurysm

Epidemiology The prevalence of abdominal aortic aneurysms at autopsy ranges from 0.6 to 1.0% in modern series (46). The prevalence of such aneurysms in screening studies of people older than 65 years is approximately 4 to 9% in men but significantly less in women. In the general population, the frequency is not known for certain because of differences in populations and results among various screening studies. The only known risk factors for arteriosclerotic abdominal aneurysms are hypertension, arteriosclerosis in other vessels, family history of abdominal aneurysm, and rarely, previous dissection. Recent research has shown abnormalities occurring in the aortic wall as well, but what initiates these abnormalities is unknown.

The mortality of untreated abdominal aneurysms is high. The only unselected series of nonoperative patients found a 33% mortality rate at 1 year and an 81% mortality rate at 5 years after the diagnosis of aneurysm (47). A 5-year mortality rate of 64 to 90% was found in a larger number of series of patients who did not undergo operation because of too high a risk or patient refusal (48–55) (Fig. 22.4). In comparison, the 5-year mortality for patients undergoing elective aneurysm repair was 40 to 63% (Fig. 22.4). The survival curves for operated patients are consistently better than—and do not overlap with—those of nonoperated patients or autopsy series. The survival of patients in operated series falls about midway between that of unoperated patients and an aged-adjusted, normal population (Fig. 22.4). The primary cause of late death was coronary artery disease. Late complica-

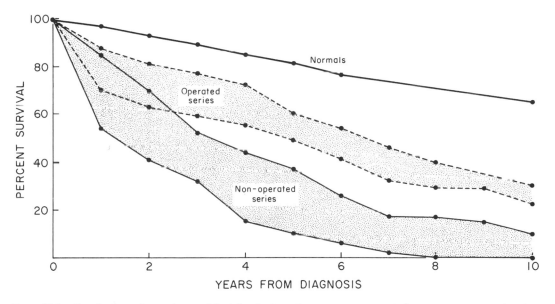

Figure 22.4. Survival rate for patients with abdominal aortic aneurysms: operated versus nonoperated series. (Data from Baker AG Jr, Roberts B, Berkowitz HD, et al. Risk of excision of abdominal aortic aneurysms. Surgery 1970;68:1129–1134; Crawford ES, Saleh SA, Babb JW, et al. Infrarenal abdominal aortic aneurysm. Ann Surg 1981;193:699–709; Darling RC, Messina CR, Brewster DC, et al. Autopsy study of unoperated addominal aortic aneurysms: the case for early resection. Cardiovasc Surg 1976;56:II-161–II-164; DeBakey ME, Crawford ES, Cooley DA, et al. Aneurysm of abdominal aorta: analysis of results of graft replacement therapy one to eleven years after operation. Ann Surg 1964;160:622–638; Esselstyn CB Jr, Humphries AW, Young JR, et al. Aneurysmectomy in the aged? Surgery 1970;67:34–39; Estes JE Jr. Abdominal aortic aneurysm: a study of one hundred and two cases. Circulation 1952;II:258–264; Foster JH, Bolasny BL, Gobbel WG Jr, et al. Comparative study of elective resection and expectant treatment of abdominal aortic aneurysm. Surg Gynecol Obstet 1969;129:1–9; Gore I, Hirst AE Jr. Arteriosclerotic aneurysms of the abdominal aorta: a review. Prog Cardiovasc Dis 1973;16:113–150; Hicks GL, Eastland MW, DeWeese JA, et al. Survival improvement following aortic aneurysm resection. Ann Surg 1975;181:863–869; Klippel AP, Butcher HR Jr. The unoperated abdominal aortic aneurysm. Am J Surg 1966;111:629–631; MacVaugh H III, Roberts B. Results of resection of abdominal aortic aneurysm. Surg Gynecol Obstet 1961;113:17–23; Schatz IJ, Fairbairn JF II, Juergens JL. Abdominal aortic aneurysm. A reappraisal. Circulation 1962;26:200–205; Szilagyi DE, Elliott JP, Smith RF. Clinical fate of the patient with asymptomatic abdominal aortic aneurysm and unfit for surgical treatment. Arch Surg 1972;104:600–606; Szilagyi DE, Smith RF, DeRusso FJ, et al. Contribution of abdominal aortic aneurysmectomy to prolongation of life. Ann Surg 1966;164:678–697; Voorhees AB Jr, McAllister FF. Long term results following resection of arteriosclerotic abdominal aortic aneurysms. Surg Gynecol Obstet 1963;117:355–358.)

tions of aneurysm repair (e.g., infection, graft failure) are rare, however, and represent only approximately 1% of late mortality.

A converse approach can be taken by examining autopsy series for the percentage of unoperated patients dying because of their aneurysm rather than another cause. On autopsy, the major cause of death in patients with aneurysm is the aneurysm itself (25–50%) rather than another cause with the aneurysm remaining intact. Other causes of death in patients with an intact aneurysm at autopsy include cardiac related, renal related, respiratory failure, stroke, and cancer (56, 57).

Although no randomized series has been performed, improved survival for patients undergoing *elective* resection of known aneurysms is strongly supported by the consistently improved survival rate of electively operated patients in all series (Fig. 22.4). Retrospective data indicating that the aneurysm is the most common cause of death in these patients also supports this idea.

There is no accepted medical treatment for abdominal aortic aneurysms. Preliminary data suggest that cessation of smoking, control of hypertension, and use of β-blockers may help to slow the progression of aneurysm size, but there are no data on reducing the risk of rupture. These methods suggested make sense, particularly for patients who are not surgical candidates or have small aneurysms

(≤4 cm) being followed serially, but there are insufficient data to definitively recommend them. They are not a substitute for surgery.

The lack of a reliable parameter to predict aneurysm rupture with a high degree of accuracy is a major deterrent to deferring operation and following these patients. No clinical or laboratory finding can predict the chances of aneurysm rupture, or signify that an impending rupture that will occur within a short period of time, with enough certainty to be clinically useful.

The one factor that has been found to consistently predict rupture is aneurysm size. Those larger than 7 cm have a 50% or greater risk of rupture, with approximately one-quarter occurring during the first year after diagnosis (58). Aneurysms between 4 to 7 cm have an approximately 25% risk of rupture (56, 58). In terms of aneurysm size alone, most surgeons currently recommend surgery for those 6 cm or larger and follow-up for those 4 cm or smaller; aneurysms of 5 cm remain a gray area.

In one study, in which ultrasonography was performed every 3 months, small aneurysms (<6 cm) grew an average of 0.4 cm per year. There was considerable individual patient variation, from 0 to 0.6 cm, and sudden, asymptomatic, large increases in size occurred in nine patients (19%). Fourteen patients (29%) required resection because of the development of symptoms or a sudden increase in aneu-

Table 22.9.   Operative Mortality for Elective Abdominal Aneurysm Repair

Study Period[a]	Operative Mortality			No. of Studies	Reference
	Median	Mean	Range		
1952–60	11%	13%	0–50%	21	46
1960–70	12%	11%	0–20%	14	46, 48
1970–	5%	5%	2.5–6%	3	59, 60, 183, 184-186

[a]Dates refer to when the series was collected and not date of publication. Series spanning more than one decade were placed in the decade in which most patients were operated on or, if evenly divided, into the later decade.

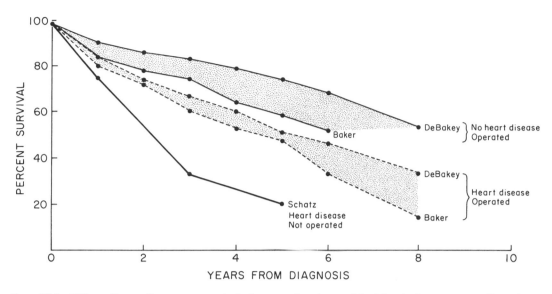

Figure 22.5. Effect of heart disease on survival of operated patients with abdominal aneurysms. (Data from Baker AG Jr, Roberts B, Berkowitz HD, et al. Risk of excision of abdominal aortic aneurysms. Surgery 1970;68:1129–1134; Gore I, Hirst AE Jr. Arteriosclerotic aneurysms of the abdominal aorta: a review. Prog Cardiovasc Dis 1973;16:113–150, 1973; Roger VL, Ballard DJ, Hallett JW, et al. Influence of coronary artery disease on moribidity and mortality after abdominal aortic aneurysmectomy: a population-based study, 1971–1987. J Am Coll Cardiol 1989;14:1245–1252; Schatz IJ, Fairbairn JF II, Juergens JL. Abdominal aortic aneurysm. A reappraisal. Circulation 1962;26:200–205.)

rysm size after being followed from 3 months to 5 years. Thus, when followed by serial ultrasonography for a short period of time, only a few patients had aneurysms rupture unexpectedly. Many patients had to undergo operation for increased aneurysm size or symptoms, however, and a significant number of patients developed unexpected, asymptomatic changes in size between ultrasound examinations.

The risk of aneurysm rupture must be compared with that of surgery. The risk of elective surgery decreased from 11% in the period from 1952 to 1960 to 5% in one current series (Table 22.9). More dramatic than the average figures in Table 22.9 is that many series in the period from 1952 to 1960 had a mortality rate that ranged from 25 to 50%, whereas after 1970, the mortality rate ranged from 2.5 to 6%. Operative mortality is lower for patients without heart disease (Fig. 22.5), and medical complications are a major proportion of postoperative complications—and therefore the risk of surgery.

The "cause" of perioperative death in elective aneurysm surgery provides the best insight regarding risk factors, despite the difficulty in assessing causes of deaths in patients with multiple problems (Table 22.10). The major cause of postoperative mortality is cardiac disease (59). Most series label most cardiac deaths as resulting from myocardial infarction without providing sufficient data to separate these from other cardiac-related causes of death. The rate of both pulmonary and renal deaths have decreased greatly since 1970 (32, 62); pulmonary causes of death have included pneumonia, respiratory failure, and pulmonary embolism. Preoperative renal failure and surgical complications greatly increase the chances of postoperative renal failure (62–64). Postoperative stroke accounted for approximately 12% of deaths, although several recent series (32, 60, 65) have reported no deaths due to stroke. As Table 22.10 illustrates, most deaths have been due to medical causes of cardiac, cerebrovascular, pulmonary, or

Table 22.10.   Medical Causes of Postoperative Mortality in Elective Aneurysm Repair: Literature Review 1955–1980[a]

Cause	Percentage of Deaths[b]	
	Range	Median
Cardiac (all)	20–100	40
Arrhythmia/arrest	3–25	—[c]
MI	12–100	34
CHF	3–50	—[c]
Cerebrovascular (stroke)	0–25	12
Pulmonary (including pneumonia)	6–41	12
PE and phlebitis	2–18	8
Renal	10–50	25
Surgical and miscellaneous	?	?

[a]Derived from Refs. 32, 48, 49, 50, 57, 59, 60, 61, 65, 183, 187–196.
[b]Total exceeds 100% because of multiple causes of death.
[c]Too few studies for accurate median.

renal complications, not surgical technique.

The frequency of postoperative medical complications (Table 22.11) is less certain. Many series do not state whether only nonfatal or all complications are reported. There is a relative ranking of problems this is similar to that with mortality, but there are two exceptions. Pulmonary complications are relatively more common than pulmonary deaths, primarily because of the occurrence of atelectasis. Gastrointestinal bleeding has been a frequent complication but has been only infrequently listed as the major or contributing cause of death. Certain gastrointestinal complications, including pancreatitis, jaundice, mesenteric infarction, and gastric dilatation, are rare.

A similar perspective on risk factors is provided by examining the concomitant medical problems in patients presenting for elective abdominal aneurysm repair (Table 22.12). Information on causes of mortality or morbidity after operation must be interpreted with caution because of widely varying criteria for diagnosis, retrospective assessment of cause of

death, and combined elective and ruptured aneurysm statistics in many series.

The role of coronary artery disease as the major risk factor of operation is consistently shown by its high prevalence in patients with aneurysm and its frequency as a cause of mortality and morbidity. Pre-existing clinical heart disease increases the risk of cardiac complications during aneurysm repair (60, 66, 67). The severity of heart disease as determined by the New York Heart Association classification increases the operative risk (48, 67).

The evaluation of patients for elective aneurysm repair emphasized cardiac evaluation because of the predominant role of heart disease in determining operative risk. Other important risk factors are pulmonary, renal, and cerebrovascular disease.

Diagnostic Activities and Approaches A comprehensive history, physical examination, and database of laboratory test results on admission are necessary in patients with aneurysm because of the common occur-

Table 22.11.   Postoperative Complications in Elective Abdominal Aneurysm Repair: Literature Review 1955–1980[a]

	Percentage of Patients	
	Range	Median
Cardiac (all)	2–47	9
Arrhythmia/arrest	1–14	4
MI	1–15	4
CHF	2–37	—[b]
Cerebrovascular (stroke)	0–11	1
GI bleeding[c]	1–5	2
Pulmonary	2–56	9
PE and phlebitis	1–11	1
Renal	1–13	6

[a]Derived from Refs. 32, 48, 49, 50, 59–61, 65, 183, 185, 187–196.
[b]Too few studies and widely varying results to give meaningful estimates of median.
[c]Less frequent GI complications were jaundice, pancreatitis, mesenteric infarction and gastric dilatation.

Table 22.12.   Preexisting Medical Problems in Patients Undergoing Elective Abdominal Aneurysm Repair: Literature Review 1955–1980[a]

	Percentage of Patients	
	Range	Median
Cardiac (all)	23–56	40
Angina	14–21	15
MI (± angina)	18–47	22
CHF	3–16	—[b]
Valvular heart disease	1–3	2
Hypertension	28–54	43
Cerebrovascular (all)	3–25	8
Stroke	3–7	5
Diabetes	7–22	9
Pulmonary	18–50	—[b]
Renal	3–22	7

[a]Derived from Refs. 32, 48, 58–60, 65, 66, 183, 187–192.
[b]Too few studies and too widely scattered results to estimate a meaningful average.

rence of multisystem disease and the risk to multiple organ systems during surgery (68). Spirometry should be performed on patients with pulmonary risk factors (see Chapter 6) due to the risk of pulmonary complications. A measurement of creatinine clearance is helpful to document baseline renal function in patients with renal disease or an elevated serum creatinine level.

During the patient workup, attention should be given to any signs indicating concomitant, undiscovered malignancy, because this occurs in a significant number of patients (69). The preoperative evaluation should focus on cardiovascular disease, which is the major risk factor for aneurysm surgery. The clinical evaluation should include a measure of functional capacity (70).

Noninvasive tests are useful in patients for whom the existence or severity of cardiac disease is uncertain clinically (see Chapter 11). Data indicate dipyridamole–thallium stress tests are predictive of postoperative cardiac complications in patients with aneurysm (70, 71). Electrocar-

diographic (ECG) treadmill stress tests also have comparable accuracy in predicting postoperative complications (70). Dobutamine stress echocardiography has comparable accuracy to treadmill or dipyridamole stress tests (70), but there is less published experience with this technique. A positive ECG, dipyridamole–thallium, or dobutamine-echocardiographic stress test usually should be considered along with the clinical evaluation in arriving at perioperative decisions and not in isolation (i.e., the sole criterion for decision making). Expert opinion no longer recommends use of routine stress tests to detect asymptomatic cardiac disease in all patients at low risk for aneurysm surgery without findings of coronary disease on clinical evaluation (e.g., history, physical examination, ECG, chest radiography) and good functional status (70).

Noninvasive evaluation of left ventricular function (e.g., MUGA scan) is useful in evaluating operative risk when there is a question regarding impaired left ventricular function, but it is not needed routinely. An ejection fraction of below 35% has represented high risk in preliminary studies (72, 73). However, aortic surgery has been performed on such patients with an acceptable mortality rate (72).

The results of noninvasive studies, including MUGA scans and dipyridamole–thallium stress tests, should serve as additional important information in assessing risk. However, they should be considered with the clinical evaluation, not in isolation as the sole basis for deciding on surgery or cardiac catheterization.

The role of coronary angiography, coronary angioplasty, and coronary artery bypass graft surgery in symptomatic patients is uncertain because of lack of controlled data showing that prior bypass surgery decreases the operative mortality. The results of uncontrolled studies are conflicting; conclusions have been reached that *routine* coronary angiography is indicated in all patients (74), in some patients (77–79), or is not indicated at all

(75, 76). Most patients considered to be high risk (as determined by coronary angiography) have symptomatic coronary disease clinically, preoperative cardiac risk factors, or poor functional capacity (70, 75, 76, 79). The operative risk in patients with a prior coronary artery bypass graft surgery is low, at 2 to 4% (74, 77, 78, 79). Aneurysm surgery has been performed after coronary angioplasty with acceptable complication rates. Few patients have been studied, however, and the timing of aneurysm surgery after percutaneous transluminal coronary angioplasty is uncertain in terms of risk of restenosis (80). Until randomized, controlled trials yield a definitive answer, coronary angiography is not routinely indicated before repair of aortic aneurysm or in asymptomatic patients. The decision in symptomatic patients should be made on the basis of clinical, laboratory, and noninvasive data regarding severity of the coronary disease as well as the local experience (70, 191).

Catheterization is indicated in some moderate and all severe cases of congestive failure due to potentially correctable causes, especially valvular heart disease. The more precise assessment of the degree of failure and left ventricular function provided by catheterization allows more precise estimation of how the patient's cardiac function will tolerate aneurysm surgery, although only qualitative guidelines can be given for first performing valvular surgery.

The treatment of patients with cerebrovascular disease undergoing aneurysm surgery is controversial. Most of the controversy regarding prophylactic carotid endarterectomy has centered on surgery for aneurysms and peripheral vascular disease. This subject is reviewed in detail in Chapter 19.

Consideration of carotid endarterectomy should be limited to patients at high risk of stroke due to symptomatic, transient ischemic attacks or high-grade stenoses, or to patients with asymptomatic bruits and high-grade stenosis (≥70%) as documented by ultrasonography, who have been shown to receive a long-term benefit from endarterectomy in recent, randomized trials (see Chapter 19). The indication in these circumstances is the patient's clinical disease, not surgical prophylaxis. The decision for patients with transient ischemic attacks or asymptomatic, high-grade stenosis is the relative priority of the two necessary surgical procedures rather than preoperative prophylaxis. In most cases, it is desirable to perform endarterectomy first, because the aneurysm repair can be done after a relatively brief wait and an asymptomatic aneurysm does not increase the risk of carotid surgery. If the aneurysm is symptomatic, however, the decision is more difficult and must be individualized depending on the risk of rupture and the local surgical experience.

Patients with chronic renal failure have undergone aortic aneurysm surgery. The risk in these patients is increased, however, especially in those patients with creatinine levels greater than 4 mg/dL (63, 64). Baseline assessment of renal function and possible use of a Swan-Ganz catheter to tightly control intravascular volume should be considered. Planning should be done for possible perioperative hemodialysis in patients with creatinine levels greater than 4 mg/dL (64), and the effect on renal failure should be considered when making decisions regarding radiographic studies requiring dye, including computed tomography, aortic angiography, and cardiac catheterization, particularly if multiple dye studies may be needed.

Postoperative Treatment Postoperatively, the major treatable problems are cardiac, pulmonary, and renal complications. The only problem precipitating stroke in this period that can be prevented is hypotension.

Patients undergoing aneurysm surgery usually are placed in an intensive care unit postoperatively and undergo intensive monitoring of cardiac rhythm, blood pressure, fluid intake and urine output, and often, central venous or pulmonary arterial pressures. Patients with significant preoperative coronary artery disease probably should be monitored for at least 3 to 5 days after surgery because of the risk of myocardial infarction and cardiac death extending to this time.

Despite growing experience, indications for Swan-Ganz pulmonary artery catheterization in surgery for aortic aneurysm are not firmly established (81–86). A Swan-Ganz catheter is indicated in the less-common aneurysms that extend above the renal arteries because of the larger hemodynamic changes that occur with cross-clamping the suprarenal aorta. The hemodynamic response to infrarenal cross-clamping during surgery is larger in patients with coronary disease (82–84). Both indications for and use of Swan-Ganz catheterization in all patients with coronary disease vary widely between centers, and no general recommendation can be given. Most centers tend to use Swan-Ganz catheters in high-risk cardiac patients. Recent data from retrospective studies about increased mortality rates with use of Swan-Ganz catheters have further fueled this controversy.

Special Considerations

Age The effect of age on mortality from surgery for aortic aneurysm is important, because aneurysm is a disease of elderly patients. From 10 to 20% of aneurysm surgery is performed on patients older than 70 years.

Patients from 70 to 80 years old generally have been considered to be very high risks for aneurysm repair, both because of their age and the major extent of the surgery. Earlier experience suggested that these patients had a very high rates of complications and mortality (49, 87).

DeBakey et al. (66) showed that patients aged from 60 to 69 years had an 11% operative mortality rate, and that patients aged from 70 to 90 years had a similar, 12% operative mortality rate. Several recent series (87–91) showed that

elective resection could be done in selected, good-risk patients older than 75 to 80 years with a 5% mortality rate, which is quite comparable to those of other age groups. The rates of postoperative cardiac, renal, and respiratory complications also are comparable to those in younger patients, and survival curves for operated patients are close to those of the general population. Patients not undergoing surgery have a 50% mortality rate at 1 year, which is approximately equally split between ruptured aneurysm and cardiac disease as the cause.

Current results suggest that age greater than 70 to 80 years alone does not markedly raise a patient's operative risk and is not a contraindication. Most authors note that it is important to consider the "physiologic" rather than the "chronologic" age of the patient. If the criteria of surgical expertise, patient condition, and lack of significant major organ disease (particularly cardiac disease) are met, it is reasonable to offer elective surgery to patients older than 80 years because of the risk of rupture within a short period of time and the reasonable, 6- to 10-year life expectancy of this group.

Ruptured Abdominal Aortic Aneurysms Rupture of an abdominal aortic aneurysm is an acute emergency that leaves no time for preoperative medical evaluation. Postoperatively, the most common cause of death is a progressive decline manifested by hypotension and multiple organ failure. Although different series (92–97) may classify this decline as due to surgery, hypotension, arrhythmia, myocardial infarction, or renal failure, the courses of decline from these causes are similar in its characteristics. The major approach to these patients is surgical repair of the aneurysm and postoperative maintenance of blood pressure. Cardiac and renal complications should be anticipated during treatment, and most patients will require central venous or pulmonary arterial pressure monitoring because of hypotension. Daily, routine monitoring of renal function (e.g., creatinine level, urine output), ECGs, and cardiac isoenzyme measurements should be performed as well. In contrast to elective cases, complications that occur with ruptured aneurysms are more closely related to those of preoperative shock and operative course rather than to those of pre-existing disease.

The most important consideration regarding ruptured aneurysm is prevention. Operative technique has improved markedly in the last 20 years, but this has had little effect on the high mortality rate of patients with ruptured aneurysm.

Mesenteric Ischemia and Infarction
Ischemia of the bowel is a rare complication of surgery for aneurysm (98–100). The colon is involved more frequently than the small bowel in ischemia after aneurysm resection.

The typical presentation of bowel ischemia after aneurysm surgery is the onset of bloody diarrhea, abdominal pain, and hypotension. The ischemic bowel also may present as hypotension without other signs or apparent causes. Other atypical presentations are gastric dilation, vomiting with or without coffee grounds, abdominal distention and ileus, diarrhea without blood, and fever. Incorrect diagnoses made most frequently are myocardial infarction (hence the reason for medical consultation) and diarrhea, which often has been attributed mistakenly to antibiotic colitis, postoperative bowel dysfunction, and tube feedings.

The workup when this complication is suspected depends on what tests are permitted by the patient's condition. Sigmoidoscopy is helpful, as the rectum and sigmoid colon are often—but not always—involved (98). The diagnosis also can be suggested by barium enema, and repeat laparotomy often is necessary.

Coincidental Malignancy Because of the age of this patient population, an unsuspected malignant lesion is found in 3 to 5% of those presenting for elective aneurysm replacement (69, 101–103). The occurrence of both unsuspected carcinoma and an aneurysm raises the question of which lesion has surgical priority.

There is no absolute rule on which lesion should be repaired first, but general guidelines are available (69, 101–103). The risk of aneurysm rupture should be evaluated on the basis of aneurysm size and symptomatology. The extent of the malignancy should be assessed in terms of the risk for spread over an interval period and whether metastases preclude cure and shortening longevity. Surgical considerations are which surgery will allow a more rapid recovery and a shorter time interval to the second operation. The surgeon often will want to remove an abdominal malignancy (usually carcinoma of the colon) first so that he or she is not working with potentially infective material near a newly placed graft.

Gastrointestinal Bleeding Gastrointestinal bleeding occurs in 0 to 3% of aneurysm replacements. The most usual cause of lower gastrointestinal bleeding or melena is intestinal ischemia. Upper gastrointestinal bleeding usually is related to stress gastritis.

Jaundice after Aneurysm Repair Jaundice occurs infrequently after elective aneurysm repair (60). Both the literature and my experience indicate that jaundice usually occurs in patients with multiple possible causes, and that it is generally not possible to specify a single cause. The causes of jaundice in this setting are similar to those in other operations (see Chapter 13). Severe, sustained hypotension and multiple transfusions commonly occur and may be more frequent causes of jaundice in aneurysm surgery.

Profound jaundice can occur after surgery for ruptured aortic aneurysms. The most likely cause in this setting is hypotension and shock. These patients have a high mortality rate because of severe ischemic damage to the other organs (104).

Liver dysfunction and jaundice may be a manifestation of sepsis in either elective surgery or repair of ruptured aneurysm. Infection should be sought in any patient with unexplained hepatic abnormalities.

Graft Infection Early postoperative infection of aortic replacement grafts occurs in from 1 to 3% of patients (105). Presenting symptoms include fever, distal embolization, and gastrointestinal bleeding from aortoenteric fistulae.

Infection is documented by obtaining positive blood cultures. Usually, blood cultures that are obtained from venous samples are adequate to discover graft sepsis. Occasionally, however, arterial blood samples will produce positive cultures when cultures of venous samples are negative.

Cultures obtained at the time of operation from the aneurysm or the abdominal cavity may be positive in up to 20% of patients; only a few of these patients will develop early or late infection (105). No specific factor is predictive of which patients with positive operative cultures will develop sepsis. Prophylactic antibiotics usually are administered (see Chapter 17).

Cataract Surgery

Epidemiology Consultation with an internist often is requested on patients undergoing cataract surgery because of their advanced age and multiple concomitant diseases. Outpatient cataract surgery generally is well tolerated. Unplanned admissions following cataract surgery usually are not related to pre-existing medical conditions, and they usually are not caused by medical complications (106). Cataract surgery can be performed under either local or general anesthesia. The only absolute indications for general anesthesia are poor patient co-operation, coughing, inability to lie still due to discomfort, and certain more complicated procedures.

The overall mortality rate from cataract surgery has been reported as from 0.005 to 0.05% depending on the center and the type of anesthesia used. If only patients older than 65 years are considered, however, mortality has been reported as from 0.01 to 0.2% (107–109) (Table 22.1). There was one death in 20,000 cataract extractions under local anesthesia (0.005%) reported in one series (107), and the risk is similar for local and general anesthesia (107–110).

Operative manipulation and several adrenergic drugs administered intraocularly can affect the patient's blood pressure and pulse rate during cataract surgery (110–117) (Table 22.13). Manipulation of or pressure on the eye may produce bradycardia (i.e., oculocardiac reflex), which is potentiated by underlying conduction system disease or hypoxia (111). This reflex is not fully prevented by preoperative atropine, but it can be abolished by use of retrobulbar block with lidocaine.

The pupil is dilated during surgery through topical administration of adrenergic agents (e.g., epinephrine, phenylephrine). Agents that produce miosis (e.g., acetylcholine) also may be administered postoperatively. In my experience, these rarely produce significant changes in blood pressure, pulse rate, or systemic complications; however, sympathetic agents occasionally produce marked hypertension and tachycardia. Similarly, acetylcholine and timolol have produced bradycardia, hypotension, or bronchospasm in occasional patients (110–118) (Table 22.13).

Diagnostic Activities and Approaches Most patients tolerate cataract surgery well, even in the presence of moderately severe, chronic cardiac or pulmonary disease. I do not consider moderately severe coronary disease to be a contraindication to this operation if the patient's disease is stable and more than 6 months have passed since myocardial infarction.

The operation should be performed

Table 22.13.   Selected Reported Side Effects of Ophthalmologic Drops[a]

Type (Drugs)	Reaction
1. Adrenergic (Phenylephrine)	HTN[b] (severe)
	Coronary spasm; MI
	Cardiac arrest
	Subarachnoid hemorrhage and HTN
(Epinephrine)	PVCs
	HTN
2. Beta-Blocker (Timolol)	Bradycardia
	Hypotension
	Syncope
	CHF
	Bronchospasm
	CNS
3. Cholinergic (Pilocarpine)	Cholinergic symptoms
4. Anticholinergic (Atropine)	CNS (confusion, hallucination)
	SVT
5. Anticholinesterase (Echothiopate)	Anticholinesterase toxicity
	Cardiac arrest
6. Carbonic anhydrase inhibitors	CNS
	Constitutional
	GI

[a]Table includes examples of side effects selected from case reports; numerous other possible reactions exist based on pharmacology of these agents.
From references 111–118.
[b]Abbreviations: HTN, hypertension; MI, myocardial infarction; CHF, congestive heart failure; CNS, central nervous system; SVT, supraventricular tachycardia; GI, gastrointestinal.

under local anesthesia in high-risk patients, because this poses no additional problems to the surgeon in most cases and probably lowers the operative risk to the patient. General anesthesia should be considered in patients who are very anxious about undergoing this surgery under local anesthesia; the small risk from general anesthesia may be preferable to the stress of anxiety. Increases in blood pressure and pulse rate due to topical drugs usually produce no symptoms and can be managed by withholding additional amounts of adrenergic agents. Short-acting antihypertensive agents (e.g., nitroprusside, trimethaphan) can be used when marked hypertension, accompanied by symptoms, develops. The short-acting esmolol or, alternatively, propranolol can be used for tachycardia. Atropine can be given for bradycardia, especially when accompanied by hypotension. Short-acting agents are preferable as the duration of action for most intraocular agents is brief. Use of drugs to reverse side effects resulting from topical anticholinergic or b-blocking agents rarely is required if careful monitoring of the patient's vital signs is performed and mydriatic agents are used in as small a dose as necessary.

Cholecystectomy

Epidemiology Treatment of gallbladder disease in cardiac patients has long been controversial. No adequate, recent study is available on the incidence of coronary artery disease among patients undergoing cholecystectomy. A 1955 report, however, found 100 patients with coronary artery disease (2%) among 5891 patients undergoing cholecystectomy (119).

Most studies on the medical complications of cholecystectomy were done in the 1950s and 1960s. These studies reported a mortality rate of 3 to 10% in patients with ischemic heart disease, and cardiac problems were implicated in 33 to 70% of perioperative deaths (119, 120). Studies from this era, however, are not necessarily applicable to current techniques.

The increased risk of cholecystectomy in cardiac patients is comparable to that of other major intra-abdominal procedures. An increased risk for cholecystectomy over that of other major abdominal procedures has not been shown in modern studies.

Cholecystectomy carries significantly increased morbidity and mortality rates in patients with chronic obstructive lung disease. Cholecystectomy shares this risk with other upper abdominal procedures, the increased risk due to the closeness of the procedure to the diaphragm with resulting atelectasis and hypoventilation. In one study (121), the risk of significant pulmonary complications or death was

20% in patients undergoing upper abdominal procedures, compared with 9% in patients undergoing lower abdominal procedures. Total pulmonary morbidity was 5% in patients undergoing upper abdominal procedures and 2.5% in those undergoing other types of operations.

Currently, there are insufficient data to show whether laparoscopic cholecystectomy carries a different risk of medical complications than the standard operation in patients with cardiac or pulmonary disease.

Diagnostic Activities and Approaches Patients with ischemic heart disease requiring surgery are at a significantly increased risk during cholecystectomy; the increase in risk is less well documented for other types of heart disease. Spirometry should be performed on patients undergoing cholecystectomy who have any history of smoking, lung disease, or cardiac disease because of the high incidence of atelectasis and hypoventilation due to the upper abdominal incision.

Treatment Principles Most patients should receive pulmonary therapy to prevent atelectasis. This is especially important in patients with both cardiac and pulmonary disease.

A common clinical dilemma is the need for cholecystectomy in patients with moderate to severe cardiac or pulmonary disease. The occurrence of symptomatic cholelithiasis and cholecystitis present a significant risk of developing recurrent episodes and complications (e.g., Gram-negative sepsis) that may exceed 20 to 50% over a short period of time. Patients with cardiopulmonary disease poorly tolerate these complications of gallbladder disease and emergency surgery. Thus the clinical dilemma is that the high risk of operating often equals or exceeds the high risk of not operating.

Moderate to severe ischemic heart disease should be optimally controlled with use of b-blockers and nitrates. Patients who remain at high risk due to recent myocardial infarction or unstable angina may warrant cardiac catheterization, bypass surgery, or use of an intra-aortic balloon pump.

Cholecystotomy is an acceptable alternative procedure for high-risk cardiac patients. It can be performed under local anesthesia and with lower operative risk. Some surgeons do not favor cholecystotomy, however, as 20% of patients will require cholecystectomy because of recurrent symptoms due to obstruction of the common bile duct. Even so, the operation does work well for most patients, and many of those requiring reoperation will have their medical condition improve or will die of other causes in the interval.

Treatment with oral chenodeoxycholic acids is not helpful in acutely symptomatic patients because of the delay until stones dissolve; its effectiveness in preventing symptomatic attacks is uncertain. Gallstone lithotripsy is not widely used at present, has not been shown to prevent symptomatic recurrences, and usually requires use of general anesthesia.

Laparoscopic cholecystectomy is the newest alternative to standard surgery, but there are insufficient data to know whether its use changes the medical risk of surgery. Laparoscopic surgery cannot be done for technical reasons in some complicated cases such as those with abscess or adhesions.

ERCP can relieve common duct obstruction, which often resolves the emergency and allows medical stabilization, or it can be done first to allow for later laparoscopic surgery. However, ERCP does not solve other problems of gallbladder disease (e.g., acute cholecystitis). While more alternatives to standard surgery now exist, the problem of medically high-risk patients remains unresolved and a difficult clinical issue.

In summary, gallstones that are clearly symptomatic have a high risk of complications over a relatively short period of time, and these complications are poorly tolerated by patients with severe cardiac disease. Some patients with moderate to severe cardiac disease can be optimally treated medically to prepare them for surgery. Some are candidates for cardiac catheterization, and the remainder should be considered for alternative procedures. Only the few patients with end-stage heart disease should not be considered for any treatment.

Patients with mild to moderate pulmonary disease usually can undergo cholecystectomy, and pre- and postoperative pulmonary therapy is important. Patients with severe pulmonary disease present a difficult clinical problem, however. Cholecystotomy may not lower the risk as much as in cardiac patients, because the same subcostal incision is used.

Special Considerations The problems posed by cholecystectomy in patients older than 65 years are discussed on page 543.

Dental Procedures and Surgery

Epidemiology The major consideration in cardiac patients undergoing dental procedures is anesthesia. The most common concern is arrhythmia, but other possible complications include angina, myocardial infarction, congestive failure, and sudden death. Local anesthesia presents the problems of using small quantities of epinephrine with the local anesthetic and the effect of anxiety and pain on the cardiac problem. Patients with valvular or septal lesions require prophylaxis for subacute bacterial endocarditis.

Death has occurred during dental anesthesia in both young, healthy patients and in those with cardiac disease. The risk of mortality from general dental anesthesia is estimated as from 1 in 250,000 to 1 in 850,000 (122–124). The risk from local anesthesia for dental work is not known, but it is thought to be lower than that for general anesthesia (122). The cause of most deaths in the setting of dental anesthesia remains speculative (122, 123).

In one study (123), deaths during general dental anesthesia presented in two ways. Respiratory symptoms often associated with airway problems tended to occur "early" in anesthesia. Sudden cardiovascular collapse most often occurred during recovery from anesthesia and without any symptoms; the cause of these deaths remains obscure. "Early" respiratory arrest accounted for 60% of deaths; "later" cardiovascular collapse of unknown cause accounted for 40%.

Deaths during dental anesthesia have been attributed to fainting in the sitting position, arrhythmia, halothane, local injection of adrenalin, aspiration, medication errors, hypotension, and cardiac arrest (124–126). The first manifestation noticed by the dentist most often is hypotension, but data on whether the initiating cause is a primary hypotensive event, arrhythmias, or respiratory arrest are lacking (124–126).

Numerous reviews have discussed the management of dental procedures in patients with cardiovascular disease (127, 128). Very limited experience (129) indicates that minor dental procedures can be done under local anesthesia with monitoring in the peri–myocardial infarction period without high risk, but more studies are necessary. Experience limited to 20 patients with coronary artery disease (130) indicated that 1:100,000 epinephrine used with lidocaine for local dental anesthesia did not produce a 1 mm or greater ST-segment depression on a computerized ambulatory monitor. Other studies found lesser degrees of ST-segment depression ($\geq$0.5 mm) with epinephrine and stressful dental procedures (130).

Arrhythmias are common in both healthy and cardiac patients undergoing dental procedures. The incidence of arrhythmia is similar for local (mean, 22%) and general (mean, 25%) anesthesia (Tables 22.14 and 22.15).

Under general anesthesia, the most common arrhythmias are nodal rhythm and premature ventricular contractions (PVCs) (Table 22.16). Complex PVCs are more common than simple PVCs. Supraventricular arrhythmias and premature atrial contractions are less frequent.

Table 22.14. Arrhythmias with Dental Procedures: General Anesthesia

Study	Number	Number of Patients with Arrhythmias (%)
Ryder, 1970	243	71 (29%)
Christenson, 1959		(18%)
Christenson, 1961[a]	417	(9%)
Kaufman, 1966	40	20 (50%)
Meyer, 1966	23	3 (13%)
Tolas, 1967	52	8 (15%)
Tuohy, 1968		(27%)
Rollmon, 1968		(18%)
Fisch, 1969[a]	103	44 (43%)
Alexander, 1971	203	84 (41%)
Miller, 1970	102	76 (75%)[a,b]
Ryder, 1971	544	129 (39%)
Forbes, 1960	100	13 (13%)
Rafel, 1972	55	0 (0%)
Gotta, 1976	109	46 (42%)
Ostroff, 1977	21	12 (50%)
Auscoll, 1954	109	20 (18%)
Hanna, 1983	30	13 (43%)
Mean		25%[c]
Median		18%[c]
Range		0–50%

[a]Reporting number of procedures rather than patients and/or numbers of arrhythmias rather than number of patients with arrhythmias.
[b]Includes sinus tachycardia.
[c]Excluding sinus tachycardia.
[d]Derived in part from Refs. 135, 136, 197–206.

High-grade arrhythmias (e.g., transient ventricular tachycardia, heart block) were seen in only a small percentage of patients. No reported patient had sustained high-grade arrhythmias or died during monitoring in the combined series of over 2000 patients.

The types of arrhythmias seen under local anesthesia differ from those seen with general anesthesia (Table 22.16). Simple PVCs are more common than complex PVCs, and premature atrial contractions are more frequent than nodal rhythm. Transient second- and third-degree heart block have been observed, but no instances of ventricular tachycardia, cardiac arrest, or death have been reported.

The effect of general dental anesthesia on blood pressure has not been well documented. Sinus tachycardia frequently occurs, however, with pulse rates exceeding 100 bpm in 10 to 40% of patients.

Many experimental studies have examined the effect of local anesthesia, with or without epinephrine, on blood pressure and pulse rate under well-controlled circumstances (131–134). Local anesthesia with epinephrine produces a small rise in blood pressure (systolic, 1–6 ± 7 mm Hg; diastolic, 0.5–3.0 ± 4 mm Hg) and pulse rate (1–5 ± 5 bpm). A spectrum of changes occurs among individual patients, including a significant number with no alter-

Table 22.15. Arrhythmias with Dental Procedures: Local Anesthesia[a]

Study	Number	Epinephrine	Patients with Arrhythmia (%)	Comment
Ryder, 1970	97	Yes	9 (9%)	Fainting 3 (30%)
Rafel, 1972	49	Some	0 (0%)	
Williams, 1963	63	Yes	15 (29%)	Cardiovascular collapse
Barkin, 1978	225	Yes	36 (16%)	Oscilloscope without printout
Hughes, 1966	77	Yes	25 (32%)	
Hughes, 1966	31	Yes	15 (48%)	
Mean			22%	
Median			16%	
Range			0–48%	

[a]Derived in part from Refs. 135, 198.

Table 22.16. Type of Arrhythmias with Dental Anesthesia[a]

	Number of Series	PAC	SVT	Simple PVC	Complex PVC	V-Tach	V-Fib	Nodal	2–3° Heart Block	Sinus Bradycardia and Other Brady-arrhythmias	Compli-cations
Local anes-thesia	5	21% (0–40%)	0% (0%)	47% (47–48%)	13% (7–20%)	0% (0%)	0% (0%)	6% (0–20%)	5% (0–13%)	22% (11–13%)	Syncope Collapse, 3 patients
General anes-thesia	11	3% (8–13%)	4% (0–25%)	14% (0–96%)	38% (0–58%)	9% (0–66%)	0% (0%)	24% (0–78%)	0.3% 0–3%	16% 12–23%	?

[a]Partially derived from Refs. 135, 197–207.

ation in their vital signs. In most patients, use of small amounts of epinephrine with the local anesthetic does not seem to cause a major additional increase in blood pressure or pulse rate (135). Evidence suggests that use of epinephrine results in lower blood pressure and pulse rate because of better anesthesia and control of pain. Use of mild sedation may block the rise in systolic blood pressure in hypertensive, but possibly not normotensive, patients.

In summary, the literature suggests, on average, that epinephrine causes little change in vital signs during dental procedures. Similar changes in blood pressure and pulse rate result from anxiety and pain. The mean figures, however, do not reflect a small number of patients who may have large increases in blood pressure and pulse rate.

Preoperative Treatment A frequent question is which cardiac patients undergoing dental work should be hospitalized or have the work performed in a same-day surgical center. Hospitalization or an outpatient surgical center provide the advantage of better blood pressure control and ECG monitoring, availability of an anesthesiologist for monitoring while the dentist is performing the procedure, and availability of medical personnel should complications arise.

Indications for hospitalization include moderate to severe angina, recent myocardial infarction, or significant arrhythmias. In most instances, dental work on patients with mild angina or who experienced myocardial infarction more than 6 months previously and have no major residual compromise usually can be done in the office under local anesthesia. Patients with ischemic heart disease requiring general anesthesia should have the work done in a hospital or same-day surgical center, though this is a conservative approach. Very anxious patients requiring extensive, painful procedures also should have the work done in a hospital or outpatient surgical unit, because anxiety-induced stress alters blood pressure and pulse rate as much as anesthesia does. Patients with valvular heart disease or congestive failure can be treated under local anesthesia as outpatients, but those with severe disease are exceptions. Prophylaxis for bacterial endocarditis prophylaxis should be given to patients with valvular heart disease; even parenteral antibiotics can now be given on an outpatient basis.

The recent advent of same-day surgical units raises the question of whether dental procedures in cardiac patients can be done in these units with resultant cost savings. Reported experience with dental patients is lacking, but experience with other types of surgery in patients with ischemic heart disease demonstrates that risk extends beyond the period of anesthesia. Therefore, until further experience is documented, patients with severe ischemic heart disease, arrhythmias, and congestive failure should undergo dental work in a hospital and be observed for an adequate period of time. The hospital setting provides better backup should complications arise in high-risk patients. Intermediate-risk patients, in whom the only concerns are the availability of an anesthesiologist and monitoring, can undergo dental work in an outpatient surgical center.

When extensive dental work requiring large doses of local anesthetic agents are planned, either multiple, staged procedures over several days should be done or general anesthesia considered. Mild sedation with a benzodiazepine or short-acting barbiturate may be helpful, especially in very anxious patients. Preliminary studies indicate that β-blockers may reduce the incidence of arrhythmias during dental general anesthesia, but further research is needed (136). Elective dental surgery should be deferred after myocardial infarction. Very limited experience indicates that minor procedures can be done for emergencies if the patient is in marked pain, similar to other minor elective surgeries, but the patient should be monitored and use of epinephrine either avoided or minimized.

Intra- and Postoperative Treatment Patients manifesting arrhythmias under general anesthesia should be checked for hypoxia by measuring arterial blood gases. In general, arrhythmias under anesthesia do not require long-term drug therapy. Patients manifesting serious arrhythmias should be treated acutely and re-evaluated when stable for chronic antiarrhythmic agents. Most physicians are willing to discharge hospitalized dental patients with cardiac disease 24 hours after their procedure if no complications occur.

Special Considerations

Bacterial Endocarditis Prophylaxis
Dental procedures are a classic cause of subacute bacterial endocarditis. Except for routine examinations, prophylaxis should be provided for all dental work, including even minor procedures such as teeth cleaning, extraction of loose teeth, and gum work.

The current recommended parenteral prophylactic regimens can be given on an outpatient basis in most areas. Until definitive data are available, the decision between the more convenient oral regimens and more intensive parenteral regimens must be made on the basis of the individual patient (as outlined in Chapter 17).

Anticoagulant Therapy

Anticoagulant therapy requires special management for dental extractions. Bleeding may not occur immediately during the procedure and may be delayed for hours to several days. A number of small series have reported dental extraction without complications in patients undergoing anticoagulation (Table 22.17). These

Table 22.17. Dental Procedures in Patient's on Anticoagulant Therapy

Study	Number	Prothrombin Time (control = 14 sec)	Complications
Askey (209)	11	14–51%	None
Frank (210)	25	15–40%	None
Ziffer (211)	2	39 sec	? excessive bleeding
Behrman (212, 214)	45	18–37 sec	None
Shira (213)	18	17–51 sec	3 excessive bleeding
Scopp (215)	2	31–39 sec	2 excessive bleeding

investigators have attributed the lack of bleeding to maintaining anticoagulation in a low-therapeutic range (1.5–2 times control), and they have noted that most bleeding has been reported in patients with prothrombin times in the high-therapeutic to excessive range (≥ 2.5 times control).

The risk of stopping anticoagulant therapy for several days is small in patients with artificial heart valves (see Chapter 11). Extensive series have not been reported, however, for briefly discontinuing anticoagulation therapy for other indications.

Dental extraction presents a risk of excessive, significant bleeding, at least in some patients receiving anticoagulation therapy. Therefore I prefer to stop coumarin (Coumadin) 24 to 48 hours before planned dental procedures and, if necessary, to administer phytonadione (Aqua-MEPHYTON) to normalize the prothrombin time (i.e., to within 2 seconds of control). Coumarin may be restarted from immediately to 48 hours after the procedure depending on the extent of the procedure and perioperative bleeding. In patients at high risk for thromboembolic phenomenon, heparin may be started within 12 to 24 hours if bleeding is minimal and be continued until the prothrombin time is therapeutic from the coumarin. Discontinuing anticoagulation therapy for this short time carries a very low risk of thromboembolism and avoids bleeding.

Patients with dental and facial trauma should be treated according to the extent of their injury and trauma. The major risk is subcutaneous bleeding into the planes of the face and neck, with resulting hematoma and, possibly, airway obstruction. All patients on anticoagulation therapy who have a history of significant orofacial trauma should be hospitalized for observation, whether or not bleeding is apparent. When forceful blunt trauma or bleeding occurs, the anticoagulant should be withheld and vitamin K_1 administered. Fresh-frozen plasma may need to be administered in the presence of significant acute bleeding, major fractures, or soft-tissue trauma. A major mistake is to assume that the absence of bleeding in the emergency room is reassuring, because delayed bleeding from hours to several days after trauma represents a major risk.

Pulmonary Disease There is no reported experience with dental extractions in patients who have pulmonary disease. Most patients with mild to moderate chronic obstructive lung disease tolerate dental procedures under local anesthesia well in the outpatient setting. Patients with severe lung disease, however, may have trouble maintaining an adequate tidal volume, resulting in hypoxia, during manipulation of the mouth, but this has not been well documented. Dental work on these patients should be performed in an inpatient or same-day surgical unit. Use of general anesthesia should be avoided.

Patients with asthma are at increased risk of bronchospasm during induction or when awakening from anesthesia. The inpatient operating room or same-day surgical unit should be considered for patients with moderate to severe asthma undergoing general anesthesia, and for some patients with severe asthma undergoing local procedures. Hospitalization should be considered as well for patients with poorly compensated asthma. The major risk of bronchospasm is in the immediate postoperative period, so these patients are good candidates for same-day surgical units and do not necessarily require 24 hours of observation.

Patients with asthma should be receiving an inhaled bronchodilator before procedures are performed, even if they normally are in a stable state without bronchodilators. The bronchodilator should be taken the morning of the surgery. Theophylline and oral bronchodilators can be taken orally the morning of surgery with a sip of water, even when general anesthesia will be used.

Dental Infections The bacteriology of the oropharynx, gums, and teeth is complex (137, 138). Most aerobic and anaerobic organisms can be found in the mouth; certain unusual organisms (e.g., actinomyces, nonpathogenic aerobic and anaerobic organisms) can be found as well. In addition, certain unusual organisms, such as actinomyces and nonpathogenic bacteria (e.g., *Fusobacterium* sp.), may cause infection. The most common aerobic species isolated is *Streptococcus*. The most common anaerobic species are *Peptostreptococcus* and *Bacteroides*. Most of the commonly isolated organisms, including most *Bacteroides* sp., are sensitive to penicillin (Table 22.18).

It is important to differentiate the location of infection, because the natural history and treatment will vary accordingly. Infection may occur in the dental pulp, periodontal area, pericoronal area, mandible, maxilla, and retropharyngeal facial spaces (137). The major, life-threatening complications are bacteremia; extension to the retropharyngeal spaces, cavernous sinus, and sinuses; and Ludwig's angina.

The most important general principle is to carefully evaluate patients with dental infections for spread to the jaw (i.e., osteomyelitis), nearby structures (i.e., cellulitis, sinusitis), and facial plains of the head and neck. A careful examination of the head, neck, and throat should be performed, and in questionable cases or patients who are seriously ill, an otolaryngology consultation is suggested. Radiography of the jaw, sinuses, and soft-tissue neck often is helpful as well.

It is important to recognize two rare, life-threatening syndromes. Ludwig's angina presents with boardlike edema below the mandible, inability to close the mouth, and elevation of the tongue. Obstruction may produce difficulties in swallowing and respiration. Infection of the retropharyngeal space may be manifested by high fever, rigors, pain, trismus, dysphasia, and difficult breathing. The importance of recognizing these syndromes is the necessity for rapid, radical surgical drainage.

Minor infections limited to the area of the teeth and gums usually may be treated with oral penicillin. Routine culturing is not necessary unless the patient fails to respond. Culture should be obtained on infections that are anatomically more extensive or that occur in patients who are severely ill. It is important to obtain both aerobic and anaerobic cultures, because both types of organisms usually are involved. In patients who are seriously ill, high-dose, intravenous penicillin is the drug of choice (10–20 million U/day in divided doses). Acceptable alternatives are clindamycin or a second- or third-generation cephalosporin with anaerobic activity.

Prompt, adequate drainage is a cornerstone of therapy for dental infections, because most such infection involve localized pus. Institution of antibiotic therapy should not produce complacency toward adequate drainage. The duration of antibiotic therapy depends on the severity of infection. In most cases, 10 to 14 days of therapy are sufficient; in osteomyelitis and extensive facial infections, longer durations of therapy (i.e., 2–6 weeks) are necessary.

Table 22.18.   Microbiology of Dental Infections[a]

Organism	% of Infections Isolated (N = 31)
Aerobic	
Streptococcus	14 (45%)
Anaerobic	
Bacteroides	21 (68%)
Fusobacterium	7 (23%)
Peptostreptococcus	16 (52%)
Peptococcus	7 (23%)
Actinomyces	4 (13%)

[a]Organisms insolated from more than 10% of patients. Data from Ref. 137.

Table 22.19.   Complications of Burns Contributing to Mortality[a]

Complications	No. of Cases
Nonbacterial	
Early shock or cardiac failure	12
Glottic burns and/or inhalation of smoke	7
Carbon monoxide poisoning	2
Pulmonary edema and/or atelectasis	11
Aspiration of vomit	2
Acute renal failure	24
Pulmonary embolism	5
Hypokalemia	4
Cardiac arrest	4
Hepatic jaundice	2
Hemorrhage from duodenal ulcer	1
Acute encephalopathy	1
Acute dilation of the stomach	3
Agranulocytosis and thrombocytopenia	1
Others	12
Total	91
Bacterial	
Septicemia (including pyemia)	60
Bronchopneumonia	56
Acute pyelonephritis	16
Meningitis	2
Enterocolitis	3
Gas gangrene	1
Others	3
Total	141

[a]From Sevitt S: Death after burning. *Med Sci Law* 6:36–44, 1966, with permission.

Burns

Burn injuries and their treatment may involve complications of every organ system (Table 22.19). Most of the complications are managed through use of routine burn-care protocols by the surgeon. This section details the three complications that most commonly lead to medical consultation by the internist in pulmonary injury, infection, and stress-induced gastrointestinal bleeding. Other complications for which consultation occasionally may be requested are briefly summarized with reference to the appropriate literature.

Pulmonary Complications

Epidemiology Pulmonary complications have been reported as occurring in from 25% to over 50% of patients with extensive burns, and they contribute to over 50% of deaths resulting from burns (139–148). The multiple causes of pulmonary complications in burn patients can be divided into early and late problems. *Early problems* are caused by direct thermal injury and carbon monoxide poisoning, mainly at the time of presentation or within several days of injury. *Late complications*, which occur after 24 hours, include chemical injury to the lungs from combustion-product pneumonia, adult respiratory distress syndrome, atelectasis, pulmonary emboli, and complications of mechanical ventilation (i.e., pneumothorax).

Diagnostic Activities and Approaches Findings suggestive of direct inhalation injury are burns due to fires in enclosed spaces, facial burns, wheezing, carbonaceous sputum, and lung findings by auscultation. None of these findings is specific, however, and a significant number of patients may lack such findings. Indirect laryngoscopy should be performed as soon as possible when upper airway damage is suspected.

Carbon monoxide levels should be obtained for all patients involved in fires in closed spaces. The arterial oxygen saturation is helpful only if measured directly.

The diagnosis of inhalation injury to the lower respiratory tract and lung may be difficult to make clinically. A number of tests have been proposed for diagnosis, however, including xenon ventilation scans, bronchoscopy, and pulmonary function testing. None of these studies has been definitely established as a procedure of choice. In addition, they may be difficult to obtain in patients who are severely injured. Many patients need to be followed clinically and to receive symptomatic treatment without a firmly established diagnosis.

Treatment Principles Burned patients with upper airway injuries need to be followed closely for airway obstruction. An endotracheal tube should be used, because tracheostomy carries a significant mortality rate in burn patients. Carbon monoxide poisoning should be treated with 100% oxygen and hyperventilation.

Inhalation injury to the lower respiratory tract should be treated by use of bronchodilators and pulmonary toilet. Use of steroids, however, is controversial (145, 149). Patients requiring mechanical ventilation should receive positive end-expiratory pressure, which, especially if initiated early, may shorten the duration of symptomatic lung injury.

Infectious Complications

Epidemiology Infections remain the primary cause of burn mortality, being a significant factor in 60 to 75% of such deaths (149, 150). The most common infections are pneumonia and of the burn wound itself. Sites of intravenous and urinary tract catheterization are the next most likely infections.

Organisms infecting patients with burns are similar regardless of the burn site because of common environmental exposure and bacteremic seeding from the wound (149). The types of organisms involved have changed greatly over the past 30 years, however. Infection with group A streptococci once occurred early in the course of the burn wound; these infections now are prevented by prophylactic use of low-dose penicillin and topical antibiotics.

Infection now tends to occur after the first week as well. Predominant bacteria are Gram-negative (especially *Pseudomonas* sp.). *Staphylococcus* sp. and fungi (especially *Candida* sp.) also commonly are involved.

Diagnostic Activities and Approaches Early in the treatment of a burn, mild leukocytosis may be found secondary to the burn itself (138, 149). Leukocytosis over 20,000 cu mm favors the development of infection. Localizing symptoms and signs frequently are absent.

Atypical presentation of infections in patients with burns are frequent, as are isolated hypothermia, hypotension, hypoxia, worsening of the burn wound, are sloughing of skin grafts. In patients with possible infection, careful examination of the chest, urine, and sites of instrumentation (e.g., urinary tract, intravenous) is important in localizing the infection site. The burn wound should be cultured by quantitative biopsy, because swab cultures cannot differentiate between colonization and infection. A colony count greater than 10^5 bacteria per 1 g of tissue indicates infection of the burn wound (138).

Treatment Principles Prevention of infection is crucial, because patients with burns are immunosuppressed and do not always respond to treatment with antibiotics. Prophylactic treatment involves the application of topical antibiotics and, in many centers, prophylactic use of low-dose penicillin (1.2–2.4 million U/day) for the first 1 to 3 days. Limiting the number of and paying meticulous attention to inserting intravenous and urinary tract catheters are important. Proper attention to asepsis in caring for the patient and prevention of cross-infection in burn units are important as well. A passive vaccine shows promise in decreasing the incidence and mortality rate of infections with *Pseudomonas* sp. (149).

Infections in patients with burns must be treated early, because these immunosuppressed patients may rapidly succumb to infection. **In general, treatment of suspected infection should begin early and not wait for positive cultures.** In the common situation in which a site of infection cannot be positively identified, appropriate coverage includes an aminoglycoside antibiotic active against *Pseudomonas* sp. and a semisynthetic penicillin active against *Staphylococcus* sp.

Proper local care should include removal and culturing of catheters suspected of infection, debridement of the burn wound, surgical removal of infected veins, and pulmonary toilet. Careful attention should be given to other complications as well, especially hypoxia and hypotension.

Gastrointestinal Bleeding

Epidemiology Clinical studies have shown evidence for upper gastrointestinal bleeding and gastritis in approximately 25% of patients with large burn injuries. Less common are frank gastroduodenal ulceration, which occurs in 12 to 25% of patients, and life-threatening hemorrhage, which occurs in 5% of patients. Serial endoscopy has shown that gastric erosions are present in most large burns and occur early, within 72 hours after injury (149, 151–154). Additional risk factors for more severe gastroduodenal injury are sepsis, hypoxia, and hypotension (154). Both intensive, prophylactic antacid therapy and, possibly, H_2-receptor blockers prevent major gastrointestinal hemorrhage after burn injury.

Diagnostic Activities and Approaches There is no consensus on which patients should undergo endoscopy. Patients with bleeding sufficient to require consideration of surgery should undergo endoscopy. Endoscopy also should be performed in patients whose past history or time course of bleeding suggest pre-existing lesions not related to their burns (e.g., esophageal varices in alcoholic patients). A search for occult sepsis and disseminated intravascular coagulation should be made in the absence of known infection or respiratory insufficiency, because one of these frequently is present in patients with bleeding.

Treatment Principles Both occult and major bleeding after burns can be prevented by administration of an intensive antacid regimen, sucralfate, or possibly, cimetidine. Hourly antacids sufficient to maintain a gastric pH greater than 3.5 should be administered prophylactically to patients with burns covering more than 20 to 50% of the body surface or who have additional risk factors of sepsis and respiratory insufficiency.

Abnormalities of Liver Function After extensive burn injuries, liver enzyme levels are elevated in as many as 50% of patients. The pattern is a hepatocellular injury, with transaminase levels being the most elevated. Results of liver function tests may become elevated within 24 hours of injury, and they may take 2 to 3 weeks to return to normal. Abnormal liver function tests occurring late after the initial injury should suggest the possibility of sepsis or hypotension. Important differential diagnoses include sepsis, acalculous, cholecystitis, and pancreatitis.

Cardiovascular Complications

Epidemiology Myocardial depression occurs after second- or third-degree burns over 40 to 60% of body surface, depending on the burn depth; cardiac output may drop to one-third of previous levels (149, 150, 155). Myocardial depression results from both volume depletion and a plasma factor causing myocardial depression (149, 150, 155). Myocardial depression can lead to clinical congestive heart failure due to the massive fluid replacement that is routinely given as therapy.

Myocardial infarction sometimes occurs, usually in elderly patients with extensive burn injuries (149). Hypertension has been reported as a complication of burns in children but not in adults. Usually, hypertension after burns in adult patients can be explained by prior hypertension or fluid overload.

Diagnostic Activities and Approaches Congestive heart failure may be extremely difficult to diagnose in patients with burns. The major differential diagnoses is pulmonary burn injury and acute respiratory distress syndrome. Swan-Ganz catheterization is useful in resolving difficult cases. Patients with severe heart disease may benefit from pulmonary arterial pressure monitoring, but the risk of infection should be recognized.

Myocardial infarction also may be difficult to diagnose. The presenting symptoms often are congestive heart failure, arrhythmias, or shock, which may have many other explanations in these patients.

Neuropsychiatric Disorders Patients with large burns may present a spectrum of psychiatric complications, ranging from mild grief to psychosis. These must be differentiated from an acute, organic brain syndrome, which can follow burn injury. The organic syndrome may range from mild lethargy to delirium or coma. There are no localizing neurologic signs, but pupillary abnormalities, abnormalities of extraocular muscles, cerebellar signs, and seizures have been reported.

The organic delirium usually is seen in patients with extensive burns (i.e., exceeding 50% of the body surface). The neurologic syndrome may not begin until 2 to 3 weeks after injury. The onset may be related to sepsis, and treatment focuses on adequate therapy for the burn injury, sepsis, and any potentiating metabolic abnormalities.

Mild lethargy and confusion in patients with burns may be the presenting symptom of metabolic abnormalities or sepsis, especially early in the course. The diagnosis of delirium secondary to burn injury should not be made until other abnormalities have been excluded, especially if the features or timing of onset is atypical.

Renal and Electrolyte Complications Acute renal failure may result from hypovolemia early in the course of burns and from septicemia later (during hospitalization). Both oliguric and nonoliguric renal failure have been reported. Multiple electrolyte and acid-base abnormalities occur both because of the burn and its treatment (149). Mild to moderate hyponatremia occurs 3 to 7 days after injury. The mechanism of the hyponatremia is not firmly established, but it probably is related to fluid therapy and mobilization of burn fluid. Treatment is restriction of free water.

Electrical Injury

Epidemiology Little quantitative literature exists on the medical complications of electrical injury, which can be divided into those occurring during the hospital course and those occurring chronically, weeks to years after injury. The most frequent acute complications are cardiac arrhythmias, respiratory arrest, renal failure, and central nervous system (CNS) damage (149, 156–158). The most immediate, generalized effects of electrical injury are cardiac arrhythmia (usually ventricular fibrillation) and respiratory arrest.

After the initial resuscitation, many ECG changes have been reported, including bundle-branch block, A-V dissociation, premature atrial and ventricular beats, and sustained supraventricular and ventricular arrhythmias. Ischemic changes on the ECG have included nonspecific ST-T wave changes in most patients and changes typical of myocardial infarction in occasional patients (156, 157). Most studies have not used cardiac scans or myocardial isoenzymes to establish whether myocardial infarction has occurred. Patients with these ischemic changes have been reported to tolerate required surgical procedures without cardiac complications (156, 157).

Respiratory arrest is a contributing cause to hypoxia and cardiac arrhythmias, but other pulmonary injuries are uncommon. Occasionally, patients will suffer a localized pneumonitis and pleural effusion related to the entrance wound. As with burns, pneumonia is a frequent and important complication.

Many patients have renal damage or failure due to multiple causes. Factors implicated in renal failure have included direct electrical damage to the kidneys, the initial hypotension, tissue breakdown products, and myoglobinuria.

Damage to the nervous system includes initial coma and spinal cord injury due to current or vertebral fractures. The course of these changes is quite variable, but permanent damage is frequent, especially in the form of spinal cord lesions (156).

Submucosal hemorrhages throughout the gastrointestinal tract occur with electrical injuries, and death from hemorrhagic necrosis of the bowel, especially the colon, occasionally results. As with burns, stress-induced gastric bleeding is a frequent problem. The most frequent cause of death in patients with electrical injuries, however, is infection (156). In addition to the common sites for burns, infection of necrotic muscle is an important source of sepsis, and prompt debridement is important.

Diagnostic Activities and Approaches
Serial ECGs and continuous monitoring for arrhythmias are important. There is a lack of reported experience, but cardiac isoenzymes (MG isoenzyme of creatine phosphokinase) should be of diagnostic help. In questionable cases of cardiac injury, ^{99}Tc or thallium scans should be obtained. Renal function, urine output, electrolytes, and acid-base status should be measured frequently during the first several days, because severe acidosis is common. During the recovery period from the acidosis, profound hypokalemia may suddenly occur.

Treatment Principles Patients with electrical injuries usually present with cardiac and respiratory arrest. Resuscitation attempts should be prolonged, because complete cardiac and neurologic recovery has been reported, even in patients requiring several hours of resuscitation. There are no data, however, to establish how long monitoring should continue, but a minimum of 3 days or until the acute stage of injury has resolved is recommended. Surgery for debridement usually

should not be delayed because of possible cardiac damage, because it is required for the patient to survive and seems to carry an acceptable risk, even in the presence of ECG abnormalities (157, 158).

All patients should have sufficient amounts of intravenous fluids to maintain both blood pressure and urine flow. The amount of fluid required is highly variable, and in contrast to burn injuries, no set regimen has been established in this setting (156). Most authors recommend that mannitol be given soon after injury to reduce myoglobin-induced renal damage. Severe acidosis is common and should be treated vigorously with sodium bicarbonate. The acidosis will plateau after the first several days, followed by a period during which severe potassium depletion may occur. It therefore is important to monitor the serum potassium level frequently, not only during bicarbonate replacement therapy but for several days thereafter.

Pelvic Exenteration

Epidemiology Pelvic exenteration is an uncommon, radical surgical procedure indicated for recurrent cancer of the cervix and certain cases of rectal cancer involving the genital tract. Even on large gynecologic oncology services, the frequency of this procedure averages only one per month, which should further decrease with current radiation therapy techniques and earlier diagnosis by use of routine Pap smears. Because of the extensive nature of the procedure, most gynecologic oncologists recommend it be performed only by teams who are experienced in both the technique and the treatment of the postoperative complications most frequently seen. The 2-year survival rate for recurrent cancer of the cervix, when treated conservatively, approaches zero. With current surgical techniques and supportive care, the 2-year survival rate for those patients treated with pelvic exenteration approximates 50%, with a 2 to 13% rate of surgical mortality.

Preoperative Evaluation Proper patient selection is the key to minimizing surgical morbidity and mortality. Tumor spread beyond the pelvis, positive peritoneal cytology, or para-aortic and pelvic node involvement make successful outcome a remote possibility. Nutritional status, circulating volume, electrolyte levels, and acid-base balance must be as close to normal as possible before surgery is undertaken.

Unrelated conditions that substantially increase morbidity and mortality are impaired renal function, cardiac failure, and poorly controlled diabetes mellitus (159, 160). Many gynecologists consider these disorders to be relative contraindications to the procedure.

Preoperative evaluation should focus on the assessment of cardiac and renal function. Time should be allowed to achieve good control of diabetes mellitus. In addition, psychosocial abnormalities (e.g., mental retardation, psychosis) profoundly alter the level of patient cooperation that is necessary for successful rehabilitation and make proper postoperative stoma care improbable.

Use of central hyperalimentation both pre- and postoperatively has had a major impact on optimizing the patient's condition; preventing infection, debility, and postoperative fistulae; and on improving wound healing (161). In addition, the routine use of preoperative prophylactic antibiotics (usually an aminoglycoside plus clindamycin) also has contributed to the prevention of postoperative wound infections. Patient support groups and stomal therapists contribute crucial emotional comfort and essential practical advice as well.

Postoperative Care In a review of 296 patients at the M.D. Anderson Hospital, Rutledge et al. (159) grouped postoperative complications into early (postoperative days 1–7), intermediate (postoperative days 7–90), and late (postoperative days 90 and later) phases (Table 22.20). In the first 7 days, complications generally could be

Table 22.20. Complications of Pelvic Exenteration in 296 Patients[a]

	Number	% of Total
Early (day 1–7)		
(1) Cardiac failure, MI, pulmonary emboli, DVT, CVAs, DIC	31	33
(2) Uremia	17	20
(3) Pneumonia	18	20
(4) Sepsis (pyelonephritis, pelvic infections, peritonitis)	21	23
(5) GI bleeding	2	2
Intermediate (day 7–90)		
(1) Sepsis, pneumonia, wound infection	41	35
(2) Intestinal obstruction and fistulas	41	35
(3) Uremia, urinary fistulae, leakage, pyelonephritis	34	29
(4) Cardiovascular	2	1
Late (>90 days)		
(1) Chronic UTI	31	38
(2) Uropathy (stones, renal failure)	15	18
(3) Intestinal obstruction	13	16
(4) Stoma retraction, herniation	12	16
(5) Perineal herniation	10	12

[a]From Rutledge et al: *Am J Obstet Gynecol* 129:881, 1977. Used with permission.

categorized as primarily medical, whereas those occurring later were more likely to be surgical.

The most common medical complications are cardiac, thromboembolic, renal failure, pneumonia, sepsis, and gastrointestinal bleeding (Table 22.21). Particular treatment problems during the first postoperative week are replacement of blood and fluids as well as nutritional support. For example, the operative field has been compared to a 10%, third-degree burn, with maintenance and replacement crystalloids and colloids being calculated accordingly (162).

Table 22.21. **Complications of Pelvic Exenteration in 37 Patients at the Milton S. Hershey Medical Center, 1972–1979**[a]

	N	%
Sepsis	7	20
Wound infection	5	15
Phlebitis	4	12
Pneumonia	2	6
Hepatitis	1	3
Small bowel obstruction	5	15
Urinary and GI conduit fistulae	6	17

[a]From Curry et al.: *Gynecol Oncol* 11:119, 1981. Used with permission.

Radical Neck Surgery

Epidemiology Most internists conceive of radical neck dissection as a mutilating procedure with high surgical morbidity and mortality. However, radical neck dissection (i.e., the unilateral, en bloc removal of the lymph nodes and drainage of the neck) gives a cosmetically good result, except when combined with extensive orofacial resections or with total laryngectomy. Aggressive plastic and reconstructive techniques often can restore patients undergoing resections of the face and mandible to good physiologic function and fair cosmetic results. Average blood loss is 1 to 3 units, and the average duration of surgery is from 1 to 3 hours. An operating time of up to 10 hours, however, may be required in complicated cases (e.g., in those with previous, uncoordinated radiation therapy or "redo" operations).

The overall surgical mortality rate is 1 to 3% with unilateral radical neck dissection and 2 to 5% with bilateral radical neck dissection. Except for very old patients (>70 years), radical neck dissection is a well-tolerated procedure, with surgical morbidity and mortality rates in appropriately prepared patients approximately equal to those of other major surgical procedures in this age group (Tables 22.22 and 22.23). The major causes of increased mortality in very old

patients are aspiration pneumonia, malnutrition, and cardiovascular disease.

Older and ill patients often are advised against surgery and referred for extensive radiation therapy; this is because of the bias of many physicians that many of these patients will not outlive their primary disease. However, many patients survive long enough to present for complex surgery at an even older age. Primary radiation therapy, if uncoordinated with surgery, often compromises the ideal surgical approach and increases the surgical morbidity rate (by 30–40% in many series) by leading to extensive fibrosis, edema, disruption of tissue planes, and altered perfusion.

Diagnostic Activities and Treatment Preoperative preparation and attention to detail play major roles in decreasing surgical morbidity and mortality. Nutritional status should be restored as closely to normal as possible via either enteral or parenteral approaches. If the oropharyngeal space is to be penetrated, prior treatment of periodontal disease should be vigorously pursued and appropriate antibiotic coverage planned. Most studies report a significant decrease in postoperative infections with use of cephalosporin (1 g preoperatively, then 500 mg every 6 hours for four doses postoperatively). Alternative antibiotic regimens are clindamycin, cephalosporin (or penicillin or clindamycin) plus tobramycin. A single, preoperative dose of antibiotic followed by administration for 1 to

Table 22.22. **Operative Mortality for Radical Neck Dissection**[a]

Age	Number	
All ages	2.8%	2.8%
≤49	0/83	0%
50–59	5/211	2.4%
60–69	3/258	1.2%
70–79	6/131	4.6%
80+	6/31	19.4%

[a]From McGuirt et al: *Laryngoscope* 87:1378, 1977. Used with permission.

Table 22.23. Type of Surgical Procedure Related to Cause of Death[a]

	Pulmonary	Cardio-vascular	Multiple Stress
Jaw-neck	1	4	1
Laryngectomy-pharyngectomy	3		1
Radical neck dissection		2	1

[a]From McGuirt et al: *Laryngoscope* 87:1378, 1977. Used with permission.

3 days postoperatively has been recommended, as has continuing prophylactic antibiotics for 5 to 7 days postoperatively. However, no data prove the superiority of a two-drug regimen or of prolonged administration. In addition, patients should be fully prepared emotionally for the recovery period, as well as for any further planned plastic and reconstructive surgery.

Postoperative Treatment

Camnitz et al. (163) conveniently divided surgical complications into intraoperative, early, and late postoperative phases. Intraoperative complications are primarily mechanical and are treated by immediate surgical correction (e.g., jugular vein bleeding, air embolism, carotid sinus syndrome, carotid thrombosis, cranial and phrenic nerve injuries, pneumothorax, thoracic duct injury). The internist rarely is involved in their diagnosis or treatment.

Early postoperative complications (i.e., days 1–7) vary according to the type of surgery. With radical neck dissection alone, most complications usually are of cardiovascular origin, whereas with pharyngectomies or laryngectomies, pulmonary complications predominate (Table 22.23). With radical neck dissection alone, cough is not impaired.

When a tracheostomy is required, drying of the airway and a poor cough with retention of secretions, atelectasis, and pneumonia are constant concerns. Tracheostomy cuffs must be fully inflated when using positive-pressure breathing to avoid forcing oropharyngeal contents into the wound. Fistula formation and wound infections are more common when the oropharyngeal space has been surgically entered. With use of closed-suction drainage catheters placed in the wound at surgery, the incidence of these complications has been substantially reduced but is still frequent, occurring in 20% or more of these patients.

Postoperative agitation and irrational behavior may be due to hypoxia. Arterial blood gases should be measured, and tracheal obstruction due to hematomas or seromas should always be considered. Other causes of agitation, such as urinary retention, delirium tremens, and intensive care unit psychosis, should be considered as well.

Late complications (i.e., >30 days) often are related to tumor recurrence or surgical mishaps (e.g., jugular vein ligation, loss of skin flaps, carotid erosion). In patients undergoing total laryngectomy and treated with radiation therapy, late hypothyroidism may occur.

In summary, radical neck dissection, laryngectomies, and pharyngectomies can be safely performed, even in aged patients, with good functional and cosmetic results if there is careful preoperative preparation, avoidance of preoperative radiation therapy uncoordinated with surgery, and use of prophylactic antibiotics.

Transurethral Prostate Resection

Transurethral resection of the prostate (TURP) is among the most common operation in elderly males. The operative risk of such surgery is very small (approximately 1%), even for patients with severe, chronic disease.

Epidemiology

Several operations are performed for benign prostatic hypertrophy, including

Table 22.24. Risk of Prostate Surgery[a]

| | Mortality | | | |
	All Patients	Patients with Cardiac Disease	Total Number (Cardiac)	Cause of Mortality
Erlik, 1968	0.93%	0.96%	539 (104)	3 pulmonary emboli 1 CVA 1 pulmonary emboli and MI
–Additional cases	0%	0%	135 (27)	
Thompson, 1962		5%	192 (192)	7 MI 1 CHF 1 SBE
Skinner, 1964		2%	124 (124)	
Mebust, 1989	0.23%	.1%	3885 (952)	1 MI

[a]Derived in part from Refs. 130, 164 and 165.

transurethral, suprapubic, and less commonly, retropubic prostatectomy. Radical prostatectomy is performed for carcinoma of the prostate. TURP is the most common operation and carries a lower risk than other procedures. Suprapubic and radical prostatectomy constitute major surgeries with a cardiopulmonary risk comparable to those of major lower intraperitoneal procedures. These more extensive procedures have an increased risk of sepsis from urinary tract infection and thromboembolism compared with TURP.

Current series indicate that TURP can be performed with a less than 1% overall mortality rate. The major consideration is the existence of cardiac disease. In combined series of 674 patients studied by Erlik et al. (164) (Table 22.24), the perioperative mortality rate was not increased in patients with (0.76%) compared to those without (0.74%) cardiac disease. In another study (130), the rate of cardiac complications was not increased in patients with pre-existing heart disease compared to those without (0.5% vs. 0.5%).

A 5% mortality rate has been reported for patients undergoing TURP after myocardial infarction (165). TURP has been performed within 6 months of a myocardial infarction without a major increase in mortality, but experience is limited. Pru-

dence dictates waiting for 6 months or longer after infarction, if possible.

The major causes of postoperative mortality after TURP are infection, pulmonary emboli, and cardiac complications (166). Most of the small number of myocardial infarctions occurred late after surgery (≥5 days) in the two reported series.

The risk of thrombophlebitis has been variously estimated as being from 7 to 80% in patients undergoing all types of prostate surgery (167). Studies of only TURP have found a rate of deep vein thrombosis (DVT) of 7 to 10% by ^{125}I fibrinogen scanning and of 5% by phleborrheography (Table 22.25).

Table 22.25. Risk of Thrombophlebitis with Transurethral Prostate Resection[a]

Study	Diagnostic Study	No. with TURP	Thrombophlebitis (%)
Mays, 1971	^{131}I fibrinogen	20	2 (10%)
Nicolardes, 1972	^{131}I fibrinogen	29	2 (7%)
Crawford, 1978	Phleborheography	150	7 (5%)
Van Arsdalen	Venography	29	2 (7%)

[a]From Refs. 167, 208, 216, 217.

The incidences of fatal pulmonary emboli after *all* types of prostatectomy was 1% in the international low-dose heparin trial (168). The available data suggest that thrombophlebitis is not as frequent a complication with TURP as many clinicians believe or as with other methods of prostate surgery. The incidence of Gram-negative sepsis after TURP also is lower in current series (average, 1–8%) than with other types of prostatectomy in earlier studies (see Chapter 17) (169).

Thus, from the viewpoint of medical problems, TURP represents a relatively safe operation. Today, the feared complications of thromboembolic events, sepsis, and myocardial infarction are much lower than reported in older series, or when prostatectomy is accomplished by other methods, but still account for most of the current, small mortality.

Diagnostic Activities and Approaches The initial database for a patient should emphasize the cardiac and the pulmonary systems. Pulmonary function tests do not need to be performed routinely in the absence of any history of physical findings of *clinically* significant pulmonary disease because of the low rate of pulmonary complications. Assessment of renal function, urine culture, and often, intravenous pyelography are routinely performed by the urologist. Abnormalities of renal function need to be further investigated before surgery.

Treatment Principles

Preoperative Treatment

Transurethral prostate resection can be performed on most patients, including those with stable, severe, chronic disease. The most important concomitant disease to be considered is coronary artery disease.

Patients with recent myocardial infarction (i.e., within the past 6 months) should have TURP deferred. In patients who do not tolerate Foley catheter drainage or have repeated complications, surgery earlier than 6 months can be considered

because of the small increase in risk, though waiting a *minimum* of 6 to 12 weeks is recommended depending on the individual circumstances. Medical therapy with finasteride or an α-blocker is an alternative in some patients. Finasteride takes months to work, however, and α-blockers carry a risk of hypotension (particularly orthostatic hypotension).

Prophylaxis to prevent thromboembolic events is controversial as there are inadequate data relating specifically to prostatectomy. Elastic stockings and early ambulation should be used for all patients as general measures. Various drug regimens have been used, including low-dose heparin and aspirin, but no regimen has proved to be efficacious. Sequential compression device stockings are another alternative that does not increase the risk of bleeding risk (see Chapter 9).

Postoperative Treatment

Any new signs that suggest deep venous thrombosis warrant Doppler ultrasonography or venography because of the inaccuracy of clinical diagnoses. Postoperative fevers are a frequent occurrence, and a careful search should be made for infection, especially of the urinary tract. Prompt therapy should be instituted for suspected urinary tract infection because of the risk of Gram-negative sepsis.

Special Considerations

Cerebrovascular Disease In one study (170), cerebrovascular accidents (CVA) extended or recurred in 2 of 22 patients (10%) undergoing TURP who had a prior stroke. No information was given on the patients' conditions or the elapsed time since the previous CVA. In my own experience, the recurrence rate for CVA has not been as high, perhaps due to patient selection, allowing an adequate time to elapse since a stroke (i.e., 6–12 weeks), and a good perioperative maintenance of blood pressure. Preoperative evaluation of patients for TURP after a stroke should include an evaluation to exclude neurologic problems as a major contributing cause to difficulty with micturition.

Hyponatremia Rarely, a marked drop in the serum sodium level occurs shortly after TURP (171–173). This hyponatremia may be marked, with the sodium level falling from normal to below 120 mEq/L. The fall in serum sodium results from absorption of irrigating fluid. This problem occurred more frequently in the past, when sterile water was used as an irrigating solution (compared with current solutions that contain mannitol or sodium chloride).

The drop in serum sodium is acute and therefore often accompanied by severe symptoms, including confusion, coma, and seizures. Rarely, the major manifestation will be focal neurologic signs. A syndrome of cortical blindness due to hyponatremia after prostatectomy has been labeled the *TURP reaction*. This is not specific for prostatectomy, however, because focal signs have been reported with hyponatremia in other circumstances as well.

Electrolyte levels should be measured immediately if a patient develops new CNS or other symptoms suggestive of hyponatremia after TURP. Treatment depends on the patient's intravascular volume; because most patients will be fluid overloaded, furosemide and hypertonic saline are the usual treatment (see Chapter 12).

REFERENCES

1. Zenilman ME. Surgery in the nursing home patient. Surg Clin North Am 1994;74:63–71.
2. Djokovic JL, Hedley-Whyte J. Prediction of outcome of surgery and anesthesia in patients over 80. JAMA 1979;242:2301–2306.
3. Ziffren SE. Comparison of mortality rates for various surgical operations according to age groups, 1951–1977. J Am Geriatr Soc 1979;10:433–438.
4. Linn BS, Linn MW. Evaluation of results of surgical procedures in the elderly. Ann Surg 1982;195:90–96.
5. Rosenthal RA, Andersen DA. Surgery in the elderly. In: Andres R, et al., eds. Principles of geriatric medicine. New York: McGraw-Hill, 1985:909–932.
6. Dunlop LWE, Rosenblood LL, Lawrason L, et al. Effects of age and severity of illness on outcome and length of stay in geriatric surgical patients. Am J Surg 1993;165:577–580.
7. Dripps RD, Lamont A, Eckenhoff JE. The role of anesthesia in surgical mortality. JAMA 1961;178:261–266.
8. Goldman L. Supraventricular tachyarrhythmias in hospitalized adults after surgery. Clinical correlates in patients over 40 years of age after major noncardiac surgery. Chest 1978;73:450–454.
9. Pollock AV, Evans M. Major abdominal operations on patients aged 80 and over: an audit. BMJ 1987;295:1522.
10. Michel SL, Stevens L, Amodeo P, et al. Surgical procedures in nonagenarians. West J Med 1984;141:61–63.
11. Hosking MP, Warner MA, Lobdell CM, et al. Outcomes of surgery in patients 90 years of age and older. JAMA 1989;261:1909–1915.
12. Warner MA, Hoskin MP, Lobdell CM, et al. Surgical procedures among those ≥90 years of age. Ann Surg 1988;207:380–386.
13. Adkins RB, Scott HW. Surgical procedures in patients aged 90 years and older. South Med J 1984;77:1357–1364.
14. Denny JL, Denson JS. Risk of surgery in patients over 90. Geriatrics 1972;27:115–118.
15. Katlic MR. Surgery in centenarians. JAMA 1985;253:3139–3141.
16. Rashad KF, Goldman EJ, Graff TD, et al. Baltimore Anesthesia Study Committee: factors in geriatric anesthesia mortality. Anesth Analg 1965;44:462–648.
17. Tarhan S, Moffitt EA, Sessler AD, et al. Risk of anesthesia and surgery in patients with chronic bronchitis and chronic obstructive pulmonary disease. Surgery 1973;74:720–726.
18. Bunkey JP, Barnes BA, Mosteller F, eds. Risks and benefits of surgery. New York: Oxford University Press, 1977:223–245.
19. Marx GF, Mateo CV, Orkin LR. Computer analysis of postanesthetic deaths. Anesthesiology 1973;39:54–58.
20. Zenilman ME, Bender JS, Magnuson TH, Smith GW. General surgical care in the nursing home patient: results of a dedicated geriatric surgery consult service. J Am Coll Surg 1996;183:361–370.
21. McGuirt WF, Loevy S, McCabe BF, et al. The risk of major head and neck surgery in the aged population. Laryngoscope 1977;87:1378–1382.
22. Gross RJ, Curtis J, Brooker A. Effect of coexisting medical illness on mortality of hip fracture repair (abstract). Clin Res 1986;34:819A.
23. Reiss R, Haddad M, Deutsch A, et al. Prognostic index: prediction of operative mortality in geriatric patients by use of stepwise logistic regression analysis. World J Surg 1987;11:248–251.

24. Seymour DG, Pringle R. Post-operative complications in the elderly surgical patient. Gerontology 1983;29:262–270.

25. Keating HJ. Preoperative considerations in the geriatric patient. Med Clin North Am 1987;71: 569–583.

26. Palmberg S, Hirsjarvi E. Mortality in geriatric surgery. Gerontology 1979;25:103–112.

27. Wilder RJ, Fishbein RH. Operative experience with patients over 80 years of age. Surg Gynecol Obstet 1961;113:205–212.

28. Boyd JB, Bradford B, Watne A. Operative risk factors of colon resection in the elderly. Ann Surg 1980;192:743–746.

29. Miller R, Marlar K, Silvay G. Anesthesia for patients aged over ninety years. N Y St J Med 1977;77:1421–1425.

30. Cole WH. Medical differences between the young and the aged. J Am Geriatr Soc 1970;18: 589–614.

31. Gerson MC, Hurst JM, Hertzberg VS, et al. Cardiac prognosis in noncardiac geriatric surgery. Ann Intern Med 1985;103:832–837.

32. Gardner RJ, Gardner NL, Tarnay TJ, et al. The surgical experience and a one to sixteen year follow-up of 277 abdominal aortic aneurysms. Am J Surg 1978;135:226–230.

33. Marshall WH, Fahey PJ. Operative complications and mortality in patients over 80. Arch Surg 1964;88:896–904.

34. Marcantonio ER, Goldman L, Mangione CM, et al. A clinical prediction rule for delirium after elective noncardiac surgery. JAMA 1994;271: 134–139.

35. Francis J, Martin D, Kapoor WN. A prospective study of delirium in hospitalized elderly. JAMA 1990;263:1097–1101.

36. Del Guercio LRM, Cohn JD. Monitoring operative risk in the elderly. JAMA 1980;243:1350–1355.

37. Lewin I, Lerner AG, Green SH, et al. Physical class and physiologic status in the prediction of operative mortality in the aged sick. Ann Surg 1971;174:217–231.

38. Seymour DG, Vaz FG. Aspects of surgery in the elderly: preoperative medical assessment. Br J Hosp Med 1987;37:102–112.

39. Andersen B, Ostberg J. Long-term prognosis in geriatric surgery. J Am Geriatr Soc 1972;20: 255–258.

40. Guillen J, Aldrete JA. Anesthetic factors influencing morbidity and mortality of elderly patients undergoing inguinal herniorrhaphy. Am J Surg 1970;120:760–763.

41. Greenburg AG, Salk RP, Peskin GW. Mortality and gastrointestinal surgery in the aged. Arch Surg 1981;116:788–791.

42. Greenburg AG, Salk RP, Pridham D. Influence of age on mortality of colon surgery. Am J Surg 1985;150:65–70.

43. Mitty WF. Surgery in the aged: seventy-five years of age and over. Springfield, IL: Charles C. Thomas, 1966.

44. Panayiotis G, Ellenbogen A, Grunstein S. Major gynecologic surgical procedures in the aged. J Am Geriatr Soc 1978;26:459–462.

45. Breyer RH, Zippe C, Pharr WF. Thoracotomy in patients over age seventy years. J Thorac Cardiovasc Surg 1981;81:187–193.

46. Gore I, Hirst AE Jr. Arteriosclerotic aneurysms of the abdominal aorta: a review. Prog Cardiovasc Dis 1973;16:113–150.

47. Estes JE Jr. Abdominal aortic aneurysm: a study of one hundred and two cases. Circulation 1950;II:258–264.

48. Szilagyi DE, Smith RF, DeRusso FJ, et al. Contribution of abdominal aortic aneurysmectomy to prolongation of life. Ann Surg 1966; 164:678–697.

49. Esselstyn CB Jr, Humphries AW, Young JR, et al. Aneurysmectomy in the aged? Surgery 1970;67:34–39.

50. MacVaugh H III, Roberts B. Results of resection of abdominal aortic aneurysm. Surg Gynecol Obstet 1961;113:17–23.

51. Foster JH, Bolasny BL, Gobbel WG Jr, et al. Comparative study of elective resection and expectant treatment of abdominal aortic aneurysm. Surg Gynecol Obstet 1969;129:1–9.

52. Gliedman ML, Ayers WB, Vestal BL. Aneurysms of the abdominal aorta and its branches. A study of untreated patients. Ann Surg 1957; 146:207–214.

53. Klippel AP, Butcher HR Jr. The unoperated abdominal aortic aneurysm. Am J Surg 1966; 111:629–631.

54. Szilagyi DE, Elliott JP, Smith RF. Clinical fate of the patient with asymptomatic abdominal aortic aneurysm and unfit for surgical treatment. Arch Surg 1972;104:600–606.

55. Schatz IJ, Fairbairn JF II, Juergens JL. Abdominal aortic aneurysm. A reappraisal. Circulation 1962;26:200–205.

56. Darling RC, Messina CR, Brewster DC, et al. Autopsy study of unoperated abdominal aortic aneurysms: the case for early resection. Cardiovasc Surg 1976;56:II-161–II-164.

57. Crawford ES, Saleh SA, Babb JW, et al. Infrarenal abdominal aortic aneurysm. Ann Surg 1981;193:699–709.

58. Bernstein EF, Fisher JC, Varco RL. Is excision the optimum treatment for all abdominal aortic aneurysms? Surgery 1967;61:83–93.

59. Roger VL, Ballard DJ, Hallett JW, et al. Influence of coronary artery disease on morbidity and mortality after abdominal aortic aneurysmectomy: a population-based study, 1971–1987. J Am Coll Cardiol 1989;14:1245–1252.

60. Young AE, Sandberg GW, Couch NP. The reduction of mortality of abdominal aortic aneurysm resection. Am J Surg 1977;134: 585–590.

61. Hicks GL, Eastland MW, DeWeese JA, et al. Survival improvement following aortic aneurysm resection. Ann Surg 1975;181:863–869.

62. Porter JM, McGregor F Jr, Acinapura AJ, et al. Renal function following abdominal aortic aneurysmectomy. Surg Gynecol Obstet 1966;123: 819–825.

63. Bush JL. Renal failure following abdominal aortic reconstruction. Surgery 1983;93:107–109.

64. Cohen JR, Mannick JA, Couch NP, et al. Abdominal aortic aneurysm repair in patients with preoperative renal failure. J Vasc Surg 1986;3:867–870.

65. Levy JF, Kouchoukos NT, Walker WB, et al. Abdominal aortic aneurysmectomy: a study of 100 cases. Arch Surg 1966;92:498–503.

66. DeBakey ME, Crawford ES, Cooley DA, et al. Aneurysm of abdominal aorta: analysis of results of graft replacement therapy one to eleven years after operation. Ann Surg 1964; 160:622–638.

67. Goldman L, Caldera DC, Southwick FS, et al. Cardiac risk factors and complications in noncardiac surgery. Medicine (Baltimore) 1978;57: 357–370.

68. Hollier LH. Surgical management of abdominal aortic aneurysm in the high risk patient. Surg Clin North Am 1986;66:269–279.

69. Szilagyi DE, Elliott JP, Berguer R. Coincidental malignancy and abdominal aortic aneurysm problems of management. Arch Surg 1967;95: 402–411.

70. Committee on Perioperative Cardiovascular Evaluation for Noncardiac Surgery. Guidelines for perioperative cardiovascular evaluation for noncardiac surgery. J Am Coll Cardiol 1996;27: 910–948.

71. Cutler BS, Leppo JA. Dipyridamole thallium 201 scintigraphy to detect coronary artery disease before abdominal aortic surgery. J Vasc Surg 1987;5:91–100.

72. Kazmers A, Cerqueira MD, Zierler RE. Perioperative and late outcome in patients with left ventricular ejection fraction of 35% or less who require major vascular surgery. J Vasc Surg 1988;8:307–315.

73. Pasternack PF, Imparato AM, Bear G, et al. The value of radionuclide angiography as a predictor of perioperative myocardial infarction in patients undergoing abdominal aortic aneurysm resection. J Vasc Surg 1984;1: 320–325.

74. Hertzer NR, Beven EG, Young JR, et al. Coronary artery disease in peripheral vascular patients. Ann Surg 1984;199:223–232.

75. Yeager RA, Weigel RM, Murphy ES, et al. Application of clinically valid cardiac risk factors to aortic aneurysm surgery. Arch Surg 1986;121:278–281.

76. Golden MA, Whittemore AD, Donaldson MC, Manick JA. Selective evaluation and management of coronary artery disease in patients undergoing repair of abdominal aortic aneurysms. Ann Surg 1990;212:415–423.

77. Blombery PA, Ferguson IA, Rosengarten DS, et al. The role of coronary artery disease in complications of abdominal aortic aneurysm surgery. Surgery 1987;101:150–155.

78. Reul GJ, Cooley DA, Duncan JM, et al. The effect of coronary bypass on the outcome of peripheral vascular operations in 1093 patients. J Vasc Surg 1986;3:788–798.

79. Ruby ST, Whittemore, Couch NP, et al. Coronary artery disease in patients requiring abdominal aortic aneurysm repair. Ann Surg 1985;201:758–764.

80. Elmore JR, Hallett JW, Gibbons RJ, et al. Myocardial revascularization before abdominal aortic aneurysmorrhaphy: effect of coronary angioplasty. Mayo Clin Proc 1993;68: 637–641.

81. Pasternack PF, Imparato AM, Baumann FG, et al. The hemodynamics of β-blockade in patients undergoing abdominal aortic aneurysm repair. Circulation 1987;76(Suppl III):III-1–III-7.

82. Attia RR, Murphy JD, Snider M, et al. Myocardial ischemia due to infrarenal aortic cross-clamping during aortic surgery in patients with severe coronary artery disease. Circulation 1976;53:961–965.

83. Bush HL Jr, LoGerfo FW, Weisel RD, et al. Assessment of myocardial performance and optimal volume loading during elective abdominal aortic aneurysm resection. Arch Surg 1977;112:1301–1305.

84. Cohen JL, Wender R, Maginot A, et al. Hemodynamic monitoring of patients undergoing abdominal aortic surgery. Am J Surg 1983;146: 174–177.

85. Kalman PG, Wellwood MR, Weisel RD, et al. Cardiac dysfunction during abdominal aortic operation: the limitations of pulmonary wedge pressures. J Vasc Surg 1986;3:773–781.

86. Huval WV, Lelcuk S, Allen PD, et al. Determinants of cardiovascular stability during abdominal aortic aneurysmectomy. Ann Surg 1983;199:216–222.

87. Edmunds LH Jr. Resection of abdominal aortic aneurysms in octogenarians. Ann Surg 1967; 165:453–457.

88. O'Donnell TF Jr, Darling RC, Linton RR. Is 80 years too old for aneurysmectomy? Arch Surg 1976;111:1250–1257.

89. Roger VL, Ballard DJ, Hallett JW, et al. Influence of coronary artery disease on morbidity and mortality after abdominal aortic aneurysmectomy: a population-based study 1971–1987. J Am Coll Cardiol 1989;14:1245–1252.

90. Sterpetti AV, Schultz RD, Feldhaus RJ, et al.

Abdominal aortic aneurysm in elderly patients. Am J Surg 1985;150:772–776.

91. Cogbill TH, Landercasper J, Strutt PH, et al. Late results of peripheral vascular surgery in patients 80 years of age and older. Arch Surg 1987;122:581–586.

92. Katz DJ, Stanley JC, Zelenock GB. Operative mortality rates for intact and ruptured abdominal aortic aneurysms in Michigan: an eleven-year statewide experience. J Vasc Surg 1994; 19:804–817.

93. Ottinger LW. Ruptured arteriosclerotic aneurysms of the abdominal aorta. Reducing mortality. JAMA 1975;233:147–150.

94. Alpert J, Brief DK, Parsonnet V. Surgery for the ruptured abdominal aortic aneurysm. JAMA 1970;212:1355–1359.

95. Darling RC. Ruptured arteriosclerotic abdominal aortic aneurysms. A pathologic and clinical study. Am J Surg 1970;119:397–401.

96. Van Heeckeren DW. Ruptured abdominal aortic aneurysms. Am J Surg 1970;119:402–407.

97. Hiatt JCG, Barker WF, Machleder HI, et al. Determinants of failure in the treatment of ruptured abdominal aortic aneurysm. Arch Surg 1984;119:1264–1268.

98. Johnson WC, Nabseth DC. Visceral infarction following aortic surgery. Ann Surg 1974;180: 312–318.

99. Smith RF, Szilagyi DE. Ischemia of the colon as a complication in the surgery of the abdominal aorta. Arch Surg 1960;80:806–821.

100. Welling RE, Roedersheimer R, Arbaugh JJ, et al. Ischemic colitis following repair of ruptured abdominal aortic aneurysm. Arch Surg 1985; 120:1368–1370.

101. Tilson MD, Fief EL, Harvey M. Malignant neoplasia in patients with abdominal aortic aneurysms. Arch Surg 1984;119:792–794.

102. Lobbatok VJ, Rothenberg RE, LaRaja RD, et al. Coexistence of abdominal aortic aneurysm and carcinoma of the colon: a dilemma. J Vasc Surg 1985;2:724–726.

103. Nora JD, Pairolero PC, Nivatvongs S, et al. Concomitant abdominal aortic aneurysm and colorectal carcinoma: priority of resection. J Vasc Surg 1989;9:630–636.

104. Hermreck AS, Proberts KS, Thomas JH. Severe jaundice after rupture of abdominal aortic aneurysm. Am J Surg 1977;134:745–748.

105. Ernst CB, Campbell HC Jr, Daugherty ME, et al. Incidence and significance of intra-operative bacterial cultures during abdominal aortic aneurysmectomy. Ann Surg 1977;185: 626–633.

106. Freeman LN, Schachat SP, Manolio TA, et al. Multivariate analysis of factors associated with unplanned admission in 'outpatient' ophthalmic surgery. Ophthal Surg 1988;19: 719–722.

107. Snow JC, Sensel S. A review of cataract extraction under local and general anesthesia at the Massachusetts eye and ear infirmary. Anesth Analg 1966;45:742–747.

108. Duncalf D, Gartner S, Carol B. Mortality in association with ophthalmic surgery. Am J Ophthalmol 1970;69:610–615.

109. Lynch S, Wolf GL, Berlin I. General anesthesia for cataract surgery: a comparative review of 2217 consecutive cases. Anesth Analg 1974;53: 909–913.

110. Adler AG. Perioperative management of the ophthalmology patient. Med Clin North Am 1987;71:561–567.

111. Rongey KA, Weisman H. Hypotension following intraocular acetylcholine. Anesthesiology 1972; 36:412.

112. Solosko D, Smith RB. Hypertension following 10 percent phenylephrine ophthalmic. Anesthesiology 1972;36:187–189.

113. McReynolds WU, Havener WH, Henderson JW. Hazards of the use of sympathomimetic drugs in ophthalmology. Arch Ophthalmol 1956;56: 176–179.

114. Adler AG, McElwain GE, Merli GJ, et al. Systemic effects of eye drops. Arch Intern Med 1982;142:2293–2294.

115. Merli GJ, Weitz H, Martin JH, et al. Cardiac dysrhythmias associated with ophthalmic atropine. Arch Intern Med 1986;146:45–47.

116. Adler AG, McElwain, Martin JH. Coronary artery spasm induced by phenylephrine eyedrops. Arch Intern Med 1981;141:1384–1385.

117. Heath P, Geiter CW. Use of phenylephrine hydrochloride in ophthalmology. Arch Ophthalmol 1949;41:172–177.

118. Everitt DE, Avorn J. Systemic effects of medications used to treat glaucoma. Ann Intern Med 1990;112:120–125.

119. Alexander S, McAlpine FS. Cholecystectomy in the cardiac patient. Med Clin North Am 1966; 50:495–500.

120. Mendelsohn D Jr, Monheit R. Electrocardiographic and blood-pressure changes during and after biliary-tract surgery. N Engl J Med 1956;254:307–313.

121. Tarhan S, Moffitt EA, Sessler AD, et al. Risk of anesthesia and surgery in patients with chronic bronchitis and chronic obstructive pulmonary disease. Surgery 1973;74:720–726.

122. Consensus conference: anesthesia and sedation in the dental office. JAMA 1985;254:1073–1076.

123. Coplans MP, Carson I. Deaths associated with dentistry. Br Dent J 1982;153:357–362.

124. Brierley JB, Miller AA. Fatal brain damage after dental anaesthesia. Its nature, etiology, and prevention. Lancet 1966;ii:869–873.

125. Cardiac irregularities during dental anaesthesia. Lancet 1966;i:754.

126. Bourne JG. Deaths with dental anaesthetics. Anaesthesia 1970;25:473–481.
127. Chamberlain FL. Management of medical-dental problems in patients with cardiovascular diseases. Mod Concepts Cardiovasc Dis 1961;30:697–700.
128. Cintron A, Medina R, Reyes AA. Cardiovascular effects and safety of dental anesthesia and dental interventions in patients with recent uncomplicated myocardial infarction. Arch Intern Med 1986;146:2203–2204.
129. Cintron G, Medina R, Reyes AA. Cardiovascular effects and safety of dental anesthesia and dental interventions in patients with recent uncomplicated myocardial infarction. Arch Intern Med 1986;146:2203–2204.
130. Mebust WK, Holtgrewe HL, Cockett ATK, et al. Transurethral prostatectomy: immediate and postoperative complications: a cooperative study of 13 participating institutions evaluating 3885 patients. J Urol 1989;141:243–247.
131. Cheraskin E, Prasertsuntarasai T. Use of epinephrine with local anesthesia in hypertensive patients. III. Effect of epinephrine on blood pressure and pulse rate. JADA 1958;57:507–519.
132. Salman I, Schwartz SP. Effects of vasoconstrictors used in local anesthetics in patients with diseases of the heart. J Oral Surg 1955;13:209–213.
133. Cheraskin E, Prasertsuntarasai T. Use of epinephrine with local anesthesia in hypertensive patients. IV. Effect of tooth extraction on blood pressure and pulse rate. JADA 1959;58:61–68.
134. McCarthy FM. A clinical study of blood pressure responses to epinephrine-containing local anesthetic solutions. J Dent Res 1957;36:132–141.
135. Williams RM, Keyes M, Becker DJ, et al. Electrocardiographic changes during oral surgical procedures under local anesthesia. Oral Surg Oral Med Oral Pathol 1963;16:1270–1275.
136. Hanna MH, Heap DG, Kimberlyey PS. Cardiac dysrhythmia associated with general anaesthesia for oral surgery. Anaesthesia 1983;38:1192–1194.
137. Chow AW, Roser SM, Brady FA. Orofacial odontogenic infections. Ann Intern Med 1978;88:392–402.
138. Burke JF. Burns. In: Mandell GL, Douglas RG, Bennett JE, eds. Principles of infectious diseases. New York: John Wiley, 1979.
139. Markley K. Burn care: infection and smoke inhalation. Ann Intern Med 1979;90:269–270.
140. DiVincenti FC, Pruitt BA Jr, Reckler JM. Inhalation injuries. J Trauma 1971;11:109–117.
141. Bartlett RH, Nicole M, Travis MJ. Acute management of the upper airway in facial burns and smoke inhalation. Arch Surg 1976;111:744–749.
142. Zikria BA, Weston CC, Chodoff M. Smoke and carbon monoxide poisoning in fire victims. J Trauma 1972;12:641–645.
143. Petroff PA, Mander EW, Clayton WH. Pulmonary function studies after smoke inhalation. Am J Surg 1976;132:346–351.
144. Zawacki BE, Jung RC, Joyce J. Smoke, burns, and the natural history of inhalation injury in fire victims: a correlation of experimental and clinical data. Ann Surg 1977;185:100–110.
145. Mellins RB, Park S. Respiratory complications of smoke inhalation in victims of fires. J Pediatr 1975;87:1–7.
146. Pruitt BA Jr, Erickson DR, Morris A. Progressive pulmonary insufficiency and other pulmonary complications of thermal injury. J Trauma 1975;15:369–379.
147. Schall GL, McDonald HD, Carr LB. Xenon ventilation-perfusion lung scans. The early diagnosis of inhalation injury. JAMA 1978;240:2441–2445.
148. Moylan JA. Smoke inhalation and burn injury. Surg Clin North Am 1980;60:1533–1540.
149. Pruitt BA Jr. Other complications of burn injury. In: Artz CP, Moncrief JA, Pruitt BA, eds. Burns: a team approach. Philadelphia: WB Saunders, 1979:523–552.
150. Sevitt S. A review of the complications of burns, their origin and importance for illness and death. J Trauma 1979;19:358–369.
151. Czaja AJ, McAlhany JC, Pruitt BA Jr. Acute gastroduodenal disease after thermal injury. An endoscopic evaluation of incidence and natural history. N Engl J Med 1974;291:925–929.
152. McAlhany JC, Czaja AJ, Pruitt BA Jr. Antacid control of complications from acute gastroduodenal disease after burns. J Trauma 1976;16:645–657.
153. McElwee HP, Sirinek KR, Levine BA. Cimetidine affords protection equal to antacids in prevention of stress ulceration following thermal injury. Surgery 1979;86:620–624.
154. Czaja AJ, McAlhany JC, Pruitt BA Jr. Acute duodenitis and duodental ulceration after burns. Clinical and pathological characteristics. JAMA 1975;232:621–624.
155. Aikawa N, Martyn JAJ, Burke JF. Pulmonary artery catheterization in thermodilution cardiac output determination in the management of critically burned patients. Am J Surg 1978;135:811–817.
156. Apfelberg DB, Masters FW, Robinson DW. Pathophysiology and treatment of lightning injuries. J Trauma 1974;14:453–460.
157. Burda CD. Electrocardiographic changes in lightning stroke. Am Heart J 1966;72:521–524.
158. Rouse RG, Dimick AR. The treatment of electrical injury compared to burn injury: a review

of pathophysiology and comparison of patient management protocols. J Trauma 1978;18: 43–46.

159. Rutledge FN, Smith JP, Wharton JT. Pelvic exenteration: analysis of 296 patients. Am J Obstet Gynecol 1977;129:881–892.

160. Curry LC, Nahhas WA, Jahshan AE. Pelvic exenteration: a 7-year experience. Gynecol Oncol 1981;11:119–123.

161. Ford JH Jr, Dudan RC, Bennett JS. Parenteral hyperalimentation in gynecologic oncology patients. Gynecol Oncol 1972;1:70–75.

162. Shepherd JH, Chamber MG. Complications of gynecological cancer surgery: a review. J R Soc Med 1986;79:289–293.

163. Camnitz PS, Biggers WP, Fischer ND. Avoidance of early complications following radical neck dissection. Laryngoscope 1979;89:1553–1562.

164. Erlik D, Valero A, Birkhan J. Prostatic surgery and the cardiovascular patient. Br J Urol 1968;40:53–61.

165. Thompson GJ, Kelalis PP, Connolly DC. Transurethral prostatic resection after myocardial infarction. JAMA 1962;182:908.

166. Sheldon CA. Perioperative care of the urologic patient. Urol Clin North Am 1983;10:1–199.

167. Nicolides AN, Field ES, Kakkar VV. Prostatectomy and deep-vein thrombosis. Br J Surg 1972;59:487–488.

168. An international multicentre trial: prevention of fatal postoperative pulmonary embolism by low doses of heparin. Lancet 1975;ii:45–51.

169. Murphy DM, Flakiner FR, Carr M. Septicemia after transurethral prostatectomy. Urology 1983;22:133–135.

170. Moisey CU, Rees RWM. Results of transurethral resection of prostate in patients with cerebrovascular disease. Br J Urol 1978;50: 539–541.

171. Henderson DJ, Middleton RG. Coma from hyponatremia following transurethral resection of prostate. Urology 1980;15:267–271.

172. Sunderrajan S, Bauer JH, Vopat RL. Postransurethral prostatic resection hyponatremic syndrome. Am J Kidney Dis 1984;4:80–84.

173. Campbell HT, Fincher ME, Sklar AH. Severe hyponatremia without severe hypoosmolality following transurethral resection of the prostate (TURP) in end-stage renal disease. Am J Kidney Dis 1988;12:152–155.

174. Kohn P, Zekert F, Vormittag E, et al. Risks of operation in patients over 80. Geriatrics 1973; 28:100–105.

175. Denney JL, Denson JS. Risk of surgery in patients over 90. Geriatrics 1972;27:115–118.

176. Greenburg AG, Salk RP, Farris JM, et al. Operative mortality in general surgery. Am J Surg 1982;144:22–28.

177. Santos AL, Gelperin A. Surgical mortality in the elderly. J Am Geriatr Soc 1975;23:42–46.

178. Cogbill TH, Landerscasper J, Strutt P, et al. Late results of peripheral vascular surgery in patients 80 years of age and older. Arch Surg 1987;122:581–586.

179. Reiss R, Deutsch AA. Emergency abdominal procedures in patients above age J Gerontol 1985;40:154–158.

180. 180.Loop FD, Lytle BW, Cosgrove DM, et al. Coronary artery bypass graft surgery in the elderly. Cleve Clin J Med 1988;55:23–34.

181. Hochberg MS, Derkac WM, Conkle DM, et al. Mitral valve replacement in elderly patients: encouraging postoperative clinical and hemodynamic results. J Thorac Cardiovasc Surg 1979;77:422–426.

182. De Bono AHB, English TAH, Milstein BB. Heart valve replacement in the elderly. BMJ 1978;2:917–919.

183. Stokes J, Butcher HR Jr. Abdominal aortic aneurysms. Factors influencing operative mortality and criteria of operability. Arch Surg 1973;107:297–301.

184. McCabe CJ, Coleman WS, Brewster DC. The advantage of early operation for abdominal aortic aneurysm. Arch Surg 1981;116:1025–1029.

185. Diehl JT, Cali RF, Hertzer NR, et al. Complications of abdominal aortic reconstruction. Ann Surg 1983;197:49–56.

186. Soreide O, Lillestol J, Christense O, et al. Abdominal aortic aneurysms: survival analysis of four hundred thirty-four patients. Surgery 1982;91:188–193.

187. Friedman SA, Hufnagel CA, Conrad PW, et al. Abdominal aortic aneurysms: clinical status and results of surgery in 100 consecutive cases. JAMA 1967;200:1147–1151.

188. Couch NP, Lane FC, Crane C. Management and mortality in resection of abdominal aortic aneurysms. A study of 114 cases. Am J Surg 1970;119:408–415.

189. Gardner RJ, Lancaster JR, Tarnay TJ, et al. Five-year history of surgically treated abdominal aortic aneurysms. Surg Gynecol Obstet 1970;130:981–987.

190. Baker AG Jr, Roberts B, Berkowitz HD, et al. Risk of excision of abdominal aortic aneurysms. Surgery 1970;68:1129–1134.

191. Cannon JA, Van de Water J, Barker WF. Experience with the surgical management of 100 consecutive cases of abdominal aortic aneurysm. Am J Surg 1963;106:128–141.

192. Hall AD, Zubrin JR, Moore WS, et al. Surgical treatment of aortic aneurysm in the aged: a review of 100 patients. Arch Surg 1970;100: 455–459.

193. May AG, DeWeese JA, Frank I, et al. Surgical treatment of abdominal aortic aneurysms. Surgery 1968;63:711–721.

194. Interhospital Cardiovascular Study Group of the University of Toronto. Surgical treatment of abdominal aortic aneurysms in Toronto: a

study of 1013 patients. Can Med Assoc J 1972;107:1091–1094.

195. Vasko JS, Spencer FC, Bahnson HT. Aneurysm of the aorta treated by excision: review of 237 cases followed up to seven years. Am J Surg 1963;105:793–801.

196. Voorhees AB Jr, McAllister FF. Long term results following resection of arteriosclerotic abdominal aortic aneurysms. Surg Gynecol Obstet 1963;117:355–358.

197. Ryder W. Hazards during anesthesia or sedation for dental procedures. Proc R Soc Med 1971;64:82–83.

198. Rafel SS. Electrocardiographic changes during outpatient oral surgery. J Oral Surg 1972;30:898–899.

199. Christenson GR, Hebert CL, Driscoll EJ. Intravenous barbiturate anesthesia for dental outpatients. Anesth Analg 1961;40:77–86.

200. Ryder W. The electrocardiogram in dental anaesthesia. Anaesthesia 1970;25:46–62.

201. Fisch C, Ochler RC, Miller JR. Cardiac arrhythmias during oral surgery with halothane-nitrous-oxide-oxygen anesthesia. JAMA 1969;208:1839–1842.

202. Ostroff LH, Goldstein BH, Pennock RS. Cardiac dysrhythmias during outpatient general anesthesia—a comparison study. J Oral Surg 1977;35:793–797.

203. Driscoll EJ, Christenson GR, White CL. Physiologic studies in general anesthesia for ambulatory dental patients. Oral Surg Oral Med Oral Pathol 1959;12:1496–1514.

204. Alexander JP. Dysrhythmia and oral surgery. Br J Anaesth 1971;43:773–777.

205. Kaufman L. Unforeseen complications encountered during dental anaesthesia. Proc R Soc Med 1966;59:731–734.

206. Miller JR, Redish CH, Fisch C. Factors in arrhythmia during dental outpatient general anesthesia. Anesth Analg 1970;49:701–706.

207. Tolas AG, Allen GD, Ward RJ. Comparison of effects of methods of induction of anesthesia on cardiac rhythm. J Oral Surg 1967;25:54–59.

208. Crawford ED, Dumbadge I, Ratledge HW. Deep venous thrombosis following transurethral resection of the prostate: diagnosis by phleborheography. J Urol 1978;120:438–441.

209. Askey JM, Cherry CB. Dental extraction during dicumarol therapy. California Med 1956;84:16–17.

210. Frank BW, Dichhaus DW, Claus EV. Dental extractions in the presence of continual anticoagulant therapy. Ann Intern Med 1963;59:911–913.

211. Ziffer AM, Scopp IA, Beck J. Profound bleeding after dental extractions during dicumarol therapy. N Engl J Med 1957;256:351–354.

212. Behrman SJ. Dental surgery during continuous anticoagulant therapy. J Am Dent Assoc 1961;62:172–180.

213. Behrman SJ, Wright IS. Dental surgery during continuous anticoagulant therapy. JAMA 1961;175:483–488.

214. Shira RB, Hall RJ, Guernsey LH. Minor oral surgery during prolonged anticoagulant therapy. J Oral Surg Anesth 1962;20:93–99.

215. Scopp IW, Fredrics H. Dental extractions in patients undergoing anticoagulant therapy. Oral Surg Oral Med Oral Pathol 1958;11:470–474.

216. Mayo ME, Halil T, Browse NL. The incidence of deep vein thrombosis after prostatectomy. Br J Urol 1971;43:738–742.

217. Vanderheyden PJ, Williams RA, Sims TN. Assessment of ST segment depression in patients with cardiac disease after local anesthesia. JADA 1989;119:407–412.

218. Hallett JW, Bower TC, Cherry KJ, et al. Selection and preparation of high-risk patients for repair of abdominal aortic aneurysms. Mayo Clin Proc 1994;69:763–768.

23
Medical Illness During Pregnancy

John Botti and Luanne Thorndyke

With the dramatic changes fostered by managed care compensation and competition, the clinical roles of primary care providers and consulting specialists have become both less well defined and more interdependent regarding women who are pregnant. Nonobstetricians are providing more prenatal care to women with medical problems who have traditionally been cared for by obstetric specialists, and advances in the diagnosis and treatment of several medical conditions have enabled obstetricians to care for an increasing number of women who previously would not (or could not) attempt pregnancy. Furthermore, crisis care settings for pregnant women (e.g., the emergency room, intensive care unit) and the geographic maldistribution of obstetricians both contribute to an environment that ensures consultation by medical specialists.

A complete survey of all medical problems encountered during pregnancy is beyond the scope of a practical review. Instead, this chapter highlights the medical advances and commonly occurring problems that may require consultation by the internist or other medical specialist.

DIABETES MELLITUS
Gestational Diabetes

Gestational (i.e., class A) diabetes is diagnosed by a two-stage assessment. Approximately 3 to 5% of patients who are challenged with a 50-g, oral glucose load between 24 and 28 weeks' gestation will have a glucose value 140 mg/dL or greater. These patients should undergo a 3-hour oral glucose tolerance test after at least 3 days of an oral carbohydrate intake of 150 g or greater. Upper normal limits include: fasting, <105 mg/dL; 1 hour, <190 mg/dL; 2 hours, <165 mg/dL; 3 hours, <145 mg/dL. Fasting hyperglycemia, or any two abnormal blood glucose readings from a single test, constitutes a diagnosis of gestational diabetes (1). Approximately 1% of pregnant women develop gestational diabetes that requires dietary adjustments to achieve glycemic control and protect the fetus.

Treatment includes dietary modifications consistent with American Diabetes Association guidelines (2) and continued monitoring of blood glucose responses. The goal is to maintain a fasting blood glucose level of less than 105 mg/dL and a postprandial blood glucose level of less than 120 mg/dL. Monitoring is best accomplished with daily, multiple fingerstick blood glucose assessments at home. Failure to achieve these guidelines or a significantly elevated HbA1c level marks the patient with gestational diabetes who will need insulin therapy. Long-term follow-up for these patients is necessary, because 25% will acquire type II diabetes within 10 years after the pregnancy.

Insulin-dependent Diabetes Mellitus

Approximately 0.5% of pregnancies are complicated by preexisting diabetes. Approximately 60% of these are type I (or juvenile-onset) insulin-dependent diabetes mellitus (IDDM); the remainder are type II (noninsulin-dependent diabetes mellitus) (3). Treatment of IDDM during pregnancy represents one of the success stories of medicine, but it remains a challenge to physicians who care for pregnant women with IDDM. The course of pregnancy for a woman with poorly controlled diabetes carries risks for both mother and fetus. Diabetic ketoacidosis (DKA), reversible ocular and renal deterioration, hypertensive complications, and operative delivery represent increased maternal risks. In a woman with poorly controlled diabetes and preproliferative or proliferative retinopathy, the rapid institution of glycemic control is associated with initial deterioration of retinal function; however, most of these lesions are both minor and reversible (4). The most effective way to prevent further transient or permanent ocular damage is strict glycemic control before conception.

Thyroid dysfunction is a known autoimmune complication associated with IDDM. Free thyroxine (T_4) and thyroid-stimulating hormone (TSH) assays should be performed.

In the fetus of a mother with poorly controlled IDDM, a threefold to fivefold increased frequency of major congenital anomalies, disorders of fetal growth, premature delivery, and metabolic derangements of the newborn period represent the historical background for an increased perinatal mortality and major disability rate among survivors. The frequency of maternal and perinatal complications in preexisting IDDM can be reduced substantially, however. For the fetus, strict glycemic control before conception, which is maintained throughout the pregnancy, is associated with a reduced rate of major congenital anomalies. Optimal treatment consists of a two-pronged approach: *(a)* strict preconception care, with appropriate education, nutrition, physical activity, multiple fingerstick glucose assessments, and insulin administration to maintain daily mean blood glucose values of 100 mg/dL or less and serum glycohemoglobin values within population norms (HbA1c level less than 7%); and *(b)* maintenance and frequent review of maternal glycemic control and general health during pregnancy, coupled with ultrasonographic surveillance and electronic monitoring of the fetal heart rate (5). For most patients, a capillary glucose assessment should include a fasting sample and 2-hour postprandial samples for each of the three major meals of the day. For some, a sample taken at 2 AM may be required, as tighter control is achieved, to prevent late-night hypoglycemia. Control of blood glucose rests on a combination of nutritional guidelines and strategic insulin therapy (6). Maternal nutritional therapy should include a diet of 50 to 60% carbohydrates (mostly of the complex variety), 12 to 20% protein, and the remainder in approximately equal quantities of unsaturated, monounsaturated, and polyunsaturated fats. The daily total caloric intake may be derived from a guideline of 35 kcal/kg of ideal body mass (i.e., weight/height). Insulin is generally given as a combination of neutral protamine Hagedorn (NPH) and regular insulin before breakfast and again before supper to maintain fasting blood glucose values of less than 105 mg/dL and postprandial values of less than 120 mg/dL; for some patients, other combinations or timing of injections may be required to obtain euglycemia. When this approach is followed, the rate of major congenital anomalies rate is no greater than that in the nondiabetic population (7, 8). Furthermore, maternal hospitalization for diabetes-related renal, ocular, and hypertensive complications are less frequent. These reductions of days in hospital as well as of hospital costs for complications during pregnancy approach 30%, with savings of approximately $5 for every $1 spent on prenatal care (9).

Diabetic Ketoacidosis

The medical specialist may be consulted for diabetic ketoacidosis (DKA) during pregnancy. DKA occurs infrequently in this situation, but precipitating factors include hyperemesis and the use of β-sympathomimetic drugs or systemic glucocorticoids for the treatment of severe asthma or premature labor. Often, the patient has not complied with recommendations to increase insulin and control her dietary intake. The patient may be in an emergency room or under the care of a family physician. Prompt, effective treatment is essential to reduce the increased risk of perinatal mortality.

Treatment of DKA in a woman who is pregnant is similar to that in nonpregnant individuals. The diagnosis is made when the serum glucose level is greater than 300 mg/dL and accompanied by ketonemia. If the serum glucose is not immediately known and the patient is lethargic or comatose, a 25-mL, 50% glucose challenge should be instituted, because pregnancy is also associated with a greater frequency of hypoglycemia. Initially, attention should be paid to replenishing water ($\approx$10% body weight in liters) and electrolytes, especially potassium; to correcting acidemia, which rarely requires the use of sodium bicarbonate; and to returning the plasma glucose to physiologic concentrations with intravenous insulin. If DKA occurs after 28 weeks' gestation, the fetal heart rate should be monitored, with correction of the maternal metabolic disorder rather than delivery being the first priority. Improvement in the maternal condition is mirrored by improvement in the fetal condition if treatment is initiated early enough. Table 23.1 presents a protocol of care for the patient with DKA during pregnancy (10).

PULMONARY DISEASE

Asthma

At least 4% of women who are of reproductive age have airway hyperresponsiveness that is consistent with the diagnosis of asthma. Of the preexisting diseases affecting pregnant women, asthma may be the most common. During pregnancy, women with asthma are divided almost equally among those with disease that will worsen, improve, or remain unchanged. The potential for asthma to affect pregnancy adversely is

---

Table 23.1.   Treatment Protocol for Diabetic Ketoacidosis During Pregnancy

---

   I. *Rehydration:* (a) Infuse 1 L of 0.9% NaCl over first hour, 1 L over the next 2 hours, and continue at 250–500 mL/h until adequate urine output is reestablished and replenishment approaches 10% of body weight. (b) Change IV solution to D_5NS as serum glucose decreases to <250 mg/dL.
  II. *Electrolyte restoration:* With adequate urine output, add KCl, 20–40 mEq/L, to IV fluids. Monitor serum K^+ at 2-hour to 4-hour intervals to maintain the level in the physiologic range.
 III. *Correction of acidemia:* Administer $NaHCO_3$, 44 mEq in 250 mL of 0.45 NS over 1 hour if pH <7.10. Repeat after 1 hour if pH remains <7.10.
  IV. *Metabolic correction:* (a) Regular insulin, 0.1 U/kg IV push, plus regular insulin infusion, 5–10 U/h. (b) Double the infusion rate if serum glucose level is not decreased by 25% in 2 hours. (c) Reduce IV infusion rate to 1–2 U/h once serum glucose level is ≤150 mg/dL.
   V. *Laboratory studies:* Serum electrolytes, glucose, arterial blood gas, complete blood count, bicarbonate, urea nitrogen, ketones. Repeat as necessary.
  VI. Search for and manage underlying cause(s).
 VII. Reestablish maternal–fetal homeostasis.

Adapted from Golde SH. Diabetic ketoacidosis in pregnancy. In: Clark SL, Cotton DB, Hankins GDV, Phelan JP, eds. Critical care obstetrics. 2nd ed. Boston; Blackwell Scientific Publications, 1991;329–339.
D_5NS, 5% dextrose in normal saline; *NS,* normal saline.

often taken too lightly by both the patient and her physicians. Pregnant women with asthma are more frequently affected by hyperemesis, vaginal bleeding, pregnancy-induced hypertension and preeclampsia, and, of course, acute respiratory distress. Fetal complications include intrauterine growth restriction, prematurity, low birth weight, neonatal hypoxia, and increased perinatal mortality. Both the frequency and severity of maternal and fetal complications correlate directly with severity of the asthma. If asthma is properly controlled before and during pregnancy, however, both maternal and fetal risks appear to be minimized.

Several measures of pulmonary function are altered by physiologic, maternal pulmonary and cardiac changes during normal pregnancy. The respiratory rate and forced expiratory volume in 1 second (FEV_1) are not changed, however, and any alteration in these two variables should be considered as abnormal and needing treatment. The goals of treatment are to prevent pulmonary complications and to give birth to a healthy infant. These are accomplished by: (a) maintaining normal pulmonary function; (b) controlling symptoms, especially nocturnal symptoms; (c) maintaining normal activity and exercise levels; (d) preventing acute exacerbations; and (e) avoiding adverse effects from asthma medications (11).

Treatment of maternal asthma is predicated on our current understanding of pathophysiologic mechanisms and objective measures for the assessment and monitoring of maternal pulmonary function. The FEV_1, as obtained through spirometry, is the single most accurate measure of obstructive dysfunction; however, useful clinical information is gained by measuring changes in the peak expiratory flow rate (PEFR) with inexpensive peak-flow meters used twice daily by the patient at home. As with changes in the FEV_1, significant decreases from the personal-best PEFR should alert the physician to adjust the patient's asthma medication. Patient education should be integrated with clinical care.

Control of exacerbating factors and reduction of the inflammatory response in acute airway hyperresponsiveness are key components of therapy for during pregnancy. Reduction in the patient's exposure to allergens and other irritants (e.g., tobacco smoke, sulfites, aspirin, β-blockers) is associated with a decreased frequency of asthma attacks and a reduced need for medication. Both immunotherapy and vaccines may further reduce exacerbations. Conditions such as rhinitis, sinusitis, and gastroesophageal reflux aggravate asthma, and early and effective treatment leads to more effective asthma control.

To prevent exacerbations during pregnancy, a combination of nonpharmacologic therapy and the minimal necessary anti-inflammatory agents should be used in a program of prevention or early intervention. Unless symptoms are poorly controlled or pulmonary functions do not normalize, inhaled agents are preferable to systemic therapy. Preferred drugs for use during pregnancy are included in Table 23.2.

If the asthmatic condition is severe enough to require emergency room care or hospitalization, the maternal Pao_2 and $Paco_2$ should be monitored. If the Pao_2 is less than 60 mm Hg, there is an associated, profound decrease in the fetal oxygen saturation. Maternal hyperventilation and hypocarbia result in decreased uterine blood flow, and administration of oxygen to the mother in these circumstances may be life-saving to the fetus. In fact, monitoring the fetal heart rate responses during an asthmatic attack may serve as an indirect indicator of the success of maternal therapy.

Pneumonia

While pneumonia occurs infrequently during pregnancy, it takes on added seriousness in the context of pregnancy-

Table 23.2. **Drugs and Dosage for Asthma During Pregnancy**

Drug Class	Specific Drug	Dosage
Anti-inflammatory	Cromolyn sodium	2 puffs q.i.d.
	Beclomethasone	2–5 puffs b.i.d.–q.i.d.
	Prednisone	40 mg/day × 1 week; taper × 1 week
Bronchodilator	Inhaled β_2-agonist	2 puffs q 4 h PRN
	Theophylline	Oral dosing to serum concentration of 8–12 µg/mL
Antihistamine	Chorpheniramine	4 mg PO q.i.d. or 8–12 mg SR b.i.d.
	Tripelennamine	25–50 mg PO q.i.d. or 100 mg SR b.i.d.
Decongestant	Pseudoephedrine	60 mg PO q.i.d. or 120 mg SR b.i.d.
	Oxymetazoline	Nasal spray or drops up to 5 days for sinusitis
Cough	Guaifenesin	2 tsp PO q.i.d.
	Dextromethorphan	
Antibiotic	Amoxicillin	3-week therapy for sinusitis

Reprinted with permission from Management of Asthma During Pregnancy. Report of the Working Group on Asthma and Pregnancy. Bethesda. US Department of Health and Human Services, Public Health Services, National Institutes of Health Publication No. 93-3279A, 1993.

associated changes in respiratory physiology combined with chronic pulmonary disease, smoking, or immunosuppression (12). Empiric treatment includes intravenous, second-generation cephalosporins and erythromycin because of the high frequency of community-acquired mycoplasma pneumonia. Pregnant women with viral, protozoan, or fungal pneumonias have increased rates of serious morbidity and mortality, especially with varicella or pneumocystis carinii pneumonias. For pneumocystis pneumonia, trimethoprim/sulfamethoxazole is the agent of choice. Varicella pneumonia requires use of intravenous acyclovir, and may require an intensive care setting during treatment (13). Maternal mortality rate from varicella pneumonia ranges between 15 and 40%.

Tuberculosis

The course of tuberculosis is not worsened by pregnancy, and in the face of alleged exposure during pregnancy or with a high-risk background, skin testing should be performed. If no other risk factors are present, a pregnant woman with an intermediate strength purified protein deriva-

tive of 15 mm or greater should undergo chest radiography with shielding of the fetus. If there is no evidence for active tuberculosis, isoniazid prophylaxis may be deferred until after pregnancy. An exception to this, however, is the human immunodeficiency virus (HIV)-positive woman, who should receive therapy after the first trimester. Pregnant women with active disease should receive a combination of isoniazid, 250 to 300 mg/day; pyridoxine, 50 mg/day; rifampin, 500 to 600 mg/day; and ethambutol, 5 to 25 mg/kg up to 2.5 g daily. This combination should be continued for a minimum of 9 months. If the tuberculosis is resistant to this combination, then pyrazinamide, 2.0 to 2.5 g/day, should be considered (14, 15).

CARDIOVASCULAR DISEASE

Adaptive increases in maternal cardiac output (CO) (30–50%), plasma volumes (45–50%), and red-blood-cell volumes (25–30%) volumes and decreases in systemic vascular resistance (15–20%) during pregnancy are easily tolerated by the patient with a healthy heart. These changes may prove disabling or catastrophic, however, for women with preexisting, severe cardiac disease and limited capacity to accommodate increased end-diastolic volumes and cardiac work, either by increased myocardial contractility or, later in pregnancy, by an increased resting heart rate. Cardiovascular disorders associated with increased maternal mortality during pregnancy are noted in Table 23.3, and several general concepts about maternal cardiovascular changes should be kept in mind.

Uterine blood flow increases during pregnancy, from 2% of the CO before conception to 17% of the CO by midpregnancy. Major disruptions of maternal cardiac function may have a profound effect on fractional CO to the uterus and its contents, and maternal supine position may affect up to 10% of otherwise normal pregnancies. Vena caval return to the heart is obstructed by the gravid uterus, producing a 25 to 30% decrease in the CO. The effect of impaired CO is dramatic, including a combination of maternal hypotension, bradycardia, and syncope with fetal bradycardia (i.e., the supine hypotension syndrome). Resolution and prevention are provided by lateral recumbent position of the pregnant woman or left lateral uterine displacement off the vena cava. During labor, improvement in maternal circulating volume by use of intravenous fluids and epidural anesthesia is also effective.

The New York Heart Association functional classification for heart disease continues to be a practical yardstick for assessing risk during pregnancy. The maternal mortality rate in class I or II cardiac disease is less than 0.5%, whereas that in class III or IV disease is almost 7%. Maternal cardiac diseases may be divided into four areas: (a) congenital cardiac disease, (b) acquired cardiac disease, (c) arrhythmias, and (d) maternal cardiac arrest. Table 23.4 provides guidelines for the pharmacologic therapy of cardiac disease during pregnancy.

Congenital Cardiac Disease

Isolated atrial septal defect (ASD) and ventricular septal defect (VSD) as well as patent ductus arteriosus (PDA) are uncommonly associated with serious cardiac complications during pregnancy. If they coexist with other congenital cardiac lesions or are unusually large, these lesions may be associated with congestive heart failure or, in the case of a large VSD or PDA, with pulmonary hypertension. The potential for complications with these lesions is increased during the midperiod of the second trimester, labor and delivery, and the first week postpartum. Left-to-right shunting with VSD is the most frequent cause of congestive heart failure, requiring careful diuresis to maintain adequate antepartum uterine circulation. Surgical closure is rarely indicated during pregnancy. A small fraction of patients with ASD may have paroxysmal atrial flutter.

Treatment should be based on the ventricular rate and may include low-energy DC cardioversion, rapid atrial pacing, or pharmacologic therapy with intravenous verapamil. Alternatively, propranolol or digoxin may be used to control the ventricular rate. Once the ventricular rate has been controlled, medical cardioversion of atrial flutter can be achieved with use of

Table 23.3. Cardiovascular Disorders Associated with Increased Maternal Mortality

Aortic stenosis
Artificial valve
Coarctation of the aorta
Eisenmenger's syndrome
Marfan syndrome
Mitral stenosis, NYHA class III or IV or with
   atrial fibrillation
Myocardial infarction
Peripartal cardiomyopathy
Primary pulmonary hypertension
Tetralogy of Fallot

NYHA, New York Heart Association.

Table 23.4.   Potential Adverse Effects of Commonly Used Cardiovascular Drugs During Pregnancy

Agent	Indication	Maternal Effects	Fetal Effects	FDA Risk Category[a]
Digitalis preparations (Digoxin)	CHF, arrhythmias	Arrhythmias, conduction disturbances	Toxicity with overdosage	C
Diuretics[b]				
Loop diuretics (Furosemide)	CHF, ↑ BP, constrictive pericarditis	↓ BP, electrolyte disorders	IUGR, acute uterine blood flow reduction	C
Thiazides[b] (Hydrochlorthiazide)	Essential hypertension	↓ BP, electrolyte disorders	Thrombocytopenia, hypoglycemia, hemolytic anemia, jaundice	C
Metolazone	↑ BP, CHF	↓ BP, electrolyte disorders		B
Potassium sparing (spironolactone, triamterene)	Edema, hypokalemia	GI disturbances, hyperkalemia, hirsutism	Feminization in animals with spironolactone	C
Antihypertensives				
Vasodilators (hydralazine, isosorbide)	CHF, ↑ BP, angina, pulmonary hypertension	↓ BP, nausea, diarrhea, headache SLE syndrome	Thrombocytopenia, leukopenia	C
α-Antagonists (prazosin, terazosin, doxazosin)	↑ BP	Syncope, nasal congestion, headache, drowsiness	No well-controlled studies	B/C
β-Antagonists (propranolol, metoprolol, atenolol, labetolol)	Angina, ↑ BP, mitral valve prolapse, cardiomyopathy, arrhythmia	Bradycardia, ↓ BP, bronchospasm, uterine contractions	Hypoglycemia, bradycardia, oliguria, hypotension at delivery	C
ACE inhibitors (enalapril, captopril)	CHF, ↑ BP	Worsening renal function, ↓ BP, angioedema, hyperkalemia	Fetal renal abnormalities, increased mortality	X
Anticoagulants				
Coumadin (sodium warfarin)	Prosthetic valves, intracardiac thrombus	Hemorrhage	Congenital anomalies, hemorrhage, stillbirth	X
Heparin	Same as Coumadin	Hemorrhage, osteoporosis	Hemorrhage	B
Miscellaneous				
Cyclosporine	Cardiac transplant	Impaired immunity, ↑ BP, renal disease, hirsutism, tremor	Embryotoxicity in animals	C
Corticosteroids	Myocarditis, pericarditis, transplants	Electrolyte disturbances, osteoporosis, peptic ulcer	No known fetal effects	B

Adapted from Shabetai R. Cardiac Diseases. In: Creasy R, Resnik R, eds. Maternal • Fetal Medicine. Vol 3. Philadelphia, Saunders 1994:768–791.

ACE, angiotensin-converting enzyme; *BP,* blood pressure; *CHF,* congestive heart failure; *GI,* gastrointestinal; *IUGR,* intrauterine growth restriction; *SLE,* systemic lupus erythematosus.

[a]FDA classification for teratogenic potential of pharmaceutical agents:

  B—No evidence of human risk, but no controlled human studies.

  C—Risk to humans has not been ruled out.

  D—Positive evidence of risk to humans from human or animal studies.

  X—Contraindicated during pregnancy. Known major fetal risk.

[b]Not indicated as short-term therapy for preeclampsia.

oral quinidine or oral procainamide (16). In older women with ASD, pulmonary hypertension and pulmonary vascular disease may already be present, and pregnancy is not recommended.

Most women with uncomplicated VSD or PDA have uneventful pregnancies, and these patients differ from those with ASD only in that they rarely have arrhythmias but require antibiotic prophylaxis for infectious endocarditis. Patients with a larger VSD may have pulmonary hypertension without increased pulmonary vascular resistance. In a small fraction of patients, the increased pulmonary vascular resistance (>1200 dyne/sec per cm^{-5}) exceeds the systemic resistance, resulting in the right-to-left shunt of Eisenmenger's pathophysiology. Maternal mortality is approximately 50% and perinatal mortality exceeds 50% with this irreversible lesion. The greatest risk occurs during labor, delivery, and the puerperium. Therapeutic abortion may be the most appropriate option for pregnant patients with increased pulmonary resistance. If a patient wishes to continue with the pregnancy, however, recommendations include curtailing exercise, bed rest, anticoagulation, cesarean delivery, and permanent sterilization (17). Maintenance of pulmonary blood flow with central hemodynamic monitoring to preserve CO during anesthesia and delivery are essential.

Congenital aortic stenosis may cause severe left ventricular hypertrophy with limited cardiac response to the increased circulatory demands of pregnancy. Critical aortic stenosis during pregnancy may be treated with aortic valve replacement or repair, but prosthetic aortic valves pose problems during pregnancy because of the need for anticoagulation. Use of heparin or warfarin during pregnancy remains controversial, and prepregnancy counseling should emphasize the substantial maternal and fetal risks (18). Less severe aortic stenosis may be treated during pregnancy without surgery. The lowered systemic vascular resistance of pregnancy

affects afterload in aortic stenosis, and use of vasodilators may decrease the systemic vascular resistance to the point at which the left ventricle cannot accommodate the demand. During labor, careful invasive monitoring is necessary to ensure adequate venous return.

Mild to moderate pulmonic stenosis is well tolerated during pregnancy. More severe pulmonic stenosis (right ventricular systemic pressure, >150 mm Hg) should be treated before pregnancy is attempted. Balloon valvotomy is generally sufficient to correct pulmonic stenosis. Idiopathic pulmonic hypertension is poorly tolerated during pregnancy and may occur with chronic pulmonary embolism; because of the high maternal mortality rate, it is recommended that patients with this disorder avoid pregnancy. Women who become pregnant, however, should be counseled about the significant risk that is involved, and if an abortion is chosen, it should be performed before the end of the first trimester.

Patients with corrected tetralogy of Fallot need antibiotic protection for bacterial endocarditis; otherwise, pregnancy is generally well tolerated. Uncorrected tetralogy is usually associated with syncopal episodes, polycythemia, and increased right ventricular pressures, each contributing to the risk of maternal mortality. The patient should be counseled to obtain surgical correction before pregnancy is attempted. If corrected before pregnancy, coarctation of the aorta poses little risk. Coarctation is also associated with congenital berry aneurysm of the circle of Willis, and care should be taken to control the intrapartum blood pressure changes. Ebstein's anomaly is frequently associated with abnormal arteriovenous conduction as well as both ventricular and supraventricular arrhythmias. Surgical repair before pregnancy usually corrects the conduction defect, thus eliminating the risk of supraventricular tachycardia during pregnancy. Patients with congenital atrioventricular block are at little risk during pregnancy when treated with a rate-responsive atrioventricular pacemaker.

Acquired Heart Disease

Rheumatic heart disease, including mitral stenosis with or without aortic regurgitation, is still a major problem in Third World countries, but it may also present in childbearing women of industrialized nations. A history of rheumatic fever in a pregnant woman is a requirement for daily penicillin or an equivalent antibiotic. Atrial fibrillation is a later complication of mitral stenosis and regurgitation, and it increases the probability of an atrial thrombus or embolic stroke. The need for increased CO during pregnancy puts added stress on the rheumatic heart, which leads to an increased risk for congestive right-heart failure, infective endocarditis, pulmonary embolism, and hemoptysis. Severe mitral stenosis carries an increased risk for maternal death in the late third trimester and the puerperium as well. Therefore, women with severe mitral stenosis should be counseled about the advantages of undergoing mitral valvotomy before attempting pregnancy. If the pregnant patient has uncorrected mitral disease, she should be advised to increase bed rest, reduce strenuous activity, and restrict salt intake (19). Diuretic therapy may be necessary as well, and if the patient has atrial fibrillation, anticoagulation with heparin should be administered. Balloon valvuloplasty may be used after the first trimester to improve mitral stenosis (20). Treatment during labor and delivery should emphasize avoidance of the supine position. Epidural anesthesia or analgesia/sedation may help decrease cardiac work in response to the pain of labor and delivery. Prophylaxis for bacterial endocarditis is indicated.

True mitral valve prolapse associated with severe dysfunction of the autonomic nervous system or arrhythmia is unusual during pregnancy. Tests of thyroid function and serum catecholamine levels should be obtained if the symptoms are severe. Combinations of selective β-blockade and anxiolytic therapy are usually sufficient to maintain a normal cardiac response, but more severe disease should be treated in the same manner as mitral regurgitation.

Idiopathic peripartum cardiomyopathy usually presents in the last month of pregnancy, or up to 6 months postpartum. By definition, it is unassociated with other hypertensive or cardiac diseases (21), and it may affect previously healthy women. Associated with the onset of this uncommon disease are: (a) older age, (b) black race, (c) twin pregnancy, and (d) preeclampsia. Several mechanisms have been proposed to explain this cardiomyopathy, including autoimmune disease and viral infection, but none has successfully explained this condition. Recurrence with subsequent pregnancy has been reported to be as high as 50%, necessitating a recommendation that these patients not become pregnant again (22). Treatment of active disease includes agents used for congestive heart failure. Long-term recovery occurs in approximately 50%, and cardiac transplant may be life-saving for those who do not recover a sustaining cardiac index. These women may have successful later pregnancies (23).

Marfan's syndrome, a hereditary disorder of connective tissue, often presents with cardiac abnormalities, including mitral and tricuspid valve prolapse and regurgitation, aortic regurgitation, and dilation of the ascending aorta. Ultimately, aortic dissection and rupture may occur, especially during increased cardiodynamic stress, and the circulatory changes of pregnancy provide such a scenario for lethal aortic rupture. Women with an aortic root diameter greater than 4.0 cm are at the highest risk for aortic dissection and should be counseled about these increased risks of becoming pregnant, as should women with clinical manifestations of chest pain, aortic diastolic murmur, and severe mitral valve prolapse. Asymptomatic patients desiring pregnancy should also be counseled about the 50% probability of autosomal dominant transmission of the syndrome to their children. Transesophageal echocardiography is a highly effective tool to document early changes in the aortic root that may lead to later dissection and rupture. Surgical treatment of aortic root dilation either before or during pregnancy may be indicated if the root diameter is greater than 5.0 cm. The recent practice of using of β-blockade for Marfan's syndrome may prove to be beneficial, and β-blockade may be used in conjunction with peripheral vasodilation by hydralazine to control blood pressure during pregnancy (24).

Indications for antibiotic prophylaxis during active labor and delivery are now limited to patients with: prosthetic cardiac valves; previous bacterial endocarditis; complex cyanotic congenital heart disease; and surgically constructed systemic pulmonary shunts. The American Heart Association recommends the combination of ampicillin, 2 g intravenously, plus gentamicin sulfate, 1.5 mg/kg intravenously, starting 1 hour before anticipated vaginal or cesarean delivery and continued not more than 8 hours after delivery (25).

Cardiac Arrhythmias

Arrhythmias may be first diagnosed during pregnancy, but most antedate pregnancy. Pregnancy-associated changes in the volume of distribution of pharmacologic agents, renal and hepatic metabolism, altered drug-protein binding, and absorption from the gastrointestinal tract may alter the effectiveness of prepregnancy dosages of antiarrhythmic agents.

Both the U.S. Food and Drug Administration (FDA) classification and potential adverse effects of various antiarrhythmic agents in pregnancy are outlined in Table 23.5. Quinidine has a long record of safe use during pregnancy, and procainamide

has the added advantage of intravenous administration, thus making it the agent of choice in short-term treatment of wide-complex tachycardia (26). Of the class 1B agents, phenytoin is the only drug with a known history of teratogenic effects on the developing fetus, and it should not be used as other agents provide equivalent therapeutic effects. Experience with class 1C drugs during pregnancy has been brief, with only limited information currently available on their safe use.

β-Adrenergic blocking agents are class 2 drugs. Recent-generation, selective β-blocking agents have less β-2 effects of blocking uterine relaxation and peripheral vasodilation. Most are considered safe and effective during pregnancy. These drugs have virtually supplanted propranolol, which has been associated with the restriction of intrauterine growth (27).

Class 3 agents delay repolarization. Sotalol has superior efficacy in patients with ventricular tachyarrythmia, but it also has β-blocking properties. Amiodarone is considered to be an FDA class D agent because of adverse fetal effects, including hypothyroidism and intrauterine growth restriction. Use of this drug is restricted to pregnant patients whose arrhythmia cannot be controlled by other agents.

Calcium channel blocking (i.e., class 4) agents are effective therapy of supraventricular tachycardia. During pregnancy, agents such as verapamil should be reserved for patients whose tachycardia does not respond to other agents, including digitalis or adenosine. Adenosine has become one of the first-choice agents for paroxysmal supraventricular tachycardia (PSVT).

Premature beats in pregnant women who are otherwise healthy should be managed by reassurance and attention to reducing their use of excitatory agents, including caffeine, alcohol, and cigarettes. Generally, tachyarrhythmias causing hemodynamic problems should be converted rapidly to a normal sinus rhythm. In otherwise healthy pregnant women who

Table 23.5. **Potential Adverse Effects of Commonly Used Antiarrhythmic Drugs During Pregnancy**

Agent	Vaughn-Williams Classification	Maternal Effects	Fetal Effects	FDA Risk Category[a]
Quinidine	1A	Thrombocytopenia cinchonism, GI, arrhythmia	Thrombocytopenia	B
Procainamide	1A	GI, SLE syndrome		B
Disopyramide	1A	Arrhythmia		C
Lidocaine	1B	Anticholinergic		C
Tocainide	1B			C
Phenytoin	1B			X
Mexiletene	1B			C
Propafenone	1C	GI, tremor, arrhythmia		C
Flecanide	1C		Embryotoxic in animals	C
Propranolol	2			C
Moricizine	1	GI, dizziness, AV block, arrhythmia	Questionable effect on weight	B
Bretylium	3			C
Amiodarone	3			D
Sotalol	3			B
Calcium channel blockers	4			B/C
Adenosine	N/A			C

AV, atrioventricular; *GI,* gastrointestinal; *N/A,* not applicable; *SLE,* systemic lupus erythematosus.

[a]FDA classification for teratogenic potential of pharmaceutical agents:

   B—No evidence of human risk, but no controlled human studies.

   C—Risk to humans has not been ruled out.

   D—Positive evidence of risk to humans from human or animal studies.

   X—Contraindicated during pregnancy. Known major fetal risk.

have frequent bouts of PSVT, conversion may occur with carotid massage, facial immersion, Valsalva's maneuver, or sedation. If PSVT accompanies organic heart disease and does not respond to vagal maneuvers, digitalis preparations, β-blockade, or both may be used. Esophageal and, occasionally, endocardial pacing may be necessary for PSVT, and procainamide may be used in PSVT with preexcitation.

The most common ventricular tachycardia (VT) during pregnancy is repetitive monomorphic VT (28). Idiopathic left VT may also occur in structurally normal hearts, whereas VT with a prolonged Q-T interval is less frequent. Short-term therapy for sustained VT usually begins with intravenous lidocaine, but it may require procainamide. If the mother's con-

dition destabilizes, DC countershock of up to 400 J may be needed to convert to a normal rhythm. Pharmacologic suppression in the patient with recurrent VT should occur in a monitored setting. First-line therapy is β-adrenergic blockade; alternative agents include procainamide, quinidine, and sotalol.

Bradycardias may require permanent pacing if they are symptomatic. If asymptomatic, prophylactic pacing before labor and delivery may be beneficial (29).

Ischemic Heart Disease and Cardiac Arrest During Pregnancy

While it is uncommon during pregnancy, coronary artery disease leading to acute myocardial infarction carries a mortality rate of approximately 50% in pregnant women. Since patient history, physical examination, and electrocardiography may be insufficient to confirm the presence of coronary occlusive disease, stress echocardiography without radionucleotide imaging may be helpful in diagnosing the cause of acute chest pain during pregnancy. More invasive cardiac catheterization, angioplasty, and coronary bypass surgery may then be justified, preferably after the first trimester and appropriate counseling about exposure of the fetus to ionizing radiation and anesthesia. Fetal mortality may be increased by extensive maternal coronary bypass surgery, which should be conducted as much as possible in a normothermic, high-flow state by an experienced cardiac surgeon and with fetal monitoring (30). Congestive heart failure most often results from coronary artery disease predating the pregnancy, but it may also result from peripartum cardiomyopathy, iatrogenic use of excess intravenous volume replacement and β-adrenergic agents in the treatment of preterm labor, myocarditis, and myxedema. A chronic left ventricular ejection fraction of at least 40% in patients with a history of congestive heart failure is associated with a safe outcome of the pregnancy. Treatment of acute congestive heart failure during pregnancy is the same as that in the nonpregnant state, including digoxin, a loop diuretic, a vasodilator, potassium supplementation, and antiarrhythmics as necessary. Angiotensin-converting enzyme inhibitors are contraindicated during pregnancy, however, because of their effects on fetal renal development.

Treatment of cardiac arrest during pregnancy is in many respects no different from treatment in the nonpregnant state. Extensive protocols for cardiopulmonary resuscitation (CPR) are available in standard publications (31, 32). The basics of CPR are initiated, and then algorithms specific to the presenting problem are followed. Intravenous fluids and 100% inspired oxygen are initiated in the anticipation of other CPR events, and as with cardiac arrest outside of pregnancy, rapid return of effective maternal circulation (less than 4 minutes after witnessed arrest) is associated with the greatest chance for a good prognosis. Any delay in establishing effective resuscitation beyond 6 minutes is associated with a high rate of brain damage in both the mother and the fetus. Specific concerns during pregnancy include (a) the effect of maternal physiologic and anatomic changes on the success of resuscitative efforts; and (b) the timing of maternal response to CPR efforts on fetal injury and survival. Because of delayed gastric emptying and reduced esophageal tone during pregnancy, protection of the maternal airway should include endotracheal intubation. The size of the gravid uterus during the second half of pregnancy may impair CPR efforts, and it should be tilted to the left side to improve perfusion. If CPR does not result in a good response within 4 minutes, then the fetus should be delivered during the fifth minute after the initiation of CPR, usually by cesarean delivery. This effort may be life-saving for both the mother and the infant, with good prognosis if arrest occurs in the third trimester (33). Perimortem cesarean delivery should also be considered at the onset of cardiac arrest considering several reports of successful perinatal outcome up to 22 minutes after documented maternal cardiac arrest and unsuccessful resuscitation, especially in women who were otherwise healthy before cardiac arrest (33a). Informed consent should be obtained by the patient and family, if possible, in anticipation of cardiac arrest occurring with medical or surgical care.

If PSVT is present, adenosine may be used. For atrial fibrillation/flutter with rapid ventricular response, diltiazem is appropriate, and magnesium sulfate is the treatment of choice for torsades de pointes. If ventricular fibrillation or pulseless VT is present, cardioversion up to three times (and gradually up to 360 J) is indicated. Use of sodium bicarbonate and pure α-adrenergic agents for maternal resuscitation is controversial, however, because of potential adverse effects on the fetus.

HYPERTENSION

Approximately 10% of pregnancies are complicated by hypertension, with 70% of these clinical presentations resulting from preeclampsia and most of the remainder from chronic essential hypertension. Other causes include renal, thyroid, and autoimmune diseases. Maternal hypertension includes several categories.

Chronic hypertension is defined as hypertension that is identified either before pregnancy or before 20 weeks' gestation. Preeclampsia is diagnosed after 20 weeks' gestation when any of the following present: (a) an increase in systolic blood pressure 30 mm Hg or greater above baseline, (b) an increase in diastolic blood pressure 15 mm Hg or greater above baseline, (c) a mean blood pressure 20 mm Hg or greater than the baseline value obtained before 20 weeks' gestation; and (d) blood pressure of 140/90 mm Hg or greater or mean blood pressure of 105 mm Hg or greater. Preeclampsia that is superimposed on chronic hypertension may also occur. This is defined as an increase in one or more blood pressure parameters (30 mm Hg systolic; 15 mm Hg diastolic, or a mean arterial pressure of 20 mm Hg) from usual baseline levels with the appearance of proteinuria or generalized edema (34). Pathophysiologically, preeclampsia is characterized by vasospasm, and it is associated with end-organ damage in severe cases. The cause of preeclampsia remains uncertain, but exaggerated pressor responses to the renin-angiotensin-aldosterone system, imbalance of vasoactive autocoids (i.e., prostacyclin/thromboxane), alterations in the synthesis or activity of endothelin-1 and nitric oxide, genetic susceptibility, and immune derangements have all been proposed. The disease may actually be a family of closely associated clinical presentations, however, with either some or all of these elements involved.

The diagnosis of preeclampsia is based on clinical findings (i.e., hypertension or defined blood pressure changes, proteinuria, edema). At least 300 mg of protein per liter in a 24-hour sample of maternal urine is diagnostic of proteinuria. As many as 80% of all women have dependent edema sometime during their pregnancy, but facial and upper extremity edema unresponsive to bed rest and rapid increases in weight are more likely to occur with preeclampsia. Preeclampsia is most often divided into the categories of mild and severe, with the latter generally indicating that delivery should be performed shortly to reduce the risks of severe complications to both the mother and the fetus (Table 23.6) (35). Other indicators of severe disease include hemolysis, elevated liver enzyme levels, and low platelet count (i.e., HELLP syndrome), as well as severe fetal growth restriction.

While the definitive treatment of preeclampsia/eclampsia is delivery, the consulting internist may become involved in the care of pregnant patients with hypertension in several clinical circumstances.

Treatment of Preexisting Essential Hypertension

Baseline renal function tests, including 24-hour urine protein excretion and se-

Table 23.6. Criteria for the Diagnosis of Severe Preeclampsia

---

I. Blood pressure ≥160 mm Hg systolic or ≥110 mm Hg diastolic on two occasions at least 6 hours apart with the patient at bed rest.
II. Proteinuria ≥5 g in a 24-hour urine collection or ≥3+ on dipstick in at least two random, clean-catch samples at least 4 hours apart.
III. Oliguria (≤500 mL in 24 hours).
IV. Cerebral or visual disturbances.
V. Epigastric pain.
VI. Pulmonary edema or cyanosis.

Reprinted with permission from Hughes EC, ed. Obstetric-gynecology terminology. Philadelphia; FA Davis, 1972.

rum uric acid levels, should be performed. Both the prenatal care provider and the consulting internist should monitor the patient for evidence of superimposed preeclampsia. Evidence of severe preeclampsia or fetal compromise indicates the need for hospitalization and delivery. Treatment of moderate-degree essential hypertension (diastolic pressure, ≥100 mg Hg) before the second trimester reduces maternal and fetal risks for complications; pharmacologic treatment of milder disease is less likely to improve the outcome of pregnancy (36). Medical therapy initiated before pregnancy should be continued.

The choice of therapeutic agents for essential hypertension during pregnancy requires the consideration of both short-term and long-term effects on the fetus. Thiazide diuretics, if used effectively before pregnancy, may be continued safely. Aggressive initial use of thiazides during pregnancy is associated with reduced maternal plasma volume, reduced birth weight, and increased perinatal mortality. With the availability of several other classes of safe pharmacologic agents, thiazides have only a limited role in early maternal treatment, and they should not be used when a diagnosis of preeclampsia is made. Methyldopa, hydralazine, selective β-sympathomimetic antagonists, and calcium channel blockade, either singly or in combination, may be used to maintain a maternal systolic blood pressure of 150 mm Hg or less and diastolic blood pressure of 100 mm Hg or less. Periodic fetal imaging and biophysical surveillance are recommended because of the documented association of intrauterine growth restriction with both pregnancy hypertension and some antihypertensive medications (37). Both reserpine and angiotensin-converting enzyme inhibitors are contraindicated during pregnancy because of their potentially severe effects on neonatal respiratory and renal functions, respectively.

Medical Therapy for Severe Preeclampsia

Antihypertensive treatment is often indicated to prevent major maternal complications in hospitalized patients with severe preeclampsia. Persistent maternal diastolic blood pressures of 105 mm Hg or greater are associated with an increased risk of maternal seizure and multiple-organ injury. CO is often elevated, and this may contribute to the hypertensive clinical state. However, plasma volume is almost always contracted. Laboratory findings include an increased hematocrit value as well as plasma uric acid and creatinine concentrations. Hydralazine, 5 mg given intravenously over 2 to 4 minutes and repeated at 20-minute intervals, has been used to maintain maternal diastolic blood pressure between 90 and 100 mm Hg. Recently, labetalol and nifedipine have been used to maintain similar maternal blood pressures. Labetalol is given intravenously as a 20-mg dose and then doubled to 40 mg, and then 80 mg, at 10-minute intervals. The 80-mg dose may be repeated twice more, to a total dose of 300 mg (38). Alternatively, nifedipine, 10 to 20 mg, may be given orally and repeated at 3- hour to 6-hour intervals (39).

Patients with HELLP-associated thrombocytopenia and elevated liver enzyme levels should undergo delivery of the fetus expeditiously. Rarely, a patient will require blood-product transfusion, and infrequently, patients may experience pulmonary edema, cardiac failure, disseminated intravascular coagulation, or acute renal failure. Therapeutic responses should be individualized to the clinical situation and an intensive care setting may be required. With delivery, the arteriolar vasospasm of preeclampsia will be reversed within 24 to 48 hours and that the resultant recovery is usually rapid.

Emergency Treatment of Eclampsia

The standard treatment for eclampsia in the United States consists of administering magnesium sulfate and delivering the fetus. Magnesium sulfate is given at 4 to 6 g intravenously over 20 minutes and then continued as an infusion, 2 to 4 g/h, in 120 mL of intravenous fluid. A second, 2-g bolus may be given cautiously if seizures have not been controlled, and if after this additional dose the seizures continue, then diazepam, 2 to 10 mg; phenytoin, 10 to 15 mg/kg; or thiopental, 100 mg, may be given slowly and intravenously. Infrequently, patients with eclampsia also experience pulmonary edema, disseminated intravascular coagulation, acute renal failure, and cerebral edema. Specific treatment for these additional problems may be required even as other care is being rendered for delivery.

In many hospitals, the intensive care unit is the best place to provide the multidisciplinary care that is essential for the health of these patients. The complications of severe preeclampsia/eclampsia include severe hypertension, oliguria, thrombocytopenia, acute impairment of renal and hepatic mechanisms, and increased potential for coagulopathy. Strict attention should be given to fluid intake and output to prevent iatrogenic complications. Intravenous fluid therapy should be restricted to between 100 and 125 mL/h unless regional anesthesia is being administered; in the latter situation, infusion of 1.0 to 1.5 liters of crystalloid may be necessary to maintain a reasonable CO in the face of pharmacologic sympathectomy. A pulmonary artery catheter may be useful in patients with limited output and poorly controlled blood pressure and who may also have evidence of early cardiac failure.

In addition to the antihypertensive agents described earlier, nitroglycerin may be administered when maternal blood pressure does not respond to other agents or is elevated enough to increase the probability of a cerebrovascular event (40). Infusion is begun at 10 mg/min and titrated to the desired blood pressure by doubling the dose every 5 minutes. Development of methemoglobinemia at high doses should be assessed and avoided; the condition and progress of the patient may require transfer to a tertiary care center.

RENAL DISEASE

Patients with chronic, mild renal disease typically have good pregnancy outcomes unless the disorder is complicated by hypertension or is associated with certain autoimmune diseases. Those with moderate or severe renal disease (glomerular filtration rate, <30 mL/min.; serum creatinine level, >1.5 mg/dL; proteinuria level, >3.5 g per 24 hours) face increased risks for spontaneous abortion, preeclampsia, fetal distress, and fetal growth disorders. Ideal treatment of chronic renal disease includes prepregnancy assessment and counseling as well as normalization of maternal blood pressure. Correction of severe anemia and attention to adequate nutrition are also important. There is some evidence that a low-protein diet (0.6–0.8 g/kg) slows reduction of the glomerular filtration rate in nonpregnant patients with diabetic nephropathy (41).

Careful monitoring of blood pressure and renal function during pregnancy is advised, with the goal of achieving a more normal blood-pressure profile, stable or improved creatinine clearance, and minimal proteinuria. Uncontrolled hypertension, creatinine clearance less than 50% of normal, and proteinuria of greater than 3.5 g per 24 hours predict a poor outcome of pregnancy and may predict worsening renal disease (42). Patients with chronic anemia (hemoglobin level, <8 g/dL) may require periodic blood transfusions to reduce the risks of fetal hypoxemia. Recently, human recombinant erythropoietin has been used successfully to improve the anemia of chronic renal disease (42a).

Hemodialysis

Pregnant patients requiring hemodialysis present special problems. Control of blood pressure, fluid balance, increased hours of dialysis, and adequate nutrition are necessary to achieve a 20 to 40% chance of reproductive success. For patients who develop chronic renal failure and who require dialysis for the first time during pregnancy, chronic ambulatory peritoneal dialysis should be considered initially because of its modulated effect on both plasma volume and arterial pressure. Renal transplant patients who become pregnant and are normotensive with at least 24 months of good graft function have excellent prognosis for successful pregnancies.

Urinary Tract Infections

Urinary tract infections and urolithiasis are more prevalent during pregnancy, with an incidence of 2 to 3% and 0.1 to 0.3%, respectively. Asymptomatic bacteruria is unlikely to come to the attention of the consulting internist, because it most often is successfully treated by a 1-day to 3-day course of an oral antibiotic. Similarly, cystitis infrequently causes complications during pregnancy when treated with a 1-week course of an appropriate antimicrobial agent. Whereas short-course therapy may be sufficient for cystitis in nonpregnant women, a similar regimen is not appropriate during pregnancy, because up to 30% of these patients will fail a test of cure and remain susceptible to pyelonephritis.

Pregnant women with pyelonephritis should usually be hospitalized, because they are more susceptible to systemic complications of urosepsis compared with women who are not pregnant. Urinary tract culture and sensitivity should be obtained even in clinically evident pyelonephritis to determine sensitivities for appropriate antibiotic therapy. Intravenous hydration and systemic antibiotics should be accompanied by fetal biophysical assessment until maternal fever lysis and clinical relief have been achieved. Tetracycline and its derivatives should be avoided throughout pregnancy, and sulfonamides and nitrofurantoin should be avoided during the final 6 weeks of pregnancy. Nitrofurantoin is also contraindicated in patients with an increased risk for glucose-6-phosphate dehydrogenase deficiency.

Patients with a renal or ureteral stone typically present with hematuria, flank pain, and sterile urine, and use of ultrasonography or limited intravenous pyelography may help in diagnosis. Because of the increased co-incidence of urinary tract infection with urolithiasis, treatment with antibiotics is similar to that in patients with acute pyelonephritis, with the addition of systemic analgesia for pain relief. Segmental epidural anesthesia may be a beneficial substitution for narcotic analgesia, and it may allow for earlier ambulation. In patients who do not respond, placement of a ureteral stent or percutaneous nephrostomy may be necessary to decompress the upper urinary tract and prevent renal damage. Conventional lithotripsy is contraindicated during pregnancy.

HEMATOLOGIC DISEASE

Anemia

Gestational increase in the maternal plasma volume is associated with a comparatively smaller increase in red-blood-cell volume, resulting in physiologic hemodilution and decreased hemoglobin concentration during the second and third trimesters. A maternal hemoglobin level of less than 11 g/dL in the first trimester or less than 10.5 gm/dL after the first trimester most often reflects either a deficiency in iron stores or a combined deficiency of both iron and folic acid (43). In the latter condition, red-blood-cell indices may be deceiving. Evaluation of a peripheral blood smear, reticulocyte count (1.2–2.9%), hemoglobin electrophoresis, serum ferritin level (≥12 mg/dL), and serum folate level (≥3 ng/dL) may help to determine the need for combined replacement or other therapies based on the underlying pathophysiology. Oral iron-replacement therapy should be 60 to 120 mg of elemental iron per day in three divided doses taken 30 minutes before meals. Iron absorption may be improved by zinc supplementation (15 mg/day) as commonly found in most prenatal multivitamin supplements. Improvement in the serum ferritin or hemoglobin levels may be seen in 1 to 2 weeks, with a return to iron normal stores within 1 to 2 months.

Folate deficiency preexisting pregnancy has been associated with neural fold maldevelopment leading to open neural-tube defects (e.g., anencephaly, spina bifida). Folate deficiency occurs less frequently in the United States than in other areas of the world, but the incidence is increased in multifetal pregnancies, thus suggesting an increased nutritional requirement beyond the generally recommended 0.4 mg/day for women of reproductive age (44). Most studies have suggested daily dosing of 0.8 to 1.0 mg. Women who have experienced a previous pregnancy complicated by a fetal open neural-tube defect should have both prepregnancy and early pregnancy administration of folic acid (4 mg/day) to decrease the risk of recurrence by 75% (45).

Hemoglobinopathies

Pregnancy poses increased risks for women with sickle hemoglobinopathies, especially hemoglobin SS disease. The frequency and intensity of sickle crises appear to increase during pregnancy, as reflected in serious maternal (1%) and perinatal (>10%) mortality rates and fetal growth restriction. Hemoglobin SC disease carries lower rates of maternal and perinatal mortality, but it also requires special attention and treatment to achieve good outcome.

Evaluation of patients during a sickling crisis should include ruling out other medical causes of pain, fever, and hemolysis. Pyelonephritis is more prevalent during pregnancy in patients with SS or SC disease, and endotoxin appears to contribute to crises by accelerating the destruction of sickled cells and decreasing the erythropoietic response. The increased susceptibility of sickling patients to life-threatening pneumonia caused by *Streptococcus pneumoniae* is reduced by prophylaxis with polyvalent pneumococcal vaccine. Finally, patients with SS hemoglobinopathies are at risk for cardiopulmonary decompensation resulting from the vasculopathy caused by recurrent sickling crises. Pulmonary edema or congestive heart failure may occur more rapidly in patients with SS hemoglobinopathies who have severe preeclampsia or premature labor and are treated with intravenous tocolytic therapy. Hemoglobin concentrations should be maintained at 7 gm/dL or more, and folate supplementation (1–2 mg/day) offsets the increased marrow turnover that occurs in response to severe anemia. The goals of therapy for sickle crises are relief of symptoms, maintenance of a serum hematocrit of 24% or greater, and a hemoglobin A concentration of greater than 50%. Treatment of sickle cell crises is outlined in Table 23.7 (46).

Rarely, women with homozygous β-thalassemia become pregnant, and treatment of these patients involves maintaining sufficient circulating red-blood-cell volume (hemoglobin level, >8 g/dL) to ensure adequate fetal oxygenation. Treatment options include transfusions or recombinant erythropoietin. Deferoxamine mesylate has proved to be useful for improving both the quality and the life span of patients with β-thalassemia, but it has not been approved for use during pregnancy. If both parents are heterozygous for α-thalassemia or β-thalassemia, prepregnancy genetic counseling should be obtained. Parents may wish to obtain prenatal diagnostic studies to determine

Table 23.7. **Management of Sickle Cell Crisis During Pregnancy**

	Primary Therapy	Supportive Therapy
Acute maternal management	1. *Hydration:* warmed Ringer's lactate, 1 per 1–2 hours, then 125 mL/h.	1. Strict intake and output, without catheterization if possible. Central venous access if impending cardiac failure or preeclampsia.
	2. *Analgesia:* Acetaminophen or IV opiates based on degree of pain relief.	2. Bed rest in warm, quiet, comfortable area. Mild sedation.
	3. IV antibiotics if evidence of infection.	3. Cultures and supportive laboratory tests.
	4. *Oxygenation:* 4–6 L/min by nasal prongs.	4. Check arterial blood gas, LDH, chemistry panel.
	5. *Transfusion (warmed):* Manual transfusion if Hgb <6 gm/dL or hematocrit <15%. Partial exchange, crossmatch 6 U, washed, buffy-coat poor packed RBCs: After: Phlebotomy of 500 mL over 30 min, transfuse 2 units over 2 hours. Repeat exchange 2–4 hours later, if necessary.	5. Check hematocrit, Hgb A concentrations after equilibration (6–8 hours); goal of Hgb A ≥50%, Hct ≥25%.
Fetal management	Electronic fetal heart monitoring if potential for perinatal survival (≥24–26 weeks' gestation).	Availability of skilled pediatric personnel to assess neonate for possible complications of maternal crisis.

Reprinted with permission from Martin JM, Files JF, Morrison JC. Sickle-cell crisis. In: Clark SL, Cotton DB, Hankins GDV, Phelan JP, eds. Critical care obstetrics. 2nd ed. Boston; Blackwell Scientific Publications, 1991;212–222.
Hgb, hemoglobin; *LDH,* lactate dehydrogenase.

the probability that their child will have serious homozygous disease.

Thrombocytopenia

Maternal thrombocytopenia (≤150 K/µL or thousand/µL) occurs in 5 to 8% of pregnant women. In most, it is a normal variant of late pregnancy and relates to increased platelet turnover. Pregnant women with this finding are generally not at increased risk for bleeding. More severe thrombocytopenia may be a complication of several serious disorders of pregnancy, including preeclampsia, placental abruption, and amnionic fluid embolism.

Autoimmune thrombocytopenia (ATP) is the most common pathologic cause of thrombocytopenia during pregnancy, and in 10 to 25% of cases, it is associated with autoimmune thyroid disease. The pathophysiologic mechanism of ATP appears to be the splenic production of immunoglobulin G (IgG) platelet autoantibodies and the destruction of sensitized platelets. Generally, women with preexisting ATP who become pregnant are at low risk for complications from this disorder. If the mother has PLa1 antibodies, transplacental passage of the IgG portion may occur, thus placing the fetus at risk for thrombocytopenia. In reality, however, most of this antibody is bound in the maternal circulation, thus protecting the fetus. The assay for the antibody is not predictive of adverse fetal effects.

The optimal treatment of ATP during pregnancy is under active investigation (47, 48). If maternal ATP precedes pregnancy, there is some risk that the maternal platelet count may be less than 50,000 cells/µL, especially during the third trimester. The threshold for treatment is not uniform, however, with recommendations to initiate therapy in the range of 20,000 to 50,000 cells/µL. Treatment may include prednisone, 1 to 2 mg/kg per day, or intravenous immunoglobulin, 1 g/kg per week, until the platelet count improves (>50,000 cells/µL).

The baseline neonatal risk for thrombocytopenia is 2%, and it is independent of any maternal diagnoses involving thrombocytopenia. Use of invasive methods to diagnose fetal thrombocytopenia or the need for preemptive cesarean delivery to prevent perinatal hemorrhagic injury does not appear to be justified.

Alloimmune thrombocytopenia is a fetal condition in which maternal antiplatelet antibodies cause the destruction of fetal platelets. The diagnosis is made through a well-documented patient history of a previously affected pregnancy. Typically, the mother does not have thromboyctopenia. Invasive diagnostic procedures to determine if the current pregnancy is affected may be risky if the fetus is severely thrombocytopenic. Typically, diagnostic and therapeutic care are rendered by specialists in maternal–fetal medicine who are experienced in percutaneous sampling of umbilical blood. Treatment includes maternal intravenous immunoglobulin, 1 gm/kg every 1 to 4 weeks, and fetal or neonatal transfusion with washed, leukocyte-poor maternal or cross-matched platelets (49). Use of corticosteroids to modulate maternal immune responses has not been shown to improve fetal thrombocytopenia.

Coagulopathies

Of the coagulopathies that occur during pregnancy, factor VIII (i.e., von Willebrand's) deficiency is the most common, with an incidence of 1 in 10,000. Patient history and measurement of factor VIII: RCoF, factor VIII:C, platelet count, and bleeding time will establish the type of factor VIII deficiency as well as the need for therapy. Cryoprecipitate or fresh-frozen plasma may be used when factor VIII cofactor is less than 80% of its normal level at delivery or if a cesarean delivery is undertaken. DDAVP (1-desamino-8-D-arginine vasopressin) or pasteurized human antihemophilic factor may also be used (50); however, more severe types of von Willebrand's disease may not respond to DDAVP.

Deficiencies of antithrombin III, protein C, and protein S may be documented for the first time during pregnancy, when they are manifested by venous thrombosis. Recently, both homocysteinemia and the Leiden Factor V mutation have been implicated as relatively common causes of thrombosis, and testing for these circulating abnormalities should also be included in the testing for causes of thrombosis (50a, 50b). If the patient has a previous diagnosis of one of these deficiencies, then prophylactic heparin, 5000 U at 8-hour intervals, appears to be beneficial during the course of pregnancy. Initial treatment of venous thrombosis consists of intravenous heparin titrated to achieve an activated partial thromboplastin time that is 2.0-fold to 2.5-fold greater than the upper normal range. Once clinical improvement is observed, maintenance therapy consists of subcutaneous heparin at therapeutic doses for the remainder of the pregnancy.

GASTROINTESTINAL, HEPATIC, BILIARY, AND PANCREATIC DISEASE

Although the physiologic changes induced by a normal pregnancy on the liver are not as marked as those in other organ systems, a number of enzyme-activity tests that are used to assess liver function are altered (Table 23.8) (51), and liver diseases complicating pregnancy can be grouped into one of three categories, as

Table 23.8.   Liver Function Tests During Pregnancy

Test	Effect of Pregnancy
Enzymes	
Alkaline phosphatase	Markedly increased
Aminotransferases	Unchanged
Lactic acid dehydrogenase	Unchanged
Bilirubin	Unchanged
Proteins	
Albumin	Decreased by 1 g/dL
Globulin	Slightly increased
Ceruloplasmin	Elevated
Hormone-binding proteins	Elevated
Transferrin	Elevated
Lipids	
Triglycerides	Elevated
Cholesterol	Doubled
Clotting factors	
Fibrinogen	Elevated
Factors VII, VIII, and X	Elevated
Clotting times	Unchanged

Reprinted with permission from Cunningham FG. Williams obstetrics. 20th ed. Stamford, Conn. Appleton & Lange, 1997: 1154.

shown in Table 23.9. Hepatic diseases that are induced by pregnancy usually disappear following delivery. Those that occur coincident with pregnancy generally follow the typical course as in nonpregnant patients. When pregnancy occurs during a chronic, more severe liver disease, it is a challenge for both the consulting internist and the obstetrician.

Use of endoscopy, ultrasonography, and, in some cases, magnetic resonance imaging has revolutionized the diagnosis of gastrointestinal disorders during pregnancy. While most gastrointestinal diseases may be treated successfully by medical therapy, surgery is appropriate for acute appendicitis and nonresponsive cholecystitis/cholelithiasis. The major areas that generally involve medical consultation are described here, and additional information may be obtained from several excellent reviews (51–53).

Nausea and Vomiting of Pregnancy

Persistent nausea and vomiting are two of the most common and frustrating problems for the pregnant patient and physician alike. Almost 20% of pregnant women experience vomiting more than once daily during early pregnancy. Almost 4% have enough disruption of their fluid, electrolyte, and nutritional status to require extensive pharmacologic or intravenous therapy, and a few patients may even require peripheral alimentation.

Recently, the diagnosis of a pregnancy-associated dysphasic gastrointestinal response has been made based on gastrointestinal motility studies using electrogastrography (54). Treatment with several pharmacologic agents, including calcium antacids, selective H_1-blockers, and gastric-emptying agents appears to improve both gastric rhythm and patient symptoms. If vomiting is unrelenting and associated with symptoms of persistent abdominal pain or jaundice, other disorders, including peptic ulcer disease, biliary disease, pancreatitis, trophoblastic disease, hepatitis, and acute fatty liver, should be considered.

If a regimen of frequent small meals and feeding before arising is unsuccessful, several pharmacologic agents, either sin-

Table 23.9.   Liver Diseases Complicating Pregnancy

Diseases Induced by Pregnancy
  Hyperemesis gravidarum with associated hepatic dysfunction
  Intrahepatic cholestasis of pregnancy
  Acute fatty liver of pregnancy
  Severe preeclampsia/eclampsia with hepatocellular damage
  HELLP syndrome
Diseases Coincidental to Pregnancy
  Acute viral hepatitis
  Drug-induced hepatitis/hepatic failure
Pregnancy in Chronic Liver Disease
  Chronic active hepatitis
  Cirrhosis
  Esophageal varices
  Liver transplantation

gly or in combination, have had varying success. These include vitamin B$_6$, doxylamine, some phenothiazines, selective histamine blockers, metoclopramide, and calcium-containing antacids. Both prescribed and nonprescribed pharmaceutical agents and their effects during pregnancy are described in Table 23.10 (55). Use of electrostimulation or acupuncture to reduce nausea through manipulation of the P6 acupuncture stimulation site at the wrist is under investigation.

Inflammatory Bowel Disease

Inflammatory bowel disease (IBD) is a relatively common medical problem affecting young women who may become pregnant, and it may appear for the first time during pregnancy. Historically, pregnancy in this patient group was discouraged because of concern over the effects of maternal exacerbations on the outcome of pregnancy. More recently, however, concerns involve the optimal timing of pregnancy and both the safety of and need for treatment during pregnancy. Current evidence suggests that pregnancy does not adversely affect the course of Crohn's disease, but that it may worsen the course of ulcerative colitis in approximately one-third of patients (56–58). Between 30 and 50% of pregnant women with IBD will experience an exacerbation either during pregnancy or postpartum (59). Women with active disease at conception are more prone to exacerbation and have a worse prognosis, and although the results of some studies suggest an increased incidence of preterm delivery and fetal growth retardation has been suggested, women with IBD typically have successful pregnancies.

While not limited to IBD alone, complaints of persistent diarrhea, particularly with bleeding, crampy abdominal pain, fever, anorexia, and anemia, should heighten clinical suspicion for the diagnosis or exacerbation of IBD. Treatment is similar in both pregnant and nonpregnant patients. No increase in congenital defects

or newborn toxicity have been observed with the use of sulfasalazine (60), and newer agents containing 5-amino-2-hydroxy-benzoic acid (mesalamine) have also been used during pregnancy (61). In addition, corticosteroids appear to be well tolerated. Metronidazole has been used in nonpregnant patients to treat perianal Crohn's disease, and although it appears to be safe for the treatment of trichomoniasis during pregnancy (59, 62), more data are needed on its use in IBD. Immunosuppressive agents are generally not recommended during pregnancy.

Treatment occurs in two phases: therapy for active disease, and therapy to maintain remission. Patients with mild distal colitis (e.g., proctitis, proctosigmoiditis) may be treated with either oral or topical agents. Patients generally respond to sulfasalazine, 3 to 4 g daily in divided doses, or mesalamine, 2 to 4 g daily. Topical mesalamine is also an option, either as a suppository for proctitis or an enema for disease to the splenic flexure. Topical corticosteroids may be administered in a foam preparation for proctitis or as an enema. In patients with moderate to severe disease, prednisone, with or without topical corticosteroid enemas, is used to achieve remission.

Once remission has been achieved, corticosteroid therapy is tapered and followed by maintenance therapy with sulfasalazine, if possible. Despite the apparent safe use of sulfasalazine during pregnancy, it is judicious to use doses no larger than those clearly needed to control the disease effectively. Sulfasalazine is effective at maintaining remission in ulcerative colitis, but neither sulfasalazine nor steroids prevent the recurrence of Crohn's disease. Continuation of any medication in asymptomatic patients who are pregnant should be weighed carefully and depends on the clinical situation. Immunosuppressive drugs such as azathioprine or 6-mercaptopurine have been used as steroid-sparing agents to maintain remission in nonpregnant patients with severe disease. Experience with aza-

Table 23.10.   Safety of Prescription Gastrointestinal Drugs During Pregnancy

Drug Use	Risk Category	Potential Fetal Effects	Comments	Use in Pregnancy
Sucralfate (Carafate)	B	No evidence of teratogenicity or congenital defects		Yes
Cimetidine (Tagamet)	B	No evidence of teratogenicity or congenital defects	Predelivery prevention; aspiration pneumonitis	Yes
Omeprazole (Losec)	C	Little human data; dose-related fetal toxicity in animals	Single-dose before obstetrical anesthesia without complication (one study)	More data needed
Meclizine (Antivert)	B	Teratogenic in animals, apparently not in humans	Antiemetic-antihistamine	If strictly indicated
Promethazine (Phenergan)	C	Possible association with cardiovascular defects	Antiemetic for intractable symptoms	If strictly indicated
Metoclopramide (Reglan)	B	No association with malformations or other adverse effects	Antiemetic; prevention of aspiration during labor	Yes
Pyridoxine (Vitamin B₆)	A	No known teratogenicity or congenital defects	Supplement with RDA dose; alternative use for nausea/vomiting	Yes
Bulk-forming agents (Metamucil, Perdiem, others)	A	No known teratogenicity or congenital defects	Agents of choice for diarrhea/constipation in pregnancy	Yes
Hyperosmotic agents (Sorbitol, glycerin, lactulose)	B	No human data available; no animal teratogenicity	Minimal systemic absorption	Yes
Lubricants (Mineral oil, Haley's)	C	Hypoprothrombinemia, neonatal bleeding if used regularly	Chronic use may lead to decreased absorption of fat-soluble vitamins	No
Saline laxatives (Milk of Magnesia, Fleets)			Maternal sodium retention, electrolyte disturbances	
Stimulants (Senokot/ Senna Bisacodyl/ Dulcolax)	C	No association with malformations or other adverse effects		Yes
Antidiarrheal (Kaopectate)	C	No reports of adverse fetal outcome	Not absorbed	Yes
Loperamide (Imodium)	B	No animal terato-genicity; human data limited.	Possible association with cardiovascular defects	If strictly needed
Diphenoxylate/ atropine (Lomotil)	C	No clear association with congenital defects		If strictly needed
Bismuth subsalicylate (Pepto-Bismol)	C	Potential for fetal toxicity from subsalicylate	Use restricted to first half of pregnancy, if at all	No

Adapted from Baron TH, Ramirez B, Richter JE. Gastrointestinal motility disorders during pregnancy. Ann Intern Med 1993;118:366–375; Lewis JH, Weingold AB. The use of gastrointestinal drugs during pregnancy and lactation. Am J Gastroenterol 1985;80:912–923; Briggs GG, Freeman RK, Yaffe SJ, eds. A reference guide to fetal and neonatal risk: drugs in pregnancy and lactation. 4th ed. Baltimore: Williams and Wilkins, 1994; Moore J, Flynn RJ, Sampaio M, et al. Effect of single-dose omeprazole on intragastric acidity and volume during obstetric anesthesia. Anesthesia 1989;44:559–562; and Sahakian V, Rouse D, Sipes S, et al. Vitamin B₆ is effective therapy for nausea and vomiting of pregnancy: a randomized, double-blind placebo-controlled study. Obstet Gynecol 1991;78:33–36.
RDA, recommended daily allowance.
A—No evidence of human risk, from controlled studies in women.
B—No evidence of human risk, but no controlled human studies.
C—Risk to humans has not been ruled out.

thioprine in pregnant patients with IBD is preliminary but encouraging (63), as are data on renal transplant recipients and patients with systemic lupus erythematosus (Table 23.11).

Patients with severe, recurrent disease present a significant challenge for the consulting internist, gastroenterologist, and obstetrician. Hospitalization, intravenous corticosteroids, intravenous fluids and electrolytes, and blood products may be required. Nutritional treatment is also an important consideration, and parenteral alimentation has been used successfully in pregnant women. Stool examination for ova and parasites, clostridial toxin, and culture for enteric pathogens should be obtained to exclude complicating infections. Surgery may be required for complications such as fulminant colitis, obstruction, perforation, and toxic megacolon.

Diagnostic evaluations, including focused radiographic studies, should not be postponed if their results are likely to affect treatment significantly. If intestinal obstruction is suspected, limited radiographic examinations, including plain films of the abdomen and following administration of a soluble contrast medium, either orally or by enema, may be necessary. Abdominal surgery may be required during pregnancy to treat complications (57), particularly abscess formation and intestinal obstruction.

Cholestasis

Cholestasis of pregnancy, which is manifested by pruritis and moderate conjugated hyperbilirubinemia (2–6 mg/dL), is the second most common cause of jaundice during pregnancy after hepatitis. The disorder also affects the prothrombin time, leading to an increased propensity for bleeding. Cholestasis of pregnancy is prevalent in Chile, Scandinavia, the Mediterranean countries, Australia, Canada, Poland, and China. Premature labor is increased in the affected pregnancies, however, the mechanism for initiating premature labor is unclear. It may relate to increased transplacental transport of estrogen and progesterone metabolites that are not cleared through the enterohepatic circulation (64). Treatment consists of a combination of cholestyramine, 4 g three to four times a day, and parenteral vitamin K. These agents confer limited effective clinical responses (65). A team approach to care, including surveillance for preterm onset of labor, is essential. Ultimately, delivery of the pregnancy is associated with a complete remission of symptoms.

Cholecystitis

Gallstones are common in women, and pregnancy increases the frequency of symptomatic cholecystitis. The treatment of acute cholecystitis in pregnancy is similar to that in nonpregnant women. If conservative methods are unsuccessful, the second trimester is the optimal time for surgery to reduce the risk for premature labor and delivery.

Hepatitis

Hepatitis is the most common serious liver disease encountered during pregnancy. Of the five major types of this viral disease, hepatitis B is the most important because of its long-term maternal and neonatal consequences (66). Nausea, vomiting, headache, and malaise typically precede jaundice by 1 to 2 weeks. Serum aminotransferase levels are in the 400 to 4000 U/L range, and they do not correspond with disease severity. Complete clinical recovery usually occurs within 1 to 2 months in all cases of hepatitis A and most cases of hepatitis B and C. Treatment during pregnancy is similar to that in nonpregnant patients: rest, a well-balanced diet, and careful monitoring of liver function tests, including the prothrombin time. Premature labor may be precipitated by a fulminant course of viral hepatitis, especially in the third trimester.

Table 23.11. Drug Effects of Antirheumatic and Immunosuppressives During Pregnancy

Drug	FDA Risk Category[a]	Potential Fetal Effects	Comments	Use in Pregnancy
Aspirin (≥650 mg)	C (D after 32–34 weeks' gestation)[b]	Bleeding and CNS hemorrhage near term; perinatal mortality, IUGR, teratogenic	80 mg/day is safe in SLE with APLS, PHI, preeclampsia, IUGR	Specific medical indications
NSAIDs (Ibuprofen)	B (D after 32–34 weeks' gestation)	Reduced fetal urine output; early closure of ductus arteriosus; pulmonary hypertension; bleeding	Short-term use may not affect amniotic fluid volume, ductus	If strictly indicated
Corticosteroids (prednisone, dexamethasone, betamethasone)	B	No association with congenital defects; may hasten fetal lung maturity	Effect of high-dose, pulse therapy has not been determined	Yes
Gold	C	Crosses placenta, limited studies; no major abnormalities observed	No long-term follow-up studies of exposed fetuses available	If strictly indicated
Penicillamine	D	Fetal malformation; connective tissue defects	Limited data; <500 mg may reduce toxicity	No
Hydroxychloroquine	C	500 mg/wk not teratogenic; fetal toxicity possible with high daily doses	Hydroxychloroquine is less toxic than chloroquine; 200–400 mg/day preferred	No
Cyclosporine	C	Spontaneous abortion; premature labor; IUGR	Limited experience in renal transplant recipients suggests low teratogenicity	If indicated

Hepatitis A

Hepatitis A is occurs in less than 1 in 1000 of U.S. adults, and the fatality rate is 2 or fewer per 1000. There has been no demonstrated case of perinatal transmission. Diagnosis is established by a positive hepatitis A–immunoglobuin M (IgM) antibody test, and treatment is nutritional support and rest. The recent development of a vaccine for hepatitis A establishes preventive care as an option in this infection. Because the vaccine contains attenuated live virus, however, it should be administered no later than 3 months before anticipated conception or deferred until after the first trimester (67).

Hepatitis B

Hepatitis B, which is caused by a DNA virus, may adversely affect the outcome of pregnancy either by acute infection during pregnancy or by long-term maternal carriage of hepatitis B surface antigen (HBsAg). Maternal infection carries a fatality rate of 1% or less. Chronic infection occurs in 10 to 15% of patients, and 25% of these patients are at risk for chronic, persistent hepatitis or cirrhosis. Long-term maternal carriage, especially if the patient is HBe antigen positive, is associated with a 10 to 20% rate of fetal transmission, most of which occurs during childbirth. Neonatal transmission of hepatitis B can

Table 23.11. *(continued)* **Drug Effects of Antirheumatic and Immunosuppressives During Pregnancy**

Drug	FDA Risk Category[a]	Potential Fetal Effects	Comments	Use in Pregnancy
Chlorambucil	D	Kidney agenesis; low birth weight; multiple abnormalities	Very limited data; other treatment alternatives preferred	No
Cyclophosphamide	D	Fetal malformation; limb abnormalities (first trimester); IUGR	Limited experience in maternal cancer patients; use in second and third trimester	No
6-Mercaptopurine	D	Prematurity; IUGR; cleft palate	Limited human data	No
Methotrexate	D	Embryotoxic; facial, skeletal abnormalities; myelosuppression	Discontinue at least 3 months before conception	No
Azathioprine	D	IUGR; immunosuppression of newborn	Experience suggests low toxicity	If strictly indicated
Intravenous immunoglobulin	C	No adverse effects observed in very limited use	Crosses placenta in significant amounts when >32 weeks' gestation	APLS

Adapted from Baron TH, Ramirez B, Richter JE. Gastrointestinal motility disorders during pregnancy. Ann Intern Med 1993;118:366–375; Lewis JH, Weingold AB. The use of gastrointestinal drugs during pregnancy and lactation. Am J Gastroenterol 1985;80:912–923; Briggs GG, Freeman RK, Yaffe SJ, eds. A reference guide to fetal and neonatal risk: drugs in pregnancy and lactation. 4th ed. Baltimore: Williams and Wilkins, 1994; Moore J, Flynn RJ, Sampaio M, et al. Effect of single-dose omeprazole on intragastric acidity and volume during obstetric anesthesia. Anesthesia 1989;44:559–562; Sahakian V, Rouse D, Sipes S, et al. Vitamin B₆ is effective therapy for nausea and vomiting of pregnancy: a randomized, double-blind placebo-controlled study. Obstet Gynecol 1991;78:33–36; Orvieto R, Achiron A, Ben-Rafael Z, et al. Intravenous immunoglobulin treatment for recurrent abortions caused by antiphospholipid antibodies. Fertil Steril 1991;56:1013–1020; Marzusch K, Tinneberg H, Mueller-Eckhardt G, et al. Is immunotherapy justified for recurrent spontaneous abortion? Lancet 1992;339:1543.

APLS, antiphospholipid antibody syndrome; *CNS,* central nervous system; *IUGR,* intrauterine growth retardation; *PIH,* pregnancy-induced hypertension; *SLE,* systemic lupus erythematosus.

[a]FDA classification for teratogenic potential of pharmaceutical agents:
  B—No evidence of human risk, but no controlled human studies.
  C—Risk to humans has not been ruled out.
  D—Positive evidence of risk to humans from human or animal studies.

[b]Theoretical risk or case reports only.

be prevented by immunization of susceptible, reproductive-age women (68) before pregnancy (Table 23.12). Treating newborn children of HBsAg carriers with hepatitis B immune globulin and hepatitis B vaccine within the first 12 hours after birth reduces the risk of transmission to between 1 and 2% (69).

Hepatitis C and D

Hepatitis C accounts for 10 to 20% of U.S. cases involving acute viral hepatitis.

Previously described as non-A, non-B hepatitis, hepatitis C is caused by an RNA virus and is most common among intravenous drug abusers and patients who have received blood-component transfusions. Long-term carriage of hepatitis C is also associated with the development of cirrhosis and primary liver cancer. Both vertical and sexual transmission are less common than for hepatitis B (70, 71). The enzyme-linked immunosorbent assay (ELISA) and immunoblot assays are not

Table 23.12.   Risk Factors for Hepatitis B Virus Infection

I. History of illicit drug use
II. History of sexually transmitted disease
III. Multiple sexual partners
IV. Work in a health care or public safety field
V. Household contact with a virus carrier
VI. Work or residence in an institution for the developmentally disabled
VII. Work or treatment in a hemodialysis unit
VIII. Receipt of clotting factor concentrates for bleeding disorders

Reprinted with permission from American College of Obstetrics and Gynecology. Hepatitis in pregnancy. ACOG Technical Bulletin No. 174, 1992.

as effective as the polymerase chain reaction (PCR) to establish the diagnosis, but PCR is expensive and difficult to perform in large-scale testing situations (72). Interferon-α has some beneficial effects in stabilizing chronic active disease, but it has not yet been approved for use in pregnancy. Hepatitis D (delta) is usually a coinfection with hepatitis B and is rarely associated with vertical transmission. Methods used to prevent the transmission of hepatitis B are generally effective in preventing infection with hepatitis D.

Cirrhosis

Postnecrotic cirrhosis from hepatitis is the most common form of cirrhosis in patients who are pregnant, although in others, long-term exposure to alcohol is the most frequent cause. Cirrhosis with portal hypertension carries a high risk of maternal mortality (25–45%) from bleeding esophageal varices or hepatic failure (73). The perinatal mortality rate approaches 50%. Recently, portal-systemic shunting and sclerotherapy have been used to control variceal bleeding (73–75). Women with severe, chronic liver disease should be fully informed of the risks involved in pregnancy and advised of appropriate birth control techniques or of liver transplantation if pregnancy is desired.

The number of liver transplants involving women who then become pregnant is steadily increasing. Indications for transplant have included posthepatitis necrotic cirrhosis, primary biliary cirrhosis, primary sclerosing cholangitis, and cirrhosis in abstaining alcoholics, and the University of Pittsburgh group reported the outcome of 19 pregnancies among 17 transplanted women (76). All of these pregnancies resulted in liveborn infants and surviving mothers, but complications included hypertension, anemia, and preterm delivery.

Liver Failure

Fulminant liver failure is a rare complication of pregnancy. It may be associated with hepatitis A or B or with problems not related to hepatitis, including preeclampsia complicated by HELLP syndrome and acute fatty liver of pregnancy (AFLP). AFLP occurs in the mid to late third trimester, and it is associated with preeclampsia in 30 to 100% of cases. AFLP is infrequent (i.e., 1 in 10,000), and our understanding of this disease is limited (77, 78). Manifestations include malaise, anorexia, lethargy, tachycardia, nausea, and vomiting. Jaundice develops 1 to 3 weeks after the onset of symptoms, with right upper quadrant tenderness, ascites, and, often, fever. Associated renal dysfunction is common, and serum transaminase (AST, ALT) levels are increased, characteristically reaching peak levels of 300 to 500 U/L, which are less than those expected in acute hepatitis (i.e., 2000–4000 U/L). Serum bilirubin levels are usually less than 10 mg/dL in either AFLP or HELLP syndrome. Both diseases may be associated with leukocytosis, thrombocytopenia, elevated serum alkaline phosphatase levels, and prolonged prothrombin and activated partial thromboplastin times. Unlike hepatitis and the HELLP syndrome, AFLP frequently manifests by hypoglycemia and early, increased serum ammonia levels. Patients are usually HBsAg negative. With impaired synthesis of coagulation factors, bleeding abnormalities are common, and patients often have metabolic acidosis. The histopathologic finding of swollen, "foamy" hepatocytes from liver biopsy specimens with the staining characteristics of fatty infiltration is a hallmark of AFLP.

The clinical course of patients with AFLP is often more complicated than with acute hepatitis or the HELLP syndrome. Some clinical similarities do exist between HELLP and AFLP, including disseminated intravascular coagulation and acute renal failure, but patients with the HELLP syndrome are not hypoglycemic and rarely go into hepatic coma. Women with AFLP may ultimately die from complications of pancreatitis, gastrointestinal bleeding, disseminated intravascular coagulation, progressive renal failure, sepsis, or irreversible shock (79). Fetal death is also a frequent complication of AFLP.

Treatment of acute liver failure during pregnancy should take place in the intensive care setting of a regional hospital (80). Optimal nutrition should be maintained by use of concentrated, intravenous glucose solutions. Protein intake should be restricted, and bacterial breakdown of gut proteins to ammonia may be minimized with use of neomycin and magnesium citrate catharsis. Both electrolyte and coagulation abnormalities should be corrected promptly. Aggressive, early treatment of nosocomial infection and prevention of gastrointestinal bleeding also increase the potential for survival. For patients who continue to deteriorate despite extensive treatment, orthotopic liver transplantation may be an option.

THYROID DISEASE

Thyroid disease is common in the general population, and especially in young women. Consequently, thyroid disorders are relatively frequent during pregnancy. Although physiologic thyroid enlargement resulting from glandular hyperplasia and increased vascularity may occur in pregnancy, any goiter or nodule should be evaluated.

Pregnancy-induced changes in thyroid physiology include increased serum concentrations of binding globulin and thyroid hormone, increased renal clearance of iodine, and increased production and turnover of T_4 (81). Changes in some thyroid function tests may occur, but in most pregnant women, the serum free T_4, free triiodothyronine (T_3), and TSH are within the normal range for nonpregnant women (81–83). Direct assays for these hormones have replaced the more variable resin T_3 uptake and total T_4 index tests. In general, the measurement of free T_4 and the ultrasensitive TSH assay will provide a reasonable assessment of maternal thyroid status.

Hypothyroidism

Although hypothyroidism has been associated with successful term pregnancies (84), higher rates of both maternal and fetal complications have been reported. Maternal complications can include anemia, preeclampsia, placental abruption, and postpartum hemorrhage. Fetal complications can include low birth weight, stillbirth, abortion, and congenital anomalies (83).

The diagnosis is suspected by the usual clinical clues of cold intolerance, cool skin, coarse hair, difficulties in concentration, irritability, and paresthesias (as seen with carpal tunnel syndrome). These symptoms may also be seen in normal pregnancy, however. Overt hypothyroidism and myxedema are often accompanied by infertility; therefore, pregnancy is uncommon. The more frequent clinical scenario is the onset of symptoms in a pregnant woman who is already on thyroid-replacement therapy. The onset of congestive heart failure complicating pregnancy should always raise the possibility of occult hypothyroidism.

Primary hypothyroidism is diagnosed by an elevated TSH level and a low free T_4

or inappropriately low total T_4 level. The most sensitive indicator of primary hypothyroidism is an elevated serum TSH level. The serum T_3 level will often remain normal until the thyroid failure is severe; therefore, this is not a useful measurement. Once the diagnosis has been established, full replacement of L-thyroxine is indicated. The usual dose is 0.1 to 0.15 mg once daily, and the dosage should be adjusted at 3-week to 4-week intervals using the serum TSH level as the clinical monitor. The goals of therapy are gradual symptomatic relief and return of the TSH level to normal. Thereafter, TSH levels should be determined at least every trimester to ensure adequate replacement.

For women already receiving T_4, therapy can be safely continued throughout pregnancy. The T_4 requirement may increase by 25 to 50% during pregnancy in these women (81–85), and thyroid function should be checked every trimester to ensure adequate replacement.

Simultaneous administration of iron therapy with L-thyroxine causes a variable reduction in absorption, which may be clinically significant (86). In patients who require both T_4 and iron supplements, separation of their ingestion times by 2 or more hours is recommended, and routine thyroid function should be monitored.

The ultrasensitive TSH assay allows for detection of gland underactivity (or underreplacement) before the onset of clinical symptoms. A common clinical situation is subclinical hypothyroidism, which is characterized by an elevated serum TSH level, normal serum T_4 and T_3 levels, and a lack of clinical symptoms. Although the effects of subclinical hypothyroidism on pregnancy outcome are not clearly defined, T_4 replacement is generally recommended.

Patients with type I diabetes who develop proteinuria during gestation may be at increased risk for de novo hypothyroidism during pregnancy (87). Thyroid function tests should be obtained in these patients, particularly if their insulin requirements do not increase as expected during the second trimester and proteinuria is either present or develops.

Solitary Thyroid Nodule

Thyroid nodules are approximately four times more common in women than in men, and they present in 1 to 2% of reproductive-age women. Thyroid carcinoma is found in 8 to 17% of solitary thyroid nodules (88). It has been commonly believed that pregnancy has no effect on the natural history of thyroid cancer, and that thyroid cancer has no significant effect on pregnancy. Some evidence suggests that the incidence of thyroid cancer may be increased in pregnancy, however, and that it may have a more aggressive course in some patients (89, 90).

A thyroid nodule should be investigated as in a nonpregnant patient, with the caveat that radionuclide scans are contraindicated during pregnancy. Ultrasonography helps to visualize multiple nodules and determine their solid or cystic nature, but this modality cannot distinguish benign from malignant disease. Fine-needle aspiration (FNA) is the most important part of the evaluation and may by safely undertaken during pregnancy. The usefulness of FNA biopsies, however, depends on the experience and expertise of the cytologist, the skill of the aspirator, and the difficulty in distinguishing certain histopathologic lesions. FNA provides diagnostic information in 70 to 90% of cases; nondiagnostic biopsies should be repeated. In nonpregnant patients, the false-negative rate is approximately 1 to 11%, and the false-positive rate is approximately 1 to 8% (91).

If the biopsy specimen suggests malignancy, then surgical excision is recommended, either during the second or third trimester or after delivery. Benign nodules can be followed or suppression with L-thyroxine attempted. Although thyroid hormone suppressive therapy often shrinks diffuse or multinodular goiter in nonpregnant patients, suppression may not occur during pregnancy because of the stimulating effects of hyperestrogenemia and other factors that are operative at this time.

Hyperthyroidism

The most common cause of hyperthyroidism during pregnancy is Graves' disease. This autoimmune disorder is associated with thyroid-stimulating antibodies, which stimulate the thyroid TSH receptor and result in thyroid hyperfunction and growth. Other causes of hyperthyroidism, such as toxic nodular goiter, gestational trophoblastic disease, toxic adenoma, and Hashimoto's thyroiditis, are much less common.

Hyperemesis gravidarum and gestation trophoblastic disease may cause changes in thyroid function. The placenta produces human chorionic gonadotrophin, which has some thyrotropinlike bioactivity. The increased production of human chorionic gonadotrophin during the first trimester is associated with an increased free T_4 index, elevated free T_4 level, and variably elevated free T_3 level. This condition is transient, however, and tends to resolve in the second trimester (81). Hyperthyroxinemia is not a feature of usual morning sickness.

Mild thyrotoxicosis is difficult to diagnose, because many of the symptoms, such as dyspnea, palpitations, and heat intolerance, may also be present in normal pregnancy. The clinical findings that are not typical of pregnancy include weight loss, significant thyroid enlargement, ophthalmopathy, and myopathy.

Once hyperthyroidism is suspected, an elevated free T_4 level and depressed TSH level confirm the diagnosis. The ultrasensitive TSH assays can distinguish hyperthyroidism, but they cannot determine severity. A 24-hour radioactive iodine uptake scan, which is helpful in nonpregnant patients, is contraindicated in pregnancy because of potential damage to the fetal thyroid gland.

Graves' disease has a variable course during pregnancy. Preexisting disease tends to worsen in the first trimester and improve during the second and third trimester. Thyroid function tests should be evaluated monthly, because medical therapy can often be tapered over the course of the pregnancy. The serum free T_4 and T_3 radioimmunoassay should be used to follow the effects of treatment, because once suppressed, the TSH level may remain low for weeks to months after the patient returns to the euthyroid state. The disease may again activate during the postpartum period, and rarely, delivery can precipitate thyroid storm.

Medical therapy is the preferred initial treatment during pregnancy, and pregnancy outcome depends on whether metabolic control is achieved. Complications of untreated or uncontrolled hyperthyroidism include preeclampsia and heart failure in the mother and prematurity, stillbirth, and increased perinatal mortality in the fetus (92).

The thioamide antithyroid drugs propylthiouracil (PTU) and methimazole are the mainstays of medical treatment. Each crosses the placenta, and each may produce fetal hypothyroidism and goiter when use is continued late in pregnancy. PTU is more highly protein bound and thus tends to cross the placenta less. It also has the advantage of blocking the conversion of T_4 to T_3 in the peripheral tissues and has become the treatment of choice (83).

Use of PTU has produced good pregnancy outcomes in women who achieve clinical euthyroidism (92). Use of PTU may also be continued postpartum while nursing. The usual starting dose is 300 to 450 mg daily, although higher dosages (600–900 mg/day) may be required. Laboratory evidence of response to therapy may take 3 to 4 weeks. Once euthyroidism is achieved (i.e., a normal T_4 or TSH level), the dose should be reduced to the smallest that will control the thyrotoxicosis. Some advocate maintaining maternal T_4 levels in the mildly thyrotoxic range to ensure that the lowest effective dose is administered.

Adverse reactions to PTU affect approximately 5% of patients, and they include fever, rash, hepatitis, and dose-related neutropenia. The most serious reaction, idiopathic agranulocytosis, occurs during the first 3 months of therapy in 0.2 to 0.5% of patients, but it is reversible after stopping the PTU. An adverse reaction to one thioamide does not necessarily predict a similar reaction to the other.

β-Blocking drugs help to blunt the effects of excess thyroid hormone and to diminish the symptoms of hyperthyroidism. Their major use is to control the maternal heart rate to less than 100 beats per minute while awaiting response to thioamide therapy. Although considered to be relatively safe during pregnancy (27), their use is generally restricted to short-term therapy in preparation for subtotal thyroidectomy or treatment of thyroid storm. Newborn children of women who are treated with these drugs near delivery should be monitored for bradycardia, hypoglycemia, and other symptoms of β-blockade.

Because radioactive iodine is contraindicated in pregnancy, subtotal thyroidectomy is the alternative, definitive therapy for Graves' disease in pregnancy. The major indications for surgery are intolerance to drug therapy, the requirement for a high dosage of antithyroid medication, or noncompliance with the medical regimen. Surgery should be performed after thyrotoxicosis has been controlled medically, and it is best undertaken from the beginning of the second trimester until early in the third trimester.

True thyroid storm in pregnancy is rare. In pregnant women with untreated hyperthyroidism, heart failure is much more likely to occur, either precipitated or intensified by other complications (e.g., preeclampsia, infection, or anemia) (94). Life-threatening hyperthyroidism requires close supervision, intensive care, and, typically, additional subspecialist consultations. Treatment of thyroid storm consists 1 g of potassium iodide to inhibit the release of thyroid hormone, and 1 g of PTU (94). Propranolol, either oral or intravenous, is often needed, although it must be used cautiously during heart failure. Other supportive measures include adequate hydration, thermoregulation, oxygen, digitalis, and aggressive treatment of hypertension, anemia, and infection (if present) to reduce the cardiac workload.

Postpartum Thyroid Dysfunction

Thyroid dysfunction following delivery is common, occurring in 5 to 10% of women (82). Postpartum thyroiditis is the main cause of thyroid dysfunction during this period. As an autoimmune disorder, it can be differentiated from Graves' disease by the absence of thyrotropin-receptor antibodies and a low radioiodine uptake. Risk factors include a previous history of the disorder and a personal or family history of thyroid or autoimmune disease. Although the cause is unknown, it is characterized histologically as a destructive, lymphocytic thyroiditis that is associated with thyroid microsomal autoantibodies. High titers of microsomal autoantibodies, when measured early in pregnancy or shortly after delivery, may identify women at high risk for developing postpartum thyroiditis (95).

Table 23.13 outlines the clinical presentation of postpartum thyroiditis. The syndrome begins 1 to 4 months postpartum as glandular destruction causes the release of preformed thyroid hormone and transient thyrotoxicosis. The onset is usually abrupt, with a small, painless goiter and mild symptoms of fatigue and palpitations, which may go unrecognized by the woman and the physician. There is neither an elevated sedimentation rate nor leukocytosis. In contrast to Graves' disease, thyroid uptake is low and thyroid-stimulating antibodies are absent. Mild elevation of the free T_4 or the free T_3 level occurs, but this is transient and does not usually require treatment. β-Adrenergic blockers have been used when severe

Table 23.13.   Clinical Presentation of Postpartum Thyroiditis

Thyrotoxic Phase
  1–4 months postpartum
  Mild symptoms or asymptomatic
  Transient elevation of free T_4 or free T_3
  Low radioiodine uptake
  Negative for thyroid-stimulating antibody
Hypothyroid Phase
  4–8 months postpartum
  Symptomatic; psychiatric symptoms
  Clinically hypothyroid; goiter with lymphocytic
    infiltration
High Titers of Thyroid Microsomal Autoantibodies
  Treatment with T_4 as needed
  Recurrence of disease in subsequent pregnancy
  Long-term hypothyroidism may occur in 25%

Adapted from Lazarus JH, Othman S. Thyroid disease in relation to pregnancy. Clin Endocrinol 1991;34:91–98.

symptoms occur. Approximately two-thirds of women who develop thyrotoxicosis will return to a euthyroid state; one-third will develop hypothyroidism (83).

Between 4 and 8 months postpartum, from 2 to 5% of all women will develop overt hypothyroidism (83). Thus, women who are at risk should be evaluated regularly for goiter (sometimes painful), lack of energy, and depression. Hypothyroidism can develop rapidly, and many women will seek treatment during this phase. Replacement therapy is indicated in symptomatic patients once hypothyroidism has been confirmed, and is continued for 12 to 18 months following delivery, then gradually tapered. Women who experience postpartum thyroiditis are at risk of permanent hypothyroidism. Therefore, long-term follow-up and regular thyroid evaluation is important.

COLLAGEN VASCULAR DISEASES

Rheumatic diseases commonly affect women of childbearing age. These diseases may be active during pregnancy and require drug treatment to control their activity and symptoms. The most common, rheumatoid arthritis and systemic lupus erythematosus, as well as the recently described antiphospholipid antibody syndrome, are discussed here.

Rheumatoid Arthritis

Rheumatoid arthritis generally improves during pregnancy. In some, however, the course may worsen, and rarely, the initial disease may appear during pregnancy or postpartum. Pregnancy outcomes are relatively normal, and a remission in one pregnancy usually predicts similar results in subsequent pregnancies. Postpartum flares are common, and progression of joint disease may also occur at this time.

Since the severity of rheumatoid arthritis is almost always decreased during pregnancy, it is frequently possible to decrease or even eliminate the use of drugs that were required for control antepartum. A summary of antirheumatic drug treatments is presented in Table 23.11. Data on the use of antirheumatic drugs are limited, and many questions about the safety of such treatment during pregnancy remain.

Low-dose aspirin (80 mg/day) has been used safely during pregnancy. Larger doses of salicylates and nonsteroidal anti-inflammatory agents are generally avoided, however, particularly during late pregnancy, because of their effect on both maternal and fetal platelet function and their potential effects on the ductus arteriosus and kidney function of the fetus. Amniotic fluid volume should be monitored closely, with use of nonsteroidal anti-inflammatory drugs to prevent oligohydramnios (96).

Use of corticosteroids may continue during pregnancy, and gold salts may be an option as well. In selected patients, intra-articular injections with steroids or gold may be a safer alternative to oral medication. Use of antimalarials, immunosuppressives, and penicillamine should be avoided. Azathioprine is relatively safe, but experience with its use has been limited.

Systemic Lupus Erythematosus

Despite many studies, controversy remains as to whether pregnancy places a patient with systemic lupus erythematosus at increased risk for exacerbation (96–100). Lupus flares do occur frequently during pregnancy, but the frequency and severity of such exacerbations vary widely.

For a patient with lupus who is considering pregnancy, the optimum time to conceive is during remission; those with lupus nephropathy have a better prognosis if the disease has been inactive for 3 to 6 months before conception. Lupus nephritis is a major risk during pregnancy, and lack of previous renal involvement does not exclude the potential for kidney disease to develop during pregnancy.

Fetal outcomes in lupus include higher rates of abortion, fetal growth retardation, stillbirth, and preterm birth (100). Fetal outcomes are worse with maternal renal involvement and hypertension and in the presence of autoimmune antibodies. Antiphospholipid antibodies (i.e., anticardiolipin antibody and lupus anticoagulant) are associated with recurrent pregnancy loss as well as with maternal thrombosis, neurologic disorders, and thrombocytopenia.

Congenital heart block resulting from transplacental passage of maternal IgG anti-SSA (Ro) and anti-SSB (La) antibodies is an uncommon but serious fetal complication (97–99). In a female patient with systemic lupus erythematosus, testing for these antibodies should be performed before pregnancy. If the tests are positive, the patient should be counseled about the risks involved with pregnancy, because pharmacologic treatment does not guarantee prevention of the neonatal disorder.

Various laboratory tests have been recommended to monitor the activity of lupus during pregnancy. The sedimentation rate is not useful, however, because it is normally elevated in pregnancy (99). Low or falling levels of complement fractions, even though not always reliable, are more likely to be associated with active disease. Frequent hematologic evaluation and assessment of renal and hepatic function are also necessary.

The diagnosis of a flare in pregnant patients with lupus may be difficult, because some of the characteristic signs and symptoms (e.g., arthralgia, facial and palmar erythema, thrombocytopenia, proteinuria, anemia) may result from the pregnancy itself and not the lupus. Reliable indicators of active disease include rising levels of anti-DNA antibody, alternative-pathway hypocomplementemia, arthritis, rash, mucosal ulcers, and lymphadenopathy (97). A flare of lupus nephritis is signaled by the worsening of hypertension, proteinuria, and renal function. This may be difficult to distinguish from preeclampsia, and additional complications of both preeclampsia and lupus flare include encephalopathy, abdominal pain, and hepatic failure or infarction (97).

Hemolysis, thrombocytopenia, anemia, and leukopenia may develop. Mild thrombocytopenia (50,000–150,000 cells/µL) usually does not require treatment. Prednisone and intravenous immunoglobulin are used for severe thrombocytopenia, significant bleeding, or impending delivery.

Treatment of active lupus in pregnant patients is similar to that in nonpregnant patients, except for use of teratogenic drugs (Table 23.11). Corticosteroids are the agents of choice. Some authorities advocate the continuous use of corticosteroids following a flare throughout the duration of the pregnancy to avoid a recurrence (96), but most do not recommend prophylactic treatment either during pregnancy or after delivery. Use of the lowest possible glucocorticoid dose to control disease activity is prudent. Azathioprine is used for steroid-resistant nephropathy, but cyclophosphamide is avoided unless life-threatening complications develop (101). Use of antimalarial agents is controversial, and opinions in the rheumatologic literature are divided. Most recommend avoiding antimalarials during pregnancy. If preeclampsia cannot be definitely excluded, then treatment for both disorders is often appropriate. Involvement of a rheumatologist, perinatologist, and tertiary care center is advisable as well.

Antiphospholipid Antibody Syndrome

Several antibodies directed against negatively charged phospholipids have been described, including several anticardiolipin antibodies (i.e., immunoglobulin A [IgA], IgG, and IgM), lupus anticoagulant, and those responsible for a false-positive serologic test for syphilis. Antiphospholipid antibodies are often found in patients with systemic lupus erythematosus, but they are also found in those with other rheumatic diseases, with nonrheumatic disorders, and in healthy persons (102). Patients with lupus who have antiphospholipid antibodies are at high risk for fetal loss, thrombocytopenia, and thrombosis.

The antiphospholipid antibody syndrome is a recently described autoimmune process that is characterized by the presence of anticardiolipin antibodies in combination with recurrent thrombosis, recurrent pregnancy loss, or thrombocytopenia. Pregnant women with these antibodies are at increased risk of spontaneous abortion, stillbirths, intrauterine fetal growth restriction, preterm birth, and thrombotic events (99).

Interpretation of a positive antibody test may be complicated for several reasons:

1. Approximately 5% of all otherwise healthy, nonpregnant patients who are screened will show nonspecific antiphospholipid antibodies in low titers (99).
2. Standardization of laboratory methods is not universally consistent. Values using the ELISA assay should be reported in units and expressed as either negative, low, medium, or high positive.

3. Levels of antiphospholipid antibodies may fluctuate during pregnancy (102).
4. A significant number of women with abnormal antiphospholipid titers, but who are otherwise healthy, will have successful pregnancy outcomes (97, 99).

Thus, at present, screening for antiphospholipid antibodies is not recommended during first pregnancies in women who are otherwise healthy.

Several treatment modalities have been used in women with recurrent fetal losses associated with antiphospholipid antibodies. Improved outcomes have been demonstrated with the combination of low-dose aspirin and prednisone (20–80 mg daily) (99), and the success of treatment is measured by the suppression of lupus anticoagulant and the reversal of clotting abnormalities. Corticosteroid therapy is started as soon as pregnancy is confirmed, or even before. Aspirin, 60 to 100 mg/day, is also started and is continued throughout the pregnancy.

The combination of aspirin and heparin has also been used with some success (103, 104). Rosove et al. (104) reported a 93% rate of live births and no fetal deaths using full-dose, subcutaneous, twice-daily heparin therapy in 14 women with previous multiple pregnancy losses associated with lupus anticoagulant, anticardiolipin antibodies, or both. In addition, encouraging results from several small studies suggest that intravenous immunoglobulin therapy may be an alternative for women in whom the standard regimens fail (105–107).

Patients with antiphospholipid antibodies need close fetal and maternal surveillance. Referral for consultation with a subspecialist having rheumatology or high-risk obstetric experience is advisable. No treatment regimen has eliminated fetal loss and adverse events in pregnant women with the antiphospholipid antibody syndrome, and complications may occur from any of the treatment options discussed. Additional study is needed to further define the indications for prenatal testing, therapeutic intervention, and appropriate therapy.

INFECTIOUS DISEASES

Several infections adversely affect the outcome in pregnancy, including many sexually transmitted diseases, group B streptococcal disease, and listeriosis. In addition, pregnant women with HIV infection, bacterial vaginosis, Lyme disease, or parvovirus B19 infection have increased risks for perinatal mortality and infected newborns.

Sexually Transmitted Diseases

During pregnancy, the most frequently encountered sexually transmitted infectious agents are *Neisseria gonorrheae*, *Treponema pallidum*, *Chlamydia trachomatis*, herpes simplex virus type 2, hepatitis B virus, and HIV. Pregnancy does not alter the clinical and laboratory criteria for these diagnoses, and symptoms may be more severe for gonococcal disease and primary herpes simplex infec-

tion when they are concurrent with pregnancy. The effect of a sexually transmitted disease on fetal health is potentially catastrophic for several reasons, including bacteremia with organ effects, intrauterine growth restriction, chronic infection, or premature labor and delivery. Early diagnosis and appropriate therapy are critical to minimize risk to the fetus; treatment recommendations are outlined in Tables 23.14 to 23.16 (108). Patients with syphilis and a history of serious penicillin allergy should be referred for allergy testing and desensitization. Reduction in quantitative rapid plasma reagent (RPR) is a marker of effective treatment.

Treatment for infection with the herpes simplex virus during pregnancy is reserved for patients with systemic, life-threatening disease. Intravenous acyclovir is the agent of choice.

All pregnant women should be tested for HBsAg, and those with increased risk for acquiring the infection should be tested for hepatitis B surface antibody as well. High-risk patients with negative serology should be offered hepatitis B vaccine to prevent infection and vertical transmission.

Table 23.14.   Treatment of *Neisseria Gonorrheae* During Pregnancy

	Diagnosis	Treatment[a]
Asymptomatic, local infection	Culture positive for *N. gonorrheae*	Ceftriaxone, 250 mg IM, single dose; or Cefixime, 400 mg orally, single dose; or Spectinomycin, 2 gm IM, single dose; and Erythromycin; base, 500 mg q 6 h × 7 days or Erythromycin-ethylsuccinate, 800 mg q 6 h × 7 days
Disseminated infection	Febrile, purulent cervical discharge, pelvic/abdominal tenderness, leukocytosis	Ceftriaxone, 2 gm IV daily; or Cefotaxime, 1 gm IV q 8 h; or Ceftizoxine 1 gm IV q 8 h; or Spectinomycin, 2 gm IM, q 12 h *until afebrile for 24–48 h; then* or Cefixime, 400 mg orally b.i.d. × 7 days

[a]Based on frequency of β-lactamase producing strains.
Modified from Centers for Disease Control. Sexually transmitted disease treatment guidelines, 1993. MMWR 1993;42 (RR-14):1–102.

Table 23.15. Treatment of Syphilis During Pregnancy

Diagnosis	Treatment
Early syphilis (primary, secondary, latent <1 year); positive serology	Benzathine penicillin G, 2.4 million U IM, single injection
Chancre, rash, condyloma lata, positive FTA/ABS	
Latent syphilis >1 year; positive serology, positive FTA/ABS	Benzathine penicillin G, 2.4 million U IM weekly × 3 weeks

Modified from Centers for Disease Control. Sexually transmitted disease treatment guidelines, 1993. MMWR 1993;42 (RR-14):1–102.

Human Immunodeficiency Virus

Pregnancy complicated by infection with HIV poses formidable problems and is responsible for life-threatening infection in 15 to 35% of all infants and children who are delivered by HIV-positive women (109). Risk factors for vertical transmission include increased maternal viral load, primary infection during pregnancy, low maternal CD4 counts, advanced clinical disease, increased neopterin or β_2-microglobulin concentrations in maternal blood, and biologic/genetic variation as expressed in rapidly replicating virus.

Recent studies have documented improved protection of infants from vertical transmission by treatment of the HIV-positive pregnant woman with zidovudine (AZT). As a result, counseling and voluntary testing for HIV is strongly recommended for pregnant women (110). More extensive counseling should be undertaken to identify and modify those behaviors that increase the risk of acquiring HIV. Patients who test positive for HIV infection also need additional counseling by personnel who are experienced in working with such women. Counseling should include information on the vertical transmission rate, the 5-year mortality rate of 25 to 30% among children born to HIV-

positive mothers, the benefits of zidovudine therapy in reducing the risk of vertical transmission, and the avoidance of breastfeeding among HIV-positive women in industrialized countries.

Most maternal–infant transmission of HIV appears to occur late in pregnancy or during labor and delivery. Phase I studies have demonstrated that zidovudine is safe in mothers, crosses the placenta well, and does not appear to cause major problems in newborns when given to mothers after the first trimester (111). The Pediatric AIDS Clinical Trials Group has provided specific guidelines for treatment with zidovudine of HIV-positive women and their children during labor and the newborn period (Table 23.17).

Group B Streptococcus

The prevalence and attack rate of *Streptococcus agalactiae* during pregnancy is currently being investigated to establish the best method of preventing perinatal transmission and maternal complications. Treatment is straightforward. Either penicillin G or ampicillin is the recommended agent for prophylactic therapy or presumptive care in suspected infection. Less certain, however, is the best, most cost-effective method of detecting risk for infection in light of high carriage rates (15–40%) and low attack rates (≈1%) among infants of colonized mothers. Currently, the American College

Table 23.16. Treatment of Chlamydia Infection During Pregnancy

Diagnosis	Treatment
Positive serology or culture; mucopurulent cervical discharge, urethritis, salpingitis	Erythromycin base, 500 mg PO; *or* Erythromycin-ethylsuccinate, 800 mg PO q 6 h × 7 days

Modified from Centers for Disease Control. Sexually transmitted disease treatment guidelines, 1993. MMWR 1993;42 (RR-14):1–102.

Table 23.17.   Zidovudine Treatment Protocol for HIV Positive Women in Labor and Their Newborns

Treatment Situation	Dose	Frequency
Maternal loading dose in labor	Zidovudine, 2 mg/kg	One time (30–60 minutes)
Maintenance dose during labor	Zidovudine, 1 mg/kg	Per hour during labor
Neonatal loading dose	Zidovudine, 2 mg/kg	Immediately after birth
Neonatal maintenance dose	2 mg/kg	Daily

Reprinted with permission from Connor EM, Sperling RS, Gelber R, et al. Reduction of maternal-infant transmission of human immunodeficiency virus type 1 with zidovudine treatment. N Engl J Med 1994; 331:1173–1180.

of Obstetrics and Gynecology recommends that intravenous antibiotic treatment be provided to women in labor with any of the criteria outlined in Table 23.18 (112).

Bacterial Vaginosis

Bacterial vaginosis is the term given to the genital tract infectious disorder that is associated with transformation of the vaginal flora (primarily *Lactobacillus* sp.) to one colonized predominantly by *Gardnerella vaginalis* and other anaerobic bacteria. It is associated with a significant increase in the rates of preterm birth and perinatal mortality and morbidity, and it possibly occurs in up to 25% of all preterm births in the United States (113). The patient is generally asymptomatic. Diagnosis is made by documenting the combination of a vaginal pH of 4.5 or greater, an

Table 23.18.   Criteria for Perinatal Antibiotic Prophylaxis of Group B Streptococcus

  I. Preterm (<37 weeks) labor
 II. Previous history of an infant affected by group B streptococcus infection
III. Group B streptococcus positive urinary tract infection
 IV. Prolonged fetal membrane rupture (≥12–18 hours)
  V. Maternal febrile (>37.5° C) response in labor
 VI. Heavy maternal colonization

Modified from American College of Obstetricians and Gynecologists. Group B Streptococcal Infections in Pregnancy. ACOG Technical Bulletin No. 170, 1992.

amine or fishy odor when vaginal fluid is mixed with 0.1% KOH solution, and "clue" cells on low-power microscopic examination of the vaginal fluid. Treatment consists of either metronidazole, 375 mg orally two times a day for 1 week, or clindamycin, 300 mg twice a day for the same length of time. Successful treatment of high-risk pregnant women has been associated with improved pregnancy outcomes.

Lyme Disease

Lyme disease, an infection of the spirochete *Borrelia burgdorferi*, is caused by the bite of an infected deer tick. It is characterized by the onset of a skin lesion, erythema migrans, that is accompanied by a flulike syndrome. Neurologic symptoms and arthralgia are common. Left untreated, the disease may progress to develop cardiac, major neurologic, and rheumatologic complications. The spirochete can cross the placenta and affect the fetus, thus producing cardiac anomalies and fetal loss. Diagnosis is made by clinical criteria, because serologic tests for Lyme disease may be negative during the first few weeks of the infection. For patients with the characteristic lesion and who have been outdoors in an endemic region, treatment may be justified before hard diagnostic data are available. Early treatment consists of a 3-week course of amoxicillin, 500 mg three times a day; penicillin V, 500 mg four times a day; or erythromycin, 250 to 500 mg four times a day in patients allergic to penicillin. Intravenous therapy with penicillin G or ceftriaxone should be used in the setting of arthritic or neurologic symptoms. Some investigators believe that, in pregnancy, intravenous antibiotic therapy should be used for any clinical symptom that is referable to Lyme disease (114).

Parvovirus

Parvovirus B19, the virus responsible for the "slapped check" disease of children, is associated with increased pregnancy loss through severe anemia in the infected fetus. The mother is usually only mildly, if at all, symptomatic, with arthralgias or mild flulike symptoms. While there is no specific antiviral treatment, early recognition of exposure allows for surveillance of the fetus by ultrasonography. If there is evidence of fetal anemia, umbilical blood sampling may be undertaken, and intrauterine fetal transfusion may be necessary. For these reasons, patients who manifest evidence of the infection or who seroconvert to parvovirus B19 during pregnancy should be referred to specialists with experience in treating this disease during pregnancy.

Listeria Sp.

Listeria monocytogenes causes a potentially fatal perinatal infection, listeriosis, which most often occurs as a foodborne outbreak. Maternal manifestations are nonspecific and flulike, and many women are asymptomatic. In most cases, the initial presentation is a febrile mother in premature labor and with brown-stained amniotic fluid. Later, blood cultures are usually positive for *Listeria* sp. Therapy consists of a combination of ampicillin and gentamicin in conjunction with assessment and care of the fetus, including emergency delivery if necessary.

IMMUNIZATIONS

The combination of rapid population growth and expanded international travel has increased the opportunities for exposure to communicable diseases. The role of immunization is important to prevent maternal and fetal disease from several pathogens. Ideally, women of childbearing age should already be immunized by scheduled vaccinations or natural childhood infection against measles, mumps, rubella, tetanus, diphtheria, and poliomyelitis; however, a remote history of having acquired any of these diseases may be unreliable (115). Concerns about the safety and efficacy of immunization during pregnancy as well as the potential for adverse effects and liability are largely theoretic. Benefits outweigh the potential risks when: *(a)* the risk from the disease is high, *(b)* infection would pose a special risk to the mother or the fetus, and *(c)* the vaccine is unlikely to cause harm (116).

Specifically, combined tetanus and diphtheria (Td) toxoids are the only immunobiologic agents routinely recommended for use in susceptible, pregnant women. Women who have not been vaccinated in the past should complete the primary series, and booster doses should be given to previously vaccinated pregnant women who have not received Td booster within the last 10 years. There is no convincing evidence of risk from the immunization of pregnant women with other inactivated virus or bacteria vaccines or toxoids. Hepatitis B vaccine is recommended for pregnant women at risk for hepatitis B infection (117) and for all newborns. Specific immune globulins are protective against hepatitis B, rabies, tetanus, and varicella. Bacterial polysaccharide immune globulins may protect against *Haemophilus influenza* type B, *Neisseria meningitidis*, and *Streptococcus pneumoniae* (118), and they are indicated for those with conditions posing special medical risks (e.g., polyvalent pneumococcal vaccine for women with splenectomy, influenza vaccine for immunosuppressed conditions).

Other diseases for which immunization may be recommended during pregnancy, especially for women who travel to countries with endemic infection (119), are found in Table 23.19. Typhoid and cholera vaccines are whole-cell, killed vaccines, and they may cause systemic febrile reactions that could place the fetus at risk. In addition, the efficacy of these vaccines remains in doubt. The safety of attenuated live, oral typhoid vaccine has not yet been established, and use of this vaccine should be avoided unless an epidemic risk exists. Use of measles, mumps, and rubella (MMR) immunizations, which also consist of live attenuated virus, should also be avoided during pregnancy. Prepregnancy care should include testing for susceptibility and immunization at least 3 months before conception. Increased fetal risk from maternal immunization has never been established, and it should not be a reason to recommend abortion. If exposure occurs during pregnancy, the pregnant woman may be protected from measles and varicella, but not from rubella or mumps, by the administration of specific immune globulin. The value of varicella-zoster immune globulin (VZIG) administered to a susceptible woman exposed to chickenpox during pregnancy, especially late in the third trimester, is debated. Current recommendations are to treat the newborn with VZIG if delivered within the time frame of 5 days before to 2 days after diagnosis of infection in the mother (117). Live attenuated varicella vaccine has been approved by the FDA and may become an additional agent to protect susceptible childbearing women. Its role in immunization during pregnancy, however, has not yet been established.

REFERENCES

1. Metzger BE, and the Organizing Committee. Summary and recommendations of the Third International Workshop—Conference on Gestational Diabetes Mellitus. Diabetes 1991;40: 197–203.
2. American Diabetes Association. Principles of nutrition and dietary recommendations for individuals with diabetes mellitus. Diabetes 1979;28:1027–1030.
3. Cousins L. The California Diabetes and Pregnancy Programme. A statewide collaborative programme for the preconception and prenatal care of diabetic women. Bailliere's Clin Obstet Gynecol 1991;5:443–459.
4. Serup L. Influence of pregnancy on diabetic retinopathy. Acta Endocrinol 1986;112(Suppl 277):122–124.
5. Moore TR. Diabetes in pregnancy. In: Creasy RK, Resnik R, eds. Maternal-fetal medicine: principles and practice. 3rd ed. Philadelphia: WB Saunders, 1994:934–978.
6. Freinkel N, Dooley SL, Metzger BE. Care of the pregnant woman with insulin dependent diabetes. N Engl J Med 1985;96:313–318.
7. Fuhrmann K, Reiher H, Semmler K, et al. The effect of intensified conventional insulin therapy before and during pregnancy on the malformation rate in offspring of diabetic mothers. Exp Clin Endocrinol 1984;83:173–176.
8. Kitzmiller JL, Gavin LA, Gin GD, et al. Preconception care of diabetes. Glycemic control prevents congenital anomalies. JAMA 1991; 265:731.
9. Scheffler RM, Feuchtbaum LB, Phibbs CS. Prevention: the cost effectiveness of the California Diabetes and Prevention Program. Am J Public Health 1992;82:168–175.

Table 23.19.   Immunization of the Pregnant Traveler

Vaccine	Safety
Bacterial	
Tetanus-diphtheria	Yes
Pneumococcal	Yes
Meningococcal	Yes
Cholera	No
Typhoid	
Killed	No
Live, attenuated	Unknown
Plague	Yes
Viral	
Japanese B encephalitis	Unknown
Hepatitis A, hepatitis B	Yes[a]
Measles, mumps, rubella	No
Influenza	Yes[a]
Poliomyelitis	
Inactivated	Yes
Live, attenuated	Caution[b]
Rabies	Yes
Yellow fever	Caution[b]
Immune globulin	Yes

[a]Generally recommended after the first trimester.
[b]Use should be avoided unless the pregnant patient is in an area of major epidemic exposure.
Modified from Hill DR. Immunizations for foreign travel. Yale J Biol Med 1992; 65:293–315.

10. Golde SH. Diabetic ketoacidosis in pregnancy. In: Clark SL, Cotton DB, Hankins GDV, Phelan JP , eds. Critical care obstetrics. 2nd ed. Boston: Blackwell Scientific Publications, 1991; 329–339.

11. Management of Asthma During Pregnancy. Report of the Working Group on Asthma and Pregnancy. Bethesda US Department of Health and Human Services, Public Health Services, Bethesda National Institutes of Health Publication No. 93-3279A, 1993.

12. Rodrigues J, Neiderman MS. Pneumonia complicating pregnancy. Clin Chest Med 1992;13: 679–691.

13. Rigby FB, Pastorek JG. Pneumonia during pregnancy. Clin Obstet Gynecol 1996;39: 107–119.

14. Centers for Disease Control. Initial therapy for tuberculosis in the era of multidrug resistance. Recommendations of the Advisory Council for Elimination of Tuberculosis. MMWR 1993; 42:1–8.

15. Centers for Disease Control. Screening for tuberculosis and tuberculous infection in high-risk populations. Recommendations of the Advisory Council for Elimination of Tuberculosis. MMWR 1990;39:1–12.

16. Zipes DP. Specific arrhythmias: diagnosis and treatment. In: Braunwald E, ed. Heart disease. 5th ed. Philadelphia: WB Saunders, 1997: 640–704.

17. Shabetai R. Cardiac diseases. In: Creasy RE, Resnik R, eds. Maternal fetal medicine. Vol 3. Philadelphia: WB Saunders 1994:768–791.

18. Elkayam U. Anticoagulation in pregnant women with prosthetic heart valves: a double jeopardy. J Am Coll Cardiol 1996;27:1704–1706.

19. Szekely P, Turner R, Snaith L. Pregnancy and the changing pattern of rheumatic heart diseases. Br Heart J 1973;35:1293–1303.

20. McKay RG, Lock JE, Safian RD, et al. Balloon dilation of mitral stenosis in adult patients: postmortem and percutaneous mitral valvuloplasty studies. J Am Coll Cardiol 1987;9: 723–731.

21. Demakis JG, Rahimtoola SH, Sutton GC, et al. Natural course of peripartum cardiomyopathy. Circulation 1971;44:1053–1061.

22. Cole P, Cook F, Plappert T. Longitudinal changes in left ventricular architecture and function in peripartum cardiomyopathy. Am J Cardiol 1987;60:811–876.

23. Key TC, Resnik R, Dittrich H, et al. Successful pregnancy after cardiac transplantation. Am J Obstet Gynecol 1989;160:367–371.

24. Elkayan U, Ostrzega E, Shotan A, et al. Cardiovascular problems in pregnant women with the Marfan syndrome. Ann Intern Med 1995;123:117–122.

25. Dejani AS, Taubert KA, Wilson N, et al. Prevention of bacterial endocarditis: recommendations by the American Heart Association. JAMA 1997;277:1794–1801.

26. Page RL. Treatment of arrhythmias during pregnancy. Am Heart J 1995;130:871–876.

27. Frishman WH, Chesner M. Beta adrenergic blockers in pregnancy. Am Heart J 1988;115: 147–152.

28. Rahilly GT, Prsytowsky EN, Zipes DP, et al. Clinical and electrophysiologic findings in patients with repetitive monomorphic ventricular tachycardia and otherwise normal electrocardiogram. Am J Cardiol 1982;50:459–468.

29. Dalvi BV, Chaudhuri A, Kulkarni HL, et al. Therapeutic guidelines for congenital complete heart block presenting in pregnancy. Obstet Gynecol 1992;79:802 804.

30. Becker RM. Intracardiac surgery in pregnant women. Ann Thorac Surg 1983;36:453–458.

31. Anonymous. Guidelines for cardiopulmonary resuscitation and emergency cardiac care. Emergency cardiac care committee and subcommittees, American Hearth Assocation. JAMA 1992;268:2171–2302.

32. Cummins RO, ed. Textbook of advanced cardiac life support. 2nd ed. Dallas: American Heart Association, 1994.

33. Lindsay SL, Hanson GC. Cardiac arrest in near-term pregnancy. Anesthaesia 1987;42: 1074–1077.

33a. Lopen-Zeno JA, Carlo WA, O'Grady JP, et al. Infant survival following delayed postmortem cesarean delivery. Obstet Gynecol 1990;76: 991–992.

34. Working Group on High Blood Pressure in Pregnancy (Gifford RW, August P, Chesley LC, et al.). National High Blood Pressure Education Working Group Report on high blood pressure in pregnancy. Am J Obstet Gynecol 1990;163:1691–1695.

35. Hughes EC, ed. Obstetric-gynecologic terminology. Philadelphia: FA Davis, 1972.

36. Sibai BM, Mabie WC, Shamsa F, et al. A comparison of no medication versus methyldopa or labetalol in chronic hypertension during pregnancy. Am J Obstet Gynecol 1990;162: 960–967.

37. Butters L, Kennedy S, Rubin PC. Atenolol in essential hypertension during pregnancy. BMJ 1990;301:587–589.

38. Mabie WC, Gonzalez AR, Sibai BM, et al. A comparative trial of labetalol and hydralazine in the acute management of severe hypertension complicating pregnancy. Obstet Gynecol 1987;70:328–333.

39. Naden RP, Redman CWG. Antihypertensive drugs in pregnancy. Clin Perinatol 1985;12: 521–538.

40. Cotton DB, Longmire S, Jones MM, et al. Cardiovascular alterations in severe pregnancy induced hypertension: effects of intravenous nitroglycerin coupled with blood volume expan-

sion. Am J Obstet Gynecol 1986;154:1053–1059.

41. Zeller K, Whittaker E, Sullivan L, et al. Effect of restricting dietary protein on the progression of renal failure in patients with insulin-dependent diabetes mellitus. N Engl J Med 1991;3224:78–81.

42. Davison JM, Lindheimer MD. Renal disorders. In: Creasy RK, Resnik R, eds. Maternal fetal medicine: principles and practice. 3rd ed. Philadelphia: WB Saunders, 1994:844–864.

42a. Blagg CR. The socioeconomic impact of rehabilitation. Am J Kidney Dis 1994;24(suppl): 517–521.

43. Centers for Disease Control. CDC criteria for anemia in children and childbearing-aged women. MMWR 1989;38:400–404.

44. National Academy of Sciences, National Research Council, Food and Nutrition Board. Recommended daily allowances. 10th ed. Washington, DC: National Academy Press, 1989.

45. Centers for Disease Control. Use of folic acid for prevention of spina bifida and other neural tube defects—1983–1991. MMWR 1991;40: 513–515.

46. Martin JM, Files JF, Morrison JC. Sickle-cell crisis. In: Clark SL, Cotton DB, Hankins GDV, Phelan JP, eds. Critical care obstetrics. 2nd ed. Boston: Blackwell Scientific Publications, 1991:212–222.

47. Burrows RF, Kelton JG. Thrombocytopenia at delivery: a prospective survey of 6715 deliveries. Am J Obstet Gynecol 1990;162:731–738.

48. Samuels P, Bussel JB, Braitman LE, et al. Estimation of the risk of thrombocytopenia in the offspring of pregnant women with presumed immune thrombocytopenia. N Engl J Med 1990;323:229–233.

49. Kaufman GE, Paidas MJ. Rhesus sensitization and alloimmune thrombocytopenia. Semin Perinatol 1994;18:333–349.

50. Rick ME. Diagnosis and management of von Willebrand's syndrome. Med Clin North Am 1994;78:609–623.

50a. Wileker DE, Dudman ND. Mechanisms of thrombogenesis and accelerated atherogenesis in homocysteinaemia. Haemostasis 1989 19(suppl 1):14–23.

50b. Rosendaal FR, Koster T, Vandenbroucke JP, et al. High risk of thrombosis in patients homozygous for Factor V: Leiden (activated protein C resistance) Blood 1995;85:1504–1508.

51. Cunningham FG. Liver disease complicating pregnancy. In: Williams obstetrics. 19th ed. Stamford: Appleton and Lange, 1993;(Suppl 1):1–15.

52. Samuels P, Cohen AW. Pregnancies complicated by liver disease and liver dysfunction. Obstet Gynecol Clin North Am 1992;19: 745–763.

53. Reyes H. The spectrum of liver and gastrointestinal disease seen in cholestasis of pregnancy. Gastroenterol Clin North Am 1992;21: 905–921.

54. Koch Kl, Stern RM, Vasey M, et al. Gastric dysrhythmias and nausea of pregnancy. Dig Dis Sci 1990;35:961.

55. Lewis JH, Weingold AB. The use of gastrointestinal drugs during pregnancy and lactation. Am J Gastroenterol 1985;80:912–923.

56. Donaldson RM. Management of medical problems in pregnancy—inflammatory bowel disease. N Engl J Med 1985;312:1616–1619.

57. Miller JP. Inflammatory bowel disease in pregnancy: a review. J R Soc Med 1986;79:221–225.

58. Woolfson K, Cohen Z, McLeod RS. Crohn's disease and pregnancy. Dis Colon Rectum 1990;33:869–873.

59. Podolsky, DK. Inflammatory bowel disease. N Engl J Med 1991;325:928–937.

60. Briggs GG, Freeman RK, Yaffe SJ, eds. A reference guide to fetal and neonatal risk: drugs in pregnancy and lactation. 4th ed. Baltimore: Williams & Wilkins, 1994.

61. Habel FM, Hui G, Greenberg GR. Oral 5-aminosalicylic acid for inflammatory bowel disease in pregnancy: safety and clinical course. Gastroenterology 1993;105:1057–1060.

62. Burtin P. Safety of metronidazole in pregnancy: a meta-analysis. Am J Obstet Gynecol 1995; 172:525–529.

63. Alstead EM, Ritchie JK, Lennard-Jones JE, et al. Safety of azathioprine in pregnancy in inflammatory bowel disease. Gastroenterology 1990;99:443–446.

64. Laatikainen T, Karjalainen O, Janne O. Excretion of progesterone metabolites in urine and bile of pregnant women with intrahepatic cholestasis. J Steroid Biochem 1973;4: 641–648.

65. Reyes H. The spectrum of liver and gastrointestinal disease seen in cholestasis of pregnancy. Gastroenterol Clin North Am 1992;21: 905–921.

66. Prevention of perinatal transmission of hepatitis B virus: prenatal screening of all pregnant women for hepatitis B surface antigen. MMWR 1988;37:341–356.

67. Licensure of inactivated hepatitis A vaccine and recommendations for use among international travelers. MMWR 1995;44:559–560.

68. American College of Obstetricians and Gynecologists. Hepatitis in pregnancy. Technical Bulletin Number 174. November 1992.

69. American College of Obstetricians and Gynecologists. Immunization during pregnancy. Technical Bulletin Number 160. October 1991.

70. Thaler MM, Park CK, Landers DV, et al. Vertical transmission of hepatitis C virus. Lancet 1991;338:17–18.

71. Lam JP, McOmish F, Burns SM, et al. Infre-

quent vertical transmission of hepatitis C virus. J Infect Dis 1993;167:572–576.

72. Wejstal R, Widell A, Mansson AS, Hermodsson S, Norlcrans G. Mother-to-infant transmission of hepatitis C virus. Ann Intern Med 1992;117:887–890.

73. Schreyer P, Caspi E, El-Hindi JM, et al. Cirrhosis-pregnancy and delivery: a review. Obstet Gynecol Surv 1982;37:304–312.

74. Kochhar R, Goenka MK, Mehta SK. Endoscopic sclerotherapy during pregnancy. Am J Gastroenterol 1990;85:1132–1135.

75. Pauzner D, Wolan I, Niv D, Ber A, David MP. Endoscopic sclerotherapy in extrahepatic portal hypertension in pregnancy. Am J Obstet Gynecol 1991;164:152–153.

76. Scantlebury V, Gordon R, Tzakis A, et al. Childbearing after liver transplantation. Transplantation 1990;49:317–321.

77. Burroughs AK, Seong NH, Dojcinar DM, et al. Idiopathic acute fatty liver of pregnancy in 12 patients. Q J Med 1982;204:481–497.

78. Riely CA, Latham PS, Romero R, et al. Acute fatty liver in pregnancy. A reassessment based on findings in nine patients. Ann Intern Med 1987;106:703–706.

79. Snyder RR, Hankins GDV. Etiology and treatment of acute fatty liver of pregnancy. Clin Perinatol 1986;13:813–825.

80. Duff P. Acute fatty liver of pregnancy. In: Clark SL, Cotton DB, Hankins GDV, Phelan JP, eds. Critical care obstetrics. 2nd Ed. Boston: Blackwell Scientific Publications, 1991:484–497.

81. Burrow GN, Fisher DA, Larsen PR. Maternal and fetal thyroid function. N Engl J Med 1994;331:1072–1078.

82. Thyroid disease in pregnancy. ACOG Technical Bulletin No. 181, 1993.

83. Becks GP, Burrow GN. Thyroid disease and pregnancy. Med Clin North Am 1991;75:121–150.

84. Montoro M, Collea JV, Frasier SD, et al. Successful outcome of pregnancy in women with hypothyroidism. Ann Intern Med 1981;94:31–34.

85. Mandel SJ, Larsen PR, Seely EW, et al. Increased need for thyroxine during pregnancy in women with primary hypothyroidism. N Engl J Med 1990;323:91–96.

86. Campbell NR, Hasinoff BB, Stalts H, et al. Ferrous sulfate reduces thyroxine efficacy in patients with thyrotoxicosis. Ann Intern Med 1992;117:1010–1013.

87. Jovanovic-Peterson L, Peterson CM. De novo clinical hypothyroidism in pregnancies complicated by type I diabetes, clinical hypothyroidism, and proteinuria: a new syndrome. Am J Obstet Gynecol 1988;159:442–446.

88. Mazzaferri EL. Management of the solitary thyroid nodule. N Engl J Med 1993;328:553–559.

89. Hod M, Sharony R, Friedman S, et al. Pregnancy and thyroid carcinoma: a review of incidence, course and prognosis. Obstet Gynecol Surv 1989;44:774–779.

90. Rosen IB, Walfish PG. Pregnancy as a predisposing factor in thyroid neoplasia. Arch Surg 1986;121:1287–1290.

91. Gharib H, Goellner JR. Fine-needle aspiration biopsy of the thyroid: an appraisal. Ann Intern Med 1993;118:282–289.

92. Davis LE, Lucas MJ, Hankins GDV, et al. Thyrotoxicosis complicating pregnancy. Am J Obstet Gynecol 1989;160:63–70.

93. deleted.

94. Lowe TW, Cunningham FG. Thyroid disease in pregnancy. In: Cunningham FG, MacDonald P, Gant N, ed. Williams obstetrics. 19th ed. Stamford: Appleton & Lange, 1993;(Suppl 9):1–15.

95. Hayslip CC, Fein HG, O'Donnell VM, et al. The value of serum antimicrosomal antibody testing in screening for symptomatic postpartum thyroid dysfunction. Am J Obstet Gynecol 1988;159:203–209.

96. Floyd RC, Roberts WE. Autoimmune diseases in pregnancy. Obstet Gynecol Clin North Am 1992;19:719–732.

97. Boumpas DT, Fessler BJ, Austin HA, et al. Systemic lupus erythematosus: emerging concepts. Part 2: dermatologic and joint disease, the antiphospholipid antibody syndrome, pregnancy and hormonal therapy, morbidity and mortality, and pathogenesis. Ann Intern Med 1995;123:42–53.

98. Urowitz MB, Gladman DD, Farewell VT, et al. Lupus and pregnancy studies. Arthritis Rheum 1993;36:1392–1396.

99. Cunningham FG. Connective tissue disorders complicating pregnancy. In: Cunningham FG, MacDonald P, Gant N, eds. Williams obstetrics, 19th ed. Stamford: Appleton & Lange, 1993;(Suppl 22):1–15.

100. Lima F, Buchanan NMM, Khamashta MA, et al. Obstetric outcome in systemic lupus erythematosus. Semin Arthritis Rheum 1995;25:184–192.

101. Bermas BL, Hill JA. Effects of immunosuppressive drugs during pregnancy. Arthritis Rheum 1995;38:1722–1732.

102. Lynch A, Marlar R, Murphy J, et al. Antiphospholipid antibodies in predicting adverse pregnancy outcome. Ann Intern Med 1994;120:470–475.

103. Cowchock FS, Reece EA, Balaban D, et al. Repeated fetal losses associated with antiphospholipid antibodies: a collaborative randomized trial comparing prednisone with low-dose aspirin treatment. Am J Obstet Gynecol 1992;166:1318–1325.

104. Rosove MH, Tabsh K, Wasserstrum N, et al. Heparin therapy for pregnant women with

lupus anticoagulant or anticardiolipin antibodies. Obstet Gynecol 1990;75:630–634.

105. Spinnato JA, Clark AL, Pierangeli SS, et al. Intravenous immunoglobulin therapy for the antiphospholipid syndrome in pregnancy. Am J Obstet Gynecol 1995;172:690–694.

106. Katz VL, Thorp JM, Watson WJ. Human immunoglobulin therapy for preeclampsia associated with lupus anticoagulant and anticardiolipin antibody. Obstet Gynecol 1990;77:986–990.

107. Orvieto R, Achiron A, Ben-Rafael Z, et al. Intravenous immunoglobulin treatment for recurrent abortions caused by antiphospholipid antibodies. Fertil Steril 1991;56:1013–1020.

108. Centers for Disease Control. Sexually transmitted disease treatment guidelines, 1993. MMWR 1993;42(RR-14):1–102.

109. Peckham C, Gibb D. Mother-to-child transmission of the human immunodeficiency virus. N Engl J Med 1995;333:298–302.

110. Connor EM, Sperling RS, Gelber R, et al. Reduction of maternal-infant transmission of human immunodeficiency virus type 1 with zidovudine treatment. N Engl J Med 1994;331:1173–1180.

111. O'Sullivan MJ, Boyer PJ, Scott GB, et al. The pharmacokinetics and safety of zidovudine in the third trimester of pregnancy for women infected with the human immunodeficiency virus and their infants: phase I acquired immunodeficiency syndrome clinical trials group study (protocol 082). Am J Obstet Gynecol 1993;168:1510–1516.

112. American College of Obstetricians and Gynecologists. Group B streptococcal infections in pregnancy. ACOG Technical Bulletin No. 170, 1992.

113. Hillier SL, Nugent RP, Eschenbach DA, et al. Association between bacterial vaginosis and preterm delivery of a low birthweight infant. The Vaginal Infection and Prematurity Study Group. N Engl J Med 1995;333:1737–1742.

114. Mead PB. Bacterial, parasitic and microbial infections in the fetus. In: Reece EA, Hobbins AC, Mahoney MJ, Petrie RH, eds. Medicine of the fetus and mother. Philadelphia: JB Lippincott, 1992:376–388.

115. Immunizations Practices Advisory Committee/ Centers for Disease Control. Rubella prevention. MMWR 1984;33:301–318.

116. Centers for Diseases Control. General recommendations on immunization. Recommendations of the Advisory Committee on Immunization Practices. MMWR 1993;43(RR-1):20–21.

117. Centers for Diseases Control. Protection against viral hepatitis: recommendations of the immunization practices advisory committee. MMWR 1990;39(S-2):1–5.

118. American College of Obstetricians and Gynecologists. Immunization during pregnancy. ACOG Technical Bulletin No. 160, 1991.

119. Hill DR. Immunizations for foreign travel. Yale J Biol Med 1992;65:293–315.

24

Useful Equations for the Consultant

Richard J. Gross and William S. Kammerer

Our expanding ability to gather clinically relevant physiologic and pharmacokinetic data has led to a profusion of formulas, nomograms, and information on which to base diagnostic and therapeutic decisions. Memorization will suffice for those we use frequently; however, memory cannot always be relied on for the others, or even for the original reference sources. Throughout this book, the authors have routinely included useful equations, rules of thumb, and clinical maxims that are appropriate to their subjects. This chapter serves as a "catch-all" for additional information that may be valuable to the consulting internist. Information of this type is of great clinical usefulness, but the "whole" patient and his or her clinical situation is of equally great importance. Diagnosis and therapy "by the numbers" alone is not our intent.

The availability of portable, programmable calculators will have a major impact on this aspect of medical practice, allowing us to calculate "on our feet" drug dosage, cardiopulmonary performance, acid-base status, statistical significance, and other aspects that are relevant to diagnostic and therapeutic decisions. The traditional bulging "peripheral brain" of most internists, consisting of innumerable pearls, cryptic notes, and references, may well be on its way to extinction, replaced by the silica-chip, microcircuited, programmable calculator.

General Information

Prefix	Multiplication Factor	Symbol
deca-	10	da
hecto-	10^2	h
kilo-	10^3	k
mega-	10^6	M
deci-	10^{-1}	d
centi-	10^{-2}	c
milli-	10^{-3}	m
micro-	10^{-6}	μ
nano-	10^{-9}	n
pico-	10^{-12}	p
femto-	10^{-15}	f

Average Future Lifetime in the United States[a]

Age Interval	Number Living[b]	Average Life Expectancy	White		All Others	
			Male	Female	Male	Female
0–1	100,000	72.4	69.3	77.0	63.6	72.5
1–5	98,387	72.6	69.4	77.0	64.2	73.1
5–10	98,104	68.6	65.6	73.2	60.5	69.3
10–15	97,930	63.9	60.8	68.3	55.6	64.5
15–20	97,747	59.0	55.9	63.4	50.8	59.5
20–25	97,251	54.3	51.3	58.6	46.2	54.7
25–30	96,572	49.7	46.8	53.7	42.0	50.0
30–35	95,902	45.0	42.1	48.9	37.8	45.3
35–40	95,186	40.3	37.5	44.1	33.7	40.7
40–45	94,164	35.7	32.9	39.3	29.7	36.3
45–50	92,643	31.3	28.4	34.7	25.9	32.0
50–55	90,335	27.0	24.2	30.2	22.3	27.9
55–60	86,855	23.0	20.3	25.9	19.0	24.1
60–65	81,778	19.3	16.7	21.8	16.1	20.7
65–70	74,502	15.9	13.6	18.0	13.6	17.5
70–75	65,367	12.7	10.8	14.3	11.2	14.3
75–80	58,151	10.1	8.5	11.1	9.6	12.5
80–85	38,694	7.9	6.6	8.5	8.5	11.0
85 and up	24,137	6.2	5.2	6.5	7.1	9.4

Reprinted with permission from World almanac and book of facts, 1977. New York: Newspaper Enterprise Association, 1977.

[a]Average number of years of life remaining at beginning of age interval.

[b]Of 100,000 born alive, number living at beginning of age interval.

Years of Life Expected at Birth

Year[a]	All Races			White			Black and Other		
	Total	Male	Female	Total	Male	Female	Total	Male	Female
1920	54.1	53.6	54.6	54.9	54.4	55.6	45.3	45.5	45.2
1930	59.7	58.1	61.6	61.4	59.7	63.5	48.1	47.3	49.2
1940	62.9	60.8	65.2	64.2	62.1	66.6	53.1	51.5	54.9
1950	68.2	65.6	71.1	69.1	66.5	72.2	60.8	59.1	62.9
1960	69.7	66.6	73.1	70.6	67.4	74.1	63.6	61.1	66.3
1965	70.2	66.8	73.7	71.0	67.6	74.7	64.1	61.1	67.4
1970	70.8	67.1	74.7	71.7	68.0	75.6	65.3	61.3	69.4
1975	72.6	68.8	76.6	73.4	69.5	77.3	68.0	63.7	72.4
1976	72.9	69.1	76.8	73.6	69.9	77.5	68.4	64.2	72.7
1977	73.3	69.5	77.2	74.0	70.2	77.9	68.9	64.7	73.2
1978	73.5	69.6	77.3	74.1	70.4	78.0	68.1	63.7	72.4
1979	73.9	70.0	77.8	74.6	70.8	78.4	69.8	65.4	74.1
1980	73.7	70.0	77.5	74.4	70.7	78.1	69.5	65.3	73.6
1981	74.2	70.4	77.8	74.8	71.1	78.4	70.3	66.2	74.4
1982	74.5	70.9	78.1	75.1	71.5	78.7	70.9	66.8	74.9
1983	74.6	71.0	78.1	75.2	71.7	78.7	70.9	67.0	74.7
1984	74.7	71.2	78.2	75.3	71.8	78.7	71.1	67.2	74.9
1985	74.7	71.2	78.2	75.3	71.9	78.7	67.0	64.8	69.3
1986	74.8	71.3	78.3	75.4	72.0	78.8	70.9	66.8	74.9
1987	75.0	71.5	78.4	75.6	72.2	78.9	66.9	65.0	69.1
1988	74.9	71.5	78.3	75.6	72.3	78.9	70.8	66.7	74.8
1989	75.1	71.7	78.5	75.9	72.5	79.2	70.9	66.7	74.9
1990	75.4	71.8	78.8	76.1	72.9	79.4	71.2	67.0	75.2
1991	75.5	72.0	78.9	76.3	72.9	79.2	71.5	67.4	75.5
1992	75.5	72.1	78.9	76.4	73.0	79.5	71.7	67.5	75.8
1993	75.5	72.1	78.9	76.3	73.0	79.5	71.5	67.4	75.5
1994	75.7	72.4	79.0	76.5	73.3	79.6	71.7	67.5	75.8
1995[b]	75.8	72.6	78.9	76.5	73.4	79.6	69.8	65.4	74.0

Reprinted with permission from World almanac and book of facts, 1997. New York: World Almanac Books, 1977–1991.

[a]Data before 1940 for death-registration states only.

[b]Preliminary

Metabolic-Physiologic

---

1. Correction of metabolic acidosis:
   HCO_3^- required = base deficit (mEq/L) $\times$ 0.3 $\cdot$ (body weight in kg)
2. Correction of metabolic alkalosis:
   HCl (mEq) required = base excess (mEq/L) $\times$ 0.4 $\cdot$ (body weight in kg)
3. Correction of K^+ deficit:
   100–200 mEq K^+ for each 1 mEq decrease in serum K^+ to 3.0 mEq/L
   300–400 mEq K^+ for each 1 mEq decrease in serum K^+ below 3.0 mEq/L
   (In presence of alkalosis, serum K^+ first corrected by an increase of 0.7 mEq for each 0.1-unit elevation of pH above 7.40)
4. Uric acid clearance (1):
   $$\frac{U_{uric} \cdot P_{cr;}}{U_{cr}} \text{ normal} = 0.4, \pm 0.1; > 0.7 = \text{gout}$$
5. Correcting WBC count in traumatic spinal tap:
   $$\text{No. of WBCs introduced} = \frac{(\text{peripheral WBC}) \times (\text{RBC in CSF})}{\text{peripheral RBC count}}$$
6. CSF sugar values in patients with meningitis:
   Nondiabetic <½ blood glucose
   Diabetic <⅓ blood glucose
7. Drugs with a high sodium content:
   Carbenicillin (4.7 mEq/g)
   Penicillin G (1.7 mEq/million U)
   Ampicillin (3 mEq/g)
   Cephalothin (2.5 mEq/g)
   Kayexalate (65 mEq/16 g)
   Fleet's Phospho-soda (24 mEq/5 mL)
8. Sodium, salt, milligrams, and milliequivalents:

Milliequivalents Na$^+$ (Approximate)	Milligrams Na$^+$	Grams Salt (NaCl) (Approximate)
11	250	0.6
22	500	1.3
43	1000	2.5
65	1500	3.8
87	2000	5.0
130	3000	7.6
174	4000	10.2

9. Relative corticosteroid potencies:

Agent	Glucocorticoid Activity (Cortisol = 1)	Mineralocorticoid Activity (Cortisol = 1)	Plasma Half-life (min)
Hydrocortisone (cortisol)	1	1	90
Cortisone	0.7	0.7	30
Prednisone	4	0.7	60
Prednisolone	4	0.7	200
Methylprednisolone	5	0.5	200
Triamcinolone	5	0	200
Dexamethasone	25	0–2	300
Betamethasone	30	0	300
Fludrocortisone	10	125	30
Aldosterone	0.1	400	
Corticosterone	0.35	2	70

CSF, cerebrospinal fluid; *RBC,* red blood cell; *WBC,* white blood cell.

Renal

1. Bedside estimate of creatinine clearance:

   a. For men $= \dfrac{98 - 16 \cdot \dfrac{(Age - 20)}{20}}{P_{cr}}$

   For women, use 90% of above value

   b. $\dfrac{Ur.\ Cr.\ grams}{Serum\ Cr.\ mg\ \%} - 70$

2. Urinary diagnostic indices:

	Prerenal Azotemia	Acute Oliguric Renal Failure	Acute Nonoliguric Renal Failure	Acute Obstructive Uropathy	Acute Glomerulonephritis
Urine osmolality, mOsm/kg H_2O	518 ± 35	369 ± 20	343 ± 17	393 ± 39	385 ± 61
Urine sodium, mEq/L	18 ± 3	68 ± 5	50 ± 5	68 ± 10	22 ± 6
Urine/plasma urea nitrogen	18 ± 7	3 ± 0.5	7 ± 1	8 ± 4	11 ± 4
Urine/plasma creatinine	45 ± 6	17 ± 2	17 ± 2	16 ± 4	43 ± 7
Renal failure index[a]	0.6 ± 0.1	10 ± 2	4 ± 0.6	8 ± 3	0.4 ± 0.1
Fractional excretion of filtered sodium[b]	0.4 ± 0.1	7 ± 1.4	3 ± 0.5	6 ± 2	0.6 ± 0.2

[a] $U_{Na} \Big/ \dfrac{U_{cr}}{P_{cr}}$

[b] $U_{Na} / P_{Na} \Big/ U_{cr} / P_{cr}$

Cardiovascular

Correlation of NYHA Functional Class with Cardiopulmonary Performance[a]				
Functional class	1	2	3	4
Ejection fraction	>0.55 0.50	0.40	0.30 0.20	0.10
End diastolic left ventricular pressure				
Rest	<12 mm Hg		>12 mm Hg	
After exercise	<12 mm Hg	>12 mm Hg		
Cardiac index (rest)	>2.5 L/min/M^2		2.0	1.5
Vital capacity			−30%	−35-50%

Normal values

Cardiac index	3.5 L/min/M^2 ± 0.7
Stroke index	46 mL/min/M^2 ± 8.1
AVO$_2$ difference	4.1 vol % ± 0.6

	O$_2$ Saturation (%)
Right atrial pressure:mean <5 mm Hg	75
Pulmonary artery pressure:<32/13 mm Hg	75
Pulmonary artery wedge:mean <13 mm Hg	97
End diastolic left ventricular pressure:<12 mm Hg	95

[a] Adapted with permission from Alderman EL. Angiographic indicators of left ventricular function. JAMA 1976;235:1055–1058.

Pulmonary

Weaning from mechanical venilation:

$$f/V_T < 100$$
$$> 100$$

Predicted
80% successfully weaned
95% failed weaning

where f = respiratory frequency (breaths/minute)
V_T = tidal volume

f/V, breaths/min/L

Calculation of Loading Dose for Phenobarbital and Hydantoin

$$L.D. = \frac{V \cdot (C_D - C_O)}{F}$$

C_D = Concentration desired
C_O = Concentration observed
  F = Bioavailability
       phenobarbital, hydantoin I.V. = 1
       phenobarbital p.o.   = 0.9
       hydantoin p.o.   = 0.95
  V = Volume of distribution:
       phenobarbital = 0.60 L/Kg
       hydantoin   = 0.65 L/Kg

Aminoglycoside Dosing Guidelines

1. Calculate loading dose (LD) based on desired peak serum level

Gentamicin / Tobramycin		*Amikacin*	
LD	Peak Level	LD	Peak Level
1.5–2.0 mg/kg	4–6 µg/mL	5.0 µg/mL	10–20 µg/mL
2.0–2.5 mg/kg	6–8 µg/mL	7.5 mg/kg	20–30 µg/mL

2. Estimate patient's creatinine clearance (CrCl) from serum creatinine

$$\text{CrCl in mL/min} = \frac{(140 - \text{age})}{SCR \times 72} \times \text{wt. in kg } (\times 0.85 \text{ for females})$$

Minimum SCR
0.5 if <60 y
1.0 if >60 y

3. Determine maintenance dose (MD) and schedule using CrCl and LD according to the table below:

CrCl	*MD = Percentage of LD*	*Dosing Interval*
90	84%	q8h
80	80%	q8h
70	76%	q8h
60	84%	q12h
50	79%	q12h
40	92%	q24h
30	86%	q24h
25	81%	q24h
20	75%	q24h

Note: These guidelines are not intended for use in patients with life-threatening infections, changing renal function, marked obesity, CrCl <20 mL/min, malnutrition, hemodialysis patients, and pediatric patients.

SUGGESTED READINGS

Alderman EL. Angiographic indicators of left ventricular function. JAMA 1976;235:1055–1058.

Anderson CC, Cohn J, Whitfield GF. Filling pressures and the critically ill patient: part II. Hosp Physician 1980;(5):39–46.

Anderson CC, Whitfield GF, Cohn J. Filling pressures and the critically ill patient: part I. Hosp Physician 1980;(3):28–32.

Bennett WM, Aronoff GR, Golper TA, et al. Drug prescribing in renal failure dosing guidelines for adults. Philadelphia: American College of Physicians, 1994.

Gottlieb AJ, Zamkoff KW, Jastremski MS, et al. The whole internist catalog. Philadelphia: WB Saunders, 1980.

Jelliffe RW. Creatinine clearance: bedside estimate (letter to the editor). Ann Intern Med 1979;79:604.

Miller TR, Anderson RJ, Linas SL, et al. Urinary diagnostic indices in acute renal failure: a prospective study. Ann Intern Med 1978;89:47–50.

Powers WJ. Cerebrospinal fluid to serum glucose ratios in diabetes mellitus and bacterial meningitis. Am J Med 1981;71:217–220.

Siber LM, Whitfield GF, Nagamatsu GR, et al. Surgical risk in a patient with recent myocardial infarction. Hosp Physician 1979;(6):31–36.

Simkin PA, Hoover PL, Paxson CS, et al. Uric acid excretion: quantitative assessment from spot, midmorning serum and urine samples. Ann Intern Med 1979;91:44–47.

Yang KL, Tobin MJ. A prospective study of indexes predicting the outcome of trials of weaning from mechanical ventilation. N Engl J Med 1991;324:1445–1450.

Index

Page numbers in italics indicate figures.
Page numbers followed by a "t" indicate tables.

Compound A, 63
ABCD diagnosis of skin cancer, 529
Abdominal aortic aneurysm, 626–635
  cardiovascular disease and, *629*
  complications of, 630t
  diagnosis of, 630–632
  epidemiology of, 626–630
  mesenteric ischemia and infarction in, 634
  mortality and, *627,* 628t, 630t
  ruptured, 633–634
Abdominal surgery (*see also* Gastrointestinal
    surgery)
  respiratory effects of, *96, 96–97, 97*
  risk in elderly, 619
Abnormal Involuntary Movement Scale (AIMS),
    598
Abscess
  endocarditis prophylaxis in, 475
  intra-abdominal, 484–488, *485–486*
  liver, 297–307, 487
  pancreatic, 487
  perinephric, 500
  radiologic evaluation in, 487–488
  splenic, 487
  subphrenic, 487
  tubo-ovarian, 503
  vaginal cuff, 503
Abuse
  alcohol (*see* Alcoholism)
  elder, 597
  substance, 561, 574–575
Academic institutions, 2 (*see also* Teaching)
ACC/AHA Ad Hoc Task Force on Cardiac Catheter-
    ization, 135
ACC/AHA guidelines, 30
  for ambulatory ECG, 160
  for clinical competence in hemodynamic moni-
      toring, 137t
  endocarditis prophylaxis, 471–475, 472t, 473t,
      474t
  for exercise stress testing, 165t
  for preoperative cardiovascular evaluation, 152t
  for preoperative testing, 161t
ACE inhibitors, 570, 571t
  anesthetic interactions, 64t
  hyperkalemia and, 246
  lithium and, 573
  in pregnancy, 667t
Acetylcholinesterase inhibitors, 559
Acid-base disturbances, 264–279, 278t, 279t
  acidosis
    diabetic ketoacidosis, 332–333, 662t, 662–663
    hyperkalemic renal tubular, 343–344
    metabolic, 232, 266–271, *268,* 269t, *270,* 278t,
        279t
    respiratory, 273, 274t, 278t, 279t
  alkalosis, 273–274, 274t, 278t, 279t
    metabolic, 233, 244, 271t, 271–273, 272t, 278t,
        279t

epidemiology of, 264
  mixed, 274–277, 278t
  physiology of, 264–266, 265t
Acidosis
  diabetic ketoacidosis, 332–333, 662t, 662–663
  hyperkalemic renal tubular, 343–344
  metabolic, 232, 266–271, *268,* 269t, *270,* 278t,
      279t, 706t
  respiratory, 273, 274t, 278t, 279t
Acquired immunodeficiency disease (AIDS) (*see*
    HIV infection)
Acral lentiginous melanoma, 530
ACT (Cortrosyn) stimulation test, 342, 354
ACTH disturbances, in adrenal insufficiency,
    340–342, 343t, 355t
Activated protein C resistance, 394
Activity, surgical risk in elderly and, 621
Acute confusional state (*see* Delirium)
Acute dystonic reactions, 597
Acute fatty liver of pregnancy, 686–687
Acute functional psychosis, clinical features of,
    596t
Acute mycoplasma pneumonia, 374
Acute noncardiac pulmonary (transfusion-related)
    edema, 368
Acute renal failure (ARF) (*see also* Acid-base
    disorders; Electrolyte disorders; Renal
    failure)
  epidemiology of, 195–197, 196t
  etiology and pathogenesis of, 204–208
  evaluation of, 208–211, 209t, 211t
  in high-risk surgical procedures, 196t, 203–204
  risk factors for, 196, 196t
  treatment of, 211–217, 212t
Acute tubular necrosis, 196, 205–206, 207 (*see also*
    Renal failure)
Acyclovir, 605t
Adenosine, 670
ADH (antidiuretic hormone), 202t, 202–203,
    230–232 (*see also* Diabetes insipidus; Hy-
    ponatremia)
  syndrome of inappropriate (SIADH), 232,
      233–235, *234,* 348–351, 350t
Adjuvant systemic cancer therapy (*see* Cancer
    chemotherapy; Radiation therapy)
Adrenal insufficiency, 340–342, 343t, 355t
Adrenocorticotropic hormone (*see* ACTH)
Affective disoders (*see* Mood disorders; Psychiatric
    considerations)
AFLP (acute fatty liver of pregnancy), 686–687
Age (*see also* Elderly)
  biological versus chronological, 7, 30
  life expectancy and, 704t
  pulmonary complications and, 100
  as risk factor, 20–21
  surgical problems related to, 616t, 616–618, 617t
AICDs (automatic implantable cardiac defibril-
    lators), 176–177
AIDS (acquired immunodeficiency disease) (*see*
    HIV infection)
AIMS (Abnormal Involuntary Movement Scale),
    598

Akathisia, 598
Alanine aminotransferase test (ALT, SGPT), 298–299 (*see also* Liver disease)
Albuterol, 248t
Alcoholic hepatitis, 299, 304
Alcoholism, 557, 574–575, 580, 590–592, 686
  CAGE questionnaire for, 591
  cerebrovascular comorbidity in, 557
  hepatic cirrhosis in pregnancy, 686
  psychiatric manifestations of, 590–592
  surgical risk and, 574–575
  TAR and feather mnemonic, 591
  Wernicke's encephalopathy in, 590–591
  withdrawal states in, 580
Alcohol use, 32
Aldosterone disturbances
  low-renin hypoaldosteronism, 330
  primary hyperaldosteronism, 345–346
  selective aldosterone deficiency, 343–345, 344t
Alfentanil, 59
Alkaline gastritis (bile gastritis, reflux gastritis), 321
Alkalosis, 273–274, 274t, 278t, 279t
  metabolic, 233, 244, 271t, 271–273, 272t, 278t, 279t, 706t
Allergy (*see also* Anaphylaxis; Hypersensitivity)
  contact dermatitis in, 536
  drug fever and, 492–493, 598–599
  to drugs, 525–526
  latex, 67
  sheet, 536
Alloimmune thrombocytopenia, 679
α-Adrenergic blocking agents, 186, 348
  depressive side effects of, 570
  in pregnancy, 667t
α-β-blocking agents, 188
α-Thalassemia, 677–678
Alprazolan, 596
Altered mental status, delirium, and coma, 564
Aluminum toxicity, 591
Alzheimer's disease, 558–559
  vs. depression, 587–588
Amantadine, 597, 605t
Ambulatory electrocardiography, 158–160
Ambulatory patients
  as defined in text, 36
  diagnostic activities and approaches for, 38t, 38–39, 39t
  eligibility of, 37t
  evaluation of, 33–40 (*see also* Preoperative evaluation)
  instructions for, 39–40
  organizational issues regarding, 36–38, 38t
  treatment of, 39–40
Ambulatory surgery, anesthesia and, 58
Amebiasis, 306
Amenorrhea, in eating disorders, 594
American College of Physicians (APA), clinical competence guidelines for hemodynamic monitoring, 137t
American Diabetes Association (ADA), dietary recommendations, 81, 661
American Heart Association (AHA), endocarditis prophylaxis recommendations, 471–475, 472t, 473t, 474t (*see also* ACC/AHA guidelines)
American Medical Association (AMA), consultant responsibilities, list of, 1

American Society of Anesthesiologists (ASA)
  mortality scale of, 617
  risk classification system, 33, 55–56, 56t
American Thoracic Society, nosocomial pneumonia, diagnosis guidelines of, 494–495
Aminoglycosides (*see also* Antibiotics)
  dosing guidelines for, 708t
  hypocalcemia and, 255
  nephrotoxicity of, 197, 201, 223
Aminotransferase (AST) tests, 298–299 (*see also* Liver disease)
Amiodarone, 64t, 670
Amitriptyline (*see* Tricyclic antidepressants)
Amphetamines, 605t
Amphotericin B, 605t
  bladder wash with, 499–500
Ampicillin, 535 (*see also* Antibiotics)
Amylase:creatinine clearance test, 307
Anabolic steroids, 605t
Anaerobic cellulitis
  clostridial, 501, 521
  nonclostridial, 501
Anal cancer, 427
Analgesia
  in cancer, 439t, 440t
  epidural, 109
  in pancreatitis, 308
  patient-controlled, 61
  in pregnancy, 684t–685t
  in renal failure, 222
Anaphylaxis
  in drug reactions, 535
  transfusion-related, 368
Anemia, 74 (*see also* Blood transfusion)
  diagnosis, 361–362, 362t
  immune hemolytic, 372t, 372–374
  macrocytic, 366–367
  microcytic, 367
  postoperative, 322, 364–370
    diagnostic evaluation, 364–367, 365t
    dilutional, 365
    nosocomial, 365
    transfusion, 367–370
  in pregnancy, 676–677
  preoperative, 361–364
    autologous transfusion, 363–364
    diagnostic evaluation, 361–362, 362t
    transfusion assessment, 362–363
Anesthesia (*see also* Anesthetic agents; Preoperative evaluation)
  ASA classification of physical status, 55–56, 56t
  critical incidents in, 56–57
  dental, 638–640
  in elderly, 619
  general, 58, 94, 95
  in hip fracture, 543–544
  in hypothyroidism, 339
  ischemic side effects of, 565
  MAC (monitored anesthesia care), 58, 59
  management of, 58–59
  in myasthenia gravis, 560
  organ system effects of, 60–64
    cardiovascular system, 61–62
    kidneys, 63–64
    liver, 62
    respiratory system, 60–61
  outpatient, 58
  preoperative evaluation for, 30t, 30–32, 31t

regional, 58–59, 95
respiratory effects of, 94–95, *95*
respiratory monitoring in, 118
risks and mortality in, 55–57, 98
in same-day admissions, 58
in sickle-cell disease, 371
specific concerns with, 66–67
  latex allergy, 67
  malignant hyperthermia, 66
  plasma cholinesterase abnormality, 66–67
spinal/epidural versus general, 57–58, 98
Anesthetic agents, 59–60 (*see also individual drugs*)
antidpressants and, 576–577
drug interactions with, 64t–65t, 64–66
liver disorders related to, 303, 313–316, 314t
local, 61
in renal failure, 222–223
Aneurysm
abdominal aortic, 626–635 (*see also* Abdominal aortic aneurysm)
congenital berry of circle of Willis, 668
electroconvulsive therapy risk and, 583
Angina (*See also* Cardiovascular disease; Myocardial infarction; Myocardial ischemia)
Ludwig's, 643
Angiography
coronary, 171
endocarditis prophylaxis in, 475
Angiomatosis, bacillary, 528
Angioplasty, in abdominal aortic aneurysm, 631
Angiotensin-converting-enzyme inhibitors (*See* ACE inhibitors; Antihypertensives)
Anorexia nervosa, 592–595
Antacids, in renal failure, 224
Anthrompometric measurements, 72–74, 73t, 74t
Antiarrhythmics
in pregnancy, 670–671
teratogenicity of, 670, 671t
Antibiotic prophylaxis, 450–475 (*see also* Antibiotics *and specific drugs;* Infection)
for bacterial endocarditis, 151, 151t
human studies of, 455–458, 458t
in labor and delivery, 670
principles for use of, 455, 458t
in prosthetic heart valves, 473, 483, 511–512, 670
recommended regimens for, 459t–460t
Antibiotics (*see also* Antibiotic prophylaxis; Infection)
aminoglycoside dosing guidelines, 708t
anesthetic interactions of, 64t
in *Clostridium difficile* infection, 323
in dental infection, 643
drug fever and, 492
drug reactions to, 535–536
in gastrointestinal reflux disease, 311
hypocalcemia and, 255
nephrotoxicity of, 197, 201
preoperative, 106
in renal failure, 223–224
resistance to, 489–490
Anticholinergics
in acute dystonic reactions, 597
in akathisia, 598
anesthetics and, 576–577
contraindications, 312
delirium and, 579–580

in parkinsonism, 563
psychiatric side effects of, 605t
Anticoagulant enzymes (hirudin), 398
Anticoagulants, 32, 141–147, 389–390 (*see also specific drugs*)
anesthetic interactions with, 64t
in antiphospholipid antibody syndrome, 693
circulating, 392
dental procedures and, 641t, 641–642
in hip fracture, 544
in hip replacement, 545–546
lupuslike anticoagulation and, 395
platelet disorders and, 397–398
in pregnancy, 667t, 668
in prosthetic heart valves, 196
in renal failure, 224
in stroke, 555
Anticonvulsants, 605t (*see also specific drugs*)
anesthetic interactions with, 64t
perioperative use of, 557t, 557–558
in pregnancy, 557–558
in renal failure, 223, 224
Antidepressants
anesthetics with, 65t, 576–577
antihypertensives with, 571t
contraindications to, 312
in elderly, 595–596
in major depression, 601–604
tricyclic, 589, 595, 602–603, 605t
  anesthetics with, 576
  in elderly, 595
Antidiarrheals, in pregnancy, 682t
Antidiuretic hormone (ADH), 202t, 202–203, 230–232
syndrome of inappropriate (SIADH), 232, 233–235, *234,* 348–351, 350t (*see also* Diabetes insipidus; Hyponatremia)
Antidysrhythmics, anesthetic interactions, 64t
Antiendomysium antibody test, 322
Antihistamines, 605t
Antihypertensives, 62 (*see also specific drugs*)
anesthetics with, 64t
impotence caused by, 570
in postoperative hypertension, 185–188
in preeclampsia, 674
in pregnancy, 667t
psychotropic drugs and, 571t
in renal failure, 223
Antimalarials
in lupus erythematosus, 692–693
in pregnancy, 692–693
Antiparkinsonism drugs (*see also specific drugs*)
anesthetic interactions with, 64t
Antiperistaltic agents (*see also specific drugs*)
contraindications to, 323
Antiphospholipid antibody syndrome, 394–395 (*see also* Hypercoagulable states)
in pregnancy, 693–694
Antiplatelet therapy (*see* Anticoagulants)
Antipsychotics, 597–604 (*see also* Psychotropic drugs *and specific drugs*)
antihypertensives and, 571t
in elderly, 596–597
prolactin inhibiting factor and, 599
Antithrombin III abnormalities, 395 (*see also* Platelet disorders)
Anxiety
in HIV infection, 589

Anxiety—*Continued*
  perioperative, 573–574
  with serotonin reuptake inhibitors, 595
  vs. agitated depression, 573
Anxiolytics, 604 (*see also specific drugs*)
Aortic aneurysm, abdominal, 626–635 (*see also*
    Abdominal aortic aneurysm)
Aortic coarctation, in pregnancy, 668
Aortic dissection, in pregnancy, 669–670
Aortic regurgitation, 192
Aortic root dilation, 669–670
Aortic valve stenosis, 190–192
  in pregnancy, 668
Aortic valvuloplasty, balloon, 194–195, 697
Apheresis, therapeutic, 403–404, 404t
Apnea, obstructive sleep, 101
Appendectomy, 461
  in elderly, 626
Arrhythmias (*see* Cardiac arrhythmias)
Arterial blood gas analysis, 50, 102, 117
Arthritis
  crystal-induced, 549
  Felty's syndrome, 549–550
  rheumatoid, 547–549
    anesthetic considerations in, 550t
    in pregnancy, 691
ASA mortality scale, 617
ASA risk classification system, 55–56, 56t
Asathioprine, 685t
Ascites, 318
  malignant, 432
Ascitic fluid albumin test, 302–303, 318
Aspiration, pulmonary, 61, 100, 495–496
Aspirin, 32 (*see also* NSAIDs)
  in antiphospholipid antibody syndrome, 693
  in DVT prophylaxis, 141
  in hip fracture, 544
  in hip replacement, 546
  platelet disorders and, 399–400
  in pregnancy, 684t, 691
  psychiatric side effects of, 607t
  in renal failure, 222
Asthma
  anesthesia in, 60–61
  dental procedures in, 642–643
  in pregnancy, 663–664, 665t
  preoperative management in, 106
  pulmonary complications and, 100
Atelectasis, 481–482, 496–497
Atenolol, 187
Atheromatous lesions, in diabetes mellitus,
    533–534
Atherosclerosis, 153t, 153–154, 181 (*see also* Cere-
    brovascular disease; Myocardial ischemia)
  cerebral, 553
Athlete's foot (tinea pedis), 522–523
Atlanto-occipital subluxation, 549
Atracurium, 59, 62, 64
Atrial fibrillation, in pregnancy, 669
Atrial septal defect, in pregnancy, 666–668
Atropine, 63, 605t (*see also* Anticholinergics)
Attending physician, 3 (*see also* Referring
    physician)
AUDIT (Alcohol Use Disorders Identification Test),
    591
Autoimmune disease
  cold, 373–374
  herpes gestationis, 531–532

  of liver, 307
  in pregnancy, 691–694
    antiphospholipid syndrome, 693–694
    systemic lupus erythematosus, 692–693
  warm, 373
Autoimmune thrombocytopenia, 679
Autoimmune thrombocytopenic purpura, 398
Autologous blood transfusion, 363–364
Auto-PEEP, 120 (*see also* Mechanical respiratory
    support)
Azathioprine, 681
  in lupus erythematosus, 692
  in myasthenic crisis, 560
Azepam, 596
Azotemia (*see also* Renal failure)
  drug therapy in, 221t, 221–224
AZT (zidovidine), 695, 696t

Bacillary angiomatosis, 528
Bacitracin, 323
Bacteremia (*see* Sepsis)
Bacterial endocarditis, subacute, 469–475,
    470t–474t
Bacterial infections, 519–523, 520t (*see also*
    Infection)
  bacterial sepsis, *522,* 522–523
  cellulitis, 501, 502, 503, 519–522, *521*
  listeriosis, 697
  toxic shock syndrome, 523
Bacterial sepsis (*see* Sepsis)
Bacterial vaginosis, in pregnancy, 696
Bacteriuria, in TURP, 466
Bacteroides fragilis, 502
Balloon valvuloplasty
  aortic, 194–195
  in pregnancy, 669
Barbiturates, 605t
  anesthetic interactions with, 64t
  in renal failure (*see also specific drugs*)
Barrett's syndrome, 424 (*see also* Esophageal
    cancer)
Basal cell carcinoma, skin, 529, *529*
Bayes' theorem, 161
BCAAs (branched-chain amino acids), 86, 90
Belladonna alkaloids, 605t
Benign postoperative intrahepatic cholestasis,
    316–317
Benzodiazepine antagonists, 59–60
Benzodiazepines, 63, 304 (*see also specific drugs*)
  in alcoholism, 591
  in anxiety, 604
  contraindications in elderly patients, 596
  delirium and, 580, 581
  flumazenil in overdose, 604
  psychiatric side effects of, 605t
Benztropine, 563, 597, 598 (*see also* Anticholin-
    ergics)
Besnier, prurigo gestationis of, 531
β-Adrenergic agonists, as bronchodilators, 105–106
β-Adrenergic antagonists, 186, 348
  in akathisia, 598
  anesthetic interactions, 64t
  contraindications, 599
  depressive side effects of, 570
  in hyperthyroidism, 690
  interactions with psychotropic drugs, 571t
  in Marfan's syndrome, 670
  in preeclampsia, 674

in pregnancy, 667t, 670
psychiatric side effects of, 605t
in renal failure, 223
Beta blockers (*see* β-Adrenergic antagonists)
β-Thalassemia, 677–678
Biguanide, 332
Bile gastritis (alkaline gastritis, reflux gastritis), 321
Biliary disorders
cholestatic jaundice (cholestasis), 316–317
extrahepatic obstruction, 316
in liver disease, 312t, 312–319
postcholecystectomy syndrome, 319–320
postgastrectomy syndrome, 320–321
postoperative cholecystitis, 319
Biliary obstruction, malignant, 432–433
Binge-purge syndrome (bulimia nervosa), 592–594
Biperiden, 597
Biphosphate therapy, 254
Bipolar disorder, 600–601
Bismuth salicylate, in pregnancy, 682t
Bladder cancer, 425
Blanzapine, 600
Bleeding (*see also* Hematologic disorders)
gastrointestinal
in abdominal aortic aneurysm, 634
in burns, 646
in intubated patients, 126
intracerebral, 555
Bleeding disorders (*see* Blood transfusion; Coagulation disorders; Hemostasis)
Bleeding history, 32, 32t, 33t
Bleomycin, 409 (*see also* Cancer chemotherapy)
in pleural effusion, 430
synergistic toxicity with oxygen, 409–410
Blood glucose monitoring, 661
Blood loss
equation for calculating, 365
as surgical classification factor, 28, 28t
Blood pressure (*see also* Hypertension)
dental anesthesia and, 639–640
Blood transfusion (*see also* Hemostasis)
assessment for, 362–363
autologous, 363–364
citrate and hypocalcemia, 255
posttransfusion hepatitis, 312, 315–316
prophylactic, in sickle-cell disease, 371
reactions to, 367–370
delayed, 369
immediate, 367–368
intermediate, 368–369
massive, 369–370, 370t
Blood urea nitrogen (BUN), 48
Body mass index (BMI), 73
Body weight, 72–74, 73t, 74t
Bone marrow-fat embolism, in sickle-cell disease, 372
Borrelia burgdorferi, 523–524, *524,* 696–697
Boston Collaborative Drug Surveillance Program guidelines, 535, 535t
Bowel obstruction in cancer, 408–409
Brain metastases, 429
Breast cancer, 412–417
adjuvant systemic therapy in, 414–417, 415t, 416t, 417t
ductal carcinoma in situ (DCIS), 414
staging of, 412t, 412–413, 443–444t
surgical options in, 413–414, 414t

Breast-conservation surgery, 413t, 413–414
Bromocriptine, 562, 563
in neuroleptic malignant syndrome, 598–599
Bronchodilator therapy, preoperative, 105–106
Bronchospasm, anesthesia in, 59–60
Bruit, cervical and stroke risk, 554
Budd-Chiari syndrome, 306
Bulimia nervosa, 592–595, 602
Bulk-forming agents, 682t
Bullae, 521t (*see also* Rashes)
BUN (blood urea nitrogen), 48, 204 (*see also* Renal failure)
Bupropion, seizure risk and, 602
Burns, 644t, 644–648
candidal infection in, 491
cardiovascular complications of, 646–647
electrical injury, 647–648
gastrointestinal bleeding in, 646
infectious complications of, 645–646
neuropsychiatric disorders and, 647
pulmonary complications of (inhalation injury), 644–645
renal and electrolyte complications of, 647
renal failure and, 203–204
stress ulcers with, 310–311
Buspirone, 604
Butterfly rash, 526
Butyrophenones, anesthetics with, 576–577
Bypass
CABG (coronary artery bypass grafting), 96, 99, 171–173, 401–402, 556, 631, 672
tibial–pedal, 534

Cachexia, 72 (*see also* Malnutrition)
CAGE questionnaire, 591
Calcitonin, 253–254
salmon, 436–437
Calcium channel blockers, 188, 605t
anesthetic interactions with, 64t
drug interactions with, 601
and hostility in schizophrenia, 573
interactions with psychotropic drugs, 571t
in mania, 573
in preeclampsia, 674
in pregnancy, 670, 674
in stroke, 555
in tardive dyskinesia, 573
Calcium disturbances
hypercalcemia, 249–254, 250t, 251t, 252t, 253t, 357
malignant, 435–439 (*see also* Hyperparathyroidism)
hypocalcemia, 213, 254–258, 255t, 256t
Calcium gluconate, 257
Caloric requirements estimation, 78, 78t
Canadian Critical Care Trials Group, 135
Cancer
anal, 427
bladder, 425
breast, 412–417
adjuvant systemic therapy in, 414–417, 415t, 416t, 417t
ductal carcinoma in situ (DCIS), 414
staging of, 412t, 412–413, 443–444t
surgical options in, 413–414, 414t
cervical, 648
coincidental with abdominal aortic aneurysm, 634

Cancer—*Continued*
  colorectal, 417–419, 444t
    adjuvant therapy in, 418–419
    preoperative treatment in, 419
    staging of, 417–418, 444t
  cutaneous metastases, 530
  drugs commonly prescribed for
    symptom control, 439t, 440t, 441t, 442t
    treatment, 438t, 439t
  esophageal, 423–425
  head and neck, 427, 530–641, 650t, 651t
  hypercalcemia in, 249–250
  lung, 106–107, 419–421, 445t
    nonsmall-cell, 419–421, 445t
    small-cell, 421
  metastatic, 428–429
    brain, 429
    complications of, 429–436
      long-bone fractures, 433–434
      malignant ascites, 432
      malignant biliary obstruction, 432–433
      malignant hypercalcemia, 435–439
      malignant pleural effusion, 430–431
      neoplastic pericardial effusion, 431
      spinal cord compression, 434–435
      superior vena cava syndrome, 429–430
      ureteral obstruction, 433
    liver, 428–429
    pulmonary, 428
    resection in, 428–429
  ovarian, 427–428
  pancreatic, 425–427
  prostate, 421–423, 423t, 434t (*see also* Transure-
      thral resection of prostate (TURP))
    staging of, 421, 444t
    surgical complications in, 422–423, 423t
  rashes in, 526–527
  "second look" surgery in, 427–428
  skin, 528–530
  skin signs of internal, 530, 530t
  staging systems for, 443–445
  surgery in
    incidental, 407–411
      general considerations, 407–408, 408t
      specific problems of, 408–411
    therapeutic, 409–439, 648–654
      anal carcinoma, 427
      bladder cancer, 425
      breast cancer, 412t, 412–417, 413t, 415t,
          416t, 417t, 443t, 444t
      colorectal cancer, 417–419, 444t
      esophageal cancer, 423–425
      head and neck cancer, 427, 530–641, 650t,
          651t
      lung cancer, 419–421, 445t
      in metastatic disease, 428–429
      pancreatic cancer, 425–427
      pelvic exenteration, 648–649, 649t, 650t
      prostate cancer, 421–423, 423t, 434t
      radical neck surgery, 640–641, 650t, 651t
      transurethral prostatic resection (TURP),
          236, 466–467, 651–654, 652t
    symptom control in, 439–443
      constipation, 439–441, 441t
      cough, 442, 442t
      dyspnea, 442, 442t
      nausea, vomiting, and dyspepsia, 394t, 441–442
      pain, 439t, 440t

Cancer chemotherapy (*see also* Cancer *and specific
      cancers*)
  adverse effects of, 409–411
  M-VAC in bladder cancer, 425
Candida albicans, 449, 491, 499–500, 525 (*see also*
      Fungal infections)
Candida parapsilosis, 491
Candida tropicalis, 491, 525
Candidiasis, 537
  oral, 527, *528*
  in tuberculous, mycotic, and viral infections, 502
Capitation, 9, 17–18
Captopril, 605t
Carbamazepine, 601
Carbidopa, 597
Carbohydrate requirements estimation, 89
Carbon monoxide poisoning, 591
Carbon tetrachloride, 62
Cardiac arrest, in pregnancy, 671–673
Cardiac arrhythmias
  atrial fibrillation and stroke risk, 554
  in dental procedures, 638–639, 639t
  perioperative, 174–177
    atrial and ventricular, 174–175
    automatic implantable cardiac defibrillators
        in, 176–177
    digoxin in, 176
    with existing pacemaker, 176
    tachycardia, 174
    transvenous pacemakers in, 175–176
  in pregnancy, 670–671
    adverse drug effects, 671t
Cardiac catheterization
  endocarditis prophylaxis in, 475
  for monitoring, 133–139 (*see also* Hemodynamic
      monitoring)
Cardiac drugs, in renal failure, 223
Cardiac pacemakers, electroconvulsive therapy
      risk and, 583
Cardiac psychosis (*see* Delirium)
Cardiac risk factors, 5
Cardiac risk in anesthesia, 55–57, 56t
Cardiac Risk Index, 21
Cardiac side effects of drugs, 598
Cardiac stress testing, 154–158, 155t, 157t
      (*see also* Myocardial infarction; Myocar-
      dial ischemia; Stress testing)
Cardiac surgery
  hematologic issues in, 401–402
  renal failure, 196t, 203–204
Cardiomyopathy
  hypertrophic, 197–198
  idiopathic peripartum, 669
Cardiovascular disease (*see also specific disorders*)
  anxiety disorders in, 573
  arrhythmias, 174–177 (*see also* Cardiac arrhyth-
      mias)
  cancer chemotherapy side effects, 410
  with cerebrovascular disease, 553
  as complication of burns, 646–647
  congestive heart failure, 168–179, 177t
  coronary revascularization procedures in,
      171–174 (*see also specific procedures*)
  depression as predictor in, 573
  in eating disorders, 594
  endocarditis prophylaxis in existing, 472t
  gallbladder surgery in, 636
  Goldman Cardiac Risk Index, 156, 157t

hypertrophic cardiomyopathy, 197–198
hypocalcemia-related, 256
myocardial infarction
anesthesia and, 56, 61
electroconvulsive therapy risk and, 583
hemodynamic monitoring in, 134
in joint replacement, 546
presentation of as fever, 482
myocardial ischemia
coronary revascularization procedures in, 171–174
coronary revasculatization procedures in (see also specific procedures)
general considerations in, 153t, 153–154
in pregnancy, 671–673
preoperative clinical predictors of, 156
preoperative testing for, 154–158, 155t, 157t
ambulatory ECG, 158–160
dobutamine stress echocardiography, 169–170
left ventricular systolic function testing, 161, 161t
nuclear scintigraphy (thallium scan), 165–167
resting ECG, 158
SPECT, 167–168
stress testing, 154–158, 155t, 157t, 161–165, 162t, 163t, 164t, 165t
technetium-99m sestamibi, 168
risk and prevalence, 179t, 179–188
silent, 182
New York Heart Association functional classification, 177t
noncardiac surgery and, 150–171
assessment of patient, 149–152, 150t, 151t
consultation considerations in, 152–153
myocardial ischemia risk and prevalence, 153t, 153–170 (see also Myocardial ischemia)
in pregnancy, 665–675, 666t
acquired, 669–673
cardiac arrhythmias, 670–671, 671t
ischemic heart disease and cardiac arrest, 671–673
congenital, 666–669
effects of commonly used drugs, 670t
hypertension, 673t, 673–674
prosthetic heart valves, 196t, 196–197, 473, 483, 511–512
in psychiatric patients, 570–572, 571t
risk factors for, perioperative, 150t, 152t
surgical risk and, 621
valvular heart disease, 188–195
Cardiovascular drugs, adverse effects in pregnancy, 667t (see also specific drugs)
Cardiovascular parameters, NYHA class correlated with cardiopulmonary parameters, 707t
Cardiovascular risk assessment, 17
Cardiovascular system, anesthetic effects on, 61–62
Carotid endartarectomy, 632
ECST (European Carotid Surgery Trial), 555
NASCET (North American Symptomatic Carotid Endarterectomy Trial), 555
prophylactic, 554
stroke risk in, 553
CASS (Coronary Artery Surgery Study), 171
Cataract surgery, 635–636, 636t

Catheterization
for abscess drainage, 488
candidal infection and urinary, 491
cardiac, endocarditis prophylaxis in, 475
for hemodynamic monitoring, 87, 133–139, 623, 633 (see also Hemodynamic monitoring)
pulmonary artery, 178–179, 179t (see also Hemodynamic monitoring)
sepsis related to, 88
urinary tract infection and, 497–500, 499t, 508–509
Cauda equina syndrome, 564–565
CAVH (continuous arteriovenous hemofiltration), 216
Cefazolin, 544
Cellulitis, 519–522, 521
clostridial, 501, 521
cryptococcal, 521, 521
in diabetes mellitus, 533
nonclostridial anaerobic, 501
pelvic, 503
staphylococcal, 521
synergistic necrotizing, 502
tinea pedis (athlete's foot) and, 522–523
Cephalosporins, 224
allergy to, 535–536
Cerebrospinal fluid (CSF), glucose testing of, 706t
Cerebrovascular accident (see Stroke)
Cerebrovascular disease, 553–558 (see also Stroke)
abdominal aortic aneurysm surgery in, 632
perioperative, 556–558
preoperative, 553–556
transurethral prostatic resection risk in, 653–654
Cervical bruit and stroke risk, 554
Cervical cancer, 648 (see also Pelvic exenteration)
Charts, 3–4
Chemotherapeutic agents (see Cancer chemotherapy and specific drugs)
Chest radiography, 44t, 44–46, 45t, 101
frequency of abnormalities in, 45t
yield of preoperative, 44t
Child's classification of cirrhosis risk, 298t
Chlamydial infection, in pregnancy, 695
Chlorambucil, 685t
Chlorimipramine (see Antidepressants)
Chloroform, 62
Chlorpromazine, 589, 597
Chlorpropamide, 353–354
Cholecystectomy, 319–320
in elderly, 636–638
Cholecystitis
postoperative, 319
in pregnancy, 683
Cholecystotomy, 637
Cholestasis (cholestatic jaundice), 316–317
of pregnancy, 683
Cholestyramine, 321, 323, 683
Chondrocalcinosis, 549
Chronic obstructive pulmonary disease (COPD) (see COPD and specific diseases)
Chronic renal failure, 217–224, 245
epidemiology of, 217–218
evaluation of, 218
treatment of, 218–224
Cimetidine, 605t, 682t (see also H_2-receptor antagonists)

Circle of Willis, congenital berry aneurysm of, 668
Cirrhosis, 241, 306–307 (*see also* Liver disease)
Cisapride, 311
Cisplatin, nephrotoxicity of, 410–411
Clonidine, 186
    interactions with psychotropic drugs, 571t
Clostridial anaerobic cellulitis, 501
Clostridia perfringens cellulitis, 521
Clostridium difficile, 323
Clostridium difficile colitis, 483, 504–505
Clotrimazole, 537
Clotting studies, 47
Clozapine, 577, 599
Coagulation disorders (*see also* Hemostasis)
    evaluation of, 380–385, 381t, 382t, 383t, 384t,
        385t
    hypercoagulable states, 393t, 393–395 (*see also*
        Thromboembolic disorders)
    in liver disease, 300–301, 390
    in pregnancy, 679
    preoperative planning in, 385–386
    skin signs in, 522–523, *523*
    treatment of
        acquired, 389–393 (*see also* Disseminated in-
            travascular coagulation (DIC); Hemolysis)
        congenital, 386–389, 387t
Coagulation factors (*see* Coagulation disorders;
        Hemostasis)
Cocaine, 606t
    anesthetic interactions with, 65t
Coccidioidomycosis, 525
Codeine, 606t
Cognitive impairment (*see* Delirium; Mental
        status)
Colitis
    Clostridium difficile, 483, 504–505
    ulcerative, in pregnancy, 681–683
Collagen vascular diseases
    in pregnancy, 691–694
        antiphospholipid syndrome, 693–694
        rheumatoid arthritis, 691
        systemic lupus erythematosus, 692–693
    rashes in, 526
Colon resection, in elderly, 625–626
Colorectal cancer, 417–419
    adjuvant therapy in, 418–419
    preoperative treatment in, 419
    staging of, 417–418, 444t
Colostomy, 324–325
Coma, 564
    in hypoglycemia, 586
    myxedema, 339 (*see also* Hypothyroidism)
Compliance, 6t, 6–7, 7t
Compound A, 63
Conflict resolution, 3
Congenital aortic stenosis, in pregnancy, 668
Congenital berry aneurysm of circle of Willis, 668
Congestive heart failure, 177–179
    clinical predictors of, 177, 177t
    etiology of, 177–178
    in joint replacement, 546
    physical examination findings in, 177
    in pregnancy, 670
    preoperative testing in, 161
    in sickle cell disorders, 677
    treatment of, 178
Constipation, in cancer, 439–441, 441t
Consultant, role of, 2t

Consultation
    AMA responsibilities list, 1
    as compared with referral, 1–2
    documentation of, 3–5
    effectiveness of, 5–7, 6t, 7t
    follow-up in, 5
    initial contact, 2–3
    role in general medicine, 9
    role of internist in, 1–8
    second, 1
    timeliness of, 4
Consultation report, 3–4
Consultation request, 2
Consultation service
    as compared with primary medicine, 9
    function of general medical, 9–18
    role of internist in, 1–8
Contact dermatitis, 536
Continuous ambulatory electrocardiography,
        158–160
Continuous arteriovenous hemofiltration (CAVH),
        216
Continuous positive airway pressure (CPAP), 108
        (*see also* Mechanical respiratory support)
Continuous renal replacement therapy (CRRT),
        214–217, 216t, 217t
Continuous venous hemodialysis (CVVHD), 216
Continuous venovenous hemofiltration (CVVH),
        215, 216
Contraceptive drugs, 606t
    drug interactions of, 601
Contrast medium (*see* Radiocontrast)
Coombs' test, indirect, 369
COPD (chronic obstructive pulmonary disease)
    with lung cancer, 106
    pulmonary complications and, 99t, 99–100
Coprolalia, 587
Coronary angiography, 171
Coronary artery bypass grafting (CABG), 96, 99
    in abdominal aortic aneurysm, 96, 99, 631
    as adjunct to noncardiac surgery, 171–173
    graft infections in, 510t, 510–511
    hemostatic problems in, 401–402
    in pregnancy, 670
    prophylactic carotid endartarectomy in, 556
Corticosteroids
    in adrenal insufficiency, 342
    in asthma, 106
    in hemolytic anemia, 373
    in lupus erythematosus, 692
    in myasthenic crisis, 560
    plastic-wrap occlusion and, 537–538
    in pregnancy, 667t, 684t, 691
    prophylactic, 342
    psychiatric side effects of, 606t
    relative potencies of, 706t
    topical, 537–538, 538t
Corticotropin-releasing-hormone test, 570
Cortrosyn (ACTH) stimulation test, 342, 354
Cough
    in cancer, 442, 442t
    in postoperative respiratory management, 108
Coumarin, 642
    in hip fracture, 544
Coumarin drugs, 389–390
Coxsackie A16 virus, 524–525
CPAP (continuous positive airway pressure), 108
        (*see also* Mechanical respiratory support)

Creatinine height index, 76
Creatinine testing, 48
Critical incidents in anesthesia, 56–57
Crohn's disease (regional enteritis)
    nutritional support in, 90
    in pregnancy, 681–683
CRRT (continuous renal replacement therapy),
        214–217, 216t, 217t
Cryoglobulinemia, 374
Cryptococcal cellulitis, 521, *521*
Cryptococcosis, 525
Crystal-induced arthritis, 549
Cushing's disease, 570
    psychiatric symptoms in, 585
CVVH (continuous venovenous hemofiltration),
        215
CVVHD (continuous venous hemodialysis), 216
Cyclobenzaprine, 606t
Cyclophosphamide, 416 (*see also* Cancer chemo-
        therapy)
    in lupus erythematosus, 692
    in myasthenic crisis, 560
    in pregnancy, 685t, 692
Cyclosporine, in pregnancy, 667t, 684t
Cystectomy, 425
Cytokines, pyrogenic, 478–479

Dalteparin, 143
Dantrolene, in drug fever, 598–599
Dapsone, 606t
DDAVP
    in cardiac surgery, 401–402
    in von Willebrand's disease, 388
Deep-breathing exercises, 107–108
Deep vein thrombophlebitis (DVT), prevention of,
        109, 141–146, 397
    comparison of methods, 144, 144t
    mechanical, 144
    pharmacologic, *142*, 142–143, *143*
    principles of, 141–142
    thrombocytopenia and, 27–455
DEET (Off!), 606t
Deferoxamine mesylate, 677–678
Delirium, 564, 577–582
    after electroconvulsive therapy, 583
    clinical features of, 596t
    in elderly, 596t, 618
    evaluation of postoperative, 580t, 580–581
    organic causes of, 578t
    quiet presentation of, 578
    risk factors for, 579–580, 618t
    terminology and classification of, 577–578
    treatment of, 581–584
Dementia, 558–559, 559t
    Alzheimer's disease, 558–559, 587–588
    clinical features of, 596t
    HIV-associated, 589–590, 589–600
    multi-infarct, 558, 588
    pseudodementia of depression, 595
    psychiatric symptoms in, 587–588
    surgical risk and, 574
    vs. depression, 587–588
Denial, 573–574
Dental procedures/dental surgery, 638–644
    anesthesia in, 638–640
    anticoagulant therapy and, 641t, 641–642
    endocarditis prophylaxis in, 473t, 474t, 475, 641
    hospitalization for, 640–641

infection in, 643, 643t
    in pulmonary disease, 642–643
Dental trauma, 642
Dependency, ventilator, 126
Depression (*see also* Psychiatric issues)
    adrenocorticoid excess in, 585
    agitated vs. anxiety, 573
    electroconvulsive therapy (ECT) in, 582–583
    in HIV infection, 589
    hypertension as related to, 570
    lithium in unipolar, 601
    major, 575, 601–604
    in Parkinson's disease, 586
    perioperative, 574
    as predictor of cardiac events, 573
    pseudodementia of, 595
    SAD (seasonal affective disorder), 603–604
    surgical risk and, 574, 575
    vs. Alzheimer's disease, 587–588
Dermatitis
    contact, 536
    seborrheic, 526, 528
Dermatologic disorders, 519–540
    in AIDS/HIV, 527t, 527–528
    dermatologic consultation in, 538
    diabetic foot disorders, *533*, 533–534
    hospitalization-associated complications in,
        534–537
        contact dermatitis, 536
        drug eruptions, *534*, 534–536, 535t
        miliaria, 536
        skin infections, 537
    malignancy, 528–531, 531t
    pregnancy-associated skin reactions, *531*, 531t,
        531–532, *532*
    pruritus, 532t, 532–533 (*see also* Rashes)
    rash and fever, 519t–520t, 519–527
        infectious causes of, 519–525 (*see also*
            Infections *and specific disorders and
            lesions*)
        noninfectious causes of, 525–527
    therapy for, 537–538, 538t
Desflurane, 59, 61, 62, 63
Desipramine, 595 (*see also* Antidepressants)
Dexamethasone, 342, 429
Dexamethasone suppression test, 570, 585
Dextran, as anticoagulant, 141
Diabetes insipidus, 199t, 237, 239, 352t, 353, 354
        (*see also* ADH (antidiuretic hormone))
Diabetes mellitus, 17
    detection of occult, 47–48
    epidemiology of, 329
    foot disorders in, *533*, 533–534
    hypothyroidism in, 688
    ketoacidosis in, 332–333, 662t, 662–663
    oral hypoglycemics in, 332
    pathophysiology of, 329
    perioperative management of, 330–332, 331t
    in pregnancy, 661–663, 663t, 688
        fetal effects of, 662
        insulin-dependent (IDDM), 661–662
        ketoacidosis in, 662t, 662–663
    preoperative evaluation, 40, 329–330
    selective aldosterone deficiency in, 343
    thyroid dysfunction in, 662
Diabetic ketoacidosis, 332–333, 662–663, 663t
Dialysis
    in chronic renal failure, 218–224

Dialysis—*Continued*
  continuous arteriovenous hemofiltration (CAVH), 216
  continuous renal replacement therapy (CRRT), 214–217, 216t, 217t
  continuous venous hemodialysis (CVVHD), 216
  continuous venovenous hemofiltration (CVVH), 215, 216
  drug therapy in, 216t, 217, 217t, 221t, 221–224
  in hypercalcemia, 254
  in hyperkalemia, 248t, 249
  nutritional support in, 90
  preoperative, 63
  prophylactic, 207–208
Diarrhea
  in enteral feeding, 85
  postsurgical, 321–322, 323, 504–505
Diastolic dysfunction, 184–185 (*see also* Hypertension)
Diastolic murmur, 192
Diazepam, 580
  as compared with buspirone, 604
DIC (disseminated intravascular coagulation), 390–392, 391t
  skin signs in, 522–523, *523*
Diet (*see also* Malnutrition; Nutrition; Nutritional evaluation)
  American Diabetes Association (ADA), 81
  high-fiber, 82
  for medical conditions, 81
  supplemental, 81–83, 213–214
Diffusing capacity of lungs, 102, 103t, 104t
Digitalis, 175
  anesthetic interactions, 65t
  in pregnancy, 666, 667t
  psychiatric side effects of, 606t
  in renal failure, 223
Diltiazem, drug interactions of, 601
Diphenhydramine, 586, 597
Diphenoxylate/atropine, 682t
Dipyridamole-thallium nuclear scintigraphy, 165–167, 169t
Disseminated intravascular coagulation (DIC), 390–392, 391t
  skin signs in, 522–523, *523*
Diuretics, 82, 211–212, 246
  anesthetic interactions of, 65t
  contraindications to, 303
  lithium with, 573
  in liver disease, 303
  in malignant hypercalcemia, 436
  ototoxicity of, 212
  in postoperative hypertension, 188
  in pregnancy, 667t
  psychotropic drugs, interactions of, 571t
  in renal failure, 223
  in SIADH, 351
  thiazide
    allergy to, 536
    in nephrogenic diabetes insipidus, 354
    in preeclampsia, 674
Dobutamine stress echocardiography, 169t, 169–170, 631
Documentation, 3–4, 5
Domperidone, 562
Doxepin (*see also* Tricyclic antidepressants)
Doxorubicin, cardiac side effects of, 410
Doxycycline, 430

Drug eruptions of skin, *534,* 534–536, 535t
Drug fever, 492–493, 598–599
Drug-induced cholestasis, 317
Drug-induced hemolysis, 372
Drug-induced hepatitis, 314, 314t
Drug-induced neutropenia, 378t
Drug interactions (*see also specific drugs*)
  with anesthetic agents, 64t–65t, 64–66
  antihypertensives with psychotropic drugs, 571t
Drug rashes, 525–526
Drug-related renal syndromes, 199t
Drug use, 32
Dumping syndrome, 320–321
Dysphagia, in esophageal cancer, 424
Dyspnea, in cancer, 442, 442t
Dystonia, psychiatric symptoms in, 586–587
Dystonic reactions, acute, 597
Dystrophy, myotonic, 563

Early Breast Cancer Trialists' Collaborative Group, 414–415
Eating disorders, 592–595
Ebstein's anomaly, 668
Echocardiography
  dobutamine stress, 169t, 169–170, 631
  indications for, 193
Eclampsia/preeclampsia, 673t, 673–674
ECST (European Carotid Surgery Trial), 555
ECT (electroconvulsive therapy), 582–583
Ecthyma gangrenosa, 522
Edema
  pulmonary
    acute noncardiac (transfusion-related), 368
    in sickle cell disorders, 677
    transfusion-related (acute noncardiac pulmonary), 368
Edrophium, 559
Effusion, malignant
  pericardial, 431
  pleural, 430–431
Elderly
  abuse of, 597
  apathetic hyperthyroidism in older patients, 334
  cauda equina syndrome and cardiac surgery in, 564
  depression in, 595
  endocarditis incidence in, 471
  insomnia in, 596
  myocardial infarction presenting as fever in, 482
  orthopaedic disorders in, 541–544
  psychiatric problems in, 595–597, 596t
  psychoactive drugs in, 595
  quality of life for, 624
  SHEP (Systolic Hypertension in the Elderly) study, 573
  surgical problems in, 30, 615–637
    age-related, 616t, 616–618, 617t
    anesthesia type and, 619
    diagnostic activities and approaches to, 622–624
    gender-related, 618, 618t
    general condition and, 620–621
    general health and, 620, *621*
    overview of, 615–616, 616t
    specific organ system disease and, 621–622, 622t
    treatment principles for, 624–625

type of procedure and, *619,* 619–620, 620t, 625–637
type of surgery and, 625–637
  abdominal aortic aneurysm, 626–635
    (*see also* Abdominal aortic aneurysm)
  appendectomy, 626
  cataract surgery, 635–636, 636t
  cholecystectomy, 636–638
  colon resection, 625–626
  gynecologic procedures, 626
  hernia repair, 625
  thoracotomy, 626
  ulcer operations, 626
Elective surgery, 22
  transfusions for, 363
Electrical injury, 646–648 (*see also* Burns)
Electrocardiography (ECG)
  AHA Task Force report on, 43
  ambulatory, 158–160
  findings in psychiatric patients, 568–569
  preoperative, 42–43, 44t
  resting, 158
  yield of routine, 44t
Electroconvulsive therapy (ECT), 582–583
Electroencephalography (EEG), in delirium, 580
Electrolyte disturbances (*see also* Acid-base
    disturbances; Renal failure)
  anesthesia and, 63
  calcium
    hypercalcemia, 249–254, 250t, 251t, 252t,
      253t, 357 (*see also* Hyperparathyroidism)
      malignant, 435–439
    hypocalcemia, 254–258, 255t, 256t
  in diabetes mellitus, 330
  hyperchloremia, 343
  magnesium
    hypermagnesemia, 260–261
    hypomagnesemia, 258–260, 259t, 260t
  phosphorus
    hyperphosphatemia, 213, 258, 264, 264t
    hypophosphatemia, 261–264, 262t, 263t
  potassium
    hyperkalemia, 244–249, 245t, *247,* 248t, 343
    hypokalemia, 240–244, 242t, *243,* 301, 345
  sodium
    hypernatremia, 236–240, *238*
    hyponatremia, 211, 228–236, *231,* 231t, 233t,
      234, 348–351
    in post-TURP syndrome, 236
Electrolyte studies, 48–49
Embolism
  fat, 545
  pulmonary, 146–147, 497, 545
    in hip fracture, 541–542, 542t
    in hip replacement, 545
Emergencies, 22
Emetine, 306
Encephalopathy, 241
  hepatic, 317–318
  in vitamin B deficiency, 591
Endartarectomy, carotid (*see* Carotid endarter-
    ectomy)
Endocarditis, antibiotic prophylaxis for
  in dental procedures, 641
  in pregnancy, 668
  subacute bacterial, 469–475, 470t–474t
Endocrine disorders (*see also* Hormones)
  adrenal insufficiency, 340–342, 343t

diabetes insipidus, 351–354, 352t
diabetes mellitus, 329–334
  epidemiology, 329
  pathophysiology, 329
  perioperative management, 330–334, 331t
  preoperative evaluation, 329–330
  selective aldosterone deficiency in, 343
hypercalcemia in, 357
hyperparathyroidism, 249–254, 355–357
  (*see also* Hypercalcemia)
pheochromocytoma, 347–348
pituitary insufficiency, 354, 355t
primary hyperaldosteronism, 345–346
psychiatric symptoms in, 584–586
selective aldosterone deficiency, 343–345, 344t
syndrome of inappropriate antidiuretic hormone
    (SIADH), 232, 233–235, *234,* 348–351,
    350t (*see also* Diabetes insipidus;
    Hyponatremia)
thyroid disorders, 334–340
  hyperthyroidism, 334–337
  hypothyroidism, 337–340
Endometriosis, puerperal, 503
Endoscopic retrograde cholangiopancreatography
    (ERCP), 306, 308–309, 425
Endoscopic surgery, 98
Endotracheal intubation, 123–124 (*see also*
    Mechanical ventilatory support)
Endotracheal suctioning, 123–124
Enflurane, 63, 304
Enoxaparin, 143
Enteral nutrition, 79–85
  complications of, 85
  diet and table foods in, 79–81, *80,* 81t
  by intubation, 84–85
  in supplemental diets, 81–83, 82t
Enterobacter sp., 491 (*see also* Infection)
Enterococcus sp., 449 (*see also* Infection)
Enzymes, anticoagulant, 398
Ephedrine, 606t
Epidural analgesia, 109
Epidural anesthesia, 57–58
Epilepsy, perioperative anticonvulsants in, 557t,
    557–558
Equations, 703–709
ERCP (endoscopic retrograde cholangiopancre-
    atography), 306, 308–309, 425
Erectile dysfunction, postprostatectomy, 423, 423t
Erythema marginatum, 526
Erythema multiforme, 526
Erythema nodosum, 525
Erythrocyte abnormalities, 370–377 (*see also*
    Hematologic disorders)
  erythrocytosis, 374–377
    absolute, 375
    appropriate or inappropriate secondary,
      375–376
    polycythemia vera, 376–377
    relative, 375
  immune hemolytic anemia, 372t, 372–374
  sickle-cell hemoglobinopathies, 370–372
Erythromycin, 311, 601 (*see also* Antibiotics)
Escherichia coli, 449 (*see also* Infection)
Esophageal cancer, 423–425
Esophageal surgery, endocarditis prophylaxis in,
    474t
Esophageal varices, 305, 318–319
European Carotid Surgery Trial (ECST), 555

Euthyroid sick syndrome, 338
Euvolemia, 199, *200*
Evaluation (*see* Preoperative evaluation)
Exercise, deep-breathing, 107–108
Extrapyradmidal disorders, 560–563 (*see also*
      Parkinson's disease)
  parkinsonian syndromes, 560–563, 562t
  postoperative complications in, 563
  psychiatric symptoms in, 586
Extubation (weaning), 126–129, 127t, *128*

Facial trauma, 642
Factitious fever, 484
Factitious hyperthyroidism, 584–585
Faculty preceptors, 11
False-positive/false-negative results, 28, 50
  for hyperkalemia, 246
Famotidine (*see* H$_2$-receptor antagonists)
Fasciitis, necrotizing, 501
Fat embolism, in sickle-cell disease, 372
Fat requirements estimation, 89
Fatty acid deficiency, 87
Fatty liver, 299–300
Febrile transfusion reactions, 368–369
Felty's syndrome, 549–550
Fenfluramine, 65, 65t
Fentanyl, 64
Fetal effects (*see also* Teratogenicity)
  of asthma, 662
  of diabetes mellitus, 662
Fetal malformation (*see* Teratogenicity)
Fever
  factitious, 484
  myocardial infarction presenting as, 482
  postoperative
    causes of, 477t–478t
    diagnostic approach to, 480t, 480–484, 481t,
      482t
    epidemiology and pathophysiology of, 478–480,
      479t
    pyrogenic cytokines and, 478–479
  post-traumatic, 504
  with rash, 519–525 (*see also* Rashes)
  rheumatic, 526
FEV (forced expiratory volume) (*see* Pulmonary
    evaluation; Pulmonary function testing)
Fine-needle aspiration (FNA), 688
Fistula, tracheoesophageal, 424–425
Flow-volume loop, 115
Fludrocortisone, 342
Fluid disturbances, 199t, 228, 229t–230t (*see also*
    Electrolyte disturbances; Hypernatremia;
    Hyponatremia; Renal failure)
Fluid management
  in renal failure, 212
  in respiratory support, 126
Fluid requirements estimation, 78
Flumazenil, 59, 604
5-Fluorouracil (5-FU), 419 (*see also* Cancer chemo-
    therapy)
  in head and neck cancer, 427
  in pancreatic cancer, 426–427
Fluoxetine (*see* Serotonin reuptake inhibitors
    [SSRIs])
Fluvoxamine (*see* Serotonin reuptake inhibitors
    [SSRIs])
Folate deficiency, 677
Follow-up, 5

Formulas
  commercial diet supplements, 83
  for enteral feeding, 84–85
Fournier's gangrene, 502
Fracture
  fat embolization in, 547
  hip, 467, 541–544, 542t, 544t, 9004t
  long-bone in cancer, 433–434
  skull, 469
Framingham Heart Study, 554
Free-water excretion (*see* Hyponatremia)
5-FU (*see* Cancer chemotherapy; 5-Fluorouracil)
Functional cardiac capacity testing, 163, 164t
Fungal infections, 491–492, 537
  candidal, 449, 491, 499–500, 502, 525, *525,* 527,
    528, 538
  chlamydial, 695
  rashes in, 525
Fungemia, 491–492
Furosemide, 303

Gallbladder disease, 319–320 (*see also* Biliary
    disorders; Cholecystectomy)
  in elderly, 636–638
  in pregnancy, 683
Gallium nitrate, 254
Gangrene
  Fournier's, 502
  gas, 502
  infected vascular, 502
Gardnerella vaginalis, 696
Gas gangrene, 502
Gastrectomy, 320–321
Gastric ulcers, 126
Gastritis, bile (alkaline, reflux), 321
Gastroenterologic conditions, 297–328 (*see also*
    Gastrointestinal surgery)
  cancer (*see also* Cancer)
    anal, 427
    bowel obstruction in, 408–409
    colorectal, 417–419, 444t
    esophageal, 423–425
    metastatic, 428–436
    pancreatic, 425–427
  in eating disorders, 594–595
  gastroesophageal reflux disease (GERD),
    311–312
  liver disease, 297–307
    abscess, 297–307, 487
    anesthesia and, 303–304, 313–316, 314t
    autoimmune, 307
    biliary disorders in, 312t, 312–319
    coagulation disorders in, 300–301, 390
    diuretics in, 303
    HBaAg carriers of, 303
    high-risk patients with, 298–300
    incidence of complications with, 298, 298t,
      299t
    pathophysiology of, 297–298
    postsurgical treatment of, 305–306
    in pregnancy, 306–307, 686
    preoperative evaluation of, 298t, 298–301,
      299t
    renal function in, 301
    surgical risk and, 304–305
    treatment of, 301–303
  ostomy care, 323–325
  pancreatitis

postoperative, 308–309
preoperative, 307–308
postoperative complications, 312–328
diarrhea, 323
jaundice/hepatic disease, 312t, 312–319
postcholecystectomy syndrome, 319–320
postgastrectomy syndrome, 320–322
postoperative cholestasis, 319
recurrent ulcer, 322–323
in pregnancy
cholecystitis, 683
cholestasis, 683
drug safety of GI drugs in, 682t
inflammatory bowel disease, 681–683
ulcer disease, 309–311
peptic ulcers, 309–310
recurrent, 322–323
stress ulcers, 310–311
Gastroesophageal reflux (GERD), 311–312
Gastrointestinal bleeding
in abdominal aortic aneurysm, 634
in burns, 646
in intubated patients, 126
Gastrointestinal drugs, safety of in pregnancy, 682t
Gastrointestinal fluids, composition of, 212t
Gastrointestinal surgery (*see also* Abdominal surgery)
endocarditis prophylaxis in, 473t, 474r
infection risk in
in abdominal trauma, 464
appendectomy, 461
cholecystectomy, 461–462
lower tract (colorectal surgery), 463–464
upper tract, 462–463
Gastrostomy, 424
G-CSF, recombinant in neutropenia, 379
Gender-related surgical problems, 618, 618t
General medical consultation service (*see under* Consultation service)
Genitourinary surgery, endocarditis prophylaxis in, 473t, 474t
Gentamycin, 255
GERD (gastroesophageal reflux disease), 311–312
Geriatric population (*see* Aging; Elderly)
Gestational trophoblastic disease, 689
GGT (τ-glutamyl transpeptidase) test, 304
Gilles de la Tourette's syndrome, 587
Glasgow criteria, for pancreatitis, 308
Gleason score for prostate cancer, 422
Glucocorticoids, in hypercalcemia, 253
Glucophage (metformin), 332
Glucose-insulin infusion, 246, 248t
Glucose testing, 47–48
of CSF, 706t
τ-Glutamyl transpeptidase (GGT) test, 304
Goldman Cardiac Risk Index, 156, 157t, 182
Gold therapy, in pregnancy, 684t, 691
Gonadal deficiency, 355t
Gonococcemia, 522
Gonorrhea (*see also* Sexually transmitted diseases [STDs])
in pregnancy, 694, 694t
Gouty arthritis, 549
Granulocyte-colony-stimulating factor (*see* G-CSF)
Granulocytic leukemoid reaction, 377 (*see also* Neutrophilia)
Graves' disease, 334–337 (*see also* Hyperthyroidism; Thyroid disorders)

Guanethidine, interactions with psychotropic drugs, 571t
Gynecologic surgery (*see also* Pelvic exenteration)
in elderly, 626
infection risk in, 465–466
abdominal hysterectomy, 465–466
vaginal hysterectomy, 465
Gynecomastia, as drug side effect, 599

Hairy oral leukoplakia, in AIDS, 527, *528*
Hallucinations, in alcoholism, 591
Haloperidol, 580, 589
drug interactions, 601
Halothane, 61, 62, 63 (*see also* Anesthesia; Anesthetic agents)
liver disorders related to, 303, 313–316, 314t
Hand-foot-and-mouth disease, 524–525
Hashimoto's thyroiditis, 338–339, 690
HBsAg carriers, 303
hCG (human chorionic gonadotropin) test, 50
Headache, postanesthesia, 57
Head and neck cancer, 427, 530–641, 650t, 651t
Health food stores, 80
Heart block, congenital in lupus erythematosus, 692
Heart failure, 177–179, 212 (*see also* Congestive heart failure)
anesthesia and, 62
in hip fracture, 541–542, 542t
in joint replacement, 547
Heart valves, prosthetic, 196t, 196–197, 473, 483, 511–512, 670
Heat rash (miliaria), 536
Heat stroke, as drug side effect, 599
Height/weight measurements, 72–74, 73t, 74t
Helicobacter pylori, 309–310
HELLP syndrome, 686–687
Hematocrit, 46, 46t, 48t
Hematologic disorders, 361–406
anemia, 361–367
diagnostic evaluation of, 361–362, 362t
postoperative, 364–367, 365t
preoperative, 361–364, 362t
blood transfusion in
assessment for, 362–363
autologous, 363–364
reactions to, 367–370
erythrocyte abnormalities, 370–377
erythrocytosis, 374–377
immune hemolytic anemia, 372t, 372–374
sickle-cell hemoglobinopathies, 370–372
of hemostasis, 380–392 (*see also* Coagulation disorders; Hemostasis)
skin signs in, 522–523, *523*
leukocyte abnormalities, 377–380
lymphocytopenia, 380
lymphocytosis, 379–380
neutropenia, 378t, 378–379, 408
neutrophilia, 377–378
pancytopenia, 380, 380t
platelet disorders
diagnosis, 396, *396*
qualitative platelet dysfunction, 398–400, 399t
thrombocytopenia, 396–398, 397t
thrombocytosis, 400
in pregnancy, 675–679
anemia, 676–677
coagulopathies, 679

Hematologic disorders—*Continued*
   hemoglobinopathies, 677–678, 678t
     thrombocytopenia, 678–679
   preoperative, 46t, 46–50
   surgical treatment issues in, 401–404
     cardiac surgery, 401–402
     splenomegaly, 402–403
     therapeutic apheresis, 403–404, 404t
Hemodialysis (*see* Dialysis)
Hemodynamic monitoring, 178–179, 179t
   clinical competence and, 136, 137t
   complications of, 136, 136t
   consensus indications for, 135, 135t
   controversies about, 133–134
   historical background of, 134
   in hypercalcemia, 253
   research regarding, 134–135
Hemoglobin (Hg) tests, 46, 46t
Hemoglobinopathy
   in pregnancy, 677–678, 678t
   sickle-cell, 370–372
Hemoglobin SS disease, 677–678
Hemoglobinuria, 197
Hemolysis, 74
   as cause of anemia, 366
   delayed, 369
   disease-related, 366
   drug-induced, 366
   sepsis-induced, 366
   transfusion-related, 366
Hemolytic anemia
   autoimmune
     cold, 373–374
     warm, 373
   diagnosis of, 372, 372t
   immune, 372t, 372–374
Hemophilia, 386–388, 387t
Hemorrhage (*see* Bleeding)
Hemostasis
   coagulation disorders of
     acquired, 389–393, 391t (*see also* Dissemi-
       nated intravascular coagulation [DIC])
     congenital, 386–389, 387t
     hypercoagulable states, 393t, 393–395 (*see also*
       Thromboemobolic disorders)
     evaluation of, 380–385, 381t, 382t, 383t, 384t,
       385t
     preoperative planning for, 385–386
Heparin, 141 (*see also* Anticoagulants)
   adjusted-dose subcutaneous, 142
   in antiphospholipid antibody syndrome,
     693
   in hip replacement, 546
   intravenous, 145–146
   low-molecular-weight, 143, 555
   minidose subcutaneous, 142
   platelet disorders and, 397–398
   in pregnancy, 668
Heparinization, 391–392, 395 (*see also* Anticoagulants; Coagulation disorders)
Hepatic abscess, 487
Hepatic cirrhosis, 241
   in pregnancy, 686
Hepatic disease (*see* Jaundice; Liver disease)
Hepatic effects of anesthesia, 62
Hepatic encephalopathy, 317–318
Hepatic failure, 317–318
   in pregnancy, 686–687

Hepatitis
   A, 684
   alcoholic, 299, 304
   B, 684–685, 686t
   C and D, 685–686
   halothane, 313–314
   ischemic, 314–315
   methoxyflurane, 314
   as postoperative complication, 317–319
   posttransfusion, 315–316
   in pregnancy, 306, 683–687
   viral types of, 315
Hepatocellular dysfunction, 313 (*see also* Hepatitis;
   Liver disease)
Hernia repair, in elderly, 625
Herpes gestationis, 531–532
Herpes simplex
   in AIDS, 527, *527*
   in pregnancy, 694
High-fiber diets, 82
Hip fracture, 467, 541–544, 542t, 9004t
Hip replacement, 467–468, 544–547, 545t
Hip surgery, 141, 144
Hirudin, 398
Histoplasmosis, 525
History
   bleeding, 32, 32t, 33t
   as compared with laboratory tests, 29t
   dietary/nutrition, 72, 297
   limited, 31
   patient-completed, 25–26
   principles of taking, 29t, 29–32, 30t, 31t, 32t, 33t
   renal, 198
   telephone, 26
   transfusion, 32
HIV infection
   candidal infections in, 525, *525*
   drug skin eruptions in, 535
   mycobacterial infections in, 524
   neuropsychiatric manifestations of, 588–590
   in pregnancy, 695
   skin manifestations of, *527*, 527t, 527–528, *528*
HLA-B8 antibodies, in myasthenia gravis, 559
Hodgkin's lymphoma, 527, 532
Hoffman degradation, 62, 64
Hollander test (insulin-hypoglycemia gastric
   analysis), 323
Home management, of TPN (total parenteral
   nutrition), 87
Hormones (*see also* Endocrine disorders)
   ADH (antidiuretic hormone), 230–232, 233–235,
     234
   PTH (parathyroid hormone), 249–254 (*see also*
     Hypercalcemia)
Hospital death risk, 579
H_2 receptor antagonists, 126
   in GERD, 311
   in pancreatitis, 308
   in peptic ulcer, 310
   in recurrent ulcer, 323
Human chorionic gonadotropin (hCG) test, 50
Human immunodeficiency virus (HIV) (*see* HIV
   infection)
Hungry bone syndrome, 255
Huntingdon's disease, 586
Hydantoin, loading dose of, 708t
Hydralazine, 186
   in preeclampsia, 674

Hydrocephalus, 588
Hydroxychloroquinine, 684t
Hyperaldosteronism, primary, 345–346
Hyperalimentation, 81–83, 82t, 213–214
Hyperamylasemia, 307–308
Hyperbilirubinemia, 203, 301 (*see also* Jaundice;
        Liver disease)
Hypercalcemia, 249–254, 250t, 251t, 252t, 253t,
        357 (*see also* Hyperparathyroidism)
    of malignancy, 249–250, 436–439
Hypercarbia, 115–116
Hyperchloremia, 343
Hypercortisolism, 570
    psychiatric manifestations in, 585
Hyperemesis gravidarum, 680–681
    thyroid function and, 689
Hyperglycemia, 88–89 (*see also* Diabetes mellitus)
Hyperkalemia, 244–249, 245t, *247*, 248t, 343
Hyperkalemic renal tubular acidosis, 343–344
Hyperlipidemia, with TPN, 89
Hypermagnesemia, 260–261
Hypernatremia, 236–240, *238*
Hyperosmotic agents, 682t
Hyperparathyroidism, 249–254, 355–357 (*see also*
        Hypercalcemia)
Hyperphosphatemia, 213, 258, 264, 264t
Hypersensitivity (*see also* Allergy; Anaphylaxis)
    drug fever and, 492–493, 598–599
    latex, 67
    transfusion reactions
        anaphylactic, 368
        skin, 367–368
Hypersplenism, 402–403
Hypertension, 17, 212, 599 (*see also* Stroke)
    depression as related to, 570
    in diabetes mellitus, 330
    diastolic dysfunction in, 184–185, 194t
    as drug side effect, 598
    myocardial ischemia risk and, 181–184
    neuropsychiatric changes in, 570
    in pheochromocytoma, 347
    prevalence and risk of, 179–181, 180t
    in psychiatric patients, 570–572, 571t
    treatment of postoperative, 185–188
Hypertensive crises, 180–181
Hyperthermia, malignant, 66
Hyperthyroidism (Graves' disease), 334–337,
        689–690
    apathetic, 334
    epidemiology of, 334
    factitious, 584–585
    preoperative evaluation in, 334–336
    psychiatric manifestations of, 584–585
    thyroid storm, 336t, 336–337
Hypertrophic cardiomyopathy, 197–198
Hypervitaminosis A, 591
Hypervitaminosis E, 591
Hypervolemia, 63, 228, 229t (*see also* Electrolyte
        disturbances; Hemostasis; Hypernatremia;
        Hyponatremia; Renal failure)
Hypoalbuminuria, 72 (*see also* Malnutrition)
Hypoaldosteronism, low-renin, 330
Hypocalcemia, 213, 254–258, 255t, 256t
Hypoglycemia
    coma in, 586
    with hyperosmotic states, 586
    psychiatric symptoms in, 585–586
Hypokalemia, 240–244, 242t, *243,* 301, 345

Hypomagnesemia, 258–260, 259t, 260t
Hyponatremia, 211, 228–236, *231,* 231t, 233t, *234,*
        348–351
    in post-TURP syndrome, 236, 654
Hypophosphatemia, 258, 261–264, 262t, 263t
Hypotension, 196, 201, 301
    orthostatic, 570, 596, 603
Hypothyroidism, 337–340
    euthyroid sick syndrome, 338
    fetal and amiodarone, 670
    in Hashimoto's thyroiditis, 338–339
    as lithium side effect, 600
    myxedema coma in, 339
    in pregnancy, 687–688
    preoperative evaluation in, 338–339
    preoperative management in, 339–340
    psychiatric manifestations of, 584–585
    surgical risk in, 337–338
Hypovolemia, 228, 229t, 301 (*see also* Electrolyte
        disturbances; Hyponatremia; Renal
        failure)
    factors responsible for, 198t
Hypoxemia, 579
Hysterectomy
    abdominal, 465–466
    vaginal, 465

Iatrogenic skin complications, *534,* 534–537, 535t
        (*see also* Dermatologic disorders)
Idiopathic hypertrophic subaortic stenosis,
        197–198
Idiopathic peripartum cardiomyopathy, 669
Ileostomy, 324
Ileus, adynamic, 409
Imipramine, 65t (*see also* Antidepressants)
Immobilization, in elderly, 625
Immune hemolytic anemia, 372t, 372–374
Immunization, in pregnancy, 697–698, 698t
Immunoglobulin, intravenous, in pregnancy, 685t
Immunosuppressive drug effects in pregnancy,
        684t–685t
Impetigo herpetiformis, 532
Impotence, antihypertensives and, 570
IMV (intermittent mandatory ventilation), 121t,
        121–122
Incentive spirometry, 108
Incontinence, postprostatectomy, 423, 423t
Indirect Coombs' test, 369
Infarction (*see also* Myocardial infarction)
    mesenteric in abdominal aortic aneurysm, 634
    myocardial, 56, 61, 134, 482, 546, 583
    in stroke
        lacunar, 554
        thromboembolic, 554
Infected vascular gangrene, 502
Infection, 449–518
    of aortic replacement graft, 635
    bacterial, 519–523, 520t
        bacterial sepsis, *522,* 522–523
        cellulitis, 519–522, *521*
        Clostridium difficile, 323
        in hip fracture, 541–542, 542t
        listeriosis, 697
        toxic shock syndrome, 523
    as burn complication, 645–646
    in cancer, 409
    classification of, 453–455
        NNISS index for, 454–455, 455t

Infection—*Continued*
  SENIC index for, 454, 454t
  dental, 643, 643t
  in diabetes mellitus, 533
  in elderly, 623, 625
  endotracheal intubation and, 126
  epidemiology of, 449–450
  fungal, 491–492, 537
    candidal, 499–500
    chlamydial, 695
    rashes in, 525
  incisional wound (surgical site) infections,
      500–502
    cellulitis
      clostridial anaerobic, 501
      nonclostridial anaerobic, 501
      synergistic necrotizing, 502
    gangrene
      Fournier's, 502
      gas, 502
      infected vascular, 502
    in joint replacement, 546
    necrotizing fasciitis, 501
    necrotizing of soft tissue, 501
    pathophysiology of, 451–455, *453*
    rates by operative procedures and risk
        category, 456t–457t
    in tuberculous, mycotic, and viral infection,
        502
  mycobacterial diseases, 524
  parasitic, 306
    rickettsial diseases, 523
    spirochetal diseases, 523–524, *524*
  postoperative problems of, 476–513
    abscess (*see also* Abscess)
      intrabdominal, 484–488, *485–486*
      perinephric, 500
    atelectasis, 496–497
    bacteremia, 488–491, 490t
    candiduria, 499–500
    diarrhea, 504–505
    fever, 478–484, 479t, 480t, 481t, 482t (*see also*
        Fever)
      causes of, 477t, 478t
      drug, 492–493
    fungemia, 491–492, 637
    indwelling catheter infection, 508–509
    intravenous infusion infections, 509
    in laparoscopic surgery, 513
    pelvic infection, 503–504
    pneumonia, 493–495
    postoperative parotitis, 507–508
    pressure ulcers, 506–507
    procedure- and device-related infections,
        509–510
    prosthetic graft infections, 510t, 510–511
    prosthetic joint infections, 512–513
    prosthetic valve endocarditis, 472, 483,
        511–512
    pulmonary aspiration, 495–496
    thrombophlebitis and pulmonary embolism,
        497
    toxic shock syndrome, 503
    in trauma, 504
    urinary tract infection, 497–500, 499t
    vertebral osteomyelitis and disk space infec-
        tion, 505–506
  in pregnancy, 694–697

    bacterial vaginitis, 696
    group B streptococcus, 695–696, 696t
    HIV infection, 695, 696t
    Listeria sp., 697
    Lyme disease, 696–697
    mortality/morbidity and, 665
    parvovirus, 697
    pneumonia, 664–665
    sexually transmitted diseases (STDs), 694t,
        694–695, 695t
  preoperative respiratory, 475–476
  prophylactic antibiotics in, 450–475
    in abdominal trauma, 464
    in appendectomy, 461
    in cholecystectomy, 461–462
    effectiveness of drugs, 450, *451*
    in gynecologic surgery, 465–466
      abdominal hysterectomy, 465–466
      vaginal hysterectomy, 465
    human trials of, 455–458, 458t
    in lower gastrointestinal (colorectal) surgery,
        463–464
    in neurosurgery, 469
      clean procedures, 469
      skull fractures, 469
    in noncardiac thoracic surgery, 468
    in orthopaedics, 467–468
      fractures and clean procedures, 468
      hip fracture, 467
      total hip replacement, 467–468
    in pneumonia, 458–461
    principles for use of, 455, 458t
    reasons for and against using, 451, 452t
    recommended procedures for, 459t–460t
    in subacute bacterial endocarditis, 469–475,
        470t–474t
    timing of administration and, 452–453
    in transurethral prostatic resection (TURP),
        466–467
    type of infection prevented by, 450–451
    in upper gastrointestinal surgery, 462–463
    in vascular surgery, 464–465
  rashes in, 519–527, 520t–521t
  rate of in selected procedures, 450t
  rickettsial, 523
    in pregnancy, 696–697
  skin, 537
  surgical risk and preexisting, 621
  urinary tract (UTI), 201–202, 490, 546
    delirium and, 579
    in pregnancy, 676
  viral
    cytomegalovirus, 316
    herpes simplex, 694
    HIV, 524, 525, *525, 527,* 527t, 527–528, *528,*
        535, 588–590 (*see also* HIV infection)
    parvovirus, 697
    rashes in, 524–525
Inflammatory bowel disease
  nutritional support in, 90
  in pregnancy, 681–683
Informed consent, by psychiatric patients, 575–576
Inhalation injury, 644–645 (*see also* Burns)
Initial contact, 2
Insomnia, in elderly, 596
Insulin, 40
  continuous infusion, 330–331, 331t
Insulin-glucose infusion, 246, 248t

Insulin-hypoglycemia gastric analysis (Hollander test), 323
Insurance, capitated, 17–18
Intensive care, hemodynamic monitoring in, 133–139
Intensive care unit psychosis (*see* Delirium)
Interferon-α, 315–316
Interferons, 606t
Intermittent mandatory ventilation (IMV), 121t, 121–122
Intermittent pneumatic compression, 144
Intermittent positive-pressure breathing (IPPB), 108 (*see also* Mechanical respiratory support)
Internist, consultant role of, 1–8
Interprofessional relationships, 2–3, 5, 10, 11
Intervertebral disk space infection, 505–506
Intra-abdominal abscess, 484–488, *485–486*
Intravenous infusion infections, 509
Intubation
    for enteral feeding, 84–85
    for mechanical ventilation, 116–130 (*see also* Mechanical respiratory support)
Invasive monitoring, 133–139 (*see also* Hemodynamic monitoring)
IPPB (intermittent positive-pressure breathing), 108 (*see also* Mechanical respiratory support)
Irritable bowel syndrome, 320
Ischemia
    mesenteric in abdominal aortic aneurysm, 634
    myocardial, 153t, 153–170, 181–184 (*see also* Myocardial infarction; Myocardial ischemia)
        in pregnancy, 671–673
    peripheral nerve palsies and, 565
    postoperative localized CNS, 564
Ischemic hepatitis, 314–315
Isoflurane, 61, 62, 63–64, 304
Isoniazid, 606t
Isosorbide, 65t, 305
Isotretinoin, 606t
Itching (*see* Pruritus)

Jaundice, 203, 316–319, 432 (*see also* Hepatitis)
    after aneurysm repair, 634–635
    classification of, 312t
    in hepatic abscess, 487
    in pregnancy, 683
Jejunostomy, 424
Johns Hopkins Medical Institutions Surgical Classification System, 28, 28t
Johns Hopkins University, consultation report form, *15–16*
Joint replacements, 544–547, 545t
    infection in, 512–513
    total hip replacement, 544–547, 545t
    total knee replacement, 546

Kaposi's sarcoma, 528, *528*
K⁺ deficit equation, 706t
Ketamine, 61, 63, 94
Ketoacidosis, diabetic, 332–333, 662–663, 663t
Ketoconazole, 537
Ketorolac, 548
Kidney (*see also* Renal)
    anesthetic effects on, 63–64
Kidney stones, in pregnancy, 676

Knee replacement, 546
Korsakoff's psychosis, 591

Labetolol, 188
Laboratory evaluation
    alanine aminotransferase test (ALT, SGPT), 298–299
    aminotransferase test (AST, SGOT), 298–299
    amylase:creatinine clearance test, 307
    antiendomysium antibody test, 322
    ascitic fluid albumin test, 302–303, 318
    cardiac stress (*see* Stress testing)
    as compared with history, 29t
    corticotropin-releasing-hormone test, 570
    dexamethasone suppression test, 570, 585
    false-positive/false-negative results, 28
    glucose tolerance test, 661
    τ-glutamyl transpeptidase (GGT) test, 304
    hematologic, 361–362, 362t
    hemostatic, 401
    indirect Coombs' test, 369
    insulin-hypoglycemia gastric analysis (Hollander test), 323
    liver function tests, in pregnancy, 679–680, 680t
    for malnutrition, 75t, 75–77, 76t, 77t
    for pituitary insufficiency, 355t
    postoperative fever, 482t, 482–483
    predictive value of, 41
    principles of selecting, 32–33
    PSA (prostate-specific antigen) test, 421–422
    pulmonary function tests, 50, 101–104, 103t, 104t, 619
    reasons for outpatient, 36t
    renal, *200,* 200–201
    in renal failure, 208–211, 209t, 211t
    screening considerations in, 40–42, 41t, 42t
    specific preoperative, *42,* 42–50, 44t, 45t, 46t, 48t
    suggestions for, *34–35*
    thyroid function tests, 334–335, 337–338
        in pregnancy, 687–688
Lactation, as drug side effect, 599
Lactose-free diets, 81
Lactose intolerance, 83, 321–322
Laparoscopic surgery, 98
    infection in, 513
Laparotomy, vertical and risk, 98
Laryngectomy, 651, 651t (*see also* Radical neck surgery)
Latex allergy, 67
Laxatives
    in cancer, 441t
    in pregnancy, 682t
Lead nephropathy, 343
Lecithin therapy, in dementia, 559
Legal issues (*see* Medicolegal issues)
Leiden Factor V mutation, 679
Length of stay, 9
    in hip replacement, 545
Lentigo maligna melanoma, 529–530
Leukemia (*see also* Neutrophilia)
    chronic lymphocytic (CLL), 379–380
Leukocyte abnormalities, 377–380 (*see also* White blood cell [WBC] abnormalities)
Leukoplakia, oral "hairy" in AIDS, 527, *528*
Levodopa, 561–563, 586, 606t
    anesthetic interactions, 64t
Lidocaine, 304

Life expectancy
  age and, 704t
  at birth, 705t
Light therapy, 603–604
Listeriosis, 697
Literature, provision of, 11
Lithium
  ACE inhibitors with, 573
  anesthetics with, 65t, 577
  antihypertensives with, 571t
  in bipolar disorder, 600–601
  diuretics with, 573
  hypothyroidism induced by, 584–585
  teratogenicity of, 600
  in unipolar depression, 601
Lithium intoxication, 601
Liver, anesthetic effects on, 62
Liver abscess, 487
Liver disease, 297–307 (see also Jaundice)
  abscess, 297–307, 487
  anesthesia and, 303–304, 313–316, 314t
  autoimmune, 307
  BCAAs (branched-chain amino acids) and, 86, 90
  biliary disorders in, 312t, 312–319
  in burn injury, 646
  cirrhosis, 241
  coagulation disorders in, 300–301, 390
  diuretics in, 303
  HBaAg carriers of, 303
  high-risk patients with, 298–300
  incidence of complications with, 298, 298t, 299t
  nutritional support in, 90
  pathophysiology of, 297–298
  as postoperative complication, 312–319
    anesthesia-induced hepatitis, 313–314
    hepatitislike pattern in, 313–316
    hepatocellular dysfunction in, 313
    hyperbilirubinemia in, 313
    ischemic hepatitis, 314–315
    jaundice in, 312t, 312–319
    posttransfusion hepatitis, 315–316
  postsurgical treatment of, 305–306
  in pregnancy, 306–307, 679–680, 680t, 683–687, 686
    cirrhosis, 686
    hepatitis, 683–687
    liver failure, 686–687
  preoperative evaluation of, 298t, 298–301, 299t
  preoperative/existing, 297–307
    anesthetic effects on, 303–304
    coagulation defects with, 300–301
    evaluation in, 298–300
    HBsAG carriers of, 303
    incidence of complications with, 298, 298t, 299t
    pathophysiology of, 297–298
    postoperative treatment of, 305–306
    with pregnancy, 306–307
    renal function and, 301
    surgical effects/surgical risk in, 304–305
    treatment of, 301–303
  renal function in, 301
  surgical risk and, 304–305
  with TPN, 89
  treatment of, 301–303
Liver enzyme tests, 49
Liver function tests, in pregnancy, 679–680, 680t
Liver metastases, 428–429

Liver transplantation, in pregnancy, 686
Lobectomy, pulmonary, 106 (see also Pulmonary procedures)
Loop, flow-volume, 115
Loperamide, 682t
Lorazepam, 580, 596
Low-fat diets, 81
Low-renin hypoaldosteronism, 330
Ludwig's angina, 643
Lung cancer, 106–107
  nonsmall-cell, 419–421, 445t
  small-cell, 421
Lung-expansion maneuvers, 107–108
Lungs (see also Pulmonary)
Lung surgery, 95–97 (see also Pulmonary evaluation; Pulmonary surgery)
Lupus erythematosus, 526
  in pregnancy, 692–693
Lupuslike anticoagulant, 395
Lyme disease, 523–524, 524
  in pregnancy, 696–697
Lymphangitis, 533
Lymphocytopenia, 380
Lymphocytosis, 379–380
Lymphoma, 527
  Hodgkin's, 532
Lysine nasal vasopressin, 353

MAC (monitored anesthesia care), 58, 59
Macrocytic anemia, 366–367
Maculopapular skin eruption, 534, 534–535
Magnesium disturbances
  hypermagnesemia, 260–261
  hypomagnesemia, 258–260, 259t, 260t
Magnesium therapy, 259–260, 260t
  in eclampsia, 675
Malignancy (see Cancer; Cancer surgery)
Malignant effusion, 430–431
Malignant hypercalcemia, 249–250, 435–439
Malignant hyperthermia, 66
Malignant melanoma, 529, 529
Malnutrition (see also Nutrition; Nutritional evaluation)
  correction of, 77–79
    caloric requirements, 78, 78t
    carbohydrate and fat requirements, 79
    fluid requirements, 78
    nutritional intervention, 79–89, 80, 81t
    protein requirements, 78
  diagnosis of, 71–77, 297
  renal failure and, 213–214
  respiratory complications and, 116–117
Manganese toxicity, 591
Mania, in HIV infection, 589
Mannitol, 211–212
MAO inhibitors
  advantages and disadvantages, 603
  in anxiety, 604
  contraindications
    anesthesia, 65t, 576
    serotonin reuptake inhibitors, 600
Marfan's syndrome, pregnancy in, 669–670
Massive transfusion syndrome, 370, 370t
MAST (Michigan Alcoholism Screening Test), 591
Measles, mumps, rubella vaccine (MMR), contraindicated in pregnancy, 698
Measurements, anthropometric, 72–74, 73t, 74t
Mechanical respiratory support, 62, 115–131

abbreviations used in, 116t
additional modes of, 129–130
in apnea, 67
epidemiology of respiratory failure, 115–117
equipment and methods, 120–125, 121t
extubation and weaning, 126–129, 127t, *128,*
    708t
indications for, 117–118
information sources for, 118, 199t
problems from, 125–126
technical aspects of, 119–120
Meclizine, 682t
Medical consultation service
attributes of general, 10–11
capitated insurance and, 17–18
description of, 12–13
forms for, *13–14, 15–16*
in risk assessment, 14–17 (*see also* Risk
    assessment)
teaching role of, 10
Medication, preoperative adjustment of, 40
Medicolegal issues, 7
Melanoma
acral lentiginous, 530
lentigo maligna, 529–530
malignant, 529, *529*
metastatic, *531*
nodular, 529
Meningococcemia, 522
Mental status, 624–625
Meperidine, 580
6-Mercaptopurine, 681, 685t
Mesalamine, 681
Metabolic acidosis, 232, 266–271, *268,* 269t, *270,*
    278t, 279t, 706t
Metabolic alkalosis, 233, 244, 271t, 271–273, 272t,
    278t, 279t, 706t
Metabolic encephalopathy (*see* Delirium)
Metabolic-physiologic equations, 706t
Metal toxicity, 591
Metastatic cancer, 428–436, *531* (*see also* Cancer)
Metastatic melanoma, *531*
Metformin (Glucophage), 332
Methimazole, in hyperthyroidism, 689
Methotrexate, in rheumatoid arthritis, 548
Methoxyflurane, 63
Methoxyflurane hepatitis, 314
Methyldopa, 571t, 606t
in preeclampsia, 674
Methylphenidate, 606t
Metoclopramide, 311, 682t
Metolazone, 667t
Metoprolol, 187
Metronidazole, 306, 323
in inflammatory bowel disease, 681
METs, 163, 164t
Microcytic anemia, 367
Midzalom, 59
Miliaria (heat rash), 536
Milton S. Hershey Medical Center, consultation
    report form, 12–14, *13–14*
Mini-Mental Status test, 623
Mithramycin, 254
Mitomycin, 410
Mitral regurgitation, 190
Mitral stenosis, 189–190, 190t (*see also* Valvular
    heart disease)
pregnancy in, 669

Mitral valve prolapse, in pregnancy, 669
Mivacurium, 59, 66–67
Mixed acid-base disturbances, 274–277, 278t
MMR (measles, mumps, rubella vaccine), contrain-
    dicated in pregnancy, 698
Mobilization, in postoperative respiratory manage-
    ment, 108–109
Monitoring, hemodynamic, 133–139 (*see also*
    Hemodynamic monitoring)
Morphine, in postoperative hypertension, 188
Mortality, age and, 704t
MPTP, parkinsonian syndromes and, 561
MUGA scan, 631
Multi-infarct dementia, 558, 588
Multiphasic chemistry panels, 49
Multiple-organ failure syndrome, 487
Multiple sclerosis, psychiatric symptoms in, 587
Munchausen syndrome, 573–574
Muscle relaxants, 59, 62, 63, 66–67, 122
Myasthenia gravis, 559t, 559–560
Myasthenic crisis, 560
Mycobacterial infections, 524
Myocardial dysfunction, 177–179 (*see also* Conges-
    tive heart failure)
Myocardial infarction (*see also* Angina; Myocardial
    ischemia)
anesthesia and, 56, 61
electroconvulsive therapy risk and, 583
hemodynamic monitoring in, 134
in joint replacement, 546
presentation of as fever, 482
Myocardial ischemia (*see also* Angina; Myocardial
    infarction)
coronary revascularization procedures in,
    171–174
general considerations in, 153t, 153–154
in pregnancy, 671–673
preoperative clinical predictors of, 156
preoperative testing for, 154–158, 155t, 157t
    ambulatory ECG, 158–160
    dobutamine stress echocardiography, 169–170
    left ventricular systolic function testing, 161,
        161t
    nuclear scintigraphy (thallium scan),
        165–167
    resting ECG, 158
    SPECT, 167–168
    stress testing, 154–158, 155t, 157t, 161–165,
        162t, 163t, 164t, 165t
    technetium-99m sestamibi, 168
silent, 182
Myoglobinuria, 198t, 209, 241
Myotonic dystrophy, 563
Myxedema coma, 339 (*see also* Hypothyroidism)

Nadolol, 305
Naltrexone, 591
Narcotics (*see also* Anesthetic agents *and specific
    drugs*)
psychiatric side effects of, 606t
in renal failure, 222
Nasal surgery, toxic shock syndrome in, 503
NASCET (North American Symptomatic Carotid
    Endartarectomy Trial), 555
National Health and Nutritional Examination
    Surveys (NHANES I and II), 73, 73t, 74t
National Nosocomial Infection Surveillance System
    (NNISS), 454–455, 455t

Nausea and vomiting
  in cancer, 394t, 441–442
  in pregnancy, 680–681
Neck surgery, radical, 640–641, 650t, 651t
Necrotizing fasciitis, 501
Necrotizing infection of soft tissue, 501
Nefazodone, 602 (*see also* Serotonin reuptake
      inhibitors [SSRIs])
Neostigmine, 63
Nephrolithiasis, in pregnancy, 676
Nephropathy, lead, 343
Nephrotoxicity, 196–197, 199t (*see also* Renal
      failure)
  of anesthetics, 63
  of cisplatin, 410–411
Neuroleptic malignant syndrome, 598–599
Neurologic conditions (*see also* Neurologic
      surgery)
  anesthesia sequelae, 57–58
  cerebrovascular disorders, 553–558 (*see also*
      Stroke)
    perioperative, 556–558
    preoperative, 553–556
  dementia, 558–559, 559t
    Alzheimer's disease, 558–559, 587–588
    multi-infarct, 558
  extrapyradmidal disorders, 560–563
    parkinsonian syndromes, 560–563, 562t
    postperative complications in, 563
  myasthenia gravis, 559t, 559–560
  myotonic dystrophy, 563
  postoperative neurologic complications, 563–565,
      564t
    altered mental status, delirium, and coma,
      564
    brachial plexus trauma, 565
    cauda equina syndrome, 564–565
    delirium, 577–582, 578t (*see also* Delirium)
    localized CNS ischemia, 564
    peripheral nerve palsies, 565
    seizure, 564
  psychiatric symptoms in, 586–589
Neurologic surgery
  diabetes insipidus following, 352t, 352–353
  infection risk in
    skull fracture, 469
    slean procedures, 469
  respiratory sequelae of, 116
Neuromuscular blockade, 122 (*see also* Muscle
      relaxants)
Neuropathic ulceration, in diabetes mellitus, 533,
      533
Neuropsychiatric disorders, in burns, 647
Neutropenia, 378t, 378–379
  in cancer patients, 408
Neutrophilia, 377–378
New York Heart Association functional classifica-
      tion, 168t, 182, 666, 707t
NHANES I and II (National Health and Nutri-
      tional Examination Surveys), 73, 73t, 74t
Niacin deficiency, 591
Nifedipine, 64t, 188
  contraindications for sublingual, 188
Nitidine (*see* H$_2$-receptor antagonists)
Nitrogen balance, 76
Nitroglycerin, 61, 65t, 186, 318
  in eclampsia, 675
Nitroprusside, in renal failure, 223

Nizatidine (*see* H$_2$-receptor antagonists)
NNISS (National Nosocomial Infection Surveil-
      lance System), 454–455, 455t
Nodules, solitary thyroid in pregnancy, 688–689
Nonclostridial anaerobic cellulitis, 501
Nonsteroidal antiinflammatory drugs (NSAIDs)
      (*see* Aspirin; NSAIDs)
Nortriptyline, 65t, 595 (*see also* Antidepressants)
Nosocomial infections (*see* Infection)
NSAIDs (*see also* Aspirin)
  contraindications to, 303, 600
  hyperkalemia and, 331
  and peptic ulcer, 309, 310
  platelet disorders and, 399–400
  in pregnancy, 684t
  preoperative consideration of, 547–548
  psychiatric side effects of, 606t
  in renal failure, 222
  toxicities in rheumatologic disease, 548t
Nuclear scintigraphy
  dipyridamole-thallium, 165–167, 169t
  technetium-99m, 168
Nutrition (*see also* Nutritional disorders; Nutri-
      tional evaluation)
  clinical conditions for support, 89–91
    chronic liver disease, 90
    inflammatory bowel disease, 90
    pancreatitis, 90
    perioperative, 89–90
    renal disease, 90
  enteral, 79–85
    complications of, 85
    diet and table foods, 79–81, *80,* 81t
    by intubation, 84–85
    supplemental diets, 81–83, 82t
  estimation of requirements
    caloric requirements, 78, 78t, 89
    carbohydrate and fat requirements, 89
    fluid requirements, 78
    protein requirements, 78
  in mechanical ventilation, 127
  parenteral (TPN), 85–89
    complications of, 87–89, 88t, 89t
    indications for TPN, 87
    methods of, 85–87, 86t
  in renal disease, 90
Nutritional disorders
  in alcoholism, 590–591
  hypervitaminosis A, 591
  hypervitaminosis E, 591
  obesity, 101, 105, 116
  starvation, 591 (*see also* Nutritional disorders)
Nutritional evaluation, 71–92, 297 (*see also*
      Malnutrition; Nutrition)
  estimation of requirements, 78, 78t, 89
  rationale for, 71–72
  techniques of, 72–77
    anthropometric measurements, 72–74,
      73t, 74t
    biochemical measurements, 75t, 75–77,
      76t, 77t
    clinical and dietary history, 72
    clinical signs of malnutrition, 74–75

Obesity
  pulmonary complications and, 100–101
  respiratory complications and, 105, 116
Obesity-hyporespiratory support syndrome, 105

Obstetrics (*see* Pregnancy)
Obstruction
 biliary, malignant, 432–433
 intestinal, 408–409
 ureteral, 433
Obstructive sleep apnea, 101
Obstructive uropathy, 199t (*see also* Renal
  failure)
Octreotide, 318–319
Oliguria, 205 (*see also* Renal failure)
Omeprazole, 682t
Oncologic disorders (*see* Cancer)
Ondansetron, 59–60
Opiates, in renal failure, 222
Opioid anesthetics, 59, 61, 63, 64t–65t
Optic nerve compression, 565
Oral "hairy" leukoplakia, in AIDS, 527, *528*
Organ donors, 224–227, 225t, 226t
Organ failure syndrome, 487
Organophosphates, anesthetics with, 65t
Organ transplantation, renal, 224–228
Orthopaedic infections
 intervertebral disk space infection, 505–506
 osteitis pubis, 506
 vertebral osteomyelitis, 505–506
Orthopaedic procedures (*see also* Rheumatology)
 fat embolization, 547
 geriatric, 541–544
 hip fractures, 541–544, 542t, 544t
 infection risk in, 467–468
  fracture and clean procedures, 468
  hip fracture, 467
  total hip replacement, 467–468
 joint replacements, 512–513, 544–547, 545t
Orthostatic hypotension, 570, 596, 603
Osteitis pubis, 506
Osteomalacia, 262
Osteomyelitis, vertebral, 505–506
Ostomates, 323–325
Ostomy care, 323–325
 colostomy, 324–325
 ileostomy, 324
Ototoxicity, 212
Outpatient surgery, 33–40 (*see also* Preoperative
  evaluation)
Ovarian cancer, 427–428
Oxygenation
 adequacy of, 117
 assessment of, 119–120
Oxygen toxicity, 120
 synergistic with bleomycin toxicity, 409–410

Paget's disease of bone, 253–254 (*see also* Hypercalcemia)
Pain
 in cancer, 408, 439t, 440t
 postoperative, 61, 109
 with TPN, 89
Palsy, postoperative peripheral nerve, 565
Pamidronate, 254
Pancreatic abscess, 487
Pancreatic cancer, 425–427
Pancreaticoduodenectomy (Whipple operation),
  426
Pancreatitis
 nutritional support in, 90
 postoperative, 308–309
 preoperative/existing, 307–308

Pancytopenia, 380, 380t
Papules, pruritic urticarial of pregnancy, 531, 531t,
  532
Parasitic infections, 306
 rickettsial diseases, 523, 696–697
 spirochetal diseases, 523–524, *524*
Parathyroid disease, psychiatric manifestations in,
  585
Parathyroid hormone (PTH), 213, 249–254
  (*see also* Hypercalcemia)
Parenteral nutrition (TPN), 85–89
 complications of, 87–89, 88t, 89t
 indications for, 87
 methods of, 85–87, 86t
Parkinsonian drug side effects, 597–598
Parkinsonian syndromes, 560–563, 562t
Parkinson's disease
 electroconvulsive therapy risk and, 583
 psychiatric symptoms in, 586
Parotitis, postoperative, 507–508
Paroxetine (*see* Serotonin reuptake inhibitors
  [SSRIs])
Paroxysmal supraventricular tachycardia, 670
Partial thromboplastin time (PTT), 47, 48t
Parvovirus infection, 697
Patent ductus arteriosus, in pregnancy, 666–668
Patient base, 10
Patient-controlled analgesia, 61
Patient history (*see* History)
Patients
 ambulatory, 33–40 (*see also* Ambulatory patients)
 explanation to, 3
 geriatric (*see* Elderly)
 high-risk, 7
 with multiple problems, 7
 nutritional concerns of, 80
 values of, 21
PEEP (positive end-expiratory pressure), 120
  (*see also* Mechanical respiratory support)
Pelvic cellulitis, 503
Pelvic exenteration, 648–649, 649t, 650t
Pelvic infections, 503–504
Pelvic thrombophlebitis, septic, 503–504
Penicillamine, in pregnancy, 684t
Penicillin, 223, 643 (*see also* Antibiotic prophy-
  laxis; Antibiotics)
 allergy to, 535–536
 semisynthetic, 645
Pennsylvania State University, Milton S. Hershey
  Medical Center, 12–14, *13–14*
Percutaneous transluminal coronary angioplasty
  (PCTA), as adjunct to noncardiac surgery,
  173–174
Pergolide, 562, 586
Perinephric abscess, 500
Perioperative nutrition, 89–90
Peripartum cardiomyopathy, idiopathic, 669
Peripheral nerve palsies, 565
Peritoneovenous shunting, 433
Peritonitis, 488 (*see also* Abscess; Infection)
pH, as respiratory indicator, 115
Pharmacological stress testing, 165–167
Pharyngectomy, 651, 651t (*see also* Radical neck
  surgery)
Phenelzine, 606t
Phenobarbitol (*see also* Barbiturates)
 loading dose of, 708t
Phenothiazines, anesthetics with, 65t, 576–577

Phenoxybenzamine, 186, 348
Phentolamine, 186
Phenylephrine, 606t
Phenytoin (*see also* Anticonvulsants)
  dosage, 557t
  teratogenicity, 557–558, 670
Pheochromocytoma, 570
  psychiatric symptoms in, 586
Philadelphia chromosome, 377
Phlebitis (*see also* Thrombophlebitis)
  in enteral feeding, 85
Phlebotomy, in polycythemia vera, 376–377
Phosphate therapy, 261–262, 262t
  in hypercalcemia, 254
Phosphorus disturbances
  hyperphosphatemia, 213, 258, 264, 264t
  hypophosphatemia, 261–264, 262t, 263t
Phrenic nerve injury, 96
Physical examination, 29–33 (*see also* History)
Physiologic monitoring, 133–139 (*see also* Hemodynamic monitoring)
Physiologic stress, 14–15
Physostigmine
  contraindications to, 580
  in delirium, 580
Phytonadione, 642
Pick's disease, 588
Pitressin, 353
Plaque
  atherosclerotic, 153t, 153–154, 181, 553 (*see also* Cardiovascular disease)
  pruritic urticarial of pregnancy, 531, 531t, *532*
Plasma cholinesterase abnormality, 66–67
Plasmapheresis, in myasthenic crisis, 560
Platelet disorders, *396,* 396–400 (*see also* Coagulation disorders; Hemostasis)
  diagnosis of, 396, *396*
  qualitative platelet dysfunction, 398–400, 399t
  thrombocytopenia, 396–398, 397t
  thrombocytosis, 400
Platinol (*see* Cancer chemotherapy)
Pleural effusion, malignant, 430–431
Pneumatic compression, intermittent, 144
Pneumonectomy, 106–107 (*see also* Pulmonary surgery)
Pneumonia, 493–495
  acute mycoplasma, 374
  in hip fracture, 541–542, 542t
  postoperative, 458–461
  in pregnancy, 664–665
PNI (prognostic nutritional index), 77, 77t
Poison ivy, 536
Polyarthritis nodosa, 526
Polycythemia vera, 376–377
Porphyria, 590
Positive end-expiratory pressure (PEEP), 120 (*see also* Mechanical respiratory support)
Postcholecystectomy syndrome, 319–320
Postgastrectomy syndrome, 320–321
Postoperative complications (*see specific procedures and conditions*)
Postoperative psychosis (*see* Delirium)
Postpartum thyroid dysfunction, 690–691, 691t
Postsplenectomy thrombocytosis, 403
Posttransfusion hepatitis, 312, 315–316
Potassium chloride therapy, 241–244
Potassium deficit equation, 706t

Potassium disturbances
  hyperkalemia, 244–249, 245t, *247,* 248t, 343
  hypokalemia, 240–244, 242t, *243,* 301, 345
Potassium restriction, 213
Potassium supplementation, 82
Prazosin, 606t
Predictive value, 41
Preeclampsia/eclampsia, 673t, 673–674
Pregnancy
  alcohol consumption in, 591
  anticonvulsants in, 557–558
  cardiovascular disease in, 665–675, 666t
    acquired cardiac disease, 669–673
      cardiac arrhythmias, 670–671, 671t
      ischemic heart disease and cardiac arrest, 671–673
    congenital cardiac disease, 666–669
    effects of commonly used drugs, 670t
    hypertension, 673t, 673–674
  collagen vascular diseases in, 691–694
    antiphospholipid syndrome, 693–694
    rheumatoid arthritis, 691
    systemic lupus erythematosus, 692–693
  diabetes mellitus in, 661–663, 663t
  gastrointestinal, hepatic, and pancreatic disease in, 679–687
    cholecystitis, 683
    cholestasis, 683
    drug safety of GI drugs in, 682t
    inflammatory bowel disease, 681–683
    liver disease, 679–680, 680t, 683–687
      cirrhosis, 686
      hepatitis, 683–687
      liver failure, 686–687
  hematologic disease in, 675–679
    anemia, 676–677
    coagulopathies, 679
    hemoglobinopathies, 677–678, 678t
    thrombocytopenia, 678–679
  immunizations in, 697–698, 698t
  immunosuppressive drug effects in, 684t–685t
  infectious diseases in, 694–697
    bacterial vaginitis, 696
    group B streptococcus, 695–696, 696t
    HIV infection, 695, 696t
    Listeria sp., 697
    Lyme disease, 696–697
    parvovirus, 697
    rickettsial, 696–697
    sexually transmitted diseases (STDs), 694t, 694–695, 695t
  lithium therapy in, 600–601
  liver disease in, 306–307
  pulmonary disease in, 663–664, 665t
    asthma, 663–664, 665t
    pneumonia, 664–665
    tuberculosis, 665
  renal disease in, 675–676
  skin reactions in, *531,* 531t, 531–532, *532*
  testing for, 49–50
  thyroid disease in, 687–691
    hyperthyroidism, 689–690
    hypothyroidism, 687–688
    postpartum disorders, 690–691, 691t
    solitary thyroid nodule, 688–689
Pregnancy-related dysphasic gastrointestinal response, 680

Preoperative evaluation (*see also* Anesthesia; Laboratory tests)
of ambulatory surgical patients, 33–40, *34–35*, 37t
approach to, 22t, 22–23
endocrine
for diabetes mellitus, 329–330
thyroid, 334–336, 338–339
forms for, *26–27,* 28t, 29t, *34–35*
general principles of, 25–29
of healthy patients, 29–33, 30t, 31t, 32t, 33t
hematologic, 361–362, 362t
of hemostasis, 380–385, 381t, 382t, 383t, 384t, 385t
platelet studies, 396, *396*
of thromboembolic risk, 393t, 393–394
hepatic, 298–300
in hip fracture, 542–543
medical risks for surgical patients, 19–23
nutritional, 71–92 (*see also* Malnutrition)
rationale for, 71–72
techniques of, 72–77, 73t, 74t, 75t, 76t, 77t
principles of risk:benefit, 19–21, 20t
psychiatric issues in, 572–577
pulmonary, 101–107 (*see also* Anesthesia; Pulmonary evaluation)
renal, 198–201, 199t, *200* (*see also* Renal failure)
Pressure ulcers, 506–507
Primary hyperaldosteronism, 345–346
Prioritization of surgery, 22–23
Problem statement, 2
Procaine derivatives, 606t
Prognostic nutritional index (PNI), 77, 77t
Prolactin inhibiting factor, antipsychotics and, 599
Prolapse, mitral valve, in pregnancy, 669
Promethazine, 682t
Propranolol, 348, 598 (*see also* β-Adrenergic antagonists)
in pregnancy, 666, 670
in thyroid storm, 690
Prophylactic antibiotics, 450–475 (*see also under* Infection)
Propofol, 59, 63, 123
Propoxyphene, drug interactions, 601
Propylthiouracil (PTU), in hyperthyroidism, 689
Prostate cancer, 421–423, 423t
staging of, 421, 444t
surgical complications in, 422–423, 423t
Prostatectomy, complications of, 422–423, 423t
Prostatic resection, 236
infection risk in, 466–467
transurethral (TURP), 236, 466–467, 651–654, 652t
Prosthetic graft infections, 510–511
Prosthetic heart valves, 194, 196t, 196–197, 473, 483, 511–512, 670
Prosthetic joints, 467–468, 512–513, 544–547, 545t
Protein C resistance, 394
Protein-energy malnutrition (*see* Malnutrition)
Protein requirements estimation, 78
Protein supplementation, 82–83
Proteus sp., 491
Prothrombin time (PT), 47, 48t
Proton-pump inhibitors, 310, 323
Protriptyline (*see* Antidepressants)
Prurigo gestationis of Besnier, 531
Prurigo gravidarum, 531, *531,* 531t
Pruritic urticarial plaques of pregnancy, 531, 531t, *532*

PSA (prostate-specific antigen) test, 421–422
Pseudodementia of depression, 595
Pseudogout, 549
Pseudomembranous (*Clostridium difficile*) colitis, 504–505
Pseudomonas sp., 449 (*see also* Infection)
Psychiatric considerations (*see also* Delirium; Neurologic disorders)
anxiety disorders, 604
drug effects
of antipsychotics, 597–604
psychiatric symptoms as, 605t–607t
in elderly patients, 595–597
electroconvulsive therapy evaluation, 582–583
medical illness and
in psychiatric patients, 567–572
evaluation of, 567–569, 568t, 569t
management of, 569–572
surgical consultation, 572–577
psychiatric symptoms in, 584t, 584–591
eating disorders, 592–595
endocrinopathies, 584–586
HIV infection, 588–590
metabolic disorders, 590
neurologic illness, 586–588
nutritional diseases and alcoholism, 590–592
postoperative delirium, 577–582, 578t
preexisting psychiatric disorders, 575–577
risk factors for psychiatric complications, 573–575
Psychoactive drugs (*see also specific drugs and drug classes*)
in anxiety disorders, 604
in bipolar disorder, 600–601
in elderly, 595
general side effects of, 597–600
in major depression, 601–604
Psychosis
in elderly, 596t, 596–597
vs. HIV infection, 589
PTCA (percutaneous transluminal coronary angioplasty), 173–174
PTH (parathyroid hormone), 249–254 (*see also* Hypercalcemia)
Puerperal endometriosis, 503
Pulmonary artery catheterization, 133–139, 178–179, 179t, 623, 633 (*see also* Hemodynamic monitoring)
Pulmonary aspiration, 495–496
Pulmonary complications, 94
of burns (inhalation injury), 644–645
Pulmonary disease (*see also* Pulmonary evaluation; Pulmonary surgery)
in cancer, 409–410
dental procedures and, 642–643
in pregnancy, 663–664, 665t
asthma, 663–664, 665t
pneumonia, 664–665
tuberculosis, 665
surgical risk and preexisting, 621
Pulmonary edema
acute noncardiac (transfusion-related), 368
in sickle cell disorders, 677
Pulmonary embolism, 146–147, 496
in hip replacement, 545

Pulmonary evaluation (*see also* Pulmonary surgery, Pulmonary disease)
  preoperative testing, 101–104, 103t, 104t, 619
    arterial blood gas analysis, 102
    chest radiography, 101
    diffusing capacity, 102, 103t, 104t
    exercise capacity, 103–104
    regional lung function assessment, 102–103
    spirometry and lung volume measurement, 101–102
  risk factors for complications, 97–101
    age, 100
    duration of surgery, 101
    obesity, 100–101
    pulmonary disease, 99t, 99–100
    smoking, 98–99
    surgical and anesthetic considerations, 97t, 97–98
Pulmonary metastases, 428
Pulmonary risk assessment, 17
Pulmonary stenosis, in pregnancy, 668
Pulmonary surgery
  approach to surgical patient, 104–107
    with existing disease, 105–106
    general surgical, 104–105
    pulmonary resection candidates, 106–107
  endocarditis prophylaxis in, 474t
  postoperative management, 107–109
    cough, 108
    DVT prophylaxis, 109
    early mobilization, 108–109
    lung expansion maneuvers, 107–108
    pain reduction, 109
Pulmonary toilet, 118, 123
Pulmonary wedge pressure, 134 (*see also* Hemodynamic monitoring)
Purpura
  thrombocytopenic, 398
  in vasculitis, 526–527
Pyelonephritis, in pregnancy, 676, 677
Pyridostigmine
  anesthetic interactions, 65t
  in myasthenic crisis, 560
Pyrogenic cytokines, 478–479

Qualitative platelet dysfunction, 398–400, 399t
Quality of life, 624
Quinidine, 64t, 606t
  in pregnancy, 670

Radiation therapy
  adverse effects of, 410, 411
  in brain metastases, 429
  in breast cancer, 413
  in esophageal cancer, 424
  in head and neck cancer, 427
  in pancreatic cancer, 426–427
Radical neck surgery, 640–641, 650t, 651t
Radiocontrast, nephrotoxicity of, 197, 201
Radiography
  chest, 44t, 44–46, 45t, 101
  in renal failure, 209
Rash (*see also* Dermatologic disorders; Infection)
  butterfly, 526
  classification of, 520t–521t
  infectious causes of
    bacterial infections, 519–523, 520t
      bacterial sepsis, *522*, 522–523

      cellulitis, 519–522, *521*
      toxic shock syndrome, 523
    mycobacterial diseases, 524
    rickettsial diseases, 523, 696–697
    spirochetal diseases, 523–524, *524*
    viral diseases, 524–525
      in fungal infections, 525
  noninfectious causes of, 525–527
    collagen vascular diseases, 526
    drugs, 525–526
    malignancy, 526–527
    vasculitis, 526–527
Red blood cell (RBC) abnormalities, 370–377
    (*see also* Erythrocyte abnormalities)
Referral, as compared with consultation, 1–2
Referring physician, 1, 2–3
Reflux, gastroesophageal (GERD), 311–312
Reflux gastritis (bile gastritis, alkaline gastritis), 321
Regional enteritis (Crohn's disease), in pregnancy, 681–683
Regurgitation
  aortic, 192
  mitral, 190
Renal disease
  in burn injury, 647
  in eating disorders, 594
  lead nephropathy, 343
  in pregnancy, 675–676
Renal effects
  of anesthesia, 63–64
  of cancer chemotherapy, 410–411
Renal evaluation, 198–201, 199t, *200* (*see also* Acid-base disorders; Electrolyte disorders; Renal failure)
Renal failure
  acute (ARF)
    epidemiology of, 195–197, 196t
    etiology and pathogenesis of, 204–208
    evaluation of, 208–211, 209t, 211t
    in high-risk surgical procedures, 196t, 203–204
    risk factors for, 196, 196t
    treatment of, 211–217, 212t
  anemia in, 366
  anesthesia in, 63
  aortic aneurysm surgery in, 632
  chronic, 217–224, 245
    epidemiology of, 217–218
    evaluation of, 218
    treatment of, 218–224
  diet in, 81
  drug therapy in azotemia, 221t, 221–224
  nutritional support in, 90
  platelet disorders and, 399–400
  selective aldosterone deficiency in, 343–345, 344t
Renal failure fluid study, 208
Renal function, in liver disease, 301
Renal function tests, equations for, 707t
Renal risk
  assessment of, 17
  in drug reactions, 535
Renal stones, in pregnancy, 676
Renal transplantation
  donors, 224–227, 225t, 226t
  epidemiology, 224–225
  recipients, 227–228

Renal tubular acidosis, hyperkalemic, 343–344
Reserpine, 606t
Resident, role of, 10–11
Respiratory acidosis, 273, 274t, 278t, 279t
Respiratory complications (*see* Anesthesia; Pulmonary evaluation; Respiratory function tests)
Respiratory disorders (*see* Pulmonary disorders *and specific diseases*)
Respiratory infection, preoperative, 475–476
Respiratory quotient (RQ) values, 85–86, 86t
Respiratory support, mechanical, 115–131 (*see also* Mechanical respiratory support)
Respiratory system, anesthetic effects on, 60–61
Rhabdomyolysis, 241, 262
Rheumatic fever, 526
   prophylaxis as compared with endocarditis, 475
Rheumatic heart disease, 189–190 (*see also* Valvular deart disease)
   pregnancy in, 669
Rheumatoid arthritis, 547–549
   anesthetic considerations in, 550t
   in pregnancy, 691
Rheumatology, 547–550
   anesthetic hazards in rheumatoid arthritis, 550t
   crystal-induced arthritis, 549
   drug considerations in patients, 547–548, 548t
   Felty's syndrome, 549–550
   shoulder-hand syndrome, 550
   underlying rheumatic disease, 548–549
Rickettsial infections, 523
   in pregnancy, 696–697
Risk
   classification of, 21
   hierarchical evaluation of, 21
Risk assessment, 14–17, 19–23
Risk:benefit balance, 21
Risk factors
   cardiac, 5
   hypothyroidism as, 337–338
   for pulmonary complications, 97–101
      age, 100
      duration of surgery, 101
      obesity, 100–101
      pulmonary disease, 99t, 99–100
      smoking, 98–99
      surgical and anesthetic considerations, 97t, 97–98
Risperidone, 599–600
Rocky Mountain spotted fever, 523
Rocuronium, 59
RQ (respiratory quotient) values, 85–86, 86t

SAD (seasonal affective disorder), 603–604
Salicylates, psychiatric side effects of, 607t
Salmon calcitonin, 436–437
Salt substitutes, 246
Sarcoma, Kaposi's, 528, *528*
Schizophrenia, 573, 575, 582 (*see also* Psychiatric considerations)
Screening tests (*see* Laboratory evaluation)
Seborrheic dermatitis, 526, 528
"Second-look" surgery
   in cancer, 427–428
   in sepsis, 484
Sedatives, 122–123 (*see also* Anesthesia; Anesthetic agents)
   in renal failure, 222

Seizures
   antipsychotics and threshold, 599
   bupropion and, 602
   perioperative anticonvulsants in, 557t, 557–558
   postoperative, 564
Selective aldosterone deficiency, 343–345, 344t
Selegiline, 561–563, 586
SEMIC (Study on the Efficacy of Nosocomial Infection Control), 454, 454t
Sepsis, 488–491 (*see also* Infection)
   bacterial, *522*, 522–523
      skin lesions in, *522*, 522–523, *523*
   breakthrough bacteremia in, 489
   candidal, 525, *525*
   in cholestasis, 317
   common causes of, 490t
   in endocarditis, 469
   incidence following selected procedures, 470t
   in joint replacement, 512–513, 546
   pressure ulcers and, 507
   in toxic shock syndrome, 523
Septic pelvic thrombophlebitis, 503–504
Seroquel, 600
Serotonin reuptake inhibitors (SSRIs)
   in anxiety, 604
   anxiety with (serotonin syndrome), 595
   in major depression, 601–602
   MAO inhibitors with (fatal reaction), 600
Serotonin syndrome, 595
Sertindole, 600
Sertraline, 602 (*see also* Serotonin reuptake inhibitors [SSRIs])
Serum glutamic-oxaloacetic transaminase test (SGOT, AST), 298–299 (*see also* Liver disease)
Serum glutamic-pyruvic transminase test (SGPT, ALT), 298–299 (*see also* Liver disease)
Sevoflurane, 59, 61, 62, 63
Sexual dysfunction, antihypertensives and, 570
Sexually transmitted diseases (STDs)
   AIDS/HIV (*see* HIV infection)
   gonorrhea, 522
   in pregnancy, 694–695
      gonorrhea, 694, 694t
      herpes simplex, 694
      syphilis, 695t
   syphilis, 50
SGOT (serum glutamic-oxaloacetic transaminase, AST) test, 298–299
SGPT (serum glutamic-pyruvic transminase, ALT) test, 298–299
Sheet allergy, 536
SHEP (Systolic Hypertension in the Elderly) study, 573
Shoulder-hand syndrome, 550
Shunting, peritoneovenous, 433
SIADH (syndrome of inappropriate antidiuretic hormone), 232, 233–235, *234*, 348–351, 350t
Sickle cell disease, in pregnancy, 677–678, 678t
Sickle-cell hemoglobinopathies, 370–372
Sick role, 574
SIMV (synchronized intermittent mandatory ventilation), 121t, 121–122
Single-photon emission computed tomography (SPECT), in cardiovascular disease, 167–168

Skin cancer, 528–530
  basal cell carcinoma, 529, *529*
  squamous cell carcinoma, 529, *529*
Skin disorders (*see* Dermatologic disorders)
Sleep apnea, 101
Sleep disturbance, in elderly, 596
Smoking, 39–40
  peptic ulcer and, 309
  respiratory complications and, 98–99, 105
  reversal of effects, 99
Society of Critical Care Medicine, 122, 123
Sodium disturbances
  hypernatremia, 236–240, *238*
  hyponatremia, 211, 228–236, *231,* 231t, 233t,
    234, 348–351
    in post-TURP syndrome, 236
Sodium nitroprusside, 185–186
Sotalol, 670
Special cases, 22
SPECT (single-photon emission computed tomog-
    raphy), in cardiovascular disease,
    167–168
Spinal anesthesia, 57–58
Spinal cord compression, 434–435
Spinal tap, WBC correction equation for, 706t
Spirochetal diseases, 523–524, *524*
Spirometry, 101–102 (*see also* Pulmonary function
    testing)
  incentive, 108
Spironolactone, 303
Splenectomy, 398, 402–403
  in hemolytic anemia, 373
Splenic abscess, 487
Splenomegaly, 402–403
Splenomegaly–granulocytopenia (Felty's) syn-
    drome, 549–550
Squamous cell carcinoma, of skin, 529, *529*
Staging systems for cancer, 443–445
Staphyllococcus aureus, 449 (*see also* Infection)
Staphylococcal septicemia, 522
Stenosis (*see also* Valvular heart disease)
  aortic valve, 190–192
  idiopathic hypertrophic subaortic (hypertrophic
    cardiomyopathy), 197–198
  mitral, 189–190, 190t
  in pregnancy
    aortic valve, 668
    pulmonary, 668
Stephens-Johnson syndrome, 526
Steroids, anabolic, 605t
Still's disease, 526
Streptococcal infection (*see also* Bacterial infec-
    tions *and specific diseases;* Infection)
  in pregnancy, 695, 696t
Stress, 624–625
  physiologic, 14–15
  and rheumatoid arthritis flare, 548–549
  surgical, 62
Stress testing
  dobutamine stress echocardiography, 169t,
    169–170, 631
  exercise, 162–165
  pharmacological, 165–167
  predictors of ischemia, 156–157
  preoperative, 154, 155t, 157t, 158
  in risk stratification, 157–158
Stress ulcers, 310–311
Stridor, 125

Stroke, 553–558
  cervical bruit and risk of, 554
  classification of and prognosis, 554
  electroconvulsive therapy risk and, 582–583
  with intracerebral bleeding, 555
  lacunar infarction, 554
  perioperative, 556–558
  postoperative, 553–554
  preoperative, 553–556
  previous or TIAs, 554–556
  thromboembolic infarction, 554
Study on the Efficacy of Nosocomial Infection
    Control (SEMIC), 454, 454t
Subacute bacterial endocarditis, 469–475,
    470t–474t
Subluxation, atlanto-occipital, 549
Subphrenic abscess, 487
Substance abuse (*see also* Alcoholism)
  parkinsonian syndromes and, 561
  surgical risk and, 574–575
Succinylcholine, 66
  contraindications, 249
Sucralfate, 682t
Suctioning, endotracheal, 123–124
Sufentanil, 64
Suicide, 574, 575, 599
Sulfasalazine, 681
Sulfonylurea hypoglycemic drugs, 332
Superior vena cava syndrome, 429–430
Surgery (*see also specific procedures and disorders*)
  ADH release and, 202t, 202–203
  elective, 22
    transfusions for, 363
  hematologic issues in, 401–404
  hepatic effects of, 304
  hip and deep vein thrombophlebitis, 141, 144
  laparotomy versus laparoscopy, 98
  major as compared with minor, 28, 28t
  metabolic responses to, 202t
  organ harvesting, 224–227
  preoperative evaluation for (*see* Preoperative
    evaluation)
  prioritization of, 22–23
  pulmonary, 104–109 (*see also* Pulmonary evalu-
    ation; Pulmonary surgery)
  pulmonary risk factors and, 97–98
  renal failure and high-risk, 196t, 203–204
  in renal transplant recipients, 227–228
  respiratory effects of
    abdominal procedures, *96,* 96–97, *97*
    nonabdominal, nonthoracic procedures, 97
    pulmonary/thoracic procedures, 95–96
  "second-look," 427–428, 484
Surgical site (wound) infection, 450–475, 453t
    (*see also under* Infection)
Surgical stress, 62
Swan-Ganz catheterization, 133–139, 178–179,
    623, 633 (*see also* Hemodynamic moni-
    toring)
Synchronized intermittent mandatory ventilation
    (SIMV), 121t, 121–122
Syndrome of inappropriate antidiuretic hormone
    (SIADH), 232, 233–235, *234,* 348–351,
    350t
Synergistic necrotizing cellulitis, 502
Syphilis, in pregnancy, 695t
Systemic lupus erythematosus (SLE), 526
  in pregnancy, 692–693

Tachycardia (*see also* Cardiac arrhythmias)
  paroxysmal supraventricular, 670
  in pregnancy, 670–671
TAR and feather mnemonic, 591
Tardive dyskinesia, 587, 596, 598
Teaching
  as function of consultation service, 9–10
  methods of, 11
Technetium-99m nuclear scintigraphy, 168
Temperature (*see also* Fever)
  normal oral, 479
  postoperative normal elevation of, 47480
Teratogenicity
  of amiodarone, 670
  of antiarrhthmics, 670, 671t
  of anticonvulsants, 557–558
  of gastrointestinal drugs, 682t
  of lithium, 600–601
Tetracyclines, 224
Tetrahydroaminoacridine, 559
Tetralogy of Fallot, in pregnancy, 668–669
β-Thalassemia, 677–678
Thallium scan, 165–167, 169t
Theophylline, 607t
  preoperative, 106
Thiamine deficiency, 590
Thiamine therapy, 580
Thiazide diuretics, 536 (*see also* Diuretics)
  contraindications, 303
  in nephrogenic diabetes insipidus, 354
  in preeclampsia, 674
  in pregnancy, 667t
Thiopental, 63
Thioridazine, 597
Thoracic surgery (*see also* Coronary artery bypass
      grafting [CABG]; Pulmonary surgery)
  endocarditis prophylaxis in, 474t
  noncardiac, infection risk in, 468
  risk in elderly, 619
Thoracoscopic surgery, 98
Thoracotomy
  in elderly, 626
  with lung resection, 96
  without lung resection, 95–96
Thrombocytopenia, 396–398, 397t
  alloimmune, 679
  autoimmune, 678–679, 679
  in pregnancy, 678–679
Thrombocytopenic purpura
  autoimmune, 398
  thrombotic, 398
Thrombocytosis, 400
  postsplenectomy, 403
Thromboembolic disorders, 141–147 (*see also* spe-
      cific disorders; Anticoagulants; Coagula-
      tion disorders; Platelet disorders)
  antiphospholipid antibody syndrome and,
      394–395
  deep vein thrombophlebitis, septic pelvic,
      503–504
  deep vein thrombophlebitis (DVT), 109, 144–146,
      497
  deep-vein thrombophlebitis (DVT)
    in hip replacement, 545
    prophylaxis, 109
    in TURP, 672t
  diagnostic approach to, 393t, 393–394
  embolism

bone marrow-fat in sickle-cell disease, 372
  pulmonary, 146–147, 497, 545
  in hip replacement, 545
  postsplenectomy thrombocytosis, 403
  prevention of, 109, 141–144, *142, 143,* 144t, 397
  prosthetic heart valves and, 196 (*see also*
      Prosthetic heart valves)
  septic pelvic thrombophlebitis, 503–504
  stroke, 554–556
  thrombophlebitis
    deep vein (*see* Deep vein thrombophlebitis
        [DVT])
    in hip replacement, 545
  in transurethral prostatic resection, 652t
Thrombotic thrombocytopenic purpura, 398
Thymectomy, in myasthenia gravis, 560
Thyroid disease
  diabetes mellitus and, 662
  in eating disorders, 594
  hyperthyroidism (Graves' disease), 334–337,
      689–690
    apathetic, 334
    epidemiology of, 334
    factitious, 584–585
    preoperative evaluation in, 334–336
    psychiatric manifestations of, 584–585
    thyroid storm, 336t, 336–337
  hypothyroidism, 337–340
    euthyroid sick syndrome, 338
    in Hashimoto's thyroiditis, 338–339
    myxedema coma in, 339
    preoperative evaluation, 338–339
    preoperative management in, 339–340
    surgical risk in, 337–338
  in pregnancy, 687–691, 690t, 690–691
    hyperthyroidism, 689–690
    hypothyroidism, 687–688
    postpartum disorders, 690–691, 691t
    solitary thyroid nodule, 688–689
  psychiatric symptoms in, 584–585
Thyroidectomy, hypocalcemia with, 255
Thyroid function tests, in pregnancy, 687–688
Thyroid hormone
  in depression, 596
  psychiatric side effects of, 607t
Thyroiditis
  Hashimoto's, 338–339, 690
  postpartum, 690–691, 691t
Thyroid nodule, in pregnancy, 688–689
Thyroid storm, 336t, 336–337
  in pregnancy, 690
TIAs (transient ischemic attacks), 554–556
Tibial–pedal bypass, 534
Tinea pedis (athlete's foot), 522–523
TIPS (transjugular intrahepatic portosystemic
      shunt), 305, 319
Tissue plasminogen activator (tPA), in stroke, 555
TNM staging system, 417, 444–445
Topical medications, 537–538, 538t
Total hip replacement, 467–468, 544–547, 545t
Total parenteral nutrition (TPN), 87–89, 88t, 89t
(Gilles de la) Tourette's syndrome, 587
Toxicity, oxygen, 120
Toxic shock syndrome, 503, 523
tPA (tissue plasminogen activator), in stroke, 555
TPN (total parenteral nutrition), 87–89, 88t, 89t
Tracheal/endotracheal complications, 125–126
Tracheostomy tubes, 124–125

Transfusion history, 32
Transfusion-related (acute noncardiac pulmonary) edema, 368
Transient ischemic attacks (TIAs), 554–556 (*see also* Cerebrovascular disease; Stroke)
Transjugular intrahepatic portosystemic shunt (TIPS), 305, 319
Transplantation
  liver in pregnancy, 686
  renal, 224–228
Transurethral resection of prostate (TURP), 236, 466–467, 651–654, 652t
Tranylcypromine, 607t
Trauma
  dental, 642
  infection in, 504
  respiratory sequelae of cranial, 116
  stress ulcers with, 310–311
Trazodone, 595, 602 (*see also* Serotonin reuptake inhibitors (SSRIs))
Treadmill testing (*see* Stress testing)
Tricyclic antidepressants (*see under* Antidepressants)
Tridil, 318
Trigeminal nerve compression, 565
Trihexyphenidyl, 563, 597, 598 (*see also* Anticholinergics)
Trimethoprimsulfamethoxazole, 535
TSH (thyroid-stimulating hormone) test, 334–335
Tuberculosis
  candidal infection in, 502
  in pregnancy, 665
Tubes
  endotracheal, 123–124
  tracheostomy, 124–125
Tubo-ovarian abscess, 503
TURP (transurethral resection of prostate), 236, 466–467, 651–654, 652t
Tzanck test, 524

Ulceration, in diabetes mellitus, 533, *533*
Ulcerative colitis
  nutritional support in, 90
  in pregnancy, 681–683
Ulcer operations, in elderly, 626
Ulcers, 309–311
  anastomatic, 321
  gastric, 126
  peptic, 309–310
  pressure, 506–507
  recurrent, 322–323
  stress, 310–311
Ultrasonography, as stroke risk indicator, 554–555
Uremia (*see* Renal failure)
Ureteral obstruction, 433
Uric acid clearance equation, 706t
Urinalysis, 48
  for glucose, 47
  in renal failure, 209
Urinary indices in acute renal failure, 210t
Urinary osmolality, 237–239, *238*
Urinary tract infections (UTIs), 201–202, 490, 497–500, 499t
  after TURP, 466
  candidal, 499–500
  delirium and, 579
  in joint replacement, 546
  perinephric abscess in, 500

Urine abnormalities, 198t (*see also* Electrolyte disorders; Fluid disorders; Renal failure)
Urologic conditions
  postprostatectomy incontinence, 423, 423t
  ureteral obstruction in cancer, 433
Urologic surgery, endocarditis prophylaxis in, 473t, 474t
Uropathy, 199t
  obstructive (*see also* Renal failure)
Urticaria, 520t (*see also* Rash)
U.S. Food Guide Pyramid, 80, *80*

Vaccination, in pregnancy, 697–698, 698t
Vaginal cuff abscess, 503
Vaginal delivery, endocarditis prophylaxis in, 475
Vaginosis, bacterial, in pregnancy, 696
Valves, prosthetic heart, 194, 196t, 196–197, 471, 473, 483, 511–512, 670
Valvular heart disease, 188–195
  evaluation in, 192t, 192–194
  in pregnancy, 666–669
  prevalence and risk, 188–189
  specific types of, 189–192
  treatment of, 194–197, 196t, 471, 473, 483, 511–512, 670
Valvuloplasty
  balloon aortic, 194–195
  balloon in pregnancy, 669
Vascular gangrene, infected, 502
Vascular surgery, infection risk in, 464–465
Vasculitis, 526–527
Vasodilators, 65t
  with psychotropic drugs, 571t
Vasomotor nephropathy (*see* Acute tubular necrosis)
Vasopressin, 305, 318
  lysine nasal, 353
Vasopressors, 599
Vecuronium, 59
Venlafaxine, 601 (*see also* Serotonin reuptake inhibitors [SSRIs])
Ventilation, assessment of, 117–118
Ventilation-perfusion scanning, 146
Ventilator dependency, 126
Ventilators (*see also* Mechanically assisted ventilation)
  types of, 121t, 121–122
  volume-limited, 121
Ventilatory failure (hypercarbia), 115–116
Ventricular septal defect, in pregnancy, 666–668
Ventricular systolic function testing, 161
Verapamil, 64t, 666 (*see also* Calcium channel blockers)
  contraindications, 601, 670
Vertebral osteomyelitis, 505–506
Vesicles, 521t (*see also* Rashes)
Viral infections
  cytomegalovirus, 316
  herpes simplex, 694
  HIV, 524, 525, *525, 527,* 527t, 527–528, *528,* 535, 588–590 (*see also* HIV infection)
  parvovirus in pregnancy, 697
  rashes in, 524–525
Vitamin B$_2$ deficiency, 590
Vitamin B$_3$ deficiency, 591
Vitamin C deficiency, 74

Vitamin deficiencies, 74–75 (*see also* Malnutrition)
Vitamin D therapy, 257–258
Vitamin excess, 591
Vitamin K deficiency, 389, 394
Vitamin K therapy, 301, 683
Volume depletion, 200t, 200–201 (*see also* Hyponatremia)
Volume disorders, 301
Volume overload, after transfusion, 369
von Willebrand's disease, 388–389, 679

Warfarin, 141, 142–143, 389–390, 395 (*see also* Anticoagulants)
  in hip replacement, 546
  in pregnancy, 668
WBC (white blood cell count), 46–47
Weaning, from mechanical ventilation, 126–129, 127t, *128*
Wegener's granulomatosis, 526
Weight gain
  as lithium side effect, 600
  tricyclic antidepressants and, 603
Weight/height measurements, 72–74, 73t, 74t
Weight loss
  in eating disorders, 594–595
  postsurgical, 322
Wernicke-Korsakoff syndrome, 580, 591

Wernicke's encephalopathy, 590–591
Whipple operation (pancreaticoduodenectomy), 426
White blood cell abnormalities, 377–380
  lymphocytopenia, 380
  lymphocytosis, 379–380
  neutropenia, 378t, 378–379
    in cancer patients, 408
  neutrophilia, 377–378
  pancytopenia, 380, 380t
Wilson's disease, 590
Withdrawal states, 580
Wooden chest sign, 563
Worcester Heart Attack Study, 134
Work-up (*see* History; Physical examination)
Wound classification, 453t, 454t, 455t (*see also* Infection)
Wound (surgical site) infections, 450–475 (*see also* Infection)

Xerosis, 532
X-ray (*see* Radiography *and specific procedures*)

Zidovudine (AZT), 695, 696t
Zinc toxicity, 591
Ziprosirosidine, 600
Zollinger-Ellison syndrome, 323

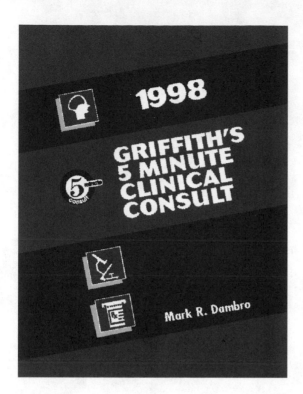